Assessment and Multimodal Management of Pain

AN INTEGRATIVE APPROACH

Assessment and Multimodal Management of Pain

AN INTEGRATIVE APPROACH

Maureen F. Cooney, DNP, FNP-BC, RNBC, AP-PMN, ACHPN
Pain Management Nurse Practitioner, Educator and Consultant
Westchester Medical Center
Valhalla, New York

Ann Quinlan-Colwell, PhD, RNBC, CNS, AHNBC
Clinical Nurse Specialist
Pain Management Educator and Consultant
Wilmington, North Carolina
Pain Management Clinical Nurse Specialist
New Hanover Regional Medical Center
Wilmington, North Carolina

ELSEVIER

Elsevier
3251 Riverport Lane
St. Louis, Missouri 63043

ASSESSMENT AND MULTIMODAL MANAGEMENT OF PAIN:
AN INTEGRATIVE APPROACH

ISBN: 978-0-323-53079-8

Notice

Library of Congress Control Number: 2020946357

Senior Content Strategist: Sandra Clark
Senior Content Development Manager: Luke Held
Content Development Specialist: Sarah Vora
Publishing Services Manager: Julie Eddy
Project Manager: Grace Onderlinde
Design Direction: Brian Salisbury

Printed in the United States of America

Last digit is the print number: 9   8   7   6   5   4   3   2   1

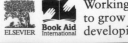

We would like to dedicate this work to all people who experience pain and the clinicians who care for them; and to all who have contributed to the field of pain management through their passion and tireless efforts in research, education, leadership, and advocacy.

Reviewers

Scotty Bethune, Physical Therapist
New Hanover Regional Medical Center
Wilmington, North Carolina

David A. Bray, R. Ac. & R.TCMP, Dipl. C.H.(NCCAOM)
Doctor of Oriental Medicine
Internal Medicine
Guangzhou University of Traditional Chinese Medicine
Guangzhou, China
Toronto, Ontario, Canada

Virginia Brendlen, MS, RN (retired)
Durham, North Carolina

LaVonne E. Couch, PT, CSCS
Program Director, Physical Therapist Assistant Program
Rowan College Gloucester County
Glassboro, New Jersey

Janette (Jan) Elliott, RN-BC, MSN, AOCN
Clinical Nurse Specialist
VA Palo Alto Pain Clinic
Palo Alto, California

Joan Farrenkopf, MFA, CST, LMBT, RYT
Healing Arts Network
New Hanover Regional Medical Center
Wilmington, North Carolina

Kimberly Galentine, PTA
New Hanover Regional Medical Center
Wilmington, North Carolina

Diane Glowacki, MSN, RN, CNS, CNRN-CMC
Clinical Nurse Specialist
Critical Care/Med-Surg
Mercy Hospital of Buffalo
Buffalo, New York

Robert W. Hutchison, PharmD, BCACP
Associate Professor of Pharmacy Practice
Pharmacy Practice
Texas A&M University, College of Pharmacy
Round Rock, Texas

Karen Isaacs, MD
Coastal Family Medicine
NHRMC Physician Group
Wilmington, North Carolina

Helen S. Kane, RN, MSN, MBA, CCRN
Clinical Nurse Specialist
Nursing
Thomas Jefferson University Hospital
Philadelphia, Pennsylvania

Jennifer E. Lee, PhD, MA
Assistant Professor
Psychology and Nursing
Mount Mercy University and the University of Iowa
Cedar Rapids, Iowa

Judith D. McLeod, RNC, DNP, CPNP
Dean of Nursing, Pediatric Nurse Practitioner
School of Nursing
California Southern University
Costa Mesa, California

Rajavi S. Parikh, DO
New Hanover Regional Medical Center
Wilmington, North Carolina

Jongbae Jay Park, KMD, PhD, Dipl OM, LAc
Associate Professor
Department of Anesthesiology
Duke University School of Medicine
Durham, North Carolina

Joy Susan Pendergrass, MSN, MEd, FNP-BC
Nurse Practitioner/Pain Consultant
Consultant
Independent Practitioner/Consultant
Fernandina Beach, Florida

Christy Seckman, DNP, RN
Goldfarb School of Nursing
St. Louis, Missouri

Meera K. Shah, PharmD, AAHIVP
Clinical Pharmacist
Hepatology and Infectious Disease
University of Kansas Health Systems
Kansas City, Kansas

Tara C. Shaw, RN, MSN
Assistant Professor
Nursing
Goldfarb School of Nursing at Barnes Jewish College
St. Louis, Missouri

Paula Denise Silver, BS Biology, PharmD
Medical Instructor
Medical Assisting/LPN/RN
ECPI University: School of Health Science
Newport News, Virginia

Linda Wilson, PhD, RN, CPAN, CAPA, BC, CNE, CHSE, CHSE-A, ANEF, FAAN
Assistant Dean for Special Projects, Simulation and CNE Accreditation
College of Nursing and Health Professions
Drexel University
Philadelphia, Pennsylvania

Robin Ye
Registered Pharmacist–State of Illinois
Doctor of Pharmacy (PharmD)
Board Certified Pharmacotherapy Specialist (BCPS); Basic Life Support (BLS)
Clinical Pharmacist
Inpatient Pharmacy
NorthShore University HealthSystem–Glenbrook Hospital
Glenview, Illinois

Contributors

Timothy J. Atkinson, PharmD
Clinical Pharmacy Specialist, Pain Management
Pharmacy Service
VA Tennessee Valley Healthcare System
Murfreesboro, Tennessee

Sue Ballato, MBA, RN, CHCQM-PS & RM, FABQAURP
Administrator
Clinical Outcomes
New Hanover Regional Medical Center
Wilmington, North Carolina

Jeffrey J. Bettinger, PharmD
Pain Management Clinical Pharmacist
Saratoga Hospital Medical Group
Saratoga, New York

Kathleen Broglio, DNP, ANP-BC, ACHPN, CPE, FPCN
Nurse Practitioner, Section of Palliative Medicine
Associate Professor, Geisel School of Medicine at
Dartmouth
Dartmouth-Hitchcock Medical Center
Lebanon, New Hampshire

Ann Quinlan-Colwell, PhD, RNBC, CNS, AHNBC
Clinical Nurse Specialist
Pain Management Educator and Consultant
Wilmington, North Carolina
Pain Management Clinical Nurse Specialist
New Hanover Regional Medical Center
Wilmington, North Carolina

Maureen F. Cooney, DNP, FNP-BC, RNBC, AP-PMN, ACHPN
Nurse Practitioner
Pain Management
Westchester Medical Center
Valhalla, New York
Adjunct Associate Professor
Lienhard School of Nursing
Pace University, College of Health Sciences
New York, New York
Instructor of Anesthesiology
Anesthesia
New York Medical College
Valhalla, New York

Meredith W. Crumb, BS, PharmD
Clinical Pharmacist
VA Tennessee Valley Healthcare System
Nashville, Tennessee

Geralyn Datz, PhD, MSCP
President
Behavioral Medicine
Southern Behavioral Medicine Associates PLLC
Hattiesburg, Mississippi

Emily Davis, RN, MSN, ACNP
Nurse Practitioner
Department of Anesthesiology
Duke University
Durham, North Carolina

Debra Drew, MS, ACNS-BC (retired), RN-BC (retired)
Retired Clinical Nurse Specialist, Pain Management
Maplewood, Minnesota

Michele Erich, MM, CCLS, MT-BC
Music Therapist/Child Life Specialist
Healing Arts Network
New Hanover Regional Medical Center
Wilmington, North Carolina

Gregory Scott Firestone, MHA, RT(R)
Director
LEAN Strategies
New Hanover Regional Medical Center
Wilmington, North Carolina

Jeffrey Fudin, BSPharm, PharmD, DAIPM, FCCP, FASHP, FFSMB
President and Director
Scientific and Clinical Affairs
Remitigate Therapeutics
Delmar, New York
Clinical Pharmacy Specialist (WOC)
Stratton VA Medical Center
Albany, New York
Adjunct Associate Professor
Western New England University College of Pharmacy
Springfield, Massachusetts

Adjunct Associate Professor of Pharmacy Practice & Pain Management
Albany College of Pharmacy & Health Sciences
Albany, New York

Carla R. Jungquist, PhD, ANP-BC, FAAN
Assistant Professor
School of Nursing
University at Buffalo
Buffalo, New York

Courtney Kominek, PharmD
Clinical Pharmacy Specialist-Pain Management
Pharmacy
Harry S. Truman Memorial Veterans' Hospital
Columbia, Missouri

Susan O'Conner-Von, PhD, RN-BC, CHPPN, CNE
Associate Professor
School of Nursing
University of Minnesota
Minneapolis, Minnesota
Director of Graduate Studies
Center for Spirituality and Healing
University of Minnesota
Minneapolis, Minnesota

Shalvi B. Parikh, MBBS
Former Research Assistant
Department of Anesthesia
Division of Pain Medicine
Westchester Medical Center
Valhalla, New York

Christine Peltier, DNP, RN-BC, FNP-BC
Nurse Practitioner
M-Health, Fairview
Minneapolis, Minnesota

Thien C. Pham, AS, BS, PharmD
Clinical Pharmacy Specialist-Pain Management
Pharmacy
VA Long Beach Healthcare System
Long Beach, California

Eva Pittman, MSN, RN-BC
LEAN Strategies Coach
LEAN Strategies Department
New Hanover Regional Medical Center
Wilmington, North Carolina

Mena Raouf, PharmD, BCPS
Clinical Pharmacy Programs Coordinator–Pain Management
Kaiser Permanente
Federal Way, Washington

Nitin K. Sekhri, MD
Medical Director of Pain Management
Anesthesiology
Westchester Medical Center
Valhalla, New York
Assistant Professor
Anesthesiology
New York Medical College
Valhalla, New York

Erica L. Wegrzyn, BS, PharmD
Clinical Pharmacy Specialist, Pain Management
Stratton VA Medical Center
Albany, New York
Adjunct Faculty
Western New England University College of Pharmacy
Springfield, Massachusetts
Albany College of Pharmacy & Health Sciences
Albany, New York

Elsa Wuhrman, DNP, FNP,BC
Nurse Practitioner and Assistant Professor of Nursing at CUIMC
Pain Management/Anesthesiology
Columbia University Irving Medical Center
New York, New York

Clinical Scenario Contributors

Cindy Kerwick

Denise Kuhn

Brian Quinlan

Foreword

It is hard for me to believe that nearly 30 years have passed since Margo McCaffery and I began writing and publishing together. It has been 21 years since the publication of our first book on pain management and nearly 10 years since the publication of our last. When Margo died and I retired, I worried that there might never be another comprehensive, clinically-focused book to guide clinicians in their efforts to manage pain. I see now that my worries were unfounded as I look at this wide-ranging, thorough work by Maureen Cooney and Ann Quinlan-Colwell. Cooney and Quinlan-Colwell are leading front-line pain management experts, and their knowledge of the literature and expertise at the bedside can be felt throughout the book. Further, the book represents the importance of a multidisciplinary approach to pain management with multiple specialist contributors providing content. The content of the book offers something for everyone, from the novice to the expert pain manager.

This comprehensive, evidence-based book emphasizes that the foundation of successful pain management is a multidisciplinary commitment to conduct a thorough assessment of the patient's unique pain experience followed by the implementation of an individualized multimodal analgesia plan that combines appropriate analgesics and integrative approaches. As you read the pages of this superb text, you will understand that this was the secret to success in achieving optimal pain control in the past, is still today, and will be in the future.

One has only to read the table of contents to appreciate the impressive scope of Cooney and Quinlan-Colwell's book. The physiology of pain, its numerous adverse effects, and the barriers to managing them are described. Misconceptions related to pain and pain management are corrected. The authors address the spiritual, emotional, and cultural aspects of the pain experience and explain the ethical framework for managing pain. State-of-the-art assessment tools and practical guidance for assessment in all populations, including those who present assessment challenges, are provided. The need for clinicians to address their knowledge deficits and biases while assessing and managing pain in the person with opioid use disorder is stressed.

The authors dissect the scientific literature to support the application of multimodal analgesia in a wide variety of clinical settings and patient populations throughout the book. Several chapters focus on the pharmacological management of pain with a presentation of the science behind the use of the various analgesic groups, specific therapies, and interventional approaches. The authors demonstrate a commitment to ensuring safe pain control through prevention and management of side effects.

Advances in the field of integrative pain management are underscored with emphasis on achieving optimal functional and quality of life goals through the practical application of nonpharmacological therapies, such as relaxation, energy therapies, meditation, and exercise. The scientific evidence for use of other important nonpharmacological methods, such as caregiver empathy and compassion, aromatherapy, diet, and mirror therapy, is presented. Guidance on how to maximize the effectiveness of cognitive behavioral techniques in combination with analgesics is offered. Where appropriate, cautions on the use of nonpharmacological methods are included.

The comprehensive nature of the book is evident with chapters ranging from the use of botanicals and herbs to establishing institutional commitment to pain management. The reader is given an opportunity to apply key points to case scenarios in nearly every chapter in the book. Extensive reference lists and an abundance of pain management resources are provided.

In closing, I want to recognize the authors' commitment to the field of pain. Writing a book such as the one Cooney and Quinlan-Colwell have written here is a personal sacrifice that demonstrates a dedication to those who experience pain and the clinicians who manage it. A book such as this is the culmination of years of intense focused work. The years spent writing represent significant time away from family members and friends. Writing a book is often a lonely pursuit that requires long hours of thinking, researching, organizing, and then finding the right words to convey the message. These hours are often late at night and in addition to other full time work, as was the case of both Cooney and Quinlan-Colwell. Thoughts of the book and the next sentence to write or rewrite invade the author's mind at work and even during sleep. It is a 24-hours-a-day, 7-days-a-week obsession. Readers of this book owe Maureen Cooney and Ann Quinlan-Colwell great thanks for the opportunity to benefit from their sacrifice.

Chris Pasero, MS, RN-BC, FAAN (Retired)

Acknowledgments

It has been a great honor to write this book. Although many family members, friends, and colleagues supported and assisted us in innumerable ways, there are a few whose support we want to acknowledge.

Ann greatly appreciates the incalculable support, patience, encouragement, home management, and computer troubleshooting of her best friend, partner, and husband Clancy. She would also like to acknowledge her sons John-Michael and Brian and granddaughter Lili Agnes who always remind her to see things from a different perspective. Ann is always indebted to her father, Bob Daly, who taught her compassion, empathy, and to remember that every person "is doing the best they can do today." She also expresses deep appreciation to many professional mentors. In particular the experience of being taught, encouraged, and supported by Dr. Mona Shattell with writing and revising manuscripts was invaluable while writing the various chapters of this book.

Ann Quinlan-Colwell, PhD, RNBC, CNS, AHNBC
317 Gregory Road
Wilmington, NC 28405
Phone: 910-632-4486
E-mail: aqcl@earthlink.net

Maureen is grateful for the support of her children, Joseph, Meghan, and Patrick, who have taught her much from their own life journeys. Sharing priceless time with parents on one end of the age spectrum, and her granddaughter Olivia, on the other end, has given Maureen the gift of seeing life through many lenses while writing this book. Humor, encouragement, and the wisdom of dear friends and colleagues have been much appreciated. She is especially grateful for the support of one colleague who guided her entry into the world of pain management nursing and another who never doubted her ability to accomplish her goals and has provided her with the guidance and encouragement needed to sail her ship safely out of the harbor.

Maureen F. (Fennessy) Cooney, DNP, FNP-BC, RNBC, AP-PMN, AHPCN
197 Mt. Airy Rd West
Croton on Hudson, NY 10520
Phone: 914-260-8295
Email: Maureen.F.Cooney@gmail.com

We wish to express our deep gratitude to our numerous colleagues who coauthored, reviewed, and otherwise contributed to this book. Their insights, knowledge, and hard work were invaluable.

Finally, there are no words that can describe our appreciation for the guidance, support, and encouragement from Chris Pasero who provided the opportunity to create this book.

Contents

1 The Evolution of Pain Assessment and Multimodal Analgesia as an Integrative Pain Management Approach, 1

Ann Quinlan-Colwell and Maureen F. Cooney

Incidence and Prevalence of Pain, 2
Historical Perspective of Multimodal Pain Management, 2
Pain Assessment as the Foundation of Multimodal Analgesia, 4
Evolution of an Integrative Multimodal Approach for Pain Management (Multimodal Analgesia) (Multimodal Treatment), 5
Drivers for Integrative, Multimodal, Opioid-Sparing Approaches, 8
Future Challenges and Opportunities for Multimodal Analgesia Within an Integrative Approach, 10
References, 15

2 Importance of Multimodal Pain Management, 19

Ann Quinlan-Colwell

Physiologic Complications of Unrelieved Pain, 19
Psychosocial Implications of Unrelieved Pain, 20
Role of Multimodal Analgesia in the Perioperative Setting, 22
Role of Multimodal Analgesia in the Management of Chronic Pain, 22
Ethical Considerations, 22
Clinical Application, 24
Key Points, 25
Case Scenario, 25
References, 25

3 Physiology of Pain, 28

Maureen F. Cooney and Shalvi B. Parikh

Theories of Pain, 28
Other Models, 30
Classifications of Pain, 31
Pain Physiology and Pathophysiology, 35
Special Conditions, 45
Key Points, 46

Case Scenario, 46
References, 46

4 Barriers to Effective Pain Management, 50

Ann Quinlan-Colwell

Patient Barriers, 50
Clinical Application, 52
Fear, 52
Fear of Side Effects, 52
Health Care Literacy, 53
Family, 53
Access Issues, 54
Provider Barriers, 55
System Barriers to Effective Pain Management, 56
Opportunities, 57
Key Points, 57
Case Scenario, 58
References, 58

5 Introduction to Pain Assessment, 61

Maureen F. Cooney

Importance of Pain Assessment, 61
Classification of Pain, 62
Roles of the Health Team in Pain Assessment, 64
Timing and Frequency of Pain Assessment, 64
Key Points, 70
Case Scenario, 70
References, 71

6 Pain Assessment in Cognitively Intact Adults, 73

Maureen F. Cooney and Debra Drew

Accurate Pain Assessment, 73
Pain Assessment, 73
Components of a Comprehensive Pain Assessment, 76
Conducting the Pain Assessment, 84
Tools for Assessing Pain, 85
Key Points, 109
Case Scenario, 109
References, 109
Appendix 6-1, 113
Appendix 6-2, 119

7 Pain Assessment of Patients Who Cannot Self-Report Pain, 120

Debra Drew and Ann Quinlan-Colwell

Pain Assessment of Patients Who Cannot Self-Report Pain, 120
Pain Assessment in Critically Ill Adults Who Cannot Self-Report Pain, 124
Patients With Delirium Who Cannot Self-Report Pain, 125
Patients With Dementia Who Cannot Self-Report Pain, 125
The Checklist of Nonverbal Pain Indicators (CNPI), 129
Patients With Intellectual Disabilities Who Cannot Self-Report Pain, 129
Patients at the End of Life Who Cannot Self-Report Pain, 131
Newer Trends in Pain Assessment for Patients Who Cannot Self-Report Pain, 131
Cautions, 132
Key Points, 132
Case Scenario, 132
References, 133

8 Assessment of Factors Affecting Pain and Affected by Pain, 136

Ann Quinlan-Colwell

Sleep, 136
Anxiety and Depression, 146
Family Assessment, 158
Financial Assessment, 158
Key Points, 158
Case Scenario, 159
References, 159

9 Basic Concepts Involved with Administration of Analgesic Medications, 163

Maureen F. Cooney and Ann Quinlan-Colwell

Patient Considerations, 163
Route Selection, 167
Analgesic Dosing Considerations, 181
Key Points, 190
Case Scenario, 191
References, 191

10 Nonopioid Analgesic Medications, 195

Meredith W. Crumb, Timothy J. Atkinson, and Maureen F. Cooney

Aspirin and Nonsteroidal Antiinflammatory Drugs, 195
Multimodal Use of Nonopioid Analgesics, 214
Key Points, 215
Case Scenario, 215
References, 216

11 Opioid Analgesics, 222

Maureen F. Cooney, Mena Raouf, Jeffrey J. Bettinger, Erica L. Wegrzyn, and Jeffrey Fudin

Section 1, 223
Opioid Pharmacology, 223
Opioid Receptors, 224
Factors Affecting Drug Response, 226
Opioid Classes, 232
Key Points, 236
Section 2, 236
Opioid Selection, 236
Key Points, 269
Section 3, 269
Opioid Dosing Practices, 269
Tapering and Discontinuing Opioid Therapy, 287
Key Points, 289
Case Scenario, 289
References, 291

12 Common Unintended Effects of Opioids, 303

Ann Quinlan-Colwell and Maureen F. Cooney

Constipation, 306
Xerostomia (Dry Mouth), 311
Opioid-Induced Nausea and Vomiting, 312
Pruritus, 314
Urinary Retention, 319
Hypogonadism, 321
Sedation, 323
Myoclonus, 325
Opioid-Induced Hyperalgesia, 326
Physical Dependence on Opioids, 327
Opioid Tolerance, 328
Immune Suppressing Effect of Opioids, 328
Key Points, 329
Case Scenario, 329
References, 329

13 Preventing Opioid-Induced Advancing Sedation and Respiratory Depression, 337

Carla R. Jungquist and Ann Quinlan-Colwell

Opioids and Respiratory Function, 338
Advancing Sedation and Opioid-Induced Respiratory Depression, 338
Identification of the Risk Factors, 339
Associated Pharmacologic Factors, 342
Strategizing to Improve Safety for Patients at Risk, 347
Assessing the Patient for Risk, 347
Procedures for Intermittent Nursing Assessment for All Patients on Opioids: Level of Sedation, 348
Procedures for Intermittent Nursing Assessment for All Patients on Opioids: Respiratory Status, 351
Interventions After Assessment, 353
Summary, 353
Key Points, 353
Case Scenario, 354

Acknowledgments, 354
References, 354

14 Opioid Use Disorder, 360

Ann Quinlan-Colwell and Maureen F. Cooney

Substance Use Disorder and Opioid Use Disorder, 361
Caring for Patients With Pain and Opioid Use Disorder, 363
Treatment of Opioid Use Disorder, 365
Pain and Opioid Use Disorder: Acute Care Setting, 369
Strategies to Reduce Risk, 376
Key Points, 377
Case Scenario, 379
References, 379

15 Coanalgesic Medications, 384

Courtney Kominek and Maureen F. Cooney

Medication Selection, 386
Gabapentinoids, 389
Antidepressants, 394
Alpha-Adrenergic Receptor Agonists, 398
Corticosteroids, 401
N-Methyl-D-Aspartate Receptor Antagonists, 403
Sodium Channel Blockers: Lidocaine and Mexiletine, 409
Muscle Relaxants, 412
Dronabinol, Nabilone, and Cannabidiol, 416
Other Coanalgesic Medications, 418
Key Points, 418
Case Scenario, 419
References, 419

16 Topical Analgesics for the Management of Acute and Chronic Pain, 429

Elsa Wuhrman, Maureen F. Cooney, and Thien C. Pham

Benefits of Topical Analgesics, 429
Types of Topical Analgesics, 431
Compound Analgesics, 441
Key Points, 443
Case Scenario, 443
References, 444

17 Patient-Controlled Analgesia, 447

Ann Quinlan-Colwell

General Concepts, 447
Optimize Safety Within the Patient-Controlled Analgesia Process, 449
Prescription Components, 455
Routes of Administration, 458
Patient Assessment and Monitoring to Optimize Safety, 462
Evaluating Equipment to Optimize Patient Safety, 464
Authorized Agent–Controlled Analgesia, 465
Key Points, 468
Case Scenario, 468
References, 468

18 Regional Analgesia, Local Infiltration, and Pain Management, 474

Maureen F. Cooney, Christine Peltier, and Ann Quinlan-Colwell

Neuraxial Analgesia, 475
Regional Analgesia, 510
Regional Analgesia Infusion Systems, 518
Local Infiltration Analgesia, 520
Additional Analgesic Procedures Involving Use of Local Anesthetics, 524
Key Points, 525
Case Scenario, 526
References, 526

19 Interventional Approaches, 533

Nitin K. Sekhri, Emily Davis, Ann Quinlan-Colwell, and Maureen F. Cooney

Anatomy of the Central Nervous System, 533
Spinal Pain, 533
Diagnostic Imaging, 537
Spinal Injections, 538
Implantable Therapies, 543
Key Points, 554
Case Scenario, 554
Acknowledgement, 555
References, 555

20 Exercise and Movement, 560

Ann Quinlan-Colwell

Fear of Pain With Movement, 561
Exercise-Induced Hypoalgesia, 564
Movement, 564
Dance Movement Therapy, 565
Exercise, 566
Tai Chi, 569
Yoga, 570
Physical Therapy, 571
Patient Education for All Exercise and Movement, 576
Key Points, 576
Case Scenario, 576
References, 578

21 Distraction and Relaxation, 586

Michele Erich, Ann Quinlan-Colwell, and Susan O'Conner-Von

Distraction, 586
Relaxation, 591
Progressive Muscle Relaxation, 594
Music Therapy, 596
Animal-Assisted Therapy, 600
Guided Imagery, 603
Autogenic Training, 604
Key Points, 605
Case Scenario, 605
References, 606

22 Cognitive-Behavioral and Psychotherapeutic Interventions as Components of Multimodal Analgesic Pain Management, 613

Geralyn Datz and Ann Quinlan-Colwell

Integrative, Interdisciplinary, and Multimodal Pain Treatment, 613
Interdisciplinary Pain Rehabilitation or Functional Restoration Programs, 615
Cognitive-Behavioral Therapy, 617
Evidence Supporting Cognitive-Behavioral Therapy for Pain Management, 622
The Activating Event Belief Consequence Model, 624
Acceptance and Commitment Therapy, 625
Biofeedback (Applied Psychophysiology), 626
Mindfulness-Based Stress Management and Mindfulness-Based Cognitive Therapy, 627
Psychoeducation, 630
Key Points, 631
Case Scenario, 631
References, 631

23 Energy Healing Therapies or Biofield Therapies as Components of Multimodal Analgesic Pain Management, 636

Ann Quinlan-Colwell and Susan O'Conner-Von

Reiki, 637
Therapeutic Touch, 638
Healing Touch, 642
Acupuncture, 642
Auricular Acupuncture, 644
Acupressure, 647
Key Points, 648
Case Scenario, 648
References, 648

24 Manual Therapies for Pain Management, 652

Ann Quinlan-Colwell

Manual Therapy, 652
Osteopathy, Osteopathy Manual Medicine, or Osteopathic Manipulative Therapy, 653
Craniosacral Therapy, 654
Massage Therapy, 655
Reflexology, 659
Chiropractic Practice, 664
Myofascial Trigger Point Therapy, 666
Muscle Energy Technique, 667
Fascial Distortion Model, 667
Key Points, 668
Case Scenario, 668
Acknowledgments, 668
References, 668

25 Spirituality as a Component of Multimodal Pain Management, 673

Susan O'Conner-Von and Ann Quinlan-Colwell

Spirituality, 673
Prayer, 674
Meditation, 675
General Cautions and Precautions Regarding Meditation, 682
Key Points, 683
Case Scenario, 683
References, 684

26 Natural Products: Supplements, Botanicals, Vitamins, and Minerals as a Component of Multimodal Pain Management, 687

Ann Quinlan-Colwell

Dietary Supplements, 688
Botanicals and Herbs, 688
Pharmaconutrients: Nutritional Modulators of Pain, 702
Supplements, 707
Vitamins, 716
Key Points, 723
Case Scenario, 723
References, 723

27 Additional Nonpharmacologic Interventions as Components of Multimodal Pain Management, 738

Ann Quinlan-Colwell

Aromatherapy, 739
Caring, Empathy, and Compassion by Caregivers, 742
Crossing Hands and/or Arms Over the Midline, 743
Dietary Choices, 745
Environmental Modifications, 747
Hypnosis, 749
Mirror Therapy or Mirror Visual Feedback Therapy, 751
Obesity and Weight Management, 754
Static Magnet Therapy, 756
Temperature Modalities, 756
Alternating or Contrasting Temperature Therapy, 759
Valsalva Maneuver, 760
Key Points, 761
Case Scenario, 761
References, 762

28 Improving Institutional Commitment for Effective Multimodal Pain Management, 770

Ann Quinlan-Colwell, Sue Ballato, Greg Scott Firestone, and Eva Pittman

Organizational Commitment to Quality and Pain Management, 770

Organizational Initiatives to Support Quality of Safe and Effective Multimodal Pain Management, 772
Quality Improvement, 781
Clinical Nursing Efforts to Support Organizational Initiatives, 787
Education of Clinicians, 789
Future Opportunities for Improvement, 790
Key Points, 790

Case Scenario, 792
References, 792

Appendix: Terminology, 797

Index, 830

Assessment and Multimodal Management of Pain

AN INTEGRATIVE APPROACH

Chapter 1 The Evolution of Pain Assessment and Multimodal Analgesia as an Integrative Pain Management Approach

Ann Quinlan-Colwell, Maureen F. Cooney

CHAPTER OUTLINE

Incidence and Prevalence of Pain, pg. 2

Historical Perspective of Multimodal Pain Management, pg. 2

Growth in Pain Research, pg. 3

Early National Efforts to Address Pain, pg. 3

Pain Assessment as the Foundation of Multimodal Analgesia, pg. 4

Evolution of an Integrative Multimodal Approach for Pain Management (Multimodal Analgesia) (Multimodal Treatment), pg. 5

Early Support for Multimodal Analgesia, pg. 5

The Increase in Opioid Prescribing, pg. 5

Rise in Opioid-Related Complications, pg. 7

Resurgence of Support for Integrative, Multimodal, Opioid-Sparing Approaches, pg. 7

Drivers for Integrative, Multimodal, Opioid-Sparing Approaches, pg. 8

Professional Organizations, pg. 8

Centers for Disease Control and Prevention Guidelines, pg. 9

The Joint Commission, pg. 9

Enhanced Recovery After Surgery Society Guidelines, pg. 9

Institute of Medicine Report, pg. 10

National Pain Strategy, pg. 10

Future Challenges and Opportunities for Multimodal Analgesia Within an Integrative Approach, pg.10

References, pg. 15

IN 1968, Margo McCaffery, a pioneer in pain management nursing taught: "Pain is whatever the experiencing person says it is, existing whenever he/she says it does" (McCaffery, 1968). From a similar perspective, in 1979, the International Association for the Study of Pain (IASP) defined pain as, "an unpleasant sensory and emotional experience associated with actual or potential tissue damage, or described in terms of such" (IASP, 1979, p. 250). Both of these definitions underscore pain as a completely subjective experience with no mechanism to objectively measure or quantify it (Aydede, 2017; Nahin, 2015). In the mid-17th century, Descartes theorized the relationship between a painful stimulus, such as a foot near a flame, results in a process similar to a cord ringing a bell in the brain, with that process resulting in the person perceiving pain (Fig. 1.1) (Moayedi & Davis, 2013). Although since the time of Descartes the knowledge and understanding of pain has dramatically evolved, the actual perception of pain can still be fully understood only by the person experiencing it.

Despite health care clinicians having responsibility to ease pain and suffering along with advances in knowledge and analgesic medications, pain continued to be inadequately managed through the end of the last century (Yaster, Benzon, & Anderson, 2017). More than a decade ago, in *Guides to the Evaluation of Permanent Impairment,* the American Medical Association (AMA) representatives wrote:

The traditional and outdated biomedical approach assumes that all pain symptoms have a specific cause and attempts to eradicate the cause directly by rectifying the presumed pathophysiology. However, chronic pain can rarely be understood by linear, nociceptive mechanisms. There is often an absence of documented physical relationship between pain and pathophysiology (Rondinelli, Genovese, Brigham, & AMA, 2008, p. 32).

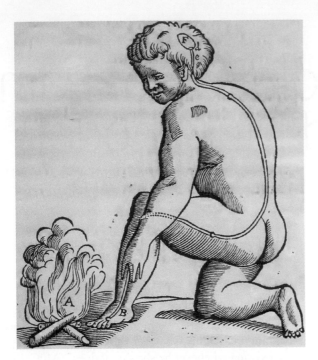

Fig. 1.1 | Drawing by Louis La Forge based on Descartes' description of *Treatise of Man* (1664). (Out of copyright.)

In this introductory chapter, an overview is presented, including brief description of the evolution of pain being understood as a complex multidimensional experience, the importance of assessing pain, and why an integrative approach of managing pain with multimodal analgesia is the safest and most effective way to support people to best control pain.

Incidence and Prevalence of Pain

Pain is primarily a universal experience occurring among humans and other animals. Even rodents with somatosensory cortex lesions who experienced *asomaesthesia*, or the inability to recognize physical sensations, experienced pain at least through the inflammatory process even when they were not able to process the sensations somatosensorily (Uhelski, Davis, & Fuchs, 2012). The small number of people who are diagnosed with a true painlessness disorder either have a Mendelian genetic trait or an abnormal development of pain receptor neurons (Nahorski, Chen, & Woods, 2015a; Nahorski, et al., 2015b). Although acute pain is a protective response to trauma or inflammation, when unrelieved it is harmful and can evolve into chronic pain (Chapman & Vierck, 2017).

In 1982, Khatami & Rush wrote: "Chronic pain is a perplexing problem that costs billions of dollars annually in the United States alone. It affects family relations, job performance, emotional well-being, and even the doctor-patient relationship" (Khatami & Rush, 1982, p. 45). Unfortunately, these words are surprisingly still accurate as a description of chronic pain 35 years later. For many reasons, despite the universality of the pain experience, it is not possible to obtain accurate data on the incidence and prevalence of pain. The challenges of collecting such data include the subjective nature of pain, numerous definitions of pain, methodologic issues, and infrequent research involving epidemiologic studies of pain (Henschke, Kamper, & Maher, 2015). This is complicated by different people not only experiencing pain differently but also understanding it and describing it differently. The same challenges exist for collecting data regarding acute pain. However, this is complicated by acute pain having a more elusive nature, which results in most acute pain data being reported only for postoperative and trauma pain (Rzewuska, Ferreira, McLachlan, Machado, & Maher, 2015).

In a 2015 National Institutes of Health (NIH) report, it was estimated that 126 million adults in the United States experienced pain at some point during the previous 3 months, with 25.3 million (11.2%) reporting chronic daily pain (Nahin, 2015). In addition, in 2015, chronic pain was again described as causing clinical, social, and financial challenges, with an estimated cost of more than $34 billion annually in Australia and between $560 and $635 billion annually in the United States (Henschke et al., 2015). These figures do not include the loss of productivity incurred by people living with pain (Dale & Stacey, 2016). The following year, it was estimated that approximately half of people in Europe experienced at least one episode of pain, with a 19% prevalence of chronic pain (Macfarlane, 2016).

The situation regarding acute pain is similar, with more than 80% of people reporting pain after surgery and approximately 75% reporting moderate, severe, or extreme pain (Chou et al., 2016). Approximately half of all patients report inadequately controlled postoperative pain (Polomano, Dunwoody, Krenzischek, & Rathmell, 2008). Despite many publications about acute pain after surgery, rigorous research is needed to ascertain the prevalence and evidence to support guidelines and recommendations for safe and effective multimodal management (Gordon, et al., 2016).

There is increasing awareness that unrelieved acute pain results in chronic pain (Choinière, et al., 2014). This is estimated to be as prevalent as 30% after some surgical procedures (e.g., herniorrhaphy, thoracotomy, limb amputation, mastectomy) (Lovich-Sapola, Smith, & Brandt, 2015). Additional research is needed to better understand the extent to which acute pain is experienced and to more fully understand the evolution of acute pain to chronic pain and how to prevent that from occurring after both surgical and trauma pain situations (Bendayan, Ramírez-Maestre, Ferrer, López, & Esteve, 2017; Chapman & Vierck, 2017; Lovich-Sapola et al., 2015; Shipton, 2014).

Historical Perspective of Multimodal Pain Management

The work of anesthesiologist John Bonica, who is considered the father of modern pain management, was instrumental in the development and advancement of multidisciplinary pain management (Tompkins, Hobelmann, & Compton, 2017). Bonica, while working with injured soldiers in World War II, recognized that despite the use of regional anesthetic techniques, many of the soldiers did not have adequate pain relief and developed chronic pain (Tompkins et al., 2017). He reached out to colleagues in the fields of psychiatry, neurology, and orthopedics and noted that when his patients were seen by consultants from those specialties, pain and functional outcomes improved. In the 1950's based upon his experiences, Bonica developed the first multidisciplinary pain clinic, which was opened in Tacoma, Washington, and relocated to the University of Washington in Seattle in the 1960s (Loeser, 2017). The treatment included multidisciplinary and integrative interventions such as physical therapy, occupational therapy, and a variety of psychologic and cognitive approaches (Gatchel, McGeary, McGeary, & Lippe, 2014; Parris, & Johnson, 2014) (see Chapters 20, 21, 22). Pharmacologic approaches were also provided, but contrary to usual practice, scheduled medication administration, rather than as-needed (prn) dosing, was employed (Tompkins et al., 2017). The patients in the multidisciplinary clinic had significant improvements in outcomes, including return to employment. Studies of patient outcomes in the multidisciplinary clinic compared to single discipline treatment, usual medical care, or no treatment, showed improved outcomes were an effect of the coordinated biopsychosocial approach to care provided in the multidisciplinary setting (Tompkins et al., 2017). As study results were disseminated, multidisciplinary programs were developed throughout the country and many of Bonica's integrative approaches to pain management were adopted (Tompkins et al., 2017).

Multidisciplinary pain clinics continued into the 1990s. Although this type of clinic still exists, the following factors contributed to the decline in the use of this approach in the United States (Tompkins et al., 2017)

- Changes in insurance reimbursement practices from bundled services to a fee-for-service model resulted in financial losses in multidisciplinary clinics.
- The introduction of managed care changed payment structures and *carved out,* or stopped, reimbursement for services such as physical therapy if the service was provided in the multidisciplinary clinic.
- Academic medical centers, which often provided multidisciplinary pain clinics, closed the clinics because of financial losses associated with managed care.
- The growth of anesthesia-based pain fellowship training programs increased the focus on procedure-based care rather than multidisciplinary care.

Growth in Pain Research

Bonica was a major contributor to the development of pain research and progress in the field of pain management in the latter half of the 20th century (Loeser, 2017). He published numerous studies that demonstrated the extent, severity, and impact of pain on a worldwide level. Bonica's work was instrumental in the formation of the American Pain Society (APS) and the IASP. His efforts encouraged a new focus on the study of pain, and over the years new pain theories were published, scientific inquiry into the field of pain expanded, and significant growth in the understanding of pain processes and pathways occurred. The identification of peripheral and central pain pathways led to great interest in pharmaceutical research and the development of different classes of analgesic agents such as the nonsteroidal antiinflammatory medications (Tompkins et al., 2017).

Early National Efforts to Address Pain

As scientific efforts to improve understanding and treatment of pain evolved, there was growth in awareness of continued undertreatment of pain as a health care problem. This awareness led to an initiative by the NIH to form a consensus development conference to address the issues and challenges associated with the need for an integration of approaches to pain management (NIH, 1986). Expert health professionals, including biomedical researchers, physicians, dentists, psychologists, nurses, and others, along with representatives of the general public, were brought together on May 19 to 21, 1986 to address the following questions (NIH, 1986):

- In what way should pain be assessed?
- In what ways should medications be used in an integrated pain management approach?
- How should nonpharmacologic approaches be used in an integrated pain management approach?
- What role does the nurse have in an integrated pain management approach?
- What are the future directions for pain management research?

As an outcome of the conference, participants reached consensus in response to these questions (NIH, 1986). It was agreed that pain is an important and complex phenomenon, and accurate pain assessment facilitates classification of pain and establishment of treatment objectives. It was also recognized that the management of pain is challenging, because although pain may be well assessed, many variables and barriers, including personal attitudes and lack of knowledge of health care providers, may interfere with adequate treatment. The pivotal role of the nurse in the assessment and management of pain was recognized. Agreement was reached that the nursing role in pain management was expected to increase with an integrated approach involving the multidisciplinary health care team is necessary.

The importance of both pharmacologic and nonpharmacologic therapies in treating different types of pain was identified, and it became evident that no single modality is appropriate for the treatment of most people in pain. The experts concluded the treatment of pain and the assessment of response to treatment require an individualized approach and appreciation for the multiple factors that have an impact on each person's pain experience and that future pain research needed to explore these many factors. The consensus group recognized "an integrated approach to the assessment and management of pain brings greater options to individuals seeking the alleviation of pain" (NIH, 1986, para. 47).

As national awareness of the problem of poorly managed pain continued to grow after the 1986 NIH consensus conference, research efforts and interest in the need for clinical improvements also increased. In 1992 the Agency for Healthcare Policy and Research (AHCPR; now the Agency for Health Care Research and Quality [AHRQ]) published the first clinical practice guideline for pain management (Berry et al., 2001). This guideline addressed pain management in patients undergoing operative or medical procedures and trauma. Subsequently, in 1994 the AHCPR released a guideline for the management of cancer pain. The developers of the 1992 guideline, like those on the NIH consensus panel, acknowledged the undertreatment of pain, recognized the complexity and subjective nature of pain, and supported the need for frequent accurate pain assessments, with the patient's self-report (when possible) as the primary source of assessment. The 1992 guideline also emphasized the need for a collaborative, interdisciplinary approach to pain, an individualized proactive pain treatment plan, the use of pharmacologic and nonpharmacologic therapies to control pain, and the need for a formalized institutional approach to acute pain management (AHCPR, 1992).

Pain Assessment as the Foundation of Multimodal Analgesia

One of the outcomes of the NIH consensus conference was agreement about the importance of the assessment of pain. It was recognized that pain assessment needs to include diagnostic evaluation and clarification of the goals of care. Assessment should be specific to the type of pain, the cause of the pain, and the characteristics of the person affected by pain. In the mid-1980s, most assessment tools were based on the chronic pain model and were often tools used in research, not clinical practice (NIH, 1986). The McGill Pain Questionnaire, a multidimensional tool developed by Melzack (1975), was introduced in 1975 to measure the sensory-discriminative, motivational-affective, and cognitive-evaluative dimensions of pain in the evaluation of pain therapies. Few valid and reliable tools were available for the assessment of acute pain. Unidimensional tools were mostly used in research to measure pain intensity to determine effectiveness of pharmacologic and other pain interventions. For example, the visual analogue scale (VAS), introduced in 1964, and the numerical rating scale (NRS), introduced after the VAS, were initially used to compare effectiveness of analgesics to placebo (Noble et al., 2005).

In 1999 inadequate assessment of pain and pain relief was identified as the most significant factor contributing to the undertreatment of pain in U.S. hospitals (Max, Payne, Edwards, Sunshine, & Inturrisi, 1999). Recognition of the importance of pain assessment led to the introduction of the phrase *pain as the fifth vital sign* by the APS and adoption of this concept by the Veterans Health Administration in their national pain strategy (Berry et al., 2001). Many embraced the use of this phrase in efforts to ensure pain would be assessed on a routine basis akin to vital signs (e.g., pulse, respiration, blood pressure). The introduction of standards for pain assessment and management by the Joint Commission on Accreditation of Healthcare Organization (JCAHO; now the Joint Commission [TJC]) in 2000 furthered the adoption of practices to facilitate routine pain assessment. However, use of the phrase *pain as the fifth vital sign* was eventually challenged and mostly abandoned, because critics opined that unlike vital signs that are objective, pain is a subjective experience and complex phenomenon that may require assessment more or less frequently than the need for vital sign measurement (Pasero, Quinlan-Colwell, Rae, Broglio, & Drew, 2016).

Optimal pain management and appropriate multimodal analgesia depend on appropriate assessment and reassessment (Chou et al., 2016). The growth in the number of unidimensional and multidimensional tools for the assessment of acute and chronic pain is the result of the cumulative efforts of the many individuals and organizations that have advocated, over the years, to improve care of patients with pain. Recent initiatives to improve pain assessment practices include the development of tools that promote a social interaction, such as the multifaceted Clinically Aligned Pain Assessment (CAPA) tool, which requires a conversation between clinician and patient to address five domains affected by pain (Topham & Drew, 2017). Many pain assessment tools have undergone psychometric testing and are intended for use in different patient populations, in patients with varied clinical conditions, and in different clinical settings. Refer to Chapters 5, 6, and 7 for in-depth information related to pain assessment.

A critical concept when assessing pain from an integrative perspective is that the pain experience involves more than just an intensity rating; thus assessment of pain must also involve additional components (Pasero et al., 2016). Emphasis is placed on the need to assess the impact of pain on an individual's function. Although function has been assessed as a component of some of the multidimensional tools used in chronic pain assessment, it is only recently gaining attention as a dimension that may be incorporated in the acute pain assessment. Frequent reassessment of pain and function are critical to facilitate optimal pain control, ensure patient safety, and gain the information needed to revise the analgesic plan of care for patients in the acute care setting (Chou, et al., 2016) and those being treated for chronic pain in primary care settings (Anderson, Zlateva, Khatri, & Ciaburri, 2015). Several of the 2018 TJC pain standards include the need for consideration of function in establishing pain treatment goals and assessing responses to multimodal pain relief measures (TJC, 2017).

As pain assessment practices and tools continue to evolve, it is essential to recognize that an accurate pain assessment is fundamental to all efforts to alleviate pain. Continued efforts to emphasize the importance of pain assessment and develop practices and tools that support accurate pain assessment are necessary for the implementation of safe and effective integrative, multimodal pain management approaches.

Evolution of an Integrative Multimodal Approach for Pain Management (Multimodal Analgesia) (Multimodal Treatment)

Early Support for Multimodal Analgesia

Although clinical care and treatment lagged behind the scientific understanding of pain, awareness of the value of multimodal analgesia evolved slowly. Identification of opioid receptors in the brain and spinal cord in the 1970s led to research that demonstrated the benefits of adding opioids to local anesthetic epidural solutions a decade later (Kehlet & Dahl, 1993). During the 1980s, experts researched the phenomenon of poorly controlled acute postoperative pain and began to employ treatment approaches that included combinations of systemic NSAIDs with opioids. The use of opioids and local anesthetics in epidural solutions expanded, and the addition of the alpha-2 agonist clonidine to epidural solutions was introduced (Kehlet, 1989; Kehlet & Dahl, 1993). Likewise, in the 1980s, interest began to develop in the use of nonopioid analgesics and tricyclic antidepressants along with opioids to improve pain relief for patients with cancer (Richlin, Jamron, & Novick, 1987).

One of the first uses of the term *multimodal analgesia* in the pain-related literature was by Khatami and Rush in their February 1982 article describing the multimodal treatment program used in a pilot study with five people living with chronic pain and in the 1-year follow-up of a subsequent study (n = 23) using the same psychology-based multimodal approach (Khatami & Rush, 1978; Khatami & Rush, 1982). Their studies were based on the hypotheses that there are both interpersonal and intrapersonal determinants involved with chronic pain and chronic pain could be better controlled by addressing symptoms, stimuli, and social system alterations. Their hypothesis was consistent with the earlier multidimensional model developed by Melzack and Casey (1968). The results of the 1-year follow-up study by Khatami and

Rush included reports of significantly less pain, anxiety, and depression with less analgesic use among the participants who completed their program (n = 14) compared with those who only partially completed their program.

Nearly a decade later, Kehlet (1989) advocated to proactively use combinations of analgesic medications as well as nonpharmacologic interventions to alleviate what he referred to as *surgical stress*. Subsequently, Kehlet and Dahl (1993) introduced the terms *multimodal analgesia* and *balanced analgesia* as a method for treating postoperative pain. The concept of using multimodal analgesia in the management of postoperative pain continued to slowly grow in use and acceptance during the 1990s (Doyle & Bowler, 1998; Michaloliakou, Chung, & Sharma, 1996; Peduto, Ballabio, & Stefanini, 1998; Sukhani & Frey, 1997).

Today, a multimodal treatment approach continues to be the most effective way to help control chronic pain (Dale & Stacey, 2016). Multimodal treatment was recently defined by the IASP as being "the concurrent use of separate therapeutic interventions with different mechanisms of action within one discipline aimed at different pain mechanisms" (IASP, 2017). This definition is consistent with the concepts of integrative health care and multimodal analgesia. As information confirms the likelihood of acute pain progressing to chronic pain, a multimodal approach for acute pain is also advocated (Chou et al., 2016; Lovich-Sapola et al., 2015) (Fig. 1.2).

It is important to distinguish polypharmacy from multimodal analgesia. Polypharmacy occurs when multiple medications are prescribed when they are not necessary and/or are not indicated (Maher, Hanlon, & Hajjar, 2014). Multimodal analgesia is the intentional use of two or more medications (and/or nonpharmacologic interventions) with various mechanisms of action that act in different locations on the pain pathway (Buvanendran & Kroin, 2009). Therefore appropriate assessment of pain is critical in determining the particular multimodal analgesia components appropriate to safely and effectively control for each patient.

The Increase in Opioid Prescribing

On an international level, the World Health Organization (WHO), recognizing the prevalence and incidence of cancer pain in developed and developing countries, proclaimed the treatment of pain as a universal right, and developed cancer pain treatment guidelines. These guidelines, referred to as the *WHO Analgesic Ladder,* consist of a three-step approach ranging from the use of nonopioids, to weak opioids, and to strong opioids depending on the patient's pain level and response to treatment (WHO, 1986). The WHO Analgesic Ladder supports the use of a multimodal approach to cancer pain management, with recommendation for the use of nonopioid analgesics and adjuvant agents at every step in the ladder (Ventafridda, Tamburini, Caraceni, & Naldi, 1987).

Broad-Spectrum Analgesics

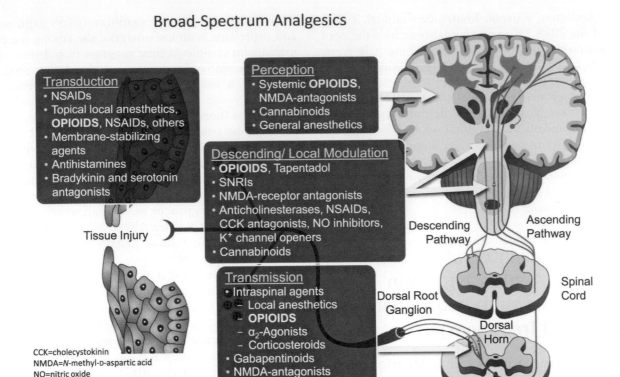

Fig. 1.2 | The sites of action of broad-analgesics. Targeting multiple distinct components in the pain-signaling pathway—transduction, transmission, perception, and modulation—is increasingly viewed as offering additive, perhaps even supra-additive (synergistic) pain reduction. Coadministration of the α2-receptor agonist clonidine along with an opioid, for example, may yield significantly greater analgesic effects when compared with either agent alone. Although the neural pathways that govern pain are yet to be fully elucidated, a balanced analgesic approach using multiple agents with unique modes of action is thought to reduce the peripheral and central sensitization and inflammation that often characterize chronic pain disorders. Adapted from D.J. Kelly, M. Ahmad, S.J. Brull, Preemptive analgesia I: physiological pathways and pharmacological modalities, Can J Anaesth, 48 (2001). In Gudin J. Opioid therapies and cytochrome interactions. J Pain Symptom Manage 2012; 44(6 Suppl), S4-S14

During the 1980s the use of opioids to treat cancer pain, particularly near the end of life, expanded in the United States as a result of advocacy by palliative care experts. Awareness of the WHO Analgesic Ladder increased, and guidelines were slowly adopted in clinical practice. Initiatives in the 1990s led to the expansion of multimodal approaches beyond the treatment of cancer pain to chronic noncancer pain. Experts called for the use of pharmacologic and nonpharmacologic approaches, but controversy existed about the use of opioids to treat chronic noncancer pain (Portenoy, 1996). Until then, opioids were rarely used for chronic noncancer pain because of concerns about the risks of tolerance, addiction, side effects, and impact on function. Clinical experience demonstrated that the benefits of long-term opioid use in the treatment of cancer pain markedly outweighed the presumed risks. Based on this experience and with heightened awareness of the inadequate treatment of chronic noncancer pain, experts in the pain community began to debate and consider the use of opioids in this population (Large & Schug, 1995; Portenoy, 1996; Turk, Brody, & Okifuji, 1994).

In 1990 the president of the APS brought attention to the problems of inadequate pain assessment and treatment and outlined necessary improvement measures. These measures included a call for the therapeutic use of opioids along with reassurance about the low risks for addiction (Baker, 2017). Limited available data demonstrated a low incidence of addiction in patients on opioid therapy for noncancer pain, but well-designed studies were lacking. Russell Portenoy, an expert palliative care physician, wrote "controlled clinical trials of long-term opioid therapy are needed, but the lack of these trials should not exclude empirical treatment (with opioids) when medical judgment supports it and therapy is undertaken with appropriate monitoring" (Portenoy, 1996, p. 212).

When concern about opioid use in patients with noncancer pain was raised, the 1980 Porter and Jick study was often cited as attesting to the safety of using opioids and the low risk for developing a substance use disorder (Compton & Volkow, 2006; Iles, Catterall, & Hanks, 2002; Kowal, 1998; Porter & Jick, 1980; Portenoy & Foley, 1986; Rich, 2001). This reference was cited more than 600 times between 1980 and 2017 (Leung, Macdonald, Stanbrook, Dhalla, & Juurlink, 2017). In actuality the frequently cited study, which reported that only 4 patients among nearly 12,000 developed addiction after being treated with opioids, was reported in a letter of five sentences to the editor, with no supporting documentation, (Porter &

Jick, 1980). All of the patients whose medical records were reviewed received opioids for a -limited period in an acute care setting. Years later, Dr. Jick shared that he never intended for the information to be generalized (Hawkins, 2017). This experience is important and serves to remind clinicians of their responsibility to critically evaluate reported data and assess whether it is appropriate to generalize the information to different populations.

Opioid use increased significantly in the 1990s and early 2000s. The rise in use has been attributed to many factors including pain management expert support, an increased focus on the importance of pain management by health care providers and the general public, addition of pain management standards by TJC in 2000, efforts to optimize patient satisfaction with pain control on Hospital Consumer Assessment of Healthcare Providers and Systems (HCAHPS) surveys, and increased availability and marketing of new opioid preparations such as extended-release oxycodone (Tompkins et al., 2017).

Rise in Opioid-Related Complications

As opioid use increased, complications of opioid use also increased in health care and community settings. The use of opioids to treat acute pain has been associated with serious opioid-related adverse events, including respiratory depression and death (Gupta et al., 2018; Lee et al., 2015; Weingarten, Warner, & Sprung, 2017). A number of agencies, including the TJC and the Institute for Safe Medication Practices (ISMP), issued warnings about the increase in serious complications of prescription opioid use, including oversedation, respiratory depression, seizures, and death (TJC, 2012; Institute for Safe Medication Practices, 2007). In a sentinel event alert, TJC addressed the safe use of opioids in the hospital setting and recommended the use of "an individualized multimodal treatment plan . . . (that) combines strategies such as psychosocial support, coordination of care, the promotion of healthful behaviors, nonpharmacologic approaches, and nonopioid pain medications" (TJC, 2012).

The rise in opioid availability also has been associated with a marked increase in problems of opioid abuse and diversion. The marked increase in opioid-related complications, including the rise in opioid use disorders and opioid-related deaths, has led to the recognition that the national opioid crisis in the United States is a real public health concern, with almost 20,000 deaths reported during 2014 (White, 2017). Many local, state, and national efforts have been developed to address the individual and societal problems associated with inappropriate use of prescribed and nonprescribed opioids and the problems associated with opioid use disorders. In response to this crisis, numerous states and institutions have placed limitations on the quantities of opioids that can be prescribed (Martin, Laderman, Hyatt, & Krueger, 2016). Clinicians are now finding themselves being held legally responsible for negative effects of opioids, including opioid abuse (Savarese &

Tabler, 2017). With heightened awareness of the risks for opioid-related complications, opioids continue to have a role in pain management when used cautiously and with monitoring for effectiveness and unintended effects.

Resurgence of Support for Integrative, Multimodal, Opioid-Sparing Approaches

An increased interest in multimodal, opioid-sparing approaches has emerged in recent years. Using the various pharmacologic and nonpharmacologic interventions in a coordinated integrative approach facilitates pain control that is patient specific and evidence based, incorporating complementary therapies (e.g., relaxation, cognitive behavioral therapy, energy work) in conjunction with traditional allopathic health care options (e.g., medications, interventions) through therapeutic relationships to facilitate healing of the entire person (Ring & Mahadevan, 2017; Sundberg et al., 2014; Twillman, 2017). This approach can be traced to Aristotle, who thought each person is a seamless composite of mind, body, and spirit; however, that perspective was eclipsed by the Cartesian split of body (medicine) and mind-spirit (church) (Rakel & Weil, 2018). Integrative health care allows for pain to be addressed from physical, cognitive, emotional, spiritual, and psychologic perspectives appropriate for the individual person experiencing the pain in the manner in which it is being experienced in collaboration with clinicians who work with patients from an evidence-informed position (Rosenthal & Lisi, 2014) (Table 1.1). From this viewpoint, pain management is planned through shared, evidence-based decision making with the patient to optimize wellness and function consistent with the goals and values of the individual patient (Twillman, 2017).

An integrated, multimodal approach for pain management is used with increased frequency to control pain with various causes in a diversity of settings. In the postoperative arena, multimodal analgesia is often used as a preventive intervention to minimize or prevent acute postoperative pain and the development of chronic pain (Rosero & Joshi, 2014). The authors of an extensive systematic review that included patients undergoing abdominal, orthopedic, gynecologic, cosmetic, spinal, urologic, cardiothoracic, and gastric bypass surgeries, discussed the various modes of analgesia regarding the particular surgeries (Gritsenko, Khelemsky, Kaye, Vadivelu, & Urman, 2014). The authors of another systematic review reported that topical nonsteroidal antiinflammatory drugs (NSAIDs) may be effective as a part of multimodal analgesia after a variety of abdominal, gynecologic, and skin grafting surgeries (Brubaker, Kendall, & Reina, 2016). An integrated multimodal approach is effective for sparing opioids in managing pain among trauma patients (Sullivan, Lyons, Montgomery, & Quinlan-Colwell, 2016). In France a multimodal approach is strongly recommended in the guidelines for caring for patients with chest trauma (Bouzat et al., 2017).

Table 1.1 | Themes of Integrative Health Care Applied to Multimodal Analgesia

Integrative Health Care Theme	Application to Multimodal Analgesia
Combined use of complementary and conventional (allopathic, traditional Western) health care with representatives of a variety of health care disciplines contribute to providing care of the patient.	Traditional allopathic health care is used in conjunction with complementary nonpharmacologic interventions by clinicians with specialized preparation to best control pain through a multimodal approach to optimize safe pain management.
Integrative health care is patient centered.	Not only is the focus of care on the patient but the patient is actively involved in planning and implementing pain management interventions that are specific to the individual needs, values, lifestyle, and preferences.
An integrative approach considers the person as a whole being including body, mind, emotions, and spirit.	Pain is understood to be a multifaceted experience involving all aspects of the person, including body, mind, emotion, and spirit. Effective management must consider all of these aspects and provide a variety of interventions appropriate for the individual person.
Interprofessional collaboration is a key component of integrative health care.	Clinicians from various conventional health care disciplines (e.g., anesthesia, neurology, nursing, psychology, physical therapy, etc.) coordinate with clinicians from complementary modalities (e.g., energy modalities, movement therapy, music therapy, herbalists, pet therapy, etc.) coordinate their activities to optimize helping the person to best control pain in a safe manner.
Integrative care is evidence based or evidence informed (using information from research and the interpretation of data to guide practice[a]).	Approaches, interventions, and treatments used are based on evidence, and the evidence informs and guides a multimodal analgesic approach to managing pain.
Health determinants and environment are important considerations in integrative health care.	An integrative approach to pain management considers the particular environment and lifestyle of the person with pain and any barriers that limit which interventions can be used.
Focus is on optimal health and wellness.	Rather than focusing on cure, integrative health care focuses on optimizing health and wellness. The goal is to support the person to be as well as possible while controlling pain with a variety of interventions in a safe and effective manner to function at the highest level possible.
Relationship between the various health care providers with the patient is important.	Effective pain management is based on a compassionate therapeutic relationship in which respect and informed decision making support the person with pain to best control pain and function at the highest level possible.

[a] Data from Brown, C., & Rogers, S. (2014). Measuring the effectiveness of knowledge creation as a means of facilitating evidence-informed practice in early years settings in one London borough. *London Review of Education, 12*(3), 245–260.
Based on Rosenthal, B., & Lisi, A. J. (2014). A qualitative analysis of various definitions of integrative medicine and health. *Topics in Integrative Health Care, 5*(4). ID 5.4004.

Drivers for Integrative, Multimodal, Opioid-Sparing Approaches

Professional Organizations

Through position statements and clinical practice guidelines, a number of professional organizations have issued recommendations for the use of multimodal analgesia. In 2016 the APS, the American Society of Regional Anesthesia and Pain Medicine, and the American Society of Anesthesiologists collaborated to develop guidelines for postoperative pain management (Chou et al., 2016). The committee strongly recommended multimodal regimens of analgesia, which they found is supported by high-quality evidence. In those guidelines, multimodal analgesia is defined as "the use of a variety of analgesic medication and techniques that target different mechanisms of action with the peripheral and/or central nervous system (which might also be combined with nonpharmacologic interventions) might have additive or synergistic effects and more effective pain relief compared with single-modality interventions" (Chou et al., 2016, p. 136). The committee clarified that the particular components of a multimodal regimen need to be individualized for the patient considering the surgical procedure and setting (Tables 1.2 and 1.3).

In 2009 the American Society for Pain Management Nursing (ASPMN, 2009) issued a call to revolutionize pain care in the United States, noting an organizational belief that a multimodal and balanced approach to managing pain is crucial to rectify the undertreatment of pain. This was followed in 2015 with a commitment to further advance pain management among patients with chronic pain through multimodal approaches (ASPMN, 2015). In position statements addressing pain in various situations, ASPMN endorsed maximizing multimodal analgesia, including nonpharmacologic interventions, nonopioid analgesics, and opioids (Czarnecki et al., 2011; Jarzyna et al., 2011; Oliver et al., 2012; Pasero et al., 2016).

The IASP, an organization formed under the leadership of John Bonica, has had a long history of supporting multidisciplinary approaches to pain management. In carrying out its mission to "bring together scientists, clinicians, health-care providers, and policymakers to stimulate and support the study of pain and to translate that knowledge into improved pain relief worldwide" (IASP, 2018), the IASP has provided many resources and supported numerous initiatives to educate health professionals about pain mechanisms and the management of pain. One of the IASP's educational initiatives includes the publication of the IASP Taxonomy, which aids health providers in sharing a common language and understanding of terms related to pain. As mentioned earlier, as a result of the work of the IASP Multimodal Pain Therapy task force, the term *multimodal treatment* was clarified and defined in 2017.

Centers for Disease Control and Prevention Guidelines

In 2016 the Centers for Disease Control and Prevention (CDC) published "A Guideline for Prescribing Opioids for Chronic Pain." The guideline was developed to assist primary care providers to prescribe opioids appropriately in the treatment of chronic noncancer pain (Dowell, Haegerich, & Chou, 2016). The goal of this initiative was to reduce opioid-related risks, including opioid use disorder, overdose, and death (Dowell et al., 2016). The CDC publication has resulted in some controversy because questions have been raised related to the lack of transparency in guideline development, potential bias against opioids on the part of some guideline authors, and concerns about barriers to appropriate opioid access (Schatman & Ziegler, 2017). Despite the controversy, the guideline supports the use of multimodal approaches and endorses nonpharmacologic interventions and nonopioid analgesics as the preferred treatments for chronic pain (Dowell et al., 2016). When opioids are necessary, the CDC recommends the concomitant use of nonpharmacologic and nonopioid analgesic measures. Thus the CDC guidelines reaffirm the support for multimodal analgesia that was introduced by Khatami and Rush over three decades earlier. Subsequent to publication of the guidelines, CDC representatives discussed the importance of understanding the population addressed with those guidelines, the need for development of nonopioid analgesia, the importance of basing decisions on supporting evidence, and respecting the need for some patients to continue with higher dose opioids (Dowell, Haegerich, & Chou, 2019).

The Joint Commission

With increasing awareness of the national crisis associated with opioid use disorder, various groups and organizations have been singled out as having contributed to the crisis.

TJC's emphasis on pain management and development of pain standards has been cited as a contributing factor to the widespread opioid problem. In response to this criticism, in 2011, the following was added to the standards:

Both pharmacologic and nonpharmacologic strategies have a role in the management of pain. The following examples are not exhaustive, but strategies may include the following: Nonpharmacologic strategies: physical modalities (for example, acupuncture therapy, chiropractic therapy, osteopathic manipulative treatment, massage therapy, and physical therapy), relaxation therapy, and cognitive behavioral therapy; Pharmacologic strategies: nonopioid, opioid, and adjuvant analgesics. (Baker, 2017, p. 6)

The 2018 TJC pain standards have undergone significant revisions that have resulted in an increased emphasis on the need for safety in opioid prescribing, patient education, and multimodal pharmacologic and nonpharmacologic approaches to pain (Baker, 2017).

Enhanced Recovery After Surgery Society Guidelines

The growing adoption of the Enhanced Recovery After Surgery (ERAS) Society guidelines is a significant driver for the use of multimodal analgesia. ERAS guidelines provide a multimodal, evidence-based approach to preoperative, intraoperative, and postoperative care for the purpose of improving surgical outcomes (Beverly, Kaye, Ljungqvist, & Urman, 2017). Early ERAS guidelines were applied to the care of patients undergoing colorectal surgery. Since then, guidelines have been developed for the care of patients undergoing a variety of major surgical procedures (Beverly et al., 2017). Surgical pathways that adopt the ERAS guidelines address the need for well-controlled postoperative pain because it is recognized that inadequate postoperative pain control and excessive opioid use may interfere with the goals of ERAS initiatives and delay return of bowel function, oral intake, mobilization, and discharge and may increase readmission rates (Tan, Law, & Gan, 2015). The guidelines include the use of multimodal, opioid-sparing approaches to reduce opioid-related side effects. These approaches are initiated preoperatively, often with the use of acetaminophen, celecoxib, and gabapentin, are employed intraoperatively with the use of regional anesthetic and analgesic techniques and opioid-sparing anesthetics and continued postoperatively with continued use of scheduled nonopioids, regional techniques, and opioids on an as-needed basis. In many hospitals, multimodal analgesia is a standard component in ERAS plans of care (Montgomery & McNamara, 2016).

Institute of Medicine Report

In 2010 the Institute of Medicine (IOM; now the National Academy of Medicine), in response to a directive from the U.S. Department of Health and Human Services (DHHS) issued through the NIH, "conducted a study to assess the state of the science regarding pain research, care, and education and to make recommendations to advance the field" (National Research Council, 2011, p. 20). The report, issued a year later, identified pain as a public health problem and summarized many of the challenges in the assessment and treatment of chronic pain. Throughout the report, multiple statements addressed the importance of multidisciplinary and multimodal approaches to pain assessment and treatment.

National Pain Strategy

After the publication of the IOM report, the DHHS requested the Interagency Pain Research Coordinating Committee (IPRCC) to coordinate efforts to address the recommendations in the IOM report and develop the National Pain Strategy (NPS). Experts from private and public organizations worked collaboratively to formulate the NPS, which was published in 2015. Among the many statements in the NPS that support the use of multimodal analgesia is one that states, "effective pain care must emphasize shared decision making, informed pain assessment, and integrated, multimodal, and interdisciplinary treatment approaches that balance effectiveness with safety" (IPRCC, 2015, p. 16). The impact of this initiative has yet to be realized because the national opioid crisis has overshadowed efforts focused on pain relief.

Passage of the Comprehensive Addiction and Recovery Act of 2016 (CARA) resulted in the DHSS formation of the Pain Management Best Practices Inter-Agency Task Force (Task Force) to address acute and chronic pain in the context of the opioid crisis (U.S. Department of Health and Human Services, 2019). The Task Force included representatives from the U.S. Department of Defense and the U.S. Department of Veterans Affairs with the Office of National Drug Control Policy, as well as non-federal representatives from the general public and professionals from diverse disciplines and views, including experts in areas related to pain management, pain advocacy, addiction, recovery, substance use disorders, mental health, minority health, and more. The Task Force finalized a report in 2019 that stressed the importance of individualized patient-centered care, based on a biopsychosocial care model, in the diagnosis and treatment of acute and chronic pain. This detailed report emphasizes the importance of pain and risk assessment and strongly supports the use of multidisciplinary and multimodal approaches to acute and chronic pain, including use of medications, interventional approaches, and physical therapies (U.S. Department of Health and Human Services, 2019).

Future Challenges and Opportunities for Multimodal Analgesia Within an Integrative Approach

Perhaps at no time has the evolution of knowledge, perspective, and interventions regarding pain been so rapid and so diverse as it has been during the last two decades, particularly since the beginning of the 21st century. However, challenges to effective pain management continue. These include (1) to use the knowledge gained to most effectively help patients who are suffering each day with pain, (2) to minimize the occurrence of unrelieved pain, (3) to continue to gain information to better understand pain processes, (4) to educate clinicians about new advances within the realm of an integrative multimodal approach for better managing pain in patient-focused partnerships, and (5) to continue to search for the safest and most effective interventions for pain management.

Sadly, many of the multimodal options are not available for many people. Some areas may not have providers who are knowledgeable in multimodal analgesia. In other areas there is a scarcity of multimodal treatment providers, particularly those who provide nonpharmacologic interventions. Nonopioid components of multimodal treatment may be cost prohibitive to people who are underinsured or uninsured (Dale & Stacey, 2016) (see Chapter 4). Technology offers an opportunity to incorporate nonpharmacologic interventions in a cost-effective and easily accessible manner for people living with chronic pain to use to self-manage pain as part of an integrative multimodal approach (Heapy et al., 2015).

An important factor for the future is increasing support for rigorous research with good methodology. Research is needed to investigate the multimodal analgesic benefit of existing medication combinations (Dahl et al., 2014), and the investigation of new analgesic medications and their role within a multimodal plan of care is welcomed. The benefits of the various nonpharmacologic interventions for managing pain and their role in a multimodal analgesic plan of care is needed. One of the most important areas of future research is to further explore ways in which an integrative approach with multimodal analgesia can be used to effectively manage postoperative pain (Rosero & Joshi, 2014; Vadivelu et al., 2014) and minimize the development of chronic pain (Clarke et al., 2015). Using multimodal analgesia in a preventive manner to prevent chronic pain in infants and children is an area in which there is scant research, and is much needed (Friedrichsdorf, 2016). Additional research is needed to explore the use of technology and the effectiveness of technologic applications as components of integrative multimodal analgesic plans of care (Heapy et al., 2015). Finally, perhaps there needs to be a reevaluation of the concepts of evidence-based practice and the goals of research in pain management, keeping a focus on safety (Robinson, 2016) and quality of life.

Table 1.2 | Options for Components of Multimodal Therapy for Commonly Performed Surgeries

Type of Surgery	Systemic Pharmacologic Therapy	Local, Intraarticular or Topical Techniques[a]	Regional Anesthetic Techniques[a]	Neuraxial Anesthetic Techniques[a]	Nonpharmacologic Therapies[b]
Thoracotomy	Opioids[c]		Paravertebral block	Epidural with local anesthetic (with or without opioid), or intrathecal opioid	Cognitive modalities TENS
	NSAIDs[d] and/or acetaminophen				
	Gabapentin or pregabalin[d]				
	IV ketamine[e]				
Open laparotomy	Opioids[b]	Local anesthetic at incision	Transversus abdominis plane block	Epidural with local anesthetic (with or without opioid), or intrathecal opioid	Cognitive modalities TENS
	NSAIDs[d] and/or acetaminophen	IV lidocaine infusion			
	Gabapentin or pregabalin[d]				
	IV ketamine[e]				
	IV lidocaine				
Total hip replacement	Opioids[c]	Intraarticular local anesthetic and/or opioid	Site-specific regional anesthetic technique with local anesthetic	Epidural with local anesthetic (with or without opioid), or intrathecal opioid	Cognitive modalities TENS
	NSAIDs[d] and/or acetaminophen				
	Gabapentin or pregabalin[d]				
	IV ketamine[e]				
Total knee replacement	Opioids[c]	Intraarticular local anesthetic and/or opioid	Site-specific regional anesthetic technique with local anesthetic	Epidural with local anesthetic (with or without opioid), or intrathecal opioid	Cognitive modalities TENS
	NSAIDs[d] and/or acetaminophen				
	Gabapentin or pregabalin[d]				
	IV ketamine[e]				
Spinal fusion	Opioids[c]	Local anesthetic at incision		Epidural with local anesthetic (with or without opioid), or intrathecal opioid	Cognitive modalities TENS
	Acetaminophen[b]				
	Gabapentin or pregabalin[d]				
	IV ketamine[e]				

Continued

Table 1.2 | Options for Components of Multimodal Therapy for Commonly Performed Surgeries—Cont'd

Type of Surgery	Systemic Pharmacologic Therapy	Local, Intraarticular or Topical Techniques[a]	Regional Anesthetic Techniques[a]	Neuraxial Anesthetic Techniques[a]	Nonpharmacologic Therapies[b]
Cesarean section	Opioids[c]	Local anesthetic at incision	Transversus abdominal plane block	Epidural with local anesthetic (with or without opioid), or intrathecal opioid	Cognitive modalities TENS
	NSAIDs[d] and/or acetaminophen				
CABG	Opioids[c]				Cognitive modalities TENS
	Acetaminophen				
	Gabapentin or pregabalin[d]				
	IV ketamine[e]				

[a] Intraarticular, peripheral regional, and neuraxial techniques typically not used together.
[b] Use as adjunctive treatments.
[c] Use IV PCA when parenteral route needed for more than a few hours and patients have adequate cognitive function to understand the device and safety limitations.
[d] May be administered preoperatively.
[e] On the basis of panel consensus, primarily consider for use in opioid-tolerant or otherwise complex patients.
NOTE: Blank cells indicate techniques generally not used for the procedure in question.
CABG, Coronary artery bypass grafting; *IV*, intravenous; *NSAIDs*, nonsteroidal antiinflammatory drugs; *PCA*, patient-controlled analgesia; *TENS*, transcutaneous electrical nerve stimulation.
Chou, R., Gordon, D. B., de Leon-Casasola, O. A., Rosenberg, J. M., Bickler, S., Brennan, T., . . . & Griffith, S. (2016). Management of postoperative pain: A clinical practice guideline from the American Pain Society, the American Society of Regional Anesthesia and Pain Medicine, and the American Society of Anesthesiologists' Committee on Regional Anesthesia, Executive Committee, and Administrative Council. *The Journal of Pain, 17*(2), 131–157.

Table 1.3 | Summary of Interventions for Management of Postoperative Pain

Intervention	Suggested Use	Comments	Contraindications and Cautions
Nonpharmacologic therapies		Might require preoperative education and patient training for optimal results	
Transcutaneous electrical nerve stimulation	Consider as an adjunct to other postoperative pain management treatments	Typically applied at incision site	Pacemaker or implanted defibrillator, lymphedema, broken skin
Cognitive modalities	Consider as an adjunct to other postoperative pain management treatments	Includes guided imagery and other relaxation methods, hypnosis, intraoperative suggestions, and music	None, caution in patients with history of psychosis
Systemic pharmacologic therapies			
Acetaminophen and NSAIDs	Use as component of multimodal analgesia	Reduces use of postoperative opioids No clear difference between IV and oral administration	Acetaminophen: hepatotoxicity NSAIDs: gastrointestinal bleeding and ulceration, cardiovascular events, renal dysfunction NSAIDs contraindicated in patients who undergo coronary artery bypass surgery

Table 1.3 | Summary of Interventions for Management of Postoperative Pain—cont'd

Intervention	Suggested Use	Comments	Contraindications and Cautions
		Celecoxib usually dosed at 200–400 mg 30 min to 1 h preoperatively and then 200 mg bid postoperatively	
		Acetaminophen usually dosed at 500–1000 mg PO or IV q6h	
		Some observational evidence of association between high-dose NSAIDs and nonunion in spinal fusion and surgery for fractures, and between NSAID use and anastomotic leak in intestinal surgery	
Oral opioids	Use as component of multimodal analgesia	Oral is the preferred route for patients who can take oral medications	Respiratory depression, potential for addiction and abuse, sedation, nausea and vomiting, constipation
Patient controlled IV analgesia with opioids	Use when the parenteral route is needed for postoperative systemic analgesia for more than a few hours	Avoid basal infusion of opioids in opioid-naive adults	See Oral opioids
Gabapentin and pregabalin	Consider as a component of multimodal analgesia, primarily studied in patients who underwent major surgery, opioid-sparing	Gabapentin doses vary; in trials usually dosed at 600–1200 mg 1–2 h preoperatively, 600 mg postoperatively (single or multiple doses)	Dizziness, sedation; reduced dose with renal dysfunction
		Pregabalin doses vary; in trials usually dosed at 100 or 300 mg preoperatively or 150 or 300 mg preoperatively followed by the same dose 12 h later	
		Higher doses might be more effective, but also might be associated with increased sedation	
Ketamine IV	Consider as a component of multimodal analgesia, in patients who undergo major surgery, opioid-sparing	Dosing varies widely, consider preoperative bolus of 0.5 mg/kg followed by an infusion at 10 mcg/kg per min intraoperatively, with or without a postoperative infusion at a lower dose	Patients with history of psychosis Hallucinations, nightmares, dissociative symptoms
		Limited evidence for use in children	
Lidocaine IV	Consider as a component of multimodal analgesia in patients who undergo open and laparoscopic abdominal surgery	Dosing varies, consider induction dose of 1.5 mg/kg followed by 2 mg/kg per h intraoperatively	Conduction block Dizziness, seizures, bradycardia
Local, intraarticular, and topical therapies			

Continued

Table 1.3 | Summary of Interventions for Management of Postoperative Pain—cont'd

Intervention	Suggested Use	Comments	Contraindications and Cautions
Local anesthetic infiltration	Use local anesthetic infiltration at incision site for surgical procedures for which there is evidence showing benefit (*examples:* cesarean section, laparotomy, and hemorrhoid surgery)	Clinicians should be knowledgeable regarding specific local anesthetic infiltration techniques	See Lidocaine IV; also local pain, infection, bleeding
Intraarticular local anesthetic and/or opioid	Use intraarticular injections for surgical procedures for which there is evidence of benefit (*examples:* hip, knee, and shoulder surgery)	Clinicians should be knowledgeable regarding specific intraarticular injection techniques.	See Lidocaine IV and Oral opioids; also local pain, infection, bleeding; potential chondrolysis with intraarticular shoulder injections
		Caution with use of continuous intraarticular bupivacaine in shoulder surgery because of association with chondrolysis	
Topical local anesthetics	No recommendations for use in adult postoperative pain. Use suggested in combination with penile nerve block in infants undergoing circumcision.	4% Liposomal lidocaine or eutectic mixture of local anesthetics, lidocaine and procaine	See Lidocaine IV; also local pain, infection, bleeding, rash
Peripheral regional and neuraxial analgesic therapies			
Peripheral regional anesthetic techniques	Use as part of multimodal analgesia for surgical procedures for which there is evidence of benefit (*examples:* thoracotomy, lower or upper extremity surgery, hemorrhoid surgery, circumcision)	Clinicians should be familiar with specific regional anesthetic techniques	See Lidocaine; also potential for falls
		Use continuous over single injection techniques when longer duration of analgesia is required	
Neuraxial analgesia (epidural with local anesthetic [with or without opioids] or intrathecal opioid)	Use for major thoracic, abdominal, cesarean section, and lower extremity surgery	No clear difference between continuous infusion with epidural catheter versus single dose of intrathecal morphine	See Lidocaine and Oral opioids; also motor weakness and risk of falls

bid, Twice per day; *IV,* intravenous; *NSAIDs,* nonsteroidal inflammatory drugs; *PO,* orally.
NOTE: Table data are not listed in order of preference or strength of evidence. The choice of treatments must be made on the basis of comprehensive patient assessment and the available evidence with consideration of multiple factors, including individual risk factors for adverse events, comorbidities, cost, patient response; combinations of medications and techniques are often indicated. Doses are for typical adults.
From Chou, R., Gordon, D. B., de Leon-Casasola, O. A., Rosenberg, J. M., Bickler, S., Brennan, T., . . . & Griffith, S. (2016). Management of postoperative pain: A clinical practice guideline from the American Pain Society, the American Society of Regional Anesthesia and Pain Medicine, and the American Society of Anesthesiologists' Committee on Regional Anesthesia, Executive Committee, and Administrative Council. *The Journal of Pain, 17*(2), 131–157.

References

Agency for Health Care Policy and Research (AHCPR). (1992, Feb.). AHCPR clinical practice guidelines, No. 1. Acute pain management: Operative or medical procedures and trauma. Rockville, MD. Retrieved from https://www.ncbi.nlm.nih.gov/books/NBK52150/ (Accessed February 04, 2018).

American Society for Pain Management Nursing (ASPMN). (2009). *ASPMN statement of support: A call to revolutionize pain care in America.* Retrieved from http://www.aspmn.org/Documents/StatementofSupportACalltoRevolutionizeChronicPainCareinAmericaFINAL_2_.pdf. (Accessed January 29, 2018).

American Society for Pain Management Nursing (ASPMN). (2015). *Multimodal therapies to manage pain: More than just opioids.* Retrieved from http://www.aspmn.org/Documents/Advocacy%20Positions%20Statements/Multimodal%20Therapies%20to%20Manage%20Pain%20-%20More%20Than%20Just%20Opioids%20%206-17-2015%20final.pdf#search=multimodal%20therapies. (Accessed 29 January 2018).

Anderson, D., Zlateva, I., Khatri, K., & Ciaburri, N. (2015). Using health information technology to improve adherence to opioid prescribing guidelines in primary care. *The Clinical Journal of Pain, 31*(6), 573–579.

Aydede, M. (2017). Defending the IASP definition of pain. *The Monist, 100*(4), 439–464.

Baker, D. W. (2017). *The Joint Commission's pain standards: origins and evolution.* Oakbrook Terrace, IL: The Joint Commission. Retrieved from https://www.jointcommission.org/assets/1/6/Pain_Std_History_Web_Version_05122017.pdf.

Bendayan, R., Ramírez-Maestre, C., Ferrer, E., López, A., & Esteve, R. (2017). From acute to chronic back pain: Using linear mixed models to explore changes in pain intensity, disability, and depression. *Scandinavian Journal of Pain, 16,* 45–51.

Berry, P. H., Chapman, C. R., Covington, E. C., Dahl, J. L., Katz, J. A., Miaskowski, C., & McLean, M. J. (2001). Pain: current understanding of assessment, management, and treatments. National Pharmaceutical Council and the Joint Commission for the Accreditation of Healthcare Organizations, VA, USA, b44.

Beverly, A., Kaye, A. D., Ljungqvist, O., & Urman, R. D. (2017). Essential elements of multimodal analgesia in enhanced recovery after surgery (ERAS) guidelines. *Anesthesiology Clinics, 35*(2), e115–e143.

Bouzat, P., Raux, M., David, J. S., Tazarourte, K., Galinski, M., Desmettre, T., … Savary, D. (2017). Chest trauma: First 48 hours management. *Anaesthesia Critical Care & Pain Medicine, 36*(2), 135–145.

Brown, C., & Rogers, S. (2014). Measuring the effectiveness of knowledge creation as a means of facilitating evidence-informed practice in early years settings in one London borough. *London Review of Education, 12*(3), 245–260.

Brubaker, L., Kendall, L., & Reina, E. (2016). Multimodal analgesia: A systematic review of local NSAIDs for non-ophthalmologic postoperative pain management. *International Journal of Surgery, 32,* 158–166.

Buvanendran, A., & Kroin, J. S. (2009). Multimodal analgesia for controlling acute postoperative pain. *Current Opinion in Anesthesiology, 22*(5), 588–593.

Chapman, C. R., & Vierck, C. J. (2017). The transition of acute postoperative pain to chronic pain: an integrative overview of research on mechanisms. *The Journal of Pain, 18*(4), 359.e1–359.e38.

Choinière, M., Watt-Watson, J., Victor, J. C., Baskett, R. J., Bussières, J. S., Carrier, M., … Racine, M. (2014). Prevalence of and risk factors for persistent postoperative nonanginal pain after cardiac surgery: a 2-year prospective multicentre study. *Canadian Medical Association Journal, 186*(7), E213–E223.

Chou, R., Gordon, D. B., de Leon-Casasola, O. A., Rosenberg, J. M., Bickler, S., Brennan, T., … Griffith, S. (2016). Management of Postoperative Pain: a clinical practice guideline from the American Pain Society, the American Society of Regional Anesthesia and Pain Medicine, and the American Society of Anesthesiologists' Committee on Regional Anesthesia, Executive Committee, and Administrative Council. *The Journal of Pain, 17*(2), 131–157.

Clarke, H., Poon, M., Weinrib, A., Katznelson, R., Wentlandt, K., & Katz, J. (2015). Preventive analgesia and novel strategies for the prevention of chronic post-surgical pain. *Drugs, 75*(4), 339–351.

Compton, W. M., & Volkow, N. D. (2006). Major increases in opioid analgesic abuse in the United States: concerns and strategies. *Drug & Alcohol Dependence, 81*(2), 103–107.

Czarnecki, M. L., Turner, H. N., Collins, P. M., Doellman, D., Wrona, S., & Reynolds, J. (2011). Procedural pain management: A position statement with clinical practice recommendations. *Pain Management Nursing, 12*(2), 95–111.

Dahl, J. B., Nielsen, R. V., Wetterslev, J., Nikolajsen, L., Hamunen, K., Kontinen, V. K., … Mathiesen, O. (2014). Post-operative analgesic effects of paracetamol, NSAIDs, glucocorticoids, gabapentinoids and their combinations: a topical review. *Acta Anaesthesiologica Scandinavica, 58*(10), 1165–1181.

Dale, R., & Stacey, B. (2016). Multimodal treatment of chronic pain. *Medical Clinics, 100*(1), 55–64.

Dowell, D., Haegerich, T. M., & Chou, R. (2016). CDC guideline for prescribing opioids for chronic pain—United States, 2016. *JAMA, 315*(15), 1624–1645.

Dowell, D., Haegerich, T., & Chou, R. (2019). No shortcuts to safer opioid prescribing. *New England Journal of Medicine, 380*(24), 2285–2287.

Doyle, E., & Bowler, G. M. (1998). Pre-emptive effect of multimodal analgesia in thoracic surgery. *British Journal of Anaesthesia, 80*(2), 147–151.

Friedrichsdorf, S. J. (2016). Prevention and treatment of pain in hospitalized infants, children, and teenagers: From myths and morphine to multimodal analgesia. In *Proceedings of the Pain 2016: Refresher Courses, 16th World Congress on Pain, Yokohama, Japan, 23–30 September 2016 (pp. 309–319).* Washington, DC: International Association for the Study of Pain, IASP Press.

Gatchel, R. J., McGeary, D. D., McGeary, C. A., & Lippe, B. (2014). Interdisciplinary chronic pain management: past, present, and future. *American Psychologist, 69*(2), 119.

Gordon, D. B., de Leon-Casasola, O. A., Wu, C. L., Sluka, K. A., Brennan, T. J., & Chou, R. (2016). Research gaps in practice guidelines for acute postoperative pain management in adults: findings from a review of the evidence for an American Pain Society Clinical Practice Guideline. *The Journal of Pain, 17*(2), 158–166.

Gritsenko, K., Khelemsky, Y., Kaye, A. D., Vadivelu, N., & Urman, R. D. (2014). Multimodal therapy in perioperative analgesia. *Best Practice & Research Clinical Anaesthesiology*, 28(1), 59–79.

Gupta, K., Prasad, A., Nagappa, M., Wong, J., Abrahamyan, L., & Chung, F. F. (2018). Risk factors for opioid-induced respiratory depression and failure to rescue: A review. *Current Opinion in Anesthesiology*, 31(1), 110–119.

Hawkins, D. (2017). How a short letter in a prestigious journal contributed to the opioid crisis. (Accessed February 13, 2018).

The Washington Post. (June 2, 2017). Retrieved from https://www.washingtonpost.com/news/morning-mix/wp/2017/06/02/how-the-opioid-crisis-traces-back-to-a-five-sentence-scholarly-letter-from-1980/?utm_term=.75a96083e5a5.

Heapy, A. A., Higgins, D. M., Cervone, D., Wandner, L., Fenton, B. T., & Kerns, R. D. (2015). A systematic review of technology-assisted self-management interventions for chronic pain. *The Clinical Journal of Pain*, 31(6), 470–492.

Henschke, N., Kamper, S. J., & Maher, C. G. (2015). The epidemiology and economic consequences of pain. *Mayo Clinic Proceedings*, 90(1), 39–147.

Iles, S., Catterall, J. R., & Hanks, G. (2002). Use of opioid analgesics in a patient with chronic abdominal pain. *International Journal of Clinical Practice*, 56(3), 227–228.

Institute for Safe Medication Practices. (Feb. 22, 2007). High alert medication feature: reducing patient harm from opiates. In *Acute Care ISMP Safety Alert!*. Available at https://www.ismp.org/newsletters/acutecare/articles/20070222.asp. (Accessed February 10, 2018).

Interagency Pain Research Coordinating Committee. (2015). *National Pain Strategy: a comprehensive population health-level strategy for pain*. Washington, DC: Department of Health and Human Services. Available at https://iprcc.nih.gov/sites/default/files/HHSNational_Pain_Strategy_508C.pdf. (Accessed January 29, 2018).

International Association for the Study of Pain (IASP). (1979). Pain terms: a list with definitions and notes on usage: recommended by the IASP subcommittee on taxonomy. *Pain*, 6(3), 247–252.

International Association for the Study of Pain (IASP). (2017). *Task Force on Multimodal Pain Treatment Defines Terms for Chronic Pain Care*. International Association for the Study of Pain. https://www.iasp-pain.org/PublicationsNews/NewsDetail.aspx?ItemNumber=6981&navItemNumber=643. (Accessed January 5, 2018).

International Association for the Study of Pain. (December 14, 2017). *Taskforce on multimodal pain treatment defines terms for chronic pain care*. IASP Publication and News. Available at https://www.iasp-pain.org/PublicationsNews/NewsDetail.aspx?ItemNumber=6981. (Accessed February 10, 2018).

International Association for the Study of Pain. (2018). *Mission and Vision*. Available at https://www.iasp-pain.org/Mission?navItemNumber=586. (Accessed February 10, 2018).

Jarzyna, D., Jungquist, C. R., Pasero, C., Willens, J. S., Nisbet, A., Oakes, L., ... Polomano, R. C. (2011). American Society for Pain Management Nursing guidelines on monitoring for opioid-induced sedation and respiratory depression. *Pain Management Nursing*, 12(3), 118–145.

Joint Commission. (2012). *Sentinel event alert issue 49: safe use of opioids in hospitals*. (August 8, 2012).

Joint Commission. (2017, June 19). *Prepublication Requirements. Standards Revisions related to pain assessment and management*. Retrieved from https://www.jointcommission.org/assets/1/18/HAP_Pain_Jan2018_Prepub.pdf.

Kehlet, H. (1989). Surgical stress: the role of pain and analgesia. *British Journal of Anaesthesia*, 63(2), 189–195.

Kehlet, H., & Dahl, J. B. (1993). The value of "multimodal" or "balanced analgesia" in postoperative pain treatment. *Anesthesia & Analgesia*, 77(5), 1048–1056.

Khatami, M., & Rush, A. J. (1978). A pilot study of the treatment of outpatients with chronic pain: Symptom control, stimulus control and social system intervention. *Pain*, 5(2), 163–172.

Khatami, M., & Rush, A. J. (1982). A one year follow-up of the multimodal treatment for chronic pain. *Pain*, 14(1), 45–52.

Kowal, N. (1998). What is the issue? pseudoaddiction or undertreatment of pain. Nursing. *Economics*, 17(6), 348–349.

Large, R. G., & Schug, S. A. (1995). Opioids for chronic pain of non-malignant origin: caring or crippling. *Health Care Analysis*, 3(1), 5–11.

Lee, L. A., Caplan, R. A., Stephens, L. S., Posner, K. L., Terman, G. W., Voepel-Lewis, T., & Domino, K. B. (2015). Postoperative opioid-induced respiratory depression: A closed claims analysis. *Anesthesiology: The Journal of the American Society of Anesthesiologists*, 122(3), 659–665.

Leung, P. T., Macdonald, E. M., Stanbrook, M. B., Dhalla, I. A., & Juurlink, D. N. (2017). A 1980 letter on the risk of opioid addiction. *New England Journal of Medicine*, 376(22), 2194–2195.

Loeser, J. D. (2017). John J. Bonica: born 100 years ago. *Pain*, 158(10), 1845.

Lovich-Sapola, J., Smith, C. E., & Brandt, C. P. (2015). Postoperative pain control. *Surgical Clinics*, 95(2), 301–318.

Macfarlane, G. J. (2016). The epidemiology of chronic pain. *Pain*, 157(10), 2158–2159.

Maher, R. L., Hanlon, J., & Hajjar, E. R. (2014). Clinical consequences of polypharmacy in elderly. *Expert Opinion on Drug safety*, 13(1), 57–65.

Martin, L., Laderman, M., Hyatt, J., & Krueger, J. (2016). *Addressing the opioid crisis in the United States. IHI Innovation Report*. Cambridge, MA: Institute for Healthcare Improvement.

Max, M. B., Payne, R., Edwards, W. T., Sunshine, A., & Inturrisi, C. E. (1999). *Principles of analgesic use in the treatment of acute pain and cancer pain* (4th ed.). Glenview, IL: American Pain Society.

McCaffery, M. (1968). *Nursing practice theories related to cognition, bodily pain, and man-environment interactions*. Los Angeles: University of California Print Office.

Melzack, R. (1975). The McGill Pain Questionnaire: major properties and scoring methods. *Pain*, 1(3), 277–299.

Melzack, R., & Casey, K. L. (1968). Sensory, motivational and central control determinants of pain: a new conceptual model. In D. Kenshalo (Ed.), *International symposium on the Skin Senses* (pp. 423–435). Springfield: CC Thomas.

Michaloliakou, C., Chung, F., & Sharma, S. (1996). Preoperative multimodal analgesia facilitates recovery after ambulatory laparoscopic cholecystectomy. *Anesthesia & Analgesia*, 82(1), 44–51.

Moayedi, M., & Davis, K. D. (2013). Theories of pain: from specificity to gate control. *Journal of Neurophysiology*, 109(1), 5–12.

Montgomery, R., & McNamara, S. A. (2016). Multimodal pain management for enhanced recovery: reinforcing the shift from traditional pathways through nurse-led interventions. *AORN Journal, 104*(6), S9–S16.

Nahin, R. L. (2015). Estimates of pain prevalence and severity in adults: United States, 2012. *The Journal of Pain, 16*(8), 769–780.

Nahorski, M. S., Chen, Y. C., & Woods, C. G. (2015a). New Mendelian disorders of painlessness. *Trends in Neurosciences, 38*(11), 712–724.

Nahorski, M. S., Al-Gazali, L., Hertecant, J., Owen, D. J., Borner, G. H., Chen, Y. C., ... Robinson, M. S. (2015b). A novel disorder reveals clathrin heavy chain-22 is essential for human pain and touch development. *Brain, 138*(8), 2147–2160.

National Research Council. (2011). *Relieving Pain in America: A Blueprint for Transforming Prevention, Care. Education, and Research*. Washington, DC: The National Academies Press. Retrieved from https://www.nap.edu/catalog/13172/relieving-pain-in-america-a-blueprint-for-transforming-prevention-care. (Accessed January 30, 2018).

National Institutes of Health. (1986, May). *The Integrated Approach to the Management of Pain*. NIH Consensus Statement. Retrieved from https://consensus.nih.gov/1986/1986PainManagement055html.htm. (Accessed February 10, 2018).

Noble, B., Clark, D., Meldrum, M., Ten Have, H., Seymour, J., Winslow, M., & Paz, S. (2005). The measurement of pain, 1945–2000. *Journal of Pain and Symptom Management, 29*(1), 14–21.

Oliver, J., Coggins, C., Compton, P., Hagan, S., Matteliano, D., Stanton, M., ... Turner, H. N. (2012). American Society for Pain Management nursing position statement: pain management in patients with substance use disorders. *Pain Management Nursing, 13*(3), 169–183.

Parris, W., & Johnson, B. (2014). *The history of pain medicine*. In *Practical Management of Pain*. (pp. 3–9). St. Louis, MO: Mosby, Inc.

Pasero, C., & McCaffery, M. (2010). *Pain Assessment and Pharmacologic Management E-Book*. St. Louis: Elsevier.

Pasero, C., Quinlan-Colwell, A., Rae, D., Broglio, K., & Drew, D. (2016). American Society for Pain Management Nursing position statement: Prescribing and administering opioid doses based solely on pain intensity. *Pain Management Nursing, 17*(3), 170–180.

Peduto, V. A., Ballabio, M., & Stefanini, S. (1998). Efficacy of Propacetamol in the treatment of postoperative pain morphine-sparing effect in orthopedic surgery. *Acta Anaesthesiologica Scandinavica, 42*(3), 293–298.

Polomano, R. C., Dunwoody, C. J., Krenzischek, D. A., & Rathmell, J. P. (2008). Perspective on pain management in the 21st century. *Pain Management Nursing, 9*(1), 3–10.

Portenoy, R. K. (1996). Opioid therapy for chronic nonmalignant pain: a review of the critical issues. *Journal of Pain and Symptom Management, 11*(4), 203–217.

Portenoy, R. K., & Foley, K. M. (1986). Chronic use of opioid analgesics in non-malignant pain: report of 38 cases. *Pain, 25*(2), 171–186.

Porter, J., & Jick, H. (1980). Addiction rare in patients treated with narcotics. *The New England Journal of Medicine, 302*(2), 123.

Rakel, D., & Weil, A. (2018). Philosophy of integrative medicine. In D. Rakel (Ed.), *Integrative Medicine*. (4th Ed). Philadelphia, PA: Elsevier. pp. 2-11.e1.

Rzewuska, M., Ferreira, M., McLachlan, A. J., Machado, G. C., & Maher, C. G. (2015). The efficacy of conservative treatment of osteoporotic compression fractures on acute pain relief: a systematic review with meta-analysis. *European Spine Journal, 24*(4), 702–714.

Rich, B. A. (2001). Prioritizing pain management in patient care. Has the time come for a new approach? *Postgraduate Medicine, 110*(3), 15–17.

Richlin, D. M., Jamron, L. M., & Novick, N. L. (1987). Cancer pain control with a combination of methadone, amitriptyline, and non-narcotic analgesic therapy: a case series analysis. *Journal of Pain and Symptom Management, 2*(2), 89–94.

Ring, M., & Mahadevan, R. (2017). Introduction to Integrative Medicine in the Primary Care Setting. *Primary Care: Clinics in Office Practice, 44*(2), 203–215.

Rondinelli, R. D., Genovese, E., Brigham, C. R., American Medical Association. (2008). *Guides to The Evaluation of Permanent Impairment* (6th Ed.). Chicago, IL: American Medical Association.

Rosero, E. B., & Joshi, G. P. (2014). Preemptive, preventive, multimodal analgesia: what do they really mean? *Plastic and reconstructive surgery, 134*(4S-2), 85S–93S.

Rosenthal, B., & Lisi, A. J. (2014). A qualitative analysis of various definitions of integrative medicine and health. *Topics in Integrative Health Care, 5*(4). ID 5.4004.

Savarese, J. J., & Tabler, N. G. (2017). Multimodal analgesia as an alternative to the risks of opioid monotherapy in surgical pain management. *Journal of Healthcare Risk Management, 37*(1), 24–30.

Schatman, M. E., & Ziegler, S. J. (2017). Pain management, prescription opioid mortality, and the CDC: is the devil in the data? *Journal of Pain Research, 10*, 2489.

Shipton, E. A. (2014). The transition of acute postoperative pain to chronic pain: Part 2–Limiting the transition. *Trends in Anaesthesia and Critical Care, 4*(2), 71–75.

Sukhani, R., & Frey, K. (1997). Multimodal analgesia approach to postoperative pain management in ambulatory surgery. *Techniques in Regional Anesthesia and Pain Management, 1*(2), 79–87.

Sullivan, D., Lyons, M., Montgomery, R., & Quinlan-Colwell, A. (2016). Exploring Opioid-Sparing Multimodal Analgesia Options in Trauma: A Nursing Perspective. *Journal of Trauma Nursing, 23*(6), 361–375.

Sundberg, T., Hök, J., Finer, D., Arman, M., Swartz, J., & Falkenberg, T. (2014). Evidence-informed integrative care systems: The way forward. *European Journal of Integrative Medicine, 6*(1), 12–20.

Tan, M., Law, L. S. C., & Gan, T. J. (2015). Optimizing pain management to facilitate Enhanced Recovery After Surgery pathways. *Canadian Journal of Anesthesia/Journal Canadien d'Anesthésie, 62*(2), 203–218.

Tompkins, D. A., Hobelmann, J. G., & Compton, P. (2017). Providing chronic pain management in the "Fifth Vital Sign" Era: Historical and treatment perspectives on a modern-day medical dilemma. *Drug and Alcohol Dependence, 173*, S11–S21.

Topham, D., & Drew, D. (2017). Quality Improvement Project: Replacing the Numeric Rating Scale with a Clinically Aligned Pain Assessment (CAPA) Tool. *Pain Management Nursing, 18*(6), 363–371.

Turk, D. C., Brody, M. C., & Okifuji, E. A. (1994). Physicians' attitudes and practices regarding the long-term prescribing of opioids for non-cancer pain. *Pain, 59*(2), 201–208.

Twillman, R. (2017). Defining integrative pain management. *The Pain Practitioner*, 27(4), 4.

Uhelski, M. L., Davis, M. A., & Fuchs, P. N. (2012). Pain affect in the absence of pain sensation: evidence of asomaesthesia after somatosensory cortex lesions in the rat. *PAIN®*, 153(4), 885–892.

U.S. Department of Health and Human Services (2019). Pain Management Best Practices Inter-Agency Task Force Report: Updates, Gaps, Inconsistencies, and Recommendations. Retrieved from U. S. Department of Health and Human Services website: https://www.hhs.gov/ash/advisory-committees/pain/reports/index.html. (Accessed February 26, 2020).

Vadivelu, N., Mitra, S., Schermer, E., Kodumudi, V., Kaye, A. D., & Urman, R. D. (2014). Preventive analgesia for postoperative pain control: a broader concept. *Local and Regional Anesthesia*, 7(1), 17–22.

Ventafridda, V., Tamburini, M., Caraceni, A., De Conno, F., & Naldi, F. (1987). A validation study of the WHO method for cancer pain relief. *Cancer*, 59(4), 850–856.

Weingarten, T. N., Warner, L. L., & Sprung, J. (2017). Timing of postoperative respiratory emergencies: when do they really occur? *Current Opinion in Anesthesiology*, 30(1), 156–162.

White, P. F. (2017). What are the advantages of non-opioid analgesic techniques in the management of acute and chronic pain? *Expert Opinion on Pharmacotherapy*, 18(4), 329–333.

World Health Organization. (1986). *Cancer Pain Relief*. World Health Organization. https://apps.who.int/iris/handle/10665/43944. (Accessed February 10, 2018).

Yaster, M., Benzon, H. T., & Anderson, T. A. (2017). "Houston, We Have a Problem!": The Role of the Anesthesiologist in the Current Opioid Epidemic. *Anesthesia & Analgesia*, 125(5), 1429–1431.

Chapter 2 Importance of Multimodal Pain Management

Ann Quinlan-Colwell

CHAPTER OUTLINE

Physiologic Complications of Unrelieved Pain, pg. 19

Psychosocial Implications of Unrelieved Pain, pg. 20

    Anxiety, pg. 20

    Depression, pg. 21

    Agitation, pg. 21

Role of Multimodal Analgesia in the Perioperative Setting, pg. 22

Role of Multimodal Analgesia in the Management of Chronic Pain, pg. 22

Ethical Considerations, pg. 22

    Ethical Principles, pg. 23

    Autonomy, pg. 23

    Beneficence, pg. 23

    Nonmaleficence, pg. 23

    Doctrine of Double Effect, pg. 24

    Justice, pg. 24

    Veracity, pg. 24

    Fidelity, pg. 24

Clinical Application, pg. 24

Key Points, pg. 25

Case Scenario, pg. 25

References, pg. 25

MULTIMODAL analgesia (MMA) needs to be the foundation of all analgesic plans of care because it is the right thing to do. This chapter will discuss several reasons why MMA is the recommended method of providing optimal safe and effective pain management. The discussion will start with the underlying ethical principles supporting MMA as the optimal way to provide safe and effective pain management. This will be followed with a discussion of the need to prevent untoward physiologic effects of unrelieved or poorly relieved pain and then the need to prevent adverse psychosocial effects of unrelieved or poorly relieved pain. The role of MMA in the acute perioperative setting, and with chronic pain, will be introduced. Finally, ethical principles and their application to multimodal pain management will be discussed.

Physiologic Complications of Unrelieved Pain

Acute pain is a symptom that alerts the person that some event (e.g., trauma, surgery, inflammation) that the body perceives is harmful or potentially harmful has occurred (Kent et al., 2017; Sessle, 2011). Through the complex process of nociception, acute pain activates a physiologic stress response that stimulates the sympathetic nervous system and the central nervous system to alert the body of potential or real injury. See Chapter 3 for discussion of the nociception process. This response also initiates protection to prevent further harm and lessen pain. Acute pain is treatable, and in the normal process as healing occurs, it decreases over a short period, often 1 week, but generally within 30 days, and then resolves completely (Kent et al., 2017; Schug, 2011; Sessle, 2011).

When acute pain is poorly managed and not adequately relieved, damaging physical effects can occur in many body systems (Table 2.1). Catabolic metabolic activity can result in hyperglycemia, muscle breakdown, and delayed wound healing (Barr, Gilles, Puntillo, Ely, & Roman, 2013; Koneti & Jones, 2016). The immune system can be negatively affected by suppression of natural killer cell activity (Barr et al., 2013). Pulmonary complications result from insufficient breathing and coughing (Koneti & Jones, 2016; Zalon, 2014). Poorly managed pain limits general movement and participation in activities such as ambulation and physical therapy that are needed to recover optimally (Koneti & Jones, 2016; Zalon, 2014). As a result, the duration of stay in an intensive care unit (ICU) and/or hospital can be prolonged and readmission is likely to occur with inadequately controlled pain (American Society for Anesthesiology [ASA], 2012; Barr et al., 2013).

Studies repeatedly show unrelieved acute pain can result in the progression to chronic pain (McGreevy, Bottros, & Raja, 2011; Trevino, Essig, deRoon-Cassini, Brasekm, & Litwack, 2014). The estimates for this development range from 20% (Sessle, 2011) up to 50% (Roe & Sehgal, 2016), with chronic pain occurring after a wide

Table 2.1	Harmful Effects of Unrelieved Pain
Domains Affected	**Specific Responses to Pain**
Endocrine	↑ Adrenocorticotrophic hormone (ACTH), ↑ cortisol, ↑ antidiuretic hormone (ADH), ↑ epinephrine, ↑ norepinephrine, ↑ growth hormone (GH), ↑ catecholamines, ↑ renin, ↑ angiotensin II, ↑ aldosterone, ↑ glucagon, ↑ interleukin-1, ↓ insulin, ↓ testosterone
Metabolic	Gluconeogenesis, hepatic glycogenolysis, hyperglycemia, glucose intolerance, insulin resistance, muscle protein catabolism, ↑ lipolysis
Cardiovascular	↑ Heart rate, ↑ cardiac workload, ↑ peripheral vascular resistance, ↑ systemic vascular resistance, hypertension, ↑ coronary vascular resistance, ↑ myocardial oxygen consumption, hypercoagulation, deep vein thrombosis
Respiratory	↓ Flows and volumes, atelectasis, shunting, hypoxemia, ↓ cough, sputum retention, infection
Genitourinary	↓ Urinary output, urinary retention, fluid overload, hypokalemia
Gastrointestinal	↓ Gastric and bowel motility
Musculoskeletal	Muscle spasm, impaired muscle function, fatigue, immobility
Cognitive	Reduction in cognitive function, mental confusion
Immune	Depression of immune response
Developmental	↑ Behavioral and physiologic responses to pain, altered temperaments, higher somatization, infant distress behavior, possible altered development of the pain system, ↑ vulnerability to stress disorders, addictive behavior, and anxiety states
Future pain	Debilitating chronic pain syndromes: postmastectomy pain, postthoracotomy pain, phantom pain, postherpetic neuralgia
Quality of life	Sleeplessness, anxiety, fear, hopelessness, ↑ thoughts of suicide

↓, Decreased; ↑, increased.

From Pasero, C., & McCaffery, M. *Pain assessment and pharmacologic management* (p. 11), St. Louis, MO: Mosby. Data from Cousins, M. (1994). Acute postoperative pain. In P. D. & Wall, R. Melzack (Eds.), *Textbook of pain* (3rd. ed). New York, NY: Churchill Livingstone; Kehlet, H. (1998). Modification of responses to surgery by neural blockade. In M. J. Cousins, & P. O. Bridenbaugh (Eds.), *Neural blockade*. Philadelphia, PA: Lippincott-Raven; Mcintyre, P. E., & Ready, L. B. (1996). *Acute pain management: A practical guide*, Philadelphia, PA: Saunders. © 2004, Pasero C. May be duplicated for use in clinical practice.

variety of surgical procedures. Interestingly, patients who recalled having pain while being a patient in an ICU were 38% more likely to develop chronic pain (Barr et al., 2013). This recollection of pain may further support the premise that chronic pain can evolve from poorly managed acute pain. The exact mechanisms by which acute pain transitions to chronic pain are not known, but most likely there are multiple factors involved (Brevik, 2017; Chapman & Vierck, 2017; Kent et al., 2017).

The proposed multifactorial basis underlying the experience of acute pain transitioning to chronic pain underscores the importance of using a variety of options supported by MMA to manage acute pain and hopefully minimize or prevent the development of chronic pain. When possible, MMA can be used as a primary prevention using a multimodal approach with preemptive analgesia before surgery and/or intraoperatively. It also can be used postoperatively or after trauma using multiple nonopioid, opioid, and nonpharmacologic interventions (ASA, 2012; McGreevy et al., 2011; Sullivan, Lyons, Montgomery, & Quinlan-Colwell, 2016).

Psychosocial Implications of Unrelieved Pain

Anxiety

Anxiety is considered a normal response to stressful events and in some situations can be advantageous by alerting the person to prepare to pay attention to what is occurring (American Psychiatric Association [APA], 2017). Comparable to the difference between acute pain being a warning to pay attention to harmful stimuli compared to chronic pain being a persistent disorder, acute anxiety calls the person to be alert, while anxiety disorders involve a disproportionate level of distress, fear, or anxiety and are associated with common mental health disorders (APA, 2017). Anxiety commonly results when there is fear or a lack of clarity (Chlan & Halm, 2013), which can occur when patients experience pain they did not expect. When postoperative patients have an expectation they will not have pain or that pain would be much less than what is actually experienced, they report that experiencing the higher level of pain makes them afraid that something went wrong during surgery.

There can be a circular relationship between anxiety and pain, with each causing the other to increase in intensity (Chlan & Halm, 2013; Quinlan-Colwell, 2012). Anxiety also affects the perception of pain (Pinto et al., 2011). It is thought the perceived intensity of pain increases with anxiety. With anxiety, there may be an expectation that greater levels of pain intensity will occur, and this may be accompanied with increased attention to painful sensations (Quinlan-Colwell, 2012). Anxiety does not cause pain, but anxiety can lead to pain being perceived more intensely, which can then lead to greater anxiety or fear of pain (see Chapter 22).

The nonpharmacologic aspects of MMA can be particularly helpful with managing anxiety. Education of patients and families is an important nonpharmacologic tool and is critical to allay worry and fears. When surgery is elective, preoperative education that provides reasonable expectations for pain and pain control is desirable (APS, 2016). Relaxation, breathing, cognitive-behavioral therapy (CBT), and problem solving can help manage anxiety and pain (Quinlan-Colwell, 2012). See Chapters 21 and 22 for in-depth discussion about these interventions as part of a multimodal approach of pain management.

Depression

Depression is "a common mental disorder characterized by sadness, loss of interest or pleasure, feelings of guilt or low self-worth, disturbed sleep or appetite, feelings of tiredness, and poor concentration" (WHO, 2017). Unrelieved pain can cause or increase depression and the associated risk for suicide (Bendayan, Ramírez-Maestre, Ferrer, López, & Esteve, 2017; Sessle, 2011). The depression and pain relationship is strong and complex. Although it is not clear exactly how depression and pain interact, Linton and Bergbom (2011) suggest catastrophizing and emotion regulation may be involved. Complicating the situation is that often there is a lack of assessment of both pain and depression (see Chapter 8). This is particularly unfortunate because it is known that when depression is treated early, people with musculoskeletal pain showed improvement in pain control as well (Linton & Bergbom, 2011). CBT is a nonpharmacologic intervention with established success when used with depression and pain (Eccleston, Morley, & Williams, 2013). See Chapter 22 for discussion of CBT interventions as part of an MMA plan of care.

MMA is most appropriate for addressing the relationship of pain coexisting with depression and anxiety. A variety of antidepressant medications (see Chapter 15) and mind-body interventions, including CBT (see Chapters 20 through 27), can be used in an MMA plan of care. The nonpharmacologic interventions discussed previously regarding anxiety can be helpful with depression as well.

Agitation

Agitation can be caused or increased with unrelieved pain and is associated with increased adverse outcomes (Barr et al., 2013). Burk and colleagues defined agitation as "excessive restlessness, or non-purposeful physical activity thought to be caused or exacerbated by pain, endotracheal tube irritation or other unpleasant events" (Burk, Grap, Munro, Schubert, & Sessler, 2014, p. 296). Controlling pain and improving patient comfort with an MMA approach, including nonsedating and nonpharmacologic interventions, is preferable to using sedating medication (Barr et al., 2013).

Unrelieved or poorly managed pain also negatively affects sleep, quality of life, relationships, and employment (Sessle, 2011). There is a reciprocal interaction between pain and these manifestations (Fig. 2.1). Assessment of each of these is important when assessing pain. See Chapter 8 for assessing pain-related symptoms.

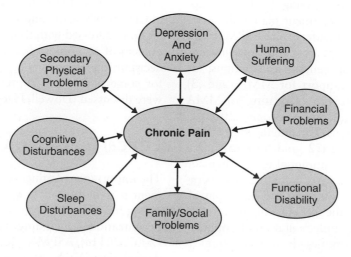

Fig. 2.1 | Reciprocal Effect. (Copyright Ann Quinlan-Colwell, 2011.)

Role of Multimodal Analgesia in the Perioperative Setting

Many of the professional organizations whose members work to control pain in the hospital setting have issued statements and guidelines supporting the use of MMA in the perioperative setting (American Academy of Pain Medicine, 2014; APS, 2016; ASA, 2012; American Society for Pain Management Nursing, 2010; Enhanced Recovery After Surgery Society, 2012; Joint Commission, 2012). The American Society for Anesthesiology (2012) recommended that whenever possible multimodal pain management, including the following, should begin preoperatively:

1. A focused history of pain
2. Physical examination
3. Development of a plan for pain control
4. Management of current medications that could cause withdrawal if abruptly stopped
5. Interventions to adequately control pain and anxiety that exist before surgery
6. MMA medications before surgery
7. Education of patient and family that includes nonpharmacologic methods

The ASA (2012) also endorsed multimodal perioperative interventions such as neuraxial analgesia with and without opioids, patient-controlled analgesia using systemic opioids, peripheral regional analgesia (e.g., intercostal block, incision infiltration, nonopioid analgesia) (see Chapters 10 and 18) and nonpharmacologic interventions (see Chapters 20 through 27).

The APS panel on the management of postoperative pain recommended MMA including both pharmacologic and nonpharmacologic methods. The panel stressed the importance for it to be individualized to the patient, condition, procedure, and setting (APS, 2016). These recommendations are consistent with the 2012 recommendations made by the Joint Commission (TJC; 2012) in the Sentinel Alert *Safe Use of Opioids in Hospitals*. Similarly, the American Society for Pain Management Nursing (ASPMN) supports an individualized MMA treatment plan to improve pain control and ensure patient safety. The ASPMN also addresses the need (1) to improve education of clinicians regarding MMA, including the benefits and options; (2) for organizations to provide support for MMA; and (3) to encourage and support nurses in advocating for MMA (Pasero, Quinlan-Colwell, Rae, Drew, & Broglio, 2016).

Consistent with these positions, The Enhanced Recovery After Surgery (ERAS) Society 2012 guidelines call for a perioperative pathway that is multimodal to best manage several aspects of perioperative care, including postoperative nausea and vomiting, gut function, and pain control. The ERAS Society discusses the benefits of multimodal medication approach and the implementation of nonpharmacologic interventions and minimally invasive surgical techniques.

Role of Multimodal Analgesia in the Management of Chronic Pain

Professional organizations have also advocated for a multimodal approach to helping patients living with chronic pain. The American Pain Society noted patients should be educated that opioids are only one part of MMA plans of care, which include nonopioid medications, nonpharmacologic interventions, addressing psychosocial issues and function (APS, 2009). The American Academy of Pain Medicine (AAPM, 2014) issued several position statements regarding chronic pain management. One specifically advocated for patients with chronic pain to have health insurance coverage for multidisciplinary pain management, including MMA. Some of the other position papers from that organization have addressed the use of opioids (AAPM, 2013a) and complementary therapies for people living with chronic pain (AAPM, 2011b). The CDC guidelines (CDC, 2016) and the national pain strategy (AAPM, 2016b) provided guidelines for referring patients to a pain management specialist (AAPM, 2016c) and supported research to investigate using cannabinoids to treat pain (AAPM, 2013b). The American Chronic Pain Association (ACPA, n.d.) is the organization representing people living with chronic pain. The ACPA issued an endorsement policy on their website that supports using a balanced multimodal approach to manage pain, improve wellness, and facilitate greater quality of life.

The statements by these organizations were timely. In 2016, the challenge of effectively managing pain and avoiding misuse of opioids was highlighted by the Centers for Disease Control and Prevention (CDC, 2016). Since that time, what has been called the opioid crisis or opioid epidemic has drawn great concern and attention. The CDC (2016) issued guidelines specifically addressing prescribing opioids for treatment of chronic noncancer pain. Those guidelines encouraged the use of nonopioid medications, coanalgesics, and nonpharmacologic interventions to manage pain while minimizing the use of opioids for chronic noncancer pain management. As noted in Chapter 1, in 2019, additional guidelines were issued by representatives of CDC in which the importance of understanding the population addressed with those guidelines, the need for development of non-opioid analgesia, the importance of basing decisions on supporting evidence, and respecting the need for some patients to continue with higher dose opioids were discussed (Dowell, Haegerich, & Chou, 2019).

Ethical Considerations

The importance of ethical considerations in pain management is underscored by the number of statements advocating for ethical pain management made by professional organizations, including statements from the AAPM (2007, 2011a), ASPMN (2010), and the American Nurses Association (ANA, 2015a).

Two provisions in the Code of Ethics of the ANA are particularly applicable to ethical pain management. The first provision states "the nurse practices with compassion and respect for the inherent dignity, worth, and unique attributes of every person" (ANA, 2015a, p. 1). The third provision states that "the nurse promotes, advocates for, and protects the rights, health, and safety of the patient" (ANA, 2015a, p. 9). See Chapter 27 for a discussion of compassion as part of MMA.

It is important to differentiate between morals and ethics. *Morals* are the personal beliefs, opinions, and guidelines that evolve from the process using ethical principles to consider and resolve issues, challenges, and dilemmas (Rich, 2013a). *Ethics* is "a systematic approach to understanding, analyzing, and distinguishing matters of right and wrong, good and bad, and admirable and deplorable as they relate to the well-being of and the relationships among sentient beings" (Rich, 2013a, p. 4).

Ethical Principles

Ethical principles are taken from the broader moral theories and provide a basis for resolving complex challenges or dilemmas (Grace, 2014). The ethical principles involved in pain management include autonomy, beneficence, justice, nonmaleficence, veracity, and fidelity.

Capacity is not an ethical principle, but it is a critical condition of autonomy. Although each state has particular legal regulations to determine the capacity of an individual, four aptitudes are generally evaluated to determine if a person has the capacity to be autonomous. These require the person being able to (1) understand pertinent data and ideas, (2) understand the particular health condition and prognosis, (3) be rational and able to use judgment, and (4) be able to accurately convey to others what is decided (Sessums, Zembruzuska, & Jackson, 2011). When the patient has capacity, it is recognized the ethical principle of autonomy takes precedence over other principles. Regarding pain management, this means when patients have capacity, the report of pain will be accepted as the patient states it. Having capacity to use the principle of autonomy also means the patient has a right to participate in decisions about which analgesia is used to treat pain, when they need to receive analgesia, and what side effects they are willing to tolerate.

Autonomy

Autonomy, or respect for autonomy, is the duty to respect, support, and advocate for individuals and their right to self-determination (i.e., to make decisions for themselves regarding their health care) (Post & Blustein, 2015; Quinlan-Colwell, 2014; Rich, 2013b). People with capacity need to be free to be involved in decisions that affect their lives and well-being. They need to be able to be free to choose and act without the control or undue influence of others or external pressures or impingements

(Quinlan-Colwell, 2014). They have the right to develop world views, beliefs, and goals and for those to be respected (Rich, 2013b). Clinicians are obligated to provide adequate information for patients to be able to make well-informed decisions (Quinlan-Colwell, 2014). Autonomy of vulnerable patients is easily violated, and clinicians have a duty to not only respect their autonomy but also to advocate for them to fully participate in decision making and receive optimal pain management.

Often patients have learned that a specific medication works well for them and they request to be given it. Clinicians need to listen to patients' reasons for wanting or not wanting to have a certain medication or wanting to or not wanting to participate in a certain therapy. MMA enables and facilitates using individualized analgesic plans of care specific for the needs of each patient. A certain medication may be the most effective treatment, but if it causes nausea in a person who detests feeling nauseous, the person has the right to refuse it. Many patients may benefit from water aerobics, but if the patient is fearful of being in water, that must be respected and the plan of care revised.

This is an area that can be challenging. Too often when a patient requests a certain medication, particularly an opioid, by name, the person is labeled as "drug seeking." That phrase implies the person does not have legitimate pain and just wants drugs. Dr. Susan O'Conner-Von cautions that people are reaching out to find relief from pain and are trying to find comfort. To more accurately describe this and to replace the disparaging term, she coined the phrase *comfort seeking* (Quinlan-Colwell & O'Conner-Von, 2014).

Beneficence

Beneficence is the duty to do good and avoid harm (Rich, 2013b), with consideration for what the person values and wants while balancing benefits against harmful effects (Quinlan-Colwell, 2014). With pain management, it can be challenging to help patients control their pain as effectively as they desire while keeping them as safe as possible. An MMA approach is key when working to achieve that balance, because a variety of medications and nonpharmacologic interventions can be used to maximize benefit while minimizing the side effects of any one medication.

Nonmaleficence

Nonmaleficence is the obligation to do no harm (Rich, 2013b). Harm often can be, at least temporarily, necessary during the care of patients; therefore harm is qualified as being no intentional harm that occurs either because of action or inaction by clinicians (Grace, 2014). With pain management, harm can occur by administering a nonsteroidal antiinflammatory drug to a patient with a known history of gastrointestinal bleeding. Harm also can occur when pain medicine is withheld from a patient who is alert and awake, reporting pain, and requesting pain medicine. Harm to a patient can occur when a patient feels judgement or prejudice. Harm can be done to patients when there is inadequate assessment of pain, sedation, and other side effects, resulting in inappropriate administration of medications causing adverse events.

With the variety of pain-relieving interventions available, MMA is an excellent way to reduce the risks of doing harm. It is important for nurses to be aware of the various options available in a multimodal plan of care to educate the patient and family. It is also important to know what other options are available from an MMA perspective and to appropriately advocate for patients to receive options that may be beneficial for them.

Doctrine of Double Effect

The doctrine of double effect recognizes "that an action that causes a serious adverse effect that has been foreseen – including death – may be morally justified if the intention behind the action was to do good" (Reynolds, Drew, & Dunwoody, 2013, p. 173). The doctrine holds that when an action is done with good intention, it is still a moral act even if the side effects are a negative outcome (White, Willmott, & Ashby, 2011). This principle is the basis for resolving dilemmas of providing good pain relief at the end of life. Even when administering high-dose opioids for pain relief may hasten death in a terminally ill patient, it is morally appropriate to administer the opioids because the *intention* is to provide comfort and relieve pain. To do otherwise would be doing harm to the dying person by causing unnecessary pain and suffering.

Justice

Justice is the ethical principle that supports that all patients receive appropriate treatment and high-quality care with fair allocation of health care resources and burdens without partiality (Post & Blustein, 2015; Rich, 2013b). Fairness is "minimizing health difference" (Guindo, et al., 2012, p. 2) to achieve equitable distribution without discrimination (Post & Blustein, 2015). Related is the concept of utility, which is maximizing good for the most people (Guindo et al., 2012; WHO, 2015).

People with similar conditions should be treated in similar manners, and those with different conditions should be treated differently (Quinlan-Colwell, 2014). When treating individuals with abdominal pain, all patients should be assessed using the tools most appropriate to their cognition and condition. All patients with pancreatitis would be treated similarly with consideration for their analgesic needs and limitations posed by allergy, intolerance, or comorbidities. Likewise, patients who are opioid tolerant most likely will have different analgesic needs from those who are opioid naive. MMA facilitates an individualized approach while standardizing the need for optimal safe and effective pain management (Pasero et al., 2016).

Veracity

Veracity is the obligation to tell the truth (Grace, 2014; Pierce, 2013) and to not deceive another person. It is not limited to interaction between the clinician and the patient. Veracity also involves being correct, complete, and unbiased when communicating information with other clinicians about patients (Grace 2014). This principle supports open communication between clinicians and patients to discuss various options available in a multimodal approach to managing pain. It also is a basic tenet for never administering placebos to patients who are in pain (Arnstein, Broglio, Wuhrman, & Kean, 2011).

Fidelity

Fidelity is the ethical principle that involves keeping commitments and promises. It is based on caring, honesty, advocacy, allegiance, confidentiality, and commitment to patients (ANA, 2015a; Pierce, 2013; Grace, 2014; Pinar & Peksoy, 2016). On a daily basis, fidelity is carried out by ensuring patient confidentiality. This principle can be challenged when patients do not want family members to know about a prognosis or event during hospitalization and have the clinician promise not to tell. In such a situation, the clinician can support both the patient and family by maintaining patient confidentiality while encouraging the patient to talk honestly with the family (ANA, 2015b).

Applying these ethical principles to pain management can be challenging, and there are times when one principle may conflict with another. When this happens, the conflict will need to be resolved. An example is when respecting a patient's autonomy may conflict with the principles of beneficence and nonmaleficence. Such conflict can occur when a patient who is lethargic and sedated wants to have more opioid medicine and to have no pain, but the nurse knows that doing so is not safe for the patient. When conflict such as this occurs, the process of utility is used to resolve the conflict.

Utility is "weighing costs and benefits and acting in such a way as to maximize benefits over costs" (Stewart, 2010, p. 3). If a patient specifically requests additional opioids be administered even though the patient is sedated and falling asleep while talking, the nurse must use utility to weigh the benefit of respecting the patient's wishes and autonomy with risking the patient's safety. The prudent decision is to keep the patient safe. MMA is helpful by providing nonsedating nonopioid and nonpharmacologic options to improve pain control without increasing sedation and compromising safety. Part of the resolution is educating the patient and family about how MMA works, why it is effective, and the need to balance pain relief with safety.

Clinical Application

Mr. Roberts is a 76-year-old man who recently underwent vascular surgery on his right leg. After surgery, he received intravenous hydromorphone for pain relief. He was confused and responded in very brief statements or single words. His family reported that he had not been like that before the surgery, and they were very concerned that his changes in mental status were due to the pain medicine. Initially, they wanted it all to be stopped and encouraged him not to complain of pain. However, whenever he moved or was turned he grimaced and sometimes made sounds that seemed to indicate he was in pain. The nurses and other clinicians were concerned that Mr. Roberts had pain that was not being addressed and that he was suffering unnecessarily (beneficence and nonmaleficence).

An ethics consult was obtained. The physician, nurse, and social worker on the ethics team met with the family and nurse leader, physician, and pain management clinician. Concerns were expressed by all present (veracity). It was clear that everyone wanted what was best for Mr. Roberts. The pain management clinician suggested acetaminophen be prescribed on a scheduled basis (650 mg qid around the clock) and low-dose oxycodone be available on an as-needed basis (prn) (e.g., 2.5–5 mg qid prn). These interventions seemed to be helpful, but Mr. Roberts continued to grimace when his right leg was moved or dressings were changed. The pain management clinician recommended oxycodone 2.5 mg qid be administered on a scheduled basis. The family and health care team agreed. Mr. Roberts was more comfortable, became less confused, and eventually was able to participate in physical therapy and return home.

Key Points

- MMA is the right thing to do for patients in pain.
- Ethics are an important consideration in pain management.
- It is important to control acute pain well to minimize development of chronic pain.
- Unrelieved pain can have negative effects in the body.
- Unrelieved acute pain can complicate recovery and impair rehabilitation.
- Unrelieved pain has negative psychosocial consequences.
- MMA can optimize pain control and limit adverse effects.
- MMA is the safest and most effective way to manage both acute and chronic pain.

Case Scenario

Maria is a 53-year-old woman who works as a waitress. Her husband died, and she has three adult children who live near to her. She manages her diabetes and high blood pressure with a reasonable diet and exercise. Last night she was walking home from the restaurant where she works and was assaulted by three men. This morning she had surgery to repair a liver laceration. She also has two fractured ribs and multiple bruises, cuts, and abrasions. Now she is in postanesthesia care unit and is quiet but guarding her chest and abdomen. She has difficulty moving even with assistance.

1. What ethical concerns might there be in caring for Maria?
2. How would you address them?
3. What physical complications could develop if her pain is not well managed?
4. What psychosocial complications could develop if her pain is not well managed?
5. How can MMA be utilized in Maria's care?

References

American Academy of Pain Medicine (AAPM). (2007). *The American Academy of Pain Medicine Ethics Charter*. Chicago, IL: American Academy of Pain Medicine.

American Academy of Pain Medicine (AAPM). (2011a). *AAPM Position Statement on Ethical Practice of Pain Medicine*. American Academy of Pain Medicine. http://www.painmed.org/press/position-statements/. (Accessed February 26, 2018).

American Academy of Pain Medicine (AAPM). (2011b). *AAPM Position Statement on Complementary and Alternative Medicine*. http://www.painmed.org/press/position-statements/. (Accessed February 26, 2018).

American Academy of Pain Medicine (AAPM). (2013a). *AAPM Speaks on the Use of Opioids in the Treatment of Chronic Pain*. American Academy of Pain Medicine. http://www.painmed.org/press/position-statements/ (Accessed February 26, 2018).

American Academy of Pain Medicine (AAPM). (2013b). *AAPM Position on Research into the Use of Cannabinoids for Medical Purposes*. American Academy of Pain Medicine. http://www.painmed.org/press/position-statements/. (Accessed February 26, 2018).

American Academy of Pain Medicine (AAPM). (2014). *Narcotics use in orthopedic trauma patients*. http://www.painmed.org/library/research/postoperative/effect-of-a-multimodal-pain-regimen-on-pain-control-patient-satisfaction-and-narcotic-use/. (Accessed February 26, 2018).

American Academy of Pain Medicine (AAPM). (2016a). *AAPM Statement on the CDC Guideline for Prescribing Opioids for Chronic Pain*. American Academy of Pain Medicine. http://www.painmed.org/press/position-statements/. (Accessed February 26, 2018).

American Academy of Pain Medicine (AAPM). (2016b). *AAPM Statement on the Release of the National Pain Strategy*. American Academy of Pain Medicine. http://www.painmed.org/press/position-statements/. (Accessed February 26, 2018).

American Academy of Pain Medicine (AAPM). (2016c). *For the Primary Care Provider: When to Refer to a Pain Specialist*. American Academy of Pain Medicine. http://www.painmed.org/press/position-statements/. (Accessed February 26, 2018).

American Chronic Pain Association (ACPA). (n.d.). Endorsement Policy. Retrieved from: https://theacpa.org/Endorsement-Policy (Accessed February 26, 2018).

American Nurses Association (ANA). (2015a). *Short Definitions of Ethical Principles and Theories Familiar Words, What Do They Mean?*. http://www.nursingworld.org/MainMenuCategories/EthicsStandards/Resources/Ethics-Definitions.pdf. (Accessed February 8, 2018).

American Nurses Association (ANA). (2015b). *American Nurses Association Position Statement on Risk and Responsibility In Providing Nursing Care.* http://www.nursingworld.org/DocumentVault/Position-Statements/Ethics-and-Human-Rights/RiskandResponsibility.pdf. (Accessed February 26, 2018).

American Pain Society (APS). (2009). Clinical guidelines for the use of chronic opioid therapy in chronic noncancer pain. *The Journal of Pain*, 10(2), 113–130. https://doi.org/10.1016/j.jpain.2008.10.008.

American Pain Society (APS). (2016). Guidelines on the management of postoperative pain: management of postoperative pain: a clinical practice guideline from the American Pain Society, the American Society of Regional Anesthesia and Pain Medicine, and the American Society of Anesthesiologists' Committee on Regional Anesthesia, Executive Committee and Administrative Council. *The Journal of Pain*, 17(2), 131–157.

American Psychiatric Association (APA). (2017). *Anxiety disorders: What are anxiety disorders?*. Retrieved from https://www.psychiatry.org/patients-families/anxiety-disorders/what-are-anxiety-disorders. (Accessed February 8, 2018).

American Society for Anesthesiology (ASA). (2012). Practice guidelines for acute pain management in the perioperative setting. *Anesthesiology*, 116(2), 248–273.

American Society for Pain Management Nursing. (2010). *Optimizing the treatment of pain in patients with acute presentations.* Retrieved from http://www.aspmn.org:Pages:-positionpapers.aspx. (Accessed February 8, 2018).

Arnstein, P., Broglio, K., Wuhrman, E., & Kean, M. B. (2011). Use of placebos in pain management. *Pain Management Nursing*, 12(4), 225–229.

Barr, J., Gilles, F., Puntillo, K., Ely, W., & Roman, J. (2013). Clinical practice guidelines for the management of pain, agitation, and delirium in adult patients in the intensive care unit. *Critical Care Medicine*, 41(1), 263–306.

Bendayan, R., Ramírez-Maestre, C., Ferrer, E., López, A., & Esteve, R. (2017). From acute to chronic back pain: using linear mixed models to explore changes in intensity, disability, and depression. *Scandinavian Journal of Pain*, 16(1), 45–51.

Brevik, H. (2017). Analyzing transition from acute back pain to chronic pain with linear mixed models reveals a continuous chronification of acute back pain. *Scandinavian Journal of Pain*, 16(1), 146–147.

Burk, R., Grap, M. J., Munro, C. L., Schubert, C. M., & Sessler, C. N. (2014). Agitation onset, frequency, and associated temporal factors in the adult critically ill. *American Journal of Critical Care*, 23(4), 296–304.

Centers for Disease Control and Prevention (CDC). (2016). CDC guideline for prescribing opioids for chronic pain—United States, 2016. *Morbidity and Mortality Weekly Report*, 65(1), 1–49. Retrieved from: https://www.cdc.gov/mmwr/volumes/65/rr/rr6501e1.htm. (Accessed February 8, 2018).

Chlan, L., & Halm, M. A. (2013). Does music ease pain and anxiety in the critically ill? *American Journal of Critical Care*, 22(6), 528–532.

Chapman, C. R., & Vierck, C. J. (2017). The transition of acute postoperative pain to chronic pain: an integrative overview of research on mechanisms. *The Journal of Pain*, 18(4), 359.e1–359.e38.

Dowell, D., Haegerich, T., & Chou, R. (2019). No shortcuts to safer opioid prescribing. *New England Journal of Medicine*, 380(24), 2285–2287.

Eccleston, C., Morley, S. J., & Williams, A. C. (2013). Psychological approaches to chronic pain management: evidence and challenges. *British Journal of Anesthesia*, 111(1), 59–63. https://doi.org/10.1093/bja/aet207.

Enhanced Recovery After Surgery (ERAS) Society. (2012). Guidelines for perioperative care in elective rectal/pelvic surgery: Enhanced Recovery After Surgery (ERAS) Society recommendations. *Clinical Nutrition*, 31(6), 801–816.

Grace, P. J. (2014). Philosophical foundations of applied and professional ethics. In P. J. Grace (Ed.), *Nursing Ethics and Professional Responsibility in Advanced Practice.* (2nd ed.) (pp 3–44). Burlington, MA: Jones & Bartlett Learning.

Guindo, L. A., Wagner, M., Baltussen, R., Rindress, D., van Til, J., & Kind, P. (2012). From efficacy to equity: literature review of decision criteria for resource allocation and healthcare decision making. *Cost Effectiveness and Resource Allocation*, 10(9), 2–13. http://www.resource-allocation.com/content/10/1/9. [Downloaded 02/24/17].

Joint Commission. (2012). Safe use of opioids in hospitals. *The Joint Commission Sentinel Event Alert*, 49, 1–5.

Kent, M. L., Tighe, P. J., Belfer, I., Brennan, T. J., Bruehl, S., & Terman, G. (2017). The ACTTION-APS-AAPM Pain Taxonomy (AAAPT) multidimensional approach to classifying acute pain conditions. *The Journal of Pain*, 18(5), 479–489.

Koneti, K. K., & Jones, M. (2016). Management of acute pain. *Surgery*, 34(2), 84–90.

Linton, S. J., & Bergbom, S. (2011). Understanding the link between depression and pain. *Scandinavian Journal of Pain*, 2(2), 47–54. https://doi.org/10.1016/j.sjpain.2011.01.005.

McGreevy, K., Bottos, M. M., & Raja, S. N. (2011). Preventing chronic pain following acute pain: risk factors, preventive strategies and their efficacy. *European Journal of Pain Supplement*, 5(2), 365–372.

Pasero, C., Quinlan-Colwell, A., Rae, D., Drew, D., & Broglio, K. (2016). Prescribing and administering opioid doses based solely on pain intensity. *Journal of Pain Management Nursing*, 17(3), 170–180.

Pierce, A. G. (2013). Ethics: what it is, what it is not and what the future may bring. In A. G. Pierce & J. A. Smith (Eds.), *Ethical and legal issues for doctoral nursing students: A textbook for students and reference for nurse leaders* (pp. 1–33). Lancaster, PA: DEStech Publications. 2013.

Pinar, G., & Peksoy, S. (2016). Simulation-based learning in healthcare ethics education. *Creative Education*, 7, 131–138. https://doi.org/10.4236/ce.2016.71013.

Pinto, P. R., McIntyre, T., Almeida, A., & Arújo-Soares, V. (2011). The mediating role of pain catastrophizing in the relationship between presurgical anxiety and acute postsurgical pain after hysterectomy. *Pain*, 153(1), 218–226. https://doi.org/10.1016/j.pain.2011.10.020.

Post, L. F., & Blustein, J. (2015). *Handbook for Health Care Ethics Committees* (2nd Ed). Baltimore, MD: John Hopkins University Press.

Quinlan-Colwell, A. (2012). *Pain Management for Older Adults: A Clinical Guide for Nurses*. New York: Springer Publishing Company.

Quinlan-Colwell, A. (2014). Making an ethical plan for treating patients in pain. *Dimensions of Critical Care Nursing*, 33(2), 91–95.

Quinlan-Colwell, A., & O'Conner-Von, S. (2014). *Shifting the paradigm. Southern Pain Society Newsletter, Summer 2014, (2-3)*.

Reynolds, J., Drew, D., & Dunwoody, C. (2013). American Society for Pain Management Nursing Position Statement: Pain management at the end of life. *Pain Management Nursing, 14*(3), 172–175.

Rich, K. L. (2013a). Introduction to ethics (pp 3-32). In J. B. Butts & K. L. Rich (Eds.), *Nursing Ethics Across the Curriculum and Into Practice* (3rd ed.). Sudbury, MA: Jones and Bartlett Publishers.

Rich, K. L. (2013b). Introduction to bioethics and ethical decision making (33-66). In J. B. Butts & K. L. Rich (Eds.), *Nursing Ethics Across the Curriculum and Into Practice* (3rd ed.). Sudbury, MA: Jones and Bartlett Publishers.

Roe, M., & Sehgal, A. (2016). Pharmacology in the management of chronic pain. *Anesthesia and Intensive Care Medicine, 17*(11), 548–551.

Schug, S. A. (2011). 2011—the global year against acute pain. *Anaesthesia Intensive Care, 39*, 11–14.

Sessle, B. J. (2011). Unrelieved pain: a crisis. *Pain Research Management, 16*(6), 416–420.

Sessums, L. L., Zembruzuska, H., & Jackson, J. L. (2011). Does this patient have medical decision-making capacity? *Journal of the American Medical Association, 306*(4), 420–427.

Stewart, R. S. (2010). Telling patients the truth. *The Online Journal of Health Ethics, 6*(1), 1–10. https://doi.org/10.18785/ojhe.0601.08.

Sullivan, D., Lyons, M., Montgomery, R., & Quinlan-Colwell, A. (2016). Exploring opioid-sparing multimodal analgesia options in trauma: a nursing perspective. *Journal of Trauma Nursing, 23*(6), 361–375.

Trevino, C. M., Essig, B., deRoon-Cassini, T., Brasekm, K., & Litwack, K. (2014). Predictors of chronic pain in traumatically injured hospitalized adult patients. *Journal of Trauma Nursing: The Official Journal of the Society of Trauma Nurses, 21*(2), 50–56. https://doi.org/10.1097/JTN.0000000000000032.

White, B., Willmott, L., & Ashby, M. (2011). Palliative care, double effect and the law in Australia. *Internal Medicine Journal, 41*(6), 485–492.

World Health Organization (WHO). (2017). *Health topics: Depression.* Retrieved February 26, 2017. http://www.who.int/topics/depression/en/.

World Health Organization (WHO). (2015). *Global health ethics key issues.* Luxembourg, Belgium: World Health Organization.

Zalon, M. L. (2014). Mild, moderate and severe pain in patients recovering from major abdominal surgery. *Pain Management Nursing, 15*(2), e1–12. https://doi.org/10.1016/j.pmn.2012.03.006.

Chapter 3 Physiology of Pain

Maureen F. Cooney, Shalvi B. Parikh

CHAPTER OUTLINE

Theories of Pain, pg. 28

Gate Control Theory of Pain, pg. 28

The Neuromatrix Theory of Pain, pg. 29

Gain Control Theory, pg. 29

Other Models, pg. 30

Biopsychosocial Model, pg. 30

Fear Avoidance Model, pg. 31

Classifications of Pain, pg. 31

Classification Based on Duration, pg. 31

Classification Based on Mechanism, pg. 31

Pain Physiology and Pathophysiology, pg. 35

Physiologic Processing of Pain, pg. 35

Abnormal Processing of Pain: Neuropathic Pain and Hypersensitization, pg. 41

Neuroinflammation and Immune System, pg. 43

Special Conditions, pg. 45

Central Pain, pg. 45

Chronic Regional Pain Syndrome, pg. 45

Key Points, pg. 46

Case Scenario, pg. 46

References, pg. 46

THE International Association for the Study of Pain (IASP) has addressed the complex nature of pain as "an unpleasant sensory and emotional experience associated with, or resembling that associated with, actual or potential tissue damage" (Raja et al., p. 2, 2020). Keeping this definition in mind, it is necessary to consider that pain is a multidimensional phenomenon, often associated with a painful sensation or stimulus, but also greatly influenced by one's thoughts, emotions, social factors, and behaviors (Herndon et al., 2016). The response to pain may be highly individualized. The management of pain requires a well-planned, multimodal approach to address the multidimensionality of pain and the complex pathways, receptors, and mediators involved in the pain experience. The purpose of this chapter is to provide foundational content related to pain physiology and pathophysiology to support the use of multimodal pharmacologic and nonpharmacologic pain management approaches.

Theories of Pain

Over the centuries, there have been many attempts to explain pain. Early people believed in a spiritual, religious, or mystical basis of pain. For some, pain was seen as a punishment for a transgression. Early beliefs about pain, such as those from ancient Egypt, Persia, and China held that pain was an emotion, not a sensation (Heydari et al., 2015). The ancient Chinese conceptualized pain as the imbalance of two forces, the yin (a negative passive force) and the yang (a positive active force) (Khan, Raza, & Khan, 2015). Aristotle described pain as an emotion, like joy, and considered the heart to be the source of all pain (Khan et al., 2015). It was not until the 17th century that Descartes proposed a specificity theory of pain, which moved the center of pain from the heart to the brain and introduced early concepts of pain pathways (Aronoff, 2016). The work of Descartes influenced experiments on the anatomy and physiology of pain that have led to the development of modern pain theories. Theories, such as pattern theory and others, which evolved in the latter half of the 20th century, refined the understanding of the role of the brain and the central nervous system (CNS) in pain processing (Moayedi & Davis, 2013).

Gate Control Theory of Pain

In 1965 Melzack and Wall proposed the gate control theory of pain, which contains conceptual components that continue to provide the basis for current research and theory development (Katz & Rosenbloom, 2015). The gate control theory, illustrated in Fig. 3.1, highlights the role of spinal and cerebral mechanisms in acute and chronic pain (Melzack & Wall, 1965; Steeds, 2016). According to this theory, both nonpainful (nonnociceptive) impulses by large myelinated nerve fibers and painful (nociceptive) impulses by smaller fibers provide input into the dorsal column, the substantia gelatinosa (SG), and a group of cells called transmission cells. A gating mechanism, consisting of a complex excitatory and inhibitory interneuron network, was thought to exist within the SG of the dorsal horn. It was theorized that activation of large fibers (A-beta), which transmit nonnoxious cutaneous sensations such as light touch, vibration, and proprioception,

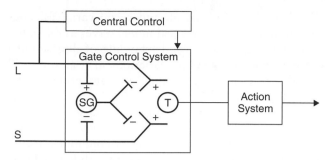

Fig. 3.1 | Gate Control Theory. *L,* large afferent nerve fibers; *S,* small afferent nerve fibers; *T,* transmission cells in the spinal cord. (Modified from Melzack R. [1991]. The gate control theory 25 years later: New perspectives on phantom limb pain [pp. 9–21]. In M. R. Bond, J. E. Charlton, & C. J. Woolf [Eds.], *Pain research and therapy: Proceedings of the VI World Congress on Pain.* Amsterdam: Elsevier.

actively inhibit the SG cells and close the *gate* to prevent pain sensation transmission to the CNS. Conversely, the *gate* was thought to open when nociceptive input by the small-diameter C axon fibers reaches a level or threshold that exceeds the ability of the large fibers to inhibit the noxious. As a result, pathways in the spinal cord are activated that lead to the experience of pain (Dowlati, 2017; Melzack & Wall, 1965; Steeds, 2016).

The concept of gate control theory has been applied clinically in pain therapies such as transcutaneous electrical nerve stimulation (TENS), spinal cord stimulation, application of heat or cold therapies, massage, and acupuncture (Czarnecki & Turner, 2018). For example, TENS involves the use of electrical current to selectively stimulate the large diameter A-beta nerve fibers in the skin over an area of pain so that transmission of pain impulses by the small-diameter nerve fibers will be inhibited (Johnson, Paley, Howe, & Sluka, 2015). Gate control theory also can be used to explain the relief of pain associated with rubbing or massaging a painful area. The Helfer skin tap technique is another example of the application of gate control theory. This technique involves the practice of lightly and repetitively tapping the skin near the intended site of an intramuscular injection and has been shown to reduce the pain associated with intramuscular injections (Arora, 2015). To the contrary, intense nonpainful stimuli also may be perceived as pain if the gates are "opened" through segmental pain facilitation from the brain, as seen in complex regional pain syndrome (CRPS) and phantom limb pain (Sluka & Clauw, 2016).

The Neuromatrix Theory of Pain

After the development of the gate control theory, Melzack (1999) later described the neuromatrix theory of pain, which proposes that a genetically determined matrix of neurons, produces characteristic nerve-impulse patterns in the body that influence pain. The neuromatrix is described as a widely distributed neural network in the brain that generates characteristic "neurosignature"

patterns of nerve impulses, leading to a multidimensional experience of pain (Melzack, 1999). The neural network consists of somatosensory, limbic, and cognitive components (Dowlati, 2017). According to this theory, the output patterns of the neuromatrix activate perceptual, homeostatic, and behavioral systems after injury, pathologic condition, or chronic stress (Melzack, 2001, 2005). These neurosignature patterns also can be triggered without any discernible sensory stimuli as in the case of phantom limb pain. The widely distributed neural network in the brain, and not the direct sensory input, is responsible for the perception of pain. Melzack emphasized that the neuromatrix is genetically determined and modified by physical and psychological stressors, which provides an explanation for the chronic physical and psychological stress associated with chronic pain (Cardenas Fernandez, 2015).

Gain Control Theory

In the years after developing the gate control theory of pain, Wall also came to a greater understanding of the processes and mechanisms involved in pain. He began development of gain control theory, which includes the possibility of increasing or decreasing the sensitivity of nociception at the peripheral, spinal, and central levels (Treede, 2016). This proposed theory, not formalized because of Wall's death before completion, continues to support the concepts in gate control theory, but expands it in proposing that, in addition to the intraspinal regulation of pain (dorsal horn and SG), other processes, including peripheral (prespinal) and supraspinal (descending) gain control mechanisms, are involved, and the dorsal horn is responsible for integrating all of these pain signals (peripheral, intraspinal, and supraspinal).

In this expansion on gate control theory, Wall theorized that gain control mechanisms work together to increase the sensitivity of the nociceptive system to significant stimuli and reduce the sensitivity to stimuli that are not actually problematic or significant. When gain control mechanisms are functioning appropriately, insignificant stimuli are disregarded and pain is not perceived. However, in the presence of lesions or diseases involving the peripheral, intraspinal, or supraspinal mechanisms, heightened responses to insignificant stimuli (sensitization or wind-up) or insensitivity (fatigue) to significant stimuli may result. For example, in the patient with a severe traumatic injury to an extremity, although healing has taken place months earlier, pain out of proportion to what might be expected might be reported when a subcutaneous injection is administered. The brainstem has a major role in exerting gain control that is triggered by both ascending and descending signals. Further identification of the multiple signaling pathways involved in gain control are expected to provide opportunities for the continued development of mechanism-based multimodal pain therapies (Treede, 2016).

Other Models

The biomedical model is used in many pain theories, including those discussed previously, to explain the pain experience. In this model, pain is described as a response to pathologic biological processes, and treatment is directed at the pathophysiologic processes (Lall & Restrepo, 2017). The biomedical understanding of pain has grown significantly in recent decades, particularly with the contributions from research in the field of genetics. However, the biomedical theories fail to adequately address the individual variability in pain or responses to pain treatment. The IASP inclusion of both sensory and emotional responses to actual or potential tissue damage in the definition of pain (Raja et al., 2020) supports the consideration of more comprehensive models than the biomedical model to explain the pain experience.

Biopsychosocial Model

The biopsychosocial model is based on the philosophical work of Engel (1977) in which alterations in health are viewed holistically, recognizing that health is influenced by biological, psychological, and social variables. Engel recognized that the biomedical model serves as the pathophysiologic basis for the understanding of disease but it does not explain individual variations in response to illness. The biopsychosocial model of pain proposes that pain is determined by "complex and bidirectional interactions among biological, psychological and social factors" (Fillingim, 2015, p. 357). The biopsychosocial model of pain has been applied to a variety of conditions, including chronic nonmalignant pain, recurrent abdominal pain, cancer treatment–related pain, and specific chronic pain conditions such as temporomandibular pain and chronic low back pain. For example, Waddell (1987) proposed a biopsychosocial model for low back pain when he observed that despite technologic advances in the recognition and treatment of low back disorders, there was an increase in the rate of low back disability. He described low back disability as an illness that results from the interrelatedness of biological, psychological, and social factors, and it is associated with distress and illness behaviors that are disproportionate to identifiable pathologic conditions (Lall & Restrepo, 2017). Fig. 3.2 provides a schematic drawing of the biopsychosocial model of pain.

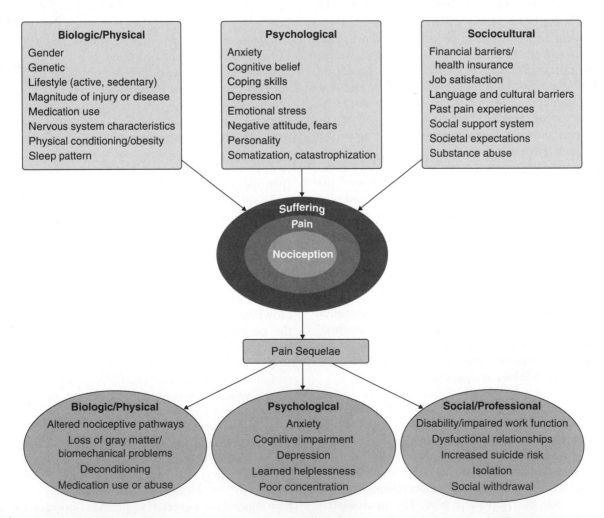

Fig. 3.2 | Biopsychosocial Model of Pain. (Cohen, S. P., & Raja, S. N. [2016]. Pain. In: L. Goldman, & A. I. Schafer [Eds.], *Goldman-Cecil Medicine* [25th ed., p. 136]. Philadelphia, PA: Saunders.

Fear Avoidance Model

The fear avoidance model of pain was originally introduced by Lethem, Slade, Troup, and Bentley (1983) in an attempt to explain why some people with musculoskeletal pain subsequently develop chronic pain syndromes. Like the biopsychosocial model of pain, the fear avoidance model acknowledges the existence of an initial biological pain cause, but chronic pain develops as a result of psychological factors. This model has been used to explain how psychological variables, such as fear, influence pain intensity and interfere with participation in activities (Vlaeyen, Crombez, & Linton, 2016). In the fear avoidance model, fear of pain is the focus, and this fear may lead to either confrontation or avoidance behaviors. When the fear is confronted, the pain will gradually resolve. When the fear results in avoidance and withdrawal behaviors, the fear will result in exaggerated avoidance behaviors, which may result in functional disabilities (Vlaeyen et al., 2016). The fear of intense pain may result in constant preoccupation with pain and hypervigilance related to any pain threat, so that even low-intensity pain sensations are perceived as unbearable and disabling (Gatchel, Neblett, Kishino, & Ray, 2016). Chronic pain may develop when pain-related fear and avoidance behaviors persist after the injury has healed. Avoidance behaviors may become persistent and continue to support the pain-related fear. They may negatively affect quality of life because they involve negative affect and the restriction of activities that were once important to the person (Vlaeyen & Linton, 2012).

Classifications of Pain

Pain can be classified in a number of ways, and there are gaps and areas of overlap in the categories that continue to be refined. Sometimes pain is categorized by location such as back pain or chest pain. Categorization by intensity requires that the patient provide a ranking of pain severity, often using words such as mild, moderate, severe, and very severe or a numerical rating (e.g., 4 on a scale of 0–10) based on a numerical rating scale such as scales described in Chapter 6. Other frequently used classifications are based on cause, disease, or pathophysiology and include categories such as postoperative pain, cancer pain, inflammatory pain, musculoskeletal pain, and ischemic pain. Pain that has an unknown cause is referred to as idiopathic or functional pain. Most commonly, pain is classified by duration and the mechanism of pain. Further elaboration on classification of pain according to duration and mechanisms follow in subsequent paragraphs, and additional information related to definitions and classifications of pain is provided in Chapter 5.

Classification Based on Duration

The classification of pain based on duration includes:

- *Acute pain:* Usually lasts up to 7 days but may have a duration of up to 3 to 6 months depending on the duration of the healing process.

- *Chronic or persistent pain:* Usually described as lasting for more than 3 to 6 months or beyond the course of an acute illness/cause (Kent et al., 2017).
- *Breakthrough pain:* Spontaneous or provoked transient increase in pain that occurs despite relatively well-controlled background pain (Herndon et al., 2016).

Acute pain is a normal response to tissue injury or inflammation and results from activation of the peripheral and central pain processes described later in this chapter. Acute pain usually has an identifiable cause and generally resolves as the source of pain progressively heals (Kent, 2017). Acute pain is associated with unpleasant sensations, and is often accompanied by physiologic, psychological, and behavioral responses.

Chronic pain, sometimes referred to as persistent pain, is a complex, multidimensional phenomenon that is not well understood, yet has significant impact on the physical, psychological, social, and economic condition of patients and their loved ones. It is not simply the continuation of an acute pain episode. Chronic pain may cause changes in brain activation patterns that are different from the patterns associated with acute pain (Groh, Krieger, Mease, & Henderson, 2018). Chronic pain is defined as pain that persists beyond the expected time for healing. Although this definition has gained general acceptance, because of individual variability and difficulty in defining the time of normal healing, 3 to 6 months is suggested as the general time frame that delineates the transition from acute to chronic pain (Herndon et al., 2016).

Chronic postsurgical pain (CPSP) or persistent postsurgical pain (PPSP) is a subcategory of chronic pain that is defined as the persistence of pain at least 3 months after the surgical procedure (Pozek, Beausang, Baratta, & Viscusi, 2016). CPSP may follow a number of different surgical procedures, and many risk factors, including severity of acute postoperative pain in the first days after surgery, have been described (Schug & Bruce, 2017). CPSP is the subject of much interest, as researchers attempt to elucidate the risk factors, the mechanisms involved, and interventions to prevent and treat the conversion from acute to chronic pain.

Breakthrough pain (BTP) is defined by the National Cancer Consortium Network (NCCN, 2017) as pain that is episodic and not controlled with an existing, regularly scheduled opioid pain regimen. Breakthrough pain may be incident (occurring as a result of an activity or an event); related to "end of dose failure," in which the pain escalates at the end of the dosing interval from the regularly scheduled opioid; or uncontrolled persistent pain, in which the dose of the opioid is not adequate to treat the pain (NCCN, 2017).

Classification Based on Mechanism

Pain may be described based on the mechanism that results in the experience of pain. The most common mechanisms of pain are nociceptive and neuropathic processes.

Table 3.1 summarizes the characteristics of nociceptive and neuropathic pain. In some situations, pain occurs as a result of a combination of both mechanisms and is referred to as mixed pain. Table 3.2 provides a summary of nociceptive and neuropathic sources of acute and chronic pain. Table 3.3 provides classifications of common pain conditions.

Nociceptive Pain

Nociceptive pain is the normal response of an intact nervous system to a noxious stimulus or tissue injury. It arises from actual or threatened damage to nonnerve tissue from the activation of the nociceptors (Herndon et al., 2016). It is an alarm that warns against threatening tissue damage. Nociception is the physiologic

---

Table 3.1 | Categorization of Neuropathic And Nociceptive Pain

Clinical Characteristic	Neuropathic Pain	Nociceptive Pain
Etiology	Nerve injury or peripheral or central sensitization	Tissue or potential tissue damage
Descriptors	Lancinating, shooting, electrical-like, stabbing	Throbbing, aching, pressure-like
Sensory deficits	Frequent (e.g., numbness, tingling, pricking)	Infrequent and, if present, in nondermatomal or non-nerve distribution
Motor deficits	Neurologic weakness may be present if motor nerve affected	May have pain-induced weakness
Hypersensitivity	Pain frequently evoked with nonpainful (allodynia) or painful (exaggerated response) stimuli	Uncommon except for hypersensitivity in the immediate area of an acute injury
Character	Distal radiation common	Distal radiation less common; proximal radiation frequent
Paroxysms	Exacerbations common and unpredictable	Exacerbations less common and associated with activity
Autonomic signs	Color changes, temperature changes, swelling, or sudomotor (sweating) activity occurs in one third to one half of patients	Autonomic signs uncommon in chronic nociceptive pain

From Cohen, S.P. & Raja, S.N. (2016) Pain. In: Goldman, Schafer AI (eds) *Goldman-Cecil Medicine, 25th ed.* Elsevier Saunders, Philadelphia, p 135.

Table 3.2 | Physiologic Sources of Nociceptive and Neuropathic Acute and Chronic Pain

Physiologic Structure	Characteristics of Pain	Sources of Acute Postoperative Pain	Sources of Chronic Pain Syndromes
Nociceptive Pain (Normal Pain Processing)			
Somatic Pain			
Cutaneous or superficial: Skin and subcutaneous tissues	Sharp, burning, pricking (well localized)	Incisional pain, pain at insertion sites of tubes and drains, wound complication, orthopedic procedures, skeletal muscle spasms, inflammation	Bony metastases, osteoarthritis and rheumatoid arthritis, low back pain, peripheral vascular diseases
Deep somatic: Bone, muscle, blood vessels, connective tissues	Dull, aching, cramping (localized and diffuse)		
Visceral Pain			
Organs and the linings of the body cavities	Poorly localized diffuse, deep cramping or splitting, sharp, stabbing	Chest tubes, abdominal tubes and drains, bladder distention or spasms, intestinal distention	Pancreatitis, liver metastases, colitis, appendicitis

Table 3.2 | Physiologic Sources of Nociceptive and Neuropathic Acute and Chronic Pain—Cont'd

Physiologic Structure	Characteristics of Pain	Sources of Acute Postoperative Pain	Sources of Chronic Pain Syndromes
Neuropathic Pain (Abnormal Pain Processing)			
Peripheral or central nervous system: Nerve fibers, spinal cord, and higher central nervous system	Poorly localized shooting, burning, tingling, fiery, shock-like, sharp, painful numbness, pins and needles sensation	Phantom limb pain, postmastectomy pain, nerve compression	Human immunodeficiency virus–related pain, diabetic neuropathy, chemotherapy-induced neuropathies, cancer-related nerve injury, radiculopathies

From Ellison, D. L. (2017). Physiology of pain. *Critical Care Nursing Clinics of North America, 29*(4), 397–406, Table 2.

Table 3.3 | Classification and Prevalence of Common Pain Conditions

Neuropathic		Nociceptive		MIXED
Peripheral[a]	**Central**	**Somatic**	**Visceral**	
Peripheral neuropathy (1%–3%)	Central poststroke pain (8%)	Arthritis (25%–40% in people > 40 y)	Endometriosis (10% in women of reproductive age)	Headache (15% for migraine, 20%–30% for tension type)
Postherpetic neuralgia (annual incidence 0.1%–0.2%)	Spinal cord injury (30%–50%)	Myofascial pain (5%–10%)	Irritable bowel syndrome (5%–15%)	Cancer[b] (lifetime prevalence 30%–40%)
Chronic postsurgical pain (5%–20% after surgery)	Multiple sclerosis (25%)	Fibromyalgia[c] (2%–4%)	Interstitial cystitis (0.2%–1% of women)	Low back pain[d] (point prevalence 10%–30%)
Phantom limb pain (30%–60%)	Parkinson's disease (10%)	Connective tissue disorders (0.2%–0.5%)	Ulcers, gastritis, esophagitis (3%–9%)	Neck pain[d] (annual incidence 20%–30%)
Trigeminal neuralgia (0.01%)	Seizure disorder (1%–3%)	Burn pain[e] (annual incidence of burns requiring hospitalization 0.01%)	Cholecystitis, appendicitis	Ischemic pain[f]
Radiculopathy, spinal stenosis (3%-10%)				
Complex regional pain syndrome (0.03%, 3%–20% after orthopedic surgery)				
Nerve entrapment syndromes (e.g., carpal tunnel, thoracic outlet, meralgia paresthetica; 2%–4%)				

From Cohen, S. P., & Raja, S. N. (2016) Pain. In L. Goldman, & A. I. Schafer (Eds.), *Goldman-Cecil Medicine* (25th ed, p. 135). Philadelphia, PA: Saunders.
[a]Prevalence rates represent proportion of patients with condition who develop pain.
[b]Neuropathic pain occurs in 20%–50% of cases and may be secondary to tumor invasion, surgery, chemotherapy, and radiation treatment.
[c]Some cases may represent a variant of central pain.
[d]Neuropathic pain may accompany nociceptive pain in 10%–35% of cases.
[e]Third-degree burns are often associated with neuropathic pain.
[f]Typically nociceptive, but long-standing pain may result in ischemic neuropathy.

process in which neural pathways in the spinal cord and brain are activated by a stimulus, usually mechanical, chemical, or thermal, that is damaging or likely to damage normal tissue. Nociceptors are free nerve endings of sensory nerve fibers that respond selectively to the noxious stimuli. Nociceptors are not uniform or homogeneous. They differ depending on their anatomic locations and functions. Nociceptors may be classified according to the type of stimuli to which they respond. Mechanoreceptors respond to stimulation from mechanical forces (lacerations, contusions, or pressure); chemoreceptors respond to chemical stimuli (acids, toxins, inflammatory mediators, ischemia); and thermoreceptors respond to temperature-related stimuli (burns, frostbite). Nociceptors are located throughout the body in skin, musculoskeletal tissues, vasculature, and viscera. The intensity of pain that is perceived with nociception will be influenced by the location, number, and type of nociceptors that are activated. These receptors respond to a broad range of stimuli through their transducer receptors and ion channels. Box 3.1 provides a list of different types of nociceptors.

Nociceptive pain is often divided into somatic or visceral pain. *Somatic pain* is pain that arises from stimulation of nociceptors in cutaneous and musculoskeletal tissues. It is associated with arthritic joint pain, myofascial pain (fibromyalgia pain), and external wound injuries and may be described as sharp, dull, and aching (Ellison, 2017; Herndon et al., 2016). It is usually well-localized or may manifest in a dermatomal pattern. *Visceral* pain arises from the activation of nerve fibers that innervate solid or hollow internal organs in response to distention,

inflammation, and ischemia. The pain from activation of visceral nociceptors is transmitted by the A-delta and C fibers and travels with autonomic afferent fibers along the same ascending tracts of the spinal cord as somatic pain (Steeds, 2016). Visceral pain is often poorly localized and may be associated with aching, cramping, colicky, pressure, or throbbing qualities. It is sometimes referred to a different location. Appendicitis and pancreatitis are examples of conditions usually associated with visceral pain.

Acute nociceptive pain generally occurs only in the presence of noxious stimulus and is relieved after the stimulus is removed. Nociceptive pain usually responds to multimodal interventions, including nonopioid and opioid medications.

Neuropathic Pain

Neuropathic pain is defined as pain that results from, or is a direct outcome of, a lesion or disease that affects the somatosensory system (Jensen et al., 2011). It is often chronic, resulting from damaged or abnormally functioning nerves in the peripheral nervous system (PNS) or CNS (Kerstman, Ahn, Battu, Tariq, & Grabois, 2013). Peripheral neuropathic pain is associated with conditions that involve damaged or abnormally functioning peripheral nerves. Postherpetic neuralgia, diabetic neuropathy, and alcohol-induced peripheral neuropathy are examples of peripheral neuropathic pain conditions (Zeng, Alongkronrusmee, & van Rijn, 2017). Central pain is a subtype of neuropathic pain that requires a primary lesion in the CNS (Cohen & Raja, 2016). Poststroke pain and spinal cord lesions are associated with central pain. With neuropathic pain, pain is not conducted through the usual nociceptive pathways because of damage in the nervous system. As explained in subsequent sections, in neuropathic pain, ectopic impulses occur without undergoing the normal process of transduction (Cohen & Mao, 2014; Ossipov, Morimura, & Porreca, 2014). Whereas nociceptive pain is the response of a normal somatosensory system to abnormal stimuli, neuropathic pain results from an abnormal somatosensory system that has been affected by a lesion or disease (Gilron, Baron, & Jensen, 2015) .

Neuropathic pain is usually described as burning, tingling, stabbing or shooting, or electric shock–like pain and may be accompanied by some degree of local weakness and numbness. Sensory loss with or without hypersensitivity in the innervated area is often associated with neuropathic pain. It also may be associated with motor and autonomic dysfunction. Severe neuropathic pain is often characterized by the following (Steeds, 2016):

- Hypersensitivity to painful stimuli—hyperesthesia
- Hypersensitivity to non-painful tactile stimuli—allodynia
- Pain of abnormal severity—hyperalgesia
- Pain of abnormal or prolonged duration—hyperpathia

Box 3.1 | Types of Nociceptors

SMALL MYELINATED A DELTA NOCICEPTORS:

Type I (high-threshold mechanical receptors):
respond to mechanical and chemical stimuli but have high heat thresholds (>50 degrees C.). Mediate *first* pain to pinprick.

Type II (very high mechanical threshold):
respond to lower heat thresholds but have very high mechanical threshold. Mediate *first* acute pain response to noxious heat.

UNMYELINATED C FIBERS:

Polymodal nociceptors: respond to noxious mechanical, thermal, and chemical stimuli.

Silent nociceptors: mechanically insensitive, heat responsive. Can develop mechanical sensitivity in the presence of inflammation.

Hudspith, M. J. (2016). Anatomy, physiology and pharmacology of pain. *Anaesthesia and Intensive Care Medicine, 17*(9), 425 -430.

Because damaged neurons have the capacity to regenerate and repair themselves, the nervous system adapts to injury, but as a result it may abnormally rewire its response to stimulation (Jensen & Finnerup, 2014). The pain associated with damaged nerves may be due to this abnormal nerve regeneration or other pathophysiologic processes. Neuropathic pain can lead to long-term changes in the nerve pathways (neuroplasticity) and abnormal processing of sensory stimuli (Ellison, 2017).

Because neuropathic pain occurs more often after injury to major nerves, the prognosis for recovery is often poor, resulting in chronic pain conditions. It has been estimated that 20% to 25% of all chronic pain has a neuropathic cause (Cohen & Raja, 2016). It is poorly responsive to usual analgesic interventions (Cohen & Mao, 2014; van Hecke, Austin, Khan, Smith, & Torrance, 2014) and requires a multimodal pain management plan that includes both pharmacologic and nonpharmacologic approaches.

Mixed Pain States

The term *mixed pain* is frequently used in the literature to describe pain states that are characterized by both nociceptive and neuropathic pain components. Mixed pain is usually associated with chronic pain conditions, and during an assessment, patients may report qualities of pain that are associated with both nociceptive and neuropathic pain. The treatment of mixed pain is challenging because of the need to address complex pain mechanisms. Cancer pain and low back pain are commonly mentioned conditions associated with mixed pain, although other painful conditions such as ischemic pain and migraine also may have nociceptive and neuropathic components (Cohen & Raja, 2016).

Pain Physiology and Pathophysiology

Physiologic Processing of Pain

Pain physiology involves a complex system of impulse transmission through peripheral nerves and ascending and descending spinal pathways, as shown in Fig. 3.3. The normal processing of noxious stimuli, or nociception, involves four physiologic processes: transduction, transmission, perception, and modulation. See Fig. 3.4 for schematic representation of nociception and Table 3.4 for a summary of these processes.

Transduction

The normal pain pathway includes activation of nociceptors in response to noxious stimuli (mechanical, chemical, or thermal) causing sodium and potassium action potential changes along the primary afferent sensory nerve fibers (first-order neurons) (McEntire et al., 2016). This process, transduction, is the first step in the pain experience and can be simply described as involving the

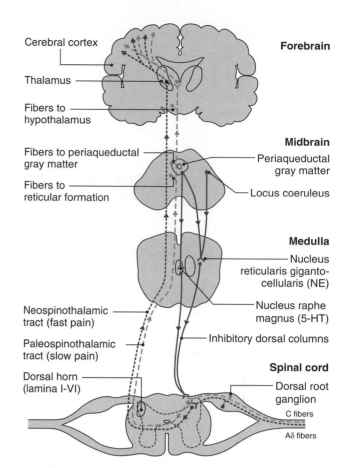

Fig. 3.3 | Spinal and Supraspinal Pain Pathways. *Black broken line,* A δ fibers (fast); *gray broken line,* C fibers (slow); *black solid line,* descending inhibitory tracts; *5 HT,* 5 hydroxytryptamine; *NE,* norepinephrine. (From Hudspith, M. J. [2016]. Anatomy, physiology and pharmacology of pain. *Anaesthesia and Intensive Care Medicine, 17*[9], 425–430.)

conversion of noxious stimuli into electrical activity in the sensory neurons when the strength of the noxious stimuli exceeds a threshold level. The electrical impulse travels along the axons of two major types of afferent nerve fibers, A-delta and C fibers (Table 3.5). The A-delta fibers are high-threshold (requiring strong stimuli), thinly myelinated fibers that are the first to respond to pain and are associated with rapid, pricking, and well-localized pain. The C-fibers are unmyelinated and are associated with pain that is slow, dull, diffuse, and aching. In addition, low-threshold A-beta fibers, which are highly myelinated and rapid, carry light touch and pressure sensations (Ellison, 2017). These nerve fibers conduct a depolarization wave that is carried to their cell bodies in the dorsal root ganglia outside the spinal cord and ultimately form synapses with excitatory or inhibitory interneurons in the dorsal horn.

With tissue injury, nociceptors may become sensitized by the release of the proinflammatory mediators (Tracey, 2017). This mixture of substances, including bradykinin, histamine, prostaglandin, and substance P, has been described as an "inflammatory soup" (Kelleher, Tewari, &

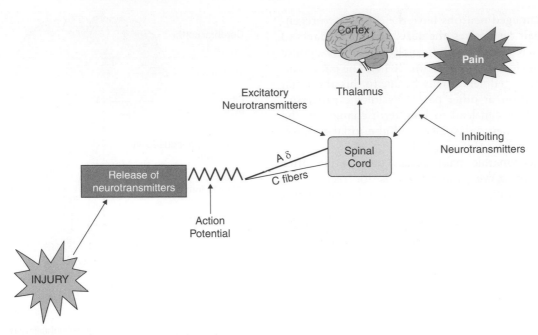

Fig. 3.4 | **Schematic Representation of Nociception.** (From Czarnecki, M., & Turner, H. [2018]. *Core curriculum for pain management nursing.* St. Louis, MO: Elsevier.)

Table 3.4	Nociception: The Neural Processing of Noxious Stimuli			
Transduction	**Transmission**	**Perception**	**Modulation**
Conversion of energy from one form to another	Primary afferent nerves carry impulse via Aδ and C fibers (nerve axons) from periphery to spinal cord	End result of neural activity of pain transmission	Inhibitory mechanisms
Starts at periphery when a noxious stimulus causes tissue damage		Conscious awareness of pain	Local and descending processes in multiple sites from periphery to cortex, and more importantly in spinal cord
Primary nociceptive fibers (afferents) are activated	**Aδ fibers:** Larger, myelinated, fast conduction, "first pain" **C fibers:** Smaller, unmyelinated, slow conduction: "second pain" Aβfibers: largest fibers, myelinated, fast conduction. Respond to touch, vibration, movement, do not normally transmit pain	Requires activation of higher brain structures (thalamus, limbic system)	Involves release of numerous neurochemicals which include: Endogenous opioids, serotonin, norepineprhine
Numerous excitatory substances are released and facilitate further nociceptor activation. These substances, collectively labeled as "inflammatory soup" include: • Prostaglandins • Bradykinin • Substance P • Serotonin • Histamine	Afferent information passes through dorsal root ganglia (DRG) to spinal cord where it synapses in dorsal horn and connects to the "second order" neurons. In the dorsal horn, incoming stimuli are modulated through complex neurophysiologic and neurochemical mechanisms. Aδ and C fibers release a variety of neurotransmitters including glutamate, neurokinins, and substance P. Glutamate binds to NMDA receptor and promotes pain transmission, Dorsal horn modulation involves local, segmental, and descending systems.	Generates a network of cortical and subcortical gray matter	

Table 3.4 | Nociception: the neural processing of noxious stimuli—cont'd

Transduction	Transmission	Perception	Modulation
Ion movement (Ca++, Na+, K+) generate action potential	The stimulus is continued from the spinal cord via multiple ascending pathways to the brainstem and higher cortical levels	Includes process that influence movement, emotions, and drives related to pain	

Modified from Figure I-2 Nociception: "Normal" pain transmission. Pasero, C. (2004). Pathophysiology of neuropathic pain. *Pain Management Nursing, 5*(4 Suppl. 1), 3–8. https://doi.org/S1524904204001018 [pii] pp. 4–5]

Table 3.5 | Characteristics of Primary Afferent Nerve Fibers

Fiber Type	A-Delta (Finely Myelinated)	C (Unmyelinated)
Fiber diameter	2–5 μm	<2 μm
Conduction velocity	5–15 m/s	0.5–2 m/s
Distribution	Body surface, muscles, joints	Most tissues
Pain sensation	Rapid, pricking, well localized	Slow, diffuse, dull, aching
Position of synapse within dorsal horn of spinal cord	Laminae I and V	Lamina II (substantia gelatinosa)

From Steeds, C. E. (2016). The anatomy and physiology of pain. *Surgery, 34*(2), Table 1.

McMahon, 2017). Table 3.6 summarizes some of the inflammatory mediators. Many other mediators originate from local tissues, immune cells, and nociceptors themselves that are also involved in nociceptor sensitization and transduction. When the nociceptors are activated, they release these compounds that are involved in further activation of additional nociceptors. Recent research has led to the identification of receptors/channels involved in inflammation, such as the transient receptor potential channels (TRPCs). There are two principle TRPC receptors/channels, TRPV1 and TRPA1, that detect noxious, inflammatory stimuli. The first, TRPV1, located on C fiber nociceptors, is activated by heat, capsaicin, and acid and is associated with more pain than normal in response to heat stimuli (thermal hyperalgesia) and spontaneous inflammatory pain (Guan, Hellman, & Schumacher, 2016). The second, TRPA1, has been identified as the main gatekeeper of inflammatory processes. Both play a major role in the development and maintenance of inflammatory pain.

The chemical specialization of nociception involving transduction (as well as transmission) is illustrated in Fig. 3.5. Increased identification of the various substances involved in nociceptor sensitization has provided opportunities for the use and continued development of various analgesics that are included in a multimodal pain management plan. For example, antiinflammatory agents reduce transduction by their peripheral actions, which inhibit cyclooxygenase (COX) isoenzymes and the production of prostaglandins (see Chapter 10). Local anesthetics, including topically administered agents such as lidocaine, reduce transduction by blocking the sodium channels involved in action potential generation (see Chapters 15, 16, 18, and 19). Anticonvulsant medications, such as gabapentin and OXcarbazepine, can reduce nociceptive transduction by altering the flux of other ions such as calcium and potassium (see Chapter 15). Capsaicin initially activates TRPV1 receptors, causing initial sensation of burning, and then desensitizes them, resulting in pain relief (Fattori, Hohmann, Rossaneis, Pinho-Ribeiro, & Verri, 2016). These and other analgesics that affect transduction are further described in Chapters 10, 15, 16, 18, and 19.

Transmission

Transmission, the second step in nociception, involves the conduction of the action potential from the periphery to the dorsal route ganglia and on to the dorsal horn of the spinal cord, where the primary order neurons (the A-delta and C-fibers) synapse with the excitatory or inhibitory second order neurons (interneurons) in the SG of the spinal cord and continue along multiple ascending pathways in the CNS (Ellison, 2017). Of note, in addition to the forward (antegrade) transmission of the pain signal from the dorsal route ganglia to the dorsal horn and to the higher centers in the CNS, nociceptors, at the dorsal route ganglia, can also send a retrograde (backward) signal back to the periphery. This retrograde signal is transmitted through calcium channel activity, which releases substance P and

Table 3.6 | Inflammatory Mediators

Mediator	Source	Tissue Target	Receptor	Somatic Target
Bradykinin	Immune cells, plasma	Blood vessels, nociceptors	Bradykinin type 1 and 2 receptors (B1R, B2R)	Thermal, mechanical
Prostaglandin	Microglia, nociceptors	Nociceptors	EP_1, EP_2, EP_{3B}, EP_{3C}, EP_4, DP_1, and DP2, receptors	Thermal, mechanical, chemical
Serotonin	Immune cells	Nociceptors	5-HT1A, 2A, 2B, 3, 4, 7	Thermal, mechanical, chemical
ATP	Microglia, nociceptors	Nociceptors, immune cells, microglia	P2X2, 3, 4, 7	Thermal, mechanical
NGF	Immune cells, nociceptors	Immune cells, nociceptors	TrkA, GPR30	Thermal, mechanical
Substance P	Nociceptors	Immune cells, blood vessels, nociceptors	NK1R	Thermal, mechanical
Glutamate	Microglia, nociceptors	Nociceptors	mGluR1, mGluR2/3, mGluR5	Thermal, mechanical
Serine proteases	Immune cells, nociceptors	Nociceptors	PAR1, PAR2, PAR4	Thermal, mechanical
CGRP	Nociceptors	Blood vessels, nociceptors, endothelial cells	Calcitonin receptor-like receptor (CRLR), receptor activity-modifying protein 1 (RAMP1)	Thermal, mechanical
Endothelin	Endothelial cells	Blood vessels, nociceptors	ET_AR, ET_BR	Thermal, mechanical, chemical

A cumulative list of known inflammatory mediators that modulate peripheral nociceptor sensitivities to somatosensory stimulation. As listed, the inflammatory mediator is released from its source(s) and targets a specific cell type to activate the noted receptor isoform(s), stimulating the identified signaling pathway to sensitize the associated somatosensation.

From Jeske, N. A. (2015). Peripheral scaffolding and signaling pathways in inflammatory pain. *Progress in Molecular Biology and Translational Science, 131*, 31–52. https://doi.org/10.1016/bs.pmbts.2014.11.016 [doi]

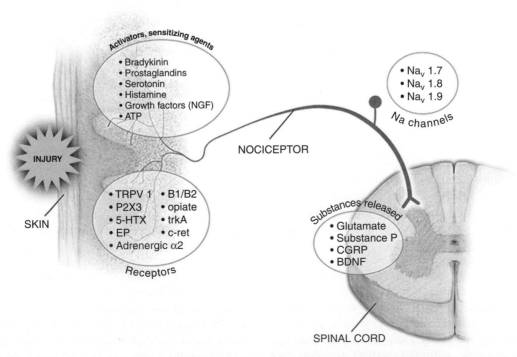

Fig. 3.5 | Chemical specialization of nociceptive sensory neurons divided into activators and sensitizing agents, receptors, sodium channels, and released substances. *ATP*, Adenosine triphosphate; *BDNF*, brain-derived neurotrophic factor; *CGRP*, Calcitonin gene related peptide; *NGF*, nerve growth factor. (From Puopolo, M., & Mendell, L. M. [2017]. Nociceptors: The gateway to pain. *Reference module in neuroscience and biobehavioral psychology.* New York, NY: Elsevier.)

other neurotransmitters that cause neurogenic inflammation and peripheral sensitization (Hudspith, 2016).

There are three types of second order neurons in the dorsal horn:

- *Nociceptive-specific neurons:* Respond to high threshold noxious stimuli
- *Wide dynamic range (WDR) neurons:* Respond to a wide range of stimuli
- *Low-threshold neurons:* Respond only to stimuli that are not harmful (Steeds, 2016)

Noxious stimuli that reach the dorsal horn cause voltage-sensitive calcium channels to open and trigger the release of neurotransmitters or neuromodulators that are involved in excitatory and inhibitory mechanisms of pain (Bourne, Machado, & Nagel, 2014).

- Glutamate, an amino acid, is the major excitatory neurotransmitter released onto spinal neurons by the primary order neurons. It plays a key role in activating receptors on central neurons that cause rapid depolarization. If the impulses are strong enough, even before the impulse reaches the brain, the individual will have a reflexive response that causes withdrawal from the painful stimuli.
- With high intensity or prolonged nociceptor activation in response to injury or inflammation, sufficient amounts of glutamate are released to cause activation of *N*-methyl-D-aspartate (NMDA) receptors. Calcium entry through these glutamate-NMDA–activated channels is responsible for sensitization of the CNS (Hudspith, 2016). NMDA receptor activation has been implicated in the development of chronic pain (Puopolo & Mendell, 2017).
- Substance P is an excitatory neurotransmitter found on C fibers that increases the transmission of pain.
- Other excitatory neurotransmitters include nitric oxide, cholecystokinin, calcitonin gene-related peptide, vasoactive intestinal peptide, and nitric oxide.
- Inhibitory neurotransmitters are also involved in transmission processes.
- Endogenous opioids such as dynorphin, enkephalin, beta endorphin, as well as norepinephrine, serotonin, somatostatin, and γ-aminobutyric acid (GABA) are among the inhibitory neurotransmitters that block pain transmission in the CNS (Ellison, 2017).

Fig. 3.6 summarizes neurochemicals involved in transmission. Many multimodal analgesic interventions target the neurotransmitters involved at the level of the dorsal horn. For example, opioids block the release of neurotransmitters, particularly substance P, at the spinal level (see Chapter 11).

From the dorsal horn, the second order neurons transmit the pain signal to the contralateral (opposite) side of the horn and the signal travels up the spinal cord. The spinal cord is composed of interconnected layers of gray matter, called Rexed laminae, that are surrounded by white matter. The 10 layers are numbered from the posterior aspect to the anterior aspect of the cord and are arranged in a butterfly shape that is depicted in Fig. 3.7. Laminae I to III contain the SG, the layers in which many of the sensory afferent nerve fibers at the dorsal horn terminate. A-delta sensory fibers end in lamina I and V, and C fibers terminate in lamina II (Steeds, 2016).

The pain stimulus in the spinal cord is transmitted by the ascending spinothalamic and spinoreticular tracts to the brainstem and thalamus. The thalamus functions as a relay station, sending somatosensory information to key cortical and subcortical structures in the brain: the insula, the anterior cingulate cortex, and the prefrontal cortex. These brain centers play major roles in pain perception (Ellison, 2017; Steeds, 2016).

Perception

Perception is the conscious awareness of pain in higher brain centers after neural transmission of noxious stimuli. It is the end result of the nervous system's response to noxious stimuli that integrates awareness, cognition, and emotions associated with pain. Various areas in the brain are involved in perception, as follows:

- The thalamus, anterior cingulate, and sensorimotor and insular corti are regions in the brain activated by the action potentials from the spinothalamic tracts to perceive localized unpleasant sensations (Grossberg, Palma, & Versace, 2016).
- The hypothalamus and amygdala are activated by action potentials from the spinobulbar tract to perceive intensity of acute pain (Grossberg, Palma, & Versace, 2016).
- The anterior cingulate gyrus of the limbic system is responsible for the emotional experience of pain (Grossberg, Palma, & Versace, 2016).
- Tectum located behind the midbrain enhances reflexes and acquired behavior patterns (Grossberg, Palma, & Versace, 2016).
- Basal ganglia are responsible for sensory discrimination of pain, affect, cognition, modulation of nociceptive information, and sensory gating to higher motor areas (Wright, 2015).

Functional magnetic resonance imaging (fMRI) and positron emission tomography (PET) are used for mapping these areas of brain during perception of nociceptive impulses. These imaging techniques have also been useful in examining other perception-related phenomena. Pain catastrophizing, a phenomenon that involves magnification, helplessness, and rumination about pain (Rice, Parker, Lewis, Kluger, & McNair, 2017), appears to activate pain centers in the brain (Craner, Sperry, & Evans, 2016). Similarly, brain imaging techniques have shown that intense emotional suffering and observing others in pain can trigger the perception of physical pain (Lamm, Decety, & Singer, 2011).

Nonpharmacologic pain management approaches such as cognitive-behavioral therapy, relaxation, distraction, meditation, and imagery may positively affect the experience

Class	Chemical	Comments
Amines	Noradrenaline 5-HT	Involved with descending modulation of pain
Endogenous opioid peptides	Enkephalins β-Endorphin	Produced in cell body and transported to nerve terminal. Widespread in CNS, but especially in sites associated with pain. Bind to opioid receptors with inhibitory effect
Nonopioid peptides	Substance P	Widespread especially in DRG of C fibers. Associated with inflammation.
	Galanin	Widespread. Involved with antinociception
	Cholecystokinin and others	Occur in DRG, dorsal horn, and spinal tracts. May be involved with visceral pain. Become depleted in nerve injury
Excitatory amino acids	Glutamate	Act on NMDA and non-NMDA receptors. Involved in development, memory, and neuronal plasticity
Inhibitory amino acids	GABA Glycine	Regulate behavior associated with non-noxious stimuli
Others	Cannabinoids	CB1 receptors in SC and on primary afferent neurons: involved in antinociception.
	Nitric oxide	In sensory neurons and dorsal horn. Involved in peripheral and central sensitization. Linked with NMDA activity

CNS, central nervous system; DRG, dorsal root ganglia; NA, noradrenaline; NMDA, N-methyl- d -aspartate; 5-HT, 5-hydroxytryptamine; GABA, γ-aminobutyric acid.

Fig. 3.6 | Chemicals Involved in Pain Transmission (From Steeds, C. E. [2016]. The anatomy and physiology of pain. *Surgery, 34*[2], 55.)

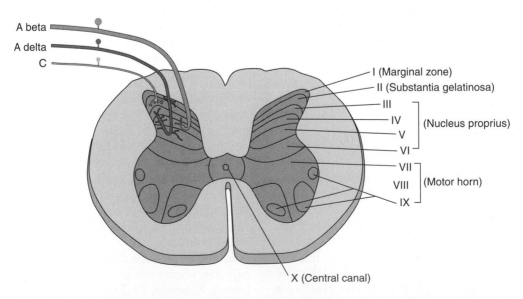

Fig. 3.7 | Dorsal Horn and Rexed Laminae. (From Czarnecki, M., & Turner, H. [2018]. *Core curriculum for pain management nursing.* St. Louis, MO: Elsevier.

of pain. Although the mechanisms by which these interventions provide pain relief are not well understood and require further research, functional and structural MRI, and other studies have identified brain locations and mechanisms involved in pain perception and modulation (Volz, Suarez-Contreras, Portilla, & Fregni, 2015; Zeidan et al., 2011). Many nonpharmacologic techniques are included as multimodal analgesic interventions and are further described in Chapters 20 to 27.

Modulation

Modulation, which is sometimes viewed as the last process in nociception, involves the alteration (either increase or decrease) of pain stimuli, which affects the perception of pain. Although pain may be modulated at every level from the periphery to the cortex (as evidenced by the effects of multimodal interventions along the pain pathway) modulation often refers to processes involving the descending nociceptive pathway from the activated midbrain to the dorsal horn of spinal cord (Ellison, 2017).

Neurons of the descending pain pathway release inhibitory neurotransmitters, including serotonin and norepinephrine, which modulate the perception of pain. The descending pathways include the periaqueductal gray (PAG) and the nucleus raphe magnus (NRM) in the brainstem and the dorsal horn of the spinal cord. The PAG is rich in opioid receptors and receives inhibitory messages from the higher centers in the cortex and hypothalamus. Dopaminergic activity in the PAG has been found to support the opioid receptor activity in this area (Tobaldini et al., 2017). PAG neurons project this inhibitory input to the NRM, which contains serotonergic neurons. The NRM then continues the downward projection to the spinal cord and the superficial and deep dorsal horn laminae (Kwon, Altin, Duenas, & Alev, 2014). At the dorsal horn of the spinal cord, these descending inhibitory mechanisms from the higher centers in the CNS may further modulate (reduce) the pain signal transmission.

At the dorsal horn, the descending pain modulation system inhibits pain by activating the endogenous opioid system and alpha-2 receptors that attenuate the function of the primary order neurons (the A-delta and C-fibers) (Kwon et al., 2014). Most of the dorsal horn opioid receptors are presynaptic (located on the terminal end of the A-delta and C-fibers), and the majority of the alpha-2 receptors are located on the postsynaptic dendrites (Hudspith, 2016; Zhang, Bao, & Li, 2015). As a result, spinal opioid and alpha-2 agonists produce analgesia by inhibiting glutamate and other excitatory pain mechanisms at the dorsal horn level. Other inhibitory processes have been identified at the dorsal horn. For example, GABA is expressed by inhibitory interneurons in the dorsal horn and also has pain inhibitory activity at the level of the spinal cord (Hudspith, 2016).

Identification of a number of descending inhibitory pathways has provided opportunities for the use of multimodal interventions that can be used to modulate pain.

Because serotonin and norepinephrine inhibit pain, antidepressant medications such as the serotonin-norepinephrine inhibitors (SNRIs) are used in pain treatment plans because they inhibit the reuptake of these neurotransmitters, thus leaving them available in the synapses (Aronoff, 2016). Baclofen, a medication that acts as a CNS depressant and skeletal muscle relaxant, is also used in pain modulation because of its ability to activate $GABA_B$ receptors and produce analgesia (see Chapter 15) (Malcangio, 2018). Various nonpharmacologic approaches, such as TENS (Chapter 20) and acupuncture (Chapter 23), are thought to modulate pain in part by activation of the endogenous opioid system (Fan et al., 2017; Vance, Dailey, Rakel, & Sluka, 2014). Other nonpharmacologic techniques, mentioned in the section on pain perception, also may have a role in pain modulation.

Abnormal Processing of Pain: Neuropathic Pain and Hypersensitization

Abnormal pain processing, often associated with neuropathic pain, is a result of peripheral or central sensitization mechanisms, as shown in Table 3.7. With abnormal processing of pain there is a shift in sensory pathways to an increased state of excitation and a loss of inhibition at the levels of the periphery, spinal cord, and/or brain (Colloca et al., 2017).

Peripheral Mechanisms and Neuropathic Pain

Peripheral mechanisms involved in neuropathic pain may develop when noxious stimuli damage peripheral epidermal nerve endings and keratinocytes and cause them to become hyperexcitable (Keppel Hesselink, Kopsky, & Bhaskar, 2016). The following processes contribute to the development of peripheral neuropathic pain:

- Damaged peripheral nociceptors may have a lowered threshold for firing, have a greater than normal response to noxious stimuli, and respond to stimuli that are not normally painful.
- Damaged tissue and cells release excitatory inflammatory mediator substances, such as bradykinin, adenosine triphosphate, histamine, prostaglandins, leukotrienes, cytokines, nerve growth factor (NGF), serotonin, and prostaglandin E2, which increase peripheral sensitization to stimuli (Steeds, 2016).
- NGF acts on C fibers to express the TrkA receptor, which is a key component of peripheral sensitization.
- The area of sensory space that causes the nociceptors to respond (the receptive field) is increased, and areas distant from the inflammatory field also can be affected. Normally silent nociceptors become active and develop sensitivity (Hudspith, 2016).
- Sprouting of damaged nerves and formation of neuromas from exposed demyelinated neuronal membrane cause ectopic nerve impulses (Steeds,

Table 3.7 | Mechanisms of Peripheral and Central Neuropathic Pain

Peripheral Mechanisms	Central Mechanisms
Peripheral sensitization initiated by release of substances from damaged cells (e.g., prostaglandins, bradykinin, serotonin, norepinephrine, substance P)	Central sensitization (hyperexcitability of central neurons) initiated by prolonged binding of neurotransmitters (e.g., glutamate, substance P)
Alteration in ion channel expression	NMDA receptor activation and influx of intracellular calcium
Collateral sprouting	Lowered threshold for nerve conduction
Recruitment of "silent" nociceptors	Increased response to stimuli
Ephaptic conduction	Enlarged receptor field
Lowered threshold for nerve depolarization → spontaneous ectopic neuronal discharges	Collateral sprouting Coupling between sensory and central nervous systems
Coupling between sensory and central nervous systems	Central disinhibition
Clinical signs: Primary hyperalgesia, burning pain, dysesthesias, paresthesias, allodynia	Clinical signs: Secondary hyperalgesia, allodynia, sympathetically maintained pain

NMDA, N-methyl-D-aspartate.

From Pasero C, McCaffery M. (2011). *Pain assessment and pharmacologic management* (p. 7). St. Louis, MO: Mosby. Data from Adler, J. E., Nico, L., VandeVord, P., et al. (2009). Modulation of neuropathic pain by glial-driven factor. *Pain Med, 10*(7), 1229–1236; Argoff, C. E., Albrecht, P., Irving, G., et al. (2009). Multimodal analgesia for chronic pain: Rationale and future directions. *Pain Medicine, 10*(Suppl 2), S53–S66; Beydoun, A., & Backonja, M. M. (2003). Mechanistic stratification of antineuralgic agents. *Journal of Pain Symptom Management, 25*(Suppl. 5), S18–S30; Bridges, D., Thompson, S. W. N., & Rice, A. S. C. (2001). Mechanisms of neuropathic pain. *British Journal of Anaesthesia, 87*(1), 12–26; Carlton, S. M. (2009). NMDA receptors revisited: Hope floats. *Pain, 146*(1–2), 1–2; Dickenson, A. H., Matthews, E. A., & Suzuki, R. (2002). Neurobiology of neuropathic pain: Mode of action of anticonvulsants. *European Journal of Pain, 6*(Suppl. A), 51–60; Mao, J., & Chen, L. L. (2000). Gabapentin in pain management. *Anesthesia & Analgesia, 91*(3), 680–687; Pasero, C. (2004). Pathophysiology of neuropathic pain. *Pain Management Nursing, 5*(4), 3–8. © 2004, Pasero C. May be duplicated for use in clinical practice.

2016). Neuromas are often found on limb amputation sites, leading to phantom limb phenomenon. Neuromas can be caused by diabetes and other progressive neurologic diseases, chemotherapy, neurotoxicity, and trauma.

Other peripheral mechanisms may be involved in neuropathic pain.

- Upregulation (an increase) of alpha-adrenergic receptors in damaged neuronal membranes may reduce the depolarization threshold of nociceptive nerves (causing them to have action potentials with less than normal amounts of stimuli) and cause abnormally severe pain (hyperalgesia) with thermal and mechanical stimuli.
- An increase in sodium channels along the neuronal membrane of damaged nerves may generate an impulse in the absence of stimulus (Colloca et al., 2017).
- Potassium and calcium channels undergo changes. TRPV1 is a calcium-permeable channel found in peripheral nociceptive neurons that primarily mediates heat hyperalgesia. Damage to peripheral nerves can reduce the activation threshold of TRPV1 to heat and low pH, and lead to peripheral sensitization and continuing pain (Treede, 2016).
- An abnormal excitatory process called cross talk or ephaptic conduction takes place among nerves, which creates chemically mediated connections between nerve fibers and abnormal activation of nociceptive

neurons (Deutch & Roth, 2014). Cross talk may take place between the sensory nerves, which are normally involved in nociception, and the sympathetic nerves in the same nerve bundle, which are not normally involved in nociception. Cross talk may contribute to the development of sympathetically mediated pain (e.g., CRPS) and respond to treatment with local anesthetic sympathetic nerve blocks (Pasero & McCaffery, 2011).

Central Mechanisms and Neuropathic Pain

Central mechanisms play a significant role in the development and maintenance of neuropathic pain. When a lesion or disease affects peripheral nerves, cellular and molecular changes are generated in the CNS and in the peripheral nerves. The barrage of impulses from the peripheral nerves on the CNS is responsible for producing ectopic firing in the dorsal route ganglia and the development of central sensitization, a key phenomenon seen in neuropathic pain (Aronoff, 2016). Simply stated, central sensitization is the increased responsiveness of neurons in the CNS to peripheral nerve input. With central sensitization, changes occur in central neurons, along with alterations in the inhibitory interneurons and descending pathways.

Many of the same chemical mediators that are involved in the sensitization of peripheral nerves are also involved in the sensitization of the CNS.

- Increased input from the peripheral nociceptors causes the second order nerves in the dorsal root ganglion to be sensitized by substance P and glutamate, the excitatory neurotransmitter associated with NMDA receptors.

- Neurochemical changes mediated by NMDA, nitric oxide, and neurokinins increase the ectopic activity and spinothalamic signaling and therefore lower the nociception threshold and spread the pain signals (Steeds, 2016).
- NMDA receptor activation leads to increased calcium channel activity, lowering the pain threshold (Patel, Montagut-Bordas, & Dickenson, 2018).
- Loss of nerve growth factor plays a major role in the pathophysiology of hypersensitization (Djouhri, 2016).

Central sensitization is often associated with a phenomenon known as pain wind-up, which may occur with repeated activation of the dorsal horn by peripheral nociceptors. Repeated stimulation of afferent C fibers of peripheral nerves, at a constant intensity, causes activation of dorsal horn neurons in the spinal cord to increase in magnitude and duration (Woda et al., 2017). If more than one stimulus arrives at the dorsal route ganglia while a previous stimulus is still discharging, the ongoing activity is augmented and a stronger response is created. With wind-up, there is increased release of neurotransmitters that strengthens excitatory pathways in the CNS. Changes in the wide dynamic range cells in the dorsal horn result in lowered thresholds for excitation, NMDA receptor activation with glutamate release, sustained depolarization, and ultimate malfunction and destruction of central inhibitory mechanisms. Wind-up is thought to contribute to the pain associated with fibromyalgia (Staud, Weyl, Riley, & Fillingim, 2014).

Another phenomenon seen in the central response to neuropathic pain is neuroplasticity, in which prolonged nociception leads to changes and reorganization in the subcortical, somatosensory, and motor cortex structures and central sensitization (Aronoff, 2016). These reorganizations may cause somatosensory and spatial remapping and rewiring, as is often seen in phantom limb pain after limb amputation. Cortical reorganization also may be involved in chronic low back pain and other neuropathic pain conditions. Many psychological conditions such as distress, depression, and anxiety related to chronic pain can cause neuroplastic changes in the brain and increase central sensitization (Aronoff, 2016). The use of non-pharmacologic multimodal therapies such as cognitive-behavioral therapy (Chapter 22), physical therapy (Chapter 20), visual training, and meditation (Chapter 25) alter the perception of pain largely through the brain's ability to undergo neuroplasticity (Ropero Pelaez & Taniguchi, 2016).

Normally, the neurons in the dorsal horn undergo strong intraspinal inhibitory control by the GABA interneurons. However, in some cases, peripheral nerve injury may lead to the suppression and death of these inhibitory interneurons. As a result, there is abnormal excitability of central neurons and generation of abnormal nociceptive signals, which are interpreted as pain by the brain (Kim et al., 2017; Ngernyam, Jensen, Auvichayapat, Punjaruk, & Auvichayapat, 2013). A more complex interaction involving GABA and the lamina I neurons has been found to exert an excitatory effect, rather than the normal inhibitory effect, on the lamina I neurons. This dysfunction in GABA pathways is the reason for the use of GABAergic medications such as baclofen to relieve neuropathic pain. Another phenomenon seen with central sensitization is the activation of immune cells, the spinal cord glia, that release brain-derived neurotrophic factor (BDNF) and cause changes in the lamina I neurons. The involvement of the glia in the function of the lamina I neurons is an illustration of the interconnectedness between the nervous system and the immune system.

Neuroinflammation and Immune System

In the past, the immune system and the nervous system were thought to operate independently of each other. However, as a result of intense research in recent years, there is greater awareness of the roles and interconnectedness of the immune and neurologic systems and their contributions to the experience of pain. Communication back and forth between nociceptor sensory neurons and cells of the immune system has been found to be involved in the regulation of pain and inflammation (Pinho-Ribiero, Verri, & Chio, 2017). The brain modulates the immune system, and the immune system modulates the nervous system. Both systems work together to protect the body. The nervous system signals the presence of injury or threats of damage, and the immune system provides protection through the inflammatory response. The immune system is also involved in tissue repair. Although the relationship between the nervous system and immune system serves very vital functions, in some cases there are negative pain-related outcomes. This reciprocal relationship between the neurons and immune cells in the CNS is thought to be a key contributor to the development of a number of chronic pain conditions (Vardeh, Mannion, & Woolf, 2016).

As stated previously, the PNS and CNS play major roles in pain. However, the earlier simplistic explanation of the role of A-delta and A-beta nociceptor neurons, and C-fiber neurons in pain physiology has evolved into a greater understanding that nociceptors are highly diverse and have distinct molecular expression patterns of ion channels, growth factor receptors, G protein–coupled receptors, and neuropeptides. The interactions between neuronal and immunologic systems is demonstrated by the discovery that immune cells play a critical role in the release of molecular mediators, including lipids, inflammatory cytokines, and immune-derived growth factors that sensitize the nociceptor sensory neurons

(Pinho-Ribeiro, Verri, & Chiu, 2017). Reciprocally, specific nociceptor subtypes have been found to have receptors for these immune molecular mediators, which results in the conduction of neuroimmune signaling.

The inflammatory process involves different types of immune-mediating cells. These cells include leukocytes (neutrophils and lymphocytes), macrophages, mast cells, and glial cells (including microglia), as well as other immunocompetent cells (astrocytes, oligodendrocytes, and others) (Chavan, Pavlov, & Tracey, 2017; Grace, Hutchinson, Maier, & Watkins, 2014). Leukocytes, macrophages, and mast cells are readily recognized by most clinicians for their roles in the inflammatory process. Glial cells, consisting of macroglia and microglia, are immune cells that are located in the PNS and CNS. In recent years, the role of glial cells in the inflammatory process and in pain modulation and amplification has been the focus of much research interest.

In the PNS, Schwann cells are glial cells that produce the myelin sheath around axons. Satellite glial cells are part of the PNS support system, located in the dorsal root and trigeminal ganglia, and are involved in sensory nerve processing (Cairns, Arendt-Nielsen, & Nacerdote, 2015). Satellite cells may be involved in the release of glutamate, the excitatory neurotransmitter that plays a major role in pain transmission. The immune system plays a role in the regulation of peripheral pain sensitization. Neuroinflammatory changes have been identified in the sensory ganglia and nerves themselves.

Microglia, the smallest glial cells, act as the sentinels, or the macrophages of the CNS (Franco & Fernandez-Suarez, 2015). In the CNS, microglia are the immune cells that contribute to maintaining pain sensitivity through the release of proinflammatory cytokines and other inflammatory mediators. These mediators serve varied functions and have been found to have a major impact on the initiation and maintenance of neuropathic pain. Microglia are distributed throughout the CNS and respond to a wide-range of disturbances in the nervous system, including peripheral nerve injury, and cause peripheral immune cell infiltration by releasing cytokines and other inflammatory mediators (Grace et al., 2014). Peripheral nerve injury leads to nociceptive input to the spinal cord, and the nociceptor neurons express and release inflammatory mediators into the cord. The microglia are the first immunocompetent cells to respond to the release of mediators from peripheral nerve injury. They respond by producing cytokines such as tumor necrosis factor-alpha (TNF-α), interleukin-1beta, and BDNF, which further sensitize neurons and promote the release of more inflammatory mediators (Aronoff, 2016; Vardeh et al., 2016). In some cases, the microglia remain in a heightened, activated state and continue to express inflammatory mediators that may result in neuropathic pain and lead to central sensitization and the development of chronic pain (Pinho-Ribeiro et al., 2017).

The development of chronic pain is more complex than the heightened activation of the microglia, although the microglia play a major role. When pain is prolonged, repetitive nociceptive signaling in the dorsal horn leads to the death of inhibitory neurons that would normally modulate pain, and nociceptive input into the spinal cord is no longer opposed. The brainstem also decreases descending inhibitory modulation. The unopposed nociceptive impulses in the dorsal horn are amplified by the microglia, and along with C-fiber changes and other mechanisms, result in changes in the architecture, or a condition known as neuroplasticity, which is associated with central sensitization and chronic pain (Pozek et al., 2016).

Continued and increased research in this area of neuroinflammation is yielding greater understanding of chronic pain states and treatment. A major area of research interest is the relationship between the opioid system and immune function. Studies have shown that opioid receptors are expressed by peripheral immune cells, and when opioids such as morphine are administered, changes can occur in immune signaling. These interactions are complicated and result in varied effects from different opioids: immunosuppression, immunostimulation, and mixed effects (Liang, Liu, Chen, Ji, & Li, 2016). Opioids also have been found to have an effect on immune cells in the CNS. Morphine has been shown to stimulate the microglia to produce cytokines, which may lead to a reduction in the analgesic effect of morphine (Cairns et al., 2015). This area is one of great interest because further research may aid in an increased understanding of the phenomena of tolerance and opioid-induced hyperalgesia (Grace et al., 2014).

Activation of microglia has been implicated in the development of many chronic pain conditions, including fibromyalgia (Kosek et al., 2015; Littlejohn, 2015) and immunologically induced fatigue (Yasui et al., 2014). Researchers are working to identify the specific immune cells and mediators that are involved in different diseases. As understanding of the interactions between neurons and immune cells increases, and as identification of the immune mediators involved in painful inflammatory conditions such as rheumatoid arthritis and inflammatory bowel disease is increased, it may be possible to develop improved treatments for these conditions. An outcome of recent clinical trials is that bioelectronic devices, which use electrons as a therapeutic intervention, have been developed and successfully used to modulate the inflammatory response in patients with rheumatoid arthritis and inflammatory bowel disease (Chavan et al., 2017).

The complexities of neuroinflammation are well beyond the scope of this book, but it is of value to appreciate the existing and future value of research in this area that may have significant implications for the understanding of pain, particularly neuropathic pain, and the transition from acute to chronic painful conditions. It is possible that the continued focus on this field of neuroinflammation will lead to the development of new treatment options and pharmacologic interventions that will aid in the management of neuropathic and chronic pain.

Special Conditions

Central Pain

Central pain results from a lesion or disease that directly affects the somatosensory system of the CNS. Many conditions can contribute to central pain, and commonly associated conditions include central poststroke pain, multiple sclerosis (MS), and spinal cord injury. Poststroke pain has been strongly associated with thalamic strokes, but strokes in other areas of the brain also may be associated with central pain (Singer, Conigliaro, Spina, Law, & Levine, 2017). Although central pain may have a variety of causes, it is associated with a number of common features, including the following (Gilron et al., 2015):

- Some degree of dysfunction of the spinothalamic pathways that leads to changes in pinprick and temperature sensation and hypersensitivity in areas of the body affected by the CNS lesion.
- Allodynia, hyperalgesia, and/or hyperpathia in areas affected by the CNS lesion because of hyperexcitability in the CNS.
- Pain qualities that are often described as icy, burning, and lancinating pain.

Multimodal approaches, including pharmacologic agents and electrical and other interventional procedures may be employed in the management of central pain (Moreno-Duarte et al., 2014; Siniscalchi, De Sarro, & Gallelli, 2014).

Chronic Regional Pain Syndrome

CRPS is a chronic neurologic pain condition that may develop after trauma or injury (often orthopedic) to a limb. This complex condition is an area that continues to be highly investigated because there is still much to be learned about its pathophysiology, prevention, and treatment. It is associated with severe pain and hyperalgesia disproportionate to the inciting injury, sensory alterations, and significant autonomic, motor, and trophic changes. Specific criteria, The Orlando Criteria for CRPS and The Budapest Clinical Diagnostic Criteria for CRPS, have been developed to aid in the diagnosis of this syndrome. Table 3.8 provides a summary of the Budapest Criteria. CRPS has been categorized as CRPS type I and CRPS type II.

CRPS type I is not associated with identified nerve damage, and the region of pain does not follow a pattern of nerve distribution; thus, based on the definition, the pain in type I is not categorized as neuropathic pain. CRPS type I is associated with edema of the extremity (usually distal), changes in skin color and temperature, abnormal sudomotor activity in the painful region, allodynia, and hyperalgesia (Goh, Chidambaram, & Ma, 2017).

CRPS type II has many of the same qualities as CRPS type I, but the symptoms occur in the region of the extremity that is associated with the distribution of the nerve or nerve branches associated with the injury.

The pathophysiology of CRPS is complex. The acute phase, often referred to as the warm phase, is associated with a highly exaggerated inflammatory response that may last for months. During this time there are multiple inflammatory mediators that sensitize the PNS and CNS and cause the release of mediators that result in endothelial dysfunction and vascular changes (Birklein & Schlereth, 2015). After the inflammatory phase, the syndrome transitions into a cold phase in which there is excessive sympathetic nervous system activity, which is responsible for allodynia, nondermatomal sensory deficits, pallor, cyanosis, sweating, and coolness of the affected area. This phase

Table 3.8 | Budapest Clinical Diagnostic Criteria for Chronic Regional Pain Syndrome[a]

Criteria	Case
1. Continuing pain that is disproportionate to any inciting event.	+
2. Must report at least one symptom in three (clinical diagnostic criteria) or four (research diagnostic criteria) of the following categories:	
• *Sensory:* Hyperesthesia or allodynia	+
• *Vasomotor:* Temperature asymmetry, skin color changes, or skin color asymmetry	−
• *Sudomotor or edema:* Edema, sweating changes, or sweating asymmetry	+
• *Motor or trophic:* Decreased range of motion, motor dysfunction (weakness, tremor, or dystonia), or trophic changes (hair, nails, or skin).	+
3. Must display at least one sign at time of diagnosis in two or more of the following categories:	
• *Sensory:* Hyperalgesia (to pinprick) or allodynia (to light touch, deep somatic pressure, or joint movement)	+
• *Vasomotor:* Temperature asymmetry, skin color changes, or skin color asymmetry	−
• *Sudomotor or edema:* Edema, sweating changes, or sweating asymmetry	+
• *Motor or trophic:* Decreased range of motion, motor dysfunction (weakness, tremor, or dystonia), or trophic changes (hair, nails, or skin)	+

[a]Endorsed by the International Association for the Study of Pain and validated by Harden et al.
From Saltık, S., Sözen, H. G., Basgul, S., Karatoprak, E. Y., & Içağasıoğlu, A. (2016). Pregabalin treatment of a patient with complex regional pain syndrome. *Pediatric Neurology, 54*, 88–90, Table 1, p.89.

is associated with neuronal plasticity and reorganization within the CNS (Birklein & Schlereth, 2015).

The management of CRPS is optimized with a multidisciplinary and multimodal approach. Physical and occupational therapies are the first-line treatment. Because CRPS is often associated with anxiety and depression, and possibly other psychological factors, participation in psychological therapy (see Chapter 20) that offers training in cognitive-behavioral therapy (Chapter 22), relaxation skills, coping skills, and biofeedback (Chapter 22) may aid in coping and recovery from this condition (Goh et al., 2017). Pharmacologic management requires a multimodal approach and may include a variety of nonopioid analgesics such as anticonvulsants, alpha-$_2$ agonists, bisphosphonates, calcitonin, subanesthetic ketamine, nonsteroidal antiinflammatory agents, and corticosteroids (Chevreau, Romand, Gaudin, Juvin, & Baillet, 2017; Orhurhu, Orhurhu, Bhatia, & Cohen, 2019; Williams, Guarino, & Raja, 2018). (See Chapters 10, 15, 16.). Interventional procedures, including sympathetic blocks, neuromodulation techniques, and, in extreme cases, sympathectomy and/or limb amputation, may be required (Williams, Guarino, & Raja, 2018) (see Chapters 18 and 19). Growth in the understanding of the pathophysiology of CRPS may lead to future treatment options and interventions involving immunomodulation, the use of hyperbaric oxygen treatments and botulinum toxin-A, and plasma exchange (Goh et al., 2017).

Key Points

- Pain perception is the result of multiple physiologic, psychological, and social factors as described in the biopsychosocial model of pain.
- The gate control theory of pain has been instrumental in providing the framework for an explanation of most pain-related phenomena.
- Pain is classified in many ways. It is commonly classified by duration and mechanism.
- Nociceptive pain is the normal processing of the nervous system to tissue damage. Subcategories include somatic pain originating from skin, muscles, bones, and soft tissues and visceral pain from activation of nerve fibers in the organs and hollow viscera.
- Neuropathic pain results from damage or lesions of nerves, is often seen as pathologic pain, and is commonly associated with chronic pain.
- Nociception involves transduction, transmission, perception, and modulation.
- Peripheral and central mechanisms are involved in the processing of nociceptive and neuropathic pain.
- Multiple ascending and descending processes in the peripheral and central nervous systems are involved in the modulation of nociceptive impulses.
- There have been major advances in understanding of the roles and interconnections of the nervous system and the immune system in the pathophysiology of pain.

- Neuromodulators, neurotransmitters, immune mediators, inflammatory mediators, and other endogenous chemical mediators are involved in all aspects of nociception and in peripheral and central sensitization.
- Increased understanding of the complex processes involved in the experience of pain has been instrumental in the development of a variety of multimodal approaches to pain management.

Case Scenario

Mr. S presents in the outpatient pain practice with a 1-year history of low back pain, which was precipitated by lifting heavy bags in his job at a mason supply company. He requests a prescription for an opioid because he was told by a coworker that his chronic pain should be treated with opioid therapy. During the visit, the clinician obtains a thorough history of Mr. S's pain, as part of a comprehensive assessment and physical examination. The clinician orders several different nonopioid medications and recommends follow-up imaging of his spine and a possible procedure if his pain does not improve. Mr. S is frustrated and overwhelmed and comes to you asking for an explanation for this complicated approach to his simple low back pain problem. He is annoyed that the clinician asked so many questions that had "nothing to do" with his pain.

1. What classifications can be used to describe Mr. S's pain?
2. What explanation do you give Mr. S for the types of pain he may be experiencing?
3. What rationale do you give for the extensive history that the provider obtained from Mr. S?
4. What is the rationale for the use of multiple different medications and possible invasive procedures to treat Mr. S's pain?
5. What nonpharmacologic home-based approaches can be recommended to Mr. S, and what is the theoretical basis for the use of these approaches?

References

Aronoff, G. M. (2016). What do we know about the pathophysiology of chronic pain? Implications for treatment considerations. *Medical Clinics of North America*, *100*, 31–42.

Arora, S. (2015). Helfer's Skin Tap Technique for IM Injection Pain. *International Journal of Nursing Science Practice and Research*, *1*(2), 19–20.

Birklein, F., & Schlereth, T. (2015). Complex regional pain syndrome-significant progress in understanding. *Pain*, *156*. https://doi.org/10.1097/01.j.pain.0000460344.54470.20. *Suppl 1*, S94-103. doi.

Bourne, S., Machado, A. G., & Nagel, S. J. (2014). Basic anatomy and physiology of pain pathways. *Neurosurg Clin N Am*, *25*, 629–638.

Cairns, B. E., Arendt-Nielsen, L., & Sacerdote, P. (2015). Perspectives in pain research 2014: neuroinflammation and glial cell activation: the cause of transition from acute to chronic pain? *Scandinavian Journal of Pain*, 6, 3–6.

Cardenas Fernandez, R. (2015). The neuromatrix and its importance in pain neurobiology. [La neuromatrix y su importancia en la neurobiologia del dolor]. *Investigacion Clinica*, 56(2), 109–110.

Chavan, S. S., Pavlov, V. A., & Tracey, K. J. (2017). Mechanisms and therapeutic relevance of Neuro-immune communication. *Immunity*, 46(6), 927–942.

Chevreau, M., Romand, X., Gaudin, P., Juvin, R., & Baillet, A. (2017). Bisphosphonates for treatment of complex regional pain syndrome type 1: a systematic literature review and meta-analysis of randomized controlled trials versus placebo. *Joint Bone Spine*, 84(4), 393–399.

Cohen, S. P., & Mao, J. (2014). Neuropathic pain: Mechanisms and their clinical implications. *BMJ (Clinical Research Ed.)*, 348, f7656. https://doi.org/10.1136/bmj.f7656 [doi].

Cohen, S. P., & Raja, S. N. (2016). Pain. In L. Goldman, & A. I. Schafer (Eds.), *Goldman-Cecil Medicine (25th ed.*, pp. 2517–2522). Philadelphia: Saunders.

Colloca, L., Ludman, T., Bouhassira, D., Baron, R., Dickenson, A. H., Yarnitsky, D., et al. (2017). Neuropathic pain. *Nature Reviews Disease Primers*, 3, 17002. https://doi.org/10.1038/nrdp.2017.2.

Craner, J. R., Sperry, J. A., & Evans, M. M. (2016). The relationship between pain catastrophizing and outcomes of a 3-week comprehensive pain rehabilitation program. *Pain Medicine (Malden, Mass.)*, 17(11), 2026–2035. https://doi.org/pnw070 [pii].

Czarnecki, M. L., & Turner, H. (2018). *Physiology of pain. Core curriculum for pain management nursing* (3rd ed., p. 132). St. Louis, MO: Elsevier.

Deutch, A. Y., & Roth, R. H. (2014). Pharmacology and Biochemistry of Synaptic Transmission: Classical Transmitters. In J. H. Byrne, R. Heidelberger, & M. N. Waxham (Eds.), *From Molecules to Networks: An Introduction to Cellular and Molecular Neuroscience* (3rd ed., p. 208). San Diego, CA: Elsevier.

Djouhri, L. (2016). PG110, A humanized anti-NGF antibody, reverses established pain hypersensitivity in persistent inflammatory pain, but not peripheral neuropathic pain, rat models. *Pain Medicine (Malden, Mass.)*, 17(11), 2082–2094. https://doi.org/pnw007 [pii].

Dowlati, E. (2017, May). Spinal Cord Anatomy, Pain, and Spinal Cord Stimulation Mechanisms. In *Seminars in Spine Surgery*. Philadelphia, PA: WB Saunders.

Ellison, D. L. (2017). Physiology of pain. *Crit Care Nurs Clin North Am*, 29(4), 397–406.

Engel, G. L. (1977). The need for a new medical model: A challenge for biomedicine. *Science (New York, N.Y.)*, 196(4286), 129–136.

Fan, A. Y., Miller, D. W., Bolash, B., Bauer, M., McDonald, J., Faggert, S., et al. (2017). Acupuncture's role in solving the opioid epidemic: Evidence, cost-effectiveness, and care availability for acupuncture as a primary, non-pharmacologic method for pain relief and management-white paper 2017. *Journal of Integrative Medicine*, 15(6), 411-425. https://doi.org/S2095-4964(17)60378-9 [pii].

Fattori, V., Hohmann, M. S., Rossaneis, A. C., Pinho-Ribeiro, F. A., & Verri, W. A. (2016). Capsaicin: current understanding of its mechanisms and therapy of pain and other pre-clinical and clinical uses. *Molecules*, 21(7), 844.

Fillingim, R. B. (2015). Heritability of catastrophizing: The biopsychosocial model in action. *Pain*, 156(3), 357–358. https://doi.org/10.1097/01.j.pain.0000460338.16353.8e [doi] p.357.

Franco, R., & Fernandez-Suarez, D. (2015). Alternatively activated microglia and macrophages in the central nervous system. *Progress in Neurobiology*, 131, 65–86.

Gatchel, R. J., Neblett, R., Kishino, N., & Ray, C. T. (2016). Fear-avoidance beliefs and chronic pain. *The Journal of Orthopaedic and Sports Physical Therapy*, 46(2), 38–43. https://doi.org/10.2519/jospt.2016.0601.

Gilron, I., Baron, R., & Jensen, T. (2015). Neuropathic pain: Principles of diagnosis and treatment. *Mayo Clinic Proceedings*, 90(4), 532–545. https://doi.org/10.1016/j.mayocp.2015.01.018 [doi].

Goh, E. L., Chidambaram, S., & Ma, D. (2017). Complex regional pain syndrome: A recent update. *Burns & Trauma*, 5. https://doi.org/10.1186/s41038-016-0066-4. 2-016-0066-4. eCollection 2017. [doi].

Grace, P. M., Hutchinson, M. R., Maier, S. F., & Watkins, L. R. (2014). Pathological pain and the neuroimmune interface. *Nature Reviews. Immunology*, 14(4), 217.

Groh, A., Krieger, P., Mease, R. A., & Henderson, L. (2018). Acute and chronic pain processing in the thalamocortical system of humans and animal models. *Neuroscience*, 387, 58–71. S0306-4522(17)30695-4 [pii].

Grossberg, S., Palma, J., & Versace, M. (2016). Resonant cholinergic dynamics in cognitive and motor decision-making: Attention, category learning, and choice in neocortex, superior colliculus, and optic tectum. *Frontiers in Neuroscience*, 9, 501. https://doi.org/10.3389/fnins.2015.00501.

Guan, Z., Hellman, J., & Schumacher, M. (2016). Contemporary views on inflammatory pain mechanisms: TRPing over innate and microglial pathways. *F1000Research*, 5, F1000 Faculty Rev-2425. eCollection 2016. https://doi.org/F1000 Faculty Rev-2425 [pii].

Herndon, C. M., Arnstein, P., Darnall, B., Hartrick, C., Lyons, M., & Sehgal, N. (2016). *Principles of Analgesic Use*. Chicago, Ill: American Pain Society.

Heydari, M., Shams, M., Hashempur, M. H., Zargaran, A., Dalfardi, B., & Borhani-Haghighi, A. (2015). The origin of the concept of neuropathic pain in early medieval Persia (9th-12th century CE). *Acta Medico-Historica Adriatica AMHA*, 13(Suppl 2), 9–22.

Hudspith, M. J. (2016). Anatomy, physiology and pharmacology of pain. *Anaesthesia & Intensive Care Medicine*, 17(9), 425–430.

Jensen, T. S., & Finnerup, N. B. (2014). Allodynia and hyperalgesia in neuropathic pain: Clinical manifestations and mechanisms. *The Lancet Neurology*, 13(9), 924–935. https://doi.org/10.1016/S1474-4422(14)70102-4.

Jensen, T. S., Baron, R., Haanpää, M., Kalso, E., Loeser, J. D., Rice, A. S., et al. (2011). A new definition of neuropathic pain. *Pain*, 152(10), 2204–2205. https://doi.org/10.1016/j.pain.2011.06.017.

Johnson, M. I., Paley, C. A., Howe, T. E., & Sluka, K. A. (2015). Transcutaneous electrical nerve stimulation for acute pain. *The Cochrane Database of Systematic Reviews*, (6):CD006142. doi(6), CD006142. https://doi.org/10.1002/14651858.CD006142.pub3 [doi].

Katz, J., & Rosenbloom, B. N. (2015). The golden anniversary of Melzack and Wall's gate control theory of pain: Celebrating 50 years of pain research and management. *Pain Research & Management*, 20(6), 285–286.

Kelleher, J. H., Tewari, D., & McMahon, S. B. (2017). Neurotrophic factors and their inhibitors in chronic pain treatment. *Neurobiology of Disease, 97,* 127–138. (Pt B). S0969-9961(16)30071-7 [pii].

Kent, M. L., Tighe, P. J., Belfer, I., Brennan, T. J., Bruehl, S., Brummett, C. M., … Edwards, D. (2017). The ACTTION–APS–AAPM Pain Taxonomy (AAAPT) multidimensional approach to classifying acute pain conditions. *Pain Medicine, 18*(5), 947–958.

Keppel Hesselink, J. M., Kopsky, D. J., & Bhaskar, A. K. (2016). Skin matters! the role of keratinocytes in nociception: A rational argument for the development of topical analgesics. *Journal of Pain Research, 10,* 1–8. https://doi.org/10.2147/JPR.S122765.

Kerstman, E., Ahn, S., Battu, S., Tariq, S., & Grabois, M. (2013). Neuropathic pain. *Handbook of Clinical Neurology, 110,* 175–187. https://doi.org/10.1016/B978-0-444-52901-5.00015-0.

Khan, M. A., Raza, F., & Khan, I. A. (2015). Pain: History, culture and philosophy. *Acta Medico-Historica Adriatica : AMHA, 13*(1), 113–130.

Kim, H. R., Han, J. Y., Park, Y. H., Kim, B. J., Yang, W., & Kim, S. (2017). Supernumerary phantom limb in a patient with basal ganglia hemorrhage - a case report and review of the literature. *BMC Neurology, 17*(1). https://doi.org/10.1186/s12883-017-0962-7. 180-017-0962-7.

Kosek, E., Altawil, R., Kadetoff, D., Finn, A., Westman, M., Le Maître, E., … Lampa, J. (2015). Evidence of different mediators of central inflammation in dysfunctional and inflammatory pain—interleukin-8 in fibromyalgia and interleukin-1 beta in rheumatoid arthritis. *Journal of Neuroimmunology, 280,* 49–55.

Kwon, M., Altin, M., Duenas, H., & Alev, L. (2014). The role of descending inhibitory pathways on chronic pain modulation and clinical implications. *Pain Practice : The Official Journal of World Institute of Pain, 14*(7), 656–667. https://doi.org/10.1111/papr.12145.

Lall, M. P., & Restrepo, E. (2017). The biopsychosocial model of low back pain and patient-centered outcomes following lumbar fusion. *Orthopedic Nursing, 36*(3), 213–221. https://doi.org/10.1097/NOR.0000000000000350.

Lamm, C., Decety, J., & Singer, T. (2011). Meta-analytic evidence for common and distinct neural networks associated with directly experienced pain and empathy for pain. *Neuroimage, 54*(3), 2492–2502.

Lethem, J., Slade, P. D., Troup, J. D., & Bentley, G. (1983). Outline of a fear-avoidance model of exaggerated pain perception-I. *Behaviour Research and Therapy, 21*(4), 401–408. 0005-7967(83)90009-8 [pii].

Liang, X., Liu, R., Chen, C., Ji, F., & Li, T. (2016). Opioid system modulates the immune function: a review. *Translational perioperative and pain medicine, 1*(1), 5.

Littlejohn, G. (2015). Neurogenic neuroinflammation in fibromyalgia and complex regional pain syndrome. Nature reviews. Rheumatology, *11*(11), 639–648.

Malcangio, M. (2018). GABA$_B$ receptors and pain. *Neuropharmacology, 136,* 102–105. (Pt A). doi:S0028-3908(17)30218-6 [pii].

McEntire, D. M., Kirkpatrick, D. R., Dueck, N. P., Kerfeld, M. J., Smith, T. A., Nelson, T. J., et al. (2016). Pain transduction: A pharmacologic perspective. *Expert Review of Clinical Pharmacology, 9*(8), 1069–1080. https://doi.org/10.1080/17512433.2016.1183481.

Melzack, R. (1999). From the gate to the neuromatrix. *Pain,* (Suppl 6), S121–S126.

Melzack, R. (2001). Pain and the neuromatrix in the brain. *Journal of Dental Education, 65*(12), 1378–1382.

Melzack, R. (2005). Evolution of the neuromatrix theory of pain. the Prithvi Raj Lecture: Presented at the Third World Congress of the World Institute of Pain, Barcelona 2004. *Pain Practice, 5*(2), 85–94. https://doi.org/PPR5203 [pii].

Melzack, R., & Wall, P. D. (1965). Pain mechanisms: A new theory. *Science (New York, N.Y.), 150*(3699), 971–979.

Moayedi, M., & Davis, K. D. (2013). Theories of pain: From specificity to gate control. *Journal of Neurophysiology, 109*(1), 5–12. https://doi.org/10.1152/jn.00457.2012.

Moreno-Duarte, I., Morse, L. R., Alam, M., Bikson, M., Zafonte, R., & Fregni, F. (2014). Targeted therapies using electrical and magnetic neural stimulation for the treatment of chronic pain in spinal cord injury. *NeuroImage, 85,* 1003–1013. https://doi.org/10.1016/j.neuroimage.2013.05.097. Pt 3. [doi].

National Comprehensive Cancer Network. (2017). NCCN Guidelines Version 2.2017. *Adult Cancer Pain.* PAIN-E page 4. Retrieved January 16, 2018 from https://www.nccn.org/professionals/physician_gls/pdf/pain.pdf.

Ngernyam, N., Jensen, M. P., Auvichayapat, N., Punjaruk, W., & Auvichayapat, P. (2013). Transcranial direct current stimulation in neuropathic pain. *Journal of Pain & Relief. Suppl* 3, 001. https://doi.org/001 [pii].

Orhurhu, V., Orhurhu, M. S., Bhatia, A., & Cohen, S. P. (2019). Ketamine infusions for chronic pain: a systematic review and meta-analysis of randomized controlled trials. *Anesthesia & Analgesia, 129*(1), 241–254.

Ossipov, M. H., Morimura, K., & Porreca, F. (2014). Descending pain modulation and chronification of pain. *Current Opinion in Supportive and Palliative Care, 8*(2), 143–151. https://doi.org/10.1097/SPC.0000000000000055 (doi).

Pasero, C., & McCaffery, M. (2011). *Pain Assessment and Pharmacologic Management.* St. Louis, MO: Mosby.

Patel, R., Montagut-Bordas, C., & Dickenson, A. H. (2018). Calcium channel modulation as a target in chronic pain control. *British Journal of Pharmacology, 175*(12), 2173–2184. https://doi.org/10.1111/bph.13789 (doi).

Pinho-Ribeiro, F. A., Verri, W. A., & Chiu, I. M. (2017). Nociceptor sensory neuron–immune interactions in pain and inflammation. *Trends in Immunology, 38*(1), 5–19.

Pozek, J. P., Beausang, D., Baratta, J. L., & Viscusi, E. R. (2016). The acute to chronic pain transition: Can chronic pain be prevented? *The Medical Clinics of North America, 100*(1), 17–30. https://doi.org/10.1016/j.mcna.2015.08.005.

Puopolo, M. & Mendell, L.M. (2017). Nociceptors: the gateway to pain. Reference module in neuroscience and biobehavioral psychology. New York, NY: Elsevier. https://doi.org/10.1016/B978-0-12-809324-5.03129-1.

Raja, S. N., Carr, D. B., Cohen, M., Finnerup, N. B., Flor, H., Gibson, S., & Song, X. J. (2020). The revised International Association for the Study of Pain definition of pain: concepts, challenges, and compromises. *PAIN.* (In press) https://doi.org/10.1097/j.pain.0000000000001939.

Rice, D. A., Parker, R. S., Lewis, G. N., Kluger, M. T., & McNair, P. J. (2017). Pain catastrophizing is not associated with spinal nociceptive processing in people with chronic widespread pain. *The Clinical Journal of Pain, 33*(9), 804–810. https://doi.org/10.1097/AJP.0000000000000464 (doi).

Ropero Pelaez, F. J., & Taniguchi, S. (2016). The gate theory of pain revisited: Modeling different pain conditions with a parsimonious neurocomputational model. *Neural Plasticity, 2016*. https://doi.org/10.1155/2016/4131395 (doi).

Saltık, S., Sözen, H. G., Basgul, S., Karatoprak, E. Y., & Içağasıoğlu, A. (2016). Pregabalin treatment of a patient with complex regional pain syndrome. *Pediatric neurology, 54*, 88–90.

Schug, S. A., & Bruce, J. (2017). Risk stratification for the development of chronic postsurgical pain. *Pain Reports, 2*(6), e627.

Singer, J., Conigliaro, A., Spina, E., Law, S. W., & Levine, S. R. (2017). Central poststroke pain: A systematic review. *International Journal of Stroke: Official Journal of the International Stroke Society, 12*(4), 343–355. https://doi.org/10.1177/1747493017701149.

Siniscalchi, A., De Sarro, G., & Gallelli, L. (2014). Central Post-stroke Pain and Pharmacological Treatment: Work in Progress. *SOJ Neurol, 1*(1), 1–2.

Sluka, K. A., & Clauw, D. J. (2016). Neurobiology of fibromyalgia and chronic widespread pain. *Neuroscience, 338*, 114–129. S0306-4522(16)30236-6 [pii].

Staud, R., Weyl, E. E., Riley, J. L., 3rd, & Fillingim, R. B. (2014). Slow temporal summation of pain for assessment of central pain sensitivity and clinical pain of fibromyalgia patients. *PloS One, 9*(2). https://doi.org/10.1371/journal.pone.0089086.

Steeds, C. E. (2016). The anatomy and physiology of pain. *Surgery, 34*(2), 55.

Tobaldini, G., Reis, R. A., Sardi, N. F., Lazzarim, M. K., Tomim, D. H., Lima, M. M. S., et al. (2017). Dopaminergic mechanisms in periaqueductal gray-mediated antinociception. *Behavioural Pharmacology, 29*(2 & 3, Special Issue), 225–233. https://doi.org/10.1097/FBP.0000000000000346 [doi].

Tracey, W. D., Jr. (2017). Nociception. *Current Biology: CB, 27*(4), R129–R133. S0960-9822(17)30069-6 [pii].

Treede, R. D. (2016). Gain control mechanisms in the nociceptive system. *Pain, 157*(6), 1199–1204. https://doi.org/10.1097/j.pain.0000000000000499.

van Hecke, O., Austin, S. K., Khan, R. A., Smith, B. H., & Torrance, N. (2014). Neuropathic pain in the general population: A systematic review of epidemiological studies. *Pain, 155*(4), 654–662. https://doi.org/10.1016/j.pain.2013.11.013.

Vance, C. G., Dailey, D. L., Rakel, B. A., & Sluka, K. A. (2014). Using TENS for pain control: The state of the evidence. *Pain Management, 4*(3), 197–209. https://doi.org/10.2217/pmt.14.13.

Vardeh, D., Mannion, R. J., & Woolf, C. J. (2016). Toward a Mechanism-Based approach to pain diagnosis. *The Journal of Pain, 17*(9), T50–T69.

Vlaeyen, J. W., & Linton, S. J. (2012). Fear-avoidance model of chronic musculoskeletal pain: 12 years on. *Pain, 153*(6), 1144–1147. https://doi.org/10.1016/j.pain.2011.12.009.

Vlaeyen, J. W., Crombez, G., & Linton, S. J. (2016). The fear-avoidance model of pain. *Pain, 157*(8), 1588–1589. https://doi.org/10.1097/j.pain.0000000000000574.

Volz, M. S., Suarez-Contreras, V., Portilla, A. L. S., & Fregni, F. (2015). Mental imagery-induced attention modulates pain perception and cortical excitability. *BMC Neuroscience, 16*(1), 15.

Waddell, G. (1987). 1987 Volvo Award in Clinical Sciences. A new clinical model for the treatment of low-back pain. *Spine, 12*(7), 632–644.

Williams, K., Guarino, A., & Raja, S. N. (2018). Complex regional pain syndrome. In *In Essentials of Pain Medicine* (pp. 223–232). Elsevier.

Woda, A., Blanc, O., Voisin, D. L., Coste, J., Molat, J. L., et al. (2017). Bidirectional modulation of windup by NMDA receptors in the rat spinal trigeminal nucleus. *European Journal of Neuroscience Wiley 2004, 19*(8), 2009–2016.

Wright, S. (2015). *The neuropsychophysiology of pain. Pain management in nursing practice* (pp. 33–54). Los Angeles, CA: Sage Publications.

Yasui, M., Yoshimura, T., Takeuchi, S., Tokizane, K., Tsuda, M., Inoue, K., & Kiyama, H. (2014). A chronic fatigue syndrome model demonstrates mechanical allodynia and muscular hyperalgesia via spinal microglial activation. *Glia, 62*(9), 1407–1417.

Zeidan, F., Martucci, K. T., Kraft, R. A., Gordon, N. S., McHaffie, J. G., & Coghill, R. C. (2011). Brain mechanisms supporting the modulation of pain by mindfulness meditation. *Journal of Neuroscience, 31*(14), 5540–5548.

Zeng, L., Alongkronrusmee, D., & van Rijn, R. M. (2017). An integrated perspective on diabetic, alcoholic, and drug-induced neuropathy, etiology, and treatment in the US. *Journal of Pain Research, 10*, 219.

Zhang, X., Bao, L., & Li, S. (2015). Opioid receptor trafficking and interaction in nociceptors. *British Journal of Pharmacology, 172*(2), 364–374. https://doi.org/10.1111/bph.12653.

Chapter 4 Barriers to Effective Pain Management

Ann Quinlan-Colwell

CHAPTER OUTLINE

Patient Barriers, pg. 50

Misconceptions, pg. 50

The Meaning of Pain, pg. 50

Culture and Beliefs, pg. 51

Clinical Application, pg. 52

Past Experiences With Pain, pg. 52

Patient Expectations of Pain and Pain Control, pg. 52

Fear, pg. 52

Fear of Side Effects, pg. 52

Fear of Substance Abuse or Misuse, pg. 53

Health Care Literacy, pg. 53

Family, pg. 53

Access Issues, pg. 54

Finances, pg. 54

Transportation, pg. 54

Residential Area, pg. 54

Provider Barriers, pg. 55

Culture, pg. 55

Perception, pg. 55

Education, pg. 55

Clinician Experience, pg. 56

Golden Rule Versus Platinum Rule, pg. 56

System Barriers to Effective Pain Management, pg. 56

Culture of the Organization, pg. 56

Continuing Education of Clinicians, pg. 56

Time, pg. 57

Insurance Coverage, pg. 57

Opportunities, pg. 57

Key Points, pg. 57

Case Scenario, pg. 58

References, pg. 58

PAIN can be thought of as a conundrum. On the one hand pain is a universal experience, with a very small minority of people who never experience pain, but on the other hand it is uniquely experienced by the individual through the lens of personal experiences, societal influences, and culture (Leknes & Bastian, 2014; Todd & Incayawar, 2013). This contributes to the widely accepted definition of pain being "whatever the experiencing person says it is. Existing whenever he/she says it does" (McCaffery, 1968).

This chapter will explore the various barriers that interfere with the assessment, treatment, and control of pain. Barriers that arise from the perspectives of the patient, the clinician, and systems will be discussed.

Patient Barriers

Each patient is an individual whose world view, understanding, and experience of pain is unique and contributes to pain being a highly subjective biopsychosocial experience (Moseley & Butler, 2015). Among other factors, the experience is influenced by misconceptions, beliefs, culture, past experiences with pain, health care literacy, fear, anxiety, expectations, and access issues.

Misconceptions

Despite increased information about pain during the past decade, many misconceptions persist among patients, family members, and clinicians. These misconceptions are major barriers to adequate pain control (Table 4.1). It is important for clinicians to listen to patients in order to learn what misconceptions they may believe and then to educate patients with evidence based information and dispel misconceptions.

The Meaning of Pain

Pain can be universally understood and at the same time is highly personal. Many factors affect the meaning of pain, including personal beliefs, past experiences, and culture. This highly personal context makes it challenging for pain to be understood by anyone other than the person experiencing it. Acute pain usually has a clear cause or

Table 4.1 | Misconceptions

Misconceptions	Correction
Reports of pain distract physician from more important things.	Physicians and other clinicians need to know about pain to best provide care. Acute pain is a symptom and needs to be addressed.
Clinicians know when patients have pain.	Pain is a subjective experience, and no one else knows when it is experienced or what it feels like other than the person experiencing it.
Patients over rate their pain.	Because pain is a subjective experience the intensity of pain is whatever the experiencing describes.
Pain medicine should be prescribed based on actual body weight.	Pain medicine is best described according to the type of pain, previous history of pain medication, previous response to pain medication and doses.
If pain medicine is used early, it will not work later, when it is really needed.	Administering pain medication early will help the person control pain. It may be helpful to begin pain medication preemptively or preoperatively to better control pain.
People who can sleep, laugh, play cards, and visit do not have pain or do not have much pain.	People cope with pain in many different ways. Distraction, including humor, can be effective coping mechanisms. Patients with chronic pain learn to sleep despite pain.
You get addicted if you take opioids.	Although patients may develop dependence or misuse opioids, they are not the majority of patients. This concern provides an opportunity for assessment of risk and education.
Pain is weakness leaving the body.	This is not true.
Pain is inevitable with . . . (aging, cancer)	Although pain is a common symptom with many disorders and diseases, it often can be avoided with preventive interventions and it can often be controlled.
The pain is not significant enough or severe enough to try to find help for it.	Acute pain is a symptom and needs to be assessed to determine the cause. Unrelieved acute pain can lead to chronic pain.
Older adults do not experience as much pain as younger adults.	There is no evidence to support this. In addition, as people age, they may develop conditions such as arthritis that are painful.
People who abuse opioids or other substances do not really have pain and are just drug seeking.	People with substance use disorders experience pain and may experience hyperalgesia with increased sensitivity to pain and may develop tolerance.

From Baker, O'Connor, & Krok-Schoen, 2014; Burner et al., 2014; Cogan et al., 2013; Paskins, Sanders, & Hassell, 2014; Quinlan-Colwell, 2012; Stein et al., 2016; Syrjala et al. 2014.

reason, and thus the meaning of the pain may be more standard. Acute pain also is generally seen to have an anticipated end such as healing from surgery. Conversely, chronic pain often does not have a clear cause and frequently there is no predictable end (Roe & Sehgal, 2016). People who live with chronic pain may also experience suffering that is the consequence of helplessness, hopelessness, and/or anxiety (Ballantyne & Sullivan, 2015). Although pain-relieving options exist many older adults consider chronic musculoskeletal pain to be part of aging that needs to be endured (Burner, et al., 2014).

Culture and Beliefs

Culture includes background, values, beliefs, attitudes, language, meanings, motivations, and learned behaviors that are shared by a particular group of people in society. It also includes shared experiences and often a shared religious or spiritual foundation within that society (Al-Harthy, Ohrbach, Michelotti, & List, 2016). The culture of the person has an impact on his or her perception of pain, response to pain (behavior), and management of pain. Culture is the matrix through which people understand and interpret their experiences, including pain and pain management (Cox & Taua, 2016).

In some cultures not being able to tolerate pain is considered a weakness, whereas in other cultures pain leads to the person receiving support and care from others (Leknes & Bastian, 2014). These are two very different cultural responses not only to pain but also to the way the person exhibits behavior in response to pain.

To provide care that is culturally safe, the clinician needs to respect the autonomy of the patient and family and interact with them from their cultural perspectives (Cox & Taua, 2016). That can be challenging if the patient is from a culture that values *stoicism* with admiration for bearing pain in a heroic manner (Leknes & Bastian, 2014) and the clinician comes from a culture in which that is a totally foreign concept. A similar challenge occurs when the situation is reversed.

Atonement may seem similar to stoicism but is quite different. Rather than admiring the ability to bear pain, the person may consider suffering and tolerating pain as an opportunity to *atone for* or "pay for" what the person perceives as past sins or transgressions (Leknes & Bastian, 2014) (see Clinical Application).

Clinical Application

An illustration of this would be an elderly woman suffering with terminal cancer who refuses to accept any pain medication until she thinks she has suffered enough to make up for her sins. She may never reveal what her sins were, but she may be adamant that she believes she needs to suffer pain commensurate with the severity of the sins. In a situation such as this, it is difficult for clinicians to know the woman must have significant unrelieved pain while not accepting any intervention to relieve the pain. Despite much education from the nurses about pain management options, she may remain adamant that for her to have a peaceful death, it is necessary for her to atone in this way. Her autonomy will likely challenge the clinician's compassion and ethical concept to do no harm. Yet, if she is competent and makes it clear her cultural concept of doing no harm is for them to respect her need to atone for her sins, they need to respect her position and continue to educate and support her (see Chapter 2).

Past Experiences With Pain

For some people living with chronic pain, their past experiences of pain not only affect the current experience of pain but also have an impact on day-to-day living with a fear of experiencing pain again as severe as it had been on other occasions. Some people who have had unrelieved pain may be more attentive to signs of pain escalating in severity (see Chapter 8). For them, even when the current pain intensity is manageable, there is an underlying anticipation of worsening pain that negatively affects their quality of life (Evers, 2015). This anticipation or fear may limit participation in enjoyable or rehabilitative activities (see Chapters 20 and 24).

Patient Expectations of Pain and Pain Control

Expectation, what a person subjectively anticipates will happen and what the consequences will be, is influenced by culture, past experiences, pain, and emotional state (Sjskatte, Røe, Fagerland, & Granan, 2017, p.1). When the actual experience of pain or pain control meets or is better than expected, the person will theoretically be more satisfied (Waljee, McGlinn, Sears, & Chung, 2014). When pain is worse than expected or pain control does

not meet what is expected, the person will theoretically be less satisfied or dissatisfied (Waljee et al., 2014).

Investigators of studies on whether patients with positive expectations about the ability to control pain were more satisfied with pain control reported inconsistent results. Some patients with positive expectations had lower than expected postoperative pain intensity, whereas others had more severe postoperative pain than they expected (Waljee et al., 2014). This difference may be at least in part related to the subjective quality of pain and rating pain on an intensity scale. Another factor that can affect expectations is the degree of optimism with which the person views the situation, with more optimistic people reportedly experiencing less pain (Hanssen, Vancleef, Vlaeyen, & Peters, 2014).

Fear

Fear can be a significant barrier to adequate pain management. (Fear of pain with potential movement or activity and the fear avoidance model will be discussed in Chapter 20.) Not only can fear limit assessment and treatment options but fear itself can increase pain (Aslaksen, & Lyby, 2015). People can resist acknowledging pain or fear for a variety of reasons. Fears may be related to their physical condition, including fear that the pain means the disease is getting worse, more tests are needed, or changes in medications are needed. Fears may be about self-image, including aging or being less active and agile. Active people may fear that they will no longer be able to participate in usual activities, hobbies, activities of daily living, or even living independently. Some may fear not being able to participate in a long anticipated event such as a wedding or graduation.

Fear of Side Effects

Fear of side effects of medications is commonly reported by people with a variety of diagnoses in various populations worldwide. Patients have reported fear of side effects while in critical care units (Batiha, 2014), recovering postoperatively after cardiac surgery (Cogan et al., 2013), living with various forms of osteoarthritis (Alami et al., 2011; Burner et al., 2014; Paskins, Sanders, & Hassell, 2014), living with various cancer diagnoses (Barratt, Klepstad, Dale, Kaasa, & Somogyl, 2015; Saifan, Bashayreh, Batiha, & AbuRuz, 2015; Syrjala et al., 2014), living in a long-term-care facility as an older adult (Long, 2013), and living with a variety of nonmalignant chronic painful conditions (Jouini et al., 2014). Common side effects that are particularly distressing to patients include nausea, vomiting, constipation, and pruritus (itching) (Barratt et al., 2015; Jouini et al., 2014). For some patients the side effect is less tolerable than suffering with pain (Saifan et al., 2015).

Unfortunately, too many patients do not know that side effects can be prevented or effectively managed. Many side effects are dose related, and the side effects can be lessened or better managed with multimodal analgesia (MMA). As a method of pain control that intentionally uses a variety of pharmacologic and nonpharmacologic interventions, with MMA it is possible to use lower doses of any one medication, thus incurring fewer side effects (Sullivan, Lyons, Montgomery, & Quinlan-Colwell, 2016).

Fear of Substance Abuse or Misuse

Fear of substance abuse or misuse of opioid medications is a substantial fear and barrier to good pain control expressed by many people with acute pain (Cogan et al., 2013), chronic nonmalignant pain (Alami et al., 2011; Paskins et al., 2014), and cancer-related pain (Baker, O'Connor, & Krok-Schoen, 2014; Paice & Von Roenn, 2014; Syrjala et al., 2014). In a 2014 survey of 379 patients awaiting surgery, nearly one-third (31%) strongly believed that "it is easy to become addicted to pain medication" (Cogan et al., 2013). The fear is not confined to patients but also is a fear held by family members concerned that their loved one could misuse or abuse medications ("become addicted") (Paice & Von Roenn, 2014) (see Chapter 14)

Fear of Appearing To Be Drug Seeking

Fear of appearing to be *drug seeking* and being judged as such is a real concern for many patients (Syrjala et al., 2014). One woman with cancer and active gastrointestinal bleeding delayed going to the emergency department (ED) because she was taking oxycodone to control her cancer pain and did not want to be accused of *drug seeking* because she had heard clinicians talk about other patients *drug seeking*. Tragically, this woman waited too long and did not survive the night (author personal report, 2015). Dr. Susan O'Connor-Von teaches that people are actually seeking comfort so the term *drug seeking* needs to be replaced with the term *comfort seeking* to more accurately describe what is happening (Quinlan-Colwell & O'Conner-Von, 2014).

Health Care Literacy

Health care literacy is an important concern with pain management because not all patients are able to procure and process the basic information about their health and management of pain, locate services, and identify clinicians and agencies to help them do so (Institute of Medicine [IOM], 2011). Health care literacy is an important factor in patient autonomy and decision making regarding pain and pain management. The relationship between health care literacy and patient empowerment is complex. People who have high health care literacy but low empowerment may be inordinately dependent on health care providers. Conversely, people who have low health care literacy but high levels of empowerment may make risky health care selections (Schultz & Nakamoto, 2013). Gender and culture are thought to influence health care literacy. It is suggested that women are more willing to discuss pain (Shea & McDonald, 2011) and are more articulate in describing pain and Caucasian patients are likely to be assertive, have higher expectations for pain to be controlled, and ask for more "potent" analgesics (Johnson, Richardson, & Kridli, 2014).

Research about health care literacy as a barrier to effective pain management is skewed because people with low health care literacy are less likely to be approached for or participate in research studies. One small study (n = 139) did assess pain awareness and knowledge of pain medications. The results showed that people with lower health care literacy had less knowledge about pain medications, pain management providers, and nonpharmacologic options to manage pain (Devraj, Herndon, & Griffin, 2013).

People with lower health care literacy also are reportedly less likely to be approached, participate in, or continue with nonpharmacologic interventions such as cognitive-behavioral therapy (CBT) (Campbell, 2011). However, a small study among people who belonged to a lower socioeconomic group in a rural area found that education and CBT were effective. Not only were the interventions effective but also the people who participated in the CBT portion of the trial had greater knowledge and less depression at the end of the study despite more people dropping out of that group (Thorn et al., 2011). It is likely that the success of the interventions was due in large part to the study staff being sensitive to the culture and literacy limitations of the participants (Campbell, 2011).

An important part of an MMA plan of care is patient education. It is clear from the Thorn et al. study that clinicians can be most effective in teaching when education is tailored specifically to the individual patient and family and/or designate support person.

Family

Concern for family members may lead to underreporting of pain. This is most dramatically seen among the American Indian population in which many subscribe to the "concept of tolerated illness." From that perspective not only should the needs of family and others take priority over one's own health but also negative health consequences should be dealt with stoically (Cross & Day, 2015). It is also seen among individuals in other ethnic groups. The desires of the patient can be a barrier to pain management because they can prevent the clinician from accurately assessing and appropriately controlling pain. Patients may have a specific self-image and may desire to be perceived by others consistent with that self-perception. If that self-perception is to be healthy, capable, and independent, the person may resist any endorsement of pain because it is contrary to "who they are." Another barrier occurs when patients desire to be perceived by clinicians as "good patients," which the person may consider contrary to reporting pain (often viewed as "complaining") or "bothering" hospital staff (i.e., asking for pain medicine).

Although little literature exists on this topic, it is seen frequently in clinical work that family caregivers will ignore their own health during the caretaking process. It is not unusual to work with a family and find that the designated caregiver has not been reporting his or her own pain and then the caregiver is subsequently diagnosed with a disease process that surely is painful. This was seen in the elderly man who was caring for his wife of over 50 years. Initially he rebuked efforts to be evaluated. His response was always "I'm just a little tired." When evaluated, he was diagnosed with a malignancy and died before his wife. His concern for her overshadowed his ever-increasing pain (author experience).

Access Issues

Access to care is an important barrier to good pain management for many people living with pain. These barriers include financial constraints, limitations in transportation, and the area in which the person resides.

Finances

Often people have financial limitations that limit their ability to control their pain, and frequently they do not share that information with clinicians. Health care can be costly. Many people do not have insurance, and even those who do often have costly copays. The best of medications will not be effective if the person cannot afford to pay for the prescription. For many older adults, they must choose between paying for food or paying for pain medication (Quinlan-Colwell, 2012). Financial constraints limit the ability to participate in nonpharmacologic therapies such as exercise and physical activity (Park, Manotas, & Hooyman, 2013), yoga (Combs & Thorn, 2014), self-management, and support groups (Matthias et al., 2016).

Transportation

Inadequate, unreliable, or unavailable transportation presents a real and challenging barrier for many people, especially those who are older, live in rural areas, or are members of a lower socioeconomic group (Smith et al., 2017; Syed, Gerber, & Sharp, 2013). African Americans are more likely to encounter transportation barriers when trying to access health care (Bhimani et al., 2017). Transportation difficulties can result in missed appointments, inadequate access, or delays in health care or medications (Syed, Gerber, & Sharp, 2013).

Telemedicine is an option for providing health care to underserved geographic and socioeconomic populations (IOM, 2012; Kahn, 2015). Technologic advances also have promise for bringing nonpharmacologic interventions such as exercise programs, yoga, peer support, mindfulness meditation, and CBT options to people who are socioeconomically challenged and who can benefit from MMA.

Residential Area

The neighborhood where people live may be a barrier in several ways. Pain management specialists and clinics tend to be located in urban areas (Eaton et al., 2012). Lower socioeconomic areas generally have less access to health care (Thomas, 2014), which requires people to travel outside of their neighborhood. Not only does this involve transportation issues but it also necessitates that people need to navigate an environment and systems that are foreign to them. Pharmacies in lower socioeconomic areas often do not carry medications used to treat pain (Stein, Alcaraz, Kamson, Fallon, & Smith, 2016).

It is often challenging to pursue self-care activities and healthy behaviors in lower socioeconomic neighborhoods. Environmental stressors often exist (Thomas, 2014), and these can make it more challenging to effectively manage pain. Self-care activities, such as getting daily exercise by walking, can be difficult in many neighborhoods where African Americans live because they are considered not to be "walkable" (Bhimani et al., 2017). A recent study reported that the walkability of a neighborhood not only affects the ability to get daily exercise and help manage pain but also can affect the development of pain in adolescents who are at risk for developing chronic pain. The proximity to parks and walkability of neighborhoods were correlated with how frequently pain was experienced and to what degree activities were limited (Schild, Reed, Hingston, Dennis, & Wilson, 2016).

Programs such as the Self-Management of Osteo-Arthritis in Veterans (SeMOA) intervention can be an effective way to overcome some of the barriers. The SeMOA used monthly telephone calls to work with African American veterans who were diagnosed with osteoarthritis to improve their pain control. The intervention was successful in two ways. There was an 89% completion rate, and the veterans perceived the intervention effective in helping them better manage their pain (Bhimani et al., 2017).

The University of Washington in Seattle, Washington has a telehealth system to assist with outreach to rural areas. The university has expanded it to include a TelePain intervention that uses video case conferences between pain specialists and community clinicians and a web-based instrument for reporting patient outcomes. The program enables patients to receive specialized pain management care and for community providers to consult with university-based pain specialists (Eaton et al., 2012).

In Wilmington, North Carolina, the New Hanover Regional Medical Center created a Community Paramedics Program. Patients who are considered at high risk for readmission to the hospital, have access issues, or are thought to need additional follow-up are visited by a group of paramedics on a regular basis. An additional benefit of this program is the paramedics develop a positive relationship with the patients, their families, and the community.

Schools that provide chiropractic education often operate community-based clinics. Frequently the clinics are located apart from the school, in low socioeconomic areas. The students provide care that is free for people who are uninsured or underinsured (Kaeser, Hawk, Anderson, & Reinhardt, 2016). These examples of community outreach are exciting and encouraging opportunities for providing MMA pain management to people who traditionally have limited options for controlling pain.

Provider Barriers

Culture

Clinicians also have unique cultural backgrounds with the same categories of characteristics and challenges as do patients. It is not uncommon for the culture of clinicians to be different from that of the patients for whom they care. In the United States, this difference is not confined to people born in other countries. There are often many cultural differences among people living in the same neighborhood. Rachel Gooberman-Hill (2015) cautions that the relationship between culture and pain is complex rather than straightforward and for that reason stereotypes need to be avoided.

To effectively interact with patients who have different backgrounds and cultures, it is important for clinicians to first assess and acknowledge their own backgrounds and culture, including any preconceived notions, prejudices, and biases they may hold (Cox & Taua, 2016). This can be challenging because prejudices and biases may be explicit or implicit. Explicit prejudice, bias, or stereotyping is a negative attitude or prejudgment that is made consciously. Implicit prejudice, bias, or stereotyping is essentially unconscious and results over time through learning and is more likely to be seen among clinicians (Rodriguez & Green, 2013). It is suggested that often clinicians may deny any explicit negative beliefs but may exhibit implicit negative attitudes and behaviors (Hirsh, Hollingshead, Ashburn-Nardo, & Kroenke, 2015). Bias, prejudice, and stereotyping are not limited to race or ethnicity. Negative behaviors are frequently seen as barriers to effective pain management in patients who have a current or even historical substance use disorder.

Clearly the topic of this contradiction between what is implicitly believed versus what is explicitly exhibited is complicated and challenging. It is important for clinicians to develop a practice to frequently introspectively review their innermost feelings, opinions, and behaviors toward people who are different from them and consider how these interfere with providing the most effective pain management. Contracting to have honest explorations of feelings and meanings of behavior with a trusted peer is one way to develop a foundation for an introspective practice.

Perception

The initial perception of the patient by the clinician can be a related barrier. One nurse educator who worked in the ED for many years illustrates this barrier when educating new ED nurses by suggesting that if he sought treatment in an ED where he was not known, his care could be very different if he arrived reporting back pain dressed in a suit after being at church rather than reporting back pain dressed in shorts and a T-shirt after working in the yard and having had a beer or two (Holtvoight, 2016). Studies have shown that when physicians lack trust in a patient, they are more reluctant to prescribe opioids for that person. The lack of trust may arise from a variety of sources ranging from the patient not having a primary care provider to the patient not *seeming* honest about pain reports (Johnson et al., 2014).

Education

Minick et al. (2012) reported that expert recommendations are not consistently adhered to by clinicians. It is not clear if the lack of adherence is due to lack of education or to other reasons; however, adequate education of health care clinicians about pain assessment and management remains insufficient and ineffective (Athlin, Carlsson & Gunningberg, 2015; Bement & Sluka, 2015; Fishman et al., 2013). A 2016 review of the literature continues to report that knowledge of pain management is inadequate among nurses and physicians (Ung, Salamonson, Hu, & Gallego, 2016).

It may be surprising that oncology physicians generally reported inadequate pain management education while they were medical students. In a national survey assessing oncologists' beliefs of how effectively they manage patients' pain, they rated themselves fairly high (7 on a scale of 0–10). When the same oncologists selected treatment options for pain, less than 40% selected options consistent with recommendations of pain management specialists (Paice & Von Roenn, 2014). In another survey, less than 20% of physicians were satisfied with the education about pain. A positive note from the same survey is that oncology physicians graduating more recently reported receiving better pain education (Kwon, 2014).

Similar to the oncology physicians, at the time of more recent graduation ED physicians reported improvement in pain education. Physicians working in EDs with more experience and those not specifically trained in emergency medicine were less likely to prescribe pain medicine than those who are trained in that specialty and were newer to the profession (Johnson et al., 2014). A recent study in Sweden among ED nurses concluded that nurses working in the ED need more education about pain and pain assessment (Athlin et al., 2015).

Inadequate pain education is not limited to nurses and physicians. A recent survey of physical therapy schools revealed that 31 contact hours was the average number taught regarding pain and most of the respondents considered that inadequate (Bement & Sluka, 2015). An interprofessional group of clinicians developed a template for core competencies including pain to be taught across the health care spectrum to prelicensure candidates (Fishman et al., 2013). It is not surprising that studies show education, particularly targeted and specialized education, improves clinicians' knowledge and attitudes about pain (Moceri & Drevdahl, 2014). Although the curricula of schools for health care professionals are full, adequate and effective education about pain will remove a key barrier for clinicians to provide pain management and ensure that pain management is safe and effective (Fishman et al., 2013; Kwon, 2014).

Clinician Experience

Because education about pain is so often inadequate, clinicians often base clinical pain management decisions on intuition and their own experiences, both personal and professional. This is seen internationally and across professional disciplines (Boissoneault et al., 2016; Hampton, Cavalier, & Langford, 2015: Hollingshead, Meints, Middleton, Free, & Hirsh, 2015; Moceri & Drevdahl, 2014; Wøen & Bjørk, 2013). Depending on the impact of these experiences of the individual clinician, this may be positive, negative, or mixed for patients. In accordance with the *Theory of Reasoned Action*, clinicians are more likely to act in a certain manner if they think the results will be positive and it is acceptable to peers (Trail-Mahan, Mao, & Bawel-Brinkley, 2013). The effect of peer pressure on clinicians' professional behavior, including use of established clinical guidelines (Twycross & Chambers, 2015), may be significant. This proposition has potential for improving professional knowledge about pain and requires further investigation.

Similarly, the culture of the health care organization and what are considered positive results influences what is beneficial or problematic for patients in pain. If a person living with pain wants to use complementary therapies but the clinicians in the organization or community have limited and negative experiences, the person is likely to receive negative feedback and no support. If, however, the clinicians have had a variety of positive experiences, they will be more apt to support and encourage the person to include a variety of complementary therapies in their analgesic plan of care (Trail-Mahan et al., 2013). In doing so, the clinician will be working with the patient to control pain using a multimodal approach.

Golden Rule Versus Platinum Rule

Many clinicians were raised to follow the *Golden Rule*, which states, "do unto others as you would have them do unto you." The *Platinum Rule* on the other hand advises, "do unto others as they wish you would do unto them" (Geller, 2015). The latter is more culturally sensitive and culturally safe than the former and better enables clinicians to address the needs and concerns of others (Geller, 2015). The Platinum Rule also is consistent with the ethical principle of autonomy. Thus it has the same caveat that if what the patient desires is dangerous or not safe, the clinician must educate the person and work to ensure safety. See Chapter 2 for more information on autonomy.

System Barriers to Effective Pain Management

Ensuring safe and effective pain management is an ethical imperative. It also significantly contributes to positive financial benefit to health care institutions. Unrelieved pain with increased lengths of hospital stay, undesirable outcomes, and poor patient satisfaction is costly. Organizational improvements based on data regarding pain-related knowledge and attitudes collected within the particular organization is beneficial for patients, clinicians, and the organization (Schreiber et al., 2014).

Culture of the Organization

When peer pressure serves as a barrier to high-quality pain management, there is a negative impact on the culture of the organization that needs attention and impetus for change beginning with the highest level of the system (Twycross & Chambers, 2015). Changing culture and behavior is a process that requires an appreciation of the complexity of the organization and requires time, commitment, and perseverance (Stevans et al., 2015).

When diversity or cultural education specifically focuses on the bonding characteristics of particular ethnic groups, there may be an unintentional stereotyping of the group. Rather, education that is patient focused encourages each patient to be evaluated and treated as an individual (Rodriguez & Green, 2013). These are important considerations when health care systems are evaluating options for diversity training or other educational efforts within an organization.

Continuing Education of Clinicians

As noted previously, inadequate education about multimodal pain management is a clear void in professional educational programs. This translates to a lack of knowledge about managing pain in the clinical setting. A systems approach that encourages and supports pain management education for all clinicians is an imperative.

This education should include competency-based programs; support for attendance at professional conferences addressing pain management; and availability of current evidence-based guidelines, standards, and literature (Jarzyna et al., 2011). Pioneering education efforts are needed and when successful should be shared and disseminated. One innovative education strategy using small group discussions with nurses in a critical care setting was successful in improving knowledge and decreasing biases (Lewis, Corley, Lake, Brockopp, & Moe, 2015).

Time

Time can be a system barrier that evolves into a barrier for individual clinicians (Paskins, Sanders, & Hassell, 2014). Thorough assessment and education take time. It can be more time consuming to develop a multimodal plan of care rather than just prescribe a single, monotherapy medication (Perry, VanDenKerkhof, Wilson & Tripp, 2017). Administration of pain medications by nurses is also time consuming (Pizzi, Chelly, & Marlin, 2013; Riemondy, Gonzalez, Gosik, Ricords, & Schirm, 2016). Pain is a symptom rather than a primary diagnosis, so the time involved in assessment, planning, treatment, and administration are often not considered by administrators. The investment of time in assessment, patient education, and collaboration with other clinicians (e.g., pharmacist, physical therapist, other specialists) contributes to more effective MMA and better pain control for patients.

Insurance Coverage

Insurance coverage is a broader, more general health care system barrier both when people are uninsured and when they are underinsured. In studying data collected by the American Cancer Society on 4707 people who survived cancer, lack of health care insurance to cover treatment of pain was the most common system barrier to effective pain management (Stein et al., 2016).

Health insurance coverage for residents of 38 U.S. states increased between 2010 and 2016, with 20.4 million fewer people uninsured in 2016 compared with 2010. Yet, 28.2 million, or 8.8%, of people in those states remained uninsured in 2016. Although that was a reduction from the 13.3% of Americans who were uninsured prior to the Affordable Care Act in 2013, The U.S. Census Bureau reported approximately 2 million Americans were uninsured in 2018 (Galewitz, 2019). Adults who were poor or near poor, those who lived in rural areas (Eaton et al., 2012), and those who were Hispanic or non-Hispanic black were considerably more likely to be uninsured (Martinez, Zammitti, & Cohen, 2016). Inadequate insurance is another barrier that is more frequently seen among African Americans (Bhimani et al., 2017). Lack of insurance is also common among temporary and unauthorized migrant people in the United States (Martinez-Donate et al., 2014).

Related to this is that people in minority groups tend to seek health care through EDs more frequently than their non-Hispanic white counterparts (Johnson et al., 2014). When patients with chronic illness, such as sickle cell disease, are uninsured or underinsured, they may not regularly see a primary provider or specialist, which can lead to seeking pain relief through the ED (Lopez, Davis, Trice, Webb, & Martin, 2016). Delays in pain management in the ED have been reported to be related to Medicaid insurance (Stang et al., 2014). Patients with Medicaid coverage and African American patients seen in the ED were less likely to receive parenteral analgesia for treatment of reports of pain (Johnson et al., 2014). African American patients in general were less likely to have adequate analgesia in one study (Minick et al., 2012; Tsai et al., 2012). They were also found to wait longer to receive analgesia, more likely to receive nonopioid medications, and less likely to have their pain reassessed (Johnson, et al., 2014; Tsai, 2012). Lack of insurance can also lead to inappropriate or dangerous pain management. In one study of older adults, misuse and illegal procurement of opioids by the older adults was found to be related to lack of insurance. In that study, older adults with insurance coverage were more than three times more likely to see a single physician and not use illegally obtained opioids (Levi-Minzi, Surratt, Kurtz, & Buttram, 2013)

Opportunities

Clearly many barriers exist that limit or prevent patients receiving effective pain assessment and optimal management of acute and chronic pain. Opportunities include assessing personal beliefs/biases, improving clinician and patient education, evaluating the culture and priorities of organizations, as well as advocating for improvements in health care coverage and access to appropriate multimodal options for all people living with pain.

Key Points

- Pain is a biopsychosocial experience that is both universal and unique for the individual experiencing pain.
- People living with pain experience personal, environmental, clinician, and system barriers to achieving safe and effective pain management.
- Practice the Platinum Rule: Do unto others as *they* would have you do unto *them*.
- On a regular basis clinicians need to introspectively review their feelings, opinions, and behaviors toward people who are different.
- Health care systems need to assume responsibility to reduce bias and increase education of clinicians.
- Clinicians need to advocate for the removal of barriers to effective pain management.

Case Scenario

Dina is a 27-year-old, single, overweight, mixed-race woman who has three small children. She has Medicaid insurance coverage. Dina graduated from high school but rarely reads and only watches television for entertainment. She is disabled related to her chronic back pain from a work-related accident when a box fell on her while working at a fast food restaurant. She does not use her car because she cannot afford the insurance for it and needs to depend on friends and relatives for transportation to a clinic that is 37 miles from her home. She does not want to use medication but she does not know how to use "those nonmedicine things."

1. What personal barriers can you identify for Dina?
2. What biases do you think clinicians might have that will interfere with managing Dina's pain?
3. What multimodal options could benefit Dina and help her better manage her pain?
4. What education would be helpful for Dina to receive?

References

Al-Harthy, M., Ohrbach, R., Michelotti, A., & List, T. (2016). The effect of culture on pain sensitivity. *Journal of Oral Rehabilitation*, *43*(2), 81–88. https://doi.org/10.1111/joor.12346.

Alami, S., Boutron, I., Desjeux, D., Hirschhorn, M., Meric, G., Rannou, F., & Poiraudeau, S. (2011). Patients' and practitioners' views of knee osteoarthritis and its management: a qualitative interview study. *PLoS ONE*, *6*(5), e19634. https://doi.org/10.1371/journalpone.0019634.

Aslaksen, P. M., & Lyby, P. S. (2015). Fear of pain potentiates nocebo hyperalgesia. *Journal of Pain Research*, *8*(10), 703–710.

Athlin, A. M., Carlsson, M., & Gunningberg, L. (2015). To receive or not to receive analgesics in the emergency department: the importance of the pain intensity assessment and initial nursing assessment. *Pain Management Nursing*, *16*(5), 743–750.

Baker, T., O'Connor, M., & Krok-Schoen, J. (2014). Experience and knowledge of pain management inpatients receiving outpatient cancer treatment: what do older adults really know about their cancer pain? *Pain Medicine*, *15*(1), 52–60. https://doi.org/10.1111/pme.12244.

Ballantyne, J. C., & Sullivan, M. D. (2015). Intensity of chronic pain – the wrong metric? *New England Journal of Medicine*, *373*(22), 2098–2099.

Barratt, D. T., Klepstad, P., Dale, O., Kaasa, S., & Somogyl, A. A. (2015). Innate immune signaling genetics of pain, cognitive dysfunction and sickness symptoms in cancer patients treated with transdermal fentanyl. *PLoS One 2015*, *10*(9), e0137179. https://doi.org/10.1371/journal.pone.0137179.

Batiha, A.-M. (2014). Pain management barriers in critical care units: a qualitative study. *International Journal of Advanced Nursing Studies*, *3*(1), 1–5.

Bement, M. K. H., & Sluka, K. A. (2015). The current state of physical therapy pain curricula in the United States: a faculty survey. *The Journal of Pain*, *16*(2), 144–152. https://doi.org/10.1016/j.jpain.2014.11.001.

Bhimani, R. H., Cross, L. J. S., Taylor, B. C., Meis, L. A., Fu, S. S., & Burgess, D. J. (2017). Taking ACTION to reduce pain: ACTION study rationale, design and protocol of a randomized trial of a proactive telephone based coaching intervention for chronic musculoskeletal pain among African Americans. *BMC Musculoskeletal Disorders*, *18*, 15. https://doi.org/10.1186/s12891-016-1363-6.

Boissoneault, J., Mundt, J. M., Bartley, E. J., Wandner, L. D., Hirsh, A. T., & Robinson, M. E. (2016). Assessment of the influence of demographic and professional characteristics on health care providers' pain management decisions using virtual humans. *Journal of Dental Education*, *80*(5), 578–587.

Burner, T., Abbott, D., Huber, K., Stout, M., Fleming, R., & Burns, E. (2014). Shoulder symptoms and function in geriatric patients. *Journal of Geriatric Physical Therapy*, *37*(4), 154–158.

Campbell, L. C. (2011). Addressing literacy as a barrier in delivery and evaluation of cognitive-behavioral therapy for pain management. *Pain*, *152*(12), 2679–2680.

Cogan, J., Ouimette, M. F., Vargas-Schaffere, G., Yegin, Z., Deschamps, A., & Denault, A. (2013). Patient attitudes and beliefs regarding pain medication after cardiac surgery: barriers to adequate pain management. *Pain Management Nursing*, *15*(3), 574–579.

Combs, M. A., & Thorn, B. E. (2014). Barriers and facilitators to yoga use in a population of individuals with self-reported chronic low back pain: a qualitative review. *Complementary Therapies in Clinical Practice*, *20*(4), 268–275.

Cox, L., & Taua, C. (2016). Cultural safety: cultural considerations. In C. Jarvis, H. Forbes, & E. Watt (Eds.), *Jarvis's Physical Examination and Health Assessment*. (2nd ed., pp. 38–58). Chatswood Australia, NSW: Elsevier.

Cross, S., & Day, A. (2015). American Indians' response to physical pain: functional limitations and help-seeking behaviors. *Journal of Social Work in Disability & Rehabilitation*, *14*, 176–191.

Devraj, R., Herndon, C. M., & Griffin, J. (2013). Pain awareness and medication knowledge: a health literacy evaluation. *Journal of Pain & Palliative Care Pharmacotherapy*, *27*(1), 19–27. https://doi.org/10.3109/15360288.2012.751955.

Eaton, L. H., Gordon, D. B., Wyant, S., Theodore, B. R., Meins, A. R., & Doorzrenbos, A. Z. (2012). Development and implementation of a telehealth-enhanced intervention for pain and symptom management. *Contemporary Clinical Trials*, *38*(2), 213–220. https://doi.org/10.1016/j.cct.2014.05.005.

Evers, E. R. (2015). *TMD Revisited: appreciating the work of illness, the balancing of risks, and the construction of moral identity involved in dealing with chronic pain. (Dissertation for Doctor of Philosophy)*. The University of Arizona Graduate School, School of Anthropology.

Fishman, S. M., Young, H. M., Arwood, E. L., Chou, R., Herr, K., & Strassels, S. A. (2013). Core competencies for pain management: results of an interprofessional consensus summit. *Pain Medicine*, *14*(7), 971–981.

Galewitz, P. (2019). Breaking a 10 year streak, the number of uninsured Americans rises. *KHN Kaiser Health News*. September 10, 2019. https://khn.org/news/number-of-americans-without-insurance-rises-in-2018/ (Accessed March 9, 2020).

Geller, S. E. (2015). Seven life lessons from humanistic behaviorism: how to bring the best out of yourself and others. *Journal of Organizational Behavior Management, 35*(1-2), 151–170. https://doi.org/10.1080/01608061.2015.1031427.

Gooberman-Hill, R. (2015). Ethnographies of pain: culture, context and complexity. *British Journal of Pain, 9*(1), 32–35.

Hampton, S. B., Cavalier, J., & Langford, R. (2015). The influence of race and gender on pain management: a systematic literature review. *Pain Management Nursing, 16*(6), 968–977.

Hanssen, M. H., Vancleef, L. M. G., Vlaeyen, J. W. S., & Peters, M. L. (2014). More optimism, less pain! The influence of generalized and pain-specific expectations on experienced cold-pressor pain. *Journal of Behavioral Medicine, 37*(1), 47–58.

Hirsh, A. T., Hollingshead, N. A., Ashburn-Nardo, L., & Kroenke, L. (2015). The interaction of patient race, provider bias, and clinical ambiguity on pain management decisions. *The Journal of Pain, 16*(6), 558–568.

Hollingshead, N. A., Meints, S., Middleton, S. K., Free, C. A., & Hirsh, A. T. (2015). Examining influential factors in providers' chronic pain treatment decisions: a comparison of physicians and medical students. *BMC Medical Education, 15*, 164. https://doi.org/10.1186/s12909-015-0441-z.

Holtvoight, J. (Emergency Department Nurse Educator) in discussion with author April, 2016.

Institute of Medicine (IOM). (2011). *Relieving pain in America: A blueprint for transforming prevention, care, education, and research*. Washington, DC: The National Academies Press.

Institute of Medicine. (2012). *The role of telehealth in an evolving health care environment*. Washington, DC: National Academies Press.

Jarzyna, D., Junguist, C. R., Pasero, C., Willens, J. S., Nisbet, A., & Polomano, R. C. (2011). American Society for Pain Management Nursing Guidelines on monitoring for opioid-induced sedation and respiratory depression. *Pain Management Nursing, 12*(3), 118–145.

Johnson, M., Richardson, K., & Kridli, S.A.-O. (2014). Disparities in pain management in the Emergency Department: an integrative review. *Open Journal of Nursing, 04*(08), 608–619.

Jouini, G., Choinè, M., Martin, E., Perreault, S., Berbiche, D., Lussier, D., ... Lalande, L. (2014). Pharmacotherapeutic management of chronic noncancer pain in primary care: lessons for pharmacists. *Journal of Pain Research, 7*, 163–173.

Kahn, J. M. (2015). Virtual visits – confronting the challenges of telemedicine. *New England Journal of Medicine, 372*(18), 1684–1685.

Kaeser, M. A., Hawk, C., Anderson, M. L., & Reinhardt, R. (2016). Community-based free clinics: opportunities for interprofessional collaboration, health promotion, and complex care management. *Journal of Chiropractic Education, 30*(1), 25–29.

Kwon, J. H. (2014). Overcoming barriers in cancer pain management. *Journal of Clinical Oncology, 32*(16), 1727–1733. https://doi.org/10.1200/JCO.2013.52.4827.

Leknes, S., & Bastian, B. (2014). The benefits of pain. *Review of Philosophy and Psychology, 5*, 57–70.

Levi-Minzi, M. A., Surratt, H. L., Kurtz, S. P., & Buttram, M. E. (2013). Under treatment of pain: a perception for opioid misuse among the elderly? *Pain Medicine, 14*(11), 1719–1729. https://doi.org/10.1111/pme.12189.

Lewis, C. P., Corley, D. J., Lake, N., Brockopp, D., & Moe, K. (2015). Overcoming barriers to effective pain management the use of professionally directed small group discussions. *Pain Management Nursing, 16*(2), 121–127.

Long, C. O. (2013). Pain management education in long-term care: It can make a difference. *Pain Management Nursing, 14*(4), 220–227.

Lopez, Davis, Trice, Webb, & Martin. (2016). Case 3: sickle cell crisis. In M. L. Martin, S. L. Heron, L. Moreno-Walton, & A. W. Jones (Eds.), *Diversity and Inclusion in Quality Patient Care* (pp. 213–218). Switzerland: Springer.

Martinez-Donate, A. P., Zhang, X., Rangel, M. G., Hovell, M., Simon, N. J., & Guendelman, S. (2014). Healthcare access among circular and undocumented Mexican migrants: results from a pilot survey on the Mexico-US border. *International Journal of Migration and Border Studies, 1*(1), 57–108. https://doi.org/10.1504/IJMBS.2014.065069.

Martinez, M. E., Zammitti, E. P., & Cohen, R. A. (2016). Health insurance coverage: early release of estimates from the National Health Interview Survey, January-September 2016. In *National Health Interview Survey Early Release Program*: National Center for Health Statistics. https://www.cdc.gov/nchs/data/nhis/earlyrelease/insur201702.pdf.

Matthias, M. S., Kukla, M., McGuire, A. B., Damush, T. M., Gill, N., & Blair, M. J. (2016). Facilitators and barriers to participation in a peer support intervention for veterans with chronic pain. *Clinical Journal of Pain, 32*(6), 534–540.

McCaffery, M. (1968). *Nursing practice theories related to cognition, bodily pain, and man-environment interactions.* Los Angeles, CA: University of California at Los Angeles Students' Store.

Minick, P., Clark, P., Dalton, J., Horne, E., Greene, D., & Brown, M. (2012). Long-Bone Fracture Pain Management in the Emergency Department. *Journal of Emergency Nursing, 38*, 211–217. https://doi.org/10.1016/j.jen.2010.11.001.

Moceri, J. T., & Drevdahl, D. J. (2014). Nurses' knowledge and attitudes toward pain in the Emergency Department. *Journal of Emergency Nursing, 40*(1), 6–12.

Moseley, G. L., & Butler, D. S. (2015). Fifteen Years of Explaining Pain - The Past, Present and Future. *Journal of Pain, 16*(9), 807–813. https://doi.org/10.1016/j.jpain.2015.05.005.

Paice, J. A., & Von Roenn, J. H. (2014). Under-or overtreatment of pain in the patient with cancer: how to achieve proper balance. *Journal of Clinical Oncology, 32*(16), 1721–1726.

Park, J., Manotas, K., & Hooyman, N. (2013). Chronic pain management by ethically and racially diverse older adults: pharmacological and nonpharmacological pain therapies. *Pain Management, 3*(6), 435–454.

Paskins, Z., Sanders, T., & Hassell, A. B. (2014). Comparison of patient experiences of the osteoarthritis consultation with GP attitudes and beliefs to OA: a narrative review. *BMC Family Medicine, 15*, 46.

Perry, J., VanDenKerkhof, E. G., Wilson, R., & Tripp, D. A. (2017). Development of a guided internet-based psycho-education intervention using cognitive behavioral therapy and self-management for individuals with chronic pain. *Pain Management Nursing, 18*(2), 90–101.

Pizzi, L. J., Chelly, J. E., & Marlin, V. (2013). Nursing time study for the administration of a PRN oral analgesic on an orthopedic postoperative unit. *Pain Management Nursing, 15*(3), 603–608.

Quinlan-Colwell, A. (2012). *Pain Management for Older Adults: A Clinical Guide for Nurses.* New York: Springer Publishing Company.

Quinlan-Colwell, A., & O'Conner-Von, S. (2014). Shifting the paradigm. Southern Pain Society Newsletter, Summer 2014, (2-3).

Riemondy, S., Gonzalez, L., Gosik, K., Ricords, A., & Schirm, V. (2016). Nurses' perceptions and attitudes toward use of oral patient-controlled analgesia. *Pain Management Nursing,* 17(2), 132–139.

Rodriguez, F., & Green, A. R. (2013). Implicit and explicit ethnic bias among physicians. In M. Incayawar & K. H. Todd (Eds.), *Culture, Brain, and Analgesia: understanding and managing pain in diverse populations* (pp. 159–167). New York: Oxford University Press.

Roe, M., & Sehgal, A. (2016). Pharmacology in the management of chronic pain. *Anesthesia and Intensive Care Medicine,* 17(11), 548–551.

Saifan, A., Bashayreh, I., Batiha, A.-M., & AbuRuz, M. (2015). Patient-and family caregiver – related barriers to effective cancer pain control. *Pain Management Nursing,* 16(3), 400–410.

Schild, C., Reed, E. A., Hingston, T., Dennis, C. H., & Wilson, A. C. (2016). Neighborhood characteristics: Influences on pain and physical function in youth at risk for chronic pain. *Children,* 3(4), 35. https://doi.org/10.3390/children3040035.

Shea, M., & McDonald, D. D. (2011). Factors associated with increased pain communication in older adults. *Western Journal of Nursing Research,* 33(2), 196–206.

Schreiber, J. A., Cantrell, D., Moe, K. A., Hench, J., McKinney, E., & Brockopp, D. (2014). Improving knowledge, assessment and attitudes related to pain management: evaluation and intervention. *Pain Management Nursing,* 15(2), 474–481.

Schultz, P. J., & Nakamoto, K. (2013). Health literacy and patient empowerment in health communication: the importance of separating conjoined twins. *Patient Education and Counseling,* 90(1), 4–11.

Sjskatte, S., Røe, C., Fagerland, M. W., & Granan, L.-P. (2017). Expectations of pain and functioning in patients with musculoskeletal disorders: a cross-sectional study. *BMC Musculoskeletal Disorders,* 18(1), 48. https://doi.org/10.1186/s12891-016-1386-z.

Smith, M. L., Prohaska, T. R., MacLeod, K. E., Ory, M. G., Eisenstein, A. R., & Satariano, W. A. (2017). Non-emergency medical transportation needs of middle-aged and older adults: a rural-urban comparison in Delaware, USA. *International Journal of Environmental Research and Public Health,* 14(2), 174. https://doi.org/10.3390/ijerph14020174.

Stang, A. S., Hartling, L., Fera, C., Johnson, D., & Ali, S. (2014). Quality indicators for the assessment and management of pain in the emergency department: a systematic review. *Pain Research Management,* 19(6), 179–190.

Stein, K. D., Alcaraz, K. I., Kamson, C., Fallon, E., & Smith, T. G. (2016). Sociodemographic inequalities in barriers to cancer pain management: a report from the American Cancer Society's Study of Cancer Survivors-II (SCS-II). *Psycho-Oncology,* 25(10), 1212–1221.

Stevans, J. M., Blise, C. G., McGee, J. C., Miller, D. L., Rockar, P., & Delitto, A. (2015). Evidence-Based Practice Implementation: Case Report of the Evolution of a Quality Improvement Program in a Multicenter Physical Therapy Organization. *Physical Therapy,* 95(4), 588–599. https://doi.org/10.2522/ptj.20130541.

Sullivan, D., Lyons, M., Montgomery, R., & Quinlan-Colwell, A. (2016). Exploring opioid-sparing multimodal analgesia options in trauma: a nursing perspective. *Journal of Trauma Nursing,* 23(6), 361–375.

Syed, S. T., Gerber, B. S., & Sharp, L. K. (2013). Traveling towards disease: transportation barriers to health care access. *Journal of Community Health,* 38(5), 976–1003. https://doi.org/10.1007/s10900-013-9681-1.

Syrjala, K. L., Jensen, M. P., Mendoza, M. E., Yi, J. C., Fisher, H. M., & Keefe, F. J. (2014). Psychological and behavioral approaches to cancer pain management. *Journal of Clinical Oncology,* 32(16), 1703–1711. https://doi.org/10.1200/JCO.2013.54.4825.

Thomas, B. (2014). Health and health care disparities: the effect of social and environmental factors on individual and population health. *International Journal of Environmental Research and Public Health,* 11(7), 7492–7507. https://doi.org/10.3390/ijerph110707492.

Thorn, B., Day, M. A., Burns, J., Kuhajda, M. C., Gaskins, S. W., & Cabbil, C. (2011). Randomized trial of group of cognitive behavioral therapy compared with a pain education control for low-literacy rural people with chronic pain. *Pain,* 152(12), 2710–2720.

Todd, K. H., & Incayawar, M. (2013). Relevance of pain and analgesia in multi-cultural societies. In M. Incayawar & K. H. Todd (Eds.), *Culture, Brain, and Analgesia: understanding and managing pain in diverse populations* (pp. 1–8). New York: Oxford University Press.

Trail-Mahan, T., Mao, C. L., & Bawel-Brinkley, K. (2013). Complementary and alternative medicine: nurses' attitudes and knowledge. *Pain Management Nursing,* 14(4), 277–286. https://doi.org/10.1016/j.pmn.2011.06.0014.

Tsai, C., Sullivan, A., Gordon, J., Kaushal, R., Magid, D., Blumenthal, D., & Camargo, A. (2012). Racial/Ethnic Differences in Emergency Care for Joint Dislocation in 53 US EDs. *The American Journal of Emergency Medicine,* 30, 1970–1980. https://doi.org/10.1016/j.ajem.2012.04.023.

Twycross, A., & Chambers, C. T. (2015). Why aren't clinical guidelines used in practice? What we learned from our twitter chat. *Pediatric Pain Letter,* 17(2), 27–34. www.childpain.org/ppl.

Ung, A., Salamonson, Y., Hu, W., & Gallego, G. (2016). Assessing knowledge, perceptions and attitudes to pain management among medical and nursing students: a review of the literature. *British Journal of Pain,* 10(1), 8–21.

Waljee, J., McGlinn, E. P., Sears, E. D., & Chung, K. C. (2014). Patient expectations and patient-reported outcomes in surgery: a systematic review. *Surgery,* 155(5), 799–808. https://doi.org/10.1016/j.surg.2013.12.015.

Wøen, H., & Bjørk, I. T. (2013). Intensive care pain treatment and sedation: nurses' experiences of the conflict between clinical judgement and standardized care: an explorative study. *Intensive and Critical Care Nursing,* 29(3), 128–136.

Chapter 5 Introduction to Pain Assessment

Maureen F. Cooney

CHAPTER OUTLINE

Importance of Pain Assessment, pg. 61

Classification of Pain, pg. 62

    Differentiation of Acute From Chronic Pain, pg. 63

    Assessment of Pain Mechanisms, pg. 63

Roles of the Health Team in Pain Assessment, pg. 64

Timing and Frequency of Pain Assessment, pg. 64

    Discrepancies in Pain Assessment, pg. 65

    Hierarchy of Pain Assessment: Assessing Pain in Patients Who Cannot Self-Report, pg. 67

Key Points, pg. 70

Case Scenario, pg. 70

References, pg. 71

the cause is unclear. The assessment of pain is challenging for health professionals because of its subjective sensory and affective dimensions and because individuals experience and respond to pain in their own unique ways. Accurate and thorough assessments of pain require health care providers to address the challenges posed by complex patient care environments, limitations of pain assessment tools, and other patient, provider, system, and societal barriers.

To appropriately assess pain, an understanding of basic pain-related concepts is needed. This chapter provides an overview of basic information needed for accurate pain assessment, such as the classification of types of pain, the role of the health team in pain assessment, timing and frequency of pain assessment, and the hierarchy of pain assessment. The chapter highlights the importance of pain assessment and some of the challenges to the assessment of pain. It lays the foundation for the following two chapters, which describe pain assessment in patients who are cognitively intact and who are cognitively impaired.

PAIN is a common reason for people to seek health care, yet it is often underrecognized, inadequately assessed, and undertreated. Even mild to moderate pain may be distressing for the individual because it may trigger a host of consequences, including fears of worsening pain, fears of the significance of pain, concerns about one's ability to meet daily responsibilities, concerns about interference with enjoyable events, and interruptions and cancellations in one's plans. Over 50 years ago, Margo McCaffery defined pain as "what the experiencing person says it is, existing whenever he says it does" (McCaffery, 1968). In the years since the publication of that definition, McCaffery, Chris Pasero, and others have strongly advocated for improvements in safe and effective pain care. Numerous publications related to pain and other educational initiatives have been developed to inform health care providers about the subjective nature of pain and the importance of pain assessment and pain management.

The awareness of the unpleasant nature of pain and increased focus on pain education, research, and development of regulatory standards, policies, and expanded treatment modalities have not eliminated the challenges posed by the subjective nature of pain, particularly when

Importance of Pain Assessment

The assessment of pain is essential to an understanding of the cause of pain, the impact of pain on function and quality of life, and the identification of strategies to aid in the selection of the most appropriate modalities to manage pain. Thorough pain assessment provides the foundation for development of an effective multimodal pain management plan of care. Nurses, because of their roles in providing ongoing care at the bedside, are most often the health professionals involved in pain assessment. Nurses regularly assess their patients as part of usual patient care, and pain assessment is an essential component of that process. Physicians, nurse practitioners, physician assistants, therapists, pharmacists, and other members of the health team also have roles in pain assessment. The aims of pain assessment are summarized in Box 5.1.

The importance of pain assessment is reflected by the measures regulatory agencies, including the Centers for Medicare and Medicaid Services (CMS) and the Joint Commission (TJC), have taken to develop standards that require pain assessment (Baker, 2016; Centers for Medicare & Medicaid Services, HHS, 2016; Joint Commission,

---

Box 5.1 Aims of Pain Assessment

- Ascertain that pain exists
- Aid in identifying the cause of pain
- Accurately understand the characteristics of pain
- Acquire information to guide pain management options
- Identify possible barriers to managing pain
- Identify comorbidities
- Identify ways to relieve pain and reduce disability

Modified from Quinlan-Colwell, A. (2012). *Pain management for older adults: A clinical guide for nurses.* New York: Springer Publishing Company.

2017; Radnovich et al., 2014). The 2018 standards published by TJC (2017) identify pain assessment and pain management as organizational priorities for hospitals and require that hospitals have criteria for screening, assessment, and reassessment of pain that consider the patient's age, condition, and cognitive ability. Pain management guidelines and position statements published by professional organizations, including the American Society for Pain Management Nursing (ASPMN), also emphasize the importance of pain assessment.

Classification of Pain

Accurate pain assessment is essential to determine the cause and understand the characteristics of pain. Pain is categorized in a variety of ways. The International Association for the Study of Pain (IASP; 2011) developed a comprehensive taxonomy of pain in 1979, which was most recently revised in 2011. Other groups have attempted to refine this classification system to address gaps in the IASP taxonomy and incorporate evidence from the growing body of pain research. One group, composed of representatives from the Analgesic, Anesthetic, and Addiction Clinical Trial Translations, Innovations, Opportunities, and Networks (ACTTION), APS, and American Academy of Pain Medicine (AAPM) proposed a multidimensional taxonomy for acute pain in 2017. This taxonomy, the ACTTION-APS-AAPM Acute Pain Taxonomy (AAAPT), followed publication of the ACTTION-APS Chronic Pain Taxonomy in 2014 (Kent et al., 2017). Recognizing that the understanding of pain is dynamic and evolving, the acute pain taxonomy group noted the future possibility of formulating a single pain taxonomy that addresses the dimensions of both acute and chronic pain (Kent et al., 2017).

The multidimensional acute pain classification system proposed by the AAAPT classifies acute pain according to the following dimensions: core criteria, common features, modulating factors, impact or functional consequences, and putative pathophysiologic pain mechanisms (Kent et al., 2017).

- Core criteria include identification of the event that precipitated the pain, timing of the onset of pain, location and type of tissue involved, and related diagnostic and procedural interventions.
- Common features characterize acute pain according to quality, duration and other time-related aspects, physical distribution of the pain, and recovery expectations.
- Modulating factors are other variables such as comorbidities (including opioid tolerance) and biopsychosocial and sociodemographic aspects that may influence acute pain.
- Impact or functional consequences refer to the physical, psychological, social, and functional outcomes resulting from acute pain.
- Putative pathophysiologic pain mechanisms are the neurobiological processes that are involved in all phases of acute pain and include genetic and mechanism-based characteristics that may guide treatment (Kent et al., 2017).

The multidimensional chronic pain classification system includes five dimensions that are similar to the acute pain system: core diagnostic criteria; common features; common medical and psychiatric comorbidities; neurobiological, psychosocial, and functional consequences; putative neurobiological and psychosocial mechanisms; risk factors; and protective factors (Fillingim et al., 2014).

- Core diagnostic criteria include signs and symptoms of chronic pain, diagnostic testing, and differential diagnosis.
- Common features are the dimensions that characterize or describe the pain, such as the timing, location, and quality.
- Common medical comorbidities include the medical diagnoses that often occur with the chronic pain condition. For example, osteoarthritis is often associated with chronic low back or joint pain.
- Neurobiological, psychosocial, and functional consequences include the impact of chronic pain on each of these dimensions. For example, chronic pain may interfere with mood, quality of sleep, social interactions, and self-care activities.
- Putative neurobiological and psychosocial mechanisms, risk factors, and protective factors increase the risk for, contribute to, or protect against worsening of the chronic pain condition (Fillingim et al., 2014).

Thorough examination of these taxonomies is beyond the scope of this chapter; however, the dimensions of core criteria and common features, which include the temporal aspects of pain, are instrumental in providing the differentiation of acute pain from chronic pain.

Differentiation of Acute From Chronic Pain

An important element of pain assessment is to obtain the history of when pain began, what may have caused it, and how long it has persisted. This information is needed to determine whether pain is acute or chronic (persistent) and may aid in determining whether pain is nociceptive, neuropathic, or mixed.

Acute pain is a physiologic response to tissue damage, such as damage resulting from surgery, trauma, and tumor invasion, and usually resolves as the tissue damage heals (Herndon et al., 2016). Acute pain is a result of activation of nociceptors and results in pain processing through the peripheral and central nociceptive pain processes described in Chapter 3. It is protective because it serves as a warning of disease or injury, and although usually time limited, it may become pathologic (Kent et al., 2017). More traditional descriptions of acute pain are that it usually has an identifiable cause such as a surgical incision, is of short duration, and is self-limiting because it resolves along with the healing process (usually in 3–6 months) (Kent et al., 2017). The AAAPT adopted the following time-based definition of acute pain, which distinguishes it from chronic pain:

Acute pain lasts for up to 7 days, but may be further qualified by the following (Kent et al., 2017):

1. Its duration is affected by the type and severity of the underlying cause of the pain.
2. It is common for acute pain to be extended beyond the 7 days to 30 days.
3. It is common for acute pain to last up to, but not beyond, 90 days after the initial onset or injury.
4. Understanding of pain mechanisms is inadequate at this time to link the duration of pain to specific physiologic mechanisms.

If not controlled, acute pain can have a negative impact on quality of life, function, and recovery (Chou et al., 2016). The severity of acute postoperative pain in the first days after surgery is one of the risk factors for the development of persistent postsurgical pain (Schug & Bruce, 2017). The assessment of acute pain is necessary to guide treatment that will facilitate recovery and possibly interrupt the progression from acute to chronic pain (Pergolizzi, Raffa, & Taylor, 2014). During the pain assessment, it is important to assess for complications of inadequate pain relief and intervene to improve pain control. Chapter 8 provides additional information related to the impact of inadequate pain control.

Assessment of acute pain also includes a physical examination for sources of pain and assessment of physiologic and behavioral indicators of acute pain. Physical signs of acute pain include autonomic nervous system responses such as hypertension, tachycardia, mydriasis, diaphoresis, pallor, shallow respirations, and behavioral indicators that include agitation, facial grimacing, and splinting or guarding (Cox, 2018). However, the absence of physical signs of acute pain does not negate the existence of acute pain.

Chronic pain is a complex, multidimensional phenomenon that is poorly understood, yet has significant impact on the physical, psychological, social, spiritual, and economic condition of patients with chronic pain and their loved ones. It is defined as pain that persists beyond the expected time for healing, and may be further defined by categories such as musculoskeletal, neuropathic, headache, or myofascial chronic pain (Dworkin et al., 2016). According to the AAPT, chronic pain is categorized by organ system and anatomic structure, with a separate category for disease-related pain, such as cancer pain or sickle cell pain that is not categorized elsewhere (Dworkin et al., 2016). Headaches are not addressed in the AAPT taxonomy, because there is a separate taxonomy for headache classification, the International Classification of Headache Disorders (ICHD) (Olesen, 2014). In assessing chronic pain, a physical examination and an assessment of the duration of pain and the other dimensions identified in Chapter 6 provide valuable information. Assessment of the dimensions of function and the impact of pain on quality of life are also of major importance.

Assessment of Pain Mechanisms

The pain assessment is instrumental in determining the mechanism or type of pain the patient is experiencing. The pain assessment may be a component of a comprehensive patient assessment that also includes an appropriate physical and psychological assessment and, in some cases, diagnostic testing. During the pain assessment, the patient's description of the quality of pain may provide insight into the cause and type of pain and therefore guide the most appropriate multimodal pharmacologic and nonpharmacologic treatment interventions. It is important to allow the patient sufficient time to provide detailed descriptions of the quality of the pain. Sometimes patients need examples of words that describe pain so they can choose the adjectives that allow them to express the pain experience. The pain descriptors may be useful in determining whether the patient is experiencing nociceptive, neuropathic, or mixed type pain. Chapter 3 provides additional information related to pain mechanisms.

Nociceptive pain is pain resulting from actual or threatened damage to tissue (other than nerve tissue) that results in activation of the nociceptors (Herndon et al., 2016). Nociceptive pain occurs with a normally functioning nervous system (La Cesa et al., 2015). Adjectives such as *throbbing, aching,* and *pressure* are often used to describe nociceptive pain. When nociceptive pain results from an injury or disease affecting somatic structures such as skin, muscle, tendons and ligaments, bone, and joints, it is referred to as *somatic* pain (Herndon et al., 2016). Somatic pain is usually well localized and results from chemical, thermal, mechanical, or multiple types of stimulation of the nociceptors. *Visceral pain,* another type of nociceptive pain, results from internal organ dysfunction and may be related to inflammation, ischemia, capsular or organ distention (e.g., renal stones, cholecystitis), or functional disease (e.g., irritable bowel syndrome) (Herndon et al., 2016). In contrast to somatic pain, visceral pain is usually diffuse and poorly localized, may be referred to other areas (e.g., cardiac pain may be referred to the arm or jaw), and may be associated with excessive autonomic reflexes and emotional responses (Herndon et al., 2016).

Neuropathic pain is defined as pain that results from, or is an outcome of, a lesion or disease that affects the somatosensory system (Jensen et al., 2011). It can result from damaged or abnormally functioning nerves in the peripheral or central nervous systems. Examples of peripheral neuropathic pain conditions include postherpetic neuralgia, diabetic neuropathy, and alcohol-induced peripheral neuropathy (Zeng, Alongkronrusmee, & van Rijn, 2017). Treatment-induced peripheral neuropathies are associated with traditional chemotherapies and radiation therapy in the management of a variety of cancer conditions. Newer treatments, such as the biologic and immunologic therapies used in the management of some cancers and other disease processes, are also associated with neuropathic pain (Stone & DeAngelis, 2016). Common causes of central pain are poststroke pain and spinal cord lesions or injuries. It has been estimated that 20% to 25% of all chronic pain is neuropathic (Cohen & Raja, 2016). Neuropathic pain is often associated with numbness and tingling, especially when present in a dermatomal or nerve distribution. Adjectives such as "burning," "shooting," and "electrical" are more likely to be associated with neuropathic pain.

Mixed pain, as the name implies, is pain that has both nociceptive and neuropathic components (Cohen & Raja, 2016). Cancer pain, low back pain, and ischemic pain are often associated with mixed type pain. In assessing pain, descriptors of one type of pain may initially be readily recognized, but with further assessment, characteristics of both nociceptive and neuropathic, or mixed pain, may be identified.

In addition to nociceptive, neuropathic, and mixed types of pain, other pain mechanisms have been identified. *Inflammatory pain,* although commonly involved in nociceptive pain, is sometimes categorized as a specific type of pain. It results from the activation and sensitization of nociceptors by inflammatory mediators (Ronchetti, Migliorati, & Delfino, 2017). Injury to tissues and immune cells may result in the release of inflammatory mediators which activate nociceptor terminals and set forth processes involving bidirectional communication between nociceptor sensory neurons and immune cells. These processes may result in both peripheral and central sensitization (Pinho-Ribeiro, Verri, & Chiu, 2017). Inflammatory pain is sometimes identified as infectious pain because inflammatory mediators may be released in response to the presence of sterile or infectious pathogens (Vardeh, Mannion, & Woolf, 2016). Recently, it has been shown that, independent from the immune response, gram-negative and gram-positive bacteria can directly activate nociceptors (Vardeh, Mannion, & Woolf, 2016). Inflammatory mediators generate pain because they irritate or sensitize the nerves leading to structural and functional changes in the nociceptor terminals.

Roles of the Health Team in Pain Assessment

All members of the health team who interact with patients have a role in the assessment of pain. In the acute care setting, physicians, nurses, nurse practitioners, and physician assistants are usually directly responsible for pain assessment. Other team members, including physical, occupational, speech, and other therapists; patient care assistants; nutritionists; and phlebotomists, assist in identifying and addressing pain. In most settings, nurses, because of their professional preparation and close patient contact, are in the best position to identify patients in pain. They are usually responsible for the assessment of pain, implementation of pain management interventions, and subsequent reassessment of the patient.

Other health care providers screen for pain during interactions with patients and notify the appropriate health care provider to facilitate a pain assessment if pain is not controlled. For example, physical and occupational therapists ensure that patients have adequate pain control before starting a therapy session and notify the nurse if pain is not controlled at any point in the session so an assessment and intervention can be provided. Patient care assistants, during their direct patient care activities, screen for pain and alert the nurse for a pain assessment if pain is reported or suspected. In settings other than acute care, other health care providers may have a more direct role in pain assessment. When the interdisciplinary team participates in pain assessment, the accuracy of the assessment is optimized by the use of a consistent approach, the same assessment tool, and communication and documentation of findings in a way that is readily accessed by all (Booker & Herr, 2016).

Timing and Frequency of Pain Assessment

Inpatient pain assessment and reassessment practices are usually governed by individual health care organization policies that identify the required timing, minimum frequency, and parameters of the pain assessment. Regulatory agencies such as TJC and individual state departments of health have standards that guide policy development. However, it is not possible to identify pain assessment timing and frequency practices that are safe and appropriate for all patients. Just as pain is an individual experience, the timing and frequency of assessment and reassessment, in addition to meeting the minimum standards required by the policies of the organization, are individualized based on the patient's condition, type of pain and pain level, and pain intervention.

Acute pain, in particular, is dynamic and therefore requires frequent assessments of intensity and quality to ensure appropriate multimodal therapies are used and doses of medications are adjusted as needed. For example, a patient with a fractured tibia before fracture reduction may initially require a multimodal approach including intravenous opioids and nonopioids, but once the fracture is reduced, it may be possible to use the oral route, reduce the opioid dose, and optimize nonopioid interventions because the pain level may have improved.

Patients are screened for pain, assessed when pain occurs, and reassessed after every pain-related intervention to determine the effectiveness of the intervention, identify adverse effects, and intervene when necessary. For postsurgical patients, pain assessments in the immediate postoperative period should be very frequent, and as pain improves the time between assessments may lengthen (Radnovich et al., 2014). After analgesic administration, reassessment is needed when the medication has reached its peak effect, requiring the nurse to recognize the time of peak effect of medications. In many cases, reassessment after an intravenous opioid occurs within 15 to 30 minutes after administration; whereas for many oral medications and nonpharmacologic interventions, reassessment may occur within 45 to 60 minutes after administration. Particular attention to the need for assessment and reassessment of patients receiving opioids is specifically addressed in Chapter 13. The use of a multimodal analgesic plan reduces risks for adverse effects while optimizing pain relief.

In the outpatient setting, screening for pain and assessment, if pain is present, should occur with each visit. When sending patients home on the same day of surgery, or shortly after, the patient and significant others need to know what to expect about postoperative pain and its intensity, probable trajectory, and duration (Radnovich et al., 2014). Education related to acute pain treatment, particularly multimodal interventions, is necessary and must include teaching about medications and their expected effects and possible side effects. When patients are discharged with prescriptions for opioids, education of patients and family members related to safe opioid use, storage, and disposal is necessary. Reassessment of pain and the effects of interventions may take place in follow-up visits, or in some situations phone call follow-ups may be appropriate.

For patients with chronic pain, pain assessment and reassessment generally take place during regularly scheduled and emergency office visits. With increasing availability of electronic and internet-based resources for patients and providers, alternative ways of assessing and reassessing pain are likely to evolve, especially in geographic areas where patients have limited access to health care resources. The outpatient chronic pain assessment should include an assessment of the pain and the impact of pain on the patient's activities. Assessment should include discussion on the interventions the patient uses to manage chronic pain, their effectiveness, and any problems associated with their use. During the assessment of chronic pain, it is important to identify opportunities for the use of a multimodal pain management approach and address any potential barriers. Assessment of the patient's

functional status is important, particularly regarding activities of daily living. A more detailed discussion of the pain assessment is presented in Chapters 6 and 7.

Discrepancies in Pain Assessment

Discrepancies between patients' and clinicians' assessments of pain have been identified as major contributors to inadequate pain relief. These discrepancies are often the result of barriers to adequate pain management, many of which are identified in Chapter 4. At times, clinicians question the accuracy of the patient's self-report of pain intensity. When incongruence exists between the patient's report and the observations of the clinicians, the management and documentation of the patient's pain level may not correspond to the patient's self-report. For example, consider the scenario of the 24-year-old woman who presents in the emergency department (ED) with abdominal pain and nausea, reporting a pain intensity level of 8 out of 10 on the numeric rating scale (NRS). When observed, the patient is noted to be texting on her cell phone and appears to be resting comfortably in bed, talking with her two friends who are at her bedside.

There are multiple possible explanations for this scenario. The patient may not understand the use of the NRS and may be too embarrassed to ask for further explanation and simply selects a number to answer the staff's questions. She may have very severe pain but is able to obtain some relief through distraction with her phone. She may feel the need to "act normally" in front of her friends. Her pain level may be fluctuating and is reduced in the short interval in which she is observed. Of concern is that health providers may regard the patient's behavior as not reflective of very severe pain and not respond promptly or appropriately to address it. The incongruence between patient self-report of pain intensity and the clinicians' observations of behavior may lead clinicians to inaccurate assessment and documentation, provide inappropriate pain management, and set up a situation in which distrust develops between the patient and providers. Possible sources of error in pain assessment are listed in Box 5.2.

Many clinicians report that they were taught to "believe" the patient's report of pain. This directive creates discomfort for some, especially when clinicians observe patient behaviors that are not what they expect from a patient with a particular pain intensity level. It may be helpful to remember that one's own expectations are influenced by many factors and the patient's pain intensity level is subjective and also multidimensional. Patient responses to pain can sometimes be controlled, and there is no evidence to link pain intensity level with a particular response or level of function. Perhaps clinicians would feel less discomfort when a patient's pain intensity level differs from the clinician's impression if clinicians are taught to "accept" a patient's self-report, clarify and ensure the patient understands what that level indicates,

Box 5.2 | Potential Sources of Inaccurate Pain Assessment

- Patient and/or clinician personal characteristics, experience, knowledge, attitudes (including bias), and other barriers, may result in underestimation or overestimation of pain.
- Vague, ambiguous, or poorly understood questions about pain may lead to inaccurate or incomplete patient responses.
- Lack of time, urgency of the patient's condition, severity of pain, setting, and competing priorities may lead to errors in pain assessment.
- Use of pain assessment tools that are not understood by the patient, including the use of tools that are not understood because of language or sensory barriers,

or the use of medical terms in patients with low health literacy, may lead to errors in pain assessment.
- Use of pain assessment tools that are not evidence-based or have not been validated for use in the patient population being assessed may result in inaccurate pain assessment.
- Pain assessment may be inaccurate if patients are unable (for various reasons) to provide accurate, clear, and complete information about their pain.

Modified from Box 44.7 in Cooney, M. F. (2017). Pain management. In P. A. Potter, A. G. Perry, P. Stockert, & A. Hall. *Fundamentals of nursing* (9th. ed.). St. Louis, MO: Elsevier.

and then address the pain with interventions that are individually selected to provide multimodal pain care that is both safe and effective. A particular pain intensity level does not dictate a particular pain intervention. If a patient's pain level is reported as 10 on a 0 to 10 NRS, this does not mandate administration of high doses of intravenous opioids. Many factors must be considered in the selection of the most appropriate management strategy. This issue of dosing to a particular number on an NRS is dangerous and is addressed further in Chapter 9.

An equally challenging situation occurs when the clinician expects the patient to have a high pain intensity level, yet the patient denies pain or reports a very minimal pain level. Consider the situation in which the patient has had a large open abdominal surgery, and on the day after surgery reports pain as minimal with an intensity level of 1 on an NRS 0 to 10. The nurse may note that the patient is not coughing, is lying very still, and has stayed in the same position for most of the shift, yet despite explanations of

the NRS, continues to rate pain as minimal. In this type of scenario, it is helpful to recognize that the patient's expectations and response to pain may differ from the nurse's expectations. The nurse's expectations of the patient's pain experience are based on influences such as personal and clinical experiences, knowledge, culture, and beliefs, which may not be shared by the patient.

There are many reasons why a patient's self-report may be different from what the clinician would expect. Culture has an impact on the meaning of pain to an individual, and influences verbal reports, behaviors, expressions of pain, and coping responses. Patients may be at increased risk for inadequate treatment of pain when health care providers do not recognize cultural influences in the pain assessment. Cultural influences are included among the barriers presented in Chapter 4 that affect pain assessment and treatment. Box 5.3 summarizes strategies that may be used to assess pain in culturally diverse populations.

Box 5.3 | Strategies for Assessing Pain in Culturally Diverse Patient Populations

- Use pain assessment tools that are culturally appropriate and written in the patient's own native language.
- Assess the patient's health literacy level to provide pain-related education using strategies that are most appropriate to the patient.
- Recognize that patients' responses to pain and pain assessment may be varied and affected by cultural influences. In some cultures, stoicism is highly valued and the expression of pain may be unacceptable.
- Accept that patients' communication styles may be influenced by culture. Some will rely primarily on verbal communication, whereas others will use

mostly nonverbal communication to send and receive information about pain.
- In some cultures, pain and suffering are closely tied to religious beliefs and should be endured to enter heaven or have a rewarding after-life.
- Examine one's own cultural background and beliefs about pain and pain management to facilitate a nonjudgmental approach to the patient with pain.

Modified from Box 44.4 in Cooney, M. F. (2017). Pain management. In P. A. Potter, A. G. Perry, P. Stockert, & A. Hall. *Fundamentals of nursing* (9th. ed.). St. Louis, MO: Elsevier.

Stoicism is a highly valued quality in some cultures and some patient populations, particularly the elderly, may highly value stoicism, resulting in the absence of pain behaviors and, at times, minimization of patient self-reports of pain (Crowe et al., 2017). Pain also may be underreported for other cultural or religious reasons, and despite patient education about the importance of pain control, patients may continue to underreport pain. Fear of consequences of pain treatment may contribute to the underreporting of pain. Patients may fear that pain treatments will result in distressing side effects or may be concerned that opioid use will result in opioid use disorder. Others may not report pain because of wanting to be a "good patient" and not burden the nurse who is already busy caring for others. Health literacy may have an effect on the ability of patients to understand and use pain assessment tools to communicate their pain experience. To obtain an accurate pain assessment, the clinician must take the time to explore the patient's understanding of pain and understanding of the questions being asked about pain. Explanations of terms and pain assessment tools, education about the consequences of untreated pain, and exploration of concerns related to pain and pain treatment are necessary to obtain accurate pain assessments and provide appropriate multimodal pain management interventions.

In a study by Dequeker, Van Lancker, and Van Hecke (2018) that included examination of agreement between nurses and hospitalized patients in the assessment of pain intensity and the identification of barriers to pain management, moderate agreement was found between nurses' and patients' assessment of pain intensity. Nurses who used a pain scale to assess pain had greater agreement with patients' pain intensity ratings. Among the 351 patients who participated, 38% were reluctant to report pain and 40% reported difficulty with the assessment of pain intensity, although only 12.6% of nurses identified patients' difficulty. The results of this study illustrate the importance of assessing patients' abilities to use pain scales and providing appropriate education about the importance of reporting pain.

In a study, 1643 patients at eight Veterans Affairs medical facilities completed a survey that included reporting of a pain score on the NRS. Health technicians were required to screen these patients for pain and document the results in the electronic medical record (EMR) on the same day. The EMR scores were found to be significantly lower than the patients' surveys (Goulet et al., 2013). Another interesting finding was that when survey NRS scores were high, NRS scores were less likely to be recorded in the EMR. The findings of this survey are similar to findings in studies that were done in the early 2000s in which providers were found to document lower pain intensity ratings than those reported by patients.

Ruben, Blanch-Hartigan, and Shipherd (2018), in two meta-analyses of pain assessment accuracy that included 90 peer-reviewed articles published from 1894 until 2016, reported that health care providers (physicians and nurses) significantly underestimated patient's pain and caretakers (parents and others) were more likely to overestimate pain. Health care providers significantly underestimated acute pain, although chronic pain was not significantly underestimated or overestimated. Older adults and males were more likely to have pain underestimated.

In a systematic literature search by Ruben, van Osch, and Blanch-Hartigan (2015), 60 studies from 1982 to 2014 that met inclusion criteria were analyzed for health care providers' pain assessment accuracy. The majority of studies were conducted in the United States (45%) and included adult patients (72%); 72% involved nurses' accuracy of assessments and 53% measured accuracy of physicians' assessments. Of the studies, 77% reported moderate to good accuracy of providers' pain assessment.

Many of the studies that examined the accuracy of physicians' and nurses' assessments of pain were done in the 1990s and early 2000s in the United States. More recent studies in other countries show that differences between patients' self-report of pain and health professionals' assessment of pain continue to exist. For example, Pierik, Ijzerman, Gaakeer, Vollenbroek-Hutten, and Doggen (2017) published the results of a prospective study of 539 adult patients with musculoskeletal pain who were admitted to an ED in the Netherlands. In most cases (63%), nurses documented pain scores that were lower than the scores provided by patients. Women, patients with lower educational levels, and those who had taken analgesics before presenting in the ED were at higher risk to be rated as having less pain than pain level that was self-reported.

Although few recent studies have been conducted in the United States related to the accuracy of pain assessment, it cannot be assumed that the increase in attention to the management of pain in recent years, the focus on patient satisfaction with pain management, and educational and research initiatives have eliminated the risks of underassessment. Certain patient populations, particularly those prone to bias, such as the elderly, the very young, the cognitively impaired, those with substance use disorders, and minority groups may continue to experience underestimations of pain and infrequent or inadequate assessments. As patient advocates and health care providers, there is an obligation to continue to work toward ensuring that every patient receives an appropriate and accurate pain assessment.

Hierarchy of Pain Assessment: Assessing Pain in Patients Who Cannot Self-Report

It is widely recognized that pain is a subjective experience, and thus the patient's self-report of pain, whenever possible, should be used as the basis for the pain assessment. Only a patient self-report can provide an assessment of pain intensity. However, there are situations in which an individual may be unable to provide a self-report of pain.

Those at extremes in age (the very young and elderly with limited cognitive and/or communication abilities), the critically ill, the developmentally disabled, and others who are unable to communicate are recognized as people at high risk for the underassessment and subsequent undertreatment of pain. Much of the work in developing a consistent approach to the assessment of pain in those who are unable to self-report has come from research with these groups; for adults, a large body of literature related to the assessment of pain in cognitively impaired and nonverbal older adults and critically ill noncommunicative patients can be found. Chapter 7 provides more detail related to the assessment of pain in patients who are cognitively impaired.

The publication of the hierarchical approach to the assessment of pain by the American Society for Pain Management Nursing in the organization's position statement (Herr, Coyne, McCaffery, Manworren, & Merkel, 2011) provides guidance to clinicians in the assessment of pain in patients who are unable to provide a self-report. The position statement, updated in 2019, based on the results of numerous studies and publications, is readily accessible on the organization's website and includes specific considerations for pain assessment in the following subpopulations who may be unable to self-report: neonates, infants, toddlers, and young children, critically ill, unconscious patients, older adults with advanced dementia, those with intellectual disabilities, and those who are at the end of life (Herr, Coyne, Ely, Gélinas, & Manworren, 2019). The use of the hierarchy (Box 5.4) continues to be recommended as the approach to pain assessment in vulnerable patient populations (Gélinas, 2016; Harris et al., 2016; Herr et al., 2019; Manworren & Stinson, 2016).

The hierarchy, summarized in Box 5.4, provides guidance for health care providers to determine the next best method to use in the assessment of pain for vulnerable patient populations. The hierarchy begins with the need for clinicians to be aware of potential causes of pain. There are many pathological conditions which result in pain and many iatrogenic causes of pain such as diagnostic testing, procedures, needle procedures, and patient mobilization. In large and international studies of patients in critical care units, turning, endotracheal suctioning, chest tube removal, wound drain removal, wound care, and arterial line insertion were identified as among the most painful procedures (Puntillo, White, Morris, & Perdue, 2001; Puntillo et al., 2014). Awareness of potential sources of pain allows clinicians to proactively anticipate and employ nonpharmacologic and pharmacologic preemptive measures (Herr et al., 2019).

The patient's self-report of pain should be elicited whenever possible (Herr et al., 2019). The self-report may include the use of any of the self-report techniques or tools described in Chapter 6. The use of tools such as the NRS should not negate the need for a more detailed discussion about the patient's pain. In a qualitative study of postoperative patients who used the NRS to report pain, patients reported that the NRS makes it easier to communicate pain to health care providers, but a dialogue about pain is crucial to clarify the individual interpretation of the pain ratings and pain relief goals (Eriksson, Wikström, Årestedt, Fridlund, & Broström, 2014). If the use of the tools is not possible, a simple communication strategy such as a nod or shake of the head, vocalization of yes or no, hand grasp, eye blink, or other recognizable gesture in response to questioning about the presence of pain is accepted as a form of pain self-report (Herr et al., 2019).

Box 5.4 | Hierarchy of Pain Assessment Techniques

1. Be aware of possible sources of pain. Assess patient's condition and/or exposure to painful procedures, including diagnostic tests, and, if appropriate, assume pain is present.
2. Attempt to obtain the patient's self-report of pain, the single most reliable indicator of pain.
3. Observe for behavioral indicators of pain (e.g., facial expressions, crying, restlessness, and changes in activity). Use reliable, evidence-based behavioral assessment tools appropriate for the selected patient population.
4. Obtain information from a surrogate who knows the patient well (e.g., a parent, spouse, or caregiver) to obtain information about underlying painful pathologic conditions or behaviors that may indicate pain.
5. Conduct an empiric analgesic trial, starting with nonpharmacological and/or nonopioid multimodal

analgesics at the lowest analgesic doses. Add low doses of short-acting opioids if no improvement in pain behaviors. Cautiously adjust doses or discontinue the trial based on assessment of behavioral response. If there is a reduction in pain behaviors with an analgesic trial, it can be used to develop a pain treatment plan.

NOTE: Vital signs and other physiologic indicators (diaphoresis, pallor, pupillary changes) are the least sensitive indicators of pain, and changes may indicate the presence of other pathologic conditions. The use of vital signs and other physiologic signs may indicate that the patient requires further assessment.

Modified from Herr, K., Coyne, P. J., Ely, E., Gélinas, C., & Manworren, R. C. (2019). Pain assessment in the patient unable to self-report: clinical practice recommendations in support of the ASPMN 2019 position statement. *Pain Management Nursing, 20*(5), 404–417.

Box 5.5 | Behavioral Indicators of Effects of Pain

VOCALIZATIONS

- Moaning
- Crying
- Gasping
- Grunting

FACIAL EXPRESSIONS

- Grimace
- Clenched teeth
- Wrinkled forehead
- Tightly closed or widely opened eyes or mouth
- Lip biting

BODY MOVEMENT

- Restlessness
- Immobilization

- Muscle tension
- Increased hand and finger movements
- Pacing activities
- Rhythmic or rubbing motions
- Protective movement of body parts
- Grabbing or holding a body part

SOCIAL INTERACTION

- Avoidance of conversation
- Focus only on activities for pain relief
- Avoidance of social contacts
- Reduced attention span
- Reduced interaction with environment

From Potter, P. A., Perry, A. G., Stockert, P., & Hall, A. (2013). *Fundamentals of nursing* (8th. ed.). St. Louis, MO: Elsevier.

When patients are unable to provide a self-report of pain, a valid alternative approach to pain assessment is observation for pain behaviors (Herr et al., 2019). Behaviors such as those summarized in Box 5.5 may indicate the presence of pain. Although there are many different behavioral responses to pain, changes in facial expression, particularly in patients with dementia, have been shown to be the most sensitive and specific nonverbal responses to pain (Hadjistavropoulos et al., 2014). Other frequently observed pain behaviors include vocalizations of pain (e.g., moaning, crying, groaning), body movements (e.g., rocking, flailing, writhing, posturing, limping, rubbing), and diminished movements (e.g., guarding, immobilizing, bracing). Many of these behavioral signs, as well as facial expression, have been incorporated into behavioral pain assessment tools, such as those described in Chapter 7. Although there are many behavioral pain assessment tools, tools vary in validity and reliability (Herr et al., 2019). At times, pain behaviors may indicate another source of distress, such as psychological or emotional distress (Herr et al., 2019). It is also necessary for clinicians to understand that in situations where pain behaviors are not present, pain may still exist. Sleep or sedation does not equate with absence of pain (Herr et al., 2019). Patients who are paralyzed will have limited ability to display pain behaviors. Others, for a variety of reasons, including severe brain damage, the use of medications that limit body movements, and some movement-limiting disease states, may be unable to display pain behaviors (Arbour & Gélinas, 2014; Coleman et al., 2015).

The ability of the clinician to interpret patient behaviors as indicative of pain is further enhanced by the next step in the hierarchy, the proxy report. Information from family members, caregivers, and others who know the patient well may help the clinician recognize behaviors that may be more subtle or more specific to that individual. For example, one caregiver of a patient with severe intellectual disabilities reported that the patient often tapped his thigh when he was in pain.

Proxy reports by family members of patients who are critically ill are in moderate agreement with patient self-report of pain (Puntillo et al., 2012). However, although proxy reports may be helpful in the recognition of pain behaviors, there may be discrepancies between patients' self-reports of pain and the recognition of pain by care providers and clinicians. Awareness of potential biases is important when significant others provide input about a patient's pain. Biases of the proxy or surrogate (significant others or health care providers) may influence the observer's interpretation of the patient's behavior and result in overestimation or underestimation of pain behaviors. Factors such as race, likability, and uncertainty about the patient's motivations for displaying pain behaviors may result in underestimation of pain (Hadjistavropoulos et al., 2007). Underestimation of pain bias has been shown to be increased in observers who have clinical experience with those in pain, and similar results have been found in experiments in which observers are overexposed to pain expression in others (Grégoire, Coll, Tremblay, Prkachin, & Jackson, 2016). To reduce risks of underestimation of pain, it is recommended to use a combination of assessment techniques, including awareness of potential sources of pain, observation for pain behaviors, input from family members or other care providers, and assessment of patient response to pain treatment (Herr et al., 2019).

The final step in the hierarchy of pain assessment techniques is to empirically use an analgesic trial. This step is used to determine whether or not pain is the cause of behaviors (Herr et al., 2019). An empiric analgesic trial is initiated when behaviors indicate the presence of pain or when behaviors continue despite measures to promote comfort and attention to basic needs (Herr et al., 2019). The analgesic trial is developed based upon an assessment of the patient and potential causes for pain. Empiric analgesic interventions include the use of multimodal nonpharmacologic and pharmacologic measures. Nonopioid and opioid medications may be initiated at low doses and carefully titrated based on changes in patients' responses. Doses may need to be increased until a therapeutic effect is seen, side effects are noted, or no benefit is noted despite all other adjustments (Herr et al., 2011; Herr et al., 2019). If the assessment indicates neuropathic pain may be present, a multimodal plan which includes neuropathic medications may be helpful (Herr et al., 2019). If pain behaviors do not improve with an empiric analgesic plan, other reasons for behaviors should be considered. If behaviors improve, the results of the analgesic trial may be used as the basis for the pain treatment plan.

Physiologic indicators of pain such as changes in blood pressure and heart rate are omitted from the hierarchy of pain assessment techniques because, although they may indicate adverse effects of severe pain, they are not valid for discriminating pain from other sources of distress (Gélinas, 2016). Often, clinicians in acute care settings expect to see vital sign changes when patients report severe pain or when assessing pain in critically ill patients who cannot give a pain report. However, a substantial number of studies in the early 2000s, many in patients in intensive care and emergency department settings, have failed to demonstrate a clear correlation between physiologic indicators and pain levels. For example, in a retrospective, observational study of 1063 adults who presented in triage at EDs with verifiable pain conditions such as renal calculi, fractures, crush injuries, and amputations, no clinically significant associations were found between self-reported pain scores and vital signs (Marco, Plewa, Buderer, Hymel, & Cooper, 2006). In a study of 105 postoperative cardiothoracic surgery patients in the ICU, patients were observed during three intervals (while unconscious and mechanically ventilated, conscious and mechanically ventilated, and after extubation) during a painful procedure and 20 minutes after the procedure (Arbour & Gélinas, 2010). The researchers in this study reported that vital signs did not consistently correlate with pain, and they recommended that vital signs be used only as cues to further assess pain, especially when behavioral indicators are not available (Arbour & Gélinas, 2010). In a more recent study of 125 postoperative patients in the intensive care unit (ICU) who underwent cardiac surgery who were assessed during painful (mediastinal tube removal) and nonpainful (noninvasive blood pressure measurement) procedures, vital signs were not found to be specific to pain (Boitor, Fiola, & Gélinas, 2016).

Vital sign changes are occasionally helpful, but, especially in critically ill patients, these measures are often influenced by factors other than pain, such as medications, mechanical ventilation, change in level of consciousness, and patients' illnesses or surgeries. In critically ill patients, behavioral indicators have been found to provide more valid information for pain assessment than physiologic indicators (Gélinas, 2016). Vital signs should only be used as indicators for the need for pain assessment.

Key Points

- Pain assessment is the foundation of an effective multimodal pain management plan.
- Pain assessment provides information needed for the classification of pain.
- Pain may be classified by location, duration, mechanism, and intensity.
- Acute pain is often protective and usually resolves within a predictable period.
- Chronic pain is complex and multidimensional and has a negative impact on the person's function and quality of life.
- The hierarchy of pain assessment is a useful tool in guiding the assessment of patients who cannot self-report pain.
- Behavioral signs of pain should not be relied on to refute or discredit the patient's report of pain, but may provide additional information to supplement the patient's self-report.
- Vital signs and other physiologic indicators are poor indicators of the presence or absence of pain, and should not be relied on to verify or refute the presence of pain. They may provide cues to indicate the need for assessment of pain.
- Clinicians need to be aware their own biases may lead to inaccurate assessments of patients' pain.
- Clinicians need to recognize and work to minimize patient, clinician, and system barriers that may have a negative impact on the accuracy of pain assessment.

Case Scenario

Mrs. R., a 76-year-old with early dementia with limited knowledge of English, was admitted to a medical floor for workup of severe abdominal pain with vomiting that began 2 days ago. She has had several admissions in the past 2 years for similar pain which resulted in lengthy admissions and detailed workups, without a definite diagnosis to explain the pain.

1. What questions need to be asked to determine the type of pain that Mrs. R. is experiencing?
2. How can the pain hierarchy be used to assess Mrs. R.?

3. What are the potential obstacles to the pain assessment for this patient?
4. What strategies can be used to engage other members of the health care team in the assessment and management of Mrs. R.'s pain?

References

Arbour, C., & Gélinas, C. (2010). Are vital signs valid indicators for the assessment of pain in postoperative cardiac surgery ICU adults? *Intensive and Critical Care Nursing*, 26(2), 83–90.

Arbour, C., & Gélinas, C. (2014). Behavioral and physiologic indicators of pain in nonverbal patients with a traumatic brain injury: An integrative review. *Pain Management Nursing*, 15(2), 506–518.

Baker, D. W. (2016). Statement on pain management: understanding how Joint Commission standards address pain. *Joint Commission Perspectives*, 36(6), 10–12.

Boitor, M., Fiola, J. L., & Gélinas, C. (2016). Validation of the Critical-Care Pain Observation Tool and vital signs in relation to the sensory and affective components of pain during mediastinal tube removal in postoperative cardiac surgery intensive care unit adults. *Journal of Cardiovascular Nursing*, 31(5), 425–432.

Booker, S. Q., & Herr, K. A. (2016). Assessment and measurement of pain in adults in later life. *Clinics in geriatric medicine*, 32(4), 677–692.

Centers for Medicare & Medicaid Services (CMS), HHS. (2016). Medicare Program: Hospital Outpatient Prospective Payment and Ambulatory Surgical Center Payment Systems and Quality Reporting Programs; Organ Procurement Organization Reporting and Communication; Transplant Outcome Measures and Documentation Requirements; Electronic Health Record (EHR) Incentive Programs; Payment to Nonexcepted Off-Campus Provider-Based Department of a Hospital; Hospital Value-Based Purchasing (VBP) Program; Establishment of Payment Rates Under the Medicare Physician Fee Schedule for . . . . *Federal register*, 81(219), 79562.

Chou, R., Gordon, D. B., de Leon-Casasola, O. A., Rosenberg, J. M., Bickler, S., Brennan, T., ... Griffith, S. (2016). Management of Postoperative Pain: a clinical practice guideline from the American Pain Society, the American Society of Regional Anesthesia and Pain Medicine, and the American Society of Anesthesiologists' committee on regional anesthesia, executive committee, and administrative council. *The Journal of Pain*, 17(2), 131–157.

Cohen, S. P., & Raja, S. N. (2016). In Lee Goldman & Andrew I. Schaefer (Eds.), *in Goldman-Cecil Medicine, Twenty-Fifth Edition*. Elsevier Saunders.

Coleman, R. M., Tousignant-Laflamme, Y., Ouellet, P., Parenteau-Goudreault, É., Cogan, J., & Bourgault, P. (2015). The use of the bispectral index in the detection of pain in mechanically ventilated adults in the intensive care unit: A review of the literature. *Pain Research and Management*, 20(1), e33–e37.

Cox, D. (2018). Pain taxonomy in M. Czarnecki & H. Turner (Eds.), *Pain Core Curriculum* (p. 84). St. Louis, MO: Elsevier

Crowe, M., Gillon, D., Jordan, J., & McCall, C. (2017). Older peoples' strategies for coping with chronic non-malignant pain: A qualitative meta-synthesis. *International Journal of Nursing Studies*, 68, 40–50.

Dequeker, S., Van Lancker, A., & Van Hecke, A. (2018). Hospitalized patients' vs. nurses' assessments of pain intensity and barriers to pain management. *Journal of Advanced Nursing*, 74, 160–171. https://doi.org/10.1111/jan.13395.

Dworkin, R. H., Bruehl, S., Fillingim, R. B., Loeser, J. D., Terman, G. W., & Turk, D. C. (2016). Multidimensional diagnostic criteria for chronic pain: introduction to the ACTTION–American Pain Society Pain Taxonomy (AAPT). *The Journal of Pain*, 17(9), T1–T9.

Eriksson, K., Wikström, L., Årestedt, K., Fridlund, B., & Broström, A. (2014). Numeric rating scale: patients' perceptions of its use in postoperative pain assessments. *Applied nursing research*, 27(1), 41–46.

Fillingim, R. B., Bruehl, S., Dworkin, R. H., Dworkin, S. F., Loeser, J. D., Turk, D. C., ... Freeman, R. (2014). The ACTTION-American Pain Society Pain Taxonomy (AAPT): an evidence-based and multidimensional approach to classifying chronic pain conditions. *The Journal of Pain*, 15(3), 241–249.

Gélinas, C. (2016). Pain assessment in the critically ill adult: recent evidence and new trends. *Intensive and Critical Care Nursing*, 34, 1–11. Available at http://www.sciencedirect.com.ezproxy.liberty.edu/science/article/pii/S0964339716000215.

Goulet, J. L., Brandt, C., Crystal, S., Fiellin, D. A., Gibert, C., Gordon, A. J., ... Justice, A. C. (2013). Agreement between electronic medical record-based and self-administered pain numeric rating scale: clinical and research implications. *Medical Care*, 51(3), 245.

Grégoire, M., Coll, M. P., Tremblay, M. P. B., Prkachin, K. M., & Jackson, P. L. (2016). Repeated exposure to others' pain reduces vicarious pain intensity estimation. *European Journal of Pain*, 20(10), 1644–1652.

Hadjistavropoulos, T., Herr, K., Prkachin, K. M., Craig, K. D., Gibson, S. J., Lukas, A., & Smith, J. H. (2014). Pain assessment in elderly adults with dementia. *The Lancet Neurology*, 13(12), 1216–1227.

Hadjistavropoulos, T., Herr, K., Turk, D. C., Fine, P. G., Dworkin, R. H., Helme, R., ... Chibnall, J. T. (2007). An interdisciplinary expert consensus statement on assessment of pain in older persons. *The Clinical Journal of Pain*, 23, S1–S43.

Harris, J., Ramelet, A. S., van Dijk, M., Pokorna, P., Wielenga, J., Tume, L., ... Ista, E. (2016). Clinical recommendations for pain, sedation, withdrawal and delirium assessment in critically ill infants and children: an ESPNIC position statement for healthcare professionals. *Intensive Care Medicine*, 42(6), 972.

Herndon, C. M., Arnstein, P., Darnall, B., Hartrick, C., Lyons, M., & Sehgal, N. (2016). *Principles of analgesic use*. Chicago, IL: *American Pain Society*.

Herr, K., Coyne, P. J., Ely, E., Gélinas, C., & Manworren, R. C. (2019). Pain assessment in the patient unable to self-report: clinical practice recommendations in support of the ASPMN 2019 position statement. *Pain Management Nursing*, 20(5), 404–417.

Herr, K., Coyne, P. J., McCaffery, M., Manworren, R., & Merkel, S. (2011). Pain assessment in the patient unable to self-report: position statement with clinical practice recommendations. *Pain Management Nursing*, 12(4), 230–250.

International Association for the Study of Pain. (2011). IASP taxonomy background. Available at https://www.iasp-pain.org/Education/Content.aspx?ItemNumber=2051&navItemNumber=576

Jensen, T. S., Baron, R., Haanpaa, M., Kalso, E., Loeser, J. D., Rice, A. S., et al. (2011). A new definition of neuropathic pain. *Pain, 152*(10), 2204-2205. doi:10.1016/j.pain.2011.06.017 [doi].

Joint Commission. (2017). R3 Report Issue 11: Pain assessment and management standards for hospitals. Available at https://www.jointcommission.org/-/media/tjc/documents/resources/patient-safety-topics/sentinel-event/r3_report_issue_11_pain_assessment_8_25_17_final.pdf?db=web&hash=-938C24A464A5B8B5646C8E297C8936C1

Kent, M. L., Tighe, P. J., Belfer, I., Brennan, T. J., Bruehl, S., Brummett, C. M., ... Edwards, D. (2017). The ACTTION–APS–AAPM Pain Taxonomy (AAAPT) multidimensional approach to classifying acute pain conditions. *Pain Medicine, 18*(5), 947–958.

La Cesa, S., Tamburin, S., Tugnoli, V., Sandrini, G., Paolucci, S., Lacerenza, M., ... Truini, A. (2015). How to diagnose neuropathic pain? The contribution from clinical examination, pain questionnaires and diagnostic tests. *Neurological Sciences, 36*(12), 2169–2175.

Manworren, R. C., & Stinson, J. (2016, August). Pediatric pain measurement, assessment, and evaluation. *Seminars in Pediatric Neurology, 23*(3), 189–200.

Marco, C. A., Plewa, M. C., Buderer, N., Hymel, G., & Cooper, J. (2006). Self-reported pain scores in the emergency department: lack of association with vital signs. *Academic Emergency Medicine, 13*(9), 974–979.

McCaffery, M. (1968). *Nursing Practice Theories Related to Cognition, Bodily Pain, and Man-environment Interactions.* Los Angeles, CA: University of California at Los Angeles Students' Store.

Olesen, J. (2014). Problem areas in the international classification of headache disorders. *Cephalalgia, 34*(14), 1193–1199.

Pergolizzi, J. V., Raffa, R. B., & Taylor, R. (2014). Treating acute pain in light of the chronification of pain. *Pain Management Nursing, 15*(1), 380–390.

Pierik, J. G., Ijzerman, M. J., Gaakeer, M. I., Vollenbroek-Hutten, M. M., & Doggen, C. J. (2017). Painful discrimination in the emergency department: Risk factors for underassessment of patients' pain by nurses. *Journal of Emergency Nursing, 43*(3), 228–238.

Pinho-Ribeiro, F. A., Verri, W. A., Jr., & Chiu, I. M. (2017). Nociceptor sensory neuron–immune interactions in pain and inflammation. *Trends in immunology, 38*(1), 5–19.

Puntillo, K. A., Max, A., Timsit, J. F., Vignoud, L., Chanques, G., Robleda, G., ... Ionescu, D. C. (2014). Determinants of procedural pain intensity in the intensive care unit. The Europain® study. *American Journal of Respiratory and Critical Care Medicine, 189*(1), 39–47.

Puntillo, K. A., Neuhaus, J., Arai, S., Paul, S. M., Gropper, M. A., Cohen, N. H., & Miaskowski, C. (2012). Challenge of assessing symptoms in seriously ill intensive care unit patients: can proxy reporters help? *Critical Care Medicine, 40*(10), 2760.

Puntillo, K. A., White, C., Morris, A. B., & Perdue, S. T. (2001). Patients' perceptions and responses to procedural pain: results from Thunder Project II. *American Journal of Critical Care, 10*(4), 238.

Radnovich, R., Chapman, C. R., Gudin, J. A., Panchal, S. J., Webster, L. R., Pergolizzi, J. V., Jr. (2014). Acute pain: effective management requires comprehensive assessment. *Postgraduate Medicine, 126*(4), 59–72.

Ronchetti, S., Migliorati, G., & Delfino, D. V. (2017). Association of inflammatory mediators with pain perception. *Biomedicine & Pharmacotherapy, 96*, 1445–1452.

Ruben, M. A., Blanch-Hartigan, D., & Shiperd, J. C. (2018). To know another's pain: a meta-analysis of caregivers' and healthcare providers' pain assessment accuracy. *Annals of Behavioral Medicine, 52*(8), 662–685. https://doi.org/10.1093/abm/kax036.

Ruben, M. A., van Osch, M., & Blanch-Hartigan, D. (2015). Healthcare providers' accuracy in assessing patients' pain: A systematic review. *Patient Education and Counseling, 98*(10), 1197–1206.

Schug, S. A., & Bruce, J. (2017). Risk stratification for the development of chronic postsurgical pain. *Pain Reports, 2*(6), e627.

Stone, J. B., & DeAngelis, L. M. (2016). Cancer-treatment-induced neurotoxicity—focus on newer treatments. *Nature Reviews Clinical Oncology, 13*(2), 92.

Vardeh, D., Mannion, R. J., & Woolf, C. J. (2016). Toward a mechanism-based approach to pain diagnosis. *The Journal of Pain, 17*(9), T50–T69.

Zeng, L., Alongkronrusmee, D., & van Rijn, R. M. (2017). An integrated perspective on diabetic, alcoholic, and drug-induced neuropathy, etiology, and treatment in the US. *Journal of Pain Research, 10*, 219.

Chapter 6 Pain Assessment in Cognitively Intact Adults

Maureen F. Cooney, Debra Drew

CHAPTER OUTLINE

Accurate Pain Assessment, pg. 73

Pain Assessment, pg. 73

   Mnemonics for use in Pain Assessment, pg. 76

Components of a Comprehensive Pain Assessment, pg. 76

   Physiologic and Sensory Aspects of Pain Assessment, pg. 76

   Pain Affect, pg. 80

   Psychosocial, pg. 80

   Cognition, pg. 80

   Sociocultural Factors, pg. 81

   Environmental Factors, pg. 81

   Context of Care, pg. 82

   Pertinent History, pg. 82

   Patient Goal, pg. 84

Conducting the Pain Assessment, pg. 84

   Assessment of Acute Pain, pg. 84

   Assessment of Chronic Pain, pg. 85

Tools for Assessing Pain, pg. 85

   Clinically Important Changes, pg. 90

   Unidimensional Pain Assessment Tools, pg. 91

   Multidimensional Pain Assessment Tools, pg. 94

   Neuropathic Pain Assessment, pg. 98

   Breakthrough Pain Assessment, pg. 102

Key Points, pg. 109

Case Scenario, pg. 109

References, pg. 109

Appendix 6-1, pg. 113

Appendix 6-2, pg. 119

Accurate Pain Assessment

Accurate pain assessment is the foundation for effective clinical care and research (Gordon, 2015). Assessment is an ongoing social transaction between the patient and health care professionals that is influenced by internal and external factors influencing both parties (Gordon, 2015). An accurate assessment of pain requires the use of good communication skills, a thorough history and physical examination, and a focus on the patient's description of the pain components. The routine assessment of pain is no longer an unfamiliar practice. In the past two decades, regulatory requirements of agencies such as the Centers for Medicare and Medicaid Services (CMS) and the Joint Commission have increased the awareness of the importance of pain assessment and reassessment. However, simply asking a patient for a pain score on a numerical pain rating (NPR) scale of 0 to 10 fails to provide enough information to guide the pain management plan of care. The health provider who shows willingness to listen and discuss the pain experience with the patient is more likely to obtain an accurate pain assessment, creating an environment in which the patient feels valued and satisfied with the pain care provided. This chapter will address the assessment of pain in patients who are cognitively intact and able to provide a pain self-report.

Pain Assessment

The timing and extent of the pain assessment is influenced by factors such as the patient condition, type, severity, location, duration of pain, and organizational requirements. For example, the patient who presents in the emergency department with severe, sharp upper abdominal pain requires a prompt and focused pain assessment to permit rapid treatment and diagnostic workup. If the same patient also has chronic, controlled low back pain, the assessment of the low back pain may need to be delayed until the acute pain issues are addressed. Likewise, a particular patient presenting in an outpatient setting for postoperative follow-up of an orthopedic procedure may have a more simple and focused assessment of postoperative pain than the patient in the neurology clinic who is being treated with a variety of interventions to address chronic daily migraines. The pain assessment content in this chapter is presented to offer guidance and a variety of tools for use in the assessment of pain, but the application of this content requires adaptation to the needs of the individual patient, available resources, clinical situation, and organization.

When a patient first presents to a health care setting, hospital, skilled nursing facility, outpatient clinic, or practice, the nurse usually completes an assessment of the patient, which, in addition to inquiring about medical and surgical history, medications, nutrition, and other elements, also includes a pain history and pain assessment. Once assured that the patient can communicate in English or an interpreter is provided, the assessment proceeds with determining if the patient is a good historian and able to report reliable information. If the patient is not able, the patient is also assessed for limitations in cognitive and sensory status, communication ability, and physical condition to determine whether modifications in the pain assessment are needed. For example, if vision, speech, or hearing are significantly impaired, the use of certain pain assessment tools may not be appropriate. It is necessary to address language barriers and provide pain assessment tools that are written in the patient's language. Elderly adults, in particular, require careful assessment for any deficits that may interfere with their abilities to provide an accurate self-report of pain.

In assessing pain in the cognitively intact patient, it is necessary to ensure that the patient understands the purpose of the assessment. At times, health care providers, for a variety of reasons, ask vague questions such as "How are you feeling today?" or "Are you comfortable?" to determine if the patient is having pain. These statements may not provide sufficient cues to elicit the report of pain because some patients may not understand what is being asked and others may respond with their usual socially appropriate response to such questions. Patients, especially older adults, may deny or minimize pain because they may fear that a pain report will result in additional testing and procedures and negative responses from care providers (Booker & Herr, 2016).

During the initial assessment, it is important to determine if pain is present or is an active problem for the patient, even if not present at the time of the assessment. If pain is a concern, further information is needed to identify whether pain is acute or chronic, or if the patient with acute pain also has underlying chronic pain. It is also necessary to determine whether pain is disease related, such as in cancer pain or pain related to sickle cell disease. In many clinical situations, an electronic or paper admission database contains a section for the documentation of the initial pain assessment. Examples of the information that may be included in the initial discussion of pain are shown in Table 6.1. When pain is an active problem, additional information may be useful, and a tool such as the Initial Pain

Table 6.1	Questions About Pain To Be Included in the Routine Nursing Admission Assessment
1. Do you have any ongoing pain problems?	___ Yes ___ No
2. Do you have pain now? If yes to either of the above:	___ Yes ___ No
3. Location of pain:	_____ (body figure drawing similar to the one in Form 6.1 may be included on the assessment form to mark the location of pain)
4. Pain intensity on a scale of 0 to 10:	Now: _____ On average (usual): _____
5. What, if any, medications do you take for pain relief?	
6. What, if any, other treatment do you receive for your pain?	
7. Is your pain satisfactorily controlled now?	___ Yes ___ No

NOTE: If a pain problem is identified and is not under satisfactory control, completion of a more comprehensive pain assessment tool may be indicated.

From Pasero, C., & McCaffery, M. (2011). Pain assessment and pharmacologic management (p. 50). St. Louis, MO: Mosby. © 2011, McCaffery M, & Pasero C. May be duplicated for use in clinical practice.

Assessment Tool (Form 6.1), may be used to guide and document the assessment process. Prioritization of the patient's needs may require a prompt and brief initial pain assessment. When feasible, a comprehensive pain assessment is completed for the patient with acute or poorly controlled chronic pain to aid in the development of an appropriate treatment plan. If pain is chronic and controlled, the goal of the assessment is to determine what pain management plan has been employed so it can be continued.

Because pain is dynamic, an ongoing assessment of pain is necessary. After the initial pain assessment, patients are subsequently assessed for changes in pain and response to pain interventions. Response to pain interventions includes assessment of efficacy, adverse effects, functionality, and overall response to treatment. The follow-up assessment is usually briefer than the initial comprehensive assessment and, in the acute care setting, more focused on the physiologic and sensory components of pain, which are described in a later section. The follow-up assessment usually includes the description of the pain, pain intensity, location, duration, and aggravating and alleviating factors.

Initial Pain Assessment Tool

Date _____

Patient's Name _____ Age _____ Room _____

Diagnosis _____ Physician _____

Nurse _____

1. LOCATION: Patient or nurse mark drawing.

2. INTENSITY: Patient rates the pain. Scale used _____

Present pain: _____   Worst pain gets: _____   Best pain gets: ____   Comfort-Function goal: _____

3. IS THIS PAIN CONSTANT? _____ YES; _____ NO
   IF NOT, HOW OFTEN DOES IT OCCUR? _____

4. QUALITY: (For example: ache, deep, sharp, hot, cold, like sensitive skin, sharp, itchy) _____

5. ONSET, DURATION, VARIATIONS, RHYTHMS: _____

6. MANNER OF EXPRESSING PAIN: _____

7. WHAT RELIEVES THE PAIN? _____

8. WHAT CAUSES OR INCREASES THE PAIN? _____

9. EFFECTS OF PAIN: (Note decreased function, decreased quality of life.)
   Accompanying symptoms (e.g., nausea) _____
   Sleep _____
   Appetite _____
   Physical activity _____
   Relationship with others (e.g., irritability) _____
   Emotions (e.g., anger, suicidal, crying) _____
   Concentration _____
   Other _____

10. OTHER COMMENTS: _____

11. PLAN: _____

Form 6.1 | Initial Pain Assessment Tool. May be completed by patients or used by clinicians to interview patients. (From Pasero, C., & McCaffery, M. [2011] *Pain assessment and pharmacologic management* [p. 51]. St. Louis, MO: Mosby. © 2011, Pasero C, & McCaffery M. May be duplicated for use in clinical practice.)

Mnemonics for use in Pain Assessment

Several memory aids have been developed to assist clinicians in remembering the various components of a comprehensive pain assessment as described in the previous sections. One tool is not necessarily better than another. These nonvalidated memory aids are only intended to guide the clinician to address the dimensions of a comprehensive pain assessment, but the mnemonics often lack the cues to assess the impact of pain on physical or emotional function or sleep (Gordon, 2015). Clinicians should decide which mnemonics are most appropriate for their practice and patient populations. Examples of some mnemonic tools are listed in Table 6.2.

Table 6.2	Examples of Mnemonic Tools for Comprehensive Pain Assessment
OPQRST	**O**nset
	Provocation or **P**alliation factors
	Quality of pain
	Region and **r**adiation
	Severity or associated symptoms
	Temporal factors/timing
SOCRATES	**S**ite(s)
	Onset
	Character
	Radiation
	Associations: any other signs or symptoms associated with the pain?
	Time course
	Exacerbating/relieving factors
	Severity
WILDA	**W**ords that describe pain
	Intensity
	Location
	Duration
	Aggravating/**A**lleviating factors
OLD CARTS P	**O**nset
	Location
	Duration
	Character
	Aggravating/relieving
	Radiation
	Timing
	Severity
	Prior pain experience

From Gordon, D. B. (2015). Acute pain assessment tools: Let us move beyond simple pain ratings. *Current Opinion Anesthesiology, 28,* 565–569.

Components of a Comprehensive Pain Assessment

The comprehensive assessment of pain includes a thorough history and physical examination, followed by appropriate laboratory work and diagnostic imaging, when appropriate, to identify the cause of the pain and develop an effective and individualized pain treatment plan. This is particularly important with acute pain, which signals the need to address the source of pain. However, despite extensive efforts to assess pain, particularly with chronic pain, it may not always be possible to identify the source (Dansie & Turk, 2013). Pain assessment is more than the recording of a simple intensity score (Pasero, Quinlan-Colwell, Rae, Broglio, & Drew, 2016). Although many providers and patients think of a pain assessment as asking the patient to rate pain on a numerical rating pain scale of 0 to 10, a pain rating (intensity) scale is only one component of the pain assessment and is intended to complement the other elements that comprise a complete assessment. For the adult who can self-report, there is opportunity to communicate the sensory component and the psychologic, social, cultural, and emotional elements of the pain experience (Finka, Gates, & Montgomery, 2015). More detail related to these components is provided in Chapters 5 and 8. Because pain is a subjective experience, self-report remains the gold standard for pain assessment (Fillingim, Loeser, Baron, & Edwards, 2016).

A comprehensive pain assessment reflects the complexity of the pain experience for each individual (Turk & Melzack, 2011; Finka et al., 2015). There are a number of factors to include: physiologic and sensory, affect, psychosocial, cognition, sociocultural, environmental, pertinent medical history, pharmacologic and nonpharmacologic interventions, and the patient's goals for managing the pain. Most patients and clinicians focus first on the physiologic or sensory aspect of pain because this aspect is often what drives the patient to seek help.

Physiologic and Sensory Aspects of Pain Assessment

Location

Have the patient identify the primary and secondary (if applicable) sites of pain. This can be accomplished by asking the patient to describe or point to the site of pain either on himself or herself, the clinician, or a body diagram such as the diagram on Form 6.1.

Intensity

This component is an attempt to quantify the pain at the present time and over a certain length of time. Pain intensity can be obtained only from the patient's self-report. Sensory intensity is the most commonly assessed aspect of pain and is used in a variety of clinical settings to determine pain level and the effectiveness of pain interventions. When obtaining a patient's report of pain intensity, it is common for the patient to report pain at the time of the assessment. However, because pain is dynamic, it is also important to ask about the fluctuation in pain intensity over time. For example, when assessing a patient 18 hours after surgery, it is helpful to ask what the worst and best pain intensity ratings have been over the time since surgery to determine whether pain is improving and responding to treatment. Likewise, in the primary care setting, when assessing the patient who presented a week earlier with an acute onset of low back pain, it is important to assess for changes in the patient's functional status and pain intensity, including changes in pain in response to analgesics and physical therapy. Each site of pain may have different levels or intensities of pain. For chronic pain, the intensity rating may not be as significant as other pain dimensions, such as functional impact. Many tools or scales have been developed to aid the patient in describing the intensity of pain. These tools are described and compared later in this chapter.

Onset and Duration (Temporal Aspects)

This dimension asks when the pain started, how long it has lasted, and whether it is constant or episodic. This temporal distinction helps determine if the pain is acute or chronic. Acute pain has traditionally been defined as pain lasting for 3 to 6 months, and if persisting beyond this time interval, it is then described as chronic pain (Flor & Turk, 2015). Chronic pain also has been distinguished from acute pain as pain that continues beyond the expected period of healing (Flor & Turk, 2015). When there is a specific event that triggered the pain, it is usually possible to predict the usual duration. However, when pain has an insidious onset, as often experienced in chronic conditions such as osteoarthritis, the duration may be difficult to determine. To determine duration when there is no clear precipitating event, patients may be able to recall if pain was present at particular occasions (e.g., start of the year, last birthday, major holiday). Variability of pain and its timing during the course of the day and night should be determined so that interventions can be targeted to modify and address pain when it heightens. Patients can be taught to optimize participation in activities during time intervals when pain is usually less or well controlled.

Asking what percentage of the day a person experiences pain is a helpful way to determine whether pain is constant or episodic. The assessment of the temporal dimension includes determining if there are episodes of breakthrough pain, experienced when there is a transient increase in pain that occurs either spontaneously or in relation to a specific trigger despite relatively stable and controlled background pain (Herndon et al., 2016; Webber, Davies, Zeppetella, & Cowie, 2014). Especially for chronic pain, a daily pain diary may be a useful tool

to aid in determining timing, as well as other dimensions of pain. The diary can be as simple as a paper and pencil recording of the time pain occurred and resolved over the course of the day or as sophisticated as the use of pain assessment applications (apps) on hand-held electronic devices (Reynoldson et al., 2014). Examples of paper pain control diaries can be found in Forms 6.2 and 6.3.

Quality

This information is helpful in distinguishing the type of pain the patient is experiencing: nociceptive (somatic or visceral), neuropathic, or mixed. The words the patient uses guide the clinician in diagnosis and treatment for a specific type of pain. Somatic pain (arising from bone, muscle, skin, joint, or connective tissue) is usually well localized and described as "aching" or "throbbing." Visceral pain (arising from the visceral organs) may manifest as "deep," "dull," "aching," "crushing," or "throbbing." Neuropathic pain (resulting from an abnormal processing of sensory input by the peripheral or central nervous systems) is described as "burning," "tingling," or "shooting." Mixed pain may involve descriptors of both nociceptive and neuropathic pain.

Aggravating and Alleviating Factors

Patients can often describe what worsens and mitigates the pain. This information can help identify the source of the pain and provide insight into functional limitations (Quinlan-Colwell, 2012). The clinician asks about prescription and over-the-counter medications, herbal preparations, dietary supplements, and the effects of each in addition to nonpharmacologic interventions that may have been tried. Heat and cold, massage, repositioning, distraction, and exercise are but a few of the interventions that patients may have found helpful. Interventions that have been effective should be continued unless contraindicated. Activities or conditions that aggravate the pain should be minimized or avoided.

Effects of Pain

This information will help determine the quality of life resulting from the pain experience. Does pain interfere with sleep or rest, fulfillment of social responsibilities, or mood? Whether acute or chronic pain, it is important to assess the impact of pain on the patient's ability to function to the extent necessary to facilitate recovery or engagement in activities that promote quality of life. A concept called pain interference may be thought of as a functional consequence of pain intensity (Cook et al., 2013). Evaluation of the impact of pain on the patient's ability to function is an important dimension of the pain assessment that should be included to guide clinical decision making (Herndon et al., 2016). For the patient with acute postoperative pain, the assessment might include observation of the patient's ability to use an incentive spirometer effectively or sit at the edge of the bed for

Pain Control Diary

This is a record of how your pain medicines are working. Please keep this record until you and your nurse/doctor find the dose and frequency of medicine that provides satisfactory pain relief for you most of the time. After that, you only need to keep this record when you have problems related to your pain medicines.

Name: _____ Date: _____

GOALS Satisfactory pain rating: _____ Activities: _____

Analgesics: _____

_____

My pain rating scale:

```
        ├──┼──┼──┼──┼──┼──┼──┼──┼──┼──┤
        0  1  2  3  4  5  6  7  8  9  10
```

No   Moderate   Worst
pain   pain   possible
                                               pain

Directions: Rate your pain before you take pain medicine and 1 to 2 hours later.

Time	Pain Rating	Pain Medicine I Took	Side Effects (drowsy? upset stomach?)	Other

If pain is greater than _____, or if you have other problems with your pain medicine, call:

Nurse: Name/phone _____

Pain Practitioner: Name/phone _____

Form 6.2 | Pain Control Diary. (From Pasero, C., & McCaffery M. [2011]. *Pain assessment and pharmacologic management* [p. 116]. St. Louis, Mosby. © 2011, Pasero C, McCaffery M. May be duplicated for use in clinical practice.)

Pain Control Diary: Patient Example

This is a record of how your pain medicines are working. Please keep this record until you and your nurse/doctor find the dose and frequency of medicine that provides satisfactory pain relief for you most of the time. After that, you only need to keep this record when you have problems related to your pain medicines.

Name: _____Martin_____ Date: _Friday_____

GOALS Satisfactory pain rating: __3__   Activities: _Sleep through the night; walk around the house___

Analgesics: _ibuprofen 400 mg 8 am, 2 pm, 8 pm; duloxetine 30 mg 8 am,_

8 pm; MS Contin 100 mg 8 am, 8 pm; MSIR 30 mg every 2 hours if needed.

My pain rating scale:

```
   |----|----|----|----|----|----|----|----|----|----|
   0    1    2    3    4    5    6    7    8    9   10
  No                    Moderate                 Worst
 pain                     pain                  possible
                                                  pain
```

Directions: Rate your pain before you take pain medicine and 1 to 2 hours later.

Time	Pain Rating	Pain Medicine I Took	Side Effects (drowsy? upset stomach?)	Other
12:15 am	6	30 morphine	No	
3	6	30 morphine		can't sleep
5:15	5	30 morphine		
8	6	30 morphine + ibuprofen + morphine SR 100 mg + duloxetine		staying in bed
10	5			talk with nurse
10:30	6	morphine 45 mg morphine SR 30 mg		
12:30 pm	3			planning to nap

If pain is greater than __5__ , or if you have other problems with your pain medicine, call:

Nurse: Name/phone ___C. Adams_____555-1234_____

Pain Practitioner: Name/phone _____Jones_____555-4321_____

Form 6.3 | Pain Control Diary: Patient Example. This patient has increasing pain resulting from metastasizing cancer. He has been receiving ibuprofen tid, duloxetine bid, morphine sustained-release bid. His breakthrough dose of short-acting morphine is 30mg po q2h prn. This plan relieved his pain to the level of 3 or less and met his goals of walking around his home and sleeping through the night uninterrupted by pain. This record reveals that his pain is no longer controlled. His pain ratings are now greater than 3, and pain awakens him at night. The patient talks with the nurse at 10 a.m., reads the diary, and says that this has happened for the past 2 days. The nurse contacts the prescriber, and the morphine doses are increased by 30% to 50% to 45mg of short-acting morphine q2h and 130mg of sustained-release morphine bid. From the previous prescription, the patient has sustained-release morphine tablets 30mg on hand, and the nurse instructs the patient to take one 30-mg tablet now along with short-acting morphine 45mg, which he does at 10:30 a.m. The entry at 12:30 p.m. shows that pain is reduced to the goal of 3, and the patient can sleep. Because of the increase in pain, the patient is instructed to make an appointment to see the prescriber the next day. (From Pasero, C., & McCaffery, M. [2011]. *Pain assessment and pharmacologic management* [p. 117]. St. Louis, MO: Mosby. © 2011, Pasero C, & McCaffery M. May be duplicated for use in clinical practice.)

a period. For the patient with chronic pain, the assessment would include determining the patient's ability to perform usual activities of daily living (ADLs) or engage in social activities that are of importance to the patient.

A number of comprehensive pain assessment tools include assessment of the effects of pain. The National Institutes of Health (NIH) Patient Reported Outcome Measurement Information System (PROMIS) project was developed to improve patient outcome measurement for clinical research across all NIH institutes (Kean et al., 2016). An outcome of this project was the development of a number of static, short form instruments designed to measure pain-related outcomes (Kean et al., 2016). One of the instruments, a short form (six item) tool, measures the interference of daily activities that pain can cause.

The items on the PROMIS short form include the following (Driban, Morgan, Price, Cook, & Wang, 2015):

- Day-to-day activities
- Work around the home
- Ability to participate in social activities
- Household chores
- Things one usually does for fun
- Enjoyment of social activities

This tool has been used in clinical practice and in research and can be downloaded from the NIH website. Tools for assessment of chronic pain that address the impact on function are described later in the chapter.

Pain Affect

Pain affect is the degree of emotional arousal caused by the experience of pain and the mental state triggered by an implicit or explicit perceived threat (Hemington et al., 2017; Turk & Melzack, 2011). Risk factors such as pain catastrophizing, anxiety, and depression strongly influence the pain experience (Hemington et al., 2017). Negative affective responses to pain, such as anxiety, fear, and anger may serve an initial protective function because they cause withdrawal from the painful stimulus. However, if these responses persist over time, they can lead to interference with ADLs and cause changes in habitual modes of response to pain and/or regulatory efficiency (Turk & Melzack, 2011), and they may be associated with chronic depression and other mood disorders (Finan & Garland, 2015). Conversely, positive affect, a state of positive mood or emotions resulting in contentment, relaxation, and peacefulness is associated with health benefits and may promote behaviors that improve self-management of chronic pain (Finan & Garland, 2015). Pain affect can be described as how unpleasant or disturbing the pain makes one feel; it can be measured using an NRS or visual analogue scale (VAS) in which the end-points of the scale range from "not at all unpleasant" to "most unpleasant feeling imaginable" (Fillingim et al., 2016). Usually, pain intensity and pain affect ratings are closely related, but at times they can be independent of each other (Fillingim

| **Box 6.1** | **"ACT-UP" Acronym for Psychosocial Assessment** |

1. Activities: How is your pain affecting your life (i.e., sleep, appetite, physical activities, and relationships)?
2. Coping: How do you deal/cope with your pain (what makes it better/worse)?
3. Think: Do you think your pain will ever get better?
4. Upset: Have you been feeling worried (anxious)/depressed (down, blue)?
5. People: How do people respond when you have pain?

From Dansie, E. J., & Turk, D. C. (2013). Assessment of patients with chronic pain. *British Journal of Anaesthesia, 111*(1), 19–25.

et al., 2016). Negative pain affect may play a role in the transition from acute to chronic pain (Hemington et al., 2017). It is important to assess affect and intensity to understand the nature of the pain experience and determine the appropriate focus of treatment.

Psychosocial

A comprehensive pain assessment should include an assessment of the common psychosocial factors that have an impact on and are affected by a patient's pain. A number of screening tools, such as the Hospital Anxiety and Depression Scale (HADS), are available to aid in assessing for the presence of anxiety and depression, which may have an impact on the patient with pain (Cho et al., 2013). The Patient Health Questionnaire (PHQ-2) is a two-item easily administered tool that was adapted from the longer, nine-item Patient Health Questionnaire (PHQ-9) (Lowe, Kroenke, Herzog, & Grafe, 2004). The PHQ-2 has been found to have validity and reliability in the initial screen for major depression (Manea et al., 2016). Another brief instrument consisting of four items, PROMIS, has been shown to be valid and reliable in identifying anxiety and depression in people with chronic pain (Kroenke, Yu, Wu, Kean, & Monahan, 2014). The acronym "ACT-UP" has been offered by Dansie and Turk (2013) as a tool to guide the psychosocial screening component of the pain assessment. The "ACT-UP" acronym is detailed in Box 6.1. Further information and additional tools related to the psychosocial assessment are provided in Chapter 8.

Cognition

The patient's knowledge, attitudes, and beliefs about pain will determine the meaning of the pain for that patient. That meaning will have an impact on the plan for managing the person's pain (Finka et al., 2015). The pain experience depends in part on how one feels, thinks, and behaves during a pain episode or exacerbation of pain (Flor & Turk,

2015). During the assessment, it is important to discuss the patient's understanding of pain so that information can be provided, misconceptions can be clarified, and providers will be better informed and more understanding of the patient's knowledge and values. For example, if a patient thinks that pain is a sign of vulnerability and weakness, it will be particularly important to anticipate pain, provide education about the negative consequences of unrelieved pain, and assist the patient to discuss feelings about pain so an acceptable treatment plan can be developed.

The assessment of cognition in the patient with chronic pain may be helpful; studies have shown that patients with chronic pain have decreased areas of cognitive function, thought to be related to neuroanatomic and neurochemical changes in the brain (Baker et al., 2017; Bushnell, Čeko, & Low, 2013; Coppieters et al., 2015). Recognition of the relationship between chronic pain and cognition is reflected in the use of cognitive-behavioral therapies as first-line psychosocial treatment for chronic pain management (Ehde, Dillworth, & Turner, 2014).

It is also important to recognize that pain may affect changes in cognition that occur acutely. Delirium is characterized by a sudden onset of cognitive decline, and pain is one of the predisposing factors for the development of delirium (Tahir & Mahajan, 2016). In a study of elderly patients without dementia who underwent elective orthopedic surgery, those with preoperative pain were found to have an increased risk for postoperative delirium (Kosar et al., 2014). Pain, lack of sleep, and physiologic disease are included among risk factors for the altered mental status (Finan, Goodin, & Smith, 2013; Patel, Baldwin, Bunting, & Laha, 2014). Chapter 7 addresses the pain assessment of cognitively impaired patients.

An assessment for changes in cognition should be included in the comprehensive pain assessment. Although a few comprehensive pain assessment tools, such as PROMIS, include items related to cognition, simple interview questions and involvement of family members in history-taking will often reveal cognitive gaps that may require referral for further assessment. However, sometimes family members are unable or reluctant to share concerns about their loved one's cognitive decline. The patient assessment should include observation and determination of the patient's mental status, including orientation level, ability to communicate, and ability to understand information that is provided.

Mental Status

The Mini-Mental State Examination (MMSE) is a tool that is commonly used in clinical practice to assess cognitive state. It is a brief tool used to screen for mild cognitive impairment, dementia, and delirium. In the cognitively intact person, the short battery of 20 individual tests takes 8 minutes for completion, but in those with dementia, it may take as long as 15 minutes (Mitchell, 2013). If the individual does not successfully complete the MMSE, referral for further evaluation of cognitive status is necessary.

Sociocultural Factors

A comprehensive pain assessment includes consideration of the impact of sociocultural factors. Sociocultural influences may contribute to biases and disparities that may have an impact on the patient's ability to receive adequate pain relief. Language, socioeconomic status, ethnicity, gender, social support, and ability to access health care are important factors to consider in the pain assessment. Health care providers must be mindful of their own sociocultural background and recognize the need to determine whether the patient's background is similar or different, to optimize objectivity in the assessment process. The physical and social environments have been found to affect the pain experience. The presence of social support has been associated with lower cardiac pain, labor pain, postoperative pain, and chronic pain (Bushnell et al., 2015). Socioeconomic conditions may affect a person's ability to access and participate in pain treatment programs such as physical or cognitive-behavioral therapies. (See Chapters 20 and 22 for additional information on this topic.)

Booker and Herr (2015) stress the importance of culturally valid self-report tools, especially for culturally diverse older adults. One cannot assume that a tool validated in English will automatically translate to a valid tool in another language. Nor can it be assumed that the meaning of a color depicting pain is valid from one culture to another. Recognizing that culture, language, gender, and age affect the validity of pain assessment tools, many researchers have examined different pain assessment tools in a variety of patient populations. When selecting pain assessment tools, it is important to consider whether the tools have been validated for use in the population that best represents the patients who are being assessed.

Health Literacy

In addition to other sociocultural factors, it is important to assess the health literacy of the patient. Health literacy is defined as "the capacity of an individual to obtain, interpret and understand basic health information and services in ways that are health enhancing" (Chinn & McCarthy, 2013, p. 247). It is important to understand what the patient knows and understands about his or her condition and how best to communicate with and educate the person. In a study of pain intensity in hospitalized patients and pain management barriers and facilitators, low health literacy was found to be one of the factors associated with higher pain intensity (Van Hecke et al., 2016). Health literacy is a significant factor that needs to be addressed in the assessment process and may also be considered in the selection of appropriate pain assessment tools.

Environmental Factors

Environmental factors include the setting in which the patient receives care and the context of care. The environment includes not only the physical environment in which the patient lives, but also the availability of support and resources in that environment. The patient's living arrangements may interfere with function and prevent adequate pain management. For example, the patient with severe osteoarthritis of the hips and knees who lives in a third-floor walk-up apartment is unlikely to leave the apartment and walk to stores or go for daily walks to maintain mobility. Environmental considerations include assessment of the availability of pharmacies that stock and dispense medications that are prescribed to treat pain. The accessibility of rehabilitation services is another environmental consideration.

Context of Care

In terms of the context of care, it is important to find out whether the stage of care is curative, chronic, or palliative. An understanding of the goals of care is needed, because this will affect the pain management plan of care. For the patient who is no longer receiving curative care, an understanding of the patient's wishes in terms of balancing pain, pain treatment side effects, and function is needed. The goals of care are often dynamic. Initially, function may be of great importance because the patient prefers to remain as active and physically engaged as possible. For others, at some point the goal may shift primarily to pain reduction as the focus on function may be lessened. In some cases, particularly near the end of life, measures to provide relief of pain and other symptoms become the main focus of care, even though the risk for adverse effects may increase. For example, near the end of life, the patient and loved ones may agree that the need for pain relief may outweigh concerns related to excessive sedation from opioids and other concomitant sedating medications. (See Chapter 2 for further discussion of the doctrine of double effect.)

Pertinent History

Medical History

Pertinent medical history for pain assessment includes a patient's state of health; disease process; past medical, surgical, and mental health histories (including any history of substance use disorders); medications (opioid naïve versus opioid tolerant); nonpharmacologic interventions; past painful experiences; and responses to interventions because these could affect the current pain experience and treatment plan. Chronic obstructive pulmonary disease, obstructive sleep apnea, and pulmonary or cardiac problems are important issues that need to be considered because they may increase risks for opioid-related respiratory depression if appropriate precautions are not exercised. More information on opioid-related respiratory depression is provided in Chapter 13. Renal or hepatic insufficiency affects the choice of analgesic medication and dosing that can be used for an individual patient. For example, morphine would likely be avoided in patients with renal disease to prevent accumulation of potentially toxic morphine

metabolites. Frequent surgeries may contribute to central pain–modulatory processes that increase sensitivity to pain (Edwards et al., 2013). Medications required for medical conditions must be known so that drug-drug interactions can be avoided. Chronic opioid use affects the choice of pain interventions, medications, and dosing.

Mental Health History

The patient history should also include any history of mental health problems. Psychiatric history needs to be included in a comprehensive pain assessment because psychological factors are known to influence, and be influenced by, acute and chronic pain. The importance of including a mental health history is illustrated by the findings that in patients who have undergone joint replacement surgeries, longitudinal studies have shown that the comorbidities of anxiety and depression are associated with more postoperative pain, higher analgesic use, more complications, and poorer functional outcomes (Edwards, Dworkin, Sullivan, Turk, & Wasan, 2016). Depression has been found to be associated with higher postoperative pain ratings and is a strong predictor of chronic postsurgical pain (Ghoneim & O'Hara, 2016). As addressed previously, tools are available to assist in screening for anxiety and depression. (See Chapter 8 for further discussion of this topic.)

Substance Use Disorder Risk and History

To safely and effectively care for patients in both the acute and chronic care settings, the patient assessment includes a determination of whether there is a history of current or past substance abuse and substance use disorders (SUDs), including alcohol, tobacco, opioids, cannabis, and other substances. When there is consideration for inclusion of opioids in the treatment plan, particularly for the management of pain in the outpatient setting, an assessment of the patient's risk for opioid use disorder (OUD) is needed. Some patients with OUD receive medication-assisted treatment with medications such as methadone, buprenorphine, or naltrexone. Medication reconciliation requires verification of these medications. Prescription monitoring program reports usually do not include methadone dispensed from an opioid treatment program (OTP) or naltrexone, so it is necessary to obtain permission to contact the OTP or the buprenorphine or naltrexone prescriber to ensure accurate medication reconciliation, appropriate pain interventions, and coordination of follow-up care (Savage, 2014). Chapter 14 provides in-depth content related to the topic of OUD; because this is an important component of patient assessment, salient points are included in this section.

The substance use history is needed to identify and intervene when patients are at risk for withdrawal. Those who are not appropriately treated for alcohol or benzodiazepine withdrawal may suffer life-threatening consequences. Opioid and other substance-related withdrawals can result in significant discomfort and physiologic complications. Given the rise in the use and misuse of opioids in recent years (Center for Behavioral Health Statistics and Quality, 2016), it is necessary to screen for possible opioid use and OUD to prevent withdrawal in the acute care setting.

Generally, withdrawal can occur 6 to 12 hours after the last dose of an immediate-release opioid, peak in 36 to 72 hours, and last about 5 days. For those taking opioids with longer half-lives, such as methadone, the onset of withdrawal may be 36 to 72 hours after the last use, and although the withdrawal symptoms may be less severe, the withdrawal can last much longer (Glue et al., 2016). To recognize and prevent opioid withdrawal, the use of a tool such as the Clinical Opioid Withdrawal Scale (COWS), shown as Form 6.4, may be helpful (Wesson & Ling, 2003).

Clinical Opiate Withdrawal Scale

For each item, circle the number that best describes the patient's signs or symptoms. Rate on just the apparent relationship to opiate withdrawal. For example, if heart rate is increased because the patient was jogging just prior to assessment, the increase pulse rate would not add to the score.

Patient's Name: _____   Date and Time ____ / ____ / ____: _____

Reason for this assessment: _____

Resting Pulse Rate: _____ beats/minute *Measured after patient is sitting or lying for one minute* 0 pulse rate 80 or below 1 pulse rate 81-100 2 pulse rate 101-120 4 pulse rate greater than 120	**GI Upset:** *Over last 1/2 hour* 0 no GI symptoms 1 stomach cramps 2 nausea or loose stool 3 vomiting or diarrhea 5 multiple episodes of diarrhea or vomiting
Sweating: *Over past 1/2 hour not accounted for by room temperature or patient activity* 0 no report of chills or flushing 1 subjective report of chills or flushing 2 flushed or observable moistness on face 3 beads of sweat on brow or face 4 sweat streaming off face	**Tremor:** *Observation of outstretched hands* 0 no tremor 1 tremor can be felt, but not observed 2 slight tremor observable 4 gross tremor or muscle twitching
Restlessness: *Observation during assessment* 0 able to sit still 1 reports difficulty sitting still, but is able to do so 3 frequent shifting or extraneous movements of legs/arms 5 unable to sit still for more than a few seconds	**Yawning:** *Observation during assessment* 0 no yawning 1 yawning once or twice during assessment 2 yawning three or more times during assessment 4 yawning several times/minute
Pupil size 0 pupils pinned or normal size for room light 1 pupils possibly larger than normal for room light 2 pupils moderately dilated 5 pupils so dilated that only the rim of the iris is visible	**Anxiety or Irritability** 0 none 1 patient reports increasing irritability or anxiousness 2 patient obviously irritable or anxious 4 patient so irritable or anxious that participation in the assessment is difficult
Bone or Joint aches: *If patient was having pain previously, only the additional component attributed to opiate withdrawal is scored* 0 not present 1 mild diffuse discomfort 2 patient reports severe diffuse aching of joints/muscles 4 patient is rubbing joints or muscles and is unable to sit still because of discomfort	**Gooseflesh skin** 0 skin is smooth 3 piloerection of skin can be felt or hairs standing up on arms 5 prominent piloerection
Runny nose or tearing: *Not accounted for by cold symptoms or allergies* 0 not present 1 nasal stuffiness or unusually moist eyes 2 nose running or tearing 4 nose constantly running or tears streaming down cheeks	**Total Score** _____ The total score is the sum of all 11 items Initials of person completing assessment: _____

Score: 5-12 = mild; 13-24 = moderate; 25-36 = moderately severe; more than 36 = severe withdrawal

Form 6.4 | Clinical Opiate Withdrawal Scale. (From Wesson, D. R., & Ling W. [2003]. The Clinical Opiate Withdrawal Scale (COWS). *Journal of Psychoactive Drugs, 35,* 253–259. Form is on p. 259.)

It is also necessary to screen for OUD to prevent inadequate pain treatment resulting from underdosing of opioids during an acute pain event. Sometimes clinicians assume that patients with OUD who report higher than expected pain scores are attempting to obtain more opioids to satisfy their cravings. However, the higher pain scores are often due to complex and poorly understood physiologic processes that occur in those who are tolerant from prescribed opioid use or those who are actively using opioids illicitly. These patients often report higher pain scores, require more postoperative opioids, and use more anxiolytics than opioid-naïve individuals (Eyler, 2013).

An opioid risk assessment may be included in the pain assessment if opioids may be part of the pain treatment plan, especially if opioids will be needed after hospitalization. In conducting the risk assessment, it is necessary to first establish a rapport with the patient because the patient may be reluctant to report a history of substance abuse, especially when past disclosure resulted in untreated pain (St. Marie, 2014). Patients and clinicians are often uncomfortable with discussions related to substance abuse. To facilitate disclosure, start the assessment with questions related to tobacco or alcohol use and further explain that these assessments aid the clinician to provide safe pain management (Walsh & Broglio, 2016).

A number of opioid risk screening tools have been developed to screen for increased risk for opioid misuse when prescribing opioids for chronic pain. These tools are screening tools, not diagnostic tools, and they have not been validated for use in the acute care setting. The purpose of these screening tools is to identify patients at increased risk so that appropriate precautions may be taken, especially if chronic opioids will be required. (More detailed information on opioid risk screening and screening tools is provided in Chapter 14.)

Patient Goal

It is important for the patient, family, and health care providers to understand that an assessment of pain is only the first step in the process of addressing pain. Another important action is to determine pain relief goals. Establishing a patient goal should include not only a comfort goal (diminishing of pain intensity or other bothersome symptoms) but also functional goals (Pasero & McCaffery, 2011). The concept of identifying a comfort goal is often difficult for a person to grasp. It is not realistic for most patients to have a comfort goal of "no pain." To strive for a goal of a zero on the NRS might incorrectly suggest treatment failure, significantly increase the patient's

risk for opioid-related side effects, or set the patient up for dissatisfaction with care because that goal might not be achievable. Further clarification of the comfort goal is necessary. Discussion could include identification of a pain level that would be acceptable to the patient, permit distraction from the pain, and not interfere with concentration or ability to engage in activity or interactions that are important to the patient. Pain's effect on functional status is gaining acceptance as an important outcome measure and guide for clinical decision-making (Backonja & Farrar, 2015; Gordon, 2015). For postsurgical patients, the goals may include the ability to breathe deeply with minimal discomfort, walk to the bathroom, and participate in physical therapy. Patients with persistent/chronic pain may strive for ability to increase involvement in self-care or return to work.

Conducting the Pain Assessment

Assessment of Acute Pain

Different tools are appropriate for use in research or in the assessment of acute pain in clinical settings. Acute pain tools need to be simple and easy for the clinician and the patient to use. It is important to teach the patient and ensure that the patient is able to understand and use the tool that has been selected. Box 6.2 provides guidance in teaching patients and families how to use a pain rating scale. Unidimensional assessment tools (e.g., measuring only pain intensity) allow quick initial assessments and reassessments. They also can assist in making appropriate clinical decisions about the pain management plan. Several acute, unidimensional pain assessment tools are described later in the text and further detailed in Table 6.3.

Unfortunately, the simple tools often used in acute pain assessment are unidimensional, measuring just pain intensity. They fail to capture the complexity of the pain experience and do not address all the dimensions of pain described in a comprehensive pain assessment (Cook et al., 2013). There is a lack of reliable and validated acute pain assessment tools to guide a brief, but more comprehensive, assessment of acute pain. Gordon (2015) implores clinicians to start thinking about the limitations of acute pain assessment tools that simply measure pain intensity. She reminds us that pain assessment should be considered an ongoing process, rather than simply a tool with pain intensity scores. Multidimensional tools are often not used in the assessment of acute pain because of the time it would take to complete the assessment. However, some simpler multidimensional tools such as the Clinically Aligned Pain Assessment (CAPA) tool (Topham & Drew, 2017), which is described later in the chapter, may be considered in the assessment of acute pain because it is brief, easy to use, and permits the assessment of more than just pain intensity.

Assessment of Chronic Pain

The assessment of chronic pain must address the many dimensions of pain, including the sensory and affective components, location and distribution, and temporal aspects. Because pain is a complex, dynamic, multidimensional phenomena, efforts must be taken to ensure that the patient and health care provider are able to interact in a way that will aid the patient to express the meaning of pain and the physical, psychosocial, cultural, and environmental factors that influence the pain experience. An assessment of the impact of chronic pain on psychological functioning, mood, and quality of life is necessary (Fillingim et al., 2016). The impact of chronic pain on function includes both an assessment of physical function, or the ability to perform ADLs, and the ability to function in a designated role (Dansie & Turk, 2013). For example, the person who lives with chronic pain may be able to carry out usual self-care activities but may be unable to work as an accountant because the pain and the medications interfere with cognition.

Tools used for chronic pain assessment should be valid, reliable, and comprehensive to address the multiple dimensions affected by chronic pain. Many of the multidimensional tools incorporate elements of the unidimensional tools to assess pain intensity but also include items related to the other pain dimensions. Table 6.4 summarizes some of the tools used in the assessment of chronic pain. In assessing chronic pain, it is important to remember that the patient may become easily fatigued. It may be necessary to use tools with fewer items, or pace the assessment so the patient is able to fully participate. Some of the frequently used multidimensional tools are described in subsequent paragraphs.

Tools for Assessing Pain

Pain rating scales and tools are used in clinical practice to aid in pain assessment and determine the effectiveness of pain management interventions and changes in pain over time. There are many different pain tools available for both acute and chronic pain assessment. A quick search of the internet will yield numerous results. Despite the temptation to use some of these scales because they seem easy to use and have eye-catching colors and graphics, it is important to use scales or tools that have been tested and found to have strong reliability and validity. Reliability means that a scale has been tested and shown to produce consistent and stable results (Heale & Twycross, 2015). For example, a pain intensity scale is shown to be reliable if, when tested, it consistently measures pain intensity from one time to the next. Validity means that the tool has been tested and shown to measure that which it is intended to measure (Heale & Twycross, 2015). For pain intensity scales, it is important to select scales that are responsive to change and have shown strong ability to detect changes in the magnitude of pain. For example, a scale used to assess acute pain should be able to measure the effects of an analgesic medication. Another important consideration is to choose scales that have been shown to have validity in similar patient populations. A scale that has been validated in a population of elderly adults with osteoarthritis may not be valid for use in young adults with acute postoperative pain.

When selecting pain scales, select scales, when possible, that are culturally appropriate for the patient population and in the patient's native language. Many scales that are available on the internet have been tested in a variety of cultures and correctly interpreted into different languages. It is best to have scales that are inexpensive and easy to score and interpret. The electronic record (EMR) offers opportunities to improve the use of pain scales. When building EMR screens, it is necessary to consider the ways in which pain scales are incorporated into the EMR and the ease in which results are made visible to the caregivers. The EMR can be a helpful tool to ensure that pain scores and other assessment data are easily retrieved by clinicians. Additionally, the EMR data can be used to track a patient's pain score trajectory and pattern over time, or even access de-identified data for quality improvement purposes to benchmark and trend how well pain is managed in a particular setting.

Effective pain scales are those that are easily explained and understood by patients and clinicians. Table 6.5 summarizes pain tools that may be used by older adults as alternatives to other self-report tools that may not be easily understood. Preferred scales are brief and do not take more than a couple of minutes for completion. When appropriate, scales can be visible to optimize patients' understanding of them. They can be laminated for placement at the bedside; copied and distributed on paper; incorporated into patient education handouts; displayed on white boards, posters, or monitor screens; or accessible on bedside tablets. When preparing scales for display, do not embellish or label the scale in any way, such as including colors or adding graphics, because this will change the reliability and validity of the scale. Other considerations for the use of pain rating scales are summarized in Box 6.3.

Box 6.2 | Teaching Patients and Their Families How to Use a Pain Rating Scale

Step 1. Show the pain rating scale to the patient and family and explain its primary purpose.

Example: "This is a pain rating scale that many of our patients use to help us understand their pain and to set goals for pain relief. We will ask you regularly about pain, but any time you have pain you must let us know. We don't always know when you hurt."

Step 2. Explain the parts of the pain rating scale. If the patient does not like it or understand it, switch to another scale (e.g., vertical scale, FACES).

Example: "On this pain rating scale, 0 means no pain and 10 means the worst possible pain. The middle of the scale, around 5, means moderate pain. A 2 or 3 would be mild pain, but 7 and higher means severe pain."

Step 3. Discuss pain as a broad concept that is not restricted to a severe and intolerable sensation.

Example: "Pain refers to any kind of discomfort anywhere in your body. Pain also means aching and hurting. Pain can include pulling, tightness, burning, knifelike feelings, and other unpleasant sensations."

Step 4. Verify that the patient understands the broad concept of pain.

Ask the patient to mention two examples of pain he or she has experienced.

If the patient is already in pain that requires treatment, use the present situation as the example.

Example: What to say if the patient is not in significant pain: "I want to be sure that I've explained this clearly, so would you give me two examples of pain you've had recently?"

If the patient's examples include various parts of the body and various pain characteristics, that indicates that he or she understands pain as a fairly broad concept.

Example: The patient might say, "I have a mild, sort of throbbing headache now, and yesterday my back was aching."

Step 5. Ask the patient to practice using the pain rating scale with the present pain or to select one of the examples mentioned.

Examples: "Using the scale, what is your pain right now?" "What is it at its worst?" Or "Using the pain rating scale and one of your examples of pain, what is that pain usually?" "What is it at its worst?"

Step 6. Set goals for comfort and function/recovery. Ask patients what pain rating would be acceptable or satisfactory, considering the activities required for recovery or for maintaining a satisfactory quality of life. (Research strongly suggests that pain rating goals of 4 or more on a scale of 0 to 10 are not appropriate.)

Example: For a surgical patient: "I have explained the importance of coughing and deep breathing to prevent pneumonia and other complications. Now we need to determine the pain rating that will not interfere with this so that you may recover quickly. If you're not sure, you can guess, and we can change it later."

Example: For a patient with chronic pain or a terminally ill patient: "What do you want to do that pain keeps you from doing? What pain rating would allow you to do this?"

Table 6.3 | Comparison of Tools Commonly Used in Acute Pain Assessment

Tool	Indications	Validity/Reliability	Advantages	Disadvantages
Visual analogue scale (VAS)	Cognitively intact adults Research studies	Reliability is lower in illiterate patients (Hawker et al., 2011). Positive correlation with other self-reported measures of pain intensity (Seng, Kerns, & Heapy, 2014). Inconsistent use of anchor words may result in different patient responses.	Ratio level data with a high number of response categories make it sensitive to small changes in pain intensity.	Preprinted tools, a marking instrument, and measuring instrument are necessary. Horizontal orientation of tool produces slightly lower scores than vertically oriented tools (Hawker et al., 2011). Cognitively impaired elders make mistakes with this tool (Peters, Patijn, & Lame, 2007) Reproducibility is poor for patients with cognitive impairment, non-English speakers, immobility, and reduced visual acuity.
Verbal descriptor scale (VDS)	Literate, English speakers do better than non-literate, non-English speakers.	Validity established (Seng et al., 2014)	Some patients prefer words to numbers to describe pain intensity. Administration is either verbal or visual. Scale is quick, simple, easy to score.	Patient forced to choose a word to indicate pain intensity even if no word matches the patient's experience. Some word descriptors may be associated with affective distress rather than pain. Tool measures an ordinal scale, but the distances between descriptors are not equal, rather they are categorical.
Numerical rating scale (NRS)	Cognitively intact patients who can express pain intensity with use of an ordinal scale.	Valid, but poor reproducibility probably because of variability in use of anchor wording (Williamson & Hoggart, 2005).	Most responsive of four tools studied (Ferreira-Valente, Pais-Ribeiro, & Jensen, 2011). Applicable in most settings (Hjermstad et al., 2011). Can be administered verbally and visually. Easy to score.	Measures only pain intensity. Many patients have difficulty expressing their complex experience with a simple number. Clinicians vary the wording for the extreme pain anchor "10" (e.g., "Pain as bad as you've ever experienced" versus "Worst pain imaginable." "Scores cannot necessarily be treated as ratio data" (Jensen & Karoly, 2011, p. 28).
FACES Pain Scale-Revised (FPS-R)	Patients with ability to think abstractly.	Valid as measure of pain intensity (Ferreira-Valente et al., 2011).	More usable with adults.	Patients with diminished visual acuity may have difficulties. May measure constructs other than pain intensity and requires abstract thinking ability (Hadjistavropoulos et al., 2007).
Iowa Pain Thermometer	Developed for research, but can be used in clinical settings.	Valid and reliable tool especially in older adults (Herr, 2011).	Can be used with patients of varying levels of cognition. Some patients prefer this tool to NRS (Ware et al., 2015).	Utility in clinical settings may be limited because it uses a 13-point scale (0–12) and may not align with other common electronic scoring measures.

Continued

Table 6.3 | Comparison of Tools Commonly Used in Acute Pain Assessment—cont'd

Tool	Indications	Validity/Reliability	Advantages	Disadvantages
Clinically Aligned Pain Assessment (CAPA) tool	Any adult who can converse with clinician.	Although valid for clinical management, tool has not been validated for research in clinical studies. Author recommends use of nonparametric tests, such as Wilcoxon or Mann-Whitney test (G. Donaldson, personal communication, January 23, 2014).	No tools needed for patient. No selection of words or numbers. Uses a conversational approach. In addition to pain intensity, the tool's focus on pain's effects on functional status and sleep, helps clinical decision making.	Some clinicians prefer simplicity of obtaining a simple pain intensity score. Complete tool may not be pertinent for assessing patients who have not received any pain management intervention.

Ferreira-Valente, M. A., Pais-Ribeiro, J. L., & Jensen, M. P. (2011). Validity of four pain intensity rating scales. *Pain, 152*(10), 2399–2404; Hadjistavropoulos, T., Herr, K., Turk, D. C., Fine, P. G., Dworkin, R. H., Helme, R., . . . & Chibnall, J. T. (2007). An interdisciplinary expert consensus statement on assessment of pain in older persons. *The Clinical Journal of Pain, 23,* S1–S43; Hawker, G. A., Mian, S., Kendzerska, T., & French, M. (2011). Measures of adult pain: Visual analog scale for pain (VAS pain), numeric rating scale for pain (NRS pain), McGill Pain Questionnaire (MPQ), short-form McGill Pain Questionnaire (SF-MPQ), chronic pain grade scale (CPGS), short form-36 bodily pain scale (SF-36BPS), and measure of intermittent and constant osteoarthritis pain (ICOAP). *Arthritis Care & Research, 63*(S11), S240–S252; Herr, K. (2011). Pain assessment strategies in older adults. *The Journal of Pain, 12*(Suppl. 1), S3–S13; Hjermstad, M. J., Fayers, P. M., Haugen, D. F., Caraceni, A., Hanks, G. W., Loge, J. H., . . . & Kaasa, S. (2011). Studies comparing numerical rating scales, verbal rating scales, and visual analogue scales for assessment of pain intensity in adults: A systematic literature review. *Journal of Pain and Symptom Management, 41*(6), 1073–1093; Jensen, M. P., & Karoly, P. (2011). In D. C. Turk & R. Melzack (Eds.), *Handbook of pain assessment* (3rd ed., pp. 19–41). New York, NY: The Guilford Press; Peters, M. L., Patijn, J., & Lamé, I. (2007). Pain assessment in younger and older pain patients: psychometric properties and patient preference of five commonly used measures of pain intensity. *Pain Medicine, 8*(7), 601–610. Seng, E., Kerns, R. D., & Heapy, A. (2014). Psychological and behavioral assessment. In H. Benzon, J. Rathmell, C. Wu, D. Turk, C. Argoff, & R. Hurley (Eds.), *Practical management of pain* (5th ed., pp. 243–256). Philadelphia, PA: Mosby; Ware, L. J., Herr, K. A., Booker, S. S., Dotson, K., Key, J., Poindexter, N., . . . & Packard, A. (2015). Psychometric evaluation of the revised Iowa Pain Thermometer (IPT-R) in a sample of diverse cognitively intact and impaired older adults: A pilot study. *Pain Management Nursing, 16*(4), 475–482; and Williamson, A., & Hoggart, B. (2005). Pain: A review of three commonly used pain rating scales. *Journal of Clinical Nursing, 14,* 798–804.

Table 6.4 | Pain Assessment Tools for Chronic and Persistent Pain

Tool	Indications	Validity/Reliability	Advantages	Disadvantages
McGill Pain Questionnaire (MPQ)	Assessment of chronic pain. Generally used in outpatient settings.	Validity and reliability examined in various contexts and different patient populations (Main, 2016). SF-MPQ is valid and reliable tool (Dworkin et al., 2008).	SF-MPQ takes 2–5 min to complete, and the word choices are not as complex as in the MPQ. The intensity ranking of mild, moderate, and severe is more easily understood by patients.	Patients require a rich vocabulary to complete the MPQ tool. The long form takes 30 min to complete. Clinician availability is needed to help patients having trouble with both the longer and shorter versions of the tool.
Chronic pain grade scale (CPGS)	All musculoskeletal and low back pain.	Valid and reliable (Hawker et al., 2011).	Multidimensional tool.	Complexity of scoring. It is less useful for assessment of pain at point of care.
Short Form-36 Bodily Pain Scale (SF-36BP)	Patients who can fill out questionnaires.	Valid and reliable (Hawker et al., 2011).	Generally easy to administer and complete. Useful in making comparisons across populations for research purposes.	At point of care, a disease-specific pain measure may be more useful.

Table 6.4 | Pain Assessment Tools for Chronic and Persistent Pain—cont'd

Tool	Indications	Validity/Reliability	Advantages	Disadvantages
Brief Pain Inventory (BPI)	Patient who is able to understand the instructions within the tool's items.	Valid and reliable in a variety of clinical settings (Pasero & McCaffery, 2011).	Has been translated into several languages. Includes a body diagram for location of pain(s).	Takes 10–15 min to complete. Patients must be able to understand the instructions in each item.
Defense and Veterans Pain Rating Scale 2.0 (DVPRS)	Patient with pain who is able to understand and respond to the questions in this tool.	Valid and reliable but psychometric testing on this tool only occurred with one assessment of pain and related outcomes in military and veteran inpatients and outpatients (Polomano et al., 2016).	Promotes a dialogue about pain between provider and patient. Translated into Spanish and Vietnamese.	Links functional verbal descriptors with numerical pain intensity, although correlation between these variables has not been established.
PEG Scale	For chronic pain in patients who can understand the questions in this tool.	Validated for use in Veterans Administration ambulatory care settings (Polomano et al., 2016).	Ultra-brief and easy to use and score. Contains only three items.	Validation in other patient populations would be helpful.

Dworkin, R. H., Turk, D. C., Wyrwich, K. W., Beaton, D., Cleeland, C. S., Farrar, J. T., . . . & Kaatz, N. P. (2008). Interpreting the clinical importance of treatment outcomes in chronic pain clinical trials: IMMPACT recommendations. *The Journal of Pain, 9*(2), 105–121; Hawker, G. A., Mian, S., Kendzerska, T., & French, M. (2011). Measures of adult pain: Visual analog scale for pain (VAS pain), numeric rating scale for pain (NRS pain), McGill Pain Questionnaire (MPQ), short-form McGill Pain Questionnaire (SF-MPQ), chronic pain grade scale (CPGS), short form-36 Bodily Pain Scale (SF-36BPS), and measure of intermittent and constant osteoarthritis pain (ICOAP). *Arthritis Care & Research, 63*(S11), S240–S252; Main, C. J. (2016). Pain assessment in context: A state of the science review of the McGill Pain Questionnaire 40 years on. *Pain, 157*(7), 1387–1399; Pasero, C., & McCaffery, M. (2011). *Pain assessment and pharmacologic management.* St. Louis, MO: Mosby; Polomano, R. C., Galloway, K. T., Kent, M. L., Brandon-Edwards, H., Kwon, K. N., Morales, C., & Buckenmaier III, C. T. (2016). Psychometric testing of the defense and veterans pain rating scale (DVPRS): A new pain scale for military population. *Pain Medicine, 17*(8), 1505–1519.

Table 6.5 | Pain Intensity Tools Recommended for Use With Older Adults Who Have Difficulty With Commonly Used Self-Report Scales

Name of Measure	Reliability	Validity/Utility
Verbal Descriptor Scales (VDS), such as Iowa Pain Thermometer, or none, mild, moderate, or severe (Closs et al., 2004; Herr et al., 2007; Taylor et al., 2005)	Adequate test-retest reliability in the cognitively intact ($r = 0.67$) and those with cognitive impairment ($r = 0.50$)	Tested in acute care, nursing home, assisted-living facility, and outpatient clinic Strong positive correlation with other pain intensity scales Validated in white and African American samples Preferred by older adults, with low failure rate even in the cognitively impaired Thermometer adaptation may assist with understanding of tool Easy to explain
FACES Pain Scale–Revised FPS-R (Li, Liu, & Herr, 2007; Miro et al., 2005; Ware et al., 2006)	Acceptable to high test-retest reliability in the cognitively intact ($r = 0.62–0.89$); decreased in those with cognitive impairment ($r = 0.26–0.67$)	FPS-R tested in acute care and community dwelling; FPS tested in subacute care, pain clinic, long-term care, assisted living facility Less strong positive correlation with other pain intensity scales; may represent more than intensity Validated in white, African American, Spanish, and Chinese FPS-R preferred by many older adults; most preferred by African American, Spanish, and Asian older adults Does not require language or reading ability

As appears in Pasero, C., & McCaffery, M. (2011). *Pain assessment and pharmacologic management* (p. 96). St. Louis, MO: Mosby. © 2011, Pasero C, & McCaffery M. May be duplicated for use in clinical practice. From Closs, S. J., Barr, B., Briggs, M., Cash, K., & Seers, K. (2004). A comparison of five pain assessment scales for nursing home residents with varying degrees of cognitive impairment. *J Pain Symptom Manage, 27*, 196–205; Herr, K., Spratt, K., Garand, L., Li, L. (2007); Evaluation of the Iowa pain thermometer and other selected pain intensity scales in younger and older adult cohorts using controlled clinical pain: A preliminary study. *Pain Medicine, 8*(7), 585–600. Li, L., Liu, X & Herr, K. (2007). Postoperative pain intensity assessment: A comparison of four scales in Chinese adults. *Pain Medicine, 8*(3), 223–234; Miró, J., Huguet, A., Nieto, R., Paredes, S., & Baos, J. (2005). Evaluation of reliability, validity, and preference for a pain intensity scale for use with the elderly. *The Journal of Pain, 6*(11), 727–735; Taylor, L. J., Harris, J., Epps, C. D., & Herr, K. (2005). Psychometric evaluation of selected pain intensity scales for use with cognitively impaired and cognitively intact older adults. *Rehabilitation Nursing, 30*, 55–61; Ware, L. J., Epps, C., Herr, K., & Packard, A. (2006). Evaluation of the Revised Faces Pain Scale, verbal descriptor scale, numeric rating scale, and Iowa Pain Thermometer in older minority adults. *Pain Management Nursing, 7*(3), 117–125.

| **Box 6.3** | Selecting a Pain Rating Scale for Use in Daily Clinical Practice |

Research has established that the tool is:

- Reasonably valid and reliable.
- Developmentally appropriate. Some scales commonly used with adults (e.g., a scale of 0–10) are clearly inappropriate for use with children who cannot count. On the other hand, some scales, such as the FACES Pain Scale-Revised (FPS-R), that are appropriate for young children may be appropriate for any age group, especially cognitively impaired patients.
- Easily and quickly understood by patients who have minimal formal education.
- Brief, easily completed in no more than 2–5 minutes
- Well-liked by patients.
- Well-liked by clinicians.
- Not burdensome on clinicians.
- Quickly explained.
- Easily scored and recorded.
- Easily used with patients to set pain management goals (i.e., comfort-function goals).

- Inexpensive.
- Easily disinfected (or inexpensive enough to discard, e.g., scales that are photocopied).
- Readily available. Multiple copies are easily and inexpensively made for distribution to clinicians, patients, and their families. Easily downloaded from the internet.
- Appropriate for patients of different cultures.
- Available in various languages spoken in the clinical setting (or may be translated easily).

As appears in Pasero, C., & McCaffery, M. (2011). *Pain assessment and pharmacologic management* (p. 54). St. Louis, MO: Mosby. Modified from Hester, N. O. (1995). Integrating pain assessment and management into the care of children with cancer. In D. B. McGuire, C. H. Yarbro, & B. R. Ferrell (Eds.), *Cancer pain management.* Boston, MA: Jones and Bartlett; and Kroenke, K., Monahan, P. O., & Kean, J. (2015). Pragmatic characteristics of patient-reported outcome measures are important for use in clinical practice. *Journal of Clinical Epidemiology, 68*(9), 1085–1092. May be duplicated for use in clinical practice.

Clinically Important Changes

In interpreting patient responses to pain intensity ratings, it is necessary to understand the significance of changes in pain ratings. Especially when titrating analgesic medications, it is helpful to know the extent of change in a pain score that provides meaningful relief. Studies have been done on a number of pain scales, in patients with acute and/or chronic pain, to determine the degree of reduction in pain score that would represent a statistically significant decrease in pain intensity. In a study of the NRS, a clinical reduction of 2 points was found to be clinically relevant for a patient with mild pain but provided little or no relevance to the patient with severe pain (Cepeda, Africano, Polo, Alcala, & Carr, 2003). To further illustrate, a reduction of pain score from 4 to 2 (50% reduction) may provide relevant relief whereas a reduction from 10 to 8 (20% reduction) may not be clinically meaningful to the patient. Patients with chronic pain have reported that successful treatment of pain would require a large reduction in pain intensity, by 50% or more (Brown et al., 2008; O'Brien et al., 2010). In another study of patients with chronic pain, the degree of acceptable change in score was even higher, ranging from 44% to 75% (Thorne & Morley, 2009).

The minimum clinically important difference (MCID) is a measure that is used to interpret the clinical relevance of results of studies. In one of the only systematic reviews of the MCID in acute pain, Olsen et al. (2017) found that the MCID in acute pain varied greatly among studies and was influenced by baseline pain levels, definitions

of improvements, and study design. In this systematic review, patients with higher baseline pain required larger reductions in pain scores to perceive pain relief, yet, conversely, noted worsening of pain with smaller increases in pain scores than patients with lower baseline scores. Older studies have shown that, on acute and chronic pain scales, a 30% (approximate) decrease from baseline scores reflects a minimally clinically meaningful reduction, but it depends on baseline pain intensity.

However, in clinical practice, a statistically significant reduction in pain intensity may not equate to a meaningful reduction in pain for the patient. The most appropriate way to determine whether a pain intervention provides adequate relief is to assess the patient. With chronic pain, participants in a study indicated that a lower level of pain severity, pain impact, and interference and a higher level of activity are acceptable pain outcomes (Thorne & Morley, 2009). An interesting approach to the assessment of pain was posed by Moore, Straube, and Aldington (2013), in which it was suggested that perhaps pain measurement, particularly in chronic pain, should be as simple as determining whether the patient's pain is "no worse than mild pain." They suggest that the goal of pain interventions should be to reduce pain to the point that it is "no worse than mild pain." In acute pain, the borderline between mild and moderate pain was found to be about 30-mm on the VAS (Collins, Moore, & McQuay, 1997). Similarly, on the NRS a cut-off point between mild and moderate pain was found to be a score of 4 or more in acute postoperative patients (Gerbershagen, Rothaug, Kalkman, & Meissner, 2011). Similar cut-off points have been shown in chronic pain (Brown, Swift, & Spark, 2012). Clinical trials are needed to validate the use of "no worse than mild pain" as an appropriate way to measure the acceptability of pain interventions.

Unidimensional Pain Assessment Tools

Numeric Rating Scale

The NRS, shown in Fig. 6.1, uses numbers to rank pain intensity scores (Hawker, Mian, Kendzerska, & French, 2011). Usually, the scale is ranked 0 to 10 or 0 to 5. The patient is instructed to choose a whole number between the two anchoring points (usually 0–10 or 0–5) that best describes the intensity of pain. As illustrated in Fig. 6.1, the scale is commonly used in the horizontal version and different words may be used to anchor the ranking of pain intensity. However, the vertical form of the NRS (also Fig. 6.1) is preferred by some patients and may be used as an alternative when a patient has difficulty with the horizontal version. "No pain" is usually the term corresponding to the lowest anchor and "worst pain imaginable" is at the other extreme (Radnovich et al., 2014). Appendix 6.1 provides translations of the NRS into many languages. "Worst pain" differs from "worst pain imaginable" in that patients may compare present pain levels to

previously experienced pain or may have vivid imaginations if their life experience of pain is limited. Sometimes patients want to choose a number that falls between the whole numbers to better describe their perceived level of pain. Patients who have multiple pain sites or varying levels of pain throughout the day may "average" their multiple ratings to arrive at a measure of the collective distress they are experiencing. The NRS is popular because it is easy to use—a patient can respond verbally, behaviorally, or by writing the response. The numbers on the NRS are sometimes combined with words and placed on a horizontal or vertical line. A limitation of the NRS, like other unidimensional tools, is that for many patients, especially those with chronic pain, the NRS does not provide sufficient information to determine the impact of pain on the patient's function, quality of life, or response to pain interventions and is therefore often combined with other elements of the pain assessment.

Visual Analogue Scale

The VAS, as seen in Fig. 6.2, consists of a 100-mm (10-cm) line that can be oriented horizontally or vertically (Hawker et al., 2011). The tool is anchored at each end with words that describe the extremes of pain levels, for example, "no pain" and "worst possible pain" or

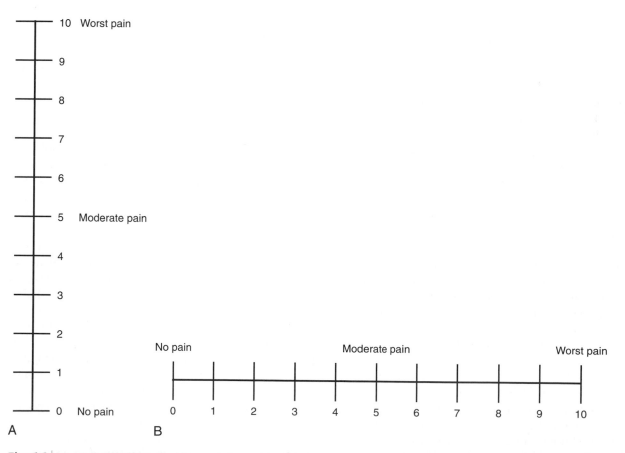

Fig. 6.1 | Numeric Rating Scale. The vertical version (A) of the numeric rating scale may be more easily understood than the horizontal version (B). (From Pasero, C., & McCaffery, M. [2011]. *Pain assessment and pharmacologic management* [p. 58]. St. Louis, MO: Mosby. The scale is in the public domain. May be duplicated for use in clinical practice.)

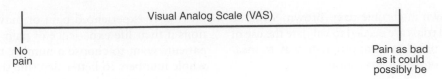

Fig. 6.2 | **(3-1) Horizontal Visual Analogue Scale.** This horizontal visual analogue scale (VAS) for rating pain intensity is a 10-cm line with word anchors. Patients are asked to mark the line. Although the VAS is frequently used in research, it is not recommended for clinical practice because scoring is time-consuming. (From Pasero, C., & McCaffery, M. [2011]. *Pain assessment and pharmacologic management* [p. 55]. St. Louis, MO: Mosby. © 2011, Pasero C, & McCaffery M. The scale is in the public domain. May be duplicated for use in clinical practice.)

"worst pain imaginable." The patient makes a mark on the line to indicate his or her level of pain intensity. The clinician measures the distance of the mark from the zero at the starting point, and determines the pain intensity by converting the millimeter (centimeter) to a whole number. For example, a mark at the 50-mm point would translate into a 5 of 10 (or 50 of 100) for pain intensity. This tool was originally designed for use in research studies, and administration is visual rather than verbal. A limitation of this instrument is that the patient has to be able to see the line clearly and hold a writing implement or point to a point on the scale that someone else can mark. Imagine the limitations of using a VAS for the patient who is just recovering from anesthesia.

Verbal Descriptor Scales

The verbal descriptor scale (VDS) or verbal rating scale (VRS) is a scale that uses words to describe pain (Finka et al., 2015). Adjectives that describe levels of pain intensity are ranked in order of severity (e.g., "no pain," "mild pain," "moderate pain," "severe pain," "extreme pain," and "the most intense pain imaginable"). There are commonly four to six anchoring words. In some versions of the VDS, each adjective is given a number that reflects the patient's pain intensity. The VDS has been shown to be effective in assessing the elderly, with and without cognitive impairments (Booker & Herr, 2016). There are major concerns with this type of tool: the patient is forced to translate a feeling into a predefined word that may not exactly fit the patient's experience (Lund et al., 2005), and adjectives have different meanings for different people (Dijkers, 2010). Caution should be taken when interpreting results of a VRS because it may measure more than pain intensity; these scales may also communicate patients' beliefs about pain and interference with function (Jensen et al., 2017). It is essential to ensure that all providers use the same descriptors and the descriptors are simple and consistent with the patient's language (Booker & Herr, 2016).

Wong-Baker FACES Pain Rating Scale

The Wong-Baker FACES pain rating scale, commonly known as the FACES scale, is widely used with pediatric patients to report pain intensity. The FACES scale was initially studied by Wong and Baker, and in 1988 they published the results of a study in which its use among 150 children aged 3 to 18 years was compared to five other pain scales (Wong & Baker, 1988). The scale features a series of faces that represent different pain levels; a happy face anchors one end and represents "no pain," and the other anchor is a face with tears, representing "most pain." FACES meets many of the criteria for selection of a pain rating scale (Fig. 6.3). Translations of the Wong-Baker FACES pain rating scale are located in Appendix 6.2. Although the original six-face (0–5) tool was intended for use in pediatrics, clinically, it is often seen on white boards in both adult and pediatric patient rooms along with the NRS. Some studies done in the late 1990s and early 2000s found that some adults preferred FACES over the NRS (Pasero & McCaffery, 2011). A criticism of the use of the FACES Pain Rating Scale in adults is that the face representing "most pain" includes tears, and tears may confound the intensity assessment because tears may represent an emotional response. Furthermore, in some cultures, crying or tears by adults is not an acceptable form of expression, and therefore, although pain might be extreme, this face might not be selected (Radnovich et al., 2014). Some practitioners have tried to simply eliminate the tears when the tool has been copied for clinical use, but this is not recommended because it could alter the validity of the tool.

FACES Pain Scale (Revised)

The FACES Pain Scale (Revised) (FPS-R) tool was developed and validated by Bieri, Reeve, Champion, Addicoat, and Ziegler (1990) in an effort to improve the assessment of pain in children who are developmentally unable (under 7 years of age) to use other pain self-report scales. The revised tool consists of six oval faces that range from a neutral visage associated with no pain to a grimacing face without tears that is meant to depict the worst pain. In the FPS-R, tears are not present in the most painful image as they are in the Wong-Baker FACES scale. This was done to increase accuracy in the measurement of pain and decrease the risk for measuring a different construct such as one that might be associated with crying, for example, fear, anger, distress, and sadness. This tool is often preferred by older adults, including those from ethnic minorities (especially African-Americans) and those with cognitive deficits mild enough to allow them to use a pain self-report tool (Herr, Bjoro, & Decker, 2006; Pasero & Herr, 2015). Reliability and validity of the FPS-R has been established in cognitively intact older adults (Stuppy, 1998; Ware, Epps, Herr, & Packard, 2006).

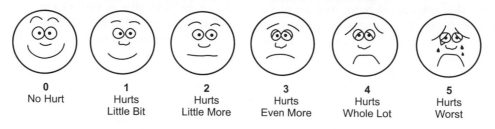

Which Face Shows How Much Hurt You Have Now?

0	1	2	3	4	5
No Hurt	Hurts Little Bit	Hurts Little More	Hurts Even More	Hurts Whole Lot	Hurts Worst

Explain to the person that each face is for a person who feels happy because he has no pain (hurt) or sad because he has some or a lot of pain. **Face 0** is very happy because he doesn't hurt at all. **Face I** hurts just a little bit. **Face 2** hurts a little more. **Face 3** hurts even more. **Face 4** hurts a whole lot. **Face 5** hurts as much as you can imagine, although you don't have to be crying to feel this bad. Ask the person to choose the face that best describes how he is feeling.

Rating scale is recommended for persons age 3 years and older.

*The **brief word instructions** under each face can also be used. Point to each face using the words to describe the pain intensity. Ask the child to choose the face that best describes own pain and record the appropriate number. Note: In a study of 148 children ages 4 to 5 years, there were no differences in pain scores when children used the original or brief word instructions. (In Wong D, Baker C: Reference manual for the Wong-Baker FACES Pain Rating Scale, Duarte, CA, 1996, City of Hope Mayday Pain Resource Center.)

Fig. 6.3 | Wong-Baker FACES Pain Rating Scale. Translations of the Wong-Baker FACES Pain Rating Scale are located in Appendix 6-2. (From Hockenberry, M. J., Wilson, D., & Winkelstein, M. L. [2005]. *Wong's essentials of pediatric nursing* [7th ed., p. 1259]. St. Louis, MO: Mosby. Used with permission. From Pasero, C., & McCaffery, M. [2011]. *Pain assessment and pharmacologic management* [p. 66–67]. St. Louis, MO: Mosby. Permission to use the FACES scale for purposes other than clinical practice can be obtained at http://www.us.elsevierhealth.com/FACES/.

The FACES-R may be accessed on the website of the International Association for the Study of Pain (IASP). In addition to the tool, the IASP provides access to instructions for use in many languages.

Iowa Pain Thermometer

The Iowa Pain Thermometer (IPT) tool, shown in Fig. 6.4, was developed at the University of Iowa, and combines words, numbers, and a diagram of a thermometer to rank pain intensity (Ware et al., 2015). The tool is oriented vertically with the bottom of the thermometer labeled as "no pain," and progressing up the thermometer, the terms are labeled "slight pain," "mild pain," "moderate pain," "severe pain," "very severe pain," and "most intense pain imaginable" (Ware et al., 2015). One of the challenges with the use of this tool is that the numerical ratings range from 0 to 13, rather than the more familiar NRS of 0 to 10.

Colored Analogue Scale

The colored analogue scale (CAS) is a pain intensity self-report tool that can be used by cognitively intact or impaired older adults to report pain (Booker & Herr, 2016). In a recent study comparing the use of the CAS, VAS, and verbally administered NRS in 150 adults with acute pain in the emergency department, it was shown that the three scales could be used interchangeably and a significant proportion of the patients (38%) preferred the CAS (Bahreini, Jalili, & Moradi-Lakeh, 2015). The CAS is a 10-cm-long triangular shape. Its width ranges from 10 mm at the lower anchor "no pain" to 30 mm at

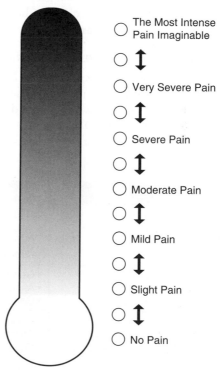

The Most Intense Pain Imaginable

Very Severe Pain

Severe Pain

Moderate Pain

Mild Pain

Slight Pain

No Pain

Iowa Pain Thermometer (IPT)

Fig. 6.4 | Iowa Pain Thermometer (IPT). (From Herr, K., Spratt, K., Spratt, K. F., Garand, L., & Li, L. [2006]. Evaluation of the Iowa Pain Thermometer and other selected pain intensity scales in younger and older adult cohorts using controlled clinical pain: A preliminary study. *Pain Management Nursing, 7*[2], 44–52. From Pasero, C., & McCaffery, M. [2011]. *Pain assessment and pharmacologic management* [p. 87]. St. Louis, MO: Mosby. May be duplicated for use in clinical practice.)

the upper anchor "worst possible pain." The color white is used to represent the absence of pain, and increases in pain intensity are shown by changes in color until the anchor of extreme pain, which is represented by the color red. Because the scale uses colors to represent pain intensity, it requires that the patient's vision allows the perception of colors. The scale can be used horizontally or vertically.

Multidimensional Pain Assessment Tools

Clinically Aligned Pain Assessment Tool

The CAPA tool (Fig. 6.5) was developed at the University of Utah to expand on the multidimensional aspects of pain assessment and link the assessment to clinical management (Topham & Drew, 2017). The CAPA tool recognizes that the pain experience is more than just pain intensity as documented by a number. The tool consists of five different parts that document level of comfort, change in pain, efficacy of pain control, and pain's effect on functioning and sleep. The patient does not verbally rank pain intensity or mark a visual tool. The tool is intended to guide a conversational approach between patient and clinician to gather categorical information. The clinician codes and documents the conversation (Gordon, 2015; Topham & Drew, 2017). The encoded responses are then used to guide more discussions with clinical team members to help develop a clinical plan for ongoing pain management.

The Defense and Veterans Pain Rating Scale 2.0

The Defense and Veterans Pain Rating Scale 2.0 (DVPRS) is a tool that was developed in recent years in response to a recognized need to improve and standardize pain assessment throughout the Department of Defense and Veteran's Health Administration Health Systems

(Buckenmaier et al., 2013) This tool incorporates the use of an NRS that is further embellished with pictures of faces, functional verbal descriptors, and color coding, which all correspond to the matched pain levels. It contains four additional questions that measure the degree to which pain interferes with usual activity and sleep, affects mood, and contributes to stress. It has undergone psychometric testing, limited to single assessment of pain and related outcomes, in military and veteran inpatient and outpatient populations and has demonstrated validity and reliability (Polomano et al., 2016). A benefit of the DVPRS is that, like the CAPA, it promotes a dialogue between the provider and the patient in assessing pain beyond a number and prompts the discussion of the impact of pain on patient function and well-being. The tool, Fig. 6.6, which has translations in Spanish and Vietnamese, is available for use in clinical practice and research on the website for the Defense and Veterans Center for Integrative Pain Management (Polomano et al., 2016). Further research on the use of this tool is needed, and there is a link on the website for health care providers to provide feedback about the use of the DVPRS.

McGill Pain Questionnaire

The long form of the McGill Pain Questionnaire (MPQ), originally published by Melzack in 1975, comprises 78 items divided into three major subscales: sensory, affective, and evaluative aspects of pain (Dansie & Turk, 2013). The MPQ is used to evaluate the effectiveness of pain interventions. The tool is also used to identify pain qualities associated with distinct neuropathic and nociceptive pain disorders (Fillingim et al., 2016). The MPQ contains a body diagram for the patient to indicate location of pain(s) and the tool has been translated into 26 different languages. A shortened version, called

Question	Response
Comfort	• Intolerable • Tolerable with discomfort • Comfortably manageable • Negligible pain
Change in Pain	• Getting worse • About the same • Getting better
Pain Control	• Inadequate pain control • Effective, just about right • Would like to reduce medication (why?)
Functioning	• Can't do anything because of pain • Pain keeps me from doing most of what I need to do • Can do most things, but pain gets in the way of some • Can do everything I need to
Sleep	• Awake with pain most of night • Awake with occasional pain • Normal sleep

Fig. 6.5 | Clinically Aligned Pain Assessment Tool (CAPA). (In Donaldson, G., & Chapman, C.R., 2013. Pain management is more than just a number. Used with permission from University of Utah. Salt Lake City, Utah.)

Defense and Veterans Pain Rating Scale

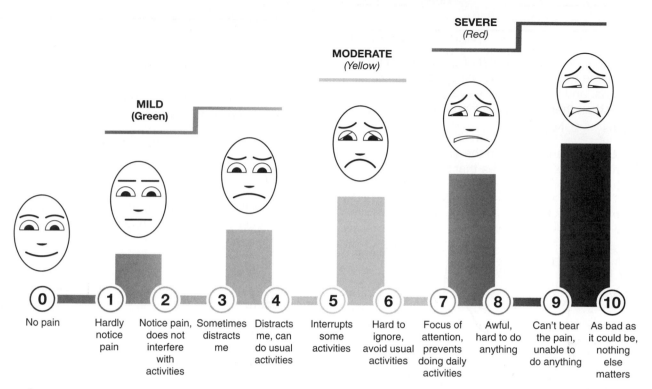

Fig. 6.6 | Defense and Veterans Pain Rating Scale (DVPRS). (Retrieved August 25, 2020 from http://www.dvcipm.org/clinical-resources/defense-veterans-pain-rating-scale-dvprs/)

the Short-Form McGill Pain Questionnaire (SF-MPQ), consists of 15 words with two subscales of pain intensity and affect (Dansie & Turk, 2013). Subsequently, the SF-MPQ was further refined and a 22-item tool, the SF-MPQ-2, was developed by Dworkin et al. (2009) and includes the most common pain descriptors and facilitates the assessment of both neuropathic and nonneuropathic pain (Lovejoy, Turk, & Morasco, 2012). The various versions of the MPQ have been examined and tested in a variety of clinical and experimental pain studies (Main, 2016).

Brief Pain Inventory

The Brief Pain Inventory (BPI) is a nine-item tool (Form 6.5) initially validated in cancer pain; it has since been validated among other clinical populations. Four of the items on the tool measure pain intensity, and the other five assess pain's interference with patient function (Kean et al., 2016). The interference scale has been used to assess responses to a variety of pain management interventions, including studies of medications and implementation of pain guidelines (Haythornthwaite, 2013). The patient is asked to score each item on a scale of 0 to 10. One item on the tool includes a body diagram that asks the patient to shade the area of pain and mark the area that hurts the most. The BPI has been translated into several different languages, and older adults have successfully used this tool.

PEG Scale

The three-item PEG Scale tool, derived from the BPI, uses the same scales and scoring and has been validated in ambulatory care settings (Kean et al., 2016; Krebbs et al., 2009). The tool's name, PEG, is derived from the constructs it measures: pain, enjoyment (of life), and general activity. This quick and easy-to-use tool, available as Form 6.6, contains one item that measures pain severity and two items that measure pain interference. This is a very useful tool, particularly in ambulatory care, given the limited amount of time available for patient visits in most ambulatory practices. Additional studies of the validity of this scale as a repeated measure and in other settings, including acute care, would be beneficial.

Functional Pain Scale

The functional pain scale (FPS) is sometimes cited in the literature on pain assessment in older adults. The FPS attempts to incorporate both subjective and objective components in the assessment of pain. It requires the patient to identify whether pain is tolerable or intolerable and is then used to determine to what extent the pain affects activities, particularly using the phone, watching TV, reading, or verbally communicating (Gloth, 2001). The scale incorporates a pain intensity rating ranging from 0 to 5. The rating component allows ease of assessing for changes in pain level (Gloth, 2001). The reliability,

Brief Pain Inventory

Date ____ / ____ / ____   Time: _____

Name: _____ _____ _____
         Last   First   Middle Initial

1) Throughout our lives, most of us have had pain from time to time (such as minor headaches, sprains, and toothaches). Have you had pain other than these everyday kinds of pain today?

   1. Yes   2. No

2) On the diagram, shade in the areas where you feel pain. Put an X on the area that hurts the most.

3) Please rate your pain by circling the one number that best describes your pain at its **worst** in the past 24 hours.

   0   1   2   3   4   5   6   7   8   9   10
   No   Pain as bad as
   pain   you can imagine

4) Please rate your pain by circling the one number that best describes your pain at its **least** in the past 24 hours.

   0   1   2   3   4   5   6   7   8   9   10
   No   Pain as bad as
   pain   you can imagine

5) Please rate your pain by circling the one number that best describes your pain on the **average**.

   0   1   2   3   4   5   6   7   8   9   10
   No   Pain as bad as
   pain   you can imagine

6) Please rate your pain by circling the one number that tells how much pain you have **right now**.

   0   1   2   3   4   5   6   7   8   9   10
   No   Pain as bad as
   pain   you can imagine

7) What treatments or medications are you receiving for your pain?

   _____

   _____

8) In the past 24 hours, how much **relief** have pain treatments or medications provided? Please circle the one percentage that most shows how much relief you have received.

   0% 10 20 30 40 50 60 70 80 90 100%
   No   Complete
   relief   relief

9) Circle the one number that describes how, during the past 24 hours, pain has **interfered** with your:

   A. General activity

   0   1   2   3   4   5   6   7   8   9   10
   Does not   Completely
   interfere   interferes

   B. Mood

   0   1   2   3   4   5   6   7   8   9   10
   Does not   Completely
   interfere   interferes

   C. Walking ability

   0   1   2   3   4   5   6   7   8   9   10
   Does not   Completely
   interfere   interferes

   D. Normal work (includes both work outside the home and housework)

   0   1   2   3   4   5   6   7   8   9   10
   Does not   Completely
   interfere   interferes

   E. Relations with other people

   0   1   2   3   4   5   6   7   8   9   10
   Does not   Completely
   interfere   interferes

   F. Sleep

   0   1   2   3   4   5   6   7   8   9   10
   Does not   Completely
   interfere   interferes

   G. Enjoyment of life

   0   1   2   3   4   5   6   7   8   9   10
   Does not   Completely
   interfere   interferes

Form 6.5 | Brief Pain Inventory. (From Pasero, C., & McCaffery, M. [2011]. *Pain assessment and pharmacologic management* [p. 53]. St. Louis, MO: Mosby. © 2011, Pasero C, & McCaffery M. May be duplicated for use in clinical practice.)

1. What number best describes your *pain on average* in the past week:

```
      0   1   2   3   4   5   6   7   8   9   10
No pain ─────────────────────────────────────── Pain as bad as
                                                 you can imagine
```

2. What number best describes how, during the past week, pain has interfered with your *enjoyment of life*?

```
              0   1   2   3   4   5   6   7   8   9   10
Does not ─────────────────────────────────────────── Completely
interfere                                             interferes
```

3. What number best describes how, during the past week, pain has interfered with your *general activity*?

```
              0   1   2   3   4   5   6   7   8   9   10
Does not ─────────────────────────────────────────── Completely
interfere                                             interferes
```

Interview version:

1. What number best describes your pain on *average* in the past week, on a scale from 0 to 10 where 0 is "no pain" and 10 is "pain as bad as you can imagine"? [0 to 10]

The following two questions ask you to describe how, during the past week, pain has interfered with your life on a "0 to 10" scale, where 0 is "does not interfere at all" and 10 is "completely interferes."

2. What number best describes how, during the past week, pain has interfered with your *enjoyment of life*? [0 to 10]

3. What number best describes how, during the past week, pain has interfered with your *general activity*? [0 to 10]

Scoring: The PEG score is the average of the 3 individual item scores. For clinical use, round to the nearest whole number.

Form 6.6 | PEG 3 Item Pain Scale. (From Krebs, E. E., Lorenz, K. A., Bair, M. J., Damush, T. A., Wu, J., Sutherland, J. M., . . . Kroenke, K. [2009]. Development and initial validation of the PEG, a 3-item scale assessing pain intensity and interference. *Journal of General Internal Medicine, 24,* 733–738.

validity, and responsiveness of this scale have been established in frail older adults (Gloth, Scheve, Stober, Chow, & Prosser, 2001). Although, at first glance, this scale may sound promising, keep in mind that, like the DVPRS, this scale attempts to link a numerical pain rating to function. There is no research to support that pain will affect the same degree of function in patients with the same pain intensity rating. An example of a problem with this scale is if the patient is able to verbally report that his or her pain rating is 5 of 5, the intensity actually must be lower, because, as this scale presumes, if pain is at a level of 5, the patient would not be able to verbalize because of the pain. It fails to take into account the fact that patients with the same pain intensity level may have different behavioral and functional responses to that level. For illustration purposes, the FPS is available in Fig. 6.7; however, readers are cautioned about the limitations of this scale.

Functional Pain Scale

0 = No Pain

1 = Tolerable (and doesn't prevent any activities)

2 = Tolerable (but does prevent some activities)

3 = Intolerable (but can use telephone, watch TV, or read)

4 = Intolerable (but can't use telephone, watch TV, or read)

5 = Intolerable (and unable to verbally communicate because of pain)

Ideally, all patients should reach a 0 to 2 level, preferably 0 to 1. It should be made clear to the respondent that limitations in function only apply if limitations are due to the pain being evaluated.

Fig. 6.7 | Functional Pain Scale (FPS). (Gloth, F. M., Scheve, A. A., Stober, C. V., Chow, S., & Prosser, J. (2001). The Functional Pain Scale: reliability, validity, and responsiveness in an elderly population. *Journal of the American Medical Directors Association, 2*[3], Table 2 on the bottom.)

Chronic Pain Grade Scale

The chronic pain grade scale (CPGS) is a multidimensional tool that is suitable for use in all chronic musculoskeletal and low back pain (Hawker et al., 2011). The tool assesses the two dimensions of pain intensity and pain-related disability. It measures the impact of persistent pain on social and work activities over time. It is an easy tool to administer because it is composed of 11 questions, but the scoring is complex because three subscale scores are used to classify subjects into 1 of 5 pain severity categories (Hawker et al., 2011).

Short-Form 36 Bodily Pain Scale

The Short-Form 36 Bodily Pain Score (SF-36 BPS) tool is one of eight subscales of the Medical Outcomes Study SF-36 questionnaire that assesses bodily pain intensity and interference of pain on normal activities (Hawker et al., 2011). With this two-item tool, the individual is asked how much bodily pain he or she had during the past 4 weeks and how much pain interfered with normal work. The SF-36 BPS has been translated and adapted for use in 50 countries. The tool and scoring instructions are available on the website of the Rand Corporation, a research company that owns the rights to the SF-36.

Neuropathic Pain Assessment

In 2008 the IASP revised the definition of neuropathic pain to state that it is "pain arising as a direct consequence of a lesion or disease affecting the somatosensory system" (Treede et al., 2008, p. 1630). Based on this definition, neuropathic pain can encompass many clinical conditions that can be categorized based on anatomic involvement (central or peripheral nervous system involvement) or cause (Gilron, Baron, & Jensen, 2015). Clinical conditions such as multiple sclerosis, diabetic peripheral neuropathy, postherpetic neuralgia, and radicular back pain are often associated with neuropathic pain. There is no single clearly diagnostic characteristic of neuropathic pain, but patients will often use words such as burning, tingling, or shooting to describe the pain (Mathieson, Maher, Terwee, de Campos, & Lin, 2015). One of the challenges is that neuropathic pain may coexist with nociceptive pain (Herndon et al., 2016).

The assessment of neuropathic pain, like all comprehensive pain assessments, includes a patient history (including history of alcohol and other substance use and toxin exposure), physical examination, and diagnostic tests when indicated (laboratory work such as electrolytes or testing for heavy metals or other toxins, and sensory testing such as nerve conduction studies and magnetic resonance imaging) (Gilron et al., 2015). At this time, the diagnosis of neuropathic pain remains challenging. For a diagnosis of neuropathic pain, the history should indicate that the patient has a relevant neurologic lesion or disease, a location/distribution of pain that is anatomically consistent with the suspected location of the peripheral or central nervous system lesion or disease, and the physical examination and diagnostic findings should support the diagnosis.

Some neuropathic pain questionnaires have been developed, but these questionnaires are mostly based on the old IASP definition of neuropathic pain, so it is important to realize that they are only one component of the assessment, and although they may be helpful, they may wrongly classify some patients and fail to identify others (Finnerup et al., 2016). The Neuropathic Pain Special Interest Group (NeuPSIG) of the IASP recommended five questionnaires for the screening of neuropathic pain (Haanpää et al., 2011). In addition to the Leeds Assessment of Neuropathic Symptoms and Signs and the Neuropathic Pain Questionnaire, which are detailed later and summarized in Table 6.6, the committee identified three other general neuropathic pain scales, available in English, that have been validated for use. The three include painDETECT, ID-Pain, and the Douleur Neuropathique 4 Questions (DN4).

Table 6.6 | Pain Assessment Tools for Neuropathic Pain

Tool	Indications	Validity/Reliability	Advantages	Disadvantages
Leeds Assessment of Neuropathic Symptoms and Signs (S-LANSS)	Screening for signs and symptoms of neuropathic pain.	Specificity and sensitivity are less robust when used in population studies.	Easy to use. Self-administered.	Better suited as a screening tool rather than an assessment tool (Weingarten et al., 2007).
Neuropathic pain scale (NPS)	Patients with signs and symptoms of neuropathic pain.	Found to be a valid and reliable tool (Galer & Jensen, 1997).	Multidimensional tool that includes a measure of pain unpleasantness.	Not all types of neuropathic pain complaints are covered in the scale's 11 items. (Fishbain et al., 2008).

From Fishbain, D. A., Lewis, J. E., Cutler, R., Cole, B., Rosomoff, H. L., & Rosomoff, R. S. (2008). Can the neuropathic pain scale discriminate between non-neuropathic and neuropathic pain? *Pain Medicine, 9*(2), 149–160; Galer, B. S., & Jensen, M. P. (1997). Development and preliminary validation of a pain measure specific to neuropathic pain the neuropathic pain scale. *Neurology, 48*(2), 332–338; and Weingarten, T. N., Watson, J. C., Hooten, W. M., Wollan, P. C., Melton, L. J., Locketz, A. J., Yawn, B. P. (2007). Validation of the S-LANSS in the community setting. *Pain, 132*(1–2), 189–194.

Leeds Assessment of Neuropathic Symptoms and Signs

The Leeds Assessment of Neuropathic Symptoms and Signs (LANSS) tool contains five items related to symptoms and two clinical examination criteria. The S-LANSS, shown in Form 6.7, is a self-report version of the LANSS, which also has been validated. The S-LANSS includes a body diagram that asks the patient to shade the painful area, and mark the one, most painful site. The diagram

---

APPENDIX

THE S-LANSS PAIN SCORE

Leeds Assessment of Neuropathic Symptoms and Signs (self-complete)

NAME_____   DATE_____

- This questionnaire can tell us about the type of pain that you may be experiencing. This can help in deciding how best to treat it.

- Please draw on the diagram below where you feel your pain. If you have pain in more than one area, **only shade in the one main area where your worst pain is.**

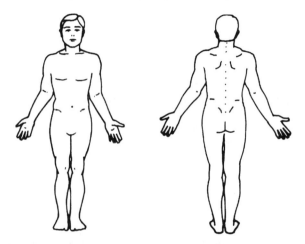

- On the scale below, please indicate how bad your pain (that you have shown on the above diagram) has been in the last week where:
  "0" means no pain and "10" means pain as severe as it could be.

NONE 0   1   2   3   4   5   6   7   8   9   10 **SEVERE PAIN**

- On the other side of the page are 7 questions about your pain (the one in the diagram).

- Think about how your pain that you showed in the diagram has felt **over the last week.** Please circle the descriptions that best match your pain. These descriptions may, or may not, match your pain no matter how severe it feels.

- Only circle the responses that describe your pain. **Please turn over.**

Form 6.7 | **The S-LANSS Pain Score.** (From Bennett, M. I., Smith, B. H., Torrance, N., & Potter, J. [2005]. The S-LANSS score for identifying pain of predominantly neuropathic origin: Validation for use in clinical and postal research. *The Journal of Pain, 6*[3], 149–158.)

is followed by seven questions that ask about the pain in the preceding week. This questionnaire is used to determine whether pain is neuropathic in origin (Bennett, Smith, Torrance, & Potter, 2005). Clinicians may prefer this tool because it is easy to administer and score. The questionnaire has been translated for use in a number of non-English versions. The psychometrics have been tested in a variety of chronic pain conditions.

S-LANSS

1. **In the area where you have pain, do you also have "pins and needles," tingling, or prickling sensations?**

   a) NO—I don't get these sensations   (0)
   b) YES—I get these sensations often   (5)

2. **Does the painful area change color (perhaps looks mottled or more red) when the pain is particularly bad?**

   a) NO—The pain does not affect the color of my skin   (0)
   b) YES—I have noticed that the pain does make my skin look different from normal   (5)

3. **Does your pain make the affected skin abnormally sensitive to touch? Getting unpleasant sensations or pain when lightly stroking the skin might describe this.**

   a) NO—The pain does not make my skin in that area abnormally sensitive to touch   (0)
   b) YES—My skin in that area is particularly sensitive to touch   (3)

4. **Does your pain come on suddenly and in bursts for no apparent reason when you are completely still? Words like "electric shocks," jumping, and bunting might describe this.**

   a) NO—My pain doesn't really feel like this   (0)
   b) YES—I get these sensations often   (2)

5. **In the area where you have pain, does your skin feel unusually hot like a burning pain?**

   a) NO—I don't have burning pain   (0)
   b) YES—I get burning pain often   (1)

6. **Gently *rub* the painful area with your index finger and then rub a non-painful area (for example, an area of skin farther away or on the opposite side from the painful area). How does this rubbing feel in the painful area?**

   a) The painful area feels no different from the non-painful area   (0)
   b) I feel discomfort, like pins and needles, tingling, or burning in the painful area that is different from the non-painful area   (5)

7. **Gently *press* on the painful area with your finger tip then gently press in the same way onto a non-painful area (the same non-painful area that you chose in the last question). How does this feel in the painful area?**

   a) The painful area does not feel different from the non-painful area   (0)
   b) I feel numbness or tenderness in the painful area that is different from the non-painful area   (3)

Scoring: a score of 12 or more suggests pain of predominantly neuropathic origin

---

Form 6.7, Cont'd

Neuropathic Pain Questionnaire

The neuropathic pain questionnaire (NPQ) consists of 12 items that include 10 items related to sensations or sensory responses and 2 related to affect (Backonja & Krause, 2003). A short form of the NPQ, Form 6.8, consists of only 3 items (numbness, tingling, and an increase in pain in response to touch). It is able to differentiate patients with neuropathic pain from those with

---

NEUROPATHIC PAIN QUESTIONNAIRE—Short Form

In order to assess and treat your pain problem, we need to thoroughly understand just exactly what type of pain you have, and how it may or may not change over time. You may have only one site of pain, or you may have more than one.

Please name the site of pain which is *most severe or disturbing* for you (e.g., arm, foot, etc.):

_____

For all of the following questions, please rate your pain at the site you just listed.
Please use the space below to describe your pain in your own words as well:

_____

Please use the items below to rate your pain as it *usually* feels. Indicate a number which represents your pain on each scale. For example, if you have no tingling pain, you would rate the first item "0". If you have the worst tingling pain imaginable, you would rate it "100". If neither of those fits your pain because it is in between, choose a number which *fits* your pain.

1Sf. Tingling Pain

0 ←——————————————→ 100   Please rate
No Tingling   Worst Tingling   your *usual* pain: _____
Pain   Pain Imaginable

2Sf. Numbness

0 ←——————————————→ 100   Please rate
No Tingling   Worst Numbness   your *usual* pain: _____
Pain   Imaginable

We are also interested in learning what circumstances cause changes in your pain. Please write the number that indicates the amount you experience each of the following:

3Sf. Increased pain due to touch

0 ←——————————————→ 100   Please rate
No Tingling   Greatest Increase   your *usual* pain: _____
Pain   Imaginable

Canonical Discriminant Function Coefficients and Structure Coefficients

Item	Canonical Discriminant Function Coefficient	Structure Coefficient
1Sf. Numbers	.017	.819
2Sf. Tingling Pain	.015	.828
3Sf. Increased Pain due to Touch	.011	.569
Constant		−1.302

TOTAL DISCRIMINANT FUNCTION SCORE: =   _____

Check one of the following boxes:

Discriminant Function Score *Below* 0: _____   Predicts **Non-Neuropathic Pain**

Discriminant Function Score *at or Above* 0: _____   Predicts **Neuropathic Pain**

Form 6.8 | The Neuropathic Pain Questionnaire-Short Form. (From Backonja, M. M., & Krause, S. J. [2003]. Neuropathic pain questionnaire: Short form. *The Clinical Journal of Pain, 19*[5], 315–316. Form is on p. 316.)

nonneuropathic pain. It can be used to monitor response to neuropathic pain treatments.

Breakthrough Pain Assessment

The National Cancer Consortium Network (NCCN) defines breakthrough pain (BTP) as pain that is episodic and not controlled with an existing, regularly scheduled opioid pain regimen (NCCN, 2020). Breakthrough pain may be incident (occurring as a result of an activity or an event); related to "end-of-dose failure," in which the pain escalates at the end of the dosing interval from the regularly scheduled opioid; or uncontrolled persistent pain, in which the dose of the opioid is not adequate to treat the pain (NCCN, 2020). Breakthrough pain is widely accepted to occur with cancer pain. For a period in the early 2000s, it was accepted that BTP is also associated with noncancer pain conditions. Currently, this is no longer fully accepted because there is inadequate evidence to support the association of breakthrough pain with noncancer conditions (Herndon et al., 2016).

Although recent publications related to breakthrough pain focus on the cancer population, patients with cancer and chronic noncancer pain may report pain that episodically exceeds the baseline pain level. This type of incident pain may be predictable (e.g., occurring after a physical therapy session), or unpredictable (e.g., sudden, unprovoked, onset of severe muscle spasm despite baseline control of knee pain). Nurses and other care providers need to assess patients for these episodes of breakthrough pain, and ensure there are interventions to eliminate, minimize, or treat them. To assess breakthrough pain, it is first essential to perform an assessment and determine that there is baseline pain that is well controlled.

To assist in the screening for breakthrough pain, Pasero & McCaffery (2011) developed a BTP screening tool, shown on Form 6.9, which contains two questions that can be placed on a form for the patient to complete or can be asked by the clinician. If screening indicates that the patient may have breakthrough pain, a more extensive assessment should take place. For breakthrough pain associated with cancer, the following tools may be helpful.

Screening Tool for Pain Flares — Breakthrough Pain (BTP)*

Instructions: We are interested in a particular type of pain you may have. Please answer the following questions:

1. Do you have pain that is:

    a. constant, almost always present, or would be present if not for the treatment you are receiving?

    _____ yes   _____ no

    b. or, do you have constant pain that is usually:

    _____ moderate pain   _____ severe pain

2. Do you have temporary flares of pain that are more intense than your constant pain?

    _____ yes   _____ no

*Note to clinician: The above questions may be placed with an existing initial pain assessment tool, such as Form 3-1 on p. 51, or the patient may complete the above form. If the patient has constant pain that is usually moderate to severe, then this needs to be controlled before addressing flares of pain. If the patient has constant pain that is usually controlled and answers yes to question 2, consider having the patient complete the form on "Assessment of Pain Flares — Breakthrough Pain (BTP)," on pp.104-105.

Form 6.9 | **Screening Tool for Pain Flares—Breakthrough Pain (BTP).** (From Pasero, C., & McCaffery, M. [2011]. *Pain assessment and pharmacologic management* [p. 103]. St. Louis, MO: Mosby. © 2011, Pasero C, & McCaffery M. May be duplicated for use in clinical practice.)

Alberta Breakthrough Pain Assessment Tool for Cancer Patients

The Alberta Breakthrough Pain Assessment Tool for Cancer Patients (ABPAT), shown in Form 6.10, was initially developed for research purposes and underwent analysis by expert panel review in which it was found to be conceptually grounded and understandable by patients and clinicians (Hagen et al., 2008). As a result,

---

TO BE COMPLETED BY PHYSICIAN OR NURSE

Instructions:

1. This module should be completed with the patient due to its complexity. The patient or clinician can answer the questions in writing, but if completed by the patient, it must be done under close supervision and help must be immediately available if required.
2. The goal is to have the patient characterize up to three distinct types of breakthrough pain. To do **this, define baseline and breakthrough pain for the patient.** Baseline pain can be defined as "the usual, steady pain you always experience." Breakthrough pain can be defined as "a brief flare-up of pain. It can be a flare-up of the usual, steady pain you always experience (your baseline pain) OR it can be a pain that is different from your baseline pain".
3. First ask the patient to describe his or her baseline pain, which may include a description of the location, severity, quality, or other features of this pain, and complete the table below.
4. Then ask how many different types of **breakthrough pains** he/she typically experiences **in a 24-hour period.** A patient may initially distinguish between breakthrough pains on the basis of any of the following variables: location, provocation, quality, etiology, or any other variable the patient feels is important.
5. Ask the patient to identify up to three of his/her **most bothersome breakthrough pains,** and complete the table below; these breakthrough pains will be the ones that are characterized.
6. Please photocopy the subsequent pages of this module to individually characterize each of the patient's three most bothersome breakthrough pains. Note that a separate Module III should be completed for each of the patient's most bothersome breakthrough pains.

Description of baseline pain	
Describe your baseline pain.	

Descriptions of distinct types of breakthrough pain	
What is your most bothersome breakthrough pain?	
What is your second most bothersome breakthrough pain?	
What is your third most bothersome breakthrough pain?	

Q2. Current breakthrough pain medications: list trade name of formulations [list generic names for all opioid and non-opioid analgesics]	Treatment Regimen		
	Route of Administration	Dose	prn Schedule

TO BE COMPLETED BY PATIENT

For which breakthrough pain are you completing this form?	

Q1. Relationship to baseline pain Is this pain a brief flare up of your baseline pain or is it a pain that is different from your baseline pain?	☐ Brief flare up of baseline pain ☐ Different from baseline pain ☐ Not sure
Q2. Last time experienced (a) When did you last have this breakthrough pain? (Please refer to your most recent breakthrough pain experience, regardless of whether or not you took medication for it).	☐ Today ☐ Yesterday ☐ Before then
(b) Beginning at what time, approximately?	

Form 6.10 | Alberta Breakthrough Pain Assessment Tool for Cancer Patients. (From Hagen, N. A., Stiles, C., Nekolaichuk, C., Biondo, P., Carlson, L. E., Fisher, K., & Fainsinger, R. (2008). The Alberta Breakthrough Pain Assessment Tool for cancer patients: A validation study using a delphi process and patient think-aloud interviews. *Journal of Pain and Symptom Management, 35*(2), 136–152. Tool is on pages 149–152.)

it is a tool that may be helpful when caring for patients with cancer who are experiencing pain. It was further examined in a multicenter study of patients with severe cancer-related pain, and its acceptability and efficacy for the assessment and characterization of cancer BTP was supported (Sperlinga et al., 2015).

Q3. Frequency (a) Approximately how many times in the past 24 hours have you had this breakthrough pain? (Please include ALL breakthrough pain experiences, regardless of whether or not you took medication for them.)	
(b) During the past 24 hours is this about the usual for you?	☐ Usual ☐ Better ☐ Worse

Q4. Intensity of pain at peak (a) When this breakthrough pain is at its worst, how would you rate this pain on a scale from 0 to 10, with 0 being "no pain" and 10 being "worst possible pain"?	
(b) How would you rate the intensity of this breakthrough pain at its worst?	☐ Mild ☐ Moderate ☐ Severe

Q5. Location Where do you feel this pain? (Please **shade in the entire area** in which you experience this pain.)	

Q6. Quality What does the pain feel like? (check ✓ all that apply)	☐ Throbbing ☐ Shooting ☐ Stabbing ☐ Sharp ☐ Cramping ☐ Gnawing ☐ Hot-Burning ☐ Aching ☐ Heavy ☐ Tender ☐ Splitting ☐ Tiring-Exhausting ☐ Sickening ☐ Fearful ☐ Punishing-Cruel ☐ Other (please describe):

Q7. Time from onset to peak intensity When you are awake, on average, how long does it usually take from the time you first feel this pain **until it is at its worst**?	☐ more than 0 and up to 10 minutes ☐ more than 10 and up to 30 minutes ☐ more than 30 minutes ☐ It's hard to say exactly when it started

Form 6.10, Cont'd

| **Q8. Time from onset to end of episode** For those pain episodes that you take breakthrough pain medication, how long does it usually take from the time you take your medication until the pain goes away? | ☐ more than 0 and up to 10 minutes ☐ more than 10 and up to 30 minutes ☐ more than 30 minutes ☐ I am not on any breakthrough pain medication |

| **Q9. Cause(s)** Is there anything that triggers this breakthrough pain? (check ✓ all that apply) | ☐ Movement in bed   ☐ Walking ☐ Standing   ☐ Sitting ☐ Coughing   ☐ Vomiting ☐ Having a bowel movement   ☐ Urinating ☐ Swallowing   ☐ Eating ☐ Touching area of skin   ☐ Breathing ☐ It recurs when I feel my scheduled pain medication wearing off ☐ No, nothing in particular triggers this pain ☐ Unsure ☐ Other (please describe): |

| **Q10. Predictability** Can you predict when your breakthrough pain will occur? | ☐ I can never predict when it will occur ☐ I can rarely predict when it will occur ☐ I can sometimes predict when it will occur ☐ I can often predict when it will occur ☐ I can always predict when it will occur |

| **Q11. General relief** Does anything help to relieve or prevent your breakthrough pain? (check ✓ all that apply) | ☐ Moving   ☐ Sitting ☐ Rolling over   ☐ Lying ☐ Urinating   ☐ Having a bowel movement ☐ Passing gas   ☐ Burping ☐ Eating   ☐ Sleeping ☐ Applying heat   ☐ Applying cold ☐ Breathing   ☐ Avoiding coughing ☐ Touching/rubbing/squeezing painful area ☐ Use of breakthrough pain medication ☐ Use of scheduled pain medication ☐ Unsure ☐ Other (please describe): |

Form 6.10, Cont'd

Q12. Relief from breakthrough pain medication In the past *24 hours*, how much relief has your breakthrough pain medication provided for this breakthrough pain?	☐ No relief ☐ Slight relief ☐ Good relief ☐ Very good relief ☐ Complete relief ☐ Not applicable: I haven't taken any breakthrough pain medication in the past 24 hours (skip questions 13-15)
Q13. Satisfaction with breakthrough pain medication In the past *24 hours*, how satisfied have you been with how well your breakthrough pain medication works for this breakthrough pain?	☐ Very satisfied ☐ Moderately satisfied ☐ Slightly satisfied ☐ Neutral ☐ Slightly dissatisfied ☐ Moderately dissatisfied ☐ Very dissatisfied
Q14. Onset of pain relief In the past *24 hours*, on average, how long has it taken for your breakthrough pain medication to **begin** to reduce your breakthrough pain? (Fill in the blank)	_____ minutes
Q15. Satisfaction with onset of pain relief In the past *24 hours*, how satisfied have you been with how fast your pain medication **begins** to reduce your breakthrough pain?	☐ Very satisfied ☐ Moderately satisfied ☐ Slightly satisfied ☐ Neutral ☐ Slightly dissatisfied ☐ Moderately dissatisfied ☐ Very dissatisfied

TO BE COMPLETED BY PHYSICIAN OR NURSE

Q1. Etiology of breakthrough pain (check ✓ all that apply)	Pain related to the site of active cancer
	Pain related to the whole body or systemic effects of the cancer disease process (e.g., muscle spasm or bedsores from debility, pain from shingles, etc.)
	Pain related to anticancer treatment (e.g., side effects of radiotherapy, chemotherapy, surgery)
	Pain caused by a concurrent disorder (e.g., osteoarthritis)
	Unknown or uncertain at this time
Q2. Inferred pathophysiology of breakthrough pain (check ✓ all that apply)	Somatic nociceptive *List damaged tissues:*
	Visceral nociceptive *List damaged tissues:*
	Neuropathic *List damaged tissues:*
	Unknown or uncertain at this time

Note: An administrative manual for the Alberta Breakthrough Pain Assessment Tool serves as a technical appendix for users, and is available by contacting the authors.

Form 6.10, Cont'd

Breakthrough Pain Assessment Tool

The Breakthrough Pain Assessment Tool (BAT) consists of 14 questions, 9 of which pertain to the pain experience, and 5 that are related to the pain treatment. This tool, Form 6.11, has had preliminary psychometric testing that supports its validity and reliability for use in adult patients with cancer-related pain (Webber et al., 2014).

Breakthrough Pain Assessment Tool-BAT

The following questions relate to your breakthrough pain over the last week. Breakthrough pain refers to the short-lived increases in your cancer pain.

Where is your breakthrough pain?
Please indicate on picture with a cross (X)

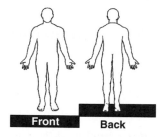

Front   Back

How often do you get breakthrough pain?
Please circle one answer

Less than once a day   1-2 times a day   3-4 times a day   More than 4 times a day

Does anything bring on your breakthrough pain?
If yes, please write down

Does anything relieve your breakthrough pain? (painkillers or other)
If yes, please write down

How long does a typical episode of breakthrough pain last?
Please circle one answer

<5 min   5-15 min   15-30 min   30-60 min   >60 min

How severe is your *worst* episode of breakthrough pain?
Please circle one number

0   1   2   3   4   5   6   7   8   9   10
No pain   Pain as bad as you can imagine

How severe is a *typical* episode of breakthrough pain?
Please circle one number

0   1   2   3   4   5   6   7   8   9   10
No pain   Pain as bad as you can imagine

Form 6.11 | Breakthrough Pain Assessment Tool (BAT). (Retrieved August 25, 2020 from http://www.cfp.ca/content/cfp/suppl/2014/12/09/60.12.1111.DC1/Breakthrough_pain.pdf)

Italian Questionnaire for Breakthrough Pain

The Italian Questionnaire for Breakthrough Pain (IQ-BTP) is a tool that has been developed to assist in the assessment of cancer and noncancer breakthrough pain. For BTP in noncancer pain, it is difficult to locate published assessment tools with good psychometrics.

This instrument has undergone testing that has shown satisfactory psychometric and validation properties for use in patients with mixed chronic pain (cancer and noncancer), but further study of its impact as a screening tool and prognostic model is needed (Dekel et al., 2016).

Breakthrough Pain Assessment Tool-BAT

The following questions relate to your breakthrough pain over the last week. Breakthrough pain refers to the short-lived increases in your cancer pain.

How much does the breakthrough pain distress you?
Please circle one number

0 1 2 3 4 5 6 7 8 9 10

Not at all   Very much

How much does the breakthrough pain stop you from living a normal life?
Please circle one number

0 1 2 3 4 5 6 7 8 9 10

Not at all   Very much

What painkillers do you take for your breakthrough pain (if any)?
Please write down type and dose of painkillers

How effective is the painkiller that you usually take for your breakthrough pain?
Please circle one number

0 1 2 3 4 5 6 7 8 9 10

Not at all   Completely
effective   effective

How long does the painkiller for your breakthrough pain take to have a meaningful effect?
Please circle one answer

No effect   0-10 min   10-20 min   20-30 min   >30 min

Do you get any side-effects from the painkiller for your breakthrough pain?
If yes, please write down type of side effect

How much do side-effects from the painkillers for your breakthrough pain bother you?
Please circle one number

0 1 2 3 4 5 6 7 8 9 10

Not at all   Very much

Form 6.11, Cont'd

Key Points

- A comprehensive assessment of pain is conducted to obtain necessary information to develop an individualized multimodal pain plan of care.
- Pain assessment of the cognitively intact adult is not simply a score on a numerical pain rating scale. A more detailed description of pain is necessary to ensure that pain is adequately assessed and managed. Mnemonics are available to guide the assessment.
- A conversational assessment of pain may be helpful in obtaining a more detailed pain description.
- A pain intensity score can only be obtained by the patient's self-report of pain.
- It is important to understand the type of pain a patient is experiencing and select tools that are appropriate for the specific type of pain.
- The same pain assessment tool should be used consistently by all providers in assessing pain of an individual patient unless a change necessitates use of a different tool.
- All members of the health care team, along with the patient and family, are partners in the assessment of pain. Communication among team members is necessary for a thorough pain assessment.
- Whenever possible, use only pain assessment scales that have been found to be reliable and validated in the patient's population.
- The impact of pain and pain interventions on the patient's function and activity should be determined when assessing the patient's pain and evaluating the patient's response to the pain plan of care.

Case Scenario

Paul is a 52-year-old English-speaking roofer who has had a 15-year history of chronic knee pain. He has tried a variety of interventions to control his pain, and was reluctant to have surgery because he does not have unemployment insurance. His pain has always been "10/10" but states he has a "high pain tolerance." He is now postoperative day 1 after a right total knee arthroplasty and he tells you that his pain is now "18/10." He appears to be drowsy and has difficulty keeping his eyes open while speaking. In reviewing his chart, you see that when asked in the presurgical setting, his pain goal was to have "no pain" after surgery. Paul's wife is at the bedside and is crying and demanding to speak to the surgeon.

- When first meeting Paul on the morning after surgery, describe the process you will use to assess his pain.
- What barriers to pain assessment do you anticipate?
- How will you assess Paul throughout the remainder of your shift?
- What pain assessment tools are most appropriate for use?
- How do you explain "pain goals" to Paul?
- How do you interact with Paul's wife?
- If Paul's pain is always a "10/10," how do you assess his response to pain interventions?
- Are there any "red flags" in Paul's history that require further assessment?
- What could have been done to create a better postoperative pain experience for Paul?

References

Backonja, M., & Farrar, J. T. (2015). Are pain ratings irrelevant? *Pain Medicine, 16*(7), 1247–1250.

Backonja, M. M., & Krause, S. J. (2003). Neuropathic pain questionnaire—short form. *The Clinical Journal of Pain, 19*(5), 315–316.

Bahreini, M., Jalili, M., & Moradi-Lakeh, M. (2015). A comparison of three self-report pain scales in adults with acute pain. *The Journal of Emergency Medicine, 48*(1), 10–18.

Baker, K. S., Georgiou-Karistianis, N., Gibson, S. J., & Giummarra, M. J. (2017). Optimizing cognitive function in persons with chronic pain. *The Clinical Journal of Pain, 33*(5), 462–472.

Bennett, M. I., Smith, B. H., Torrance, N., & Potter, L. (2005). The S LANSS score for identifying pain of predominantly neuropathic origin: validation for use in clinical and postal research. *The Journal of Pain, 6*(3), 149–158.

Bieri, D., Reeve, R. A., Champion, G. D., Addicoat, L., & Ziegler, J. B. (1990). The FACES pain scale for the self-assessment of the severity of pain experienced by children: Development, initial validation, and preliminary investigation for ratio scale properties. *Pain, 41*(2), 139–150.

Booker, S., & Herr, K. (2015). The state of "cultural validity" of self-report pain assessment tools in diverse older adults. *Pain Medicine, 16*(2), 232–239.

Booker, S. Q., & Herr, K. A. (2016). Assessment and measurement of pain in adults in later life. *Clinics in Geriatric Medicine, 32*(4), 677–692.

Brown, J. L., Edwards, P. S., Atchison, J. W., Lafayette-Lucey, A., Wittmer, V. T., & Robinson, M. E. (2008). Defining Patient-Centered, Multidimensional Success Criteria for Treatment of Chronic Spine Pain. *Pain Medicine, 9*(7), 851–862.

Brown, K. E., Swift, I., & Spark, M. J. (2012). Pain Severity Cut-Points and Analgesic Use by Community-Dwelling People for Chronic Pain. *Journal of Pharmacy Practice and Research, 42*(3), 196–199.

Buckenmaier, C. C., Galloway, K. T., Polomano, R. C., McDuffie, M., Kwon, N., & Gallagher, R. M. (2013). Original research article: Preliminary validation of the defense and veterans pain rating scale (DVPRS) in a military population. *Pain Medicine, 14*, 110–123.

Bushnell, M. C., Čeko, M., & Low, L. A. (2013). Cognitive and emotional control of pain and its disruption in chronic pain. *Nature Reviews Neuroscience, 14*(7), 502–511.

Bushnell, M. C., Case, L. K., Čeko, M., Cotton, V. A., Gracely, J. L., Low, L. A., & Villemure, C. (2015). Effect of environment on the long-term consequences of chronic pain. *Pain, 156*(0 1), S42.

Center for Behavioral Health Statistics and Quality. (2016). *Key substance use and mental health indicators in the United States: Results from the 2015 National Survey on Drug Use and Health*. Retrieved August 29, 2020 from https://www.samhsa.gov/data/sites/default/files/NSDUH-FFR1-2015/NSDUH-FFR1-2015/NSDUH-FFR1-2015.htm.

Cepeda, M. S., Africano, J. M., Polo, R., Alcala, R., & Carr, D. B. (2003). What decline in pain intensity is meaningful to patients with acute pain? *Pain*, *105*(1), 151–157.

Chinn, D., & McCarthy, C. (2013). All Aspects of Health Literacy Scale (AAHLS): developing a tool to measure functional, communicative and critical health literacy in primary healthcare settings. *Patient Education and Counseling*, *90*(2), 247–253.

Cho, C. H., Seo, H. J., Bae, K. C., Lee, K. J., Hwang, I., & Warner, J. J. (2013). The impact of depression and anxiety on self-assessed pain, disability, and quality of life in patients scheduled for rotator cuff repair. *Journal of Shoulder and Elbow Surgery*, *22*(9), 1160–1166.

Collins, S. L., Moore, R. A., & McQuay, H. J. (1997). The visual analogue pain intensity scale: what is moderate pain in millimetres? *Pain*, *72*(1), 95–97.

Cook, K. F., Dunn, W., Griffith, J. W., Morrison, M., Tanquary, J., Sabata, D., ... Gershon, R.C. (2013). Pain assessment using the NIH toolbox. *Neurology*, *80*(Suppl 3), S49–S53.

Coppieters, I., Ickmans, K., Cagnie, B., Nijs, J., De Pauw, R., Noten, S., & Meeus, M. (2015). Cognitive performance is related to central sensitization and health-related quality of life in patients with chronic whiplash-associated disorders and fibromyalgia. *Pain Physician*, *18*(3), E389–E401.

Dansie, E. J., & Turk, D. C. (2013). Assessment of patients with chronic pain. *British Journal of Anaesthesia*, *111*(1), 19–25.

Dekel, B. G. S., Remondini, F., Gori, A., Vasarri, A., Di Nino, G., & Melotti, R. M. (2016). Development, validation and psychometric properties of a diagnostic/prognostic tool for breakthrough pain in mixed chronic-pain patients. *Clinical Neurology and Neurosurgery*, *141*, 23–29.

Donaldson, G., & Chapman, C. R. (2013). Pain management is more than just a number. University of Utah Health/Department of Anesthesiology, Salt Lake City Utah.

Dijkers, M. (2010). Comparing quantification of pain severity by verbal rating and numeric rating scales. *The Journal of Spinal Cord Medicine*, *33*(3), 232–242.

Driban, J. B., Morgan, N., Price, L. L., Cook, K. F., & Wang, C. (2015). Patient-Reported Outcomes Measurement Information System (PROMIS) instruments among individuals with symptomatic knee osteoarthritis: A cross-sectional study of floor/ceiling effects and construct validity. *BMC Musculoskeletal Disorders*, *16*(1), 253.

Dworkin, R. H., Turk, D. C., Revicki, D. A., Harding, G., Coyne, K. S., Peirce-Sandner, S., & Farrar, J. T. (2009). Development and initial validation of an expanded and revised version of the Short-form McGill Pain Questionnaire (SF-MPQ-2). *PAIN®*, *144*(1), 35–42.

Dworkin, R. H., Turk, D. C., Wyrwich, K. W., Beaton, D., Cleeland, C. S., Farrar, J. T., ... Kaatz, N. P. (2008). Interpreting the clinical importance of treatment outcomes in chronic pain clinical trials: IMMPACT recommendations. *The Journal of Pain*, *9*(2), 105–121.

Edwards, R. R., Dworkin, R. H., Sullivan, M. D., Turk, D. C., & Wasan, A. D. (2016). The role of psychosocial processes in the development and maintenance of chronic pain. *The Journal of Pain*, *17*(9), T70–T92.

Edwards, R. R., Mensing, G., Cahalan, C., Greenbaum, S., Narang, S., Belfer, I., ... Jamison, R. N. (2013). Alteration in pain modulation in women with persistent pain after lumpectomy: Influence of catastrophizing. *Journal of Pain and Symptom Management*, *46*(1), 30–42.

Ehde, D. M., Dillworth, T. M., & Turner, J. A. (2014). Cognitive-behavioral therapy for individuals with chronic pain: Efficacy, innovations, and directions for research. *American Psychologist*, *69*(2), 153.

Eyler, E. C. (2013). Chronic and acute pain and pain management for patients in methadone maintenance treatment. *The American Journal on Addictions*, *22*, 75–83.

Ferreira-Valente, M. A., Pais-Ribeiro, J. L., & Jensen, M. P. (2011). Validity of four pain intensity rating scales. *Pain*, *152*(10), 2399–2404.

Fillingim, R. B., Loeser, J. D., Baron, R., & Edwards, R. R. (2016). Assessment of chronic pain: domains, methods, and mechanisms. *The Journal of Pain*, *17*(9), T10–T20.

Finan, P. H., & Garland, E. L. (2015). The role of positive affect in pain and its treatment. *The Clinical Journal of Pain*, *31*(2), 177.

Finan, P. H., Goodin, B. R., & Smith, M. T. (2013). The association of sleep and pain: An update and a path forward. *The Journal of Pain*, *14*(12), 1539–1552.

Finka, R. M., Gates, R. A., & Montgomery, R. K. (2015). Physical aspects of care; Pain and gastrointestinal symptoms. In J. Paice, & B. Ferrell (Eds.), *HPNA Palliative Nursing Manuals*. New York, NY: Oxford University Press.

Finnerup, N. B., Haroutounian, S., Kamerman, P., Baron, R., Bennett, D. L., Bouhassira, D., ... Raja, S. N. (2016). Neuropathic pain: An updated grading system for research and clinical practice. *Pain*, *157*(8), 1599.

Fishbain, D. A., Lewis, J. E., Cutler, R., Cole, B., Rosomoff, H. L., & Rosomoff, R. S. (2008). Can the Neuropathic Pain Scale discriminate between non-neuropathic and neuropathic pain? *Pain Medicine*, *9*(2), 149–160.

Flor, H., & Turk, D. C. (2015). *Chronic pain: an integrated biobehavioral approach*. Philadelphia, PA: Lippincott Williams & Wilkins.

Galer, B. S., & Jensen, M. P. (1997). Development and preliminary validation of a pain measure specific to neuropathic pain The Neuropathic Pain Scale. *Neurology*, *48*(2), 332–338.

Gerbershagen, H. J., Rothaug, J., Kalkman, C. J., & Meissner, W. (2011). Determination of moderate-to-severe postoperative pain on the numeric rating scale: A cut-off point analysis applying four different methods. *British Journal of Anaesthesia*, *107*(4), 619–626.

Ghoneim, M. M., & O'Hara, M. W. (2016). Depression and post-operative complications: An overview. *BMC Surgery*, *16*(1), 5.

Gilron, I., Baron, R., & Jensen, T. (2015). Neuropathic pain: Principles of diagnosis and treatment. *Mayo Clinic Proceedings*, *90*(4), 532–545.

Gloth, F. M. (2001). Pain management in older adults: prevention and treatment. *Journal of the American Geriatrics Society*, *49*(2), 188–199.

Gloth, F. M., Scheve, A. A., Stober, C. V., Chow, S., & Prosser, J. (2001). The Functional Pain Scale: reliability, validity, and responsiveness in an elderly population. *Journal of the American Medical Directors Association*, *2*(3), 110–114.

Glue, P., Cape, G., Tunnicliff, D., Lockhart, M., Lam, F., Gray, A., ... Howes, J. (2016). Switching opioid-dependent patients from methadone to morphine: safety, tolerability, and methadone pharmacokinetics. *The Journal of Clinical Pharmacology*, *56*(8), 960–965.

Gordon, D. B. (2015). Acute pain assessment tools: let us move beyond simple pain ratings. *Current Opinion Anesthesiology*, 28, 565–569.

Haanpää, M., Attal, N., Backonja, M., Baron, R., Bennett, M., Bouhassira, D., ... Jensen, T. S. (2011). NeuPSIG guidelines on neuropathic pain assessment. *PAIN®*, 152(1), 14–27.

Hadjistavropoulos, T., Herr, K., Turk, D. C., Fine, P. G., Dworkin, R. H., Helme, R., ... Chibnall, J. T. (2007). An interdisciplinary expert consensus statement on assessment of pain in older persons. *The Clinical Journal of Pain*, 23, S1–S43.

Hagen, N. A., Stiles, C., Nekolaichuk, C., Biondo, P., Carlson, L. E., Fisher, K., & Fainsinger, R. (2008). The Alberta Breakthrough Pain Assessment Tool for cancer patients: a validation study using a delphi process and patient think-aloud interviews. *Journal of Pain and Symptom Management*, 35(2), 136–152.

Hawker, G. A., Mian, S., Kendzerska,T., & French, M. (2011). Measures of adult pain: Visual analog scale for pain (VAS pain), numeric rating scale for pain (NRS pain), McGill pain questionnaire (MPQ), short-form McGill pain questionnaire (SF-MPQ), chronic pain grade scale (CPGS), short form-36 bodily pain scale (SF-36BPS), and measure of intermittent and constant osteoarthritis pain (ICOAP). *Arthritis Care & Research*, 63(S11), S240-S252.

Haythornthwaite, J. A. (2013). Assessment of pain beliefs, coping, and function. In S. B. McMahon, M. Koltzenburg, I. Tracey, & D. Turk (Eds.), *Wall & Melzack's Textbook of Pain*. Philadelphia, PA: Elsevier Health Sciences.

Heale, R., & Twycross, A. (2015). Validity and reliability in quantitative studies. *Evidence-Based Nursing*, 18(3), 66–67.

Hemington, K. S., Cheng, J. C., Bosma, R. L., Rogachov, A., Kim, J. A., & Davis, K. D. (2017). Beyond Negative Pain-Related Psychological Factors: Resilience Is Related to Lower Pain Affect in Healthy Adults. *The Journal of Pain*, 18(9), 1117–1128.

Herndon, C. M., Arnstein, P., Darnall, B., Hartrick, C., Hecht, K., Lyons, M., & Seghal, N. (2016). *Principles of Analgesic Use*. Chicago, Ill: American Pain Society.

Herr, K. (2011). Pain assessment strategies in older adults. *The Journal of Pain*, 12(suppl 1), S3–S13.

Herr, K., Bjoro, K., & Decker, S. (2006). Tools for assessment of pain in nonverbal older adults with dementia: a state-of-the-science review. *Journal of Pain and Symptom Management*, 31(2), 170–192.

Hjermstad, M. J., Fayers, P. M., Haugen, D. F., Caraceni, A., Hanks, G. W., Loge, J. H., ... Kaasa, S. (2011). Studies comparing numerical rating scales, verbal rating scales, and visual analogue scales for assessment of pain intensity in adults: A systematic literature review. *Journal of Pain and Symptom Management*, 41(6), 1073–1093.

Jensen, M. P., & Karoly, P. (2011). In D. C. Turk, & R. Melzack (Eds.), *Handbook of Pain Assessment* (3ʳᵈ edition, pp. 19–41). New York, NY: The Guilford Press.

Jensen, M. P., Tomé-Pires, C., de la Vega, R., Galán, S., Solé, E., & Miró, J. (2017). What determines whether a pain is rated as mild, moderate, or severe? The importance of pain beliefs and pain interference. *The Clinical Journal of Pain*, 33(5), 414–421.

Kean, J., Monahan, P. O., Kroenke, K., Wu, J., Yu, Z., Stump, T. E., & Krebs, E. E. (2016). Comparative Responsiveness of the PROMIS Pain Interference Short Forms, Brief Pain Inventory, PEG, and SF-36 Bodily Pain Subscale. *Medical Care*, 54(4), 414–421.

Kosar, C. M., Tabloski, P. A., Travison, T. G., Jones, R. N., Schmitt, E. M., Puelle, M. R., ... Reid, M. C. (2014). Effect of preoperative pain and depressive symptoms on the risk of postoperative delirium: a prospective cohort study. *The Lancet Psychiatry*, 1(6), 431–436.

Krebs, E. E., Lorenz, K. A., Bair, M. J., Damush, T. M., Wu, J., Sutherland, J. M., ... Kroenke, K. (2009). Development and initial validation of the PEG, a three-item scale assessing pain intensity and interference. *Journal of General Internal Medicine*, 24(6), 733–738.

Kroenke, K., Monahan, P. O., & Kean, J. (2015). Pragmatic characteristics of patient-reported outcome measures are important for use in clinical practice. *Journal of Clinical Epidemiology*, 68(9), 1085–1092.

Kroenke, K., Yu, Z., Wu, J., Kean, J., & Monahan, P. O. (2014). Operating characteristics of PROMIS four-item depression and anxiety scales in primary care patients with chronic pain. *Pain Medicine*, 15(11), 1892–1901.

Lowe, B., Kroenke, K., Herzog, W., & Grafe, K. (2004). Measuring depression outcome with a brief self-report instrument: Sensitivity to change of the Patient Health Questionnaire (PHQ-9). *Journal of Affective Disorders*, 81(1), 61–66.

Lovejoy, T. I., Turk, D. C., & Morasco, B. J. (2012). Evaluation of the Psychometric properties of the Revised Short-form McGill Pain Questionnaire (SF-MPQ-2). *Journal of Pain*, 13(12), 1250–1257.

Lund, I., Lundeberg, T., Sandberg, L., Budh, C. N., Kowalski, J., & Svensson, E. (2005). Lack of interchangeability between visual analogue and verbal rating pain scales: a cross-sectional description of pain etiology groups. *BMC Medical Research Methodology*, 4(5), 31.

Main, C. J. (2016). Pain assessment in context: a state of the science review of the McGill pain questionnaire 40 years on. *Pain*, 157(7), 1387–1399.

Manea, L., Gilbody, S., Hewitt, C., North, A., Plummer, F., Richardson, R., ... McMillan, D. (2016). Identifying depression with the PHQ-2: A diagnostic meta-analysis. *Journal of Affective Disorders*, 203, 382–395.

Mathieson, S., Maher, C. G., Terwee, C. B., de Campos, T. F., & Lin, C. W. C. (2015). Neuropathic pain screening questionnaires have limited measurement properties. A systematic review. *Journal of Clinical Epidemiology*, 68(8), 957–966.

Mitchell, A. J. (2013). The Mini-Mental State Examination (MMSE): An update on its diagnostic validity for cognitive disorders. In A. Larner (Ed.), *Cognitive Screening Instruments*. *Springer*. https://doi.org/10.1007/978-1-4471-2452-8_2. London.

Moore, R., Straube, S., & Aldington, D. (2013). Pain measures and cut-offs: "no worse than mild pain" as a simple, universal outcome. *Anaesthesia*, 68(4), 400–412.

National Comprehensive Cancer Network, 2020. National Comprehensive Cancer Network (2020). *NCCN Guidelines Version 1.2020, Adult Cancer Pain*, PAIN-E page 4. Retrieved August 29, 2020 from https://www.nccn.org/professionals/physician_gls/pdf/pain.pdf.

O'Brien, E. M., Staud, R. M., Hassinger, A. D., McCulloch, R. C., Craggs, J. G., Atchison, J. W., ... Robinson, M. E. (2010). Patient-Centered Perspective on Treatment Outcomes in Chronic Pain. *Pain Medicine*, 11(1), 6–15.

Olsen, M. F., Bjerre, E., Hansen, M. D., Hilden, J., Landler, N. E., Tendal, B., & Hróbjartsson, A. (2017). Pain relief that matters to patients: systematic review of empirical studies assessing the minimum clinically important difference in acute pain. *BMC Medicine, 15*(1), 35.

Pasero, C., & Herr, K. A. (2015). Practice recommendations for pain assessment by self-report with African American older adults. *Geriatric Nursing, 36*(1), 67–74.

Pasero, C., & McCaffery, M. (2011). *Pain assessment and pharmacologic management.* St. Louis, MO: Mosby.

Pasero, C., Quinlan-Colwell, A., Rae, D., Broglio, K., & Drew, D. (2016). American Society for Pain Management Nursing Position Statement: Prescribing and administering opioid doses based solely on pain intensity. *Pain Management Nursing, 17*(3), 170–180.

Patel, J., Baldwin, J., Bunting, P., & Laha, S. (2014). The effect of a multicomponent multidisciplinary bundle of interventions on sleep and delirium in medical and surgical intensive care patients. *Anaesthesia, 60*(6), 540–549.

Peters, M. L., Patijn, J., & Lamé, I. (2007). Pain assessment in younger and older pain patients: psychometric properties and patient preference of five commonly used measures of pain intensity. *Pain Medicine, 8*(7), 601-610.

Polomano, R. C., Galloway, K. T., Kent, M. L., Brandon-Edwards, H., Kwon, K. N., Morales, C., & Buckenmaier, C. T., III. (2016). Psychometric testing of the defense and veterans pain rating scale (DVPRS): a new pain scale for military population. *Pain Medicine, 17*(8), 1505–1519.

Quinlan-Colwell, A. (2012). Pain assessment in the older adult patient. In *Compact Clinical Guide to Geriatric Pain Management.* New York, NY: Springer Publishing.

Radnovich, R., Chapman, C. R., Gudin, J. A., Panchal, S. J., Webster, L. R., & Pergolizzi, J. V., Jr. (2014). Acute pain: effective management requires comprehensive assessment. *Postgraduate Medicine, 126*(4), 59–72.

Reynoldson, C., Stones, C., Allsop, M., Gardner, P., Bennett, M. I., Closs, S. J., & Knapp, P. (2014). Assessing the Quality and Usability of Smartphone Apps for Pain Self-Management. *Pain Medicine, 15*(6), 898–909.

St. Marie, B., (2014). Health care experiences when pain and substance use disorder coexist: "Just because I'm an addict doesn't mean I don't have pain." *Pain Medicine, 15,* 2075–2086.

Savage, S. R. (2014). Opioid therapy for pain. In R. K. Ries, D. A. Fiellin, S. C. Miller, & R. Saitz (Eds.), *The ASAM principles of addiction medicine* (5th ed., pp. 1500–1529). Philadelphia, PA: Wolters Kluwer.

Seng, E., Kerns, R. D., & Heapy, A. (2014). Psychological and behavioral assessment. In H. Benzon, J. Rathmell, C. Wu, D. Turk, C. Argoff, & R. Hurley (Eds.), *Practical management of pain* (5th ed., pp. 243–256). Philadelphia, PA: Mosby.

Sperlinga, R., Campagna, S., Berruti, A., Laciura, P., Ginosa, I., Paoletti, S., ... Saini, A. (2015). Alberta Breakthrough Pain Assessment Tool: a validation multicentre study in cancer patients with breakthrough pain. *European Journal of Pain, 19*(7), 881–888.

Stuppy, D. J. (1998). The Faces Pain Scale: reliability and validity with mature adults. *Applied Nursing Research, 11*(2), 84–89.

Tahir, T. A., & Mahajan, D. (2016). Delirium. *Medicine, 44*(12), 724–728.

Thorne, F. M., & Morley, S. (2009). Prospective judgments of acceptable outcomes for pain, interference and activity: patient-determined outcome criteria. *PAIN®, 144*(3), 262–269.

Topham, D., & Drew, D. (2017). Quality improvement project: Replacing the numeric rating scale with a clinically aligned pain assessment (CAPA®) tool. *Pain Management Nursing, 18*(6), 363–371.

Treede, R. D., Jensen, T. S., Campbell, J. N., Cruccu, G., Dostrovsky, J. O., Griffin, J. W., ... Serra, J. (2008). Neuropathic pain redefinition and a grading system for clinical and research purposes. *Neurology, 70*(18), 1630–1635.

Turk, D. C., & Melzack, R. (Eds.). (2011). *Handbook of pain assessment* (3rd ed.). New York, NY: The Guilford Press.

Van Hecke, A., Van Lancker, A., De Clercq, B., De Meyere, C., Dequeker, S., & Devulder, J. (2016). Pain intensity in hospitalized adults: a multilevel analysis of barriers and facilitators of pain management. *Nursing Research, 65*(4), 290–300.

Walsh, A., & Broglio, K. (2016). Pain management in the individual with serious illness and comorbid substance use disorder. In J. Pace, & D Wholihan (Eds.), *51. Nursing Clinics of North America: Palliative Care* (pp. 433–447).

Ware, L. J., Epps, C. D., Herr, K., & Packard, A. (2006). Evaluation of the revised faces pain scale, verbal descriptor scale, numeric rating scale, and Iowa pain thermometer in older minority adults. *Pain Management Nursing, 7*(3), 117–125.

Ware, L. J., Herr, K. A., Booker, S. S., Dotson, K., Key, J., Poindexter, N., ... Packard, A. (2015). Psychometric evaluation of the revised Iowa Pain Thermometer (IPT-R) in a sample of diverse cognitively intact and impaired older adults: A pilot study. *Pain Management Nursing, 16*(4), 475–482.

Webber, K., Davies, A. N., Zeppetella, G., & Cowie, M. R. (2014). Development and validation of the breakthrough pain assessment tool (BAT) in cancer patients. *Journal of Pain and Symptom Management, 48*(4), 619–631.

Weingarten, T. N., Watson, J. C., Hooten, W. M., Wollan, P. C., Melton, L. J., Locketz, A. J., & Yawn, B. P. (2007). Validation of the S-LANSS in the community setting. *Pain, 132*(1–2), 189–194.

Wesson, D. R., & Ling, W. (2003). The Clinical Opiate Withdrawal Scale (COWS). *Journal of Psychoactive Drugs, 35,* 253–259.

Williamson, A., & Hoggart, B. (2005). Pain: a review of three commonly used pain rating scales. *Journal of Clinical Nursing, 14,* 798–804.

Wong, D. L., & Baker, C. M. (1988). Pain in children: comparison of assessment scales. *Pediatric Nursing, 14*(1), 9–17.

Appendix 6-1

Translations of the Numeric Rating Scale

English

Please point to the number that best describes your pain.

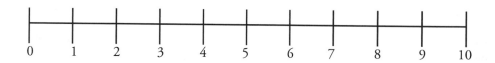

No pain   Terrible pain

Chinese*

請指出那個數字反應你痛的程度.

Please point to the number that best describes your pain.

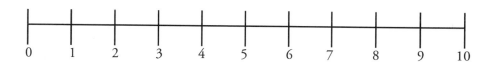

無痛   **劇痛**
No pain   Terrible pain

French†

Veuillez indiquer le chiffre qui décrit le mieux votre douleur.

Please point to the number that best describes your pain.

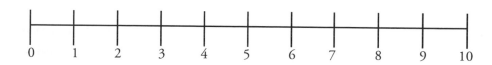

Pas de douleur   **Douleur intense**
No pain   Terrible pain

German[†]

Deuten Sie bitte zu der Zahl, die ihren Schmerzen am besten entspricht.

Please point to the number that best describes your pain.

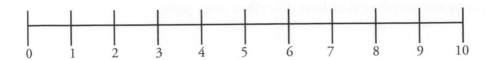

Keine Schmerzen   Fürchterliche Schmerzen

No pain   Terrible pain

Greek (modern)[†]

Παρακαλώ, δείξετε με το δάκτυλό σας τον αριθμό που δείχνει πόσο πόνο έχετε.

Please point to the number that best describes your pain.

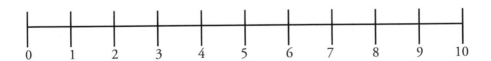

Δεν έχω πόνο   Έχω πολύ πόνο

No pain   Terrible pain

Hawaiian*

E ʻoluʻolu e kuhi i ka helu e like me ke ʻano o kou ʻeha.

Please point to the number that best describes your pain.

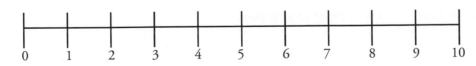

ʻAʻohe ʻeha   He ʻeha palena ʻole

No pain   Terrible pain

Hebrew†

אנא הצבע על המספר אשר מתאר במדוייק- את הכאב.

Please point to the number that best describes your pain.

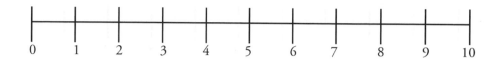

ללא כאב
No pain

כאב נורא
Terrible pain

Ilocano (spoken in the Philippines)*

Itudom man iti numero nga mangipakita nu kasano't kasakit iti marikriknam.

Please point to the number that best describes your pain.

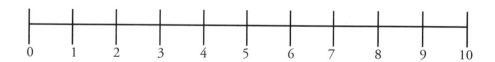

Awan ti sakit
No pain

Nasakit launay
Terrible pain

Italian*

Per piacere indica il numero che descrive meglio il tuo dolore.

Please point to the number that best describes your pain.

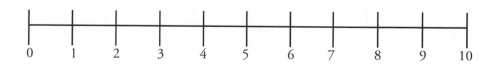

Nessun dolore
No pain

Dolore terribile
Terrible pain

Japanese[†]

痛みの強さの度合を0~10までの段階で示して下さい 。

Please point to the number that best describes your pain.

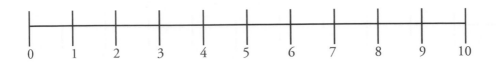

ゼロ　全く痛みがない

No pain

激痛

Terrible pain

Korean

현재 통증의 강도를 가장 잘 나타내는 번호에 표시하십시오.

Please point to the number that best describes your pain.

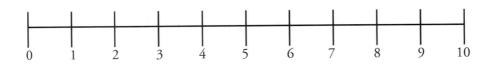

통증이 없음

No pain

통증이 너무 심함

Terrible pain

Urdu (spoken in Pakistan)[†]

برائے مہربانی اس نمبر کی طرف اشارہ کریں جو آپ کے درد کی شدت کو بہتر
طور پر بتلاتا ہے۔

Please point to the number that best describes your pain.

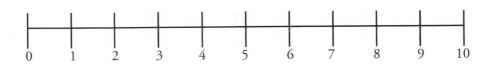

کوئی درد نہیں ہے

No pain

شدید ترین درد ہے

Terrible pain

Polish[†]

Proszę wskazać numer, który najlepiej określa jak silny jest ból.

Please point to the number that best describes your pain.

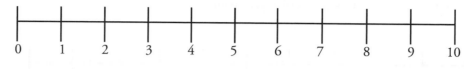

Nie mam bólu
No pain

Straszny ból
Terrible pain

Russian[†]

Пользуясь десятибалльной шкалой, укажите, пожалуйста, насколько сильно Вы чувствуете боль.

Please point to the number that best describes your pain.

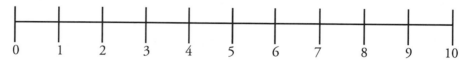

Боли нет совсем
No pain

Очень сильная боль
Terrible pain

Samoan*

Faamolemole ta'u mai le numera e faamatala ai le ituaiga tigā o loo e lagonaina.

Please point to the number that best describes your pain.

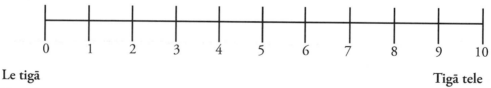

Le tigā
No pain

Tigā tele
Terrible pain

Spanish[†]

Por favor señale el número que mejor describe su dolor.

Please point to the number that best describes your pain.

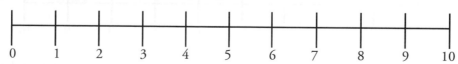

No tiene dolor
No pain

Tiene un terrible dolor
Terrible pain

Tagalog (spoken in the Philippines)†

Ituro po ninyo ang bilang na nagpapahiwatig ng tindi ng sakit.

Please point to the number that best describes your pain.

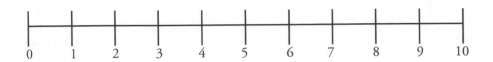

Walang sakit
No pain

Napakasakit
Terrible pain

Tongan (spoken in Tonga, an island in the south Pacific)†

I he ngaahi fika koena, fakailongai mai ai e tuunga ho felanga'aki.

Please point to the number that best describes your pain.

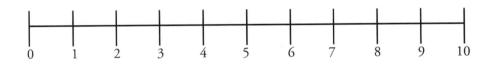

Ikai ha felanga'aki
No pain

Ikai matuuaki'e langa
Terrible pain

Vietnamese

Vui lòng chỉ ra số mô tả tốt nhất cơn đau của quý vị.

Please point to the number that best describes your pain.

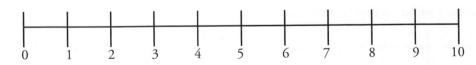

Không đau
No pain

Đau kinh khủng
Terrible pain

Appendix 6-2

Translations of Wong-Baker FACES Pain Rating Scale

Chinese

解釋給人聽用每張臉譜來代表著一個人的感覺是因爲沒有疼痛〔傷痛〕而感快樂或是因爲些許疼痛或者是許多疼痛而感傷心。第零張臉是很快樂的因爲他一點也不覺得疼痛。第一張臉只痛一丁點兒。第二張臉又痛多了一些。第三張臉痛得更多了。第四張臉是非常痛了。第五張臉是爲人們所能想像到的劇痛既使感到這樣難過，卻不一定哭出來。請這人選擇出最能代表他現在感覺的一張臉譜。此量表適用於三歲以上的人。

French

Expliquez à la personne que chaque visage représent un personne qui est heureux parce qu'elle n'a pas point du mal ou triste parce qu'il a un peu ou beaucoup du mal. **Visage 0** est trés heureux parce qu'elle n'a pas point du mal. **Visage 1** a un petit peu de mal. **Visage 2** a plus du mal. **Visage 3** a encore plus du mal. **Visage 4** a beaucoup du mal. **Visage 5** a autant mal que vous pouvez imaginer, bien que ces mauvais sentiments ne finissent pas nécessairement a vous faire pleurer. Demandez à la personne de choisir le visage qui convient le mieux avec ses sentiments.

Ces evaluations sont recommendés pour des personnes de trois ans et davantage.

Italian

Spiegare a la persona che ogni facien è per una persona che si sente felice perchè non tiene dolore oppure triste perchè ha poco o molto dolore. **Faccia O** è molto felice perchè non tiene dolor. **Faccia 1** tiene poco dolore. **Faccia 2** tiene un po più di dolore. **Faccia 3** tiene più dolore. **Faccia 4** tiene molto dolore. **Faccia 5** tiene molto dolore che non puoi immaginare però non devi piangere per tenere dolore. Domandi ala persona di scegliere quale faccia meglio descrive come si sente.

Grado scale è raccomandata a la persona di tre anni in sù.

Japanese

3歳以上の患者に望ましい。それぞれの顔は、患者の痛み (pain, hurt) がないのでご機嫌な感じ、または、ある程度の痛み・沢山の痛みがあるので悲しい感じを表現していることを説明して下さい。0＝痛みがまったくないから、とても幸せな顔をしている、1＝ほんの少し痛い、2＝もう少し痛い、3＝もっと痛い、4＝とっても痛い、5＝痛くて涙を流す必要はないけれども、これ以上の痛みは考えられないほど痛い。今、どのように感じているか最もよく表わしている顔を選ぶよう、患者に求めて下さい。

Portuguese

Explique a pessoa que cada face representa uma pessoa que está feliz porque não têm dor, ou triste por ter um pouco ou muita dor. **Face 0** está muito feliz porque não têm nenhuma dor. **Face 1** tem apenas um pouco de dor. **Face 2** têm um pouco mais de dor. **Face 3** têm ainda mais dor. **Face 4** têm muita dor. **Face 5** têm uma dor máxima, apesar de que nem sempre provoca o choro. Peça a pessoa que escolhe a face que melhor descreve como ele se sente.

Esta escala é aplicável a pessoas de tres anos de idade ou mais.

Romanian

Explică persoanei că fiecare faţă este specifică diferitelor stări fizice; o persoană este ferioita pentru că nu are nici o durere ori tristă pentru că suferă puţin sau mai mult. **Faţa 0** este foarte ferioită pentru că nu are absolut nici o durere. **Faţa 1** are un pic de durere. **Faţa 2** are ceva mai mult. **Faţa 3** suferă şi mai mult. **Faţa 4** suferă foarte mult. **Faţa 5** este greu de imaginat cât de mult suferă, căci nu trebuie neapărat să plângi, oricat de tare te-ar durea. Intreabă persoana să indice figura care-i desorie cel mai bine starea fizică.

Acest **grad de durere** este racomandat pentru persoanele de la 3 ani în sus.

Spanish

Expliquele a la persona que cada cara representa una persona que se siente feliz porque no tiene dolor o triste porque siente un poco o mucho dolor. **Cara 0** se siente muy feliz porque no tiene dolor. **Cara 1** tiene un poco de dolor. **Cara 2** tiene un poquito más de dolor. **Cara 3** tiene más dolor. **Cara 4** tiene mucho dolor. **Cara 5** tiene el dolor más fuerte que usted pueda imaginar, aunque usted no tiene que estar llorando para sentirse asi de mal. Pidale a la persona que escoja la cara que mejor describe su proprio dolor.

Esta escala se puede usar con personas de tres años de edad o más.

Vietnamese

Xin cắt nghĩa cho mỗi người, từng khuôn mặt của một người cảm thấy vui vẻ tại vì không có sự đau đón hoặc, buồn vì có chút ít hay rất nhiều sự đau đón.

Cái **mặt** với **số 0** thì rất là vui tại vì mặt ấy không có sự đau đón. **Mặt số 1** chỉ đau một chút thôi. **Mặt số 2** hơi đau hơn một chút nữa. **Mặt số 3** đau hơn chút nữa. **Mặt số 4** đau thật nhiều. **Mặt số 5** đau không thể tưởng tượng, mặc dù người ta không cần phải khóc mới cảm thấy được sự buồn khổ như thế.

Bạn hỏi từng người tự chọn khuôn mặt nào diễn tả được sự đau đón của chính mình.

Chapter 7 Pain Assessment of Patients Who Cannot Self-Report Pain

Debra Drew, Ann Quinlan-Colwell

CHAPTER OUTLINE

Pain Assessment of Patients Who Cannot Self-Report Pain, pg. 120

Pain Assessment in Critically Ill Adults Who Cannot Self-Report Pain, pg. 124

Pain Assessment and Intervention Notation Algorithm, pg. 124

Nonverbal Pain Assessment Tool, pg. 124

Adult Nonverbal Pain Score, pg. 124

Behavioral Pain Scale, pg. 124

The Critical Care Pain Observation Tool, pg. 125

Patients With Delirium Who Cannot Self-Report Pain, pg. 125

Patients With Dementia Who Cannot Self-Report Pain, pg. 125

Pain Assessment Checklist for Seniors With Limited Ability to Communicate, pg. 126

Pain Assessment in Advanced Dementia, pg. 126

The Checklist of Nonverbal Pain Indicators (CNPI), pg. 129

Patients With Intellectual Disabilities Who Cannot Self-Report Pain, pg. 129

The Revised Faces, Legs, Activity, Cries, Consolability Scale, pg. 130

The Individualized Numeric Rating Scale, pg. 130

The Non-Communicating Adult Pain Checklist, pg. 130

Patients at the End of Life Who Cannot Self-Report Pain, pg. 131

The Multidimensional Objective Pain Assessment Tool, pg. 131

The Pain Assessment in Advanced Dementia Tool, pg. 131

Newer Trends in Pain Assessment for Patients Who Cannot Self-Report Pain, pg. 131

Bispectral Index, pg. 131

Pupillary Reflex as a Physiologic Measure, pg. 132

The Nociception Level Index, pg. 132

Cautions, pg. 132

Key Points, pg. 132

Case Scenario, pg. 132

References, pg. 133

THE intent of this chapter is to explore the challenges involved when assessing people who cannot self-report pain. Conditions and situations that limit or prevent self-report are described. Tools used to assess these patients, including strengths and limitations, are described. Discussion includes how these tools can most effectively be used to manage pain.

Pain Assessment of Patients Who Cannot Self-Report Pain

The most accurate report of pain is self-report of pain by the patient (Booker & Herr, 2016). Pain assessment becomes more challenging when a patient cannot provide this most reliable method of determining the existence, location, severity, intensity, and quality of the subjective experience of pain. With many different conditions, there are several groups of people who cannot provide a self-report of their pain experience, including patients with delirium, dementia, cognitive impairment, or intellectual disabilities (IDs) and those who are critically ill or intubated.

Assessing pain accurately is important for many reasons that will be described, including providing the foundation for most effective pain management (Quinlan-Colwell, 2012). Accurate assessment forms the basis for optimal clinical care and research (Gordon, 2015). To ensure institutional standards for the assessment of pain for all patients, including those unable to self-report, the Joint Commission (TJC, 2016 p. 1,) expects the following:

- "The hospital assesses and manages the patient's pain.
- The hospital conducts a comprehensive pain assessment that is consistent with its scope of care, treatment, services, and the patient's condition.
- The hospital uses methods to assess pain that are consistent with the patient's age, condition, and ability to understand."

Although challenging, it is important to remember that many people with cognitive impairment, including dementia, are able to self-report pain. The person may not be able to describe pain in detail, though indicating the presence of pain through simple language or purposeful nonverbal communication is often possible. Appropriate pain assessment begins with asking the patient to self-report any pain by asking specific questions rather than open-ended questions. One might ask the specific question "Does your leg hurt when you move it?" rather than a more vague or difficult to comprehend question of "Do you have pain anywhere?" The person may be able to point to a painful area on his or her own body or on a sketch of a human body (Booker & Herr, 2016).

The authors of an American Society for Pain Management Nursing position paper noted that all persons with pain deserve prompt recognition and treatment (Herr, Coyne, Ely, Gélinas, & Manworren, 2019a; Herr, Coyne, Ely, Gélinas, & Manworren, 2019b). The

challenge is how a clinician assesses pain when the tools of self-report cannot be used or the clinician cannot depend on them. A framework developed to guide assessment approaches for patients who are unable to self-report was recently updated (Herr et al., 2019a; Herr et al, 2019b). This framework includes the following components:

1. Be cognizant of any factors that may be causing pain (e.g., chronic pain, recent injuries, painful procedures) (Herr et al., 2019a; Herr et al, 2019b). *Assume pain is present* (Makic, 2013a) for patients who have a painful condition, such as trauma, burns, surgery, certain types of cancer, chronic painful conditions, turning of intubated patients (Barr et al., 2013). For patients who do not have a current painful condition, it is important to consider any painful conditions before admission. Even for patients with no current or historical diagnosis indicative of pain, it is important to consider at least minimal discomfort related to being confined to bed, intravenous infusions, urinary catheters, and other medical interventions.
2. Attempt to obtain a self-report of pain perhaps through head or eye movements (Herr et al., 2019a; Herr et al, 2019b).
3. Observe the behaviors of the patient using a behavioral pain assessment tool (Herr et al., 2019a; Herr et al, 2019b). When a patient cannot use the tools described for cognitively intact adults (Chapter 6), monitor and assess behaviors of the patient using a valid observational tool (Tables 7.1 and 7.2) that

Table 7.1	Common Behavioral Tools Used for Patients in Intensive Care Units Who Cannot Self-Report Pain		
Tool With Description	**Advantages**	**Disadvantages**
Pain Assessment and Intervention Notation (PAIN) algorithm (Puntillo, Stannard, Miaskowski, Kehrle, & Gleeson, 2002) Consists of three parts: Pain assessment, the ability of patient to tolerate opioids, and guidelines for analgesic treatment.	Algorithm helps provide a systematic approach to pain assessment and guide to analgesic administration.	Too long and cumbersome for everyday practice. Reliability and validity could not be established.
Nonverbal Pain Assessment Tool (NPAT) (Klein, Dumpe, Katz, & Bena, 2010) Consists of five domains: Emotion, movement, verbal cues, facial cues, and positioning/guarding.	Interrater reliability high for verbal adults.	Not validated in noncommunicative adults.
Adult Nonverbal Pain Score (NVPS) (Odhner, Wegman, Freeland, Steinmetz, & Ingersoll, 2004) Based on FLACC scale: Contains behavioral and physiologic dimensions and autonomic indicators.	Considered valid because of correlation between NVPS and FLACC scale was high.	Based on a tool (FLACC) that was validated in children. Reliability was fair to poor when used with burn population. Physiologic data are least sensitive markers for the presence of pain. Use with caution in patients with facial burns that may affect facial expressions (Gélinas, 2016).

Table 7.1 | Common Behavioral Tools Used for Patients in Intensive Care Units Who Cannot Self-Report Pain—cont'd

Tool With Description	Advantages	Disadvantages
Behavioral Pain Scale (BPS) (Payen et al., 2001) Consists of three observational items scored from 1–4, for potential total of 12 indicating higher levels of pain.	Good interrater reliability for patients in deep sedation or in conscious sedation. Superior tool for patients in the ICU (Gélinas, 2016).	Interrater agreement varied widely: Good agreement in resting state, but poor after a painful procedure. May lack specificity in detection of pain.
Critical Care Pain Observation Tool (CPOT) (Gélinas & Johnston, 2007) Consists of four domains: Facial expressions, movements, muscle tension, and ventilator compliance. Includes vocalization for nonventilated patients. Each domain scored 0–2, with possible total score of 8 = most pain.	Sensitive and specific. Clear and easy to use. Useful for sedated patients (Gélinas, 2010; Li, Puntillo, & Miaskowski, 2008). Can be used for both ventilated and nonventilated patients. Found to be a more specific, reliable tool in nonverbal critically ill patients (Buttes, Kael, Cronin, Stocks, & Stout, 2014; Stites, 2013). Superior tool for ICU patients (Gélinas, 2016)	May have limitations for patients with chronic/persistent pain or concurrent delirium. Use with caution with patients with traumatic brain injury, because they tend to have lower CPOT scores as a result of neutral facial behaviors during usually painful turning procedures (Gélinas, 2016).

FLACC, Faces, Legs, Activity, Cries, Consolability scale; *ICU,* intensive care unit.
Adapted from Drew, D. J. & Pelitier C. H. (2018). Pain assessment. In: *Core Curriculum for Pain Management Nursing.* M. L. Czarnecki & H. N. Turner pp. 218–237.

Table 7.2 | Comparison of Tools for Assessment of Patients With Dementia

Tool and Description	Advantages	Disadvantages
Pain Assessment Checklist for Seniors with Limited Ability to Communicate (PACSLAC) (Fuchs-Lacelle & Hadjistavropoulos, 2004) 60-item checklist: Facial expressions, activity/body movements, social/personality/mood, physiologic indicators/eating, sleeping changes/vocal behaviors.	Good construct validity and reliability. 5 minutes to complete tool. Able to discriminate among painful, calm, and distressing events. Comprehensive indicators address all six pain behavior categories included in the American Geriatrics Society (AGS) guidelines (Pasero & McCaffery, 2011).	Checklist is long. Validity based on nurses' retrospective reports (Hadjistavropoulos, Herr, Turk, Fine, Dworkin, Helme, & Williams, 2007).
PACSLAC-II (Chan, Hadjistavropoulos, Williams, & Lints-Martindale, 2014) Modified version and shortened to 31 items.	Reliable, valid, able to differentiate between pain and nonpain states. Preferred by long term-care nurses and aides over PACSLAC (Chan, et al., 2014).	
Pain Assessment in Advanced Dementia Scale (PAINAD) (Warden, Hurley, & Volicer, 2003; Ersek, Herr, Neradilek, Buck, & Black, 2010) Five-item observational tool with range of 0–10: breathing, negative vocalization, facial expression, body language, consolability.	Sensitive tool for detecting pain in people with advanced dementia. Reliable and valid (Schuler et al., 2007). 5 minutes to complete tool. Has been translated into four languages. Can discriminate between groups with and without pain in long-term and acute care settings (Pasero & McCaffery, 2011).	High false positive rate with frequent detection of psychosocial distress rather than pain (Jordan, Hughes, Pakresi, Hepburn, & O'Brien, 2011). Low internal consistency may imply that a construct other than pain is being measured by some items (Hadjistavropoulos et al., 2007). Findings from the Ersek et al., 2010 study indicate that this tool warrants further study with clinical users and should be used only as part of a comprehensive approach to pain assessment.

Continued

Table 7.2 | Comparison of Tools for Assessment of Patients With Dementia—cont'd

Tool and Description	Advantages	Disadvantages
Checklist of Nonverbal Pain Indicators (CNPI) (see Fig. 7.3) (Feldt, 2000; Pasero & McCaffery, 2011) A brief observation list of six behaviors that indicate pain in nonverbal patients: Vocalizations, facial grimacing, bracing, rubbing, restlessness, and vocal complaints. Behaviors are observed at rest and with activity. Each category can be assigned a number of 0–1 for total possible score of 12.	CNPI identifies behaviors that indicate pain. It can be used as a screening tool to identify patients who are in pain. CNPI is designed for use with older, cognitively impaired adults in acute care. It provides reliable, valid determination of behaviors that indicate pain through test comparison of behaviors in verbal, cognitively intact patients compared to nonverbal, cognitively impaired patients.	It relies on observation. Potential inconsistencies are related to observer variation.
Certified Nursing Assistant Pain Assessment Tool (CPAT) (Cervo et al., 2009) 12-item tool to be used by CNAs observing pain behaviors in patients with dementia.	No evidence of content validation by experts. Tool is useful in evaluating effects of pain treatment in nursing home residents with dementia (Cervo et al., 2012).	Ability to quantify pain and measure treatment responses has not been determined.
Noncommunicative Patient's Pain Assessment Instrument (NOPPAIN) (Zwakhalen, Hamers, Abu-Saad, & Berger, 2006) Consists of four sections and combines information about pain behaviors, care conditions, and Likert scales of pain intensity.	Easy to use (Ferrari et al., 2009).	Tested with nursing assistants. Questionable whether nursing assistants can assess complex problem of pain during daily care situations (Zwakhalen et al., 2006).
Pain Assessment in Noncommunicative Elderly Persons (PAINE) (Cohen-Mansfield, 2006) Comprehensive list of pain symptoms used with systematic questioning by direct caregivers.	Valid and useful in detecting pain in persons with dementia.	

CNA, Certified nurse assistant.
Adapted from Drew, D. J. & Pelitier C. H. (2018). Pain assessment. In: *Core Curriculum for Pain Management Nursing.* M. L. Czarnecki & H. N. Turner pp. 218–237.

rates behaviors associated with pain. Some tools give number values to identified behaviors, and the values are tallied for a total score. It is important to remember that these total scores describing behavior are not in any way aligned with a self-report of pain intensity. The behavioral pain scores based on a clinician's observation of a patient's behaviors must be interpreted differently from a patient's self-report pain intensity score. The tools do not measure the same dimensions of pain as the patient self-reports. As a result, the assessment cannot include important components of location, duration, intensity, quality, causative factors, aggravating factors, alleviating options, functional limitations, and meaning of the pain to the person. Behavioral pain scales only provide the detection of pain probably being present. These tools cannot discriminate intensity such as the difference between mild, moderate, and severe levels of pain (Gélinas, 2016).

4. Seek information from family members and caregivers about the patient's history and behaviors related to pain (i.e., *proxy reporting of pain*) (Herr et al., 2019a; Herr et al, 2019b). Use *proxy reporting of pain* in combination with pain-related behaviors and pain-related changes in activity with credible information obtained from persons who know the patient well (surrogates). It is very important to remember that this is not a report by the patient but rather is the subjective understanding and interpretation by another person. No matter how close the other person is to the patient, the information is understood through the lens of their interpersonal relationship and the beliefs of the reporting person (Dion-Odom, Willis, Bakitas, Crandall, & Grace, 2015; Levine, Hoffman, Byron, Arnold, & Kondrat, 2015).

5. *Attempt an analgesic trial* when behaviors indicate pain or a pathologic condition or procedure is

likely to produce pain (Herr et al., 2019a; Herr et al, 2019b). For example, a multimodal approach of using combinations of pharmacology and complementary interventions (e.g., nonsteroidal antiinflammatory drug [NSAID], opioid, music, touch therapies, and ice) can be attempted during the postsurgical time. If behaviors improve or decrease on a behavioral tool, assume pain was a contributing factor and continue the intervention as appropriate and needed (Makic, 2013a).

In one randomized clinical trial of patients with moderate to severe dementia, the study group received a standardized stepwise protocol of analgesics: daily treatment with acetaminophen, morphine, buprenorphine transdermal patch, or pregabalin. The control group received the usual care and treatments (not specified). After 8 weeks, the study group demonstrated significantly less aggressive behaviors than did the control group, which received usual management of pain (Husebo, Ballard, Sandvik, Nilsen, & Aarsland, 2011).

It is important to minimize dependence on physiologic measures as indicators of pain. Physiologic measures such as changes in heart rate, blood pressure, and respiratory rate are not sufficiently sensitive to discriminate pain from other sources of distress. An expert panel that developed clinical practice guidelines for the management of pain, agitation, and delirium in adult patients in the intensive care unit (ICU), suggested that vital signs not be used alone for pain assessment. Vital signs should be used only as a cue to begin further assessment of pain in patients who cannot self-report their pain. (Barr et al., 2013). In addition, through the process of physiologic adaptation, patients who live with chronic pain rarely have increased physiologic changes (Di Lernia, Serino & Riva, 2016; Makic, 2013a).

Pain Assessment in Critically Ill Adults Who Cannot Self-Report Pain

Most critically ill patients will likely experience pain during their ICU hospitalization. Gélinas (2016) estimates that 30% of patients in the ICU have pain at rest and more than 50% have pain during common care procedures, such as turning, endotracheal suctioning, tube or drain removal, wound care, and arterial line insertions. Patients who cannot reliably self-report their experience of pain are at risk for undertreatment of pain (Voepel-Lewis, Zanotti, Dammeyer, & Merkel, 2010). Pain assessment of the critically ill patient may be complicated by agitation, delirium, compromised hemodynamic state, and neuromuscular-mediated physiologic responses. They also may be intubated, further reducing their ability to communicate effectively. The following tools were reviewed by several authors for use in the critical care setting (see Table 7.1).

Pain Assessment and Intervention Notation Algorithm

The Pain Assessment and Intervention Notation (PAIN) algorithm tool helps provide a systematic approach to pain assessment and analgesic administration. It consists of three parts: pain assessment, the ability of the patient to tolerate opioids, and guidelines for subsequent analgesics. The algorithmic approach provides a systematic way to assess pain and guide analgesic intervention. Reliability and validity have not been established, and it is considered long and cumbersome for everyday practice (Puntillo, Stannard, Miaskowski, Kehrle, & Gleeson, 2002).

Nonverbal Pain Assessment Tool

The Nonverbal Pain Assessment Tool (NPAT) consists of five domains: emotion, movement, verbal cues, facial cues, and positioning/guarding. In each domain there are descriptions of behavior that can be given numerical scores of 0 to 3. Although interrater reliability is high for verbal adults, the tool has not been validated in noncommunicative adults (Klein, Dumpe, Katz, & Bena, 2010).

Adult Nonverbal Pain Score

The adult Nonverbal Pain Score (NVPS) tool was based on the Faces, Legs, Activity, Cries, Consolability (FLACC) scale commonly used with children who cannot self-report pain. The NVPS contains behavioral and physiologic domains and autonomic indicators. The tool correlates with the FLACC scale and is therefore considered valid, but caution must be used in certain populations. For example, facial burns in a patient would affect the reliability of facial expressions (Gélinas, 2016). Again, it is important to remember that physiologic measures are the least sensitive markers of the existence of pain (Odhner, Wegman, Freeland, Steinmetz, & Ingersoll, 2004).

Behavioral Pain Scale

Considered a superior tool for patients in the ICU (Gélinas, 2016), the Behavioral Pain Scale (BPS) consists of three behavioral domains: facial expression, movements of upper limbs, and ventilation compliance. Each domain is scored from 1 to 4 for a potential high score of 12. The higher the score, the more likely it is that the behaviors indicate higher levels of pain. The tool was found to have good interrater reliability for patients in deep sedation or in conscious sedation. In other populations, the interrater agreement varied widely. There was good agreement for patients in a resting state, but poor agreement after a painful procedure. The tool may lack the specificity needed to detect pain (Payen et al., 2001). The BPS interprets absent upper limb movement to mean little or no pain, but in fact the absence of upper limb movement might simply reflect sedation, weakness, or paraplegia. Another criticism of this tool is the numbering system uses the number 1 as the absence of pain rather than using 0 to depict no pain.

The Critical Care Pain Observation Tool

The Critical Care in Pain Observation Tool (CPOT) was developed for the patient in a critical care setting who may or may not be on ventilation (Gélinas & Johnston, 2007). Considered sensitive and specific to detecting pain, it is also easy to use. The tool's components include facial expressions, bodily movements, muscle tension, and ventilator compliance (if applicable). For nonventilated patients, verbal vocalizations are included. Each component is scored 0 to 2 for a potential total of 8. The higher the number, the more likely the patient is in pain. The tool may have limitations for patients with chronic/persistent pain whose facial expressions and/or body movements may have been attenuated over time. Because patients with traumatic brain injury tend to have lower CPOT scores related to neutral facial behaviors, caution must be used in relying on this tool with this population (Gélinas, 2016). The CPOT has been found useful for pain assessment of sedated patients (Gélinas, 2010; Li, Puntillo, & Miaskowski, 2008; Rijkenberg, Stilma, Endeman, Bosman, & Oudemans-van Straaten, 2015).

Of the tools listed above the BPS and CPOT were considered the most valid and reliable of the pain assessment tools for the patient in the ICU who cannot self-report but whose motor function is intact and behaviors are observable (Gélinas, 2016; Payen & Gélinas, 2014; Rijkenberg et al., 2015). As the result of a small study with intubated and mechanically sedated patients (n = 72), Rijkenberg, Stilma, Bosman, van der Meer, and van der Voort (2017) concluded that although the BPS and CPOT are valid and reliable for clinical use, discriminant validation is not acceptable and needed further research.

Although no tool is perfect for all patients, each patient deserves to be assessed using the best tool for his or her condition or situation (see Table 7.1). This may require the clinician to try different tools until the most appropriate one is identified to assess the particular patient and to guide clinical decision making. Research is needed to continue to refine understanding, strengths, weaknesses, most appropriate use, and validity and reliability of these tools as well as others in development.

Patients With Delirium Who Cannot Self-Report Pain

Not only may patients with delirium be suffering with pain, but unrelieved pain is a risk factor for developing delirium (Makic, 2013b). Delirium is a mental state characterized by impaired memory and judgment, disorientation, confusion, and varying degrees of paranoia and hallucinations, due to a reversible impairment of cerebral metabolism, neurotransmitter abnormalities, or both. Delirium is transient, usually with acute onset from cerebral dysfunction and is more prevalent than may be expected. A study involving patients with trauma (n = 215) found 36% in the ICU had delirium and 11% in the intermediate care unit had delirium (Von Rueden et al., 2017). Another study found that 33% of patients with cancer (n = 81) in a Danish hospital had signs of delirium (Grandahl, Nielsen, Koerner, Schultz, & Arnfred, 2016). During acute delirium, the ability to self-report pain may be seriously compromised.

Behavioral pain scales were validated in only two studies of patients with delirium in the ICU. The Behavior Pain Scale–Non-Intubated (BPS-NI) is used with patients in the ICU who cannot report pain but who are not on mechanical ventilation (Olsen et al., 2015). Olsen and colleagues (2015) reported that the tool has good discriminant validity at rest and with painful procedures. The values were not affected by nonpainful procedures. Both the BPS-NI and CPOT appear to be valid for use in patients in the ICU who are experiencing delirium (Gélinas, 2016). Because there is continuing concern about the level of validity with behavioral scales for patients in the ICU with cognitive deficits, further research is needed to support external validity.

Patients With Dementia Who Cannot Self-Report Pain

At least 50% of people with dementia regularly experience pain, predominantly from the musculoskeletal system (Lichtner et al, 2014). Dementia is very common in older adult patients in acute hospitalizations, affecting one in four patients, and of those patients with dementia who are admitted to hospitals, 54% are admitted due to pain (Jackson et al., 2017). Although symptoms may be similar between delirium and dementia, they are different clinical situations. Dementia is the result of either exogenous or intrinsic processes affecting cerebral neurochemistry or anatomic damage to the brain (Lippmann & Perugula, 2016). Dementia proceeds with significant and progressive decline in executive functions of the brain (e.g., memory, language, judgment, attention span, social skills, and perceptual-motor functions).

With dementia unrelieved pain may be exhibited in agitated or aggressive behavior (Lichtner, et al, 2014). Persons with dementia may exhibit impaired memory and/or judgment, variable alertness, confusion/disorientation, poor social skills, and variable degrees of paranoia. Dementia is most commonly caused by neurodegenerative diseases such as Alzheimer's disease or Parkinson's disease (Corriveau et al, 2017; Owens-Walton et al, 2019). Other causes include toxins from alcohol, lead poisoning, drugs, and infections such as prion disease or acquired immunodeficiency syndrome (AIDS), neurosyphilis, or autoimmune diseases, endocrine disorders, Huntington's disease, and space-occupying lesions.

It is important to remember that older adults with mild to moderate dementia are often able to self-report pain even if they are not able to report pain intensity (Booker & Herr, 2016; Quinlan-Colwell, 2012) and unrelieved pain can increase dementia-related agitation (Quinlan-Colwell, 2012). Self-report from patients with advanced dementia is limited and sometimes unobtainable due to impaired cognitive, linguistic, and social skills. Autonomic reactions can indicate the presence of acute pain, but measures such as heart rate, blood pressure, and respiratory rate are not as useful to identify persistent pain (Hadjistavropoulos et al., 2014). In patients with dementia, pain is often associated with agitation.

One research team developed a stepwise protocol (Habiger, Flo, Achterberg, & Husebo, 2016) to treat pain, psychosis, and agitation. In that cluster-randomized clinical trial the researchers found that the pain treatment reduced agitation, aberrant motor behavior, and psychosis. They also reported use of opioid analgesics did not increase psychotic symptoms in these patients with dementia.

An expert consensus panel (Herr, Bursch, Ersek, Miller, & Swafford, 2010) reviewed 14 observational tools for use with patients with dementia and recommend the following for use:

- Abbey Pain Scale
- Checklist of Nonverbal Pain Indicators (CNPI)
- Certified Nurse Assistant Pain Assessment (CPAT)
- Disability Distress Assessment Tool (Dis DAT)
- Discomfort Behavior Scale (DBS)
- Doloplus 2
- Elderly Pain Caring Assessment 2 (EPCA-2)
- Mobilization-Observation-Behavior-Intensity-Dementia Pain Scale (MOBID)
- Nursing Assistant-Administered Instrument to Assess Pain in Demented Individuals (NOPPAIN)
- Pain Assessment Checklist for Seniors with Limited Ability to Communicate (PACSLAC)
- Pain Assessment for the Dementing Elderly (PADE)
- Pain Assessment in Advanced Dementia (PAINAD)
- Pain Assessment in Noncommunicative Elderly Persons (PAINE)
- Pain Behaviors for Osteoarthritis Instrument for Cognitively Impaired Elders (PBOICIE)

The tools with strongest conceptual and psychometric support and clinical usefulness are presented in Table 7.2. Two tools most recommended for nursing home residents with advanced dementia: were the PACSLAC and PAINAD (Herr et al., 2010) (see Table 7.2).

Pain Assessment Checklist for Seniors With Limited Ability to Communicate

The PACSLAC tool was developed by a Canadian team to enable a familiar caregiver to observe for common and subtle pain behaviors (Fuchs-Lacelle & Hadjistavropoulous, 2004) (Fig. 7.1). It consists of four subscales with a total of 60 items: facial expressions; activity/body movements; social, personality, mood, and physiologic indicators; and eating, sleeping, and vocal behaviors. Each of the 60 items are scored as 0 or 1, for a potential high score of 60. Although there are numerous items, it takes only about 5 minutes to complete. The tool is able to discriminate among painful, calm, and distressing events. Comprehensive indicators address all six pain behavior categories included in the American Geriatrics Society (AGS) guidelines of 2002 (Pasero & McCaffery, 2011). When used by caregivers, the PACSLAC is reported to have good inter-rater reliability (Cheung & Choi, 2008).

The PACSLAC-II is a modified version of the PACSLAC with only 31 items. It is still reliable and valid. This shortened version is preferred by clinicians over the original 60-item tool (Chan, Hadjistavropoulos, Williams, & Lints-Martindale, 2014; Ammaturo, Hadjistavropoulos, & Williams, 2017).

Pain Assessment in Advanced Dementia

The PAINAD tool is sensitive for detecting pain in persons with advanced dementia. It is a five-item tool that includes assessment of breathing, negative vocalization, facial expression, body movements, and consolability (Fig. 7.2). Each item is scored 0 to 2, for a total of 10 possible points (Warden, Hurley, & Volicer, 2003; Ersek, Herr, Neradilek, Buck, & Black, 2010). It is estimated to take about 5 minutes to complete. There appears to be a high false positive rate with frequent detection of psychosocial distress (Jordan, Hughes, Pakresi, Hepburn, & O'Brien, 2011), which may indicate the tool is measuring some other construct rather than pain (Hadjistavropoulos et al., 2007). One criticism of the tool concerns the inclusion of the Cheyne-Stokes breathing pattern in the first domain, which is not necessarily indicative of pain (Gregory, 2012). Named for John Cheyne and William Stokes, who described the breathing pattern in the 1800s, Cheyne-Stokes breathing consists of a pattern of very shallow, almost imperceptible breathing alternating with periods of deep breathing, and 10 to 20 seconds of apnea before the cycle is repeated. This pattern often precedes death and may be the result of increased partial pressure of carbon dioxide (pCO_2) blood concentrations, use of sedatives or opiates, cerebral vascular accidents, or other severe neurologic insults (Eldridge, 2017; Wang, Cao, Feng, & Chen, 2015).

Despite the advantages of each tool, there is still no one instrument that is ideal for assessing pain in patients with dementia (Hadjistavropoulos et al., 2014). To help guide selection of the most appropriate tool, Booker and Herr (2016) developed an algorithm for selecting the appropriate tool for patients with particular characteristics (see Table 7.3).

Indicate with a checkmark which of the items on the PACSLAC occurred during the period of interest. Scoring the subscales is derived by counting the checkmarks in each column. To generate a total pain sum all subscale totals.

Facial Expression	Present
Grimacing	
Sad Look	
Tighter Face	
Dirty Look	
Change in Eyes (squinting, dull, bright, increased eye movements)	
Frowning	
Pain Expression	
Grim Face	
Clenching Teeth	
Wincing	
Open Mouth	
Creasing Forehead	
Screwing Up Nose	

Social/Personality/Mood	Present
Physical Aggression (e.g., pushing people and/or objects, scratching others, hitting others, striking, kicking)	
Verbal Aggression	
Not Wanting To Be Touched	
Not Allowing People Near	
Angry/Mad	
Throwing Things	
Increased Confusion	
Anxious	
Upset	
Agitated	
Cranky/Irritable	
Frustrated	

Activity/Body Movement	Present
Fidgeting	
Pulling Away	
Flinching	
Restless	
Pacing	
Wandering	
Trying to Leave	
Refusing to Move	
Thrashing	
Decreased Activity	
Refusing Medications	
Moving Slow	
Impulsive Behaviours (Repeat Movements)	
Uncooperative/Resistance to Care	
Guarding Sore Area	
Touching/Holding Score Area	
Limping	
Clenching Fist	
Going Into Fetal Position	
Stiff/Rigid	

Other (Physiologic Changes/Eating Sleeping Changes/Vocal Behaviors)	Present
Pale Face	
Flushed, Red Face	
Teary Eyed	
Sweating	
Shaking/Trembling	
Cold? Clammy	
Changes in Sleep Routine (Please circle 1 or 2) 1) Decreased Sleep --------- 2) Increased Sleep During the Day	
Changes in Appetite (Please circle 1 or 2) 1) Decreased Appetite --------- 2) Increased Appetite	
Screaming/Yelling	
Calling Out (i.e., for help)	
Crying	
A Specific Sound of Vocalization For pain "ow," "ouch"	
Moaning and Groaning	
Mumbling	
Grunting	
Total Checklist Score	

Fig. 7.1 | Pain Assessment Checklist for Seniors With Limited Ability to Communicate (PACSLAC). (From Fuchs-Lacelle, S., & Hadjistavropoulos, T. [2004]. Development and preliminary validation of the pain assessment checklist for seniors with limited ability to communicate [PACSLAC]. *Pain Management Nursing, 5*[1], 37–49. The PACSLAC may not be reproduced or translated without permission. For permission to reproduce the PACSLAC contact the copyright holders [Thomas.hadjistavropoulos@uregina.ca]. The developers of the PACSLAC specifically disclaim any and all liability arising directly or indirectly for use or application of the PACSLAC. Use of the PACSLAC may not be appropriate for some patients, and the PACSLAC is not a substitute for a thorough assessment of the patient by a qualified health professional.)

The PAINAD Scale				
	0	**1**	**2**	**Score**
Breathing (independent of vocalization)	Normal	Occasional labored breathing, short period of hyperventilation	Noisy labored breathing, long period of hyperventilation, Cheyne-stokes respirations	
Negative vocalization	None	Occasional moan or groan, low level of speech with a negative or disapproving quality	Repeated trouble calling out, loud moaning or groaning, crying	
Facial expression	Smiling or inexpressive	Sad, frightened, frowning	Facial grimacing	
Body language	Relaxed	Tense, distressed pacing, fidgeting	Rigid, fists clenched, knees pulled up, pulling or pushing away, striking out	
Consolability	No need to console	Distracted or reassured by voice or touch	Unable to console, distract, or reassure	
				Total

Fig. 7.2 | PAINAD Tool. (From Warden, V., Hurley, A. C., & Volicer, V. [2003]. Development and psychometric evaluation of the Pain Assessment in Advanced Dementia [PAINAD] Scale. *Journal of the American Medical Directors Association,* 4:9–15. Developed at the New England Geriatric Research Education & Clinical Center, Bedford VAMC, MA.)

Table 7.3 | Tool Selection Algorithm for Patients With Particular Characteristics

Reliability and Ability to Self-Report Determination Process	Pain Tool Selection Process		Additional Considerations for Pain Tool Selection
Triggers to establish self-report ability: Note a diagnosis of cognitive impairment, dementia, or mental health condition. Note a condition that may interfere with verbal report (e.g., aphasia), Administer a quick, reliable mental status examination, and/or observe coherence of thoughts and verbal communication (and/or ability to explain what pain is to them). Techniques to establish reliability to self-report using pain tools: Ask older adult to pick two words that similarly describe pain from a list mixed with pain and nonpain descriptors and observe for conceptual understanding. Assess conceptual understanding on the use of a self-report pain scale by asking the person where mild and severe pain are represented on a pain scale of 0–10, then repeat this task several minutes later (should have the same or similar scores if reliably reporting pain); this also can be done by asking if 7 is more intense pain than 9 on the NRS. Use a pain screener test.	*If older adult:* Can communicate verbally or nonverbally purposefully (e.g., pointing, head nods, etc.), can self-report reliably, and is cognitively intact.	*Use a valid, reliable, and patient-preferred self-report pain scale such as:* • FPS-r • VDS • IPT-r • NRS	Congruent with patient's culture of pain expression, accurate language, and available in different languages (or can be easily translated). Accommodates patient's sensory impairments. Accommodates patient's developmental, intellectual, and cognitive level; easily understood. Easily and quickly explained to patient or observer. Easily used, scored, and recorded consistently. Can be used by interdisciplinary personnel. Easily linked to patient's comfort–function–mood goals. Meets organizational and regulatory standards. Fits with quality indicators and institutional documentation system. Can be used as data for quality improvement and evidence-based practice projects.

Table 7.3	Tool Selection Algorithm for Patients With Particular Characteristics—cont'd	
Reliability and Ability to Self-Report Determination Process	**Pain Tool Selection Process**	**Additional Considerations for Pain Tool Selection**
	Cannot consistently communicate verbally or nonverbally purposefully, cannot self-report consistently, and has fluctuating cognitive status (e.g., dementia, delirium).	Attempt self-report first by using a valid, reliable, and preferred self-report pain scale (see previous) and observational pain–behavior tool such as: • PAINAD • PACSLAC-II • Abbey Pain Scale • Doloplus-2	
	Cannot communicate verbally, cannot self-report, and is not cognitively intact.	Use an assessment protocol such as the: • Hierarchy of Pain Assessment25 • ADD • MOBID-2 and a valid, reliable observational pain–behavior tool (see previous).	

ADD, Assessment of Discomfort in Dementia Protocol; *FPS-r,* Faces Pain Scale-revised; *IPT-r,* Iowa Pain Thermometer-revised; *MOBID-2,* Mobilization-Observation-Behavior-Intensity-Dementia-2 pain scale; *NRS,* numeric rating scale; *PACSLAC-II,* Pain Assessment Checklist for Seniors with Limited Ability to Communicate; *PAINAD,* Pain Assessment in Advanced Dementia; *VDS,* verbal descriptor scale.

Booker, S. Q., & Herr, K. A. (2016). Assessment and measurement of pain in adults in later life. *Clinical Geriatric Medicine, 32*(4), 682–683.

The Checklist of Nonverbal Pain Indicators (CNPI)

The Checklist of Nonverbal Pain Indicators (CNPI) was designed to assess pain in older adults with cognitive impairment. Validity and reliability were not tested by the developers of the tool. It assesses six components believed to indicate pain. These include vocalizations, facial expressions, bracing, restlessness, massaging an area, and vocal expressions of pain (Feldt, 2000) (Fig. 7.3).

Patients With Intellectual Disabilities Who Cannot Self-Report Pain

People with intellectual disabilities (IDs) were born with cognitive impairments or developed impairments in early childhood (Herr et al., 2019a; Herr et al., 2019b). The disability continues lifelong in contrast to a cognitive impairment, which develops or occurs at any age. Generally, these individuals are defined by intelligence quota (IQ) scores. The majority of patients with ID can self-report pain, but with lower IQ scores, self-report may not be possible. An IQ score of less than 50 indicates moderate, severe, or profound impairment (Herr et al., 2019a; Herr et al., 2019b).

Although people with ID likely experience pain at a rate similar to others, they are at risk for pain not being identified or treated because of their limited ability to communicate pain (Boerlage et al., 2013; de Knegt et al., 2013). In a study in Netherlands with 356 people with ID ranging from 7 to 91 years, only 18% were assessed as having pain which was lower than expected (Boerlage et al., 2013). Not only do individual responses to pain vary greatly in this population but also their usual behaviors and the ability to distinguish between pain and other disliked sensations also vary widely (de Knegt et al., 2013). Knowledge of an individual's behaviors requires collaboration with a parent or caregiver so that pain is not overestimated or underestimated. Most behavioral pain assessment tools have been tested and used in children with IDs, but a few studies have included adults. Clinicians must select a tool that is appropriate to each individual's cognitive development and the type of pain suspected.

Proxy ratings for an individual's pain are based on reports of parents/caregivers who know the individual well. The Individualized Numeric Rating Scale (INRS) is based on a caregiver's knowledge of the family member's previous behaviors during a painful condition. Other tools that have been used to assess pain in adult patients with ID include the Checklist of Nonverbal Pain

PAIN SCALE FOR COGNITIVELY IMPAIRED, NON-VERBAL ADULTS

Checklist of Non-Verbal Pain Indicators (CNPI)		
Indicators:	With Movement	At Rest
Vocal Complaints (non-verbal expression of pain demonstrated by moans, groans, grunts, cries, gasps, sighs)		
Facial Grimaces and Winces (furrowed brow, narrowed eyes, tightened lips, dropped law, clenched teeth, distorted expression)		
Bracing (clutching or holding onto bed/chair, caregiver, or affected area during movement)		
Restlessness (constant or intermittent shifting of position, rocking, intermittent hand motions, inability to keep still)		
Rubbing (massaging affected area)		
Vocal Complaints (verbal expression of pain using words, e.g., "ouch" or "that hurts," cursing during movement or exclamation of protest, e.g., "stop" or "that's enough")		
Total Score		

Fig. 7.3 | **Checklist of Non-Verbal Pain Indicators (CNPI).** (From Feldt, K. S. [2000]. The checklist of nonverbal pain indicators [CNPI]. *Pain Management Nursing, 1*[1], 13–21.)

Indicators (CNPI), the Revised FLACC scale, INRS, and Noncommunicating Adult Pain Checklist (NCAPC).

The Revised Faces, Legs, Activity, Cries, Consolability Scale

The Revised Faces, Legs, Activity, Cries, Consolability Scale (r-FLACC) scale is a modification of the FLACC scale developed for assessing pain in children. The original tool scores the five behavioral categories from 0 to 2, with a range of 0 to 10. The revised tool allows for additional descriptors of that particular patient's observable behaviors to be included in each category. The tool is still scored 0 to 2 in each category for a possible total of 10. The revised tool allows for additional descriptors of that particular patient's observable behaviors to be included in each category. The r-FLACC can be helpful to distinguish pain from other symptoms such as spasticity (Fox, Ayyangar, Parten, Haapala, Schilling, & Kalpakjian, 2019).

The Individualized Numeric Rating Scale

The Individualized Numeric Rating Scale (INRS) is an NRS of 0 to 10 that is individualized to the patient. Built on the NRS (in which numbers ranging from 0 to 10 are placed at equidistant points on a line, with 0 equaling no pain and 10 equaling the worst pain imaginable), the nurse or parent uses the FLACC acronym (Faces, Legs, Activity, Cries, Consolability) descriptors adding to the

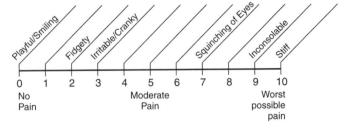

Fig. 7.4 | **Individualized Numeric Rating Scale.** (From Solodiuk, J., & Curley, M. A. Q. [2003]. Evidence based practice: Pain assessment in nonverbal children with severe cognitive impairments—The Individualized Numeric Rating Scale [INRS]. *Journal of Pediatric Nursing, 18*[4], 295–299.)

line, and patient pain behaviors that correspond to that particular patient's pain intensity (Solodiuk & Curley, 2003; Solodiuk et al., 2010). For example, a parent may assign the following words to the numbers on the NRS to describe the child's pain behaviors: playful/smiling = 0, fidgety = 2, irritable/cranky = 3, eyes shut tight = 7, inconsolable = 9, stiff = 10 (Fig. 7.4).

The Non-Communicating Adult Pain Checklist

The Non-Communicating Adult Pain Checklist (NCAPC) was developed to better capture pain behaviors of adults with intellectual and developmental disabilities by modifying the 30 items from the NCCPC down to 18 items.

The original NCCPC consisted of 30 items and scored 0 or 1 per item for a potential total of 30. Lotan, Moe-Nilssen, Ljunggren, and Strand (2010) studied 59 adults. The researchers reported that the NCAPC not only differentiated between pain and nonpain situations but was also sensitive to pain at all levels of intellectual and developmental disabilities.

Patients at the End of Life Who Cannot Self-Report Pain

Cognitive function tends to decline as disease progresses at the end of life. Estimation of delirium ranges from 26% to 62% on admission and rises to 88% in the last days and hours of life for patients admitted to palliative care programs (Hosie, Davidson, Agar, Sanderson, & Phillips, 2012). Another study showed 30% of patients entering a palliative care program were diagnosed with delirium (Kim et al., 2015). To date, a limited number of pain measurement tools have been developed and validated specifically for patients receiving palliative care regardless of clinical setting or disease trajectory.

The Multidimensional Objective Pain Assessment Tool

The Multidimensional Objective Pain Assessment Tool (MOPAT) was developed to assess acute pain in patients receiving palliative care without dementia who are unable to self-report pain, regardless of setting (e.g., acute care hospital, hospice) or whether receiving formal palliative care services (Wiegand, et al, 2018). The original tool was scored on two dimensions of pain assessed in patients: behavioral and physiologic (McGuire, Kaiser, Haisfield-Wolfe, & Iyamu, 2016). Behavioral indicators of pain include restlessness, muscle tension, frowning/grimacing, and patient sounds (e.g., moaning) scored from 0 (none or not present) to 3 (most severe) with an adjustment for patients who cannot make sounds (e.g., intubated, mechanically ventilated). Physiologic indicators of pain assessed by the original MOPAT included blood pressure, heart rate, respiratory rate, and diaphoresis, scored as no change from normal or baseline or a change from normal or baseline (McGuire et al., 2016). The hospice version of the MOPAT does not include the blood pressure item (McGuire et al., 2016). There is preliminary evidence of validity and reliability in both the acute care hospital and inpatient hospice settings (McGuire, Reifsnyder, Soeken, Kaiser, & Yeager, 2011; McGuire et al., 2016). The current version of the MOPAT is scored using only the behavioral indicators, because further work is being done on the validity of the physiologic indicators. Training on use of the MOPAT is accomplished with education modules including videotapes of pain behaviors and case scenarios (McGuire et al., 2016).

The Pain Assessment in Advanced Dementia Tool

The PAINAD (see Fig. 7.1) was also tested in older adults in long-term care and is suggested for assessing some persons at end of life (Herr et al., 2019a; Herr et al., 2019b). The absence of pain reports or pain behaviors as the patient nears death does not necessarily mean that pain has decreased or ceased, especially if pain was present when the person was cognitively intact. Treatment of pain should continue with modifications as necessary (see also Chapter 2).

Newer Trends in Pain Assessment for Patients Who Cannot Self-Report Pain

Although research has been done on using heart rate as a surrogate for nociception in sedated patients (Broucqsault-Dedrie, De Jonckheere, Jeanne, & Nseir, 2016), others contend that correlation of changes in vital signs with pain behaviors or self-reports of pain has been weak or absent (Arbour, Choiniére, Topolovec-Vranic, Loiselle, & Gélinas, 2014). Although heart rate and blood pressure increase in patients in ICUs who are exposed to painful procedures, vital signs are not considered clinically significant because sometimes vital signs do not increase with painful procedures (Gélinas, 2016). An increase in heart rate and blood pressure requires a careful assessment of all the potential reasons for the observed change. Pain may be considered one of the causes, and an analgesic trial may be warranted (see the framework to guide pain assessment [Herr et al., 2019]).

Bispectral Index

The bispectral (BIS) index is new in the arena of intensive care pain research. The BIS index is a single number that is computed from a complex algorithmic equation based on electroencephalogram (EEG) data. The index provides a number that is linked to a patient's level of consciousness. BIS values of less than 40 indicate a deep hypnotic state, and values of 40 to 60 indicate levels of general anesthesia. Two research teams found the BIS was not superior to end-tidal anesthetic gas protocols to prevent anesthesia awareness—the unintended intraoperative awareness that can result in anxiety and post-traumatic stress disorder (PTSD) (Avidan et al., 2008; Fritz et al., 2013). The primary purpose for BIS is not to measure pain, but rather for the titration of anesthetic agents during surgery, and therefore further research is needed to see if it can be used in the ICU pain assessment process. One study found that BIS values with and without neuromuscular blocks are not comparable in awake patients because the BIS algorithm requires muscle activity (Schutter, Newell, Strickland, & Barry, 2015). Currently this index can be used only in sedated patients. It would not be applicable to patients who are conscious yet unable to self-report (Gélinas, 2016).

Pupillary Reflex as a Physiologic Measure

Interest has been growing in the use of pupillary reflexes as a physiologic measure of the presence of pain. The pupil of the eye will contract on exposure of the retina to light. The pupils will also change size in response to various stimuli, such as point of fixation, effects of drugs, sudden loud noises, or emotional stimuli. Several studies showed positive correlations between pupil dilation and self-report of acute pain: in postoperative patients awakening from general anesthesia, during endotracheal suctioning and repositioning, and before dressing changes in patients with cellulitis. "Overall, these results suggest that pupillometry may potentially guide clinicians to adjust analgesia before nociceptive procedures in critically ill patients" (Gélinas, 2016, p. 8). Recently researchers in France reported from a proof of concept perspective that using pupillary reflex was not effective for assessment of pain in patients who are sedated and critically ill (Vinclair, 2019). Clearly this is an area where additional research is needed.

The Nociception Level Index

An index of nociception was tested in a preliminary validation study of 58 patients under general anesthetic. The nociception level (NoL) index is based on a nonlinear combination of physiologic changes: heart rate and heart rate variability, photoplethysmograph wave amplitude, and skin conductance. In those study patients, the NoL index responded to increased stimulus intensity and remained unchanged in response to nonnoxious stimuli. The study found that NoL was superior to any of the other indices alone. The implications for clinical practice is that NoL is an effective index for trending nociceptive states of the anesthetized patient (Edry, Recea, Dikust, & Sessler, 2016).

Cautions

All behavioral tools have two important limitations. First, it is important to remember that any score that is tallied does not equate to a self-report of pain intensity. Second, the absence of behavior does not mean there is no pain. The patient may not be exhibiting behavior for a variety of reasons, including neuromuscular blockade, sedation, or encephalopathy. When it is likely that the patient is experiencing pain but not exhibiting behaviors indicating pain, it is appropriate to assume that pain is present and implement an analgesic trial and reassess (Makic, 2013a; Herr et al, 2019).

Behavioral tools do not always assess pain. Sometimes the behaviors may be reflecting other constructs such as fear, anxiety, or delirium/dementia. Gregory (2012) contends there is no ideal behavioral tool that meets all populations' needs and that the tools are but one piece of a comprehensive pain assessment of the patient who cannot self-report the existence and experience of pain. The authors recommend supplementing the behavioral observations with knowledge of the patient's condition and information from family members who know the patient well.

Key Points

- The absence of behavior does not mean the absence of pain.
- Self-report is the most accurate assessment of pain.
- Patients with cognitive impairment may be able to report pain even if they cannot report location or intensity.
- In the absence of self-report, behavioral tools can be used to assess patient behaviors that indicate pain.
- If there are no behaviors indicating pain, but it is likely the person has pain, begin an analgesic trial.
- It is important to obtain as much historical medical information as possible from medical records and significant others.

Case Scenario

A 45-year-old man is admitted to the ICU after surgery for repair of multiple broken bones sustained in a motor vehicle accident. He is intubated and alternately sedated and awake. The team has decided to use the Critical Care Pain Observation Tool (CPOT) because the patient is having trouble communicating effectively. At rest the CPOT score is a four:

- Facial expression = 1, as evidenced by presence of frowning, brow lowering, orbit tightening, and levator contraction.
- Body movements = 1, as evidenced by the patient moving with slow cautious movements as if to protect himself.
- Muscle tension = 1, as evidenced by resistance to passive movements.
- Compliance with the ventilator = 1, as evidenced by alarms stopping spontaneously after the patient coughs.
  1. What is your assessment about the existence and intensity of this patient's pain at rest?
  2. Could these behaviors indicate something other than pain in this patient with trauma?
  3. What interventions would you consider to address your concerns for this patient's comfort level?

Later in your shift, it is time to turn this same patient. You had administered analgesics about an hour ago because of your assessment of pain at rest. Again, using the CPOT tool to gauge his comfort status, you calculate a total of 8 during the turning procedure and immediately afterward.

- Facial expression = 2, because of the presence of the features you saw earlier plus a distinct grimacing with eyes shut tight.

- Body movements = 2, because of the patient moving his limbs and thrashing about, not following commands, and striking out at staff.
- Muscle tension = 2 because of strong resistance to passive movements, appearing very tense.
- Compliance with the ventilator = 2, because of asynchrony of the ventilator from his "fighting it."
  1. What is your assessment, now, of this patient's pain during the turning process?
  2. Was the medication given 1 hour earlier adequate for this procedure?
  3. Could he be exhibiting other emotions through his change in behaviors?
  4. If you think he is having increased incidental pain, what would be some interventions that you would employ to prevent this in the future?

References

Ammaturo, D. A., Hadjistavropoulos, T., & Williams, J. (2017). Pain in Dementia: Use of observational pain assessment tools by people who are not health professionals. *Pain Medicine*, *18*(10), 1895–1907. https://doi.org/10.1093/pm/pnw265.

Arbour, C., Choiniére, M., Topolovec-Vranic, J., Loiselle, C. G., & Gélinas, C. (2014). Can fluctuations in vital signs be used for pain assessment in critically ill patients with a traumatic brain injury? *Pain Research and Treatment*, *2014*, Article ID 175794. https://doi.org/10.1155/2014/175794.

Avidan, M. S., Zhang, L., Burnside, B. A., Finkel, K. J., Searleman, A. C., Selvidge, J. A., Saager, L., Turner, M. S., Rao, S., Bottros, M., Hantler, C., Jacobsohn, E., & Evers, A. S. (2008). Anesthesia awareness and the bispectral index. *New England Journal of Medicine*, *358*(11), 1097–1108. https://doi.org/10.1056/NEJMoa0707361.

Barr, J., Fraser, G. L., Puntillo, K., Ely, E. W., Gélinas, C., Dasta, J. F., Davidson, J. E., Devlin, J. W., Kress, J. P., Joffe, A. M., Coursin, D. B., Herr, D. L., Tung, A., Robinson, B. R. H., Fontaine, D. K., Ramsay, M. A., Riker, R. R., Sessler, C. N., Pun, B., Skrobik, Y., & Jaeschke, R. (2013). Clinical practice guidelines for the management of pain, agitation, and delirium in adult patients in the intensive care unit. *Critical Care Medicine*, *41*(1), 263–306.

Boerlage, A. A., Valkenburg, A. J., Scherder, E. J., Steenhof, G., Effing, P., Tibboel, D., & van Dijk, M. (2013). Prevalence of pain in institutionalized adults with intellectual disabilities: A cross-sectional approach. *Research in Developmental Disabilities*, *34*(8), 2399–2406.

Booker, S. Q., & Herr, K. A. (2016). Assessment and measurement of pain in adults in later life. *Clinical Geriatric Medicine*, *32*(4), 677–692.

Broucqsault-Dedrie, C., De Jonckheere, J., Jeanne, M., & Nseir, S. (2016) Measurement of heart rate variability to assess pain in sedated critically ill patients: A prospective observational study. *PLOS One*. https://doi.org/10.1371/journal.pone.0147720.

Buttes, P., Keal, G., Cronin, S. N., Stocks, L., & Stout, C. (2014). Validation of the Critical-Care Pain Observation Tool in adult critically ill patients. *Dimensions of Critical Care Nursing*, *33*(2), 78–81. https://doi.org/10.1097/DCC.0000000000000021.

Cervo, F. A., Bruckenthal, P., Fields, S., Bright-Long, L. E., Chen, J. J., Zhang, G., & Strongwater, I. (2012). The role of the CNA Pain Assessment Tool (CPAT) in the pain management of nursing home residents with dementia. *Geriatric Nursing*, *33*(6), 430–438.

Chan, S., Hadjistavropoulos, T., Williams, J., & Lints-Martindale, A. (2014). Evidence-based development and initial validation of the Pain Assessment Checklist for Seniors with Limited Ability to Communicate-II (PACSLAC-II). *Clinical Journal of Pain*, *30*(9), 816–824. https://doi.org/10.1097/AJP.0000000000000039.

Cheung, G., & Choi, P. (2008). The use of the Pain Assessment Checklist for Seniors with Limited Ability to Communicate (PACSLAC) by caregivers in dementia care facilities. *The New Zealand Medical Journal*, *121*(1286), 21–29. ISSN 11758716.

Cohen-Mansfield, J. (2006). Pain assessment in noncommunicative elderly persons-PAINE. *Clinical Journal of Pain*, *22*(6), 569–575. https://doi.org/10.1097/01.ajp.0000210899.83096.

Corriveau, R. A., Koroshetz, W. J., Gladman, J. T., Jeon, S., Babcock, D., Bennett, D. A., ... Fillit, H. (2017). Alzheimer's Disease–Related Dementias Summit 2016: National research priorities. *Neurology*, *89*(23), 2381–2391.

de Knegt, N. C., Pieper, M. J., Lobbezoo, F., Schuengel, C., Evenhuis, H. M., Passchier, J., & Scherder, E. J. (2013). Behavioral pain indicators in people with intellectual disabilities: a systematic review. *The Journal of Pain*, *14*(9), 885–896.

Di Lernia, D., Serino, S., & Riva, G. (2016). Pain in the body. Altered interoception in chronic pain conditions: a systematic review. *Neuroscience and Biobehavioral Reviews*, *71*, 328–341.

Dion-Odom, J. N., Willis, D. G., Bakitas, M., Crandall, B., & Grace, P. J. (2015). Conceptualizing surrogate decision making at end of life in the intensive care unit using cognitive task analysis. *Nursing Outlook*, *63*(3), 331–340.

Edry, R., Recea, V., Dikust, Y., & Sessler, D. I. (2016). Preliminary intraoperative validation of the nociception level index: A non-invasive nociception monitor. *Anesthesiology*, *125*, 193–203.

Eldridge, L. (2017). *Cheyne-Stokes respirations and treatment*. https://www.verywell.com/Cheyne-Stokes-respirations-2249076.

Ersek, M., Herr, K., Neradilek, M. B., Buck, H. G., & Black, B. (2010). Comparing the psychometric properties of the checklist of nonverbal pain behaviors (CNPI) and the pain assessment in advanced dementia (PAIN-AD) instruments. *Pain Medicine*, *11*(3), 395–404. https://doi.org/10.1111/j.1526-4637.2009.00787.x.

Feldt, K. S. (2000). The checklist of non-verbal pain indicators (CNPI). *Pain Management Nursing*, *1*(1), 13–21. https://doi.org/10.1053/jpmn.2000.5831.

Ferrari, R., Martini, M., Mondini, S., Novello, C., Palonba, D., Scacco, C., ... Vescovo, G. (2009). Pain assessment in non-communicative patients: The Italian version of the Non-Communicative Patient's Pain Assessment Instrument (NOPPAIN). *Aging Clinical and Experimental Research*, *21*(4), 298–306.

Fox, M. A., Ayyangar, R., Parten, R., Haapala, H. J., Schilling, S. G., & Kalpakjian, C. Z. (2019). Self-report of pain in young people and adults with spastic cerebral palsy: inter-rater reliability of the revised Face, Legs, Activity, Cry, and

Consolability (r-FLACC) scale ratings. *Developmental Medicine & Child Neurology, 61*(1), 69–74.

Fritz, B. A., Rao, P., Mashour, G. A., Abdallah, A. B., Burnside, B. A., Jacobson, E., Zhang, L., & Avidan, S. A. (2013). Postoperative recovery with bispectral index versus anesthetic concentration-guided protocols. *Anesthesiology, 118*(5), 1113–1122.

Fuchs-Lacelle, S., & Hadjistavropoulos, T. (2004). Development and preliminary validation of the pain assessment checklist for seniors with limited ability to communicate (PACSLAC). *Pain Management Nursing, 5*(1), 37–49. https://doi.org/10.1016/j.pmn.2003.10.001.

Gélinas, C. (2010). Nurses' evaluations of the feasibility and the clinical utility of the critical- care pain observation tool. *Pain Management Nursing, 11*(2), 115–125. https://doi.org/10.1016/j.pmn.2009.05.002.

Gélinas, C. (2016). Pain assessment in critically ill adult: Recent evidence and new trends. *Intensive and Critical Care Nursing, 34*(1), 1–11.

Gélinas, C., & Johnston, C. (2007). Pain assessment in the critically ill ventilated adult: Validation of the critical-care pain observation tool and physiologic indicators. *Clinical Journal of Pain, 23*(6), 497–505. https://doi.org/10.1097/AJP.0b013e31806a23fb.

Gordon, D. B. (2015). Acute pain assessment tools: let us move beyond simple pain ratings. *Current Opinion in Anesthesiology, 28*(5), 565–569.

Grandahl, M. G., Nielsen, S. E., Koerner, E. A., Schultz, H. H., & Arnfred, S. M. (2016). Prevalence of delirium among patients at a cancer ward: Clinical risk factors and prediction by bedside cognitive tests. *Nordic Journal of Psychiatry, 70*(6), 413–417.

Gregory, J. (2012). How can we assess pain in people who have difficulty communicating? A practice development project identifying a pain assessment tool for acute care. *International Practice Development Journal, 2*(2), 1–22. http://www.fons.org/library/journal.aspx.

Habiger, T. F., Flo, E., Achterberg, W. P., & Husebo, B. S. (2016). The interactive relationship between pain, psychosis, and agitation in people with dementia: results from a cluster-randomised clinical trial. *Behavioural Neurology, 2016*. https://doi.org/10.1155/2016/7036415.

Hadjistavropoulos, T., Herr, K., Prkachin, K. M., Craig, K. D., Gibson, S. J., Lukas, A., & Smith, J. H. (2014). Pain assessment in elderly adults with dementia. *Lancet Neurology, 13*(12), 1216–1227.

Hadjistavropoulos, T., Herr, K., Turk, D. C., Fine, P. G., Dworkin, R. H., Helme, R., … Williams, J. (2007). An interdisciplinary expert consensus statement on assessment of pain in older persons. *Clinical Journal of Pain, 23*(1), S1–S43. https://doi.org/10.1097/AJP.0b013e31802be869.

Herr, K., Bursch, H., Ersek, M., Miller, L. L., & Swafford, K. (2010). Use of pain-behavioral assessment tools in the nursing home: Expert consensus recommendations for practice. *Journal of Gerontological Nursing, 36*(3), 18–29. https://doi.org/10.3928/00989134-20100108-04.

Herr, K., Coyne, P. J., Ely, E., Gélinas, C., & Manworren, R. C. (2019a). ASPMN 2019 Position Statement: Pain Assessment in the Patient Unable to Self-Report. *Pain Management Nursing, 20*(5), 402–403.

Herr, K., Coyne, P. J., Ely, E., Gélinas, C., & Manworren, R. C. (2019b). Pain assessment in the patient unable to self-report: clinical practice recommendations in support of the ASPMN 2019 position statement. *Pain Management Nursing, 20*(5), 404–417.

Hosie, A., Davidson, P., Agar, M., Sanderson, C., & Phillips, J. (2012). Delirium prevalence, incidence, and implications for screening in specialist palliative care inpatient settings: A systematic review. *Palliative Medicine, 27*(6), 486–498.

Husebo, B. S., Ballard, C., Sandvik, R., Nilsen, O. B., & Aarsland, D. (2011). Efficacy of treating pain to reduce behavioural disturbances in residents of nursing home with dementia: cluster randomized clinical trial. *British Medical Journal, 343*, 4065. https://doi.org/10.1136/bmj.d4065.

Jackson, T. A., Gladman, J. R. F., Harwood, R. H., MacLullich, A. M. J., Sampson, E. L., Sheehan, B., D. H. J. (2017). Challenges and opportunities in understanding dementia and delirium in the acute hospital. *PloS Medicine, 14*(3), e1002247. https://doi.org/10.1371/journal.pmed.11002247.

Joint Commission (TJC). (2016). *Joint Commission Statement on Pain Management* Retrieved from. https://www.jointcommission.org/joint_commission_statement_on_pain_management/.

Jordan, A., Hughes, J., Pakresi, M., Hepburn, S., & O'Brien, J. T. (2011). The utility of PAINAD in assessing pain in a UK population with severe dementia. *International Journal of Geriatric Psychiatry, 26*(2), 118–126. https://doi.org/10.1002/gps.2489.

Klein, D., Dumpe, M., Katz, E., & Bena, J. (2010). Pain assessment in the intensive care unit: development and psychometric testing of the nonverbal pain assessment tool. *Heart & Lung, 39*(6), 521–528. https://doi.org/10.1016/j.hrtlng.2010.05.053.

Levine, C., Hoffman, J. M., Byron, J., Arnold, R., & Kondrat, A. (2015). Surrogate decision making and truth telling in a rehabilitation case. *PM R, 7*(7), 762–769.

Li, D., Puntillo, K., & Miaskowski, C. (2008). A review of objective pain measures for use with critical care adult patients unable to self-report. *Journal of Pain, 9*(1), 2–10. https://doi.org/10.1016/j.jpain.2007.08.009.

Lichtner, V., Dowding, D., Esterhuizen, P., Closs, S. J., Long, A. F., Corbett, A., & Briggs, M. (2014). Pain assessment for people with dementia: a systematic review of systematic reviews of pain assessment tools. *BMC Geriatrics, 14*(138), https://doi.org/10.1186/1471-2318-14-138.

Lippmann, S., & Perugula, M. L. (2016). Delirium or Dementia? *Innovations in Clinical Neuroscience, 13*(9-10), 56–57.

Lotan, M., Moe-Nilssen, R., Ljunggren, A. E., & Strand, L. I. (2010). Measurement properties of the Non-Communicating Adult Pain Checklist (NCAPC): A pain scale for adults with Intellectual and Developmental Disabilities, scored in a clinical setting. *Research in Developmental Disabilities, 31*(2), 367–375.

Lotan, M., Moe-Nilssen, R., Ljunggren, A., & Strand, L. (2009). Reliability of the Non-Communicating Adult Pain Checklist (NCAPC), assessed by different groups of health workers. *Research in Developmental Disabilities, 30*, 735–745.

Makic, M. B. F. (2013a). Pain management in the nonverbal critically ill patient. *Journal of PeriAnesthesia Nursing, 28*(2), 98–101.

Makic, M. B. F. (2013b). Preventing delirium in postoperative patients. *Journal of PeriAnesthesia Nursing, 28*(6), 404–408.

McGuire, D. B., Kaiser, K. S., Haisfield-Wolfe, M. E., & Iyamu, F. (2016). Pain assessment in noncommunicative adult palliative care patients. *Nursing Clinics of North America, 51*(3), 397–431.

McGuire, D. B., Reifsnyder, J., Soeken, K., Kaiser, K. S., & Yeager, K. A. (2011). Assessing pain in nonresponsive hospice patients: Development and preliminary testing of the multidimensional objective pain assessment tool. (MOPAT). *Journal of Palliative Medicine, 14*(3), 287–292. https://doi.org/10.1089/jpm.2010.0302.

Odhner, M., Wegman, D., Freeland, N., Steinmetz, A., & Ingersoll, G. L. (2004). Assessing pain control in nonverbal critically ill adults. *Dimensions of Critical Care Nursing, 22*(6), 260–267.

Olsen, B. F., Rustøen, T., Sandvik, L., Miaskowski, C., Jacobsen, M., & Valeberg, B. T. (2015). Development of a pain management algorithm for intensive care units. *Heart & Lung: The Journal of Acute and Critical Care, 44*(6), 521–527.

Owens-Walton, C., Jakabek, D., Power, B. D., Walterfang, M., Hall, S., van Westen, D., … Hansson, O. (2019). Structural and functional MRI changes associated with cognitive impairment and dementia in Parkinson disease. *medRxiv*, 19002147.

Pasero, C., & McCaffery, M. (2011). *Pain assessment and pharmacologic management*. St. Louis, MO: Mosby.

Payen, J.-F., & Gélinas, C. (2014). Measuring pain in non-verbal critically ill patients: which pain instrument? *Critical Care, 18*(5), 554–555.

Payen, J. F., Bru, O., Bosson, J. L., Lagrasta, A., Novel, E., Deschaux, I., Lavagne, P., & Jacquot, C. (2001). Assessing pain in critically ill sedated patients by using a behavioral pain scale. *Critical Care Medicine, 29*(12), 1–11.

Puntillo, K., Pasero, C., Li, D., Mularski, R. A., Grap, M. J., & Sessler, C. N. (2009). Evaluation of pain in ICU patients. *Chest, 135*(4), 1069–1074.

Quinlan-Colwell, A. (2012). *Compact Clinical Guide to Geriatric Pain Management*. New York, NY: Springer Publishing.

Rijkenberg, S., Stilma, W., Bosman, R. J., van der Meer, N. J., & van der Voot, P. H. J. (2017). Pain measurement in mechanically ventilated patients after cardiac surgery: Comparison of the behavioral pain scale (BPS) versus critical-care pain observation tool (CPOT). *Journal of Cardiothoracic and Vascular Anesthesia, 31*(4), 1227–1234.

Rijkenberg, S., Stilma, W., Endeman, H., Bosman, R. J., & Oudemans-van Straaten, H. M. (2015). Pain measurement in mechanically ventilated critically ill patients: behavioral pain scale versus critical-care pain observation tool. *Journal of Critical Care, 30*(1), 167–172.

Schuler, M. S., Becker, S., Kaspar, R., Nikolaus, T., Kruse, A., & Basler, H. D. (2007). Psychometric properties of the German "Pain Assessment in Advanced Dementia Scale" (PAINAD-G) in nursing home residents. *Journal of the American Medical Directors Association, 8*(6), 388–395.

Schutter, P. J., Newell, S., Strickland, P. A., & Barry, J. J. (2015). Response of bispectral index to neuromuscular block in awake volunteers. *British Journal of Anaesthesia, 115*(Suppl 1), i95–i103. https://doi.org/10.1093/bja/aev072.

Solodiuk, J., & Curley, M. A. Q. (2003). Evidence based practice: Pain assessment in nonverbal children with severe cognitive impairments: The Individualized Numeric Rating Scale (INRS). *Journal of Pediatric Nursing, 18*(4), 295–299.

Solodiuk, J. C., Scott-Sutherland, J., Meyers, M., Myette, B., Shusterman, C., Karian, V. E., Harris, S. K., & Curley, M. A. Q. (2010). Validation of the Individualized Numeric Rating Scale (INRS): A pain assessment tool for nonverbal children with intellectual disability. *Pain, 150*(2), 231–236. 20363075.

Stites, M. (2013). Observational pain scales in critically ill adults. *Critical Care Nurse, 33*(3), 68–78. https://doi.org/10.4037/ccn2013804.

Vinclair, M., Schilte, C., Roudaud, F., Lavolaine, J., Francony, G., Bouzat, P., … Payen, J. F. (2019). Using pupillary pain index to assess nociception in sedated critically ill patients. *Anesthesia & Analgesia, 129*(6), 1540–1546.

Voepel-Lewis, T., Zanotti, J., Dammeryer, J. A., & Merkel, S. (2010). Reliability and validity of the Face, Legs, Activity, Cry, Consolability behavioral tool in assessing acute pain in critically ill patients. *American Journal of Critical Care, 19*(1), 55–61. https://doi.org/10.4037/ajcc2010624.

Von Rueden, K. T., Wallizer, B., Thurman, P., McQuillan, K., Andrews, T., Merenda, J., & Son, H. (2017). Delirium in trauma patients: prevalence and predictors. *Critical Care Nurse, 37*(1), 40–48. https://doi.org/10.4037/CCN2017373.

Wang, Y., Cao, J., Feng, J., & Chen, B. (2015). Cheyne-Stokes respiration during sleep: mechanisms and potential interventions. *British Journal Hospital Medicine, 76*(7), 390–396. https://doi.org/10.12968/hmed.2015.76.7.390.

Warden, V., Hurley, A. C., & Volicer, L. (2003). Development and psychometric evaluation of the pain assessment in advanced dementia (PAINAD) scale. *Journal of the American Medical Directors Association, 4*(1), 9–15. https://doi.org/10.1097/01.JAM.0000043422.31640.F7.

Wiegand, D. L., Wilson, T., Pannullo, D., Russo, M. M., Kaiser, K. S., Soeken, K., & McGuire, D. B. (2018). Measuring acute pain over time in the critically ill using the Multidimensional Objective Pain Assessment Tool (MOPAT). *Pain Management Nursing, 19*(3), 277–287.

Zwakhalen, S. M. G., Hamers, J. P. H., Abu-Saad, H. H., & Berger, M. P. F. (2006). Pain in elderly people with severe dementia: A systematic review of behavioural pain assessment tools. *BMC Geriatrics, 6*(3), 1–15. https://doi.org/10.1186/1471-2318-6-3.

Chapter 8 Assessment of Factors Affecting Pain and Affected by Pain

Ann Quinlan-Colwell

CHAPTER OUTLINE

Sleep, pg. 136

Insomnia Disorder, pg. 137

Assessment of Sleep Quality, pg. 137

Treatment of Sleep Disorders, pg. 137

Obstructive Sleep Apnea, pg. 144

Anxiety and Depression, pg. 146

Anxiety, pg. 146

Depression, pg. 149

Family Assessment, pg. 158

Financial Assessment, pg. 158

Key Points, pg. 158

Case Scenario, pg. 159

References, pg. 159

THIS chapter will explore several factors that both affect pain and are affected by pain. As discussed previously, pain is a multifaceted experience influenced by a variety of psychosocial factors (Maeoka, Hiyamizu, Matsuo, & Morioka, 2015), including anxiety, fear, and depression. Pain is also an experience that affects numerous aspects of life, including activities, function, sleep, and socialization. To best understand how the person experiencing pain is fully affected, it is important to consider several other variables as elements of the comprehensive patient assessment. This chapter includes information to support the need for an assessment of sleep, obstructive sleep apnea, anxiety, depression, family relations, and financial status. Other factors, including general history, physical examination, all current medications, all herbal products, supplements, substances used, alcohol consumption, activity, cultural influences, and system barriers (see Chapter 4) also should be considered in the patient assessment (see Chapters 6 and 7). When assessment indicates there are comorbidities or other concerns related to one of these areas, referral to a clinician who specializes in the area is warranted. If a specialist is not available, consultation with another team member may be helpful.

Sleep

Adequate restorative sleep is an essential component of being healthy (Hoey, Fulbrook, & Douglas, 2014). *Sleep health* is a frequently used but not well understood term. Buysse proposed the following definition: "sleep health is a multidimensional pattern of sleep-wakefulness, adapted to individual, social, and environmental demands, that promotes physical and mental well-being. Good sleep health is characterized by subjective satisfaction, appropriate timing, adequate duration, high efficiency, and sustained alertness during waking hours" (Buysse, 2014, p. 12).

Although pain is often considered to be the cause of interrupted sleep, the relationship between sleep and pain is now described as bidirectional and synergistic (Buysse, 2014; Koffel et al., 2016; Schrimpf et al., 2015; Tang, Goodchild, Sanborn, Howard, & Salkovskis, 2012). Several researchers have investigated the relationship between sleep and pain and have reported interesting results about the relationship. In a large study of more than 10,000 middle-aged patients (46% males and 54% females), data regarding sleep onset, sleep deficiency and frequency, and the intensity of insomnia, were correlated with increased pain sensitivity and decreased tolerance of painful stimuli (Sivertsen et al., 2015). The researchers in that work concluded that the risk for a reduction in pain tolerance is increased with disordered sleep and that additional research is needed. When the relationship among pain, sleep impairment, and anxiety was investigated among patients living with Parkinson's disease (PD) (Rana, Qureshi, Kachhvi, Rana, & Chou, 2016), the investigators found that when compared to PD patients not reporting pain, patients living with PD who reported chronic pain also had inferior quality of sleep and more anxiety (Rana, Qureshi, Kachhvi, Rana, & Chou, 2016). An even stronger relationship was reported in a smaller study with 250 veterans with chronic musculoskeletal pain, in which the researchers found that although changes in pain predicted changes in sleep, changes in sleep were more strongly predictive of changes in pain (Koffel et al., 2016).

Roehrs and Roth (2017) investigated the perspective of improving ability to manage pain by improving sleep. Their small feasibility study conducted with 53 participants who were scheduled for elective orthopedic surgery (Roehrs & Roth, 2017). The participants were randomized into two groups. One group continued to sleep as usual preoperatively. The second group extended the time they were in bed by 2 hours per night during the preoperative week. The researchers found that postoperatively the patients who had increased their time in bed preoperatively had significantly less pain and used less opioids (Roehrs & Roth, 2017). The preliminary results of another 2017 study showed a positive relationship between better sleep quality and less pain disability and conversely that inferior sleep quality may be associated with sustaining chronic pain (Johnson, Weber, McCrae, & Craggs, 2017). The findings of these studies are consistent with the belief that impaired sleep is more predictive of pain than vice versa (Finan, Goodin, & Smith, 2013; Tang et al., 2012). Recently, Slavish, Graham-Engeland, Matire, and Smyth (2017) suggested that there is actually "a vicious cycle" that occurs between chronic pain and impaired sleep or insomnia, with each seeming to make the other worse.

Insomnia Disorder

Insomnia disorder is a concept explained as a displeasure, complaint, or frustration with the amount or the quality of sleep related to falling asleep, and/or staying asleep, and/or returning to sleep after awakening, and/or awakening earlier than desired and not being able to return to sleep (American Academy of Sleep Medicine [AASM], 2014; Miller, Espie, & Kyle, 2014). In the most recent edition of *The International Classification of Sleep Disorders*, third edition, cognitive deficiencies during the day were included as part of the definition of insomnia disorder (AASM, 2014). Insomnia is reported by 24% to 35% of adults to occur occasionally and by 9% to 15% of adults to be a chronic problem (Kirwan, Pickett, & Jarrett, 2017). Insomnia is costly and is linked with fatigue, impaired quality of life, and multiple physical and psychological conditions (Reynolds & Ebben, 2017). Insomnia is also reported as a risk factor both for experiencing higher intensity of pain and for developing chronic pain (Mundt, Eisenschenk, & Robinson, 2017).

Assessment of Sleep Quality

Assessment of sleep is an important but often neglected component of pain assessment and management. Buysse (2014) advises that assessment of sleep health should include ease of falling asleep, duration of sleep, satisfaction with sleep, frequency and severity of insomnia, and restorative effect while awake. In their study Sivertsen et al. (2015)

assessed insomnia intensity and frequency with simple 4-point Likert scales using the following qualifiers:

- *Insomnia frequency:* (1) "never, or just a few times a year," (2) "1 to 3 times a month," (3) "approximately once a week," (4) "more than once a week."
- *Insomnia severity:* (1) "no complaint," (2) "little complaint," (3) "pretty much," (4) "very much."

Although these questions seem reasonable and appropriate to use in clinical practice, they have not been tested for validity, reliability, or predictive value.

The *Pittsburgh Sleep Quality Index (PSQI)* was developed in 1989. It is a 19-item tool that assesses seven aspects of sleep, including subjective quality, latency, duration, habitual efficiency, disturbances, use of medication to induce sleep, and functioning during the day (Buysse et al., 1989). It has been used in a variety of populations and countries. Among these were studies involving patients with rheumatoid arthritis (Nicassio et al., 2014), temporomandibular disorders (Rener-Sitar, John, Bandyopadhyay, Howell, & Schiffman, 2014), and Chinese women with breast cancer (Ho & Fong, 2014). Although this tool is validated and established, it was never intended to be used as an impartial tool for use by a variety of clinicians (Klingman, Jungquist, & Perlis, 2017) (Fig. 8.1).

The *Global Sleep Assessment Questionnaire (GSAQ)* is a tool used to screen for sleep disorders. It was originally tested among 212 adults with promising results (Roth et al., 2002). Although more research is needed in clinical areas, in a recent review of questionnaires used to screen for sleep, GSAQ was found to be inclusive, efficient, and appropriate for clinical use (Klingman, Jungquist, & Perlis, 2017) (Table 8.1).

The *Epworth Sleepiness Scale* is a tool used to measure sleepiness during the day and was originally tested in adults with a high internal consistency (r = 0.88) (Johns, 1991, 1992) (Fig. 8.2). Subsequently, it was determined to be a valid and reliable tool to measure sleepiness during the day in those between the ages of 12 and 18 years (Janssen, Phillipson, O'Connor, & Johns, 2017). When using the tool, the clinician asks patients to rank from 0 to 3, how easy it is for them to fall asleep in eight situations that normally allow for sleeping. Scores are tallied, and the instructions are that those within the 10 to 24 range indicate concern for disproportionate sleepiness (Mansukhani, Olson, & Ramar, 2013). The authors of a retrospective review (n = 268) reported that sensitivity was only 66% when the suggested cut-off score of 10 was used but sensitivity increased to 76% when the cut-off score was reduced to 8 (Doneh, 2015). This indicates that it may be advisable to use a cut-off score of 8 in most populations.

Treatment of Sleep Disorders

Treatment of sleep disorders can be accomplished from a variety of perspectives but are most effective when individualized to meet specific patient needs

Text continued on page 143

Pittsburgh Sleep Quality Index (PSQI)

Name _____ ID # _____ Date _____ Age _____

Instructions:

The following questions relate to your usual sleep habits during the past month *only*. Your answers should indicate the most accurate reply for the *majority* of days and nights in the past month. Please answer all questions.

1. During the past month, when have you usually gone to bed at night?

USUAL BED TIME _____

2. During the past month, how long (in minutes) has it usually take you to fall asleep each night?

NUMBER OF MINUTES _____

3. During the past month, when have you usually gotten up in the morning?

USUAL GETTING UP TIME _____

4. During the past month, how many hours of *actual sleep* did you get at night? (This may be different than the number of hours you spend in bed.)

HOURS OF SLEEP PER NIGHT _____

For each of the remaining questions, check the one best response. Please answer *all* questions.

5. During the past month, how often have you had trouble sleeping because you...

(a) Cannot get to sleep within 30 minutes

| Not during the past month ____ | Less than once a week ____ | Once or twice a week ____ | Three or more times a week ____ |

(b) Wake up in the middle of the night or early morning

| Not during the past month ____ | Less than once a week ____ | Once or twice a week ____ | Three or more times a week ____ |

(c) Have to get up to use the bathroom

| Not during the past month ____ | Less than once a week ____ | Once or twice a week ____ | Three or more times a week ____ |

(d) Cannot breathe comfortably

| Not during the past month ____ | Less than once a week ____ | Once or twice a week ____ | Three or more times a week ____ |

(e) Cough or snore loudly

| Not during the past month ____ | Less than once a week ____ | Once or twice a week ____ | Three or more times a week ____ |

(f) Feel too cold

| Not during the past month ____ | Less than once a week ____ | Once or twice a week ____ | Three or more times a week ____ |

(g) Feel too hot

| Not during the past month ____ | Less than once a week ____ | Once or twice a week ____ | Three or more times a week ____ |

(h) Had bad dreams

| Not during the past month ____ | Less than once a week ____ | Once or twice a week ____ | Three or more times a week ____ |

(i) Have pain

| Not during the past month ____ | Less than once a week ____ | Once or twice a week ____ | Three or more times a week ____ |

Fig. 8.1 | **The Pittsburgh Sleep Quality Index (PSQI).** (From Buysse, D. J., Reynolds III, C. F., Monk, T. H., Berman, S. R., & Kupfer, D. J. [1989]. The Pittsburgh Sleep Quality Index: A new instrument for psychiatric practice and research. *Psychiatry Research, 28*[2], 193–213.)

Continued

Pittsburgh Sleep Quality Index (PSQI), continued

(j) Other reason(s), please describe _____

_____

How often during the past month have you had trouble sleeping because of this?

Not during the   Less than   Once or   Three or more
past month _____   once a week _____   twice a week _____   times a week _____

6. During the past month, how would you rate your sleep quality overall?

Very good   _____
Fairly good   _____
Fairly bad   _____
Very bad   _____

7. During the past month, how often have you taken medicine (prescribed or "over the counter") to help you sleep?

Not during the   Less than   Once or   Three or more
past month _____   once a week _____   twice a week _____   times a week _____

8. During the past month, how often have you had trouble staying awake white driving, eating meals, o engaging in social activity?

Not during the   Less than   Once or   Three or more
past month _____   once a week _____   twice a week _____   times a week _____

9. During the past month, how much of a problem has it been for you to keep up enough enthusiasm to get things done?

No problem at all   _____
Only a very slight problem   _____
Somewhat of a problem   _____
A very big problem   _____

10. Do you have a bed partner or roommate?

No bed partner or roommate   _____
Partner/roommate in other room   _____
Partner in same room, but not same bed   _____
Partner in same bed   _____

If you have a roommate or bed partner, ask him/her how often in the past month you have had...

(a) Loud snoring

Not during the   Less than   Once or   Three or more
past month _____   once a week _____   twice a week _____   times a week _____

(b) Long pauses between breaths while asleep

Not during the   Less than   Once or   Three or more
past month _____   once a week _____   twice a week _____   times a week _____

(c) Legs twitching or jerking while you sleep

Not during the   Less than   Once or   Three or more
past month _____   once a week _____   twice a week _____   times a week _____

(d) Episodes of disorientation or confusion during sleep

Not during the   Less than   Once or   Three or more
past month _____   once a week _____   twice a week _____   times a week _____

(e) Other restlessness while you sleep; please describe _____

_____

Not during the   Less than   Once or   Three or more
past month _____   once a week _____   twice a week _____   times a week _____

Fig. 8.1, Cont'd

Scoring instructions for the Pittsburgh Sleep Quality Index

The Pittsburgh Sleep Quality Index (PSQI) contains 19 self-rated questions and 5 questions rated by the bed partner or roommate (done as available). Only self-rated questions are included in the scoring. The 19 self-rated items are combined to form seven "component" scores, each of which has a range of 0-3 points. In all cases, a score of "0" indicates no difficulty, while a score of "3" indicates severe difficulty. The seven component scores are then added to yield one "global" score, with a range of 0-21 points, "0" indicating no difficulty and "21" indicating severe difficulties in all areas.

  Scoring proceeds as follows:

Component 1: Subjective sleep quality

  Examine question #6, and assign score as follows:

Response	Component 1 score
"Very good"	0
"Fairly good"	1
"Fairly bad"	2
"Very bad"	3

Component 1 score: _____

Component 2: Sleep latency

1. Examine question #2, and assign score as follows:

Response	Score
≤15 Minutes	0
16-30 minutes	1
31-60 minutes	2
>60 minutes	3

Question #2 score: _____

2. Examine question #5a, and assign score as follows:

Response	Score
Not during the past month	0
Less than once a week	1
Once or twice a week	2
Three or more times a week	3

Question #5a score: _____

3. Add #2 score and #5a score:

Sum of #2 and #5a: _____

4. Assign component 2 score as follows:

Sum of #2 and #5a:	Component 2 score:
0	0
1-2	1
3-4	2
5-6	3

Component 2 score: _____

Component 3: Sleep duration

  Examine question #4, and assign score as follows:

Response	Component 3 score
>7 hours	0
6-7 hours	1
5-6 hours	2
<5 hours	3

Component 3 score: _____

Fig. 8.1, Cont'd

Component 4: Habitual sleep efficiency

(1) Write the number of hours slept (question #4) here: _____

(2) Calculate the number of hours spent in bed:

         • Getting up time (question #3): _____

         • Bedtime (question #1): _____   _____

           Number of hours spent in bed: _____

(3) Calculate habitual sleep efficiency as follows:

    (Number of hours slept/Number of hours spent in bed) × 100 = Habitual sleep efficiency (%)

         (_____ /_____) × 100 = _____ %

(4) Assign component 4 score as follows:

Habitual sleep efficiency %	Component 4 score
>85%	0
75%-84%	1
65%-74%	2
<65%	3

                                  Component 4 score: _____

Component 5: Sleep disturbances

(1) Examine questions #5b-5j, and assign scores for *each* question as follows:

Response	Score
Not during the past month	0
Less than once a week	1
Once or twice a week	2
Three or more times a week	3

                #5b score _____

                  c score _____

                  d score _____

                  e score _____

                   f score _____

                  g score _____

                  h score _____

                   i score _____

                   j score _____

(2) Add the scores for questions #5b-5j:

              Sum of 5b-5j: _____

(3) Assign component 5 score as follows:

Sum of #5b-5j	Component 5 score
0	0
1-9	1
10-18	2
19-27	3

                                  Component 5 score: _____

Component 6: Use of sleeping medication

    Examine question #7 and assign scores as follows:

Response	Component 6 score
Not during the past month	0
Less than once a week	1
Once or twice a week	2
Three or more times a week	3

                                  Component 6 score: _____

Fig. 8.1, Cont'd

Component 7: Daytime dysfunction

(1) Examine question # 8, and assign scores as follows:

Response	Score
Never	0
Once or twice	1
Once or twice each week	2
Three or more times each week	3

Question #8 score: _____

(2) Examine question #9, and assign scores as follows:

Response	Score
No problem at all	0
Only a very slight problem	1
Somewhat of a problem	2
A very big problem	3

Question #9 score: _____

(3) Add the scores for question #8 and #9:

Sum of #8 and #9: _____

(4) Assign component 7 score as follows:

Sum of #8 and #9	Component 7 score
0	0
1-2	1
3-4	2
5-6	3

Component 7 score: _____

Global PSQI Score

Add the seven component scores together:

Global PSQI Score: _____

Fig. 8.1, Cont'd

Table 8.1 | Global Sleep Assessment Questionnaire (GSAQ)

Patient Initials: _____ Date: __/__/__
Age: _____ Sex: ☐ Male ☐ Female
Height: _____ Weight: _____

Employment Status: ☐ Day shift ☐ Night shift
☐ Rotating shift
Retired: ☐ Unemployed ☐ Employed Full-time
☐ Employed Part-time ☐ Homemaker (Please check all that apply)

Over the past month, have you had a major stressful event that you feel affected your sleep? If so, please describe:

_____

INSTRUCTIONS: Please answer the questions below by writing on the line provided or by checking the box that best describes you. Please select only one answer for each question.

During the **PAST 4 WEEKS**, how often . . .

1. Did you have difficulty falling asleep, staying asleep, or feeling poorly rested in the morning?	☐ Never	☐ Sometimes	☐ Usually	☐ Always
2. Did you fall asleep unintentionally or have to fight to stay awake during the day?	☐ Never	☐ Sometimes	☐ Usually	☐ Always
3. Did sleep difficulties or daytime sleepiness interfere with your daily activities?	☐ Never	☐ Sometimes	☐ Usually	☐ Always
4. Did work or other activities prevent you from getting enough sleep?	☐ Never	☐ Sometimes	☐ Usually	☐ Always
5. Did you snore loudly?	☐ Never	☐ Sometimes	☐ Usually	☐ Always
6. Did you hold your breath, have breathing pauses, or stop breathing in your sleep?	☐ Never	☐ Sometimes	☐ Usually	☐ Always
7. Did you have restless or "crawling" feelings in your legs at night that went away if you moved your legs?	☐ Never	☐ Sometimes	☐ Usually	☐ Always
8. Did you have repeated rhythmic leg jerks or leg twitches during your sleep?	☐ Never	☐ Sometimes	☐ Usually	☐ Always

Continued

Table 8.1	Global Sleep Assessment Questionnaire (GSAQ)—cont'd

9. Did you have nightmares, or did you scream, walk, punch, or kick in your sleep?   ☐ Never   ☐ Sometimes   ☐ Usually   ☐ Always

10. Did the following things disturb your sleep: ☐ Never   ☐ Sometimes   ☐ Usually   ☐ Always
   a. Pain _____
   b. Other physical problems ___
   c. Worries _____
   d. Medications _____
   e. Other: _____ (Please specify)

11. Did you feel sad or anxious?   ☐ Never   ☐ Sometimes   ☐ Usually   ☐ Always

From Roth, T., Zammit, G., Kushida, C., Doghramji, K., Mathias, S. D., Wong, J. M., & Buysse, D. J. 2002. A new questionnaire to detect sleep disorders. *Sleep Medicine, 3*(2), 99–108. © Pharmacia Corporation 2001.

Epworth Sleepiness Scale

How likely are you to nod off or fall asleep in the following situations, in contrast to feeling just tired? This refers to your usual way of life in recent times.

Even if you haven't done some of these things recently, try to work out how they would have affected you. It is important that you answer each question as best you can.

Use the following scale to choose the most appropriate number for each situation.

	Would never nod off 0	Slight chance of nodding off 1	Moderate chance of nodding off 2	High chance of nodding off 3
Sitting and reading				
Watching TV				
Sitting, inactive, in a public place (e.g., in a meeting, theater, or dinner event)				
As a passenger in a car for an hour or more without stopping for a break				
Lying down to rest when circumstances permit				
Sitting and talking to someone				
Sitting quietly after a meal without alcohol				
In a car, while stopped for a few minutes in traffic or at a light				

Add up your points to get your total score. A score of 10 or greater raises concern: you may need to get more sleep, improve your sleep practices, or seek medical attention to determine why you are sleepy.

Fig. 8.2 | **Epworth Sleepiness Scale.** (From Johns, M. W. [1991]. A new method for measuring daytime sleepiness: The Epworth sleepiness scale. *Sleep, 14,*[6], 540–545.)

and situations. Pharmacologic interventions can be prescribed; however, the interaction with analgesic or other medications, comorbidities, patient age, and side effects must be considered. Although medications such as benzodiazepine-receptor agonists may be helpful for short periods, side effects are concerning. In addition to the risk for side effects, there is no strong evidence to support their effectiveness over long periods of time (van Straten et al., 2017). The Centers for Disease Control and Prevention (CDC) recommendations advised that concomitant use of benzodiazepines with opioids needs to be avoided whenever possible (Dowell, Haegerich, & Chou, 2016). Similarly, non-benzodiazepine receptor agonists have not been proved effective for long

Box 8.1	Good Sleep Hygiene

- Avoid caffeine and alcohol close to bedtime.
- Increase daytime activities.
- Avoid stimulation, such as electronic devices and television.
- Participate in relaxing activities, such as warm bath.
- Ensure a darkened room with limited stimulating light signals, including mobile phones and computers.

durations and they have undesirable side effects (Miller et al., 2014).

Many cognitive behavioral interventions are effective to assist patients with poor sleep health and insomnia. These range from the simple use of a white noise machine to guided muscle relaxation and include options for good sleep hygiene (Box 8.1).

Cognitive-behavioral therapy for insomnia (CBT-I) can be learned and used to alter thoughts, patterns, and behaviors involved with insomnia. The National Institutes of Health, American Academy of Pain Medicine, and American College of Physicians all endorsed the therapy (Reynolds & Ebben, 2017). It is considered the standard of care treatment for chronic primary insomnia and comparable in effectiveness to sleep medications (Finan, Buenaver, Runko, & Smith, 2014). CBT-I also is used effectively for patients who suffer with both insomnia and chronic pain (Geiger-Brown et al., 2015). Although CBT-I is not associated with reducing pain severity, it is reported to reduce pain interference and disability associated with pain (Finan, Buenaver, Runko & Smith, 2014). Typically, CBT-I requires the patient to monitor their sleep patterns and consists of the following components (Edinger, Leggett, Carney, & Manber, 2017; Finan, Buenaver, Runko & Smith, 2014; Reynolds & Ebben, 2017):

- Sleep education that includes circadian function, patterns of sleep, realistic expectations, and rationale for the various components of CBT-I.
- Therapy for sleep restriction to consolidate sleep involves limiting the time spent in bed so that time is no longer than the average amount of actual sleep time usually experienced.
- Learning to control impulses and stimuli, being sensitive to indications of being ready to fall asleep. Learning and adopting good sleep hygiene with behaviors that promote sleep.
- Altering circadian rhythm regularity and configuration.
- Cognitive therapy to manage and replace dysfunctional thinking. Because worrying is strongly predictive of not falling asleep, techniques to control and manage worry is an important part of CBT-I.
- Learning and using methods of relaxing (breathing, progressive muscle relaxation, imagery).

Obstructive Sleep Apnea

In addition to assessing for general patterns and quality of sleep, patients also need to be assessed for *obstructive sleep apnea (OSA),* which is correlated with perioperative complications and potentially longer lengths of stay (Avitsian & Galway, 2015; Chou et al., 2016; Spence, Han, McGuire, & Couture, 2015). OSA is characterized by a disturbance, reduction, or absence in breathing (airflow) for at least 10 seconds because of a physical obstruction to airflow despite ventilatory effort during sleep (Avitsian & Galway, 2015; Spence et al., 2015; Weatherspoon, Sullivan, & Weatherspoon, 2016). It is associated with snoring, nonrestorative sleep, morning headaches, cognitive impairment, and drowsiness or falling asleep during the day (Spence et al., 2015; Ward, 2015).

OSA is a concern among patients in the community with chronic pain, as well, affecting approximately 15% of people age 55 or older (Marshansky et al., 2017). As many as 84% of people with any form of sleep apnea are diagnosed with OSA compared to the other forms, central or complex sleep apnea (Avitsian & Galway, 2015). Prevalence is higher among men, with estimates ranging from 4% to 14%, than among women, with estimates ranging from 2% to 4% (Avitsian & Galway, 2015; Spence et al., 2015; Ward, 2015). These numbers are most likely underestimates because it is not known how many people are not diagnosed. OSA is higher among people with certain comorbidities such as obesity (Avitsian & Galway, 2015), hypertension, cardiovascular disorders, diabetes, anxiety, depression, and those undergoing bariatric surgery (Mansukhani et al., 2013; Spence et al., 2015). OSA also has been associated with intensifying some chronic musculoskeletal and craniofacial pain conditions (Marshansky et al., 2017).

Assessment of Sleep Apnea

Screening for OSA should routinely be done before surgery (Spence et al., 2015). *STOP-BANG* is a short, eight-question, yes or no assessment tool (Table 8.2) that is effective for evaluating patients at risk for OSA. Patients with a score of 3 or higher are determined to be at high risk for OSA (Chung, 2012; Legler, 2017). Recently the specificity of predicting OSA among patients scoring 3 or greater was improved by assessing body type being either apple-shaped or pear-shaped (Sangkum et al., 2017).

Interventions to promote safety are important when managing pain in patients with OSA. An integrative proactive and multimodal analgesic plan is essential to optimize safe and effective pain management. Box 8.2 presents strategies to reduce risk among patients with OSA.

The postoperative care of patients with OSA is important because this is a time when they may be at increased risk for apnea. Communication among all team members is essential, and the duration of postoperative monitoring may need to be increased. This is particularly important when patients have received long-acting or repeated doses

Table 8.2 | STOP-BANG

Yes	No	**Snoring?**
		Do you snore loudly (loud enough to be heard through closed doors or your bed partner elbows you for snoring at night)?
Yes	No	**Tired?**
		Do you often feel tired, fatigued, or sleepy during the daytime (such as falling asleep during driving or talking to someone)?
Yes	No	**Observed?**
		Has anyone observed you stop breathing or choking/gasping during your sleep?
Yes	No	**Pressure?**
		Do you have or are being treated for high blood pressure?
Yes	No	**Body mass index more than 35 kg/m²?**
Yes	No	**Age older than 50 years?**
Yes	No	**Neck size large? (measured around Adam's apple)** For male, is your shirt collar 17 inches or larger? For female, is your shirt collar 16 inches or larger?
Yes	No	**Sex = male?**

For general population, OSA–low risk: yes to 0-2 questions; OSA–intermediate risk: yes to 3-4 questions; or OSA–high risk: yes to 5-8 questions, yes to 2 or more of 4 STOP questions + male sex, yes to 2 or more of 4 STOP questions + BMI > 35 kg/m², or yes to 2 or more of 4 STOP questions + neck circumference 16 inches/40 cm. Property of University Health Network. Please use "About Us" for more information. http://www.stopbang.ca. Permission obtained from University Health Network. Modified from Chung, F., Yegneswaran, B., Liao, P., Chung, S. A., Vairavanathan, S., Islam, S., . . . & Shapiroet, C. M. (2008). STOP Questionnaire: A tool to screen patients for obstructive sleep apnea. *Anesthesiology, 108*, 812; Chung, F. (2012). High STOP-BANG scores indicate a high probability of obstructive sleep apnea. *British Journal of Anaesthesia,108*(5), 768–775; and Chung, F., Yang, Y., Brown, R., Liao, P. (2014). Alternative scoring models of STOP-Bang questionnaire specificity to detect undiagnosed obstructive sleep apnea. *Journal of Clinical Sleep Medicine, 10*, 951–958. From Avitsian, R., & Galway, U. (2015). Assessment and management of obstructive sleep apnea for ambulatory surgery. *Advances in Anesthesia, 33*(1), 61–75.

Box 8.2 | Obstructive Sleep Apnea Risk Reduction Precautions

- Identify patients with known or suspected OSA (use STOP-BANG score ≥ 3) (consider moderate to severe OSA if score ≥ 5).
- Minimize preoperative sedation.
- Prepare for possible difficult airway.
- Minimize use of long-acting opioids.
- Nonopioid techniques preferable. Consider multimodal analgesic techniques and regional anesthesia when possible.
- Use short-acting inhaled or intravenous anesthetics (i.e., desflurane, sevoflurane, propofol) intraoperatively.
- Ensure patient is fully conscious and cooperative and has full reversal of neuromuscular blockade before extubation.
- Use the nonsupine position for recovery.
- Resume CPAP therapy in patients with OSA.
- Consider initiating CPAP postoperatively if noncompliant with preoperative CPAP, or if patient has severe OSA, or experiences recurrent PACU respiratory events.
- Consider extended care in a monitored bed with continuous $ETCO_2$ and/or SPO_2 for moderate-to-severe OSA if postoperative opioids required and/or for recurrent PACU respiratory events.
- Educate surgeon, patient, and family on how to monitor for respiratory events postoperatively.

CPAP, Continuous positive airway pressure; $ETCO_2$, end-tidal carbon dioxide; *OSA,* obstructive sleep apnea; *PACU,* postanesthesia care unit; SPO_2, pulse oximetry/oxygen saturation; *STOP-BANG,* Snoring, Tiredness, Observed apnea, high blood Pressure, Body mass index greater than 35 kg/m², Age older than 50, Neck circumference greater than 40 cm, and male Gender.
NOTE: OSA risk reduction precautions based on published research, guidelines, and expert opinion.
From Spence, D. L., Han, T., McGuire, J., & Couture, D. (2015). Obstructive sleep apnea and the adult perioperative patient. *Journal of PeriAnesthesia Nursing, 30*(6), 528–545.

of opioids (Weatherspoon et al., 2016). The American Society of Anesthesiologists in their 2014 practice guidelines recommended the following:

- Regional analgesia
- Nonopioid analgesics
- Minimize opioid use and avoid basal infusions with patient-controlled analgesia (PCA)
- Position nonsupine with elevation of head
- Supplemental oxygen
- Noninvasive positive pressure-assisted ventilation (NIPPV) with continuous positive airway pressure (CPAP)
- Continuous pulse oximetry

Because opioids can cause the pharyngeal muscles to relax (Mansukhani et al., 2013), it is also recommended that assessment of OSA be part of assessment of patients prescribed opioids on an outpatient basis. Family members need to be educated about concerns for respiratory depression when patients with untreated or undertreated sleep apnea manage pain with opioids at home. Appropriate education and prescription of naloxone is appropriate when it is available as a preventive measure (Dowell et al., 2016).

Education is important. Patients need to be educated in the risks of untreated OSA and how to minimize the risks. These risks include obesity, cigarette smoking, alcohol, sedatives, hypnotics, and opioids (Mansukhani et al., 2013; Ward, 2015). Guidance and encouragement to help patients reduce these risks is important. Patients and families also need to be educated that patients with OSA need to be evaluated with diagnostic sleep studies and treated with appropriate interventions. To date there is no information to support nonmedical interventions to effectively manage OSA (Billings & Maddalozzo, 2013). Patients and families also need to know that snoring does not mean sound sleep, but rather indicates airway obstruction.

Anxiety and Depression

In 2013 Rogers, Kemp, McLachlan, and Blyth reported that mental and emotional suffering was reported more by patients who were being treated with opioids to manage chronic noncancer pain than those who were not being treated with opioids. Again, the relationship is not clear (Rogers et al., 2013). Some researchers think that patients who have a mental health diagnosis are more likely to be treated with prescription opioids and in higher doses than those without a mental health diagnosis and call this "adverse selection" (Howe & Sullivan, 2014). Fear of pain and thus avoidance of activities is a related concern and is discussed in Chapter 20.

Anxiety

Anxiety is defined by the American Psychological Association as "an emotion characterized by feelings of tension, worried thoughts and physical changes like increased blood pressure … usually have recurring intrusive thoughts or concerns" (APA, n.d.a.). The relationship between pain and anxiety is closely intertwined and in some ways challenging to unravel. The relationship between anxiety and pain perception has long been thought to be strong and cyclical with anxiety increasing the perception of pain and pain in turn leading to greater anxiety and depression (Gerrits, van Marwijk, van Oppen, van der Horst, & Pennix, 2015).

It is well known that patients with high anxiety and difficult to manage pain have less desirable postoperative outcomes (Hudson & Ogden, 2016). The complexity of the relationship was underscored in a study that assessed the effect of repeated painful stimulation on reports of pain intensity and anxiety. The researchers found that although reported pain intensity decreased significantly over a 3-day period, anxiety significantly increased during that time (Maeoka et al., 2015).

The investigators of a 2013 study involving 124 patients undergoing total hip arthroplasty reported a strong correlation between postoperative anxiety and postoperative acute pain. They also reported that although presurgical anxiety was most predictive of postoperative anxiety, presurgical optimism was also predictive of lower postoperative anxiety and was highly predictive of pain intensity (Pinto, McIntyre, Ferrero, Almeida, & Araújo-Soares, 2013).

Anxiety Sensitivity

Anxiety sensitivity, which is a well-known concept involved in the risk for developing and maintaining anxiety, involves fear of what will happen as a result of sensations or feelings related to anxiety (Mitchell, Riccardi, Keough, Timpano, & Schmidt, 2013). It is easy to understand how anxiety sensitivity can be involved in the pain experience. Patients who fear pain may have greater anxiety sensitivity. This relationship also seems to be cross cultural. A study done in 2016 by Velasco et al. with 203 Latinos of whom 84% were women living in the United States confirmed the interconnective relationship between pain intensity and anxiety sensitivity, which were also significantly linked to social anxiety and depressive symptoms. Similar results were reported from a recent study in Japan that involved 74 university students. Students who had higher anxiety sensitivity reported greater fear in anticipation of pain and more intense pain after a cold pressor test (Dodo & Hashimoto, 2017). In a Canadian study, women were found to have greater AS than men. Women in that study also had more pain intensity with less tolerance of both heat and cold pain (Thibodeau, Welch, Katz, & Asmundson, 2013).

Discomfort Intolerance

Discomfort intolerance is a related construct that is used to understand the ability of the person to endure physical sensations that are not comfortable for the person to experience (Mitchell et al., 2013). Discomfort intolerance is somewhat like pain intolerance but is different in scope and intensity because discomfort intolerance encompasses any uncomfortable sensation, not just truly painful sensations. The higher the discomfort intolerance score, the less able the person is to tolerate uncomfortable physical sensations and subsequently may be more inclined to perceive them as dangerous and react excessively to them. It is suggested that discomfort intolerance is correlated with anxiety sensitivity and in at least one study was found to be more common in people diagnosed with panic disorders (Mitchell et al., 2013). From this perspective, the person with high discomfort intolerance experiences pain as distressful and a danger, and, as a result, the person becomes increasingly anxious about what the pain will feel like and how intense it will become. Discomfort intolerance is also correlated with obesity, which can be modified to improve management of pain (Fergus, Limbers, Griggs, & Kelley, 2015). (See Chapter 27 for discussion of obesity and pain.) The relationship between discomfort intolerance with pain and possible relationship with pain and obesity is an area in need of research.

Pain Anxiety

Pain anxiety involves the expectation and concern that pain will occur when activities in the future are undertaken (Gyurcsik, Cary, Sessford, Flora, & Brawley, 2015). The temporal relationship is critical to the concept because this is anxiety about pain that is not occurring now but that is anticipated to occur in the future. Reports on gender difference and pain anxiety are mixed. Although there are numerous reports that discuss the relationship between pain and gender, the relationship may be affected by factors other than just gender. In a Canadian study, women experienced greater pain anxiety and greater pain intensity (Thibodeau et al., 2013). In a more recent study, men who had higher pain anxiety also had higher pain intensity and women had a higher fear of reinjuring themselves (Kreddig & Hasenbring, 2017). It is possible that the relationship between pain anxiety and pain intensity is stronger than the relationship between gender and pain intensity, or at least pain anxiety may be a strong contributing factor in the gender relationship.

Pain Catastrophizing

Pain catastrophizing is a maladaptive way of responding to pain that increases the perception of pain (Finan et al., 2018). It is characterized by predominantly negative thoughts about pain, with associated fears of moving, injury, and reinjury (Suhaimi, 2018) (see Chapters 20 and 22), rumination, and often feeling helpless (Finan et al., 2018). It is associated with chronic pain, higher pain intensity, disability, less favorable outcomes (Junghaenel, Schneider, & Broderick, 2017; Werti et al., 2014), and greater risk for misuse of opioids (Finan et al., 2018). A multidisciplinary approach is often most effective; thus evaluation by members of a multidisciplinary team is desirable (Suhaimi, 2018). In an interesting study (n = 71),

essays written by people with chronic pain were analyzed and compared with the *Pain Catastrophizing Scale;* pain catastrophizing correlated with greater use of pronouns in both first-person singular and in reference to others and with more frequent expressions of anger and sadness (Junghaenel et al., 2017).

Assessment of Anxiety

There are numerous reliable and validated tools to assess anxiety. The tools briefly described in this section can be used in a timely manner in a clinical setting.

The *General Anxiety Disorder–7 (GAD-7) scale* (Spitzer, Kroenke, Williams, & Löwe, 2006) is an effective screening tool that has demonstrated validity and reliability. The authors suggest that in addition to screening the tool can be used to assess progress with treatment. As the result of a recent systemic review and meta-analysis the authors recommended using either 8 or 9 as a cut-off score to heighten sensitivity of the tool (Plummer, Manea, Trepel, & McMillan, 2016).

The *Patient Health Questionnaire-4 (PHQ-4)* is an ultra-brief, four-item tool validated for screening anxiety and depression (Kroenke, Spitzer, Williams, & Löwe, 2009) (Fig. 8.3). It is considered an efficient screening tool for both anxiety and depression and an adequate

PHQ-4				
Over the <u>last 2 weeks</u>, how often have you been bothered by the following problems? (Use "✓" to indicate your answer)	Not at all	Several days	More than half the days	Nearly every day
1. Feeling nervous, anxious, or on edge	0	1	2	3
2. Not being able to stop or control worrying	0	1	2	3
3. Feeling down, depressed, or hopeless	0	1	2	3
4. Little interest or pleasure in doing things	0	1	2	3

Scoring

PHQ-4 total score ranges from 0 to 12, with categories of psychological distress being:

• Normal   0-2

• Mild   3-5

• Moderate   6-8

• Severe   9-12

Anxiety subscale = sum of items 1 and 2   (score range, 0 to 6)

Depression subscale = sum of items 3 and 4   (score range, 0 to 6)

On each subscale, a score of 3 or greater is considered positive for screening purposes

Fig. 8.3 | The Patient Health Questionnaire-4 (PHQ-4). The PHQ scales were developed by Drs. Robert L. Spitzer, Janet B. W. Williams, and Kurt Kroenke and colleagues. The PHQ scales are free to use. For research information, contact Dr. Kroenke at kkroenke@regenstrief.org. (From Kroenke, K., Spitzer, R. L., Williams, J. B. W., & Löwe, B. [2009]. An ultra-brief screening scale for anxiety and depression: The PHQ-4. *Psychosomatics, 50,*[6], 613–621.)

substitute for the somewhat longer GAD-7 (Kroenke et al., 2009).

The *Hospital Anxiety and Depression Scale (HADS)* is longer than the GAD-7 and PHQ-4 (Fig. 8.4). It consists of two subscales that measure anxiety (HADS-A) and depression (HADS-D). Each subscale has seven questions

and is designed to be used among hospital patients not in a psychiatric unit (Pinto, et al, 2013).

The *Pain Catastrophizing Scale* is a self-report tool with 13 items from the perspective of pain that is present or anticipated to occur (Sullivan, Bishop & Pivik, 1995). Studies are promising for a new *Daily Pain*

Hospital Anxiety and Depression Scale (HADS)

Tick the box beside the reply that is closest to how you have been feeling in the past week.
Don't take too long over your replies: your immediate is best.

D	A		D	A	
		I feel tense or 'wound up':			**I feel as if I am slowed down:**
	3	Most of the time	3		Nearly all the time
	2	A lot of the time	2		Very often
	1	From time to time, occasionally	1		Sometimes
	0	Not at all	0		Not at all
		I still enjoy the things I used to enjoy:			**I get a sort of frightened feeling like 'butterflies' in the stomach:**
0		Definitely as much		0	Not at all
1		Not quite so much		1	Occasionally
2		Only a little		2	Quite Often
3		Hardly at all		3	Very Often
		I get a sort of frightened feeling as if something awful is about to happen:			**I have lost interest in my appearance:**
	3	Very definitely and quite badly	3		Definitely
	2	Yes, but not too badly	2		I don't take as much care as I should
	1	A little, but it doesn't worry me	1		I may not take quite as much care
	0	Not at all	0		I take just as much care as ever
		I can laugh and see the funny side of things:			**I feel restless as I have to be on the move:**
0		As much as I always could		3	Very much indeed
1		Not quite so much now		2	Quite a lot
2		Definitely not so much now		1	Not very much
3		Not at all		0	Not at all
		Worrying thoughts go through my mind:			**I look forward with enjoyment to things:**
	3	A great deal of the time	0		As much as I ever did
	2	A lot of the time	1		Rather less than I used to
	1	From time to time, but not too often	2		Definitely less than I used to
	0	Only occasionally	3		Hardly at all
		I feel cheerful:			**I get sudden feelings of panic:**
3		Not at all		3	Very often indeed
2		Not often		2	Quite often
1		Sometimes		1	Not very often
0		Most of the time		0	Not at all
		I can sit at ease and feel relaxed:			**I can enjoy a good book or radio or TV program:**
	0	Definitely	0		Often
	1	Usually	1		Sometimes
	2	Not Often	2		Not often
	3	Not at all	3		Very seldom

Please check you have answered all the questions

Scoring:

Total score: Depression (D) _____   Anxiety (A) _____

0-7 = Normal
8-10 = Borderline abnormal (borderline case)
11-21 = Abnormal (case)

Fig. 8.4 | **Hospital Anxiety and Depression Scale (HADS).** (From Zigmond, A. S., & Snaith, R. P. [1983]. The Hospital Anxiety and Depression Scale. *Acta Psychiatrica Scandinavica, 16*[6], 361–370.)

Catastrophizing Scale, but additional testing and research are needed (Darnall et al., 2017).

Depression

Depression is reported to be the most common of all mental health disorders, with 17.3 million adults in the United States estimated to experience one or more episodes of major depression in 2017 (NIMH, 2019). Of those, the prevalence was greater among women than men and most frequent among those between 18 and 25 years, with the greatest frequency in that group among those who reported being of mixed race (NIMH, 2019). It is more than just feeling sad and is characterized by not having interest in or experiencing pleasure while participating in usual activities. There is often either a gain or loss in body weight, changes in sleeping patterns, low or deficient energy, difficulty in concentration, and feeling of guilt or worthlessness. There also may be suicide ideation or in other ways thinking about death (APA, n.d.b.).

Depression and pain are frequently comorbid. As discussed with sleep and anxiety, it is often challenging to determine the actual relationship, the influence of one upon the other, or any possible cause and effect between the two. Some studies have reported that depression develops as a result of chronic pain, whereas others indicate that people living with depression may be at greater risk for developing chronic pain (Okifuji & Turk, 2016). Interestingly, there does seem to be a relationship between the number of different sites where a person experiences pain and the likelihood of developing depression, with the likelihood of developing depression increasing with more locations of pain (Gerrits et al., 2014).

In a different study, the longer patients with chronic pain and no prior history of opioid use were treated with opioids, the more risk they had for developing depression (Scheerer et al., 2014). A 2015 study reported that of the 61% of the community-based Australian participants (1418) who reported depression, nearly half of them (48%) reported developing depressive symptoms after using opioids to treat chronic pain (Smith et al., 2015). These studies underscore the importance of not only assessing for depression when pain is first being treated but also periodically during the treatment of chronic pain.

Considering the impact that chronic pain can have on the quality of life, it can be considered amazing that most people who live with chronic pain do not also have comorbid depression. Yet, the data show this is not the case (Okifuji & Turk, 2016). From what we currently know it seems that the chance of experiencing comorbid depression with chronic pain is related to physical and cognitive factors as well as medications being used (Gillanders, Ferreira, Bose, & Esrich, 2013; Okifuji & Turk, 2016). In addition to "vulnerability factors" that can increase the likelihood of developing depression along with chronic pain, there are "resilience factors" that

Table 8.3	Vulnerability and Resilience Factors for Depression in Chronic Pain	
Vulnerability/Exacerbating Factors	**Resilience/Protective Factors**
Helplessness	Resourcefulness
Feelings of no self-control	Sense of control
Low self-efficacy	High self-efficacy
Catastrophizing	Optimism
Rigid thinking	Psychological flexibility
Defeated/overwhelmed	Resilient
Lack or perceived lack of social support	Availability of positive social support

From Okifuji, A., & Turk, D. C. (2016). Chronic pain and depression: Vulnerability and resilience. In M. al'Absi, & D. C. Turk (Eds.), *Neuroscience of pain, stress and emotion: Psychological and clinical implications* (pp. 181–201). San Diego, CA: Academic Press.

can help defend against that happening (Okifuji & Turk, 2016). Table 8.3 compares the "vulnerability" and "resilience" factors identified by Okifuji and Turk (2016). See Chapter 22 for discussion of pain and depression.

Assessment of Depression

Numerous reliable and valid tools are available to assess depression. The following tools can be used in a reasonable time frame within a clinical setting.

The *PHQ-9* is a simple nine-question self-report tool that is designed to take less than 5 minutes to complete. It was developed based on the *Diagnostic and Statistical Manual of Mental Disorders,* fourth edition (DSM-IV) criteria for depression and considered a valid tool for measuring the severity of depression (Kroenke, Spitzer, & Williams, 2001). Each of the nine questions can be answered as 0, indicating none or "not at all" during the last month; 1, indicating that the item was experienced "several days" during the last month; 2, indicating that it was experienced "more than half the days"; or 3, indicating that it was experienced "nearly every day" during the past month (Fig. 8.5). The *PHQ-9* is the longer version of the *PHQ-4* (see Fig. 8.3) that was previously described with anxiety.

The PHQ-9 has been validated for use with many populations and in numerous countries, including Mexico (Arrieta et al., 2017), Haiti (Marc et al., 2014), Viet Nam (Nguyen et al., 2016), and with British Sign Language (Belk, Pilling, Rogers, Lovell, & Young, 2016). An innovative adaptation of the PHQ-9 is using it in an automated telephone-based format, which was evaluated to be valid and reliable (Farzanfar et al., 2014). The telephone adaptation can be used to save time and can be used in conjunction with patients who are being evaluated via telemedicine programs.

PATIENT HEALTH QUESTIONNAIRE (PHQ-9)

NAME: _____   DATE: _____

Over the last 2 weeks, how often have you been
bothered by any of the following problems?
(use "✓" to indicate your answer)

	Not at all	Several days	More than half the days	Nearly every day
1. Little interest or pleasure in doing things	0	1	2	3
2. Feeling down, depressed, or hopeless	0	1	2	3
3. Trouble falling or staying asleep, or sleeping too much	0	1	2	3
4. Feeling tired or having little energy	0	1	2	3
5. Poor appetite or overeating	0	1	2	3
6. Feeling bad about yourself—or that you are a failure or have let yourself or your family down	0	1	2	3
7. Trouble concentrating on things, such as reading the newspaper or watching television	0	1	2	3
8. Moving or speaking so slowly that other people could have noticed. Or the opposite—being so figety or restless that you have been moving around a lot more than usual	0	1	2	3
9. Thoughts that you would be better off dead, or of hurting yourself	0	1	2	3

add columns _____ + _____ + _____

(Healthcare professional: For interpretation of TOTAL,   TOTAL: _____
please refer to accompanying scoring card).

10. If you checked off any problems, how difficult have these problems made it for you to do your work, take care of things at home, or get along with other people?	Not difficult at all	_____
	Somewhat difficult	_____
	Very difficult	_____
	Extremely difficult	_____

Fig. 8.5 | **PHQ-9 Patient Health Questionnaire–9.** (From Kroenke, K., Spitzer, R., & Williams, J. [2001]. The PHQ-9: Validity of a brief depression severity measure. *Journal of General Internal Medicine, 16*[9], 606–613. PHQ9 © Copyright Pfizer Inc. All rights reserved.)

Continued

PHQ-9 Patient Depression Questionnaire

For initial diagnosis:

1. Patient completes PHQ-9 Quick Depression Assessment.
2. If there are at least 4 ✓s in the shaded section (including Questions #1 and #2), consider a depressive disorder. Add score to determine severity.

Consider Major Depressive Disorder

• if there are at least 5 ✓s in the shaded section (one of which corresponds to Question #1 or #2)

Consider Other Depressive Disorder

• if there are 2-4 ✓ in the shaded section (one of which corresponds to Question #1 or #2)

Note: Since the questionnaire relies on patient self-report, all responses should be verified by the clinician, and a definitive diagnosis is made on clinical grounds taking into account how well the patient understood the questionnaire, as well as other relevant information from the patient. Diagnoses of Major Depressive Disorder or Other Depressive Disorder also require impairment of social, occupational, or other important areas of functioning (Question #10) and ruling out normal bereavement, a history of a Manic Episode (Bipolar Disorder), and a physical disorder, medication, or other drug as the biological cause of the depressive symptoms.

To monitor severity over time for newly diagnosed patients or patients in current treatment for depression:

1. Patients may complete questionnaires at baseline and at regular intervals (eg, every 2 weeks) at home and bring them in at their next appointment for scoring or they may complete the questionnaire during each scheduled appointment.
2. Add up ✓ by column. For every ✓ : Several days = 1, More than half the days = 2, Nearly every day = 3
3. Add together column scores to get a TOTAL score.
4. Refer to the accompanying **PHQ-9 Scoring Box** to interpret the TOTAL score.
5. Results may be included in patient files to assist you in setting up a treatment goal, determining degree of response, as well as guiding treatment intervention.

Scoring: add up all checked boxes on PHQ-9

For every ✓ Not at all = 0; Several days = 1;
More than half the days = 2; Nearly every day = 3

Interpretation of Total Score

Total Score	Depression Severity
1-4	Minimal depression
5-9	Mild depression
10-14	Moderate depression
15-19	Moderately severe depression
20-27	Severe depression

Fig. 8.5, Cont'd

The *HADS* (see Fig. 8.4), which was described earlier in regard to anxiety, also can be used to screen for depression.

The *Center for Epidemiologic Studies Depression Scale (CES-D)* is a somewhat longer tool that contains 20 questions, which are similar to the PHQ-9, are rated with a score ranging from 0 to 60, with higher scores indicating more symptoms and/or greater severity of symptoms (Radloff, 1977) (Fig. 8.6). Although the CES-D has long been used in research and practice, an evaluation done in Canada cautioned that there may be an inflation of the depression scores in women (Carleton et al., 2013). This points to the need for additional research with established tools to assess for appropriateness with different populations to identify gender, age, socioeconomic, ethnic, and cultural differences.

The *Geriatric Depression Scale (GDS)* is a 30-item instrument used to specifically assess depression in older adults (Fig. 8.7). There is a 15-item version that is comparable in efficacy (Fig. 8.8). A unique benefit of using the GDS rather than another tool with older adults is that it is designed to differentiate depression from dementia (Quinlan-Colwell, 2012).

The *Beck Depression Inventory (BDI)* is a reliable and valid tool developed in 1961 as a 21-item self-report (Beck, Steer, & Garbin, 1988; Beck, Ward, Mendelson, Mock, & Erbaugh, 1961). It is estimated to take 10 minutes to complete but does require the person have at least a fifth-grade reading level (APA, 2017).

Center for Epidemiologic Studies Depression Scale (CES-D)

Below is a list of the ways you might have felt or behaved. Please tell me how often you have felt this way during the past week.

	During the Past Week			
	Rarely or none of the time (less than 1 day)	Some or a little of the time (1-2 days)	Occasionally or a moderate amount of time (3-4 days)	Most or all of the time (5-7 days)
1. I was bothered by things that usually don't bother me.	☐	☐	☐	☐
2. I did not feel like eating; my appetite was poor.	☐	☐	☐	☐
3. I felt that I could not shake off the blues even with help from my family or friends.	☐	☐	☐	☐
4. I felt I was just as good as other people.	☐	☐	☐	☐
5. I had trouble keeping my mind on what I was doing.	☐	☐	☐	☐
6. I felt depressed.	☐	☐	☐	☐
7. I felt that everything I did was an effort.	☐	☐	☐	☐
8. I felt hopeful about the future.	☐	☐	☐	☐
9. I thought my life had been a failure.	☐	☐	☐	☐
10. I felt fearful.	☐	☐	☐	☐
11. My sleep was restless.	☐	☐	☐	☐
12. I was happy.	☐	☐	☐	☐
13. I talked less than usual.	☐	☐	☐	☐
14. I felt lonely.	☐	☐	☐	☐
15. People were unfriendly.	☐	☐	☐	☐
16. I enjoyed life.	☐	☐	☐	☐
17. I had crying spells.	☐	☐	☐	☐
18. I felt sad.	☐	☐	☐	☐
19. I felt that people dislike me.	☐	☐	☐	☐
20. I could not get "going."	☐	☐	☐	☐

SCORING: zero for answers in the first column, 1 for answers in the second column, 2 for answers in the third column, 3 for answers in the fourth column. The scoring of positive items is reversed. Possible range of scores is zero to 60, with the higher scores indicating the presence of more symptomatology.

Fig. 8.6 | Center for Epidemiologic Studies Depression Scale (CES-D). (Redrawn from Radloff, L. S. [1977]. The CES-D scale: A self-report depression scale for research in the general population. *Applied Psychological Measurement, 1,*(3), 385–401.)

Suicide Ideation

An important aspect of assessing depression is screening for suicide ideation. In the United States, prevalence of suicide rose by 28% between 2000 and 2015, with a reported 44,193 people across the life span dying (Table 8.4) (Stone et al., 2017). In 2017, deaths by suicide continued to rise to 47,173, with a 3.7% increase from the previous year (Kochanek, Murphy, Xu, Arias, 2019). There is minimal evidence to support many screening tools being able to accurately assess people at risk for suicide, with false-positive results commonly occurring among the tools rated with fair quality (O'Connor, Gaynes, Burda, Soh, & Whitlock, 2013).

The *Columbia Suicide Severity Rating Scale (C-SSRS)* is the tool with possible exception of the previously listed limitations, but evaluations of the tool vary. The approved risk assessment consists of three pages with interview questions and formal assessment (Substance Abuse and Mental Health Services Administration [SAMHSA], n.d.). The investigators of three multisite studies (n = 124; n = 312; n = 237), using the C-SSRS with adolescents and adults, concluded that it has good validity (convergent

Text continued on page 155

Geriatric Depression Scale (Long Form)

Patient's Name: _____ Date: _____

Instructions: Choose the best answer for how you felt over the past week.

No.	Question	Answer	Score
1.	Are you basically satisfied with your life?	YES / NO	
2.	Have you dropped many of your activities and interests?	YES / NO	
3.	Do you feel that your life is empty?	YES / NO	
4.	Do you often get bored?	YES / NO	
5.	Are you hopeful about the future?	YES / NO	
6.	Are you bothered by thoughts you can't get out of your head?	YES / NO	
7.	Are you in good spirits most of the time?	YES / NO	
8.	Are you afraid that something bad is going to happen to you?	YES / NO	
9.	Do you feel happy most of the time?	YES / NO	
10.	Do you often feel helpless?	YES / NO	
11.	Do you often get restless and fidgety?	YES / NO	
12.	Do you prefer to stay at home, rather than going out and doing new things?	YES / NO	
13.	Do you frequently worry about the future?	YES / NO	
14.	Do you feel you have more problems with memory than most?	YES / NO	
15.	Do you think it is wonderful to be alive now?	YES / NO	
16.	Do you often feel downhearted and blue?	YES / NO	
17.	Do you feel pretty worthless the way you are now?	YES / NO	
18.	Do you worry a lot about the past?	YES / NO	
19.	Do you find life very exciting?	YES / NO	
20.	Is it hard for you to get started on new projects?	YES / NO	
21.	Do you feel full of energy?	YES / NO	
22.	Do you feel that your situation is hopeless?	YES / NO	
23.	Do you think that most people are better off than you are?	YES / NO	
24.	Do you frequently get upset over little things?	YES / NO	
25.	Do you frequently feel like crying?	YES / NO	
26.	Do you have trouble concentrating?	YES / NO	
27.	Do you enjoy getting up in the morning?	YES / NO	
28.	Do you prefer to avoid social gatherings?	YES / NO	
29.	Is it easy for you to make decisions?	YES / NO	
30.	Is your mind as clear as it used to be?	YES / NO	
		TOTAL	

This is the original scoring for the scale: One point for each of these answers.
Cutoff: normal 0-9; mild depressives 10-19; severe depressives 20-30.

1. NO	6. YES	11. YES	16. YES	21. NO	26. YES
2. YES	7. NO	12. YES	17. YES	22. YES	27. NO
3. YES	8. YES	13. YES	18. YES	23. YES	28. YES
4. YES	9. NO	14. YES	19. NO	24. YES	29. NO
5. NO	10. YES	15. NO	20. YES	25. YES	30. NO

Fig. 8.7 | **Geriatric Depression Scale (30 Item).** (From Yesavage, J. A., Brink, T. L., Rose, T. L., et al. [1983]. Development and validation of a geriatric depression screening scale: A preliminary report. *Journal of Psychiatric Research*, 17, 37–49.)

Geriatric Depression Scale (Short Form)

Patient's Name: _____ Date: _____

Instructions: Choose the best answer for how you felt over the past week.

No.	Question	Answer	Score
1.	Are you basically satisfied with your life?	YES / *NO*	
2.	Have you dropped many of your activities and interests?	*YES* / NO	
3.	Do you feel that your life is empty?	*YES* / NO	
4.	Do you often get bored?	*YES* / NO	
5.	Are you in good spirits most of the time?	YES / *NO*	
6.	Are you afraid that something bad is going to happen to you?	*YES* / NO	
7.	Do you feel happy most of the time?	YES / *NO*	
8.	Do you often feel helpless?	*YES* / NO	
9.	Do you prefer to stay at home, rather than going out and doing new things?	*YES* / NO	
10.	Do you feel you have more problems with memory than most people?	*YES* / NO	
11.	Do you think it is wonderful to be alive?	YES / *NO*	
12.	Do you feel pretty worthless the way you are now?	*YES* / NO	
13.	Do you feel full of energy?	YES / *NO*	
14.	Do you feel that your situation is hopeless?	*YES* / NO	
15.	Do you think that most people are better off than you are?	*YES* / NO	
		TOTAL	

Scoring:

Answers indicating depression are in bold and italicized; score one point for each one selected. A score of 0 to 5 is normal. A score greater than 5 suggests depression.

Fig. 8.8 | **Geriatric Depression Scale (15 Item).** (Modified from Sheikh, J. I., & Yesavage, J. A. [1986]. Geriatric Depression Scale (GDS): Recent evidence and development of a shorter version. *Clinical Gerontology, 5*[1/2], 165–173, 1986.)

Geriatric Depression Scale (Short Form)
Self-Rated Version

Patient's Name: _____   Date: _____

Instructions: _Choose the best answer for how you felt over the past week._

No.	Question	Answer	Score
1.	Are you basically satisfied with your life?	YES / NO	
2.	Have you dropped many of your activities and interests?	YES / NO	
3.	Do you feel that your life is empty?	YES / NO	
4.	Do you often get bored?	YES / NO	
5.	Are you in good spirits most of the time?	YES / NO	
6.	Are you afraid that something bad is going to happen to you?	YES / NO	
7.	Do you feel happy most of the time?	YES / NO	
8.	Do you often feel helpless?	YES / NO	
9.	Do you prefer to stay at home, rather than going out and doing new things?	YES / NO	
10.	Do you feel you have more problems with memory than most people?	YES / NO	
11.	Do you think it is wonderful to be alive?	YES / NO	
12.	Do you feel pretty worthless the way you are now?	YES / NO	
13.	Do you feel full of energy?	YES / NO	
14.	Do you feel that your situation is hopeless?	YES / NO	
15.	Do you think that most people are better off than you are?	YES / NO	
		TOTAL	

Fig. 8.8, Cont'd

Table 8.4	Suicide by Age Group and Cause of Death Category	
Age Group (y)	**Cause of Death Category**	
10–14	3rd	
15–24	2nd	
25–34	2nd	
35–44	4th	
45–54	5th	
55–64	8th	

Stone, D. M., Holland, K. M., Bartholow, B., Crosby, A. E., Davis, S., & Wilkins, N. (2017). Preventing suicide: A technical package of policies, programs, and practices. Atlanta, GA: National Center for Injury Prevention and Control, Centers for Disease Control and Prevention.

and divergent) with high sensitivity and specificity when identifying suicide behaviors (Posner et al., 2011). Subsequently, criticisms of the C-SSRS include that by using it combinations of suicide ideation and behaviors may not be identified, instructions are flawed, and wording is ambiguous (Giddens, Sheehan, & Sheehan, 2014). When used to screen patients with severe mental illness with high risk (n = 1055), it was noted to have good psychometric properties (Madan et al., 2016).

Recently, the National Institute of Mental Health (NIMH, 2017) published the _Ask Suicide-Screening Questions_ tool. The asQ, as it is known, consists of five direct questions and reportedly has good psychometric properties. Although it is identified for use among those between 10 and 24 years of age, it could be applicable to older adults as well. Research is needed to better screen and assess for suicide ideation (Fig. 8.9).

asQ
Ask Suicide-Screening Questions

Information Sheet

Screening Youth for Suicide Risk in Medical Settings

A rapid, psychometrically sound 4-item screening tool for all pediatric patients presenting to the emergency department, inpatient units, & primary care facilities.

BACKGROUND

- In 2010, suicide became the 2nd leading cause of death for youth ages 10-24.
- In 2015, more than 5,900 American youth killed themselves.
- In the U.S., over 2 million young people attempt suicide each year. 90% of suicide attempts among youth are unknown to parents.
- Early identification and treatment of patients at elevated risk for suicide is a key suicide prevention strategy, yet high risk patients are often not recognized by healthcare providers.
- Recent studies show that the majority of individuals who die by suicide have had contact with a healthcare provider within three months prior to their death.
- Unfortunately, these patients often present solely with physical complaints and infrequently discuss suicidal thoughts and plans unless asked directly.

Suicide in the Hospital

Suicide in the medical setting is one of the most frequent sentinel events reported to the Joint Commission (JC). In the past 20 years, over 1,300 patient deaths by suicide have been reported to the JC from hospitals nationwide.

- Notably, 25% of these suicides occurred in non- behavioral health settings such as general medical units and the emergency department.
- Root cause analyses reveal that the lack of proper "assessment" of suicide risk was the leading cause for these reported suicides.

Ask directly about suicidal thoughts –
EVERY HEALTHCARE PROVIDER CAN MAKE A DIFFERENCE

Screening in Medical Settings

The emergency department, inpatient units, and primary care settings are promising venues for identifying young people at risk for suicide.

- Several studies have refuted myths about iatrogenic risk of asking youth questions about suicide, such as the worry about "putting ideas into their heads."
- Screening positive for suicide risk on validated instruments may not only be predictive of future suicidal behavior, but may also be a proxy for other serious mental health concerns that require attention.
- Non-psychiatric clinicians in medical settings require brief validated instruments to help detect medical patients at risk for suicide.

Emergency Department (ED)

- For over 1.5 million youth, the ED is their only point of contact with the healthcare system, creating an opportune time to screen for suicide risk.
- Screening in the ED has been found to be feasible (non-disruptive to workflow and acceptable to patients and their families).

Inpatient Units

- Research reveals that the majority of medical inpatients have never been asked about suicide before; however, opinion data indicate that most adolescents support screening in inpatient settings.

Primary Care/Inpatient Clinics

- Primary Care Physicians (PCPs) are often the de-facto principal mental healthcare providers for children and adolescents.
- Adolescents may be more comfortable discussing risk-taking activities with PCPs than with specialists.

Suicide Risk Screening Recommendations

- 2007 – The JC issued National Patient Safety Goal 15A, requiring suicide risk screening for all patients being treated for mental health concerns in all healthcare settings.
- 2010 & 2016 – The JC issued a Sentinel Event Alert, recommending that all medical patients in hospitals also be screened for suicide risk.

Fig. 8.9 | *Ask Suicide-Screening Questions* (asQ) tool.

asQ Development

- The ASQ was developed in 3 pediatric Emergency Departments (EDs):
  - Children's National Medical Center, Washington, DC
  - Boston Children's Hospital, Boston, Massachusetts
  - Nationwide Children's Hospital, Columbus, Ohio

- For use by non-psychiatric clinicians
- Takes less than 2 minutes to screen
- Positive screen: "yes" to any of the 4 items
- **Sound psychometric properties***

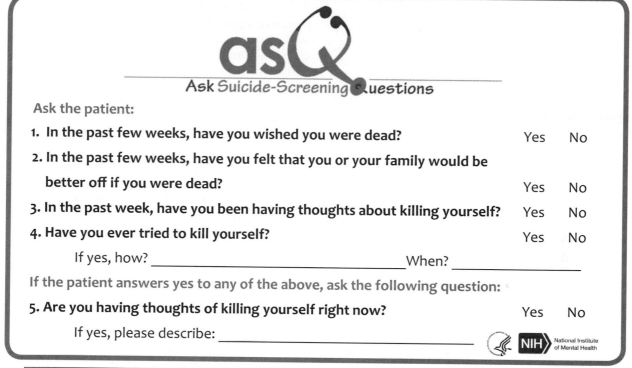

asQ

Ask Suicide-Screening Questions

Ask the patient:

1. **In the past few weeks, have you wished you were dead?** Yes No

2. **In the past few weeks, have you felt that you or your family would be better off if you were dead?** Yes No

3. **In the past week, have you been having thoughts about killing yourself?** Yes No

4. **Have you ever tried to kill yourself?** Yes No

   If yes, how? _____ When? _____

If the patient answers yes to any of the above, ask the following question:

5. **Are you having thoughts of killing yourself right now?** Yes No

   If yes, please describe: _____

National Institute of Mental Health

For description of study:
*Horowitz LM, Bridge JA, Teach SJ, Ballard E, Klima J, Rosenstein DL, Wharff EA, Ginnis K, Cannon E, Joshi P, Pao M. Ask Suicide-Screening Questions (ASQ): A Brief Instrument for the Pediatric Emergency Department. Arch Pediatr Adolesc Med. 2012;166(12):1170-1176.

After administering the asQ

- If patient answers "No" to all questions 1 through 4, screening is complete (not necessary to ask question #5). No intervention is necessary (*Note: Clinical judgment can always override a negative screen).

- **If patient answers "Yes" to any of questions 1 through 4, or refuses to answer, they are considered a positive screen. Ask question #5 to assess acuity:**

  ☐ "Yes" to question #5 = **acute positive screen** (imminent risk identified)
    - **Patient requires a STAT safety/full mental health evaluation.** Patient cannot leave until evaluated for safety.
    - Keep patient in sight. Remove all dangerous objects from room. Alert physician or clinician responsible for patient's care.

  ☐ "No" to question #5 = **non-acute positive screen** (potential risk identified)
    - **Patient requires a brief suicide safety assessment to determine if a full mental health evaluation is needed.** Patient cannot leave until evaluated for safety.
    - Alert physician or clinician responsible for patient's care.

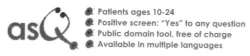

- Patients ages 10-24
- Positive screen: "Yes" to any question
- Public domain tool, free of charge
- Available in multiple languages

For more information contact:

Lisa M. Horowitz, Ph.D., M.P.H. Email: horowitzl@mail.nih.gov
Intramural Research Program, National Institute of Mental Health, NIH

Jeffrey A. Bridge, Ph.D. Email: jeff.bridge@nationwidechidlrens.org
Nationwide Children's Hospital, The Ohio State University College of Medicine

Elizabeth A. Wharff, Ph.D., M.S.W. Email: elizabeth.wharff@childrens.harvard.edu
Boston Children's Hospital, Harvard Medical School

asQ Suicide Risk Screening Toolkit **NATIONAL INSTITUTE OF MENTAL HEALTH (NIMH)**  6/13/2017

Fig. 8.9, Cont'd

Family Assessment

Support of the patient by family members is advantageous but also can be challenging. As with other factors affecting pain, it is difficult to tease out cause and effect and influence. Chronic pain can have an impact on usual roles and relationships (Riffin, Fried, & Pillemer, 2016). It may be necessary for a spouse or other family member to assume roles that were traditionally undertaken by the person now limited by pain (Shaw, Campbell, Nelson, Main, & Linton, 2013). This may cause stress, role ambiguity, and anger by the spouse or other family members and role ambiguity, frustration, and guilt by the person in pain. Readjusting to different roles that were not anticipated may take time and work. Professional assistance from behavioral health professionals may be necessary and helpful (Riffin et al., 2016).

Harmful reactions to the patient on one hand may be manifested as anger and even abuse. On the other extreme, reactions may be excessively sympathetic to the point of disabling the person experiencing pain (Shaw et al., 2013). Again, professional assistance through counseling may be helpful.

There are no specific tools validated for this purpose. Assessment can be done using organization-specific psychosocial assessment tools. Patients living with chronic pain may be vulnerable either physically or emotionally; thus it is important to assess for any signs of physical abuse and to ask if the patient is experiencing any physical or emotional abuse. Assessment needs to include physical examination and reflective listening with follow-up questions and routine psychosocial questions.

Referral to a social worker, department of social services, or adult protective services is needed if the assessment, patient reports, behaviors, or activities indicate the patient is in danger or at risk for harm.

Financial Assessment

Finances can be an important consideration for patients and providers when considering options for pain management. Pain management is expensive. In 2010 the annual cost of treating pain was estimated at between $560 and $635 billion, which surpassed the costs of treating heart disease, cancer, and diabetes (Eckard et al., 2016; Gaskin & Richard, 2012). In 2010 it was computed that out-of-pocket costs for pain management accounted for 17% of the incremental costs of medical expenditures related to pain management and was surpassed only by Medicare expenditures at 25% and private insurance at 43% (Gaskin & Richard, 2012).

In the hospital setting the scope of insurance coverage can dictate options for medical, intraoperative, and post-operative analgesia. Although there are many nonopioid types of analgesia, they may not be covered and therefore not be available to the individual patient. Some patients may have the ability and willingness to pay out of pocket, so it is important to discuss the options with the patient and family.

For patients with chronic pain, financial restrictions are often significant and limiting (Schumacher et al., 2014). In one study, 73.1% of the responders perceived pain management as a financial burden that was third only behind inadequate access to pain management specialists and unwillingness to make lifestyle changes as a barrier to effective pain management (Remster & Marx, 2011). In addition to the cost of clinician visits, medications, and treatments, there are indirect costs and financial burdens related to lost wages (Gaskin & Richard, 2012).

This is an area of health care that is particularly deficient in research or evidence-based information and poses a great opportunity for future research (Gordon et al., 2016; Schumacher, et al., 2014). At the same time, all of us working in clinical settings know that patients are limited in both pharmacologic and nonpharmacologic options because of cost and limited finances. The medication or intervention may be the most appropriate for the patient, but it is useless if the patient cannot afford it and insurance coverage is limited.

No financial specific assessment tools were found in the literature. It is recommended to open the discussion with the patient and family about a variety of options and ask about insurance coverage and other financial resources.

It is important for the clinician to be aware of the cost of pharmacologic and nonpharmacologic options in their geographic area because these can vary widely. In many areas, there may be wide variation among pharmacies in the cost of medications. In areas where there are professional schools of massage, chiropractic, yoga, or acupuncture, it may be possible for patients to have care or treatments by students at reduced rates. There are many low-cost or free options available electronically, including coloring pages, exercise instruction, and video game–based physical therapy options (Eckard et al., 2016). An inexpensive option for cognitive-behavioral therapies is reviewing with the patient the various applications on their mobile phone or electronic device that teach or guide many interventions, including yoga, meditation, guided relaxation, and tai chi, in addition to avenues of distraction, including puzzles and games.

Key Points

- Pain is often comorbid with anxiety and/or depression and/or sleep disturbances.
- Patients experiencing pain need to be assessed for anxiety and/or depression and/or sleep disturbances.

- Obstructive sleep apnea is a particular concern for patients taking sedating medications for pain management.
- Pain can have a negative impact on family and social relationships.
- Family members may behave on a continuum ranging from supportive to abusive.
- Patients living with pain need to be assessed for physical and emotional abuse.
- Finances can be stretched and limited when pain is occurring.
- Financial limitations may limit the options for managing pain that are available to the person experiencing pain.
- When assessment indicates that one of these comorbidities is present, referral to a clinician who specializes in the area is warranted.

Case Scenario

Marianna is 44-year-old married mother of two. Last year she was diagnosed with rheumatoid arthritis (RA) and treated with supplements, aspirin, as-needed ibuprofen, and occasionally corticosteroids. Now she is hospitalized with abdominal pain, nausea, and vomiting. She reports that her joint pain also seems more intense than it has been recently. She occasionally has chest pain, but all her cardiac tests have been normal. She is also frustrated because she has gained a great amount of weight.

1. In addition to her RA and pain, what comorbidities may Marianna be experiencing?
2. What assessment other than pain would you do?
3. What assessment tools would you use?
4. What type of education does she need?
5. What community resources may be available for Marianna?
6. What professionals could be consulted to assist in the care of Marianna?

References

American Academy of Sleep Medicine. (2014). *The International Classification of Sleep Disorders* (3rd Ed). Darien, IL: American Academy of Sleep Medicine.

American Psychological Association (APA). (n.d.a.). *Anxiety*. http://www.apa.org/topics/anxiety/ Retrieved 04/12/2017.

American Psychological Association (APA). (n.d.b.). *Depression*. http://www.apa.org/topics/depression/ Retrieved 05/26/2017.

American Psychological Association (APA). (2017). *Beck Depression Inventory (BDI)*. http://www.apa.org/pi/about/publications/caregivers/practice-settings/assessment/tools/beck-depression.aspx Retrieved 10/28/2017.

Arrieta, J., Aguerrebere, M., Raviola, G., Flores, H., Elliott, P., & Franke, M. F. (2017). Validity and utility of the Patient Health Questionnaire (PHQ-2) and (PHQ-9) for screening and diagnosis of depression in rural Chiapas, Mexico: A cross-sectional study. *Journal of Clinical Psychology*, 73(9), 1076–1090.

Avitsian, R., & Galway, U. (2015). Assessment and management of obstructive sleep apnea for ambulatory surgery. *Advances in Anesthesia*, 33(1), 61–75. https://doi.org/10.1016/j.aan.2015.07.001.

Beck, A. T., Steer, R. A., & Garbin, M. G. (1988). Psychometric properties of the Beck Depression Inventory: twenty-five years of evaluation. *Clinical Psychology Review*, 8(1), 77–100.

Beck, A. T., Ward, C. H., Mendelson, M., Mock, J., & Erbaugh, J. (1961). An inventory for measuring depression. *Archives of General Psychiatry*, 4(6), 561–571.

Belk, R. A., Pilling, M., Rogers, K. D., Lovell, K., & Young, A. (2016). The theoretical and practical determination of clinical cut-offs for the British Sign Language versions of PHQ-9 and GAD-7. *BMC Psychiatry*, 16. https://doi.org/10.1186/s12888-016-1078-0.

Billings, K. R., & Maddalozzo, J. (2013). Complementary and integrative treatments managing obstructive sleep apnea. *Otolaryngologic Clinics of North America*, 46(3), 383–388.

Buysse, D. J. (2014). Sleep health: Can we define it? Does it matter? *Sleep*, 37(1), 9–17.

Buysse, D. J., Reynolds, C. F., Monk, T. H., Berman, S. R., & Kupfer, D. J. (1989). The Pittsburgh Sleep Quality Index: a new instrument for psychiatric practice and research. *Psychiatry Research*, 28(2), 193–213.

Carleton, R. N., Thibodeau, M. A., Teale, M. J. N., Welch, P. G., Abrams, M. P., & Asmundson, G. J. G. (2013). The Center for Epidemiologic Studies Depression Scale: A review with a theoretical and empirical examination of item content and factor structure. *PLoS One*, 8(3). https://doi.org/10.1371/journal.pone.0058067.

Chou, R., Gordon, D. B., de Leon-Casasola, O. A., Rosenberg, J. M., Bickler, S., Brennan, T., & Griffith, S. (2016). Management of Postoperative Pain: A Clinical Practice Guideline from the American Pain Society, the American Society of Regional Anesthesia and Pain Medicine, and the American Society of Anesthesiologists' Committee on Regional Anesthesia, Executive Committee, and Administrative Council. *The Journal of Pain*, 17(2), 131–157.

Chung, R. (2012). High STOP-BANG scores indicate a high probability of obstructive sleep apnea. *British Journal of Anaesthesia*, 108(5), 768–775.

Darnall, B. D., Sturgeon, J. A., Cook, K. F., Taub, C. J., Roy, A., Burns, J. W., … Mackey, S. C. (2017). Development and Validation of a Daily Pain Catastrophizing Scale. *The Journal of Pain*, 18(9), 1139–1149.

Dodo, N., & Hashimoto, R. (2017). The effect of anxiety sensitivity on psychological and biological variables during cold pressor test. *Autonomic Neuroscience: Basic and Clinical*, 205, 72–76. https://doi.org/10.1016/j.autneu.2017.05.006.

Doneh, B. (2015). Epworth Sleepiness Scale. *Occup Med (London)*, 65, 508.

Dowell, D., Haegerich, T. M., & Chou, R. (2016). CDC guideline for prescribing opioids for chronic pain—United States, 2016. *JAMA*, 315(15), 1624–1645.

Eckard, C., Ashbury, C., Bolduc, B., Camerlengo, C., Gotthardt, J., & Horzempa, J. (2016). The integration of technology into treatment programs to aid in the reduction of chronic pain. *Journal of Pain Management Medicine*, 2(3), 1–5.

Edinger, J. D., Leggett, M. K., Carney, C. E., & Manber, R. (2017). Psychological and behavioral treatments for insomnia II: Implementation and specific populations (Chapter 86). In *Principles and Practice of Sleep Medicine* (6th ed.). Philadelphia: Elsevier.

Farzanfar, R., Hereen, T., Fava, J., Davis, J., Vachon, L., & Friedman, R. (2014). Psychometric properties of an automated telephone-based PHQ-9. *Telemedicine and e-Health*, 20(2), 115–121. https://doi.org/10.1089/tmj.2013.0158.

Fergus, T. A., Limbers, C. A., Griggs, J. O., & Kelley, L. P. (2018). Somatic symptom severity among primary care patients who are obese: examining the unique contributions of anxiety sensitivity, discomfort intolerance, and health anxiety. *Journal of Behavioral Medicine*, 41(1), 43–51.

Finan, P. H., Goodin, B. R., & Smith, M. T. (2013). The association of sleep and pain: An update and a path forward. *Journal of Pain*, 14(12), 1539–1552 (PubMed: 24290442).

Finan, P. H., Buenaver, L. F., Coryell, V. T., & Smith, M. T. (2014). Cognitive-behavioral therapy for comorbid insomnia and chronic pain. *Sleep Medicine Clinics*, 9(2), 261–274.

Finan, P. H., Carroll, C. P., Moscou-Jackson, G., Martel, M. O., Campbell, C. M., Pressman, A., … Haythornthwaite, J. A. (2018). Daily Opioid Use Fluctuates as a Function of Pain, Catastrophizing, and Affect in Patients with Sickle Cell Disease: An Electronic Daily Diary Analysis. *The Journal of Pain*, 19(1), 46–56.

Gaskin, D. J., & Richard, P. (2012). The economic costs of pain in the United States. *The Journal of Pain*, 13(8), 715–124.

Geiger-Brown, J. M., Rogers, V. E., Liu, W., Ludeman, E. M., Downton, K. D., & Diaz-Abad, M. (2015). Cognitive behavioral therapy in person with comorbid insomnia: A meta-analysis. *Sleep Medicine Reviews*, 23(1), 54–67.

Gerrits, M. M. J. G., van Marwijk, H. W. J., van Oppen, P., van der Horst, H., & Pennix, B. W. J. H. (2015). Longitudinal association of pain, and depression and anxiety over four years. *Journal of Psychosomatic Research*, 78(1), 64–70.

Gerrits, M. M., van Oppen, P., van Marwijk, H. W., Pennix, B. W., & van der Horst, H. (2014). Pain and the onset of depressive and anxiety disorders. *Pain*, 155(1), 53–59.

Giddens, J. M., Sheehan, K. H., & Sheehan, D. V. (2014). The Columbia-Suicide Severity Rating Scale (C-SSRS): Has the "Gold Standard" Become a Liability? *Innovations in Clinical Neuroscience*, 11(9-10), 66.

Gillanders, D. T., Ferreira, N. B., Bose, S., & Esrich, T. (2013). The relationship between acceptance, catastrophizing and illness representations in chronic pain. *European Journal of Pain*, 17(6), 893–902.

Gordon, D. B., de Leon-Casasola, O. A., Wu, C. L., Sluka, K. A., Brennan, T. J., & Chou, R. (2016). Research gaps in practice guidelines for acute postoperative pain management in adults: Findings from a review of the evidence for an American Pain Society Clinical Practice Guideline. *The Journal of Pain*, 17(2), 158–166.

Gyurcsik, N. C., Cary, M. A., Sessford, J. D., Flora, P. K., & Brawley, L. R. (2015). Pain, anxiety, and negative outcome expectations for activity: Do negative psychological profiles differ between the inactive and active? *Arthritis Care & Research*, 67(1), 58–64.

Ho, R. T. H., & Fong, T. C. T. (2014). Factor structure of the Chinese version of the Pittsburgh Sleep Quality Index in breast cancer patients. *Sleep Medicine*, 15(5), 565–569.

Hoey, L. M., Fulbrook, P., & Douglas, J. A. (2014). Sleep assessment of hospitalized patients: A literature review. *International Journal of Nursing Studies*, 51(9), 1281–1288.

Howe, C. Q., & Sullivan, M. D. (2014). The missing "P" in pain management: how the current opioid epidemic highlights the need for psychiatric services in chronic pain care. *General Hospital Psychiatry*, 36(1), 99–104.

Hudson, B. F., & Ogden, J. (2016). Exploring the impact of intraoperative interventions for pain and anxiety management during local anesthetic surgery: A systematic review and meta-analysis. *Journal of PeriAnesthesia Nursing*, 31(2), 118–133.

Janssen, K. C., Phillipson, S., O'Connor, J., & Johns, M. W. (2017). Validation of the Epworth Sleepiness Scale for Children and Adolescents using Rasch analysis. *Sleep Medicine*, 33, 30–35.

Johns, M. W. (1991). A new method for measuring daytime sleepiness: the Epworth sleepiness scale. *Sleep*, 14(6), 540–545.

Johns, M. W. (1992). Reliability and factor analysis of the Epworth Sleepiness Scale. *Sleep*, 15(4), 376–381.

Johnson, M., Weber, J., McCrae, C., & Craggs, J. (2017). (397) Catch 22 of insomnia and chronic pain: Exploring how insomnia and sleep impact the neural correlates of chronic pain. *The Journal of Pain*, 18(4), S73.

Junghaenel, D. U., Schneider, S., & Broderick, J. E. (2017). Linguistic Indicators of Pain Catastrophizing in Patients with Chronic Musculoskeletal Pain. *The Journal of Pain*, 18(5), 597–604.

Kirwan, M., Pickett, S. M., & Jarrett, N. L. (2017). Emotion regulation as a moderator between anxiety symptoms and insomnia symptom severity. *Psychiatry Research*, 254(1), 40–47.

Klingman, K. J., Jungquist, C. R., & Perlis, M. L. (2017). Questionnaires that screen for multiple sleep disorders. *Sleep Medicine Reviews*, 32(1), 37–44.

Kochanek, K. D., Murphy, S. L., Xu, J., & Arias, E. (2019). Deaths: final data for 2017. *National Vital Statistics Reports*, 68(9), 1–20.

Koffel, E., Kroenke, K., Bair, M. J., Leverty, D., Polusny, M. A., & Krebs, E. E. (2016). The bidirectional relationship between sleep complaints and pain: analysis of data from a randomized trial. *Health Psychology*, 35(1), 41–49. https://doi.org/10.1037/hea0000245.

Kreddig, N., & Hasenbring, M. I. (2017). Pain anxiety and fear of (re)injury in patients with chronic back pain: Sex as a moderator. *Scandinavian Journal of Pain*, 16(1), 105–111.

Kroenke, K., Spitzer, R., & Williams, J. (2001). The PHQ-9: validity of a brief depression severity measure. *Journal of General Internal Medicine*, 16(9), 606–613.

Kroenke, L., Spitzer, R. L., Williams, J. B. W., & Löwe, B. (2009). An ultra-brief screening scale for anxiety and depression: The PHQ-4. *Psychosomatics*, 50(6), 613–621.

Legler, C. D. (2017). STOP-BANG assessment and postoperative outcomes. *Journal of PeriAnesthesia Nursing*, 33(3), 330–337. https://doi.org/10.1016/j.jopan.2015.06.004.

Madan, A., Frueh, B. C., Allen, J. G., Ellis, T. E., Rufino, K. A., Oldham, J. M., & Fowler, J. C. (2016). Psychometric Reevaluation of the Columbia-Suicide Severity Rating Scale: Findings From a Prospective, Inpatient Cohort of Severely Mentally Ill Adults. *The Journal of Clinical Psychiatry*, 77(7), e867–e873.

Maeoka, H., Hiyamizu, M., Matsuo, A., & Morioka, S. (2015). The influence of repeated pain stimulation on the emotional aspect of pain: A preliminary study in healthy volunteers. *Journal of Pain Research*, 8, 431–436.

Mansukhani, M. P., Olson, E. J., & Ramar, K. (2013). Adult obstructive sleep apnea (Reference Module). *In: Neuroscience and biobehavioral psychology, from Encyclopedia of Sleep* (pp. 279–289). New York: Elsevier. https://doi.org/10.1016/B978-0-12-378610-4.00322-3.

Marc, L. G., Henderson, W. R., Desrosiers, A., Testa, M. A., Jean, S. E., & Akom, E. E. (2014). Reliability and validity of the Haitian Creole PHQ-9. *Journal of Internal Medicine*, 29(12), 1679–1686.

Marshansky, S., Mayer, P., Rizzo, D., Baltzan, M., Denis, R., & Lavigne, G. J. (2017). Sleep, chronic pain, and opioid risk for apnea. *Progress in Neuro-Psychopharmacology and Biological Psychiatry.*, 87, 234–244. Pt. B.

Miller, C. B., Espie, C. A., & Kyle, S. D. (2014). Cognitive behavioral therapy for the management of poor sleep in insomnia disorder. *ChronoPhysiology and Therapy*, 4, 99–107.

Mitchell, M. A., Riccardi, C. J., Keough, M. E., Timpano, K. R., & Schmidt, N. B. (2013). Understanding the associations among anxiety sensitivity, distress tolerance, and discomfort intolerance: A comparison of three models. *Journal of Anxiety Disorders*, 27(1), 147–154.

Mundt, J., Eisenschenk, S., & Robinson, M. (2017). (396) Severity and likelihood of chronic pain in individuals with obstructive sleep apnea and insomnia. *The Journal of Pain*, 18(4), S73.

National Institute of Mental Health (NIMH). (2017). Ask Suicide-Screening Questions—NIMH Toolkit Information Sheet. https://www.nimh.nih.gov/research/research-conducted-at-nimh/asq-toolkit-materials/asq-tool/information-sheet_155866.pdf. Accessed 8/15/2020.

National Institute of Mental Health (NIMH). (2019). Major Depression. https://www.nimh.nih.gov/health/statistics/major-depression.shtml. Accessed 8/15/2020.

Nguyen, T. Q., Banden-Roche, K., Bass, J. K., German, D., Nguyen, N. T. T., & Knowlton, A. R. (2016). A tool for sexual minority mental health research: The Patient Health Questionnaire (PHQ-9) as a depressive symptom severity measure for sexual minority women in Viet Nam. *Journal for Gay and Lesbian Mental Health*, 20(20), 173–191.

Nicassio, P. M., Ormseth, S. R., Custodio, M. K., Olmstead, R., Weisman, M. H., & Irwin, M. R. (2014). Confirmatory factor analysis of the Pittsburgh Sleep Quality Index in rheumatoid arthritis patients. *Behavioral Sleep Medicine*, 12(1), 1–12. https://doi.org/10.1080/15402002.2012.720315.

O'Connor, E., Gaynes, B. N., Burda, B. U., Soh, C., & Whitlock, E. P. (2013). Screening for and treatment of suicide risk relevant to primary care: a systematic review for the US Preventive Services Task Force. *Annals of Internal Medicine*, 158(10), 741–754.

Okifuji, A., & Turk, D. C. (2016). Chronic pain and depression: vulnerability and resilience. In M. Flaten, & M. al'Absi (Eds.), *Neuroscience of Pain, Stress and Emotion*. San Diego: Academic Press.

Pinto, P. R., McIntyre, T., Ferrero, R., Almeida, A., & Araújo-Soares, V. (2013). Predictors of acute postsurgical pain and anxiety following primary total hip and knee arthroplasty. *The Journal of Pain*, 14(5), 502–515.

Plummer, F., Manea, L., Trepel, D., & McMillan, D. (2016). Screening for anxiety disorders with the GAD-7and GAD-2: A systematic review and diagnostic meta-analysis. *General Hospital Psychiatry*, 39(2), 24–31.

Posner, K., Brown, G. K., Stanley, B., Brent, D. A., Yershova, K. V., Oquendo, M. A., … Mann, J. J. (2011). The Columbia–Suicide Severity Rating Scale: initial validity and internal consistency findings from three multisite studies with adolescents and adults. *American Journal of Psychiatry*, 168(12), 1266–1277.

Quinlan-Colwell, A. (2012). A review of pain assessment tools for use with the older adult patient. *In: Compact Clinical Guide to Geriatric Pain Management*. New York: Springer Publishing.

Radloff, L. S. (1977). The CES-D scale: a self-report depression scale for research in the general population. *Applied Psychological Measurement*, 1(3), 385–401.

Rana, A. Q., Qureshi, A. R. M., Kachhvi, H. B., Rana, M. A., & Chou, K. L. (2016). Increased likelihood of anxiety and poor sleep quality in Parkinson's disease patients with pain. *Journal of Neurological Sciences*, 369, 212–215.

Remster, E. N., & Marx, T. L. (2011). Barriers to managing chronic pain: perspectives of Appalachian providers. *Osteopathic Family Physician*, 3, 141–148.

Rener-Sitar, K., John, M. T., Bandyopadhyay, D., Howell, M. J., & Schiffman, E. L. (2014). Exploration of dimensionality and psychometric properties of the Pittsburgh Sleep Quality Index in cases with temporomandibular disorders. *Health and Quality of Life Outcomes*, 12, 10.

Reynolds, S. A., & Ebben, M. R. (2017). The cost of insomnia and the benefit of increased access to evidence-based treatment: cognitive behavioral therapy for insomnia. *Sleep Medicine Clinics*, 12(1), 39–46.

Riffin, C., Fried, T., & Pillemer, K. (2016). Impact of pain on family members and caregivers of geriatric patients. *Clinics of Geriatric Medicine*, 32(4), 663–675.

Roehrs, T. A., & Roth, T. (2017). Increasing presurgery sleep reduces postsurgery pain and analgesic use following joint replacement: a feasibility study. *Sleep Medicine*, 33(2), 109–113.

Rogers, K. D., Kemp, A., McLachlan, A. J., & Blyth, F. (2013). Adverse selection? A multidimensional profile of people dispensed opioid analgesics for persistent non-cancer pain. *PLoS One*, 8(12), e80095.

Roth, T., Zammit, G., Kushida, C., Doghramji, K., Mathias, S. D., Wong, J. M., & Buyesse, D. J. (2002). A new questionnaire to detect sleep disorders. *Sleep Medicine*, 3(2), 99–108.

Sangkum, L., Klair, I., Limsuwat, C., Bent, S., Myers, L., & Thammasitboon, S. (2017). Incorporating body-type (apple vs pear) in STOP-BANG questionnaire improves its validity to detect OSA. *Journal of Clinical Anesthesia*, 41, 126–131.

Scheerer, J. F., Svrakic, D. M., Freedland, K. E., Chrusciel, T., Balasubramanian, S., … Bucholz, K. K. (2014). Prescription opioid analgesics increase the risk of depression. *Journal of General Internal Medicine*, 29(3), 491–499.

Schrimpf, M., Liegl, G., Boeckle, M., Leitner, A., Geisler, P., & Pieh, C. (2015). The effect of sleep deprivation on pain perception in healthy subjects: a meta-analysis. *Sleep Medicine*, 16(10), 1313–1320.

Schumacher, K. L., Clark, V. L. P., West, C. M., Dodd, M. J., Rabow, M. W., & Miaskowski, C. (2014). Pain medication management processes used by oncology outpatients and family caregivers Part I: health systems contexts. *Journal of Pain and Symptom Management*, 48(5), 770–783.

Shaw, W. S., Campbell, P., Nelson, C. C., Main, C. J., & Linton, S. J. (2013). Effects of workplace, family and cultural influences on low back pain: what opportunities exist to address social factors in general consultations? *Best Practices & Research Clinical Rheumatology*, 27(5), 637-348.

Sivertsen, B., Lallukka, T., Petrie, K. J., Steingrimsdóttir, Ô. A., Stubhaug, A., & Nielsen, C. S. (2015). Sleep and pain sensitivity in adults. *Pain*, 156(8), 1433–1439.

Slavish, D., Graham-Engeland, J., Matire, L., & Smyth, J. (2017). Bidirectional associations between daily pain, affect, and sleep quality in young adults with and without chronic back pain. *The Journal of Pain*, 18(4), S73.

Smith, K., Mattick, R. P., Bruno, R., Nielsen, S., Cohen, M., & Degenhardt, L. (2015). Factors associated with the development of depression in chronic non-cancer pain patients following the onset of opioid treatment for pain. *Journal of Affective Disorders*, 184(1), 72–80.

Spence, D. L., Han, T., McGuire, J., & Couture, D. (2015). Obstructive sleep apnea and the adult perioperative patient. *Journal of PeriAnesthesia Nursing*, 30(6), 528–545.

Spitzer, R. L., Kroenke, L., Williams, J. B. W., & Löwe, B. (2006). A brief measure for assessing generalized anxiety disorder. *Archives of Internal Medicine*, 166(10), 1092–1097.

Stone, D. M., Holland, K. M., Bartholow, B., Crosby, A. E., Davis, S., & Wilkins, N. (2017). *Preventing Suicide: A Technical Package of Policies, Programs, and Practices. Atlanta, GA: National Center for Injury Prevention and Control.* Atlanta, GA: Centers for Disease Control and Prevention.

Substance Abuse and Mental Health Services Administration. (N.D.) *Columbia-Suicide Severity Rating Scale (C-SSRS)-Risk Assessment (Lifeline crisis center version).* Retrieved 10/28/2107 from https://suicidepreventionlifeline.org/wp-content/uploads/2016/09/Suicide-Risk-Assessment-C-SSRS-Lifeline-Version-2014.pdf.

Suhaimi, A. (2018). Low back pain. In D. X. Cifu, & H. L. Lew (Eds.), *Braddom's Rehabilitation Care: A Clinical Handbook* (pp. 228–237e). Philadelphia: Elsevier.

Sullivan, M. J., Bishop, S. R., & Pivik, J. (1995). The pain catastrophizing scale: development and validation. *Psychological Assessment*, 7(4), 524.

Tang, N. K. Y., Goodchild, C. E., Sanborn, A. N., Howard, J., & Salkovskis, P. M. (2012). Deciphering the temporal link between pain and sleep in a heterogeneous chronic pain patient sample: A multilevel daily process study. *Sleep*, 35(5), 675–687. https://doi.org/10.5665/sleep.1830 [PubMed: 22547894].

Thibodeau, M. A., Welch, P. G., Katz, J., & Asmundson, G. J. G. (2013). Pain-related anxiety influences pain perception differently in men and women: A quantitative sensory test across thermal pain modalities. *Pain*, 154(3), 419–426.

van Straten, A., van der Zweerde, T., Kleiboer, A., Cuijpers, P., Morin, C. M., & Lancee, J. (2017). Cognitive and behavioral therapies in the treatment of insomnia: a meta-analysis. *Sleep Medicine Reviews*, 38, 3–16.

Velasco, R. V., Bakhshaie, J., Walker, R. L., Viana, A. G., Garza, M., Ochoa-Perez, M., ... Zvolensky, M. J. (2016). Synergistic effects of pain intensity and anxiety sensitivity in relation to anxiety and depressive symptoms and disorders among economically disadvantaged Latinos in a community-based primary care setting. *Journal of Anxiety Disorders*, 43, 23–31.

Ward, C. (2015). Safe use of opioids in individuals with obstructive sleep apnea. *Pain Management Nursing*, 16(3), 411–417.

Weatherspoon, D., Sullivan, D., & Weatherspoon, C. A. (2016). Obstructive Sleep Apnea and Modifications in Sedation. *Critical Care Nursing Clinics*, 28(2), 217–226.

Werti, M. M., Burgstaller, J. M., Weiser, S., Steurer, J., Kofmehl, R., & Held, U. (2014). Influence of catastrophizing on treatment outcome in patients with nonspecific low back pain: A systematic review. *Spine*, 39(3), 263–273.

Chapter 9 Basic Concepts Involved with Administration of Analgesic Medications

Maureen F. Cooney, Ann Quinlan-Colwell

CHAPTER OUTLINE

Patient Considerations, pg. 163

    Age, pg. 163

    Genetics, pg. 166

Route Selection, pg. 167

    Oral Route, pg. 167

    Transmucosal Route, pg. 171

    Intravenous Route, pg. 173

    Subcutaneous Route, pg. 175

    Intramuscular Route, pg. 178

    Topical, pg. 178

    Transdermal, pg. 179

    Neuraxial and Peripheral Nerve Routes, pg. 181

Analgesic Dosing Considerations, pg. 181

    Equianalgesic Dosing, pg. 181

    Around-the-Clock Dosing, pg. 182

    Awakening Patients for Analgesic Administration, pg. 184

    Dosing to Pain Intensity Using Numbers or Word Descriptors, pg. 184

    Range Orders, pg. 187

    Therapeutic Duplication, pg. 190

Key Points, pg. 190

Case Scenario, pg. 191

References, pg. 191

PAIN is a multidimensional experience that is subjective and unique for each person; therefore, effective and safe pain management requires consideration of individual patient needs and responses. Medication administration is a significant component of a multimodal pain management plan used to address acute and chronic pain. To provide safe and effective pharmacologic interventions, consideration of some of the basic concepts of analgesic administration is helpful. The purpose of this chapter is to address issues related to medication administration that have specific relevance to the administration of analgesics.

Patient Considerations

Variability in individual responses to analgesics, such as development of side effects, may be attributed to multiple patient-specific factors, including age, gender, opioid tolerance, renal function, liver function, body composition, drug-drug interactions, and genetics. These individual patient-related factors require consideration when selecting and dosing analgesics to optimize effects and reduce risks for analgesic-related adverse outcomes. Many of these factors are addressed in subsequent chapters that review various classes of medications; however, age-related considerations and genetics require particular mention in this section.

Age

Older adults are among the vulnerable patients who are at particular risk for the undertreatment of pain. Undertreatment may, in part, be related to clinicians' concerns about analgesic risks, polypharmacy, and lack of knowledge about safe pain management in older adults. Risks related to analgesic medication administration may be increased in older patients because of alterations in physiologic functioning and disease. Some of the age-associated risks are outlined in Table 9.1. When possible, nonpharmacologic therapies to address pain are preferred, but when these therapies alone are not adequate, pharmacologic approaches may be included (Herndon et al., 2016).

Normal aging is associated with declining organ function, and many of the common diseases and chronic conditions seen in elderly patients also have an impact on organ function. Altered organ function, reduced cardiac output, and decreased organ perfusion may alter the pharmacodynamics (i.e., the effect of a drug on the body) and pharmacokinetics (i.e., drug absorption, distribution, metabolism, excretion) of many analgesics. Changes in liver function and reduced renal function may lead to altered metabolism

Table 9.1 | Major Categories of Risk for Pain Therapies in Older Adults

Risk Category	Mechanism	Example
Decline in organ function	Age-related decline in organ blood flow; slowing of CNS function	Altered metabolism and clearance, especially renally excreted drugs with active metabolites (e.g., morphine)
Polypharmacy	Higher prevalence of multiple comorbidities	Acute kidney injury, NSAIDs with ACE inhibitors
Pharmacokinetics	Loss of muscle mass; increased adipose tissue. Altered volumes of drug distribution	Lengthened half-life of lipophilic drugs (e.g., fentaNYL)
Drug sensitivity	Decline in cortical mass, decreased drug receptor populations	Delirium related to anticholinergic drugs (e.g., meperidine)
Frailty	Decline in physiologic reserve to respond to severe complications	Increased mortality from a fall caused by overmedication with opioids

ACE, Angiotensin-converting enzyme; *CNS,* central nervous system; *NSAIDs,* nonsteroidal anti-inflammatory drugs.
From McKeown, J. L. (2015). Pain management issues for the geriatric surgical patient. *Anesthesiology Clinics, 33*(3), 563–576.

Table 9.2 | Physiologic Changes Associated With Aging

Central nervous system	↓ Cerebral blood flow, ↓ cortical mass	Altered perception and affective expression of pain
Peripheral nervous system	↓ Blood flow, nerve damage from higher glucose levels	↓ Sensitivity to pain, temperature, touch
Cardiovascular	↓ Cardiac output	↑ Toxicity as a result of ↑ peak concentration after bolus
Gastrointestinal	↓ Gastric secretions	Impaired dissolution of some drugs, gut absorption remains normal
Hepatic	↓ Number of hepatocytes, ↓ cytochrome P450 function, ↓ synthetic function, ↓ serum protein	Impaired metabolism especially demethylation, ↑ drug-drug reactions, ↓ protein binding, ↑ free serum drug level
Renal	↓ Renal blood flow, ↓ GFR	Impaired clearance of metabolites, ↑ half-lives of renally cleared drugs
Musculoskeletal	↓ Muscle mass, ↑ adipose	↓ Water VD (i.e., ↑ dose toxicity with hydrophilic drugs); ↑ fat VD (i.e., ↑ half-life lipophilic drugs)

↓ Decreased; ↑, increased; *GFR,* glomerular filtration rate; *VD,* volume of distribution.
From McKeown, J. L. (2015). Pain management issues for the geriatric surgical patient. *Anesthesiology Clinics, 33*(3), 563–576.

and accumulation of toxic metabolites. Opioids, for example, are metabolized in the liver, many through phase I and the cytochrome P450 system. With aging, declines in cytochrome P3A4 function and other cytochrome P450 enzymes may reduce clearance of medications, such as oxyCODONE, traMADol, and methadone, thus necessitating dose reductions to prevent opioid-related adverse effects (Sekhri & Cooney, 2017). Table 9.2 describes many of the physiologic changes associated with aging that may lead to adverse reactions associated with analgesics.

To improve the safety and effectiveness of medications prescribed for the elderly, the American Geriatrics Society (AGS) published the Beers Criteria, which lists medications that are potentially problematic for use in older adults (AGS 2019 Beers Criteria Update Expert Panel, 2019). The list includes five categories: medications noted to be potentially inappropriate for most older adults; medications to be avoided in older adults with certain conditions due to medication-condition interactions by which the medication may worsen the condition; medications to be used with caution in older adults; notable

drug-drug interactions; and medications that require dose adjustment based on kidney function. Table 9.3 includes examples of analgesic-related medications that are listed among medications in the Beers Criteria.

General principles for analgesic administration in the elderly support the use of a multimodal analgesia (MMA) plan. MMA is recommended because older adults are particularly vulnerable to adverse outcomes associated with higher doses of single agents such as opioids or nonsteroidal antiinflammatory drugs (NSAIDs). A multimodal plan that includes a foundation of nonpharmacologic approaches, nonopioid analgesics, and opioids when needed as coanalgesics is preferred (Arnstein & Herr, 2017). Use of topical formulations of various agents may provide effective pain relief with fewer adverse effects (Arnstein & Herr, 2017). Interventional procedures, such as nerve blocks, epidural steroid injections, and spinal techniques (see Chapters 18 and 19),

Table 9.3 | Examples of Analgesic-Related Medications Included in the Beer's Criteria

Drug	Use	Problem	Recommendation	Alternative
Meperidine	Pain	Anticholinergic effects, delirium, neurotoxic metabolites	Avoid	Other analgesics; Use MMA, including nonpharmacologic approaches
Opioids	Pain	Increased fall risk if used with two or more other CNS-active drugs	Avoid three or more CNS-active drugs; minimize CNS active-drugs; Avoid concurrent use of opioids with benzodiazepines or gabapentin/pregabalin; avoid opioids except in situations of severe, acute pain	Initiate at lowest effective dose; Careful titration; Use other analgesics; Use MMA, including nonpharmacologic approaches
Non–COX selective NSAIDS (e.g., ibuprofen, naproxen, diclofenac)	Pain	Increased risk for GI bleeding and peptic ulcer disease in those older than 75 years or if on parenteral corticosteroids, anticoagulants, or antiplatelet medications	Avoid chronic use unless alternatives are not effective and if patient can take gastroprotective agents	Other non-opioid analgesics (acetaminophen); Use MMA, including nonpharmacologic approaches
Indomethacin	Pain	Highest risk of all NSAIDs for adverse effects. Increased risk of GI bleeding, peptic ulcer disease, and kidney injury. More likely to cause adverse CNS effects than other NSAIDS.	Avoid	Other non-opioid analgesics (acetaminophen); Use MMA, including nonpharmacologic approaches
Ketorolac	Pain	Increased risk of GI bleeding, peptic ulcer disease, and acute kidney injury	Avoid	Other non-opioid analgesics (acetaminophen); Use MMA, including nonpharmacologic approaches
Gabapentin, pregabalin	Pain	CNS adverse effects with varying levels of kidney function; Gabapentin and pregabalin are associated with increased risk of severe-sedation-related adverse effects, including respiratory depression and death if used in combination with opioids	Reduce dose; Avoid combination of gabapentin or pregabalin with an opioid unless using to transition off opioid to gabapentin or pregabalin.	Other analgesics; Use MMA, including nonpharmacologic approaches
traMADol	Pain	Risk of SIADH/hyponatremia	Use with caution	
Alpha-$_2$ agonists, (e.g., cloNIDine)	Pain; Reduction of opioid withdrawal symptoms	CNS effects, bradycardia, hypotension	Avoid as first-line agent	Use MMA, including nonpharmacologic approaches
Antihistamines (e.g., diphenhydrAMINE, hydrOXYzine, promethazine)	Opioid-related pruritus, nausea	Anticholinergic effects, constipation, sedation, confusion, delirium	Avoid	Ondansetron, nalbuphine

Continued

Table 9.3 | Examples of Analgesic-Related Medications Included in the Beer's Criteria—cont'd

Drug	Use	Problem	Recommendation	Alternative
Antispasmodics (e.g., scopolamine)	Opioid-related nausea	Anticholinergic effects	Avoid	Ondansetron
Muscle relaxants (e.g., cyclobenzaprine, methocarbamol)	Musculoskeletal pain, spasm	Anticholinergic effects, sedation, increased fracture risk, synergistic with opioids	Avoid	Local therapy, heat, cold, repositioning
Tertiary tricyclic antidepressants (e.g., amitriptyline)	Neuropathic pain	Anticholinergic effects, sedation, orthostatic hypotension, delirium, increased fall risk	Avoid; minimize number of anticholinergic medications and CNS-active drugs	DULoxetine, low-dose gabapentin
Benzodiazepines (e.g., diazePAM, LORazepam)	Anxiety, nausea	Prolonged half-lives, sedation, delirium, cognitive impairment, falls, fractures	Avoid; Avoid use of benzodiazepine with opioids	Low-dose haloperidol

CNS, Central nervous system; *COX*, cyclooxygenase; *GI*, gastrointestinal; *NSAID*, nonsteroidal antiinflammatory drug.

Data from: 2019 American Geriatrics Society Beers Criteria® Update Expert Panel, Fick, D. M., Semla, T. P., Steinman, M., Beizer, J., Brandt, N., ... & Flanagan, N. (2019). American Geriatrics Society 2019 updated AGS Beers Criteria® for potentially inappropriate medication use in older adults. *Journal of the American Geriatrics Society, 67*(4), 674-694; American Geriatrics Society 2015 Beers Criteria Update Expert Panel. (2015). American Geriatrics Society 2015 updated Beers criteria for potentially inappropriate medication use in older adults. *Journal of the American Geriatrics Society, 63*(11), 2227–2246

are multimodal strategies that may optimize comfort and eliminate or reduce the need for pharmacologic approaches. The multimodal plan must be individualized because there are situations in which the risk of a medication or procedure outweighs potential benefit or when pain is not amenable to a particular approach.

Acetaminophen has been considered a first-line analgesic for the elderly with acute and chronic mild to moderate pain, particularly with musculoskeletal pain (Abdulla et al., 2013). Although the use of acetaminophen has been recommended to improve physical function, including activities of daily living (ADLs) participation and sleep (Dentino, Medina, & Steinberg, 2017), published systematic reviews have shown limited effectiveness and increased risks (Marcum, Duncan, & Makris, 2016). Recommended maximum dosing of acetaminophen is 3 g/day, which, because of age-related decline in liver function, is less than the 4 g/day dosing restriction for younger adults (Bartoszczyk & Herr, 2016; Cornelius, Herr, Gordon, & Kretzer, 2017; Herndon et al., 2016). NSAIDs are generally avoided in the elderly because of their associated cardiovascular, gastrointestinal, renal, and cerebrovascular risks. Additionally, many elderly are on anticoagulants and other medications that pose increased risks of drug-drug interactions when NSAIDs are included. When necessary, it is recommended to use them at the lowest possible dose, for limited periods, and under medical supervision (Arnstein & Herr, 2017; Dentino et al., 2017).

When pain is not adequately addressed with nonpharmacologic approaches and acetaminophen, the addition of opioid therapy may be appropriate. As with all patients, and particularly in older adults, the decision to use opioids requires that the benefits be carefully weighed against the risks. Opioids can be used safely in older adults with

consideration of age-related pharmacokinetic changes and other factors, such as dosing and organ function. The effects of aging on absorption, distribution, metabolism, and elimination generally require lower initial dosing with careful dose and dose frequency adjustments.

Specific medication-related properties require avoidance of some opioids and make others less desirable among older adults. For example, meperidine is included in the Beers list as a medication that should not be used because of its anticholinergic effects and the risk for accumulation of neurotoxic metabolites. Morphine, although not specifically included on the Beers Criteria, has properties that require careful consideration. In a study comparing the pharmacokinetics of oral morphine over a 24-hour period in older to younger adults, older adults had decreased clearance and greater absorption of morphine with higher plasma concentrations and larger areas under the plasma-time concentration curve (Baillie, Bateman, Coates, & Woodhouse, 1989). The altered morphine pharmacokinetics may necessitate the use of lower than recommended initial doses with careful titration to reduce risks of unintended effects. Age-associated reductions in renal function increase the risk for opioid-related toxicity when medications that have active metabolites such as morphine, codeine, and oxyCODONE are used. These factors do not contraindicate the use of these medications, but require conservative initial doses, careful assessment of effects, and incremental dose titrations based on response.

Genetics

Many health care providers who work in clinical settings have observed variability in patients' individual responses to analgesic medications. Some patients may experience significant pain relief with small doses of opioids yet have side effects such as excessive sedation and respiratory depression. Others, despite significant upward titration of doses, continue to have unrelieved pain but may also experience adverse effects from high doses. Rotation to a different opioid is sometimes observed to provide pain relief with lower morphine equivalent doses than the initial opioid. The significant variability in the ways people respond to different medications is well recognized (Crews et al., 2014). Although variability in individuals' responses to analgesics may be explained by many factors, such as age, gender, culture, drug-drug interactions, environmental factors, and drug bioavailability, research has offered insight into the impact of genetics on medication effects (Dworkin, McDermott, Farrar, O'Connor, & Senn, 2014; Nielsen et al., 2015a).

Pharmacogenetics is the study of how variations or allelic difference in single genes may be responsible for variability in specific medication responses, and *pharmacogenomics* is the study of the inherited genetic differences that result in individual responses to drugs (Manworren, 2015; Ting & Schug, 2016). In the field of pain management, there is increasing interest in the role of genetics on drug targets and metabolism. Genetics have been found to influence pain and responses to pain medications (Nielsen et al., 2015a), and in recent years there has been marked growth in research in this field. As a result of research findings, changes in clinical practice have begun to emerge, because testing results may be considered in the development of individualized multimodal analgesic plans. To demonstrate the growing impact of genomic science, there are a number of guidelines that address the use of genetic testing in clinical practice (Manworren, 2015).

As awareness of the impact of genetic variability on pain and individual responses to analgesic measures increase, there may be less reliance on standard prescribing practices or order sets in which it is expected that "one size will fit all." An increase in the practice of individualizing treatment approaches may be seen in some settings as health care providers and patients recognize that not all people will have the same response to the same medication. Personalized medicine, or the more recently adopted term, *precision medicine,* involves the use of medications specifically selected for an individual patient based on the patient's genetic makeup, which influences effectiveness and metabolism of the medication (Manworren, 2015).

Many clinical and academic laboratories now offer specific genetic testing panels for pain management, focusing on liver enzymes that are involved in the metabolism of opioids. Genetic testing of these enzymes is available from major laboratories across the United States (Agarwal, Udoji, & Trescot, 2017). Blood, buccal swabs, and saliva are used in the testing, making it fairly simple and minimally invasive to obtain samples that may help guide opioid selection, particularly in the outpatient setting. Although clinical and economic benefits of genetic testing have been demonstrated in the use of cardiovascular medications, the out-comes from use of this testing in pain management have not yet been established. In addition to economic costs, ethical concerns exist about inequalities in the health care system and the role that genetics may play in further exacerbating these inequalities (Agarwal et al., 2017).

Route Selection

Analgesics may be delivered by a variety of routes, making it possible for patients who are unable to take oral medications to receive pain-relieving medications in the inpatient, outpatient, and home settings. Awareness of the various routes and specific considerations associated with them is important in ensuring safe and effective medication administration. Alternative routes provide options for multimodal analgesic administration when a different route is beneficial or when obstacles prevent the use of the more commonly used routes. Table 9.4 provides a summary of routes for analgesic administration.

Oral Route

When possible, the oral route is the preferred delivery method because it is convenient, flexible, and noninvasive. The oral route provides a slower onset of action, delayed peak time, relatively stable blood levels, and longer duration than parenterally administered doses of the same medications (Herndon et al., 2016). Analgesia from oral medications is usually less than the same dose administered parenterally because oral medications require absorption from the gastrointestinal tract and first-pass metabolism through the liver.

Oral medications are available in a variety of preparations, including liquids (solutions, suspensions, emulsions, extracts), tablets, and capsules. In recent years, progress has been made in the development of abuse-deterrent oral opioid formulations that make it difficult to crush or otherwise alter the medication, thereby reducing the risks of inhalation, intentional injection, and overdose-related deaths. Some medications are available in short-acting or immediate-release formulations that are used to treat acute, intermittent, and breakthrough pain. Longer acting agents, controlled-release or sustained-release preparations, are available to treat pain that is almost constant and predictable.

The pharmacologic properties of individual agents vary, but in general the onset of action of oral medications is usually within 45 minutes, with peak activity in 1 to 2 hours and duration of about 4 hours. Longer acting, controlled-release and sustained-release formulations of some medications are available that, because of different pharmaceutical techniques, alter the release of the active medication molecules, thereby delaying their delivery and prolonging their duration of action. The peak effect of the controlled-release or sustained-release medications may not occur for 3 to 4 hours after administration, and the

Text continued on page 171

Table 9.4 | Summary of Medication Routes

Route	Advantages	Disadvantages/Limitations	Other Considerations
Oral (PO)	Convenient, flexible, noninvasive, more stable blood levels, longer duration of action than parenteral. Short-acting and longer acting formulations of medications may be available.	Onset and peak action are not as fast as IV, so may not be ideal for very severe acute pain. Requires first-pass hepatic metabolism. Oral route may not be available or tolerated by some. Variable bioavailability.	Preferred route when possible.
Transmucosal (intranasal, oral buccal, sublingual)	Provides rapid onset of action when parenteral options are not available. Does not require first-pass metabolism.	Reduced absorption if hydrophilic medication. Shorter duration of action than oral. Rapid onset of some transmucosal opioids may be associated with increased risks for adverse drug effects, including respiratory depression and increased risk for abuse and diversion.	Includes intranasal, oral buccal, and sublingual routes. Transmucosal fentaNYL products (TIRFs) require prescribers, pharmacies, and patients to be registered in REMS program.
Rectal	Rapidly absorbed because of rich blood supply. An option when oral and parenteral routes are unavailable. Simple, easy, can be used in home care, particularly with cognitively impaired.	Many factors may interfere with absorption; potential delayed or rapid absorption therefore risks for pain undertreatment and serious adverse outcomes. Patients and caregivers may find this route objectionable. Contraindicated in thrombocytopenia, neutropenia, immunosuppression, rectal lesions/fissures, GI bleeding, diarrhea, previous colorectal surgery.	Medications placed high up in the rectum undergo first-pass metabolism. Those placed in lower rectum avoid first pass. Codeine and traMADol require first pass for active form, so placement high up in rectum is needed. Limited number of commercially available products, but some PO formulations can be used, and compounding pharmacies may offer preparations.
Vaginal	Offers an option for medication administration when alternative routes are not possible. Has been used in palliative care.	Data limited to a few older case studies. No commercially available vaginal preparations. Vaginal pH may affect efficacy. Unpredictable bioavailability. Patients and caregivers may find this route objectionable.	
Intravenous (IV)	Fastest onset and peak action with IV route. Preferred for relief of severe acute pain, such as postoperative pain and for acute pain when PO route is unavailable. Bioavailability is 100%. Often administered as bolus doses, but opioids and some nonopioid analgesics can be administered as continuous infusions. IV opioids may be administered using PCA devices.	With opioid use, rapid onset and time to peak effect may increase risks for supratherapeutic levels resulting in minor adverse drug effects such as pruritus and nausea, as well as serious effects, including respiratory depression. Risks for respiratory depression may be higher with use of continuous IV opioid infusions, particularly when pain intensity is lower and when close monitoring is not provided. Requires IV access. IV administration guidelines related to dosing and administration techniques must be followed to reduce risks for local and systemic adverse effects.	Time to peak effect and duration are affected by lipophilicity of medication. Both opioids and nonopioid analgesics are available for IV administration. Requires close monitoring for effectiveness and adverse effects, especially with opioid administration in opioid-naïve patients.

Table 9.4 | Summary of Medication Routes—cont'd

Route	Advantages	Disadvantages/Limitations	Other Considerations
Subcutaneous	Parenteral route option when IV route is inaccessible or not feasible. Mostly used for subcutaneous opioid administration. Similar bioavailability to IV administration. Provides a parenteral route for opioid administration outside the acute care setting, especially for palliative care. Bolus doses and continuous infusions may be administered via this route.	Limited data available for use of subcutaneous route in nonopioid analgesics. Requires absorption from subcutaneous tissue to central circulation and therefore lower C_{max} and longer T_{max} than IV route. Absorption depends on drug solubility, injection site, blood pressure, circulation. Volume of injectate for bolus and infusion is limited. Infusion rates > 3 mL/h may lead to edema and poor absorption. Requires high-concentration solutions for continuous infusion.	Onset 10–15 minutes. Analgesia duration 3–4 hours. Absorption may be delayed with edema and poor circulation. Avoid with coagulation disorders and near sites of inflammation or infection. Various access sites, including abdomen, thighs, buttocks, and subclavicular area. Addition of hyaluronidase to continuous infusion may allow increase in infusion rate. Change subcutaneous continuous infusion access site weekly.
Intramuscular (IM)	Only advantage is that IM route provides parenteral access for NSAIDs when IV route is unavailable.	No advantage over IV or subcutaneous routes. Painful. Potential development of abscess, hematomas. Unreliable, unpredictable absorption increases risks for undertreatment of pain; also increases risks for adverse drug effects, including respiratory depression, if a delayed peak occurs when a subsequent dose also peaks. Delayed peak effect.	Avoid use of IM route.
Topical	Topical opioid and nonopioid analgesics and adjuvants may provide effective localized pain relief with lessened systemic absorption and associated adverse effects. Fewer drug-drug interactions. Simple application.	Systemic absorption is possible in some situations; may be variable and may be difficult to determine extent of absorption. Effective dose may be difficult to determine. No commercially available opioids. Limited research on the use, effectiveness, and risks of noncommercially available products and topical medication combinations. Local skin reactions are possible.	NSAIDs, capsaicin products, steroids, and local anesthetics are commercially available. Compounding pharmacies may provide topical products containing opioids, ketamine, cloNIDine, baclofen, tricyclic antidepressants, gabapentin.
Intraarticular and periarticular injections	Injection of local anesthetics and/or opioids into joint spaces provides localized analgesia and minimal systemic effects.	Variable response because of differences in surgical technique, extent of inflammation, use of tourniquets, and medication uptake. Potential for injection site bleeding and infection. Limited well-designed studies. Risks for opioid-related adverse drug effects and local anesthetic toxicity if significant systemic absorption. Variable dose requirements.	May be injected as a single shot or continuously infused. Simple, disposable infusion devices allow patients who have undergone surgery to continue therapy at home for a limited time and facilitate easy discontinuation and removal.

Continued

Table 9.4 | Summary of Medication Routes—cont'd

Route	Advantages	Disadvantages/Limitations	Other Considerations
Transdermal (TD)	Provides route for systemic absorption of lipophilic medications such as fentaNYL, buprenorphine, and cloNIDine when enteral and parenteral options are not available or preferred. Bypasses GI tract and first-pass metabolism. Fewer GI side effects. Noninvasive. Mostly constant rate of drug delivery. May be left in place for several days at a time, thereby improving adherence.	Hydrophilic products such as morphine are not readily absorbed through the usual TD route. Most products are not appropriate for intermittent and unstable pain because medication is delivered continuously at a constant rate. Most products take several hours for medication to reach a steady state, so not indicated for acute pain. Most products take several hours after removal for medication effect to resolve. Fever, heat exposure, and increased activity may accelerate medication delivery and increase risks for adverse effects, including respiratory depression. Local skin reactions are possible.	Initial bolus doses and subsequent breakthrough medication doses may be required to provide analgesia until TD product steady state is reached and for treatment of episodes of breakthrough pain. Advances in TD drug delivery systems are being developed to facilitate delivery of hydrophilic medications. Warn patients about the risks of increased medication absorption because of the application of external heating devices (heating pads, electric blankets, hot packs) over the TD product. Prolonged cold exposure and low blood flow states may reduce medication absorption and lead to inadequate analgesia. Rotate application sites.
Neuraxial and peripheral (perineural) nerve	Neuraxial often involves administration of medications into IT or epidural space, which reduces peripheral medication side effects and allows for use of smaller doses of medication. May be single shots, bolus doses, and/or continuous infusions. May use PCA with epidural catheters. Temporary percutaneous approaches for short-term IT therapy. Implanted internal pumps and tunneled catheters for long-term IT use. Local anesthetic may be administered into areas adjacent to peripheral nerves by single shots or continuous infusions to provide targeted analgesia. Peripheral (perineural) local anesthetics provide pain relief without opioid-related side effects.	Neuraxial: Uncommon but serious complications such as spinal infections and hematoma are possible. Neuraxial and peripheral local anesthetic use poses risk for accidental vascular uptake and local anesthetic toxicity. Neuraxial local anesthetic may cause degrees of sympathetic block, which may lead to hypotension and orthostatic changes. Peripheral or neuraxial local anesthetic may cause motor block, which increases risks for falls. Lack of pain with use of local anesthetics may delay recognition of serious complications such as compartment syndrome. Inflammation and infection at catheter insertion sites are possible. Permanent IT catheters may be associated with granuloma formation.	IT medications cover the spinal cord adjacent to infusion site, allowing lowest doses of medications. Morphine, ziconitide, and baclofen are approved for IT use. Other medications are used off-label. Epidural medications may include opioids, local anesthetics, cloNIDine, ketamine, baclofen. Epidural medications only partially diffuse to the spinal cord, so dosing is higher than with IT dosing. Morphine is hydrophilic so will remain in epidural space and provide spread in CNS. Morphine may spread rostrally in the cerebrospinal fluid up to brainstem and result in delayed respiratory depression and sedation. Lipophilic fentaNYL in epidural space is readily absorbed into vascular circulation and may produce more systemic side effects than morphine. Appropriate monitoring for side effects, including local anesthetic toxicity, hemodynamic changes, motor block, and opioid-related adverse effects is necessary.

C_{max}, Maximum concentration; *CNS*, central nervous system; *GI*, gastrointestinal; *IT*, intrathecal; *NSAIDs*, nonsteroidal antiinflammatory drugs; *PCA*, patient-controlled analgesia; *REMS*, Risk Evaluation and Mitigation Strategy; T_{max}, time to maximum concentration.
©Cooney, M., Quinlan-Colwell, A. May be duplicated for use in clinical practice.

duration of action may be 8, 12, or 24 hours, depending on the medication. Because of the delayed peak effect, controlled or sustained-release medications are not appropriate for the treatment of acute pain. These formulations also are not appropriate for use in patients who have intermittent pain, because the medication effect would then be present at times when not needed, thus increasing the risks for untoward effects. A benefit of these longer acting agents is that they are not associated with the frequent peaks and troughs in medication levels often seen with regular dosing of short-acting medications. A downside of longer acting analgesics is that, as with most medications, it takes five half-lives to clear the medication, so, if a patient is experiencing an untoward response from a longer acting medication, the medication may not clear for several days.

An important concept in medication selection is that medication is most effective and associated with fewer side effects when the onset, peak action, and duration of the medication closely resemble the onset, peak, and duration of the pain. For example, pain of a severe intensity that is constant and continuous, without marked increases or decreases, might be well addressed with a sustained-release oxycodone or morphine product (and other multimodal approaches) because the long-acting medication provides a longer steady analgesic level. Pain that is episodic, increases over a short time, peaks and remains moderate to severe, and then diminishes and resolves after several hours, but recurs several times in the day, may be best managed with a short-acting medication such as HYDROmorphone. HYDROmorphone (short acting) has an onset of 30 minutes, peaks in 30 to 90 minutes, and has a duration of 4 to 5 hours, which matches well with the pattern of the patient with episodic pain. If the duration of the medication exceeds the duration of pain, the patient is vulnerable to the development of excessive sedation and may develop respiratory depression. If the pain lasts longer than the medication, pain will not be controlled, requiring an increase in dose, decrease in interval between doses, or, for the opioid-tolerant patient, the addition of a long-acting agent, in addition to nonopioid medications and nonpharmacologic interventions to ensure optimal pain care.

It is important to educate patients and caregivers about the timing of medication administration, whether medications should be taken with or without food, drug-drug interactions, and the need to take medications only as directed. Patient and family education about the importance of never crushing, cutting, dissolving, or in any other way altering sustained-release and controlled-release medications is necessary to prevent changes in the physical properties of the medication. Alteration of these medications can result in the rapid release of larger amounts of medications than desired, placing the patient at risk for serious complications. Alcohol consumption is also generally contraindicated with opioids, but particularly when long-acting agents are used, because alcohol may degrade the extended-release mechanism and cause the release

of larger doses with the associated risks for overdose (Herndon et al., 2016). If a patient's condition changes so that the patient is no longer able to swallow a medication, it is important to determine a safe, alternative route to oral medication administration. Often, the short-acting agents may be crushed, but refer to the prescriber and the product information before altering the use of an oral medication.

Transmucosal Route

Sublingual, Buccal, and Intranasal

The transmucosal route commonly refers to sublingual, buccal, and intranasal medication administration techniques, although some sources include rectal and vaginal delivery among the transmucosal routes. More commonly used transmucosal analgesics are fentaNYL, fentaNYL-like products (SUFentanil) (Porela-Tiihonen, Kokki, & Kokki, 2017), and buprenorphine.

The efficacy of transmucosal medications is related to the time the medication is in contact with the mucosa and the lipid solubility of the product. The greater the lipid solubility, the better is the absorption of the transmucosal agents. This route is a good option for patients who require rapid relief of severe pain and do not have an intravenous route for analgesic administration. FentaNYL in oral transmucosal, buccal, sublingual, and intranasal spray formulations is approved for cancer breakthrough pain in opioid-tolerant patients because the products, further described in Chapter 11, are rapidly absorbed and do not require first-pass hepatic metabolism. Transmucosal fentaNYL products have an onset of action in minutes, with a duration of action of approximately 1 to 2 hours, making them good options for cancer breakthrough pain, which often has a similar temporal pattern. The onset of the nasal spray product is faster than that of the oral transmucosal product, and the nasal spray has shown higher patient satisfaction than the oral transmucosal products. These transmucosal immediate-release fentaNYL products (TIRFs) are carefully regulated by the U.S. Food and Drug Administration (FDA) because they are particularly dangerous if not prescribed and used appropriately and pose high risk for abuse and diversion. Prescribers of TIRFs must have completed a federally required Risk Evaluation and Mitigation Strategy (REMS) program. Prescribers, pharmacies, and patients in the outpatient setting who are involved with TIRFs must be registered through the REMS program.

Naloxone, an opioid antagonist, is available in intranasal formulations. Ketorolac, an NSAID, is available as a nasal spray and is indicated for short-term management (maximum 5 days) of moderate to severe pain (Herndon et al., 2016). Ketamine intranasal formulations, available through compounding pharmacies, are gaining popularity because of their relative safety, ease of use, and efficacy, particularly in emergency medicine settings (Shimonovich et al., 2016). Several of the triptans (serotonin 5-HT[1B/1D] receptor agonists), used in the treatment of migraine headaches, are available in intranasal formulations. As advanced medication delivery systems are developed, formulations of other nonopioid analgesics, including NSAIDS such as ketorolac and meloxicam, will become available as oral transmucosal agents (Pergolizzi, Taylor, & Raffa, 2015; Rajeswari, Gowda, Kumar, Thimmasetty, & Mehta, 2015).

Rectal Route

The rectal route, a form of transmucosal medication administration, is addressed separately because it has unique considerations. Like other transmucosal formulations, rectally administered medications are rapidly absorbed into systemic circulation. The rich blood supply in the rectum facilitates rapid absorption because medications simply diffuse across a lipid membrane. A disadvantage to this route is that a number of variables affect the degree of rectal absorption, including medication formulation, presence of stool in the rectum, duration and extent of medication retention, pH of the rectal contents, presence of local inflammation, site of placement of the medication in the rectum, and differences in venous drainage in the rectosigmoid region (Bauer & Chudnofsky, 2014).

An understanding of the venous drainage of the rectosigmoid region is important as the area of venous drainage impacts peak serum concentration of medications. Medications administered high up in the rectum are delivered to an area that is drained by the superior rectal vein and are delivered directly to the liver by the portal vein and will therefore undergo first-pass metabolism. The lower rectum is drained by the inferior and middle rectal veins, which eventually drain into the vena caval system, so medications placed in the lower rectum are delivered systemically and will avoid first-pass hepatic metabolism. It is therefore important to note that medications such as codeine and traMADol that require extensive first-pass metabolism are unlikely to provide analgesia if inserted into the lower rectum.

The rectal route for analgesic administration is appropriate when patients are unable to take oral or parenteral medications. Advantages of rectal medication administration are that it is simple, inexpensive, and does not require extensive training. The route is particularly useful for pediatric and cognitively impaired patients, and patients near the end of life, but many patients and their caregivers find this route objectionable and are reluctant to use it. Disadvantages for rectal administration include the unpredictable and variable absorption through this route that poses risks for delayed or inadequate pain relief. When the rectal route is used for opioid administration, there is the potential for serious adverse outcomes when absorption is rapid, as noted in case reports of opioid overdose associated with rectal opioid administration (Bauer & Chudnofsky, 2014). The rectal route is contraindicated for those who are immunosuppressed, thrombocytopenic, or neutropenic or who have rectal lesions, lower gastrointestinal bleeding, diarrhea, fissures, inflammation, or previous colorectal surgery (Green & Tay, 2016; Kestenbaum et al., 2014).

Analgesics available for rectal administration are commonly supplied as suppositories, although other formulations may be used, including pills, capsules, and liquids. Commercially available opioid suppositories in the United States include morphine and HYDROmorphone, and other opioid suppositories (oxyCODONE and oxy-MORphone) are available outside the United States. Compounding pharmacies may provide other dosage formulations and alternative opioids, such as methadone. Oral opioid tablets can be used for rectal administration. Dosing for rectal opioids is similar to oral dosing, but because of the potential variability in absorption, initial rectal doses are usually reduced. Dose adjustments are made based on assessment of the analgesic response and presence of side effects. The effectiveness and tolerability of modified-release opioid preparations have been demonstrated, and the steady state provided with rectal use of the modified-release oral form shows good absorption, slow release, equal or greater systemic absorption, lower peak concentration, and prolonged time to peak effect. Rectal administration of modified-release oral opioid formulations is often used in palliative care, particularly when patients have stable opioid requirements. A number of studies have demonstrated the effectiveness and safety of the rectally administered controlled-release morphine products (Kestenbaum et al., 2014). Like orally administered modified-release products, these medications should not be crushed or dissolved for rectal administration.

Nonopioid analgesics that may be administered through this route include acetaminophen, aspirin, and indomethacin. Another NSAID, diclofenac, is formulated for rectal administration but may not be commercially available in the United States. A case report describing the use of rectally administered pregabalin in a patient with neuropathic pain who was unable to take oral medications demonstrated adequate serum levels and reduction of neuropathic symptoms, without significant side effects, when doses were titrated up to 300 mg tid (Doddrell & Tripathi, 2015). Table 9.5 provides examples of medications that may be administered rectally.

Gastrointestinal Stomal Route

For patients with enteral stomas who are unable to use other routes for medication administration, the stomal route may provide an option for analgesic administration. Sigmoid (left-side) ostomies are more appropriate for medication administration than right-side because right-side ostomies are usually associated with a liquid form of effluent and high transit times which prevent adequate dissolution and absorption of medication. Left-side ostomies are usually drained by veins that enter portal circulation; thus dosing of medications is similar to oral dosing. This route is rarely used because of the increased availability of alternative methods of medication administration. Few studies have been published to describe the administration of medication through the enteral stomal route (Moore, 2015).

Table 9.5 | Examples of Medications Administered by the Rectal Route

Medication	Adult Dose/Frequency	Onset	Duration	Comments
Acetaminophen	325–650 mg q4–6h or 1000 mg q6h	<1h	4–6h	Maximum dose 4 g/day
Aspirin	300–600 mg q4-6h	<1h	4–6h	Maximum 4 g/day
Indomethacin	25–50 mg q8–12h	30 min	4-6h	Maximum 200 mg/day Only available in 50-mg suppositories; may need to be cut
Morphine	5–20 mg q4h	30 min	4–6h	Individualize dose; Absorption may vary greatly; close observation for respiratory depression
HYDROmorphone	3 mg q6–8h	30 min	6–8h	Individualize dose; Absorption may vary greatly; close observation for respiratory depression

Modified from Table 26.3 in Bauer, S. J., & Chudnofsky, C. R. (2014). Alternative methods of drug administration. In J. R. Roberts & J. R. Hedges (Eds.), *Roberts and Hedges' clinical procedures in emergency medicine E-book* (pp. 469–483.e2). Philadelphia: Saunders.

Vaginal Route

There is little published literature related to the use of the vaginal route for medication administration, although this route has been used for opioid administration, mostly in palliative care situations (Kestenbaum et al., 2014). There are no commercially available analgesics for vaginal administration, but the use of other medications approved for intravaginal use has shown that vaginal pH may affect the medication efficacy.

The only available literature that describes the use of the vaginal route for opioid administration consists of case reports. An early study showed that modified-release morphine (Oramorph SR) was safe and effective when administered every 12 hours by the vaginal route to patients with cancer pain (Grauer, Bass, & Wenzel, 1992). Patients in this study reported no consistent changes from the oral route in the frequency of adverse experiences, morphine requirements, or pain intensity ratings. In a case report, a patient achieved adequate analgesia using modified-release and short-acting morphine and morphine suppositories by the vaginal route as an alternative to intravenous patient-controlled analgesia (PCA) (Ostrop, Lamb, & Reid, 1998). Unpredictable bioavailability was reported as a concern.

A later study examined the use of vaginal fentaNYL in four patients with stable cancer pain (Fisher, Stiles, Heim, & Hagen, 2006). The researchers compounded 50 mcg of fentaNYL into a suppository with a water-soluble base and administered two suppositories 1.5 to 2 hours before the patients' regularly scheduled oral opioid. No plasma fentaNYL was detected, and patients reported no discernable pain relief with this dose, so the researchers increased the dose to 200 mcg in the fourth patient. This patient reported transient mild dizziness 1 hour after administration, and although her pain intensity did not change, she required less breakthrough analgesia on that day. The researchers concluded that although their study showed that fentaNYL is absorbed vaginally, a 200-mcg dose of fentaNYL vaginally was at the low end of what would be needed for analgesic activity.

In another 2006 study, 36 opioid-naïve patients with moderate to severe cancer pain were administered 10 mg controlled-release oxyCODONE tablets intravaginally every 12 hours (Zhang, Ruan, Liu, & Yu, 2009). Of the patients, 6 experienced complete pain relief, 20 had significant relief, 4 had moderate relief, and 2 had no relief. The average time for onset of analgesia was 49 minutes, and the average duration of effect was 13.8 hours. The main reported side effect was vaginal burning, but no patients discontinued use because of side effects.

Although there are many other well-studied routes of analgesic administration, in very limited circumstances, the vaginal route may provide an access for opioid administration when other options are unavailable. As with any route or drug that has not been fully researched, other routes known to be safe and effective are preferred and recommended.

Intravenous Route

Opioid and nonopioid analgesics may be administered through the intravenous route. It is highly beneficial to have the ability to provide MMA with the use of intravenous nonopioids such as NSAIDs and acetaminophen when patients are unable to take oral medications. The intravenous (IV) route provides the fastest route for the administration and effect of opioids, and is a preferred administration technique for patients with acute postoperative pain and those who have acute pain with decreased enteral absorption. The time to peak effect and duration of activity of intravenous medications depend on the lipophilicity of the medication and its ability to cross the blood-brain barrier. Intravenous medications are 100% bioavailable.

An intravenous bolus of an analgesic means that the medication is injected usually over 1 to 2 minutes through an intravenous access. This technique is often used for very severe pain that requires rapid relief. Ketorolac may be rapidly administered intravenously to provide analgesia. An intravenous bolus of fentaNYL can enter the central venous system (CNS) in 1 to 5 minutes, whereas it may take an intravenous bolus of morphine 15 to 30 minutes to gain similar access. Product inserts or other drug references provide information to guide the speed of intravenous bolus administration. A phenomenon sometimes described as "speed shock" may be possible if the rate of intravenous medication administration is faster than recommended. Speed shock is a systemic reaction that may occur when a foreign substance is rapidly introduced into the body, as in the case of an intravenous bolus of medication (Brooks, 2017). The duration of analgesia depends on the pharmacokinetics of the agent and, to some extent, the dose. For the treatment of severe acute pain, intravenous boluses of an opioid can be repeated once the opioid has reached the expected time for the peak effect, to allow upward titration of the medication until acceptable pain relief is achieved. The use of small doses of an intravenous opioid, administered more frequently than the usual every 4 hours, allows for more stable blood levels of the opioid and better titration to meet the analgesic requirements of individual patients (Burwaiss & Comerford, 2013; Herndon et al., 2016).

Some intravenous analgesics are administered over a longer period, often referred to as an intravenous piggy-back (IVPB) or intermittent infusion. Product inserts for intravenous preparations and other drug reference resources provide guidelines for recommended administration techniques. For example, a formulation of intravenous acetaminophen is recommended to be administered over 15 minutes to prevent vein irritation associated with rapid intravenous administration yet provide optimal analgesia by providing a sufficient concentration of medication to cross into the CNS (Mallinckrodt Pharmaceuticals, 2017). A formulation of intravenous ibuprofen requires dilution and administration over 5 to 10 minutes (Cumberland Pharmaceuticals, 2016).

In some instances, prescribers order opioids to be diluted and intermittently administered over a specified period. Although not always directed to do so, nurses sometimes choose to dilute opioids and administer them over an extended period. The Institute for Safe Medication Practices (ISMP) conducted a study of nurses' intravenous medication administration practices in 2014 and found that over 83% of nurses further dilute medications that are already prepared in a form that is ready for injection (Grissinger, 2017). Opioids are among the most common medications that are further diluted. Reasons cited by nurses for additional dilution are to optimize comfort, avoid vein irritation, and allow slower administration. Nurses reported that they dilute medications, including medications provided in a prefilled syringe, and some piggy back them to another infusion (although not prescribed), to allow a slower infusion and permit observation of the patient's response to the medication (Grissinger, 2017). Although nurses may use these practices

with the intent to improve patient safety, there is no evidence that safety is enhanced. The ISMP cites multiple safety concerns associated with these practices and issued guidelines for the safe administration of intravenous push medications for adults (ISMP, 2015). Key points in the guidelines include using readily available, standardized, facility-approved intravenous push medication resources and ensuring organizational policies to guide the administration of intravenous medications. Patient safety is optimized when patients are carefully assessed and monitored, particularly during the interval when medications reach peak effect.

In some situations, an intravenous analgesic, usually an opioid, may be administered as a continuous infusion over an extended period. Because medications typically require several half-lives (often five) to reach a steady state, to prevent inadequate pain control it is usually necessary to precede the continuous infusion with intravenous boluses of the opioid, which are carefully titrated until pain is relieved. The continuous infusion, sometimes referred to as a maintenance or basal infusion, is then used to maintain analgesic levels. When PCA devices are used, the opioid may be continuously infused through the device as a solo analgesic therapy or may be used along with patient-controlled boluses. The advantage of continuous infusions is that they provide consistent blood levels of the medication, avoiding the peaks and troughs seen with intravenous bolus doses. The major disadvantage is that they may significantly increase the risks of opioid-related advancing sedation and respiratory depression, particularly in opioid-naïve patients or in patients who have variable pain levels. Studies have shown that continuous infusions fail to improve analgesia in patients with acute postoperative pain yet increase the incidence and severity of serious opioid-related adverse events, including respiratory depression (Herndon et al., 2016). The dangers associated with continuous opioid infusions require that they be used only in carefully selected patients in settings where patients can be closely monitored for adverse effects or in situations in which continuous opioid infusions are needed for comfort at the end of life (Burwaiss & Comerford, 2013).

Although opioids are the most commonly used continuous analgesic infusions, some nonopioid medications also may be continuously infused. Ketamine (described in detail in Chapter 15) is an anesthetic agent that in low, or subanesthetic, doses may be administered by intravenous bolus and/or continuous infusion to provide analgesia. Continuous intravenous infusion of lidocaine is one of the multimodal recommendations for the intraoperative and perioperative management of patients undergoing open and laparoscopic abdominal surgeries because it has been shown to reduce the duration of ileus and improve analgesia (Chou et al., 2016). Another nonopioid, ketorolac, has been shown to improve analgesia, reduce opioid consumption, and reduce side effects when administered as a continuous infusion in an MMA plan for patients who have undergone surgery, including patients who have had total knee replacements (Schwinghammer et al., 2017).

Subcutaneous Route

When a parenteral route is needed for opioid administration and the intravenous route is unavailable or not feasible, the subcutaneous route is an acceptable alternative. Although in some parts of the world, NSAIDs are regularly administered via the subcutaneous route, this route for NSAID administration in the United States is mostly limited to off-label use and clinical trials. A review of off-label use of subcutaneous ketorolac provided data that included case studies and observational studies in which subcutaneous boluses and continuous infusions were used. Subcutaneous ketorolac was found to provide analgesic benefit in cancer-related and postoperative pain, with minimal side effects, but most data were related to the use of continuous subcutaneous infusions and few reports involved subcutaneous bolus injections (Vacha, Huang, & Mando-Vandrick, 2015). In a study that compared use of intramuscular (IM) injections of ketorolac 30 mg qid for 24 hours to the use of continuous subcutaneous infusions of ketorolac 120 mg over 24 hours, the area under the curve (AUC) and half-life ($T_{1/2}$) in both arms of the study had similar values, suggesting similar bioavailability (Burdick et al., 2017).

When the subcutaneous route is selected, it is usually employed for opioid administration. In the acute care setting, this route is considered as second line to intravenous opioid administration because the speed of effect is faster with intravenous administration (Mercadante, 2016). In comparing intravenous and subcutaneous opioid administration, both have been found to provide similar efficacy and have similar side effects (Herndon et al., 2016; Mecadante, 2016). Although a large retrospective chart review of patients who received opioids in the emergency department found that more nausea, vomiting, and hypotension were noted in patients who received intravenous opioids than subcutaneous or oral opioids (Daoust, Paquet, Lavigne, Piette, & Chauny, 2015), variables such as dose and administration technique (e.g., injection rate) were not addressed.

The pharmacokinetics of medications delivered via the subcutaneous route differ from the those with the intravenous route because subcutaneous medications must undergo absorption into the central circulatory system, a phase that is not necessary with intravenous medications. The absorption phase is responsible for the decreased maximum concentration (C_{max}) and prolonged time to maximum concentration (T_{max}) seen with the subcutaneous route compared to the intravenous route. However, subcutaneous and intravenous medications have similar bioavailability because the AUC and $T_{1/2}$ are slightly higher with subcutaneous compared to intravenous medications (Arthur, 2015). Thus dosing of subcutaneous and intravenous medications is similar, yet, as always, patients must be assessed and dose adjustments based on the patient's response to the medications.

The onset of the analgesic effect of subcutaneous opioid injection usually begins in 10 to 15 minutes, and the analgesia lasts for 3 to 4 hours. However, a number of variables can affect absorption and analgesic effect. Absorption of subcutaneous medications depends on drug solubility, injection site, blood pressure, vasoconstriction, and peripheral circulation (Ripamonti & Bosco, 2015). The presence of edema, particularly anasarca, and poor peripheral circulation will limit absorption. The subcutaneous route is avoided in patients with coagulation disorders, and injection is avoided near tissue where there is inflammation, abscess, or edema (Mercadante, 2016). The subcutaneous route permits a variety of access locations, including the abdomen, thighs, buttocks, and subclavicular areas. Sites that permit the greatest mobility and fewest limitations are preferred. Fig. 9.1 illustrates common sites for subcutaneous injection.

In palliative care situations, the subcutaneous route is particularly acceptable because it allows patients who require parenteral opioids to receive them outside the acute care setting. Subcutaneous opioids may be administered by intermittent injection, or for continuous pain, continuous infusions using gravity, syringe pumps, or other systems to regulate flow rates. Subcutaneous continuous infusions are preferred in some palliative situations, particularly home care, because the subcutaneous route is associated with less infection risk than the intravenous route, involves fewer changes in catheter placement sites as subcutaneous needles or catheters may be left in longer than intravenous needles or catheters, and may be more comfortable because of fewer needlesticks (Bartz et al., 2014). Box 9.1 provides guidelines for the administration of subcutaneous infusions. Cachexia does not contraindicate the use of the subcutaneous route (Herndon et al., 2016), but the site for needle placement requires careful selection and inspection, particularly when used for continuous infusion. The dose and infusion rates need adjustment based on assessment of the patient's pain relief and presence of any side effects.

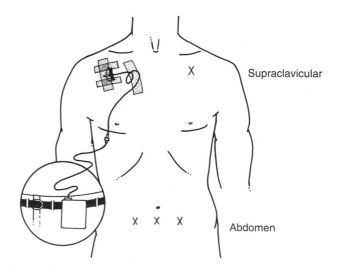

Fig. 9.1 | Subcutaneous infusion needle placement. (From Pasero, C., & McCaffery, M. *Pain assessment and pharmacologic management* [p. 401]. St. Louis, MO: Mosby.)

Box 9.1 | Guidelines for Subcutaneous Infusion

BEFORE INITIATING SUBCUTANEOUS THERAPY

- Convert current opioid dose to equianalgesic parenteral opioid dose (see Chapter 11)
- Calculate breakthrough dose (see Chapter 11)
- Breakthrough doses should be approximately 50% of hourly opioid requirement and offered as often as every 15 minutes.

SUPPLIES

- Nonsterile gloves (worn by person starting or discontinuing subcutaneous infusion)
- Commercially supplied subcutaneous needle or 27-gauge butterfly needle
- Analgesic infusion pump that can deliver in tenths of a milliliter (0.1 mL/h). Pumps used to deliver continuous infusions or PCA are usually acceptable. Ideally, the pump should be portable and lightweight. Portable disposable infusion devices also are used for subcutaneous infusion.
- Subcutaneous infusion solution (prepared by pharmacy)
- Infusion administration set
- Transparent adhesive dressing or transparent tape (nonallergic tape if patient is sensitive)
- Chlorhexidine 2% + isopropyl alcohol 70% applicator
- Four-way stopcock and additional administration set if two sites will be used

PLACING SUBCUTANEOUS NEEDLE AND INITIATING INFUSION

- A single subcutaneous infusion site can usually accept 2 to 3 mL/h.
- Highly concentrated solutions (e.g., HYDROmorphone 10 mg/mL or morphine 10 mg or more/mL are used for subcutaneous infusion.)
  1. Connect solution to administration set; follow directions for loading and programming analgesic infusion pump.
     - Verify solution concentration and analgesic infusion pump programming by independent double-check process before initiation of therapy to help ensure accuracy.
  2. Select site: Any area with a layer of subcutaneous fat is acceptable. Select the site that least interferes with mobility (ask patient about preferred sites and lying positions). Primary sites: Left or right subclavicular anterior chest wall; left, right, or center abdomen. Other sites: Upper arms, thighs, or buttocks. (Document why alternative sites are used.)

  3. Prepare skin: Clip excessive hair. Perform 30-second skin scrub with chlorhexidine applicator in circular motion from center outward. Do not wave, blow, or blow dry.
  4. Needle insertion: Use a 27-gauge butterfly needle placed at a 45- to 90-degree angle, or use a commercially supplied subcutaneous needle. (Be sure to remove introducer needle by grasping tip protruding from top of disk and pulling it straight out. The plastic catheter that surrounded the introducer needle is left in place.)
  5. Dressing: Keep site as visible as possible for assessment purposes; cover with a moisture-responsive transparent adhesive dressing. Tape may be used if patient prefers or is allergic to transparent dressing. Make a loose loop of infusion tubing and anchor with tape. Write date and time on a small piece of adhesive tape and place on edge of dressing.

DOCUMENTATION

Pain ratings; sedation levels; respiratory status; adverse effects; site; solution, including concentration and additives; biomedical number on pump if nondisposable pump is used (for risk management tracking purposes); infusion rate; PCA dose; delay; and pump history (therapy drug use). If PCA is not used, document short-acting opioid prescription for management of breakthrough pain.

MAINTAINING SUBCUTANEOUS INFUSION

- Site should be checked every 2 hours for first 8 hours, then at least twice daily (every 4 hours if the infusion rate is more than 1.7 mL/h). Home setting: Family can be instructed to check the site in the morning before the patient dresses and in the evening after undressing.
- Site inflammation, erythema, leakage, bruising, swelling, and burning indicate the need for a site change.
- Infusion site should be changed every 7 days or sooner if inflammation, leakage, or swelling occurs (rotate site in clockwise fashion, and use at least four distinct sites, if possible, to ensure healing).
- Change tubing and drug reservoirs according to institutional policy and procedure.

TROUBLESHOOTING

- Because the subcutaneous route has a slow onset, it is not acceptable for uncontrolled, severe escalating pain. The intravenous route must be used to control pain if necessary before subcutaneous infusion is initiated.

Box 9.1 | Guidelines for Subcutaneous Infusion—cont'd

Before discontinuing intravenous access, give an intravenous bolus dose equal to the hourly opioid dose the patient has been receiving to allow time for opioid absorption by the subcutaneous route and to prevent loss of pain control during the transition.

- If breakthrough pain occurs despite dose adjustments, poor absorption at the site may be the problem. Changing the infusion site may reestablish analgesia without increasing the dose.
- If possible, increase the concentration of the infusion solution when the required dose nears 2 mL/h.
- If the infusion is more than 2 mL/h, a four-way stopcock and two subcutaneous infusion sets can be used to branch the infusion from one infusion pump to two subcutaneous sites. The sites can be as close as 2 inches apart. In extreme cases (when switching to another route is not possible or death is imminent), this double-site method can be used to provide the mainstay opioid and a third site used for PCA bolus doses for management of breakthrough pain; however, the more sites used to deliver opioid, the fewer available sites for rotation. When multiple sites are used, more frequent assessment of sites is necessary (at least every 4 hours).

PREPARING FOR DISCHARGE FROM THE HOSPITAL

- As soon as possible before discharge, determine whether subcutaneous infusion will be continued at home.
- If so, determine family's willingness to maintain subcutaneous infusion in the home, because this is vital to successful therapy (see Patient Teaching).
- Make necessary referrals and contacts (e.g., home health, hospice, home infusion company, insurance company) to arrange for appropriate level of home care after discharge.
- Make arrangements with local pharmacy/infusion service for infusion pump and preparation of drug reservoirs so that the family can pick up drug reservoirs and other supplies weekly.

PATIENT TEACHING

- Provide demonstrations and verbal and written instructions on needle placement, site care, pain and adverse effect assessment, management of breakthrough pain, pump management, and documentation.
- Allow patient and family time to practice working with supplies and pump under the guidance of a clinician.
- Remind family to keep extra batteries for portable pump at home. Routine battery changes can be done once the typical battery life for the patient is determined (battery life depends on infusion rate and PCA demands).

- Provide instructions on how to obtain and store extra drug reservoirs.
- Provide family with name and number of 24-hour contact person.
- Reassure patient and family that another route can be substituted at any time if the subcutaneous route does not work.

DISCONTINUING SUBCUTANEOUS ADMINISTRATION

1. Determine need for alternative analgesia. If patient will receive short-acting oral opioids, give the first scheduled dose 1 hour before stopping the subcutaneous infusion. If the patient will receive a modified-release opioid, give the first scheduled dose 2 hours before stopping the subcutaneous infusion.
2. Turn off pump.
3. Loosen dressing and pull infusion set straight out with a swift motion. Apply pressure for 30 seconds. If the skin is intact, a dressing is not needed. If the site is excoriated, dress with triple antibiotic cream and gauze until healed.
4. Discard unused opioid solution according to institutional policy and procedure.

NOTE: The subcutaneous route of administration for the continuous infusion of opioids as opposed to intermittent injections is an alternative route for patients with persistent cancer pain who are unable to take oral medications and who do not have central venous access and for patients who experience dose-limiting adverse effects with oral opioids.
PCA, Patient-controlled analgesia.

From Pasero, C., & McCaffery, M. (2011). *Pain assessment and pharmacologic management* (pp. 402–403). St. Louis, MO: Mosby. Data from Anderson, S. L., & Shreve, S. T. (2004). Continuous subcutaneous infusion of opiates at end-of-life. *Annals of Pharmacotherapy, 38*(6), 1015–1023; Bruera, E., Brennels, C., Michaud, M., Chadwick, S., & MacDonald, R. N. (1987). Continuous SC infusion of narcotics using a portable disposable device in patients with advanced cancer. *Cancer Treatment Report, 71*(6), 635–637; Capes, D., Martin, K., & Underwood, R. (1997). Performance of a restrictive flow device and an electronic syringe driver for continuous subcutaneous infusion. *Journal of Pain Symptom Management, 14*(4), 210–217; Chaiyakunapruk, N., Veenstra, D. L., Lipsky, B. A., Saint, S. (2002). Chlorhexidine compared with povidone-iodine solution for vascular catheter-site care: A meta-analysis. *Annals of Internal Medicine, 136*(11), 792–801; Coyle, N. (1996). Cancer patients and subcutaneous infusions. *American Journal of Nursing, 96*(3), 61; Coyle, N., Mauskop, A., Maggard, J., & Foley, K. M. (1996). Continuous subcutaneous infusions of opiates in cancer patients with pain. *Oncology Nursing Forum, 13*(4), 53–57; University of Wisconsin Hospital & Clinics, Madison. (2009). Policy and procedure: Continuous subcutaneous opioid infusion. Madison, WI: University of Wisconsin Hospitals & Clinics. © 2011, Pasero, C., & McCaffery, M. May be duplicated for use in clinical practice.

High-concentration opioid formulations are used for subcutaneous continuous infusion because infusion volumes are limited in most situations. Concentrated morphine and HYDROmorphone are the more commonly used subcutaneous opioids, although fentaNYL, SUFentanil, alfentanil, and other opioids also have been used (Kestenbaum et al., 2014). HYDROmorphone may be preferable to morphine because its higher potency allows smaller volumes of fluid to be administered, an important consideration with subcutaneous infusions. If a patient's morphine requirements are high, the increased morphine concentration may be associated with problematic local histamine release (Herndon et al., 2016). Subcutaneous infusion of methadone is generally avoided because it causes skin irritation, and infusion rates beyond 2 to 3 mL/h are likely to cause local edema, infiltration, and poor absorption, which would lead to inadequate analgesia (Kestenbaum et al., 2014).

Infusion pumps with the capability of delivering in tenths of a milliliter are necessary to accommodate high-concentration/low-volume infusions. Most patients can absorb 3 mL/h, and some can absorb as much as 5 mL/h (Kestenbaum et al., 2014). The volume of infusion during subcutaneous continuous infusion can be greatly increased by the addition of hyaluronidase to the infusate. In an older study, it was found that hyaluronidase at a conventional dose of 150 units in 250 or 500 mL can permit infusion rates greater than 100 mL/h and has been shown to permit an infusion rate of 500 mL/h with subcutaneous medication boluses (Pirrello, Ting Chen, & Thomas, 2007). Breakthrough doses of subcutaneous analgesics may be provided as subcutaneous injections or PCA boluses administered by the clinician or patient (Leppert, Krajnik, & Wordliczek, 2013; McNicol, Ferguson, & Hudcova, 2015).

Successful subcutaneous administration in the home depends on the ability of the family and community health care system to manage this administration route in the home. Nursing oversight and patient/family education must be provided to ensure that sterile technique is used to establish injection sites, and all must become familiar and skilled in the use of needles, syringes, an infusion pump, and other equipment. The subcutaneous injection site must be changed at least weekly, and the potential for local tissue injury and infection at the infusion site must be monitored.

In considering subcutaneous medication delivery in the outpatient setting, in addition to availability of support services, the cost and insurance coverage must be considered. Because an infusion device and supplies are necessary, subcutaneous administration usually is more expensive than oral administration. Important points to address when establishing a plan for parenteral opioid analgesic infusion in the home include identifying the person who will assume primary responsibility for the technologic and security aspects of the infusion; educating the patient and family about pain, signs of adverse effects, and appropriate interventions; and ensuring a plan for support services and follow-up.

Intramuscular Route

The IM route is not an acceptable route for the administration of analgesics (Herndon et al., 2016; Jin et al., 2015; Kestenbaum et al., 2014). This route has numerous disadvantages and essentially no advantages. Disadvantages include painful administration, unreliable absorption with a 30- to 60-minute lag time to peak effect, and a rapid drop in action compared with oral administration (Herndon et al., 2016). Complications of repeated IM administration can result in sterile abscess and fibrosis of muscle and soft tissue (Herndon et al., 2016). Other recognized complications include nerve damage, hematoma, bleeding, cellulitis, tissue necrosis, and gangrene (Harada, Kashihara, Iwamuro, & Otsuka, 2017; Kasatkin, Urakov, Lukoyanov, 2016; Nakajima et al., 2017). The intramuscular route is a particularly poor choice for older adults and children who have decreased muscle mass.

The results of an extensive literature search by Jin et al. (2015) failed to demonstrate advantages of the intramuscular route over intravenous or subcutaneous analgesic administration. In studies comparing intravenous to intramuscular and subcutaneous to intramuscular morphine administration, the intravenous route provided faster, better, and more predictable analgesia than the intramuscular route. The subcutaneous route, although providing pain relief and side effects similar to those with the intramuscular route, was strongly preferred and more acceptable to patients. In a systematic review and meta-analysis of analgesics used in the management of renal colic, the intravenous route of administration was found to be more efficacious and less painful than the intramuscular route (Pathan, Mitra, & Cameron, 2018). The only benefit cited for intramuscular administration was that the intramuscular route for NSAID administration would allow quick and safe administration if the intravenous route was not available.

In addition to being ineffective, the intramuscular route of opioid administration is dangerous, especially for opioid-naïve patients. Unreliable absorption makes it difficult to predict peak times of the opioid administered. If doses are repeated at relatively short intervals, it is possible to exceed the effective dose, a situation that is made more likely to occur by the delay in peak effect after intramuscular injection. If injections are given in the setting of changing circulatory status (e.g., before or after a period of hypotension), intramuscular absorption may be altered, and necessitate adjustment of the dose, dosing interval, and level of monitoring to reduce risks for serious adverse events.

Topical

Topical analgesics are applied directly to the site where pain is located, and the medication is expected to have a local effect. Topical analgesics do not have a significant systemic effect because there is minimal systemic absorption. This route of analgesic administration is associated with fewer side effects and drug-drug interactions, and patients tolerate this route better than many oral medications (Peppin et al., 2015). Because of the reduced risk for systemic effects of topical analgesics, this route of administration is being viewed with great interest and receiving significant consideration.

In inflammation, studies have shown that the number of opioid receptors and opioid receptor fibers at the site of inflammation is increased, supporting the practice of topical (peripheral) application of opioids. Reduction in the number of immune cells near the inflamed site where topical morphine has been applied is thought to support the hypothesis that topical opioids are locally effective at sites of inflammation (Leppert et al., 2013). In an older systematic review, it was found that topical opioids applied to inflamed, clean wounds without excessive exudation or eschar provide pain relief generally within 1 hour and for a prolonged time, sometimes as long as 24 hours (Farley, 2011). In a more recent systematic review, topical opioids used to treat inflammatory acute postoperative pain were effective (Nielsen, Hennenberg, Schmiegelow, Friis, & Rømsing, 2015b). However, in the same review, it was reported that although statistically significant reductions in pain scores and increased time to the request for the first analgesic dose were noted with the topical opioids compared to placebo, in most studies involving acute postoperative pain, clinically significant reductions in pain were not noted.

Topical applications of opioids, including morphine, HYDROmorphone, methadone, and buprenorphine have been used over the years to treat pain associated with skin ulcerations, chemotherapy-associated mucositis, and lesions associated with calciphylaxis in patients on dialysis (Bastami, Frödin, Ahlner, & Uppugunduri, 2012; Peppin et al., 2015). In a review of opioids used to provide relief of burn pain, a limited number of studies were found that addressed the use of topical opioids, but the reviewers reported that the topical use of morphine offers a viable alternative for burn patients (Yang, Xu, & He, 2018). Although topical opioid application is simple, requires little equipment, and is thought to be associated with lower risks than systemic opioids, there are concerns about selection of the appropriate dose and drug absorption. Questions about absorption of topically applied opioids have been raised because, in some older studies of patients who received topical morphine gel, morphine metabolites were identified in the urine, leading to concerns that the topical application may actually be transdermal (Wilken, Ineck, & Rule, 2005), but these findings were not supported in other studies (Paice et al., 2008).

Many other analgesics are effectively used as topical agents. Topical agents, including local anesthetics, capsaicin, and NSAIDs, are readily available in a variety of strengths and formulations, including patches, creams, ointments, and gels. These agents can be used in an MMA plan and offer the benefit of side effect reduction because of the lack of significant systemic absorption. Compounding pharmacies can provide topical analgesics in a variety of vehicles, including sprays, ointments, and creams that consist of a single agent or combinations of several medications to provide effective MMA in a single product. For example, a compound may be formulated that contains a local anesthetic, an antiinflammatory agent, an opioid, and cloNIDine. Other agents such as tricyclic antidepressants, ketamine, gabapentin, and baclofen are also sometimes used in topical compounds. A more detailed review of topical analgesic agents is provided in Chapter 16.

Intraarticular and Periarticular Injections

Intraarticular and periarticular injections are routes of medication administration used in a multimodal plan to provide pain relief into or around joint spaces. These routes are similar to topical analgesics in that the drug effect is expected to be localized to the area of injection, with minimal systemic absorption. Opioids alone or in combination with other analgesics, usually local anesthetics, have been injected into these areas to improve postoperative pain and outcomes after joint procedures. This has become a fairly common practice and was supported by an earlier systematic review (Gupta, Bodin, Holmström, & Berggren, 2001) and continues to be supported in dose-finding studies (Gupta et al., 2015). Given the national initiatives on shortening lengths of stay associated with joint surgeries, intraarticular and periarticular injections offer effective multimodal approaches to pain control without the major systemic opioid-related risks that lead to prolonged hospital stays. These medications may be administered as a single injection or may be continuously infused through an easily removable catheter, over time, at a low rate. Special infusion devices are available that allow the patient to be discharged home with the continuation of the local anesthetic infusion. The rationale for the use of intraarticular and periarticular opioids is that intraarticular peripheral opioid receptors have been identified, and it is thought that the administration of opioids into the joint will alleviate pain without the potential for adverse effects associated with systemic administration (Green & Tay, 2016). The belief that intraarticular opioid receptors are present is supported by the observation that the injection of intraarticular naloxone reverses pain relief in patients who have received intraarticular morphine. Differences in analgesic response have been shown between individuals, and it is thought that differences in surgical technique, extent of inflammation, use of tourniquets, and medication uptake may lead to variations in response.

Transdermal

Transdermal (TD) drug delivery systems, unlike topical medications, are designed to allow the controlled absorption of medication through the skin for the purpose of systemic distribution. Medications that are more lipophilic are the most appropriate for the transdermal route because they will more readily be absorbed through the skin, which is composed of lipids and proteins. A lipid-rich intracellular pathway permits passive diffusion of highly lipophilic drugs through this and other layers. In addition to lipophilicity, other characteristics that enhance absorption include low molecular weight, solubility in water and oil, and a low melting point (Leppert et al., 2013). FentaNYL meets all of these requirements, and the transdermal fentaNYL absorption pathway and drug delivery system are illustrated in Figs. 9.2 and 9.3. In contrast, morphine is very hydrophilic and is not absorbed across intact skin.

The transdermal route offers several advantages. Transdermal medications bypass the gastrointestinal tract and first-pass hepatic metabolism. Transdermal delivery provides a noninvasive route for patients who are unable to take oral medications, is associated with fewer gastrointestinal side effects than oral medications because it bypasses the gastrointestinal tract, and pro-

vides a constant delivery of medication, thereby reducing frequent fluctuations in pain levels and the need for repeated dosing of short-acting medications.

Opioids, including fentaNYL and buprenorphine, are available in patch form for transdermal medication delivery. CloNIDine, an alpha-$_2$ agonist sometimes used as an adjunct in a multimodal plan, is also available as a transdermal patch. Transdermal patches are convenient and easy to apply and may be left in place for several days, thereby improving adherence to the analgesic treatment regimen.

The transdermal route is usually not employed for patients who have intermittent or unstable pain or patients who require rapid opioid titration because the transdermal route provides a continuous administration of medication at a constant rate. The primary disadvantages of transdermal delivery compared to other delivery methods are that the skin and other tissues act as both a barrier and a reservoir; it takes a number of hours for the medication to reach a steady state after the patch is placed (often around 12 hours), and the medication continues to enter systemic circulation for a variable period after the patch is removed. Short-acting medication often needs to be available to treat breakthrough pain that exceeds the level of analgesia provided by transdermal patches (Leppert et al., 2013). Thus transdermal fentaNYL patches are not indicated for opioid-naïve patients or for the treatment of acute postoperative pain.

Special care must be taken to assess patients for any conditions that may alter medication absorption from the patch. Fever, marked increases in physical activity, and heat exposure, as in the case of application of a heating pad or electric blanket, may accelerate medication absorption from the patch and therefore place the patient at risk for serious consequences (Green & Tay, 2016). Conditions that decrease peripheral perfusion, such as prolonged cold exposure or low blood flow states, may reduce absorption and reduce analgesia. Skin at the site

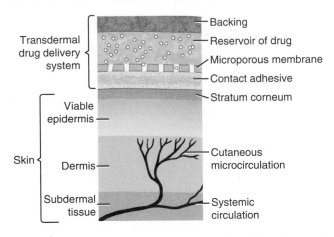

Fig. 9.2 | Transdermal fentaNYL absorption pathway.(From Pasero, C., & McCaffery, M. *Pain assessment and pharmacologic management* [p. 401]. St. Louis, MO: Mosby.)

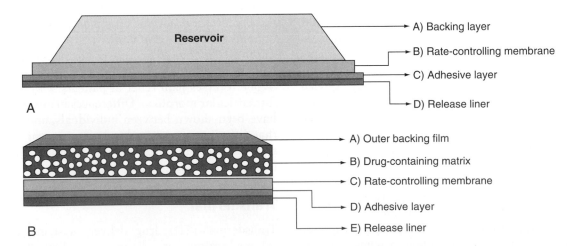

Fig. 9.3 | Transdermal fentaNYL drug delivery system. (From Pasero, C., & McCaffery, M. *Pain assessment and pharmacologic management* [p. 401]. St. Louis, MO: Mosby.)

of patch application may become irritated or inflamed, so site rotation is recommended; if the rash or skin response is severe, an alternative route may be needed.

Neuraxial and Peripheral Nerve Routes

Neuraxial and peripheral nerve approaches have increasingly been used as routes for analgesic delivery in the acute care setting. Intrathecal analgesic delivery is also available for cancer and noncancer chronic pain in outpatients with the use of implanted intrathecal pumps for chronic pain. These routes are presented in detail in Chapter 19.

Analgesic Dosing Considerations

When selecting appropriate doses of opioids and nonopioids to be used in a multimodal analgesic plan, many variables must be considered. Pain intensity and the effect of pain level on the patient's ability to participate in necessary activities are major factors in analgesic dose selection. Analgesic medication doses are intended to provide sufficient pain relief so pain does not interfere with function or quality of life, yet doses must be carefully selected to minimize risk for associated adverse drug events. Comorbidities such as pulmonary, cardiac, liver, and renal conditions necessitate adjustments in analgesic doses to reduce complications of medication administration. Analgesic dosing also requires consideration of patient age, body composition, drug-drug interactions, medication-specific variables, and other factors described in the opening paragraphs of this chapter. For opioids, consideration of prior opioid use, including determination of opioid tolerance, is important. The FDA defines an opioid tolerant patient as one who, for one week or longer, is receiving a minimum of 60 mg oral morphine/day, 25 mcg transdermal fentanyl/hour, 30 mg oral oxycodone/day, 8 mg oral hydromorphone/day, 25 mg oral oxymorphone/day, or the equianalgesic dose of another opioid. (FDA, 2015). Those who are not opioid tolerant (opioid naïve patients) are likely to require lower initial doses of medication to provide analgesia than opioid tolerant patients who are undergoing the same procedure. Opioid naïve patients may be at greater risk for opioid-related adverse effects than opioid tolerant patients (Joint Commission, 2012). For chronic opioid therapy in non cancer pain, professional and regulatory agency guidelines provide dosing recommendations, which often suggest limitations in duration of opioid therapy and the morphine equivalent daily dose.

Equianalgesic Dosing

At times, for patients who are receiving opioid therapy, it is necessary to change from one route of medication administration to another. The first-pass liver effect must be considered when changing between oral and parenteral routes to prevent underdosing or overdosing. For example, in the patient who is taking oral morphine for cancer pain, it may be necessary to transition to the intravenous route if the patient is unable to take oral medications because of severe nausea and vomiting. To prevent inadvertent undertreatment of pain or serious adverse events associated with overtreatment, it is recommended to consult equianalgesic dosing tables and monitor patients closely during the conversions. Equianalgesic dosing tables have been developed to provide dose a degree of guidance when switching between routes or medications. For example, in general, because of first-pass effect the equianalgesic ratio between oral and parenteral morphine is 3:1. Thus, if a patient required 30 mg of oral morphine for pain relief, an equianalgesic intravenous dose would be 10 mg.

Equianalgesic dosing charts are also available to guide dose selection when rotating between different types of opioids. There are several reasons why a patient may require rotation from one opioid to another. For example, if a patient who had adequate pain control on oxyCODONE is no longer able to take an oral medication, it may be necessary to rotate to a parenteral opioid or a transdermal medication. Some patients, despite dose adjustments, may develop unacceptable side effects with one opioid and require an alternative opioid. For example, with declining renal function, a patient may have significant side effects if morphine metabolites accumulate, and require rotation to an opioid such as oxyCODONE that lacks problematic metabolites. Other patients are rotated to a different opioid when they develop risks for drug-drug interactions or require increasing doses of the original opioid to experience adequate pain relief (tolerance), but the higher doses result in unacceptable side effects.

An important consideration when rotating from one opioid to another is the awareness of the concept of incomplete cross-tolerance. In other words, although a patient may have tolerance to the original opioid, it is unlikely that the patient will have the same degree of tolerance to the new opioid, therefore necessitating a reduction in the new opioid dose by at least 25% to 50% of the calculated equianalgesic dose to prevent serious adverse effects such as excessive sedation and respiratory depression (see Chapter 13). The more conservative new dose (50% of the calculated equianalgesic dose) is advised for those who require high doses of the discontinued opioid or are elderly, medically frail, or nonwhite (Smith & Peppin, 2014). Conversions involving methadone are even more complex, and guidance from one who is familiar with the unique properties of this medication is recommended.

Opioid rotation is challenging because it is important to ensure that the new opioid provides adequate pain relief but, most importantly, that serious opioid-related adverse effects are prevented. In 2009, an expert panel established a guideline for opioid rotation that involved a two-step approach for the calculation of the new opioid dose (Fine & Portenoy, 2009). It was hoped that the guideline would promote consistency and improve safety and efficacy in opioid rotation, yet concerns related to rotation practices continue. After the publication of the 2009 expert panel publication on opioid rotation, concerns and criticisms have been raised that rotation protocols and practices lack validation for efficacy and safety (Webster & Fine, 2012).

Equianalgesic tables are approximations, mostly derived from expert opinion and/or single-dose studies in patients with acute pain of noncancer origin. There is a lack of research to support a number of dose conversion ratios that are found in the tables. Although equianalgesic dosing tables are widely published and electronically available on many opioid dosing calculation applications (apps), there is significant inconsistency among tables. Different sources cite different guidelines and ratios for rotation. Thus it is not surprising that in studies comparing skill levels of practitioners when rotating a patient from one opioid to another, varying skill levels have been found (Webster & Fine, 2012). Many opioid calculators are available electronically, and can be accessed easily from a "smart" device. Caution is necessary as the electronic calculators, like the tables, lack consistency in equianalgesic dosing and do not consider individual patient characteristics, comorbidities, and drug-drug interactions.

These concerns highlight the importance of careful dose selection and monitoring during opioid rotation. It is important for prescribing clinicians to have an understanding of opioid pharmacology and a commitment to tailoring the choice of opioid and dose to the patient's individual characteristics and response. All clinicians have a role in assessment of effectiveness and identification of adverse effects during opioid rotation. Recognition of the benefits and limitations of opioid equianalgesic dosing tables along with appreciation of an individual's opioid tolerance and risks increases the likelihood that the transition from one opioid or route to another opioid or route will be accomplished without loss of pain relief or the development of opioid-related adverse effects. The use of multimodal pharmacotherapy and nonpharmacologic measures also support smooth transitions in opioid rotation. Further detail related to conversion from one opioid to another or from one route to another is provided in Chapter 11.

Around-the-Clock Dosing

Two basic goals of providing effective pain management are the prevention of pain, when possible, and the maintenance of pain at a level that allows the patient to accomplish functional or quality of life goals with relative ease. To achieve these goals, particularly for the patient who has significant pain most of the time, it may be necessary to administer an analgesic on a scheduled around-the-clock (ATC) basis, rather than as needed (*pro re nata* [prn]), to minimize the risk for gaps in analgesia. This practice is controversial and evidence of efficacy and safety is lacking. ATC dosing regimens are designed to control persistent pain, or pain that is present continuously throughout the day (Herndon et al., 2016). It has

been thought that the use of ATC analgesic administration may help minimize the undertreatment of pain in patients who are hesitant to request pain medication and eliminates delays patients encounter while waiting for caregivers to prepare and administer prn pain medication. It has been proposed that scheduled dosing, rather than prn administration, may reduce patient anxiety about medication administration delays and needing to watch the clock to ensure pain does not become unmanageable before a requested dose is delivered. However, evidence to support the use of this practice is sparse and conflicting, and while benefits may outweigh risks with ATC dosing of nonopioid analgesics, ATC dosing of opioids may increase patient risks for serious adverse effects. The use of ATC dosing requires careful consideration of the type of pain (acute, chronic, cancer, noncancer), intensity and temporal pattern of pain, comorbidities, setting, opioid tolerance, and other patient-specific factors.

In an early comprehensive review of scheduled dosing of opioids in postoperative patients, it was reported that there was inadequate evidence to support this practice (Riddell & Craig, 2003). In a 2017 systematic review of analgesic dosing in postoperative pediatric surgical (tonsillectomy) patients, researchers cited the paucity of evidence to support dosing practices and noted there was no significant difference in pain control or side effects between groups, although ATC dosing was associated with higher amounts of analgesics than prn dosing (Erskine, Wiffen, & Conlon, 2015). Recognizing the possible benefits to scheduled dosing of opioids, while concerned about potential risks, Paice, Noskin, Vanagunas, and Shott (2005) conducted a quality improvement study of scheduled versus prn opioid dosing. A parallel-design study of medical inpatients with pain from a variety of origins compared ATC scheduled opioid doses with prn opioid doses and found that those who received ATC doses experienced lower pain intensity ratings. A significantly greater percentage of the prescribed opioid was administered when it was given ATC (70.8%) compared with prn (38%). There were no differences in adverse effects between the two groups. The results of this project demonstrated that scheduled dosing was associated with decreased pain intensity, and there was no difference in adverse events between the two groups.

In 2011 Von Korff et al. (2011) published the results of a cross-sectional study of time-scheduled dosing compared to pain-contingent dosing of opioids in 2109 patients receiving chronic opioid therapy for noncancer pain in ambulatory care settings. Their initial hypothesis was that the group of patients who received time-scheduled doses would have fewer psychosocial problems associated with their opioid use and would be less concerned about their ability to control their opioid use than the pain-contingent group. The results of the study, which involved 25- to 30-minute telephone interviews and a review of pharmacy electronic drug databases of two health plans, failed to support the hypothesis. There was no significant difference in psychosocial problems between groups. Those in the time-scheduled group received substantially higher daily opioid doses than the pain-contingent group, although average pain intensity and depression levels were similar between groups. The time-scheduled group were more likely to report a background of alcohol or drug problems, were more preoccupied with opioid use, were less able to control their opioid use, had more concerns about opioid dependence, and had higher levels of opioid control concerns. The researchers concluded that more prospective and experimental research is needed to examine benefits and risks of time-scheduled and pain-contingent dosing practice. Although this is only one study with methodologic limitations, the findings that patients using pain-contingent dosing did not have poorer pain control than those on time-scheduled dosing are noteworthy, particularly because these patients did not demonstrate dose escalation and were mostly in control of their opioid use (Ballantyne, 2011).

Although ATC analgesic dosing regimens have been attributed to recommendations by the World Health Organization (WHO) in 1986 and 1997 in what has become known as the WHO Analgesic Ladder, it must be recognized that these recommendations were based on the need to address the international inadequacies in the management of cancer pain (Ballantyne, Kalso, & Stannard, 2016). The ladder was not intended to provide guidance for the management of all types of pain in all patient populations, and dosing "by-the-clock" was not recommended based on strong evidence. The use of ATC dosing of opioids for cancer pain in opioid-tolerant individuals has been recommended, based on titration of short-acting opioids to determine the optimal 24-hour dose (Herndon et al., 2016). This practice is supported in the National Comprehensive Cancer Network Adult Cancer Pain Guidelines (NCCN) (2017). NCCN advises that additional short-acting analgesic doses (breakthrough doses, supplemental doses, or rescue doses) may be needed to relieve pain that exceeds, or breaks through, the ongoing pain.

Opioid-naïve patients with acute pain are generally not appropriate candidates for the use of ATC opioid dosing. This strategy may place the patient at increased risk for opioid-related harm, including respiratory depression and death. Acute pain is often associated with variability in pain intensity levels. The use of fixed-dosing ATC opioid administration is risky, because doses might be scheduled when pain is lessened, leading to opioid levels that are unopposed by pain and the potential for opioid-related harm. If opioids are needed to treat acute pain in opioid-naïve patients, they should be provided on a prn basis using immediate-release opioid products (Herndon et al., 2016). However, regularly scheduled opioids may be beneficial for patients who are unable to provide a self-report of pain, if it is probable that pain is continuous and if patients are carefully assessed for medication effectiveness and side effects (Herndon et al., 2016).

In the acute care setting, the scheduling of ATC doses of short-acting opioids may actually result in inadequate pain treatment. Electronic medical records and computerized medication administration systems are in widespread use. A delay in ability to treat pain may occur if a patient is assessed to be too sedated to receive an opioid dose at a scheduled time or if the patient refuses the medication at that time, and the nurse appropriately withholds a dose. Later when the patient is fully awake, and reporting significant pain, the nurse may be unable to obtain the analgesic from the computerized system and it may take time to contact the prescriber to reorder medication. It is important to determine an alternative plan, specific to individual patients and health care settings, to ensure significant delays in analgesic delivery are avoided.

A major benefit of MMA plans is that it may be possible to provide ATC pain relief with reduced risks for opioid-related adverse drug events. The American Society of Anesthesiologists Task Force on Acute Pain Management, in their 2012 clinical practice guidelines for acute perioperative pain management, recommend the use of MMA, including the use of central regional analgesic, and, unless contraindicated, the use of an ATC regimen of NSAIDs, cyclooxygenase 2 (COX-2) inhibitors, or acetaminophen. Newer guidelines for the management of acute postoperative pain, developed by a multidisciplinary expert panel from several professional organizations, expand on these recommendations and call for the use of ATC nonopioid analgesics and nonpharmacologic therapies as components of MMA regimens (Chou et al., 2016). Although there is still a role for the use of opioids to address pain not controlled by ATC interventions, opioids would not be scheduled, thereby reducing related risk for adverse events and unnecessary opioid exposure.

The grave concerns about the rise in opioid use, misuse, and abuse; substance use disorders; and overdose-related deaths and the lack of evidence to support the use of chronic opioid administration for noncancer pain have led to a need to optimize non–opioid-based multimodal strategies to address acute and chronic pain. In 2016 the Centers for Disease Control and Prevention (CDC) published the "CDC Guideline for Prescribing Opioids for Chronic Pain" to guide primary care clinicians in the treatment of chronic noncancer pain. The CDC recommends the use of multimodal nonopioid and nonpharmacologic approaches to chronic pain management, and the guideline developers were unable to cite evidence to support the use of scheduled dosing of opioids for chronic noncancer pain management (Dowell, Haegerich, & Chou, 2016).

The current practices and available studies suggest the need for more research evaluating the best method for analgesic dose administration in a variety of populations and for a variety of types of pain. Until research proves otherwise, based on appropriate assessment, patient-specific nonopioid multimodal ATC pharmacologic approaches and nonpharmacologic measures are preferred for the prevention and recurrence of pain. The decision to add opioids (prn or ATC) is based on careful determination of risk versus benefit as a result of assessment of patient-specific pain, condition, and opioid-related risks.

Awakening Patients for Analgesic Administration

Nurses and other health providers sometimes wonder if patients in the hospital setting should be awakened and given pain medication and if patients in the home setting should be taught to wake themselves during their normal sleep time to take their pain medications to keep pain under control. There is very little evidence to guide the practice of awakening patients to administer analgesics, and none could be found related to this practice in opioid-naïve patients with acute pain.

The limited research available to address the question of whether patients should be awakened to receive pain medication was conducted a number of years ago and addressed the efficacy of providing a double dose of an opioid (twice the patient's usual opioid dose) versus the usual dose of an opioid at bedtime in patients with cancer pain. A double-blind, randomized, crossover study compared the two methods using morphine, and found average pain, strongest night pain, and sleep quality were slightly better in those who took a double dose compared with those who took a single dose, but the difference was not clinically significant (Dale et al., 2009). The researchers suggested that the slight difference may have been due to initial higher exposure to the M6G morphine metabolite. A previous prospective study of patients receiving palliative care found that all pain scores were worse in patients who took a double dose of opioid compared with those who took a single dose at bedtime followed by another dose 4 hours later (Todd, Rees, Gwilliam, & Davies, 2002). Further, those in the double-dose group required more breakthrough analgesia and experienced more adverse effects.

As addressed in the previous section, opioid-naïve patients are at particular risk for opioid-related adverse events, and doubling an opioid dose for no reason other than to facilitate sleep poses significant risks for respiratory depression. Such a practice contradicts current guidelines, which recommend that the lowest possible dose of an opioid that provides adequate pain relief should be used. The practice of double dosing lacks well-designed prospective studies, and it is possible that even in patients who are opioid tolerant, what is observed to be improved sleep may actually be excessive sedation as a result of the higher opioid dose. For the opioid-tolerant patient with persistent pain, a more acceptable approach to the challenge of uncontrolled nighttime pain is the use of a multimodal analgesia plan consisting of nonopioids and a long-acting, modified-release opioid, if an opioid is determined to be necessary.

More recently, studies have shown that disturbed sleep contributes to worsening of pain, and opioids interfere with normal sleep. Chapter 8 provides a more detailed review of the relationship between sleep and pain. Although inadequate pain control can negatively affect sleep, current evidence suggests it may not be appropriate to awaken a sleeping patient to administer an analgesic as the disturbance in sleep may have the unintended effect of worsening pain. In a review article that examined pain and sleep interactions, it was found that sleep disturbances are associated with pain-related discomfort and decreased pain thresholds and may contribute to hyperalgesia (Koffel et al., 2016). The authors of the review offer several different possible explanations for the reported impact of sleep disturbance on pain. Additionally, in this review the authors cite multiple studies that report the negative effects of opioids on sleep architecture. Opioids have been shown to interfere with slow wave sleep and rapid eye movement sleep.

The recent emphasis on hourly rounding on patients in the acute care setting provides the opportunity to identify, assess, and intervene for patients who may have inadequate pain relief or other concerns that are interfering with restorative sleep. The paucity of evidence to recommend awakening patients to administer pain medication, the potential for adverse effects from this practice, and the growing body of evidence that demonstrates the negative effects of sleep disturbance on pain, contribute to the following recommendations. Until research suggests otherwise, based on appropriate assessment, patient-specific nonopioid multimodal ATC pharmacologic approaches and nonpharmacologic measures are preferred to prevent episodes of awakening from sleep with severe pain. In certain situations, including at end of life, when opioids are necessary, controlled-release oral and transdermal opioid preparations for opioid-tolerant patients may alleviate pain over an extended period and permit sleep (Herndon et al., 2016). When opioids are used, an awareness of the need to assess for adverse effects and the possible impact of opioids on sleep is needed to determine whether adjustments are needed in the pain management plan.

Dosing to Pain Intensity Using Numbers or Word Descriptors

Dosing to numbers is the practice of prescribing a specific dose of a medication based only on the intensity of pain reported by the patient (Pasero, 2014; Pasero et al., 2011). Although this most frequently is associated with opioids, it is also done with nonopioid medications as well. An example of dosing to numbers using the 11-point numerical rating scale (NRS) (0–10) is: morphine 2 mg IV for pain intensity ratings 3 to 4; 4 mg for ratings 5 to 6; and 6 mg for ratings greater than 6 (von Baeyer & Pasero, 2017). Interestingly, this practice is sometimes confused with range orders (see later) because dosing to intensity involves prescribing a specific dose to be administered for more than one number on the NRS. However, the practice is very different because the specific dose is aligned with the two or more specific numbers representing pain intensity, with no consideration for any other aspects of pain or the condition of the patient. Range orders will be described and discussed in the following section.

Dosing to pain intensity using verbal descriptors is a process comparable to dosing to specific numerical descriptors. The difference is that when using verbal descriptors, words such as *mild, moderate,* or *severe* are used to determine a specific dose of medication. An example of using verbal descriptors is morphine 2 mg IV for mild pain; 4 mg IV for moderate pain; and 6 mg IV for severe pain (Pasero, Quinlan-Colwell, Rae, Broglio, & Drew, 2016). Again, there is no consideration for any aspects of the pain experience or patient condition other than pain intensity.

The practice of dosing to pain intensity, using either numbers or word descriptors, can present a threat to patient safety. It has been associated with and blamed for increases in adverse events related to opioid administration (von Baeyer & Pasero, 2017). Safe and effective pain management needs to be based on a comprehensive assessment of pain that is customized for each patient rather than only considering the single pain quality of intensity (see Chapters 5 through 8). Whenever possible this comprehensive assessment needs to include the self-report of pain intensity by the patient; however, it should not be limited to only that one parameter. When opioid orders require medication to be dosed solely according to pain intensity, nurses are led to administer opioid medications based on the single, completely subjective parameter of pain intensity reported by the patient, with no consideration of the many other factors that need to be considered when administering opioids (Table 9.6) (Pasero et al., 2016). Because experiencing pain is a multifaceted and dynamic process involving physical, cognitive, emotional factors, culture, and past experiences of pain (Ravn, Frederiksen, Skovsen, Christrup, & Werner, 2012), the practice obliterates many other considerations.

Pain intensity is only one component of this complex experience. Intensity most often is measured using either numbers or word descriptors. Using the NRS necessitates translating the complex multifaceted experience of pain into a single finite number (Castarlenas et al, 2016). That is challenging for patients to do, and it is affected by the ability of the person experiencing pain to conceptualize the intensity of the pain and then apply a subjective arbitrary number to that intensity. Since intensity is a subjective interpretation of only one aspect of the total subjective experience of pain, there is no clear commonality of a numeric intensity report among individuals.

On the surface, it may seem that using word descriptors is simpler, but it is perhaps even more confusing and even less reliable. One Danish study attempted to determine at what points *mild, moderate, and severe* correlate to numbers among people living with chronic pain. They found that even among people living with chronic pain there were no consistently accepted cut-off points

at which numbers attribute to the word descriptors. The authors of that study concluded use of these word descriptors in clinical settings is ambiguous and should be used cautiously (Boonstra, Preuper, Balk, & Stewart, 2014). Because patients who live with chronic pain can be considered experienced in assessing and rating their own pain, the findings of that study underscore the subjectivity of self-reporting pain intensity. In Germany, Gerbershagen, Rothaug, Kalkman, and Meissner (2011) compared four methods to identify a cut-off point between mild and moderate to severe pain and concluded the number 4 on the NRS is the average cut-off point between the intensities of mild and moderate to severe. The researchers of that study cautioned that their conclusion is only a guide and that "pain treatment should be tailored to individual needs" (p. 623). The investigators of another study conducted in the United States found there was significant variation in the relationship between *mild, moderate,* and *severe* and numbers corresponding to those words when patients describe pain intensity. In that study, patients who reported their pain intensity as *4* on the NRS were asked to describe that *4* with word descriptors. Some used *mild,* others used *moderate,* and still others used *severe* (Frey-Law, Lee, Wittry, & Melyon, 2014).

As pain and pain intensity are subjective, so opioid requirements and metabolism are also subjective and unique for each person. Opioid requirements are variable and not necessarily the same over time even as needed by the same person (McCaffery, Herr, & Pasero, 2011). To date there is no research that supports the idea that a specific dose of an opioid will control pain of a certain intensity for many, let alone all, patients (Table 9.7) (Pasero et al., 2016).

Dosing to pain intensity or a number representing the intensity also poses a threat to the ethical principles of beneficence *(doing good)* and nonmaleficence *(doing no harm)* (see Chapter 2). When medications are prescribed to be administered depending on a specific intensity described by either word descriptor or numerical report by the patient, the nurse may be faced with an ethical dilemma. This can occur when the nurse appropriately assesses the patient, then critically appraises that the patient is sedated and concludes it is not safe to administer the medication as prescribed based on the corresponding number or intensity the patient reported. In this situation, the nurse has three choices. The first choice is to administer the medication as prescribed based on the patient self-report of pain intensity despite knowing that it is not safe and could do serious harm. The second option, in an effort to prevent harm to the patient, is to *work around* the order. That could be done by documenting a lower pain intensity score than the patient reported and then giving either a lower dose of medication or no medication based on the fictitious lower pain intensity score, which is consistent with prescription for a lower dose of medication or no medication (Avian et al., 2016; von Baeyer & Pasero, 2017). Neither the first nor

Table 9.6 | Factors in Addition to Pain Intensity That Influence Opioid Dose Requirement

Factor	Considerations
Age	Opioids are metabolized in the liver and excreted by the kidneys either unchanged or as metabolites. Some degree of renal insufficiency occurs as a result of normal aging, making older adults susceptible to drug effects and metabolite accumulation. The need to reduce initial opioid doses and establish longer dosing intervals should be anticipated for both older adults and the very young, such as neonates and infants, who have incomplete organ development.
Quality of pain	The words patients use to describe their pain are helpful in determining the underlying pain mechanism and appropriate treatment. "Aching" or "throbbing" pain may indicate nociceptive pain, which is responsive to such analgesics as acetaminophen, nonsteroidal antiinflammatory drugs, local anesthetics, and opioids. "Burning" or "shooting" pain is associated with neuropathic pain, which is responsive to such analgesics as anticonvulsants, antidepressants, and local anesthetics.
Sedation level	Increased levels of sedation precede opioid-induced respiratory depression, making sedation assessment before and at peak effect time after opioid administration essential. Opioid dose should be reduced whenever increased sedation is detected, and monitoring of sedation level and respiratory status should be increased in frequency and intensity until sedation and respiratory status are normalized and stable.
Respiratory status	All patients are at risk for opioid-induced respiratory depression; however, patients with pulmonary compromise, such as chronic obstructive pulmonary disease or obstructive sleep apnea, are at elevated risk. Initial and ongoing assessment of patient risk for opioid-induced respiratory depression helps determine appropriate opioid dosing and level of monitoring.
Functional status	The goal of analgesic treatment is to improve the patient's ability to achieve functional goals, such as ambulation and participation in physical therapy. The patient's functional goals and activity schedule are important considerations in determining opioid dose selection and timing of administration. There may be a need for higher doses before painful activities than at bedtime. Include efficacy of opioid treatment toward goal achievement in handoff reports for continuity of care.
Tolerance	Opioid tolerance is the state of adaptation in which exposure to an opioid induces changes that result in diminution of one or more of the opioid's effects over time, making assessment of previous and current opioid use before opioid administration essential. Patients receiving long-term opioid therapy may experience decreased analgesia and side effects because of the presence of opioid tolerance.
Drug-drug interactions	When two drugs are given at the same time, one drug may alter the effect of the other drug either by changing its effectiveness or increasing its side effects. For example, concomitant administration of other sedating drugs during opioid therapy, especially benzodiazepines, increases the risk for respiratory depression.
Reaction/response to prior opioid treatment	Assessment before opioid treatment should include the patient's response to previous opioids, including analgesic efficacy and side effects. Many factors influence response to opioid analgesics. Changes in opioid or dose may be effective in patients who report a lack of efficacy or intolerable side effects with a previously prescribed opioid.
Physical and psychiatric comorbidities	Assessment before opioid administration should include the presence, severity, and treatment of comorbidities. Physical comorbidities can affect hepatic metabolism and renal excretion of opioids; psychiatric comorbidities can affect how pain is perceived and expressed; drugs used to treat comorbidities can act synergistically or in an additive manner to affect opioid analgesic efficacy and side effects.
Genitourinary status	Opioids can increase smooth muscle tone in the bladder, ureters, and sphincter, which can cause bladder spasms and urine retention. Urinary tract infections and stones can cause pain. Assessment of potential sources of pain and optimizing treatment with multimodal analgesia may help improve analgesia with the lowest effective opioid dose.
Cardiovascular status	Opioids can lower blood pressure by dilating peripheral arterioles and veins. Dehydration and hypotensive drugs can worsen postural hypotension. In addition to optimal hydration, multimodal analgesia strategies that allow the lowest effective opioid dose may be helpful in minimizing adverse cardiovascular effects.

From Pasero, C., Quinlan-Colwell, A., Rae, D., Broglio, K., & Drew, D. (2016). American Society for Pain Management Nursing Position Statement: prescribing and administering opioid doses based solely on pain intensity. *Pain Management Nursing, 17*(3), 170–180.

	Table 9.7	Strengths and Weaknesses of the Single-Item Measures of Pain Intensity

Scale	Strengths	Weaknesses
Visual analogue scale (VAS)	Easy to administer. Many ("infinite") response categories. Scores can be treated as ratio data. Good evidence for construct validity.	Some people, especially older people, have difficulty using VAS. Extra step in scoring the paper-and-pencil version can take more time and adds an additional source of error.
Numerical rating scale (NRS)	Easy to administer. Many responses categories if NRS-101 is chosen. Easy to score. Compliance with measurement task is high. Good evidence for construct validity.	Limited number of response categories if the NRS-11 is used. Scores cannot necessarily be treated as ratio data.
Verbal rating scale	Easy to administer. Easy to score. Good evidence for construct validity. Compliance with measurement task is high. May approximate ratio scaling if cross-modality matching methods (or scores developed from these methods) are used.	Can be difficult for persons with limited vocabulary. Relatively few response categories compared with the VAS or NRS-101. If scored using the ranking method, the scores do not necessarily have ratio qualities. People are forced to choose one word, even if no word on the scale adequately describes their pain intensity.

Modified from Jensen, M. P., & Karoly, P. (2011). Self-report scales and procedures for assessing pain in adults. In D. C. Turk & R. Melzack (Eds.), *Handbook of pain assessment* (3rd ed., p. 28). New York: Guilford Press; with permission.; Found in Castarlenas, E., de la Vega, R., Jensen, M. P., & Miró, J. (2016). Self-report measures of hand pain intensity current evidence & recommendations. *Hand Clinics, 32*(2016), 11–19.

second is ethically feasible, and the second option is illegal because it involves falsifying documentation in a medical record. The third option is to contact the prescribing clinician, explain the condition of the patient, and request to change the prescribed order to one that is safe for the patient. From moral, ethical, and legal perspectives, *only* the third option is acceptable.

The practice of dosing analgesia to numbers or pain intensity evolved as misconceptions and inaccurate information were shared among clinicians and administrators (Quinlan-Colwell, 2018). One of these misconceptions is that the state boards of nursing prohibit range orders because range orders require nurses to practice medicine without a license. To the contrary, no state board of nursing has endorsed the allegation that using range orders constitutes nurses practicing medicine without a license (Pasero et al., 2016). The ISMP, in 2015, qualified earlier statements they had issued, by writing that organizations should include objective criteria for dosing medications that need to be based on the symptoms of the individual and that the correct dose in a range order must be based on objective data (ISMP, 2015). Dosing to numbers is inconsistent with that requirement because the individual self-report of pain, based on pain being whatever the patient determines it to be, although critically important, is a purely subjective factor (McCaffery et al., 2011). Objective data include such patient characteristics as age, comorbidities, sedation level, respiratory status, and concurrent sedating medications (Pasero, 2014; Pasero et al., 2016). Additional objective data include patient allergies, prior history of pain, historical use of pain medications

before admission, and how the patient responded to previous doses of medication.

The practice of dosing analgesia to numbers or pain intensity is antithetical to the Institute of Medicine (IOM, now the National Institute of Medicine) advisement that quality patient care is patient centered and focused on the patient as a unique individual and includes meaningful communication with shared decisions about care (IOM, 2001). Not only is pain intensity just one component of the pain experience, prescribing a uniform dose of analgesia based on an arbitrary number or word descriptor is contrary to individualized patient-centered care. The position of The American Society for Pain Management Nursing (ASPMN) holds "that the practice of prescribing doses of opioid analgesics based solely on a patient's pain intensity should be prohibited because it disregards the relevance of other essential elements of assessment and may contribute to untoward patient outcomes" (Pasero et al., 2016, p. 170). The reader is referred to the *ASPMN Position Statement: Prescribing and Administering Opioid Doses Based Solely on Pain Intensity* for additional information and guidance on this topic.

Range Orders

A range order is a medication prescription "in which the selected dose varies over a prescribed range according to the patient's situation and status" (Pasero, 2014, p. 249). Examples of range orders are morphine 2 to 4 mg IV every 2 hours prn for pain or oxyCODONE 5 to 10 mg PO every 3 hours prn for pain (Drew et al., 2018). Range orders enable nurses to administer the most appropriate dose of medication to achieve the greatest satisfactory pain control possible while maintaining optimal patient safety (Yin, Tse, & Wong, 2015). Intrinsic in this process is assessment of the patient, clinical evaluation of patient-related information, monitoring the patient, and critical thinking by the clinician. As discussed in Chapters 1 through 4, pain is a multifaceted experience that is uniquely experienced by each patient. The response to pain medication varies in a wide range among people experiencing pain (Drew et al., 2018). Thus, the idea of one arbitrary dose of analgesia fitting all patient needs, conditions, and safety requirements is contrary to the concept that "pain is whatever the experiencing person says it is" (McCaffery, 1968).

Range orders are prescribed to provide for the particular medication dosage to be administered from within a given range of possible doses (i.e., morphine 2 to 4 mg IV), with the specific dose dependent upon assessment of pain and condition of the individual patient (Quinlan-Colwell, 2018). Prescribing analgesia by range orders is the most appropriate and safest alternative to the practice of dosing to numbers or intensity that is currently available. To date there is no data to support a particular dose of an analgesic medication safely and effectively relieving any specific pain level (Drew et al, 2018). Many medications, including analgesics, anxiolytics, antiemetics, and laxatives, are prescribed in a range manner. Throughout the world, prn analgesic medications, especially opioids, have long been prescribed in ranges with the intent to effectively manage both acute and chronic pain (Athlin, Juhlin, & Jangland, 2017; Drew et al., 2014; Pasero, 2014; Yin, Tse, & Wong, 2015). In fact, range orders are considered by many experts in pain management to be essential for the provision of individualized, safe, and effective pain management (Drew et al., 2014; Pasero et al., 2011). An important safety benefit is that range orders "enable necessary and safe adjustments to doses based on individual responses to treatment" (Drew et al 2018, p. 2018). The importance of clinicians using range orders in pain management can be appreciated from the importance placed in the Pain Management Nursing Scope and Standards competencies, in which it is advised that nurses need to assess patient responses and outcomes to medications and modify the analgesic plan of care accordingly (ASPMN, ANA, 2016). Range orders enable nurses to exemplify that competency.

When prescribed as a range order, prn analgesic medications need to be administered in doses based on thorough assessment of the patient regarding current report of pain, current level of sedation, history of pain, analgesic medications prescribed before admission if hospitalized, and response of the patient to the dose of medication previously administered. Safe administration of range orders also depends on the clinician's knowledge about the medication, including anticipated onset, peak effect, and duration of action. In addition to knowledge of the medication, various aspects of the individual patient need to be considered (Fig. 9.4). These individual characteristics include, but are not limited to, age, current health status, pain sensitivity, pain tolerance, previous experience with pain, previous opioid use, comorbidities, renal function, and hepatic function (Pasero, Quinlan-Colwell, Rae, Broglio, & Drew, 2016; Drew et al., 2018) (Box 9.2). Additional considerations include the pharmacokintetcs of the opioid and other medications being administered, particularly those with sedating effects (Drew et al., 2018). It is important for the clinician to appreciate the pharmacodynamics (the effect in the body) of all medications administered. Assessment and re-assessment of objective measures including respiratory status, sedation level, and functional status are imperative (Pasero, Quinlan-Colwell, Rae, Broglio, & Drew, 2016; Drew et al., 2018). The authors of the most recent ASPMN position paper addressing range orders advised "if partial doses are administered upon initiation of therapy wait until peak effect of the first dose has been reached before giving a subsequent dose (and) Avoid making a patient wait a full time interval after giving an additional partial dose within the allowed range" (Drew et al., 2018, p. 209). To help guide administration of range orders, Fig. 9.4 and Box 9.2 can be copied and used in the clinical setting for easy reference. A good rule of thumb when implementing range orders is to "start low and go slow," especially with children and older adults (Pasero, 2014).

Each organization needs to develop a policy to guide prescription and administration of range orders, provide guidelines for constructing range orders (i.e., a dose range and specified time interval), and provide education to clinicians. Education needs to include the following concepts (Drew et al., 2014; Drew et al, 2018; Quinlan-Colwell, 2018):

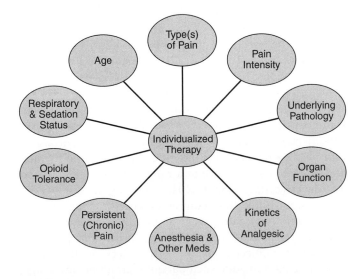

Fig. 9.4 | Individualized dose selection: "It Depends campaign." (Copyright 2013, Chris Pasero. Retrieved from https://marlin-prod. literatumonline.com/cms/attachment/2014528789/2035893778/ gr1_lrg.jpg. Accessed July 8, 2017.)

BOX 9.2 | Considerations for the Prescription and Implementation of Opioid Dose Range Orders

- Use multimodal analgesia to facilitate the administration of the lowest effective opioid dose; that is, ensure nonopioids, such as acetaminophen and nonsteroidal antiinflammatory drugs, if not contraindicated, are the foundation of the pain treatment plan for all patients with acute pain.
- Do not exceed the maximum daily dose of the nonopioids in the treatment plan.
- The maximum dose in the opioid dose range order should be at least two times but generally no more than four times the lowest dose in the range.
- An example of an acceptable opioid dose range for an adult is morphine 2 to 8 mg IV.
- Orders should specify a specific dosing interval and indication, for example, every 2 hours when necessary for pain.
- If the patient is opioid naïve, the first dose should be the lowest dose in the range order.
- Consider multiple factors, including the patient's pain intensity, age, sedation level, respiratory status, comorbidities and organ function, concurrent medications and anesthesia, presence of underlying chronic pain, whether the patient is opioid naïve or opioid tolerant, and the kinetics (i.e., onset, peak, and duration) of the opioid to be administered, when selecting a dose from a range order.
- For the very young and old, "start low and go slow."
- Anticipate a more pronounced opioid peak effect and longer duration of action in patients with hepatic or renal insufficiency.
- Recognize that comorbidities may affect the patient's response to an opioid dose, for example, patients who are debilitated or those with respiratory insufficiency are at higher risk for hypoxia.
- Recognize that concomitant administration of other sedating drugs, such as general anesthetics, sedating muscle relaxants, benzodiazepines, diphenhydrAMINE, and promethazine, have an additive effect and should be used with caution with opioid pain management therapies; systematic sedation assessment is essential, with the understanding that increased sedation precedes respiratory depression.
- Evaluate how well the patient tolerated a previous opioid dose; that is, how well did the prior dose relieve the pain, and were there any side effects?
- Contact the prescriber for alternative orders if the dose options within the prescribed range pose a threat to patient safety or are inadequate for the achievement of optimal pain control.

IV, Intravenous.

Institute for Safe Medication Practices (ISMP) Pain Scales Don't Weigh Every Risk ISMP MEDICATION SAFETY ALERT! Institute for Safe Medication Practices (2002); C. Pasero, T.E. Quinn, R.K. Portenoy, et al. Opioid analgesics C. Pasero, M. McCaffery (Eds.), Pain Assessment and Pharmacologic Management, Mosby/Elsevier, St. Louis, MO (2011), pp. 277–622; C. Pasero. Safe IV opioid titration for severe acute pain. J Perianesth Nurs, 25 (2010), pp. 314–318; C. Pasero, R.C. Manworren, M. McCaffery IV opioid range orders for acute pain management Am J Nurs, 107 (2007), pp. 52–59; D.B. Gordon, J. Dahl, P. Phillips, et al. The use of "as-needed" range orders for opioid analgesics in the management of acute pain: A consensus statement from the American Society for Pain Management Nursing and the American Pain Society Pain Manag Nurs, 5 (2004), pp. 53–58.

- A dose range of medication that should provide safe pain control and reasonable titration
- Need to avoid therapeutic duplication (see later) by qualifying when a route should be used (i.e., administer oral medications first; only administer intravenous opioids when oral medications are not effective)
- A finite range (i.e., 5 to 15 mg PO oxyCODONE every 3 hours prn)
- Consideration of the pharmacokinetics and pharmacodynamics of the medication
- Administration of medications via range orders based on a thorough assessment of the patient, including:
  - Analgesic medications used before hospitalization
  - Comorbidities that could affect absorption, metabolism, and excretion
  - Age and body habitus
  - Alertness and sedation level
  - Respiratory status
  - Report of pain including intensity
  - Response to previous doses of the medication
- Avoidance of administration of partial doses of medication at more frequent intervals
- Ensure shift to shift communication regarding dosing needs and patient responses to dosing

Clinicians are encouraged to use these educational concepts not only to guide administration but also to educate patients and their families regarding the importance of ensuring patient safety while working to successfully control pain. This also provides opportunity to educate patients and families about multimodal pain management and the importance of using a multimodal approach to safely and effectively manage pain (Quinlan-Colwell, 2018).

Several misconceptions persist about range orders. Perhaps the greatest misconception is that the Joint Commission (TJC) prohibits range orders. This is not true. TJC actually reviewed the ASPMN position statement on range orders (Drew et al., 2014). TJC standard calls for clarity and accuracy of medication orders while advocating for care that is appropriate for each patient (The Joint Commission, 2018). Another misconception is that the board of nursing prohibits range orders. In the United States, currently there are only a few states in which the board of nursing does not approve or allow for nurses to administer medications using range orders. Most boards of nursing do not prohibit range orders. Nurses are advised to always check with the individual board of nursing where they are currently practicing and verify the position of that state board. It is wise for each health care organization to have a policy stating the position of the individual organization regarding range orders and to provide education that guides the prescription, implementation, and administration of range orders. Both the policy and the related education are best when they are clear, consistent, and easy to understand.

A significant and ironic paradox exists regarding range orders. Although some organizations prohibit the use of medications to be prescribed as range orders and nurses to implementing such medication orders for hospitalized patients, the same organizations often require nurses to educate patients regarding how to take medications after discharge from the hospital. The irony is that many, if not most, analgesic medications prescribed at discharge for patients to self-administer at home are written as range orders. Actually, they are often written with two ranges (e.g., take 1 to 2 tablets every 4 to 6 hours). In these situations, nurses who are not allowed to administer medications prescribed in a range are expected to educate patients on how to self-administer medications written in that manner (Quinlan-Colwell, 2018).

The Joint Statement by the ASPMN and the APS noted that range orders enable clinicians to promote patient safety by enabling the safe and effective dosing of analgesics based on the individual needs and characteristics of each patient (Drew et al., 2014; Drew et al, 2018). The reader is referred to the 2018 position paper "'As-Needed' Range Orders for Opioid Analgesics in the Management of Pain: A Consensus Statement of the American Society for Pain Management Nursing and the American Pain Society" for additional information and guidance on this topic.

Therapeutic Duplication

In some instances the concept of therapeutic duplication has been confused with or blended with range orders (Quinlan-Colwell, 2018). Therapeutic duplication of medication prescription is totally different. It occurs when two or more medications of the same category, and/or with the same or similar indication or action, with equivalent generic components are prescribed on a prn basis (i.e., two nonsteroidal medications or two anticoagulant medications scheduled at the same time or time interval) (Andrus

& Stevenson, 2015; Clyne et al., 2015; Fusco, Paulus, Shubat, & Miah, 2015; Ross, 2017). This is generally considered to be polypharmacy, a concern for safety, and potentially inappropriate prescribing (Baysari, Westbrook, Egan, & Day, 2013; Clyne, et al., 2015). There is increased risk of intensification of side effects (Sakr, Hallit, Haddad, & Khabbaz, 2018). It can unintentionally occur when a new equivalent medication is prescribed without discontinuing the original or when more than one clinician is prescribing similar medications (Warholak, Rupp, Zale, Hines, & Park, 2015).

It is important to differentiate between therapeutic duplication and MMA. The Centers for Medicare and Medicaid Services (CMS) defined therapeutic duplication as "the use of more than one medicine from the same drug category or therapeutic class to treat the same condition" (CMS, 2017, p. 19). The distinction between therapeutic duplication and MMA prescribing is that with MMA, medications from different groups are prescribed intentionally and deliberately as part of a coordinated analgesic plan of care with directions for administration rather than prescribed in an unintentional, erroneous manner as occurs with polypharmacy.

It is also important to appreciate the difference between therapeutic duplication and range orders. Since there is a prescribing quality with therapeutic duplication that necessitates a decision to determine which medication should be administered, it is outside nursing scope of practice (Quinlan-Colwell, 2018). Choosing between two or more medications prescribed in a duplicative sense is totally different from using critical assessment to select a dose of a medication from a prescribed range depending upon and according to the situation and status of the patient.

Key Points

- Pain is a multifaceted experience that is subjective and unique for each person, and therefore effective and safe pain management requires consideration of individual patient needs and responses.
- Older adults, because of age-related changes in pharmacokinetics, comorbidities, and polypharmacy, are at increased risk for adverse drug events and require careful selection of analgesics and close monitoring for medication-related adverse effects.
- Many factors influence an individual's response to pain and analgesic interventions. Increasing awareness of the role of genetics on individual pain experiences and responses to analgesics contributes to the growth in personalized pain care.
- The oral route is the preferred route for analgesic administration, but when the oral route is not appropriate, alternative routes may be selected based on individual patient characteristics and circumstances.

- For some patients, especially older adults, an effective pain management approach may consist of nonopioid multimodal ATC medications and nonpharmacologic measures with consideration of benefits and risks to the individual patient.
- Opioids may be appropriate for use in certain patient-specific situations, after careful consideration of individual patient requirements, risks, and benefits.
- When opioids are necessary, it is preferred that they be used as prn medications on a foundation of scheduled nonopioid analgesics and nonpharmacologic interventions.
- Equianalgesic dosing charts provide estimates of the potency of one opioid compared to another or one route of an opioid compared to a different route of the same opioid.
- When rotating from one opioid to another, ensure appropriate patient monitoring to readily identify and intervene if there are signs of opioid-related adverse effects or undertreatment of pain.
- Prescribing analgesic doses based solely on intensity or a number is dangerous.
- Range orders are used internationally to provide safe and effective pain management.

Case Scenario

Sam is an 82-year-old man who lives with osteoarthritis and chronic low back pain. He has a history of coronary artery disease and had two stents placed in his heart last year. He treats his chronic pain with acetaminophen and exercise, including walking and bicycling with a recumbent bicycle. He also has a history of obstructive sleep apnea. Sam had exploratory abdominal surgery three days ago and reports "moderate" and "severe" pain in his abdomen. He is eating a regular diet and sleeps intermittently. Sometimes he is sleepy and lethargic when he asks for "pain medicine" "for moderate pain" or "for severe pain." He only has morphine prescribed as 2 mg IV for mild pain; 4 mg IV for moderate pain, and 6 mg IV for severe pain, and "HYDROmorphone 1 mg IV for moderate pain" and "2 mg IV for severe pain."

1. What patient-specific considerations need to be addressed in the management of Sam's pain?
2. What concerns do you have for his current situation and pain medication orders?
3. What medication options would be safer for Sam?
4. What obligations do the nurses have in caring for Sam?
5. What medications could be included in a multimodal analgesic plan of care for Sam?
6. What nonpharmacologic interventions could be included in a multimodal analgesic plan of care for Sam?

References

2019 American Geriatrics Society Beers Criteria® Update Expert Panel, Fick, D. M., Semla, T. P., Steinman, M., Beizer, J., Brandt, N., … Flanagan, N. (2019). American Geriatrics Society 2019 updated AGS Beers Criteria® for potentially inappropriate medication use in older adults. *Journal of the American Geriatrics Society, 67*(4), 674–694.

Abdulla, A., Adams, N., Bone, M., Elliott, A. M., Gaffin, J., Jones, D., … Schofield, P. (2013). Guidance on the management of pain in older people. *Age and Ageing, 42.* i1-57.

Agarwal, D., Udoji, M. A., & Trescot, A. (2017). Genetic Testing for Opioid Pain Management: A Primer. *Pain and Therapy, 6*(1), 93–105.

American Geriatrics Society 2015 Beers Criteria Update Expert Panel. (2015). American geriatrics society 2015 updated beers criteria for potentially inappropriate medication use in older adults. *Journal of the American Geriatrics Society, 63*(11), 2227–2246.

American Society for Pain Management Nursing, American Nurses Association (ASPPMN, ANA). (2016). *Pain Management Nursing: Scope and Standards of Practice.* Silver Spring, MD: American Nurses Association.

American Society of Anesthesiologists Task Force on Acute Pain Management. (2012). Practice guidelines for acute pain management in the perioperative setting: an updated report by the American Society of Anesthesiologists Task Force on Acute Pain Management. *Anesthesiology, 116,* 248–273.

Andrus, M. R., & Stevenson, T. L. (2015). Three-year review of pharmacy students' interventions and activities in an outpatient teaching family medicine center. *Currents in Pharmacy Teaching & Learning, 7*(2), 192–198. https://doi.org/10.1016/j.cptl.2014.11.016.

Arnstein, P., & Herr, K. A. (2017). Persistent pain management in older adults. *Journal of Gerontological Nursing, 43*(7), 20–31.

Arthur, A. O. (2015). Innovations in Subcutaneous Infusions. *Journal of Infusion Nursing, 38*(3), 179–187.

Athlin, A. M., Juhlin, C., & Jangland, E. (2017). Lack of existing guidelines for a large group of patients in Sweden: a national survey across the acute surgical care delivery chain. *Journal of Evaluation in Clinical Practice, 23,* 89–95.

Avian, A., Messerer, B., Wünsch, G., Weinberg, A., Kiesling, A. S., & Berghold, A. (2016). Postoperative paediatric pain prevalence: a retrospective analysis in a university teaching hospital. *International Journal of Nursing Studies, 62*(1), 36–43.

Baillie, S. P., Bateman, D. N., Coates, P. E., & Woodhouse, K. W. (1989). Age and the pharmacokinetics of morphine. *Age and Ageing, 18*(4), 258–262.

Ballantyne, J. C. (2011). Opioids around the clock? *Pain, 152*(6), 1221–1222.

Ballantyne, J. C., Kalso, E., & Stannard, C. (2016). WHO analgesic ladder: a good concept gone astray. *British Medical Journal, 352,* i20.

Bartoszczyk, D. A., & Herr, K. A. (2016). Managing pain in frail elders. *American NurseToday, 11*(4).

Bartz, L., Klein, C., Seifert, A., Herget, I., Ostgathe, C., & Stiel, S. (2014). Subcutaneous administration of drugs in palliative care: results of a systematic observational study. *Journal of Pain and Symptom Management, 48*(4), 540–547.

Bastami, S., Frödin, T., Ahlner, J., & Uppugunduri, S. (2012). Topical morphine gel in the treatment of painful leg ulcers, a double-blind, placebo-controlled clinical trial: a pilot study. *International Wound Journal, 9*(4), 419–427.

Bauer, S. J., & Chudnofsky, C. R. (2014). Alternative methods of drug administration. In J. R. Roberts, & J. R. Hedges (Eds.), *(2013). Roberts and Hedges' Clinical Procedures in Emergency Medicine E-Book. Chapter 26, 469-483.e2* (6th edition). Philadelphia: Saunders.

Baysari, M. T., Westbrook, J. I., Egan, B., & Day, R. O. (2013). Identification of strategies to reduce computerized alerts in an electronic prescribing system using a Delphi approach. *Studies in Health Technology and Informatics, 192,* 8–12. https://doi.org/10.3233/978-1-61499-289-9-8.

Boonstra, A. M., Preuper, H. R. S., Balk, G. A., & Stewart, R. E. (2014). Cut-off points for mild, moderate, and severe pain on the visual analogue scale for pain in patients with chronic musculoskeletal pain. *Pain, 155,* 2545–2550.

Brooks, N. (2017). *Intravenous Therapy Administration: a practical guide* (p. 70). Cumbria, United Kingdom: M&K Update Ltd.

Burdick, M., Mamelok, R., Hurliman, M., Dupuis, M., Xie, Y., Grenier, J., ... Noymer, P. (2017). Comparison of the Pharmacokinetics of Ketorolac Tromethamine After Continuous Subcutaneous Infusion and Repeat Intramuscular Bolus Injections in Healthy Adult Subjects. *Clinical Pharmacology in Drug Development, 6*(4), 343–349.

Burwaiss, M., & Comerford, D. (2013). Techniques of opioid administration. *Anaesthesia & Intensive Care Medicine, 14*(11), 491–495.

Castarlenas, E., de la Vega, R., Jensen, M. P., & Miró, J. (2016). Self-report measures of hand pain intensity current evidence & recommendations. *Hand Clinics, 32*(1), 11–19.

Centers for Disease Control and Prevention (CDC). (2016). CDC Guideline for Prescribing Opioids for Chronic Pain. Retrieved from https://www.cdc.gov/drugoverdose/prescribing/guideline.html.

Centers for Medicare and Medicaid Services (CMS). (2017) Home health quality reporting program (QRP) participant questions from in person training on November 16-17, 2016–Current as of February 2017. Retrieved March 28, 2017 from: https://www.cms.gov/Medicare/Quality-Initiatives-Patient-Assessment-Instruments/HomeHealthQualityInits/Downloads/November-2016_HH_QRP_Training_QAs.pdf.

Chou, R., Gordon, D. B., de Leon-Casasola, O. A., Rosenberg, J. M., Bickler, S., Brennan, T., ... Griffith, S. (2016). Management of Postoperative Pain: a clinical practice guideline from the American pain society, the American Society of Regional Anesthesia and Pain Medicine, and the American Society of Anesthesiologists' committee on regional anesthesia, executive committee, and administrative council. *The Journal of Pain, 17*(2), 131–157.

Clyne, B., Smith, S. M., Hughes, C. M., Boland, F., Bradley, M. C., & Fahey, T. (2015). Effectiveness of a multifaceted intervention for potentially inappropriate prescribing in older patients in primary care: a cluster-randomized controlled trial (OPIT-SCRIPT) Study. *Annals of Family Medicine, 13*(6), 545–553.

Cornelius, R., Herr, K. A., Gordon, D. B., & Kretzer, K. (2017). Acute Pain Management in Older Adults. *Journal of Gerontological Nursing, 43*(2), 18–27.

Crews, K. R., Gaedigk, A., Dunnenberger, H. M., Leeder, J. S., Klein, T. E., Caudle, K. E., ... Prows, C. A. (2014). Clinical Pharmacogenetics Implementation Consortium guidelines for cytochrome P450 2D6 genotype and codeine therapy: 2014 update. *Clinical Pharmacology & Therapeutics, 95*(4), 376–382.

Cumberland Pharmaceuticals. (2016). Caldolor product insert. Retrieved from http://www.caldolor.com/dosing-administration/.

Dale, O., Piribauer, M., Kaasa, S., Moksnes, K., Knobel, H., & Klepstad, P. (2009). A double-blind, randomized, crossover comparison between single-dose and double-dose immediate-release oral morphine at bedtime in cancer patients. *Journal of Pain and Symptom Management, 37*(1), 68–76.

Daoust, R., Paquet, J., Lavigne, G., Piette, É., & Chauny, J. M. (2015). Impact of age, sex and route of administration on adverse events after opioid treatment in the emergency department: a retrospective study. *Pain Research and Management, 20*(1), 23–28.

Dentino, A., Medina, R., & Steinberg, E. (2017). Pain in the Elderly: Identification, Evaluation, and Management of Older Adults with Pain Complaints and Pain-related Symptoms. *Primary Care, 44*(3), 519.

Doddrell, C., & Tripathi, S. S. (2015). Successful use of pregabalin by the rectal route to treat chronic neuropathic pain in a patient with complete intestinal failure. BMJ case reports, 2015, bcr2015211511.

Dowell, D., Haegerich, T. M., & Chou, R. (2016). CDC guideline for prescribing opioids for chronic pain—United States, 2016. *Journal of the American Medical Association, 315*(15), 1624–1645.

Drew, D. J., Gordon, D. B., Morgan, B., & Manworren, R. C. (2018). "As-Needed" Range Orders for Opioid Analgesics in the Management of Pain: A Consensus Statement of the American Society for Pain Management Nursing and the American Pain Society. *Pain Management Nursing, 19*(3), 207–210.

Drew, D., Gordon, D., Renner, L., Morgan, B., Swensen, H., & Manworren, R. (2014). The use of "as-needed" range orders for opioid analgesics in the management of pain: a consensus statement of the American Society of Pain Management Nurses and the American Pain Society. *Pain Management Nursing, 15*(2), 551–554.

Dworkin, R. H., McDermott, M. P., Farrar, J. T., O'Connor, A. B., & Senn, S. (2014). Interpreting patient treatment response in analgesic clinical trials: implications for genotyping, phenotyping, and personalized pain treatment. *Pain, 155*(3), 457–460.

Erskine, A., Wiffen, P. J., & Conlon, J. A. (2015). As required versus fixed schedule analgesic administration for postoperative pain in children. *Cochrane Database of Systematic Reviews, 2.*

Farley, P. (2011). Should topical opioid analgesics be regarded as effective and safe when applied to chronic cutaneous lesions? *Journal of Pharmacy and Pharmacology, 63*(6), 747–756.

FDA. (2015). Extended-release (ER) and long-acting (LA) opioid analgesics Risk Evaluation and Mitigation Strategy (REMS). Retrieved from www.fda.gov/downloads/drugs/drugsafety/postmarketdrugsafetyinformationforpatientsandproviders/ucm311290.pdf. (Accessed March 21, 2020).

Fine, P. G., & Portenoy, R. K. (2009). Establishing "best practices" for opioid rotation: conclusions of an expert panel. *Journal of Pain And Symptom Management*, 38(3), 418–425.

Fisher, K., Stiles, C., Heim, B., & Hagen, N. A. (2006). Can fentanyl be systemically absorbed when administered vaginally? A feasibility study. *Journal of Palliative Care*, 22(1), 54.

Frey-Law, L. A., Lee, J. E., Wittry, A. M., & Melyon, M. (2014). Pain rating schema: three distinct subgroups of individuals emerge when rating mild, moderate and severe pain. *Journal of Pain Research*, 7(1), 13–23.

Fusco, J. A., Paulus, E. J., Shubat, A. R., & Miah, S. (2015). Warfarin and rivaroxaban duplication: a case report and medication error analysis. *Drug Safety – Case Report*, 2(1), 5. https://doi.org/10.1007/s40800-015-0007-3.

Gerbershagen, H. J., Rothaug, J., Kalkman, C. J., & Meissner, W. (2011). Determination of moderate-to-severe postoperative pain of the numeric rating scale: a cut-off point analysis applying four different methods. *British Journal of Anaesthesiology*, 107(4), 619–626.

Grauer, P. A., Bass, J., & Wenzel, E. (1992). A feasibility study of the rectal and vaginal administration of sustained-release morphine sulfate tablets (Oramorph™) for the treatment of cancer-related pain. In Abstracts, 49th American Society of Hospital Pharmacists (ASHP) Annual Meeting (Vol. 68).

Green, C. J., & Tay, Y. C. (2016). Techniques of opioid administration. *Anaesthesia & Intensive Care Medicine*, 17(9), 454–459.

Grissinger, M. (2017). Some IV Medications Are Diluted Unnecessarily in Patient-Care Areas, Creating Undue Risk. *Pharmacy and Therapeutics*, 42(8), 490.

Gupta, A., Bodin, L., Holmström, B., & Berggren, L. (2001). A systematic review of the peripheral analgesic effects of intraarticular morphine. *Anesthesia & Analgesia*, 93(3), 761–770.

Gupta, B., Banerjee, S., Prasad, A., Farooque, K., Sharma, V., & Trikha, V. (2015). Analgesic efficacy of three different dosages of intra-articular morphine in arthroscopic knee surgeries: Randomised double-blind trial. *Indian Journal of Anaesthesia*, 59(10), 642.

Harada, K., Kashihara, N., Iwamuro, M., & Otsuka, F. (2017). Multiple abscesses caused by repetitive intramuscular injections. *Journal of General and Family Medicine.*, 18(5), 301–302.

Herndon, C. M., Arnstein, P., Darnall, B., Hartrick, C., Lyons, M., & Sehgal, N. (2016). *Principles of analgesic use*. Chicago, Ill: American Pain Society.

Institute for Safe Medication Practices. (2015). ISMP safe practice guidelines for adult IV push medications. Retrieved from http://www.ismp.org/Tools/guidelines/IVSummitPush/IVPushMedGuidelines.pdf.

Institute of Medicine (IOM). (2001). *Crossing the quality chasm: a new health system for the 21st century*. Washington, DC: The National Academies Press.

Joint Commission. (2012). Sentinel event alert issue 49: safe use of opioids in hospitals (August 8, 2012). Retrieved from https://www.jointcommission.org/-/media/deprecated-unorganized/imported-assets/tjc/system-folders/topics-library/sea_49_opioids_8_2_12_finalpdf.pdf?db=web&hash=0135F306FCB10D-919CF7572ECCC65C84. Accessed March 21, 2020.

Jin, J. F., Zhu, L. L., Chen, M., Xu, H. M., Wang, H. F., Feng, X. Q., ... Zhou, Q. (2015). The optimal choice of medication administration route regarding intravenous, intramuscular, and subcutaneous injection. *Patient Preference and Adherence*, 9, 923.

Kasatkin, A. A., Urakov, A. A., & Lukoyanov, I. A. (2016). Nonsteroidal anti-inflammatory drugs causing local inflammation of tissue at the site of injection. *Journal of Pharmacology & Pharmacotherapeutics*, 7(1), 26.

Kestenbaum, M. G., Vilches, A. O., Messersmith, S., Connor, S. R., Fine, P. G., Murphy, B., ... Muir, J. C. (2014). Alternative routes to oral opioid administration in palliative care: a review and clinical summary. *Pain Medicine*, 15(7), 1129–1153.

Koffel, E., Kroenke, K., Bair, M. J., Leverty, D., Polusny, M. A., & Krebs, E. E. (2016). The bidirectional relationship between sleep complaints and pain: Analysis of data from a randomized trial. *Health Psychology*, 35(1), 41.

Leppert, W., Krajnik, M., & Wordliczek, J. (2013). Delivery systems of opioid analgesics for pain relief: a review. *Current pharmaceutical design*, 19(41), 7271–7293.

Mallinckrodt Pharmaceuticals. (2017). Ofirmev product insert. Available at http://www.ofirmev.com/.

Manworren, R. C. (2015). Multimodal pain management and the future of a personalized medicine approach to pain. *AORN Journal*, 101(3), 307–318.

Marcum, Z. A., Duncan, N. A., & Makris, U. E. (2016). Pharmacotherapies in geriatric chronic pain management. *Clinics in Geriatric Medicine*, 32(4), 705–724.

McCaffery, M. (1968). *Nursing practice theories related to cognition, bodily pain, and man-environment interactions*. Los Angeles, CA: University of California.

McCaffery, M., Herr, K., & Pasero, C. (2011). Assessment. In C. Pasero, & M. McCaffery (Eds.), *Pain Assessment and Pharmacologic Management* (pp. 13–176). St. Louis, MO: Mosby.

McNicol, E. D., Ferguson, M. C., & Hudcova, J. (2015). Patient controlled opioid analgesia versus non-patient controlled opioid analgesia for postoperative pain. *The Cochrane Library 2014*, 2(6), CD003348.

Mercadante, S. (2016). Parenteral routes for opioid administration in cancer pain management. *European Journal of Internal Medicine*, 34, e39–e40.

Moore, S. (2015). Medication absorption for patients with an ileostomy. *British Journal of Nursing*, 24.

Nakajima, Y., Mukai, K., Takaoka, K., Hirose, T., Morishita, K., Yamamoto, T., ... Nakatani, T. (2017). Establishing a new appropriate intramuscular injection site in the deltoid muscle. *Human Vaccines & Immunotherapeutics*, 13(9), 2123–2129.

National Comprehensive Cancer Network. (2017). NCCN Clinical Practice Guidelines in Oncology: Adult Cancer Pain. Version 2.2017. Published May 10, 2017.

Nielsen, B. N., Henneberg, S. W., Schmiegelow, K., Friis, S. M., & Rømsing, J. (2015b). Peripherally applied opioids for postoperative pain: evidence of an analgesic effect? A systematic review and meta-analysis. *Acta Anaesthesiologica Scandinavica*, 59(7), 830–845.

Nielsen, L. M., Olesen, A. E., Branford, R., Christrup, L. L., Sato, H., & Drewes, A. M. (2015a). Association Between Human Pain-Related Genotypes and Variability in Opioid Analgesia: An Updated Review. *Pain Practice*, 15(6), 580–594.

Ostrop, N. J., Lamb, J., & Reid, G. (1998). Intravaginal morphine: An alternative route of administration. *Pharmacotherapy: The Journal of Human Pharmacology and Drug Therapy*, 18(4), 863–865.

Paice, J. A., Noskin, G. A., Vanagunas, A., & Shott, S. (2005). Efficacy and safety of scheduled dosing of opioid analgesics: a quality improvement study. *The Journal of Pain*, 6(10), 639–643.

Paice, J. A., Von Roenn, J. H., Hudgins, J. C., Luong, L., Krejcie, T. C., & Avram, M. J. (2008). Morphine bioavailability from a topical gel formulation in volunteers. *Journal of Pain and Symptom Management*, 35(3), 314–320.

Pasero, C. (2014). One size does not fit all: opioid dose range orders. *Journal of PeriAnesthesia Nursing*, 29(3), 246–252.

Pasero, C., Quinn, T. E., Portenoy, R., & McCaffery, M. (2011). Opioid analgesics. In C. Pasero, & M. Mc Caffery (Eds.), *Pain Assessment and Pharmacologic Management* (pp. 277–622). St. Louis, MO: Mosby.

Pasero, C., Quinlan-Colwell, A., Rae, D., Broglio, K., & Drew, D. (2016). American Society for Pain Management Nursing Position Statement: prescribing and administering opioid doses based solely on pain intensity. *Pain Management Nursing*, 17(3), 170–180.

Pathan, S. A., Mitra, B., & Cameron, P. A. (2018). A Systematic Review and Meta-analysis Comparing the Efficacy of Nonsteroidal Anti-inflammatory Drugs, Opioids, and Paracetamol in the Treatment of Acute Renal Colic. *European Urology*, 73(4), 583–595.

Peppin, J. F., Albrecht, P. J., Argoff, C., Gustorff, B., Pappagallo, M., Rice, F. L., & Wallace, M. S. (2015). Skin matters: a review of topical treatments for chronic pain. Part two: treatments and applications. *Pain and Therapy*, 4(1), 33–50.

Pergolizzi, J. V., Taylor, R., & Raffa, R. B. (2015). Intranasal ketorolac as part of a multimodal approach to postoperative pain. *Pain Practice*, 15(4), 378–388.

Pirrello, R. D., Ting Chen, C., & Thomas, S. H. (2007). Initial experiences with subcutaneous recombinant human hyaluronidase. *Journal of Palliative Medicine*, 10(4), 861–864.

Porela-Tiihonen, S., Kokki, M., & Kokki, H. (2017). Sufentanil sublingual formulation for the treatment of acute, moderate to severe postoperative pain in adult patients. *Expert Review of Neurotherapeutics*, 17(2), 101–111.

Quinlan-Colwell, A. (2018). Promoting evidenced-based practice and dispelling urban legends to achieve safer pain management. *Journal of PeriAnesthesia Nursing*, 33(1), 96–100.

Rajeswari, S. R., Gowda, T. M., Kumar, T. A., Thimmasetty, J., & Mehta, D. S. (2015). An appraisal of innovative meloxicam mucoadhesive films for periodontal postsurgical pain control: A double-blinded, randomized clinical trial of effectiveness. *Contemporary Clinical Dentistry*, 6(3), 299.

Ravn, P., Frederiksen, R., Skovsen, A. P., Christrup, L. L., & Werner, M. U. (2012). Prediction of pain sensitivity in healthy volunteers. *Journal of Pain Research*, 5, 313–326.

Riddell, R. R. P., & Craig, K. D. (2003). Time-contingent schedules for postoperative analgesia: a review of the literature. *The Journal of Pain*, 4(4), 169–175.

Ripamonti, C. I., & Bosco, M. (2015). Alternative routes for systemic opioid delivery. In E. Bruera, I. Higginson, C. F. von Gunten, & T. Morita (Eds.), *Textbook of Palliative Medicine and Supportive Care* (p. 431). Boca Raton, FL: CRC Press.

Ross, J. (2017). New Evidence on Drug Interactions: Improving Patient Safety. *Journal of PeriAnesthesia Nursing*, 32(2), 148–150.

Sakr, S., Hallit, S., Haddad, M., & Khabbaz, L. R. (2018). Assessment of potentially inappropriate medications in elderly according to Beers 2015 and STOPP criteria and their association with treatment satisfaction. *Archives of Gerontology and Geriatrics*, 78, 132–138.

Schwinghammer, A. J., Isaacs, A. N., Benner, R. W., Freeman, H., O'Sullivan, J. A., & Nisly, S. A. (2017). Continuous Infusion Ketorolac for Postoperative Analgesia Following Unilateral Total Knee Arthroplasty. *Annals of Pharmacotherapy*, 51(6), 451–456.

Sekhri, N. K., & Cooney, M. F. (2017). Opioid Metabolism and Pharmacogenetics: Clinical Implications. *Journal of PeriAnesthesia Nursing*, 32(5), 497–505.

Shimonovich, S., Gigi, R., Shapira, A., Sarig-Meth, T., Nadav, D., Rozenek, M., ... Halpern, P. (2016). Intranasal ketamine for acute traumatic pain in the Emergency Department: a prospective, randomized clinical trial of efficacy and safety. *BMC Emergency Medicine*, 16(1), 43.

Smith, H. S., & Peppin, J. F. (2014). Toward a systematic approach to opioid rotation. *Journal of Pain Research*, 7, 589–608.

The Joint Commission. (2018). *2018 Hospital Accreditation Standards*.

Ting, S., & Schug, S. (2016). The pharmacogenomics of pain management: prospects for personalized medicine. *Journal of Pain Research*, 9, 49–56.

Todd, J., Rees, E., Gwilliam, B., & Davies, A. (2002). An assessment of the efficacy and tolerability of a 'double dose' of normal-release morphine sulphate at bedtime. *Palliative Medicine*, 16(6), 507–512.

Vacha, M. E., Huang, W., & Mando-Vandrick, J. (2015). The role of subcutaneous ketorolac for pain management. *Hospital Pharmacy*, 50(2), 108–112.

von Baeyer, C. L., & Pasero, C. (2017). What nurses' workarounds tell us about pain assessment. *International Journal of Nursing Studies*, 67, A1–A2.

Von Korff, M., Merrill, J. O., Rutter, C. M., Sullivan, M., Campbell, C. I., & Weisner, C. (2011). Time-scheduled vs. pain-contingent opioid dosing in chronic opioid therapy. *Pain*, 152(6), 1256–1262.

Warholak, T. L., Rupp, M. T., Zale, A., Hines, M., Park, S. (2015). Check it out: a practical tool for improving medication safety. *Journal of the American Pharmacists Association*, 55(6), 621–625. https://doi.org/10.1331/JAPhA.2015.14280.

Webster, L. R., & Fine, P. G. (2012). Review and critique of opioid rotation practices and associated risks of toxicity. *Pain Medicine*, 13(4), 562–570.

Wilken, M., Ineck, J. R., & Rule, A. M. (2005). Chronic arthritis pain management with topical morphine: case series. *Journal of Pain & Palliative Care Pharmacotherapy*, 19(4), 39–44.

Yang, C., Xu, X. M., & He, G. Z. (2018). Efficacy and feasibility of opioids for burn analgesia: An evidence-based qualitative review of randomized controlled trials. *Burns.*, 44(2), 241–248. https://doi.org/10.1016/j.burns.2017.10.012.

Yin, H.-H., Tse, M. M. Y., & Wong, F. K. Y. (2015). Systematic review of the predisposing, enabling and reinforcing factors which influence nursing administration of opioids in the postoperative period. *Japan Journal of Nursing Science*, 12(2), 59–275.

Zhang, X., Ruan, X., Liu, C., & Yu, Z. (2009). Effect of vaginal administration of controlled-release oxycodone on cancer pain. *Chinese Journal of Cancer*, 28(7), 740–742.

Chapter 10 Nonopioid Analgesic Medications

Meredith W. Crumb, Timothy J. Atkinson, Maureen F. Cooney

CHAPTER OUTLINE

Aspirin and Nonsteroidal Antiinflammatory Drugs, pg. 195

> History, pg. 195
>
> Pharmacologic Effects, pg. 197
>
> Indications for Use, pg. 199
>
> Adverse Effects, pg. 200
>
> Nanopharmacology, pg. 205
>
> Dosing and Formulations, pg. 206
>
> Use in Special Populations, pg. 209
>
> Acetaminophen, pg. 210

Multimodal Use of Nonopioid Analgesics, pg. 214

Key Points, pg. 215

Case Scenario, pg. 215

References, pg. 216

IN clinical practice, medications used for pain management are divided into three categories: nonopioid analgesics, opioids, and adjuvants or coanalgesics. Nonopioid analgesics, the focus of this chapter, include nonsteroidal antiinflammatory drugs (NSAIDs), aspirin, and acetaminophen, which are available both over-the-counter (OTC) and by prescription. Nonopioid analgesics are widely used for the treatment of pain and fever, and NSAIDs are used for their antiinflammatory effect. In clinical practice, there are some misconceptions related to the use of nonopioid analgesics. Table 10.1 summarizes and clarifies of some of the misconceptions. Nonopioid analgesics, used without other analgesic medications, may provide effective pain relief in some conditions; they are also used in combination with other analgesic interventions in multimodal pain management plans of care. The use of nonopioid analgesics in a multimodal pain management plan has been recommended by a number of professional organizations and regulatory agencies to optimize patient comfort and reduce risks associated with opioid monotherapy (Chou et al., 2016; Dowell, Haegerich, & Chou, 2016; Joint Commission, 2012, 2017; Jungquist et al., 2020). Chapters 1 and 2 provide more detail related to the use of multimodal analgesia.

The purpose of this chapter is to describe the use of nonopioid analgesics and review each class of medications. The pharmacokinetics and pharmacodynamics, indications for nonopioid analgesic use (Box 10.1), contraindications, warnings, and potential adverse effects are described. Examples of frequently used medications, formulations, dosing ranges, and clinical considerations are provided.

Aspirin and Nonsteroidal Antiinflammatory Drugs

History

The history of aspirin, derived from willow bark, is well described by Ugurlucan et al. (2012). Extracts from the bark of the willow tree were recognized as early as 500 BCE for antipyretic, antiinflammatory, and analgesic effects (Desborough, & Keeling, 2017; Ugurlucan et al., 2012). In 1828 Johann Buchner, a professor of pharmacy, isolated bitter-tasting crystals from willow bark and named it "salicin." In 1838 Rafael Piria, an Italian chemist, further purified salicin by hydrolysis and oxidation to a more active and pure form, salicylic acid. Salicylic acid was used for inflammatory disorders, but use was limited by severe stomach irritation. In 1858 the French chemist Francis Gerhardt buffered salicylic acid with sodium and acetyl chloride, creating acetylsalicylic acid (ASA), but abandoned his research, unable to obtain improvement in gastrointestinal (GI) tolerability. During the 1870s scientists demonstrated that ASA could successfully treat rheumatoid arthritis, rheumatic fever, and gout. ASA was not stable enough for widespread use until 1897, when Felix Hoffman, a German chemist working for the Bayer Company, was involved in the development of a form of ASA from *Spirea ulmaria*, a plant that contains salicylin. The Bayer Company patented the chemical as aspirin in 1899 as a powder and then as a tablet in 1900 (Ugurlucan et al., 2012).

Worldwide, aspirin quickly became the most popular analgesic, used for backache, headache, and arthritis. A 1939 guideline in the *Annals of Rheumatic Diseases*

Table 10.1 | Misconceptions About Nonopioids

Misconception	Correction
Regular daily use of nonopioids is safe.	Adverse effects from long-term use of NSAIDs are considerably severe and life threatening. NSAIDs can cause gastric ulcers, increased bleeding time, and cardiovascular adverse events. Acetaminophen can cause hepatotoxicity.
Nonopioids are not useful analgesics for severe pain.	Nonopioids alone are rarely sufficient to relieve severe pain, but they are an important part of a multimodal analgesic plan. One of the basic principles of analgesic therapy is: Whenever pain is severe enough to require an opioid, adding nonopioids (acetaminophen and NSAID) should be considered.
It is unacceptable polypharmacy to administer an NSAID, opioid, and one or more adjuvant analgesics (e.g., local anesthetic, anticonvulsant, antidepressant) for pain control.	Analgesics within each of the three analgesic groups relieve pain by different mechanisms. It is acceptable and, in most cases, recommended multimodal analgesia to administer more than one drug if each one is for a specific purpose.
A nonopioid should not be given at the same time as an opioid.	It is safe to administer a nonopioid and opioid at the same time. Giving a dose of nonopioid at the same time as a dose of opioid poses no more danger than giving the doses at different times. In fact, many opioids are compounded with a nonopioid (e.g., Percocet [oxyCODONE and acetaminophen]).
Administering NSAIDs rectally or parenterally prevents gastric ulcers.	Regardless of the route of administration, NSAIDs inhibit prostaglandins that are necessary to maintain the protective barrier in the GI tract. Rectal or parenteral administration will only avoid the local irritation that can occur with oral administration.
Topical nonopioids are not effective analgesics.	Topical nonopioids have been shown to produce effective analgesia for mild to moderate acute or persistent (chronic) pain with a lower incidence of GI adverse effects.
Administering antacids with NSAIDs is an effective method of reducing gastric distress.	Administering antacids with NSAIDs can lessen distress but may be counterproductive. Antacids reduce the absorption and therefore the effectiveness of the NSAID by releasing the drug in the stomach rather than in the small intestine, where absorption occurs.
For patients receiving long-term treatment with NSAIDs, H_2 blockers such as cimetidine (Tagamet) provide effective protection against gastric and duodenal ulcers.	H_2 blockers at higher than standard doses may be helpful, but miSOPROStol (Cytotec) and proton pump inhibitors (PPIs) such as esomeprazole (NexIUM), lansoprazole (Prevacid), and omeprazole (PriLOSEC), are more effective and the only proven methods to reduce the occurrence of gastric and duodenal ulcers.
Gastric distress (e.g., abdominal pain) is indicative of NSAID-induced gastric ulceration.	Most patients with gastric lesions have no symptoms until bleeding or perforation occurs.
NSAIDs affect bone healing and should not be taken after orthopedic surgery.	Withdrawal of COX-2 inhibition when NSAIDs are discontinued after a short-term course (10–14 days) restores normal bone healing with no discernible effects on fracture healing (see text for exceptions and references).

COX-2, Cyclooxygenase 2; GI, gastrointestinal; H_2, histamine 2; NSAID, nonsteroidal antiinflammatory drug.
Modified from Pasero, C., & McCaffery, M. *Pain assessment and pharmacologic management* (p. 180). St. Louis, Mosby. © 2011, Pasero, C., & McCaffery, M. May be duplicated for use in clinical practice.

described the important role of aspirin therapy due to the antipyretic and analgesic activity combined with its relative harmlessness (Tegner, 1939). The GI adverse effects were well known, but in the absence of alternatives, the benefits seemed to outweigh the risks. Therapeutic doses of aspirin used during this time seem incredibly high compared to doses used in modern medicine. For example, in rheumatic fever a high therapeutic dose was 12 g (37 tablets)/day and standard dosing for rheumatoid arthritis was 5.2 g (16 tablets)/day (Farber, Yiengst, & Shock, 1949; Pinals & Frank, 1967).

In 1965 the modern age of NSAIDs began with the U.S. Food and Drug Administration (FDA) approval of indomethacin as the first nonaspirin NSAID (Drugs@FDA: Indocin, 1965). Although still demonstrating considerable GI upset, indomethacin was an enormous improvement

---

Box 10.1	Indications for Nonopioid Analgesics

- *Mild pain:* Start with a nonopioid. Acetaminophen or an NSAID alone often provides adequate relief.
- *Moderate to severe pain:* Pain of any severity may be at least partially relieved by a nonopioid. For some types of moderate pain, especially muscle and joint pain, NSAIDs alone or in combination with acetaminophen may provide adequate relief. However, an NSAID alone usually does not relieve severe pain.
- *Postoperative pain:* Perioperative use of acetaminophen and an NSAID, especially parenteral ketorolac (Toradol) when not contraindicated, should be part of a multimodal analgesic plan begun preoperatively and continued throughout the postoperative course.
- *Persistent (chronic) pain:* Various types of persistent pain, including cancer-related bone pain, osteoarthritis, and rheumatoid arthritis, are appropriate indications for an NSAID.

- *Pain that requires an opioid:* Whenever pain is severe enough to require an opioid, always consider adding a nonopioid for the following reasons:
  - Opioid dose-sparing effect (i.e., opioid dose may be lowered without decreasing pain relief. A decreased opioid dose can result in a reduction in opioid-induced adverse effects). A common example is oral or rectal acetaminophen and intravenous ibuprofen or intravenous ketorolac plus an opioid postoperatively.
  - Opioids and nonopioids relieve pain by different mechanisms.

From Pasero, C., & McCaffery, M. *Pain assessment and pharmacologic management* (p. 182). St. Louis, Mosby. © 2011, Pasero, C. & McCaffery, M. May be duplicated for use in clinical practice.

---

over aspirin in terms of reducing pill burden, acid load, and overall tolerability. In 1971 Sir John Vane, the British pharmacologist, described inhibition of prostaglandin synthesis as the mechanism of action for aspirin and NSAIDs, and won the Noble Prize in 1982 for his work (Ugurlucan, 2012). Vane's discovery sparked an NSAID research renaissance and from 1976 to 1991, yielded 15 new medications in as many years.

Lists many of the NSAIDS approved for use in the United States. Aspirin is the original NSAID and shares the same binding site as other NSAIDs, but because it has some unique characteristics, it is often classified separately from the other NSAIDs. Although there are currently more than 25 NSAIDs, they belong to more than six distinct chemical classes with significant differences in pharmacology, pharmacokinetics, and cyclooxygenase selectivity, all of which contribute to their unique efficacy and safety profile (Furst, 1994; Mitchell, Larkin, & Williams, 1995). A summary of the NSAID chemical classes is provided in Fig. 10.1.

Pharmacologic Effects

Aspirin and NSAIDs produce therapeutic effects by reducing inflammation, pain, and fever through inhibition of prostaglandin biosynthesis. Prostaglandins are involved in a variety of physiologic functions, including inflammation, pain, fever, platelet aggregation, mucosal protection in the GI tract, and regulation of renal function (Zhou, Boudreau, & Freedman, 2014). Prostaglandins are produced through the metabolism of arachidonic acid, which is illustrated in the cyclooxygenase 1 (COX-1) and COX-2 pathway in Fig. 10.2.

Aspirin and NSAIDs inhibit the biosynthesis of prostaglandins by preventing the substrate arachidonic acid from binding to the active site of COX enzymes (Waller & Sampson, 2018). There are two known isoforms of the COX enzyme, COX-1 and COX-2, each with distinct physiologic roles. A review of the actions of these enzymes and prostaglandins is helpful to understand the pharmacologic effects of aspirin and NSAIDs.

COX-1 is constitutively expressed in nearly all cells, contributes to regulation of renal and gastric blood flow, and provides a cytoprotective effect on the GI tract (Brenner & Stevens, 2018; Waller & Sampson, 2018). COX-1 is the only isoform expressed in platelets, and produces TXA_2 and PGI_2 in equal amounts, thereby maintaining a balance in platelet activity (Brenner & Stevens, 2018). COX-1 catalyzes platelet TXA_2 which facilitates platelet aggregation and hemostasis while PGI2 is a potent vasodilator and inhibitor of platelet aggregation (Brenner & Stevens, 2018; Waller & Sampson, 2018). Aspirin and NSAIDS, through inhibition of COX-1 enzymes, interfere with production of TXA_2 and PGI_2 thereby disrupting the normal balance of these prostaglandins, and increasing the potential for platelet aggregation (Brune & Patrignani, 2015).

COX-2 is expressed in the brain, kidneys, and blood vessels, the areas most susceptible to thrombotic events, and COX-2 expression can be caused by cytokine release from injury or inflammation (Waller & Sampson, 2018). COX-2 produces PGI_2 and PGE_2, but not TXA_2. In the presence of inflammation, PGE_2 is the primary prostaglandin produced; this is significant because high levels of PGE_2 inhibit aggregation and promote vasodilation (Waller & Sampson, 2018). As described in Chapter 3, PGE_2 and PGI_2 have a

Chemical Classes of
Nonsteroidal Antiinflammatory Drugs (NSAIDs) in the United States

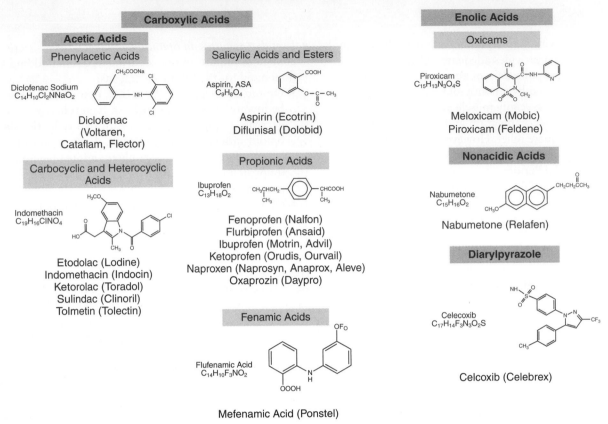

Note: Most common brand names listed. Not all inclusive.

Fig. 10.1 | **Chemical classes of nonsteroidal antiinflammatory drugs.** (Modified from Fudin, J., & Henderson, T. Chemical classes of nonsteroidal anti-inflammatories [NSAIDs] in US. Retrieved July 10, 2017, from http://paindr.com/wp-content/uploads/2014/07/NSAIDS-Chemical-Classes_2014_Shahzad-Henderson-Fudin.pdf)

significant role in inflammatory pain as they sensitize Aδ and C fiber nerve endings in peripheral tissues to the nociceptive activity of substance P, bradykinin, and serotonin (Brune & Patrignani, 2015; Waller & Sampson, 2018). Peripheral inflammation and COX-2 activity may also contribute to an increase in PGE_2 in the central nervous system and development of central hyperalgesia (Brune & Patrignani, 2015).

Aspirin

Aspirin is composed of both a reactive acetyl group of unmetabolized aspirin and the salicylate metabolite (Schrör & Voelker, 2016). Aspirin irreversibly inactivates COX-1 and suppresses production of prostaglandin H2 by the binding of aspirin's acetyl group to the active site on the COX-1 enzyme; aspirin also inhibits COX-2, but at a far slower rate than COX-1 inactivation (Mekaj, Daci, & Mekaj, 2015; Schrör, & Voelker, 2016). The irreversible inactivation of COX-1 causes aspirin to be associated with significantly higher bleeding risks than other NSAIDs because platelets cannot recover and are inhibited for their entire life cycle (7–10 days).

Some patients take aspirin for cardiac protection and also take nonaspirin NSAIDs for analgesic effects. Nonaspirin NSAIDs are reversible inhibitors of COX but may compete with aspirin for the binding site. It is important to educate patients who require aspirin for prevention of cardiac events to take it at least 30 minutes before nonaspirin NSAIDs to receive the intended cardioprotective effects (Moore, Pollack, & Butkerait, 2015).

NSAIDs

NSAIDs, like aspirin, exert their effects through the inhibition of the COX enzymes. Nonselective NSAIDs inhibit COX-1 and COX-2, and selective NSAIDs block only COX-2. The nonselective NSAIDs tend to have a greater tendency to block COX-1 then COX-2. NSAIDs vary in their degree of COX-1 and COX-2 inhibition and selectivity; familiarity with these properties can be useful to determine NSAID-related risks. Fig. 10.3 displays the relative COX-1 and COX-2 selectivity of the different NSAIDs. The extent to which an NSAID inhibits COX-1 and COX-2 accounts for its effects and adverse effects. COX-2 inhibition is responsible for the antiinflammatory

ENZYME PATHWAY: COX-1 AND COX-2

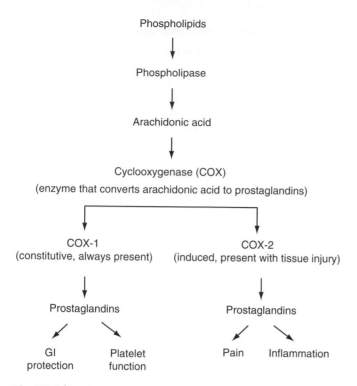

Fig. 10.2 | **Cyclooxygenase 1 (COX-1) and COX-2 enzyme pathway.** (From Pasero, C., & McCaffery, M. [2011]. *Pain assessment and pharmacologic management* [p. 6]. St. Louis, Mosby. © 2011, Pasero C, & McCaffery M. May be duplicated for use in clinical practice.)

antipyretic, analgesic, and antiinflammatory properties, which are all mediated by COX-2.

Indications for Use

Aspirin

Aspirin is rarely used for its analgesic effects because of the availability of NSAIDs with better safety profiles. Aspirin is now primarily used for cardioprotective and antiplatelet effects (Negm & Furst, 2017). Aspirin is rarely used for analgesia; therefore, content in the remaining sections of this chapter primarily address the use of nonaspirin NSAIDs.

NSAIDs

NSAIDs encompass a class of medications available OTC or by prescription that are widely used to treat inflammation, pain, and fever. Over the years, many well-designed trials have documented the analgesic benefits of NSAIDs in a variety of painful conditions. NSAIDs are included in recommendations from professional organizations for the treatment of conditions such as osteoarthritis, dental pain, and postoperative pain. For example, the American College of Rheumatology (Hochberg et al., 2012) and the Osteoarthritis Research Society International (OARSI) (McAlindon et al., 2014) offer conditional recommendations for the use of NSAIDs as a first-line analgesic for osteoarthritis. Guidelines for the management of acute postoperative pain developed by the American Pain Society (APS), American Society of Regional Anesthesia and Pain Medicine (ASRA), and American Society of Anesthesiologists' Committee on Regional Anesthesia, Executive Committee, and Administrative Council (Chou et al., 2016) cite strong recommendation with high-quality evidence for the use of multimodal analgesia, including the use of acetaminophen and/or NSAIDs for patients

and analgesic effect of NSAIDs, and COX-1 inhibition and, to some extent, COX-2 inhibition, is responsible for NSAID-related adverse effects (Brune & Patrignani, 2015). No NSAID, other than aspirin, has ever been used for its COX-1 properties; NSAIDs are exclusively used for

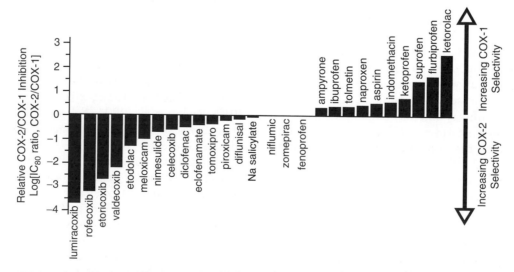

Fig. 10.3 | **Nonsteroidal antiinflammatory drug cyclooxygenase 1 (COX-1) and COX-2 selectivity.** (From Antman, E. M., DeMets, D., & Loscalzo, J. [2005]. Cyclooxygenase inhibition and cardiovascular risk. *Circulation, 112*[5], 759-770; modified from Warner, T. D., & Mitchell, J. A. [2004]. Cyclooxygenases: New forms, new inhibitors, and lessons from the clinic. *FASEB J, 18,* 790-804.)

who have no contraindications for use of these medications. A strong recommendation with moderate-quality evidence is also made for the use of a preoperative dose of celecoxib, unless contraindicated.

Most NSAIDs are indicated for relief of pain and/or inflammation in patients with rheumatoid arthritis, osteoarthritis, ankylosing spondylitis, polyarticular juvenile idiopathic arthritis, tendonitis, bursitis, acute gout, and primary dysmenorrhea. In general, NSAIDs have strong evidence for decreasing stiffness and inflammation and improving functional mobility (Zhang et al., 2010). The analgesic benefit of NSAIDS was reported by researchers in numerous studies. In a network meta-analysis involving 129 trials and 32,129 participants with knee osteoarthritis, use of intraarticular injections of hyaluronic acid or corticosteroid, nonselective NSAIDs, or a COX-2 inhibitor (celecoxib), were noted to provide clinically significant improvements in pain over a 3-month period (Bannuru et al., 2015). When 35 randomized placebo-controlled trials of NSAIDs used to treat spinal pain (neck and back) were reviewed, researchers reported NSAIDs effectively reduced pain, but small effects above placebo were reported (Machado et al., 2017). The authors of a recent systematic review, which included 36 randomized controlled trials (RCTs) and 4887 patients with acute kidney stone pain, reported that among those with normal kidney function, NSAIDs provided more effective and sustained pain relief with fewer side effects than opioids or acetaminophen (Pathan, Mitra, & Cameron, 2018).

Adverse Effects

NSAIDs are more than 90% protein bound, and because only the free fraction of circulating drug exerts its pharmacologic effect, bleeding risk increases substantially when plasma protein levels decline and more free circulating drug is available, such as with severe hepatic dysfunction. NSAIDs are nearly all metabolized through the cytochrome P450 (CYP450) system via the 2C9 isoenzyme (Brenner & Stevens, 2018). Although this pathway does not have the same drug interactions as other CYP enzymes, it has a few that are of note; for example, warfarin, a commonly used anticoagulant, is also metabolized through this pathway and may explain the increased bleeding risk when warfarin and NSAIDs are coadministered (in addition to the antiplatelet effects of NSAIDs) (Brenner & Stevens, 2018).

The adverse effects of NSAIDs have been the primary focus of NSAID research for the past 20 years. Research efforts have focused exclusively on elucidating the risk for GI bleeding and more recently on cardiovascular adverse effects. The type and degree of COX inhibition and corresponding PGI_2/TXA_2 imbalance is the preferred hypothesis surrounding many of the side effects of NSAIDs (Waller & Sampson, 2018). At higher doses, all NSAIDs lose selectivity because they will significantly inhibit both COX-1 and COX-2 and dramatically increase risk for adverse effects.

Bleeding and Gastrointestinal Adverse Effects

Bleeding risks associated with NSAIDs vary depending on the degree of COX-1/COX-2 inhibition and selectivity; familiarity with these properties can be useful to determine bleeding risk (see Box 10.2 and Fig. 10.3). The degree of COX-1 inhibition by an NSAID plays an integral role in determining a patient's bleeding risk because COX-1 inhibition directly affects platelet aggregation (Waller & Sampson, 2018). NSAIDs bind reversibly to COX-1 (unlike aspirin, which binds irreversibly) and inhibit platelet function only for the duration of binding, which is usually shorter than their duration of action. Therefore, bleeding risks are less common when NSAIDs are used intermittently than when used regularly (Waller & Sampson, 2018).

GI complications, including nausea, dyspepsia, ulceration, bleeding, and perforation, are the most common NSAID-associated adverse effects (Moore, Pollack, & Butkerait, 2015; Ofman, Maclean, Straus et al., 2002; Waller & Sampson, 2018). Normally, the COX-1 enzyme expressed in the gastric epithelial cells leads to the production of PGs (PGE_2 and PGI_2), which are responsible for maintaining GI mucosal integrity by increasing mucous production and decreasing acid production (Brenner & Stevens, 2018). The risk for GI bleeding increases as the COX-1 selectivity of specific NSAIDs increases. For example, indomethacin, with its high COX-1 selectivity, poses a greater risk for GI bleeding than ibuprofen. In a number of older studies, ibuprofen was associated with less GI-related risk than other NSAIDs (Henry et al., 1996; Lewis et al., 2002). COX-2 inhibition also plays a role in GI side effects because COX-2 may be involved in healing of gastric lesions; additionally, COX-2 inhibition may contribute to ulcer development (Brune & Patrignani, 2015).

Risk factors for NSAID-related GI complications include high NSAID dose, longer duration of NSAID therapy, older age, *Helicobacter pylori* infection, history of ulcer or ulcer complications, and concomitant use of OTC NSAIDs, low-dose aspirin, anticoagulants, or corticosteroids (Goldstein & Cryer, 2015; McGettigan & Olsen, 2017; Richy et al., 2004; Scheiman, 2016). Table 10.2 summarizes some of the risk factors for NSAID-related adverse GI events.

Strategies to mitigate GI risk include use of gastroprotective cotherapy or use of a COX-2–selective agent (Yuan et al., 2016). Cotherapy can include miSOPROStol, proton pump inhibitors (PPIs), or double-dose histamine receptor type-2 receptor antagonists (H_2RAs). MiSOPROStol 200 mcg qid (800 mcg/day) is effective but requires frequent dosing and is generally not well tolerated because of GI adverse effects, including diarrhea and abdominal pain (Goldstein & Cryer, 2015). MiSOPROStol 400 mcg is better tolerated and

| **Box 10.2** | Adverse Effects of Nonopioids and Their Treatment and Prevention |

ACETAMINOPHEN

Hepatic effects: Hepatotoxicity occurs with overdose. At recommended doses, certain individuals are also at risk. Preventive strategy is to avoid or use with caution in patients with the following:

- Malnourishment, recent fasting
- Alcoholism, regular and heavy use of alcohol
- Preexisting liver disease
- Concomitant use of other potentially hepatotoxic drugs

Renal effects: Long-term use associated with declines in GFR and chronic renal failure; dose-dependent increases in renal insufficiency.

Cardiovascular effects: Long-term use associated with elevated risk; dose-dependent increases in blood pressure.

Hematologic effects: May interfere with platelet aggregation and interact to potentiate the anticoagulant effect of warfarin (Coumadin).

NSAIDS

Gastric effects: Acute local irritation from orally administered NSAIDs can produce uncomfortable symptoms (e.g., dyspepsia) but rarely indicative of serious injury. May resolve with continued use. Treatment options:

- Lower the dose.
- Switch to another NSAID.
- Though enteric-coated NSAIDs do not reduce the risk of upper GI adverse events, they may help to relieve dyspepsia.
- Use a topical NSAID.
- Take the NSAID with food or a large glass of water.
- Antacids may reduce symptoms, but they also reduce absorption of the NSAID.
- H$_2$ antagonists (e.g., cimetidine [Tagamet], famotidine [Pepcid], raNITIdine [Zantac]) are less effective than miSOPROStol and PPIs; all can be expensive.

Systemic gastrointestinal effects: Can occur regardless of route of administration. NSAIDs interfere with PG synthesis throughout the body. PG reduction impairs the protective barrier in the GI tract and allows injury to occur. Patient may be asymptomatic until bleeding or perforation occurs.

Risk factors for NSAID-induced GI adverse effects:

- Presence of prior ulcer disease or ulcer complications
- Advanced age

- CV disease and other comorbidities
- RA
- Concomitant treatment with corticosteroids or anticoagulants (or other antiplatelet drugs)
- Use of more than one NSAID, including cardioprotective aspirin
- High NSAID doses
- Long-term NSAID use
- Use of NSAID with high risk for GI toxicity (e.g., indomethacin [Indocin], piroxicam [Feldene], sulindac [Clinoril]).
- Patient unlikely to survive a GI complication
- Gastroprotective therapies:
  - MiSOPROStol (Cytotec). Reduces the occurrence of gastric and duodenal ulcers.
  - For patients who cannot afford or tolerate miSOPROStol, use a PPI (e.g., esomeprazole [NexIUM], lansoprazole [Prevacid], and omeprazole [PriLOSEC])
- H$_2$ blockers (e.g., cimetidine [Tagamet], famotidine [Pepcid], raNITIdine [Zantac]) are less effective than miSOPROStol and PPIs.
- A single strategy such as antacids, buffered tablets, or enteric-coated tablets does not provide sufficient protection.

Cardiovascular effects: All NSAIDs carry a risk for CV adverse effects through prostaglandin inhibition; an increased risk for CV events is associated with COX-2 inhibition, whether it is produced by those drugs labeled COX-2 selective (e.g., celecoxib) or those that are nonselective inhibitors of both COX-1 and COX-2 (e.g., ibuprofen, naproxen, ketorolac), and the risk varies across drugs, even within classes.

Hematologic effects: Most nonselective NSAIDs increase bleeding time. Ibuprofen can interfere with the cardioprotective effect of aspirin, so it should be taken 30 minutes to 2 hours after aspirin intake or at least 8 hours before. Preventive strategies when bleeding is a concern:

- Use NSAIDs that have minimal or no effect on bleeding time, such as COX-2–selective NSAIDs (e.g., celecoxib) or the nonselective NSAIDs choline magnesium trisalicylate (Trilisate), salsalate (Disalcid), and nabumetone (Relafen).
- Use acetaminophen instead of an NSAID (see discussion of concomitant acetaminophen and warfarin use).

Continued

Box 10.2   Adverse Effects of Nonopioids and Their Treatment and Prevention—cont'd

- To decrease bleeding associated with operative procedures, stop aspirin therapy 1 week before surgery (see the text for exceptions), and stop most other NSAIDs 3 days before surgery. Aspirin has an irreversible effect on platelets, but other NSAIDs do not.

Renal effects: Renal insufficiency is uncommon, and acute renal failure is rare, but long-term NSAID use at high doses may cause end-stage renal disease. Preventive strategies in patients with impaired renal function:

- Avoid indomethacin.
- Consider aspirin, celecoxib, or opioid analgesia.
- Use the lowest effective dose for the shortest time needed.
- Monitor kidney function.

Cognitive effects: Mild to moderate sedation and dysfunction can occur (CNS effect). Treatment options:

- Lower the dose.
- Discontinue the NSAID.
- Switch to another NSAID.

CNS, Central nervous system; COX, cyclooxygenase; CV, cardiovascular; GFR, glomerular filtration rate; h, hour; H_2, histamine receptor type-2; MI, myocardial infarction; NSAID, nonsteroidal antiinflammatory drug; PG, prostaglandin; PPI, proton pump inhibitor; RA, rheumatoid arthritis.

From Pasero, C., & McCaffery, M. *Pain assessment and pharmacologic management* (pp. 186-187). St. Louis, Mosby. © 2011, Pasero C, McCaffery M. May be duplicated for use in clinical practice.

---

significantly reduces risk for gastric but not duodenal ulcers (Rostom et al., 2009). MiSOPROStol should not be used in pregnant women because of its abortifacient property and is not recommended for use in women of childbearing potential (Drugs@FDA: Cytotec, 2016). In general, H_2RAs are better tolerated than miSOPROStol, but although H_2RAs are effective in duodenal ulcer prevention, they have not been shown to be as effective as miSOPROStol or PPIs in preventing NSAID-induced gastric ulcers (Goldstein & Cryer, 2015). Double doses of H_2RAs and standard PPI doses have been found to be effective in preventing endoscopically detected duodenal and gastric ulcers (Scheiman, 2016).

PPIs are recommended for their gastroprotective effect in patients taking NSAIDs. A systematic review involving 12,532 participants from 31 trials demonstrated effectiveness and safety of PPIs in peptic ulcer prevention among patients requiring NSAID therapy (Yang et al., 2017). There was no significant difference in effectiveness or safety of the various PPI medications. A systematic review of strategies to reduce GI risks with NSAID use, involving 82 trials and 125,053 participants, demonstrated that selective COX-2 inhibitors along with PPIs offered the greatest protection because they were associated with the lowest GI-related toxicity, followed by selective COX-2 inhibitors without a PPI, and finally by nonselective NSAIDs along with PPIs (Yuan et al., 2016). Published studies have reported adverse outcomes related to the long-term use of PPIs, such as risk for bacterial enteric infections, osteoporosis, and dementia, but most of the studies are observational and evidence is insufficient to determine causation (Vaezi, Yang, & Howden, 2017). It is necessary to weigh the known benefits of PPIs over possible risks, and it is recommended to continue PPI use when

there is proven benefit (prevention of GI adverse effects) at the lowest effective dose (Vaezi et al., 2017).

Enteric-coated tablets or buffered preparations have not been shown to ensure adequate gastric protection (AlHajri, 2017; Scheiman, 2016). To minimize risks for NSAID-related gastric injury, it is important for clinicians to counsel patients about the need to avoid taking higher than directed NSAID doses and avoid use of concomitant prescription and OTC NSAID- and aspirin-containing products. Table 10.3 summarizes protective strategies to reduce potential for GI bleeding based on patient risk factors.

Cardiovascular Adverse Effects

Cardiovascular homeostasis is supported by the effects of COX-1 and COX-2 on the arachidonic and COX enzyme pathway. As previously described, in homeostasis, COX-1 and COX-2 activity play a significant role in maintaining a balance between promotion and inhibition of platelet aggregation.

Medications that inhibit COX-2, thereby reducing levels of PGI_2 will have prothrombotic effects, and those that inhibit COX-2 to a much greater extent than COX-1 will promote thrombosis because of a disturbance in the physiologic balance between PGI_2 and TxA_2 (Fanelli, Ghisi, Aprile, & Lapi, 2017). Although all NSAIDs inhibit COX-2 to some extent, they vary in degree of inhibition and effect on thrombosis (see selectivity index in Fig. 10.3). Those classified as COX-2–selective NSAIDs and those nonselective NSAIDs with relatively greater effects on COX-2 were thought to have more intense prothrombotic effects than others with less COX-2 selectivity (Brune & Patrignani, 2015; Patrono & Baigent, 2017).

Table 10.2 | Risk Factors for Nonsteroidal Antiinflammatory Drug–Induced Adverse Gastrointestinal Effects

Risk Factor	Comments
History of ulcers or GI events; use of antiulcer therapy for any reason	Patients with this risk factor are considered at high to very high risk for an adverse GI event.
Age 65 years or older	Risk increases with age. At age 45–64 years, 15 in 10,000 individuals will have a serious GI bleed and 2 in 10,000 will die from a GI bleed; at age 65–74 years, 17 in 10,000 will have a serious GI bleed and 3 in 10,000 will die from a GI bleed. The highest risk is in individuals age 75 and older when 91 in 10,000 will experience a GI bleed and 15 in 10,000 will die from a GI bleed.
Comorbidity (e.g., CV disease, CHF, COPD)	Individuals with CV disease are likely to take low-dose aspirin, which places them at higher risk for GI complications when NSAIDs are taken concomitantly.
Extensive or severe RA	Individuals with RA are two times more likely to develop GI complications than the general population. Pain relief from NSAIDs may be misinterpreted as disease regression; therefore, NSAID use should be in conjunction with disease-modifying therapy.
Concomitant glucocorticoid therapy, particularly in patients with RA	No increased risk of GI complications when glucocorticoids are used alone; however, used with NSAIDs may increase risk by as much as four-fold; warn patients to avoid NSAIDs during glucocorticoid therapy.
Concomitant anticoagulant therapy	Not strictly prohibited but may predispose to increased risk for GI mucosal break and hemorrhage; increase in INR may occur. INR should be monitored frequently if acetaminophen or NSAID is taken with warfarin. COX-2 selective NSAIDs, which have no effect on platelet aggregation, are best choices in such patients, if not contraindicated.
Type of NSAID	Lower risk: salsalate, magnesium choline trisalicylate, low doses of ibuprofen, naproxen,[a] etodolac, meloxicam, nabumetone, or COX-2–selective NSAIDs
	Higher risk: piroxicam,[a] sulindac, indomethacin, ketoprofen, ketorolac
Use of high-dose singular NSAIDs	Effects are dose-related; regardless of NSAID, the higher the dose, the higher the GI risk.
Use of combinations of NSAIDs, including low-dose aspirin cotherapy	Combinations of NSAIDs, including aspirin at any dose, increase GI risk (e.g., combination cardioprotective aspirin and NSAID therapies increase relative GI risk 2–4 times that of NSAIDs or aspirin alone; combination COX-2–selective NSAID plus cardioprotective aspirin provides some GI protection but substantially less than a COX-2 selective NSAID alone).
Helicobacter pylori infection	Independent and modifiable risk factor; may increase risk by two- to four-fold in regular NSAID users. Routinely test for presence in patients with high GI risk. Treat, if present, before NSAID therapy.
Excessive alcohol intake	Independent risk factor; magnitude unclear.
Cigarette smoking	Independent risk factor; magnitude unclear.

CHF, Congestive heart failure; COPD, chronic obstructive pulmonary disease; COX, cyclooxygenase; CV, cardiovascular; GI, gastrointestinal; INR, international normalized ratio; NSAID, nonsteroidal antiinflammatory drug; RA, rheumatoid arthritis.

[a]Avoid full-dose naproxen, piroxicam, and oxaprozin in older adults because of long half-life and increased risk for GI toxicity.

From Pasero, C., & McCaffery, M. *Pain assessment and pharmacologic management* (p. 192). St. Louis: Mosby. Data from Agency for Healthcare Research and Quality (AHRQ). (2007). *Choosing non-opioid analgesics for osteoarthritis: Clinician's guide.* Retrieved July 24, 2008 from http://effectivehealthcare.ahrq.gov/; American Geriatrics Society (AGS) Panel on Pharmacological Management of Persistent Pain in the Older Persons. (2009). The pharmacological management of persistent pain in older persons. *Journal of the American Geriatric Society, 57*(8), 1331-1346; Chan, F. K. L., & Graham, D. Y. (2004). Prevention of non-steroidal anti-inflammatory drug gastrointestinal complications: Review and recommendations based on risk assessment. *Alimentary Pharmacology Therapeutics, 19*(10), 1051-1061; Chan, F. K. L., Hung, L. C. T., & Suen, B. Y., Wong, V. W. S., Hui, A. J., Wu, J. C. Y., . . . Sung, J. J. Y. (2004). Celecoxib versus diclofenac plus omeprazole in high-risk arthritis patients: Results of a randomized double-blind trial. *Gastroenterology, 127*(4), 1038-1043; Fick, D. M., Cooper, J. W., Wade, W. E., Waller, J. L., Maclean, J. R., & Beers, M. H. (2003). Updating the Beers criteria for potentially inappropriate medication use in older adults. *Archives of Internal Medicine, 163*(22), 2716-2724; Gabriel, S. E.,

Jaakkimainen, L., & Bombardier, C. (1991). Risk for serious gastrointestinal complications related to use of nonsteroidal anti-inflammatory drugs: A meta-analysis. *Annals of Internal Medicine, 115*(10), 787-796; Hanlon, J. T., Backonja, M., Weiner, D., & Argoff, C. (2009). Evolving pharmacological management of persistent pain in older persons. *Pain Medicine, 10*(6), 959-961; Kurata, J. H., & Nogawa, A. N. (1997). Meta-analysis of risk factors for peptic ulcer: Nonsteroidal anti-inflammatory drugs, *Helicobacter pylori*, and smoking. *Journal of Clinical Gastroenterology, 24*(1), 2-17; Kuritzky, L., & Weaver, A. (2003). Advances in rheumatology: Coxibs and beyond. *Journal of Pain Symptom Management, 25*(2S), S6-S20; Laine, L. (2001). Approaches to nonsteroidal anti-inflammatory drug use in the high-risk patient. *Gastroenterology, 120*(3), 594-606; Laine, L., White, W. B., Rostom, A., & Hochberg, M. (2008). COX-2 selective inhibitors in the treatment of osteoarthritis. *Seminars in Arthritis and Rheumatism, 38*(3), 165-187; Solomon, D. H., Glynn, R. J., Rothman, K. J., Schneeweiss, S., Setoguchi, S., Mogun, H., . . . Stürmer, T. (2008). Subgroup analyses to determine cardiovascular risk associated with nonsteroidal anti-inflammatory drugs and coxibs in specific patient groups. *Arthritis Care Research, 59*(8), 1097-1104; Wilcox, C. M., Allison, J., Benzuly, K., Borum, M., Cryer, B, Grosser, T., . . . Simon, L. (2006). Consensus development conference on the use of nonsteroidal anti-inflammatory agents, including cyclooxygenase-2 enzyme inhibitors and aspirin. *Clinical Gastroenterology and Hepatology, 4*(9), 1082-1089. © 2011, Pasero, C., & McCaffery, M. May be duplicated for use in clinical practice.

Table 10.3 | Protective Strategies to Reduce Nonsteroidal Antiinflammatory Drug–Related Gastrointestinal Risks

Risk Level for Gastrointestinal Complications	Protective Strategy
None	Monotherapy with the least ulcerogenic agent at the lowest effective dose for the shortest duration
Low	Monotherapy with the least ulcerogenic nonselective NSAID at the lowest effective dose for the shortest duration
Moderate (advanced age or one or two risk factors)	Nonselective NSAID + proton pump inhibitor or misoprostol, or COX-2 inhibitor (celecoxib) for limited duration at lowest effective dose
High, or previous ulcer complications, or ≥ 2 risk factors	COX-2 inhibitor (celecoxib) at lowest effective dose, or nonselective NSAID + proton pump inhibitor, or *Helicobacter pylori* eradication
Previous lower gastrointestinal bleed[a]	COX-2 inhibitor (celecoxib) at lowest effective dose

COX-2, Cyclooxygenase type 2; *NSAID,* nonsteroidal antiinflammatory drug.

[a] In patients with previous NSAID-induced lower gastrointestinal bleed, more data are needed before a protective strategy can be recommended.

From Herndon, C. M., Hutchison, R. W., Berdine, H. J., Stacy, Z. A., Chen, J. T., Farnsworth, D. D., . . . Fermo, J. D. (2008). Management of chronic nonmalignant pain with nonsteroidal antiinflammatory drugs. *Pharmacotherapy, 28*(6), 788-805.

There are new studies evaluating the dose-dependent effect of COX-2–selective NSAIDs. The PRECISION trial, a randomized, multicenter, double-blind, noninferiority trial compared moderate doses of celecoxib with naproxen and ibuprofen in 24,081 patients who required these medications for osteoarthritis or rheumatoid arthritis pain and were at risk for cardiovascular disease (Nissen et al., 2016). Celecoxib was noninferior to prescription-strength naproxen and ibuprofen in primary cardiovascular outcomes of death, first occurrence of nonfatal myocardial infarction, or stroke during or within 30 days of treatment discontinuation. There was no significant difference between celecoxib and naproxen or ibuprofen in major adverse cardiovascular events (Nissen et al., 2016).

The results of the PRECISION trial support the need to avoid NSAIDs, if possible, in those with or at high risk for cardiovascular disease; if NSAIDs are required, they should be used at the lowest effective doses for the shortest length of time because risks appear to be dose and duration related (Nissen et al., 2016; Pepine & Gurbel, 2017). Naproxen has been recommended as the NSAID of choice when NSAID therapy is required for patients at risk for cardiovascular complications (Anwar, Anwar & Delafontaine, 2015). However, the results of the PRECISION trial do not support earlier recommendations that naproxen is associated with better cardiovascular outcomes than other NSAIDs (Nissen et al., 2016). The PRECISION trial results support previous study outcomes that prompted the FDA, in 2015, to issue class warnings on cardiovascular risk (FDA, 2015).

Renal Adverse Effects

NSAIDs can cause adverse renal effects because of their inhibition of renal prostaglandins, which regulate renal blood flow. NSAIDs impair prostaglandin-mediated renal vasodilation leading to vasoconstriction of the afferent arteriole that supplies blood to the kidneys. This decreases blood pressure in the kidney, which relies on pressure for adequate filtration. COX-1 and COX-2 are both constitutively expressed in the kidneys; therefore, those receiving nonselective or COX-2–selective NSAIDs have the potential for adverse renal effects (Patrono, 2016). In a systematic review of NSAIDs and acute kidney injury, a statistically significant elevated risk for acute kidney injury was found among those using nonselective NSAIDs, and a comparable but not statistically significant risk was associated with the use of specific COX-2 inhibitor (celecoxib) and nonselective medications with the most COX-2 selectivity (meloxicam and diclofenac) (Ungprasert, Cheungpasitporn, Crowson, & Matteson, 2015). In the PRECISION trial those who received ibuprofen compared to celecoxib had more serious renal effects, but the difference between naproxen and celecoxib in development of serious renal effects was insignificant (Nissen et al., 2016).

Compensatory mechanisms to improve renal blood flow include the increased production and release of renin and angiotensin II, which cause vasoconstriction of the efferent arteriole to normalize pressure at the glomerulus. (Burke, Pabbidi, Farley, & Roman, 2014). This compensatory mechanism is blocked in patients taking angiotensin-converting enzyme (ACE) inhibitors or aldosterone-receptor blocker (ARB) medications, and these patients are at higher risk for developing acute kidney injury when using concomitant NSAIDs (Prieto-García et al., 2016). The risk is increased further when patients are also taking a diuretic medication or are hypovolemic, which reduces blood volume delivered to the kidney, leading to kidney injury. Caution should be used when NSAIDs are used in combination with ACE/ARB or diuretics, especially in patients with risk factors for acute kidney injury, such as older patients or patients with diabetes, renal insufficiency, ascites, or heart failure (Dreischulte, Morales, Bell, & Guthrie, 2015; Khan, Loi, & Rosner, 2017; Prieto-García et al., 2016).

Blood Pressure Adverse Effects

NSAIDs impair prostaglandin-mediated renal vasodilation and cause sodium retention, which can lead to volume retention and subsequent increases in blood pressure. Despite this effect, increases in blood pressure are variable among NSAIDs, and elevations are usually slight (Lovell & Ernst, 2017).

Cognitive Adverse Effects

NSAIDs have received research interest because of their potential for neuroprotective effects. Although early studies demonstrated cognitive changes such as memory loss, concentration problems, confusion, and personality changes, especially in older patients who were taking nonselective NSAIDs (Goodwin & Regan, 1982; Wysenbeek, Klein, Nakar, & Mane, 1988), more recent research has focused on the potential benefits of NSAIDs in preventing cognitive decline associated with aging. Interest in NSAIDs as a pharmacologic intervention to prevent or reduce progression of cognitive decline has resulted in a number of studies. In a review of NSAIDS and Alzheimer's disease (AD), a condition associated with inflammation, Deardorff and Grossberg (2017) noted epidemiologic studies have shown a decrease in Alzheimer's disease in people who chronically take NSAIDs. Those results are not supported by RCTs. However, Deardorff and Grossberg (2017) note a decreased incidence of Alzheimer's disease in cognitively normal patients who are on long-term NSAID therapy for other indications. NSAIDs have been associated with cerebral adverse effects such as medication-overuse headaches (Peck, Roland, & Smitherman, 2018), drug-induced aseptic meningitis (Morís & García-Moncó, 2018), and lowered seizure threshold (Auriel, Regev, & Korczyn, 2014).

Hepatic Adverse Effects

Although NSAID-related liver injury is less common than other adverse effects associated with NSAID use, some risk exists, and experts advise against the use of NSAIDs in patients with cirrhosis (Klinge et al., 2018; Loy, 2017; Weersink et al., 2018). Schmeltzer et al. (2016) cite studies which show a low incidence of NSAID-related liver injury (ranges from 1 to 9 cases per 100,000 patients); however, few systematic, prospective studies have addressed the risk of NSAID-induced hepatotoxicity. In a review of registry data from the U.S. Drug-Induced Liver Injury Network (DILIN), which reports idiosyncratic drug-induced liver injury from medications and herbal and dietary supplements, 30 of 1221 DILIN cases, were attributed to eight different NSAIDs (Schmeltzer et al., 2016). The most commonly implicated NSAID was diclofenac (16/30), and in each of the 16 cases, diclofenac use was associated with hepatocellular injury (Schmeltzer et al., 2016). Based on these results, Schmeltzer et al. (2016) recommend limiting the use of diclofenac to situations in which other NSAIDs are not effective and suggest monitoring for signs of hepatotoxicity.

FDA Warnings

In 2005 the FDA released a boxed warning for all NSAIDs stating both (1) NSAIDs are associated with an increased risk for adverse cardiovascular thrombotic events, including myocardial infarction and stroke; and (2) NSAIDs may increase risk for GI irritation, inflammation, ulceration, bleeding, and perforation. These events may occur at any time during therapy and without warning (FDA, 2005). In July 2015 the FDA strengthened warnings for cardiovascular events with NSAIDs as a class effect (FDA, 2015).

Safety Summary

Research highlighting the potential adverse effects associated with NSAIDs and the issuance of warnings related to NSAIDs require clinicians to carefully assess the benefits versus risks of NSAID use for individual patients. The level of COX-2 inhibition that can be used to target pain and inflammation and decrease GI risk, while avoiding unnecessary cardiovascular risk, has yet to be elucidated. The use of a multimodal pain management plan that incorporates pharmacologic and nonpharmacologic interventions may facilitate use of lower doses of NSAIDs than would be required if NSAIDs were used as monotherapy. New NSAID approvals over the past 20 years reflect the effort to improve the safety of these medications by decreasing GI or cardiovascular toxicity. These attempts include the development of COX-2–selective inhibitors to decrease GI toxicity and the combination of gastroprotective agents with NSAIDs to decrease GI toxicity.

Nanopharmacology

Advances and innovations in the use of nanopharmacology may improve NSAID safety. Nanotechnology has become the most recent trend in NSAID production and drug approvals. Nanopharmacology involves the use of nanotechnology (technology used to create novel, very small materials using different organic and inorganic properties of materials) for the purpose of selectively delivering the active ingredients of pharmaceuticals to specific sites in the body; nanopharmacology may allow increased efficacy of medications with reduced toxicity because the medication is delivered directly to the targeted site of medication (Jain, Mehra, & Jain, 2014). A process called *micronizing* reduces drug particle size and thereby improves dissolution and absorption, leading to quicker onset of analgesia at lower than traditional doses (Maniar, Jones, Gopalakrishna, & Vangsness, 2017; Manvelian, Daniels, & Gibofsky, 2012).

Whereas absorption for typical NSAIDs is high, submicron NSAIDs have much finer particles, approximately 10 times smaller than those of conventional formulations, which have shown the ability to achieve standard peak plasma concentrations (C_{max}) with lower doses and overall systemic exposure (area under the curve). For example, submicron diclofenac can achieve similar efficacy with 35-mg rather than 50-mg strengths, and submicron indomethacin with 40 mg compared to 50 mg (Manvelian et al., 2012). Efficacy comparable with that of traditional NSAIDs has been demonstrated in clinical trials, but whether the decreased particle size will result in decreased side effects remains unclear and postmarketing studies may provide some clarity.

Dosing and Formulations

A variety of NSAIDs are available for administration by oral (tablets, capsules, liquids), intravenous, rectal, and topical routes (including gels and patches). Dosing depends on the specific NSAID and route.

Oral

Oral NSAIDs are often recommended for treatment of a variety of painful conditions, including osteoarthritis and chronic low back pain (Table 10.4) (Brune & Patrignani, 2015; Pelletier, Martel-Pelletier, Rannou, & Cooper, 2016). Oral NSAIDs are available in a variety of formulations, including tablets, enteric-coated tablets, capsules, and solutions; some, including diclofenac and naproxen, are available in short-acting and extended-release formulations (FDA, 2018). To improve GI tolerability of NSAIDs, some NSAIDs have been developed as fixed-dose combination products with H_2RAs (Altman, Bosch, Brune, Patrignani, & Young, 2015; Bello, Kent, Grahn, Ball, & Holt, 2015); limited fixed-dose NSAID and PPI combination products are available, and others are under development (Altman et al., 2015; Sostres & Lanas, 2016).

Parenteral

There are NSAID preparations that may be used parenterally (Table 10.5). Ketorolac is a prescription NSAID that is FDA approved for the treatment of moderate to severe acute pain requiring analgesia at the opioid level. The use of ketorolac is limited to a maximum of 5 days because of the potential for increasing the frequency and severity of adverse reactions, mainly the risk for bleeding (Drugs@FDA: Toradol, 2014). An intravenous formulation of ibuprofen (Caldolor) is FDA approved for the management of mild to moderate pain, the management of moderate to severe pain as an adjunct to opioid analgesics, and the reduction of fever (Drugs@FDA: Caldolor, 2016). Other intravenous NSAID formulations are under development.

Table 10.4	Common Nonsteroidal Antiinflammatory Drug Oral Formulations and Dosing[a]		
Drug	**Low Dose**	**Medium Dose**	**High or Maximum Dose**
Nonselective NSAIDs			
Diclofenac potassium	50 mg bid	50 mg tid	50 mg qid (in RA only)
Diclofenac sodium	50 mg bid	75 mg bid	50 mg qid or 100 mg SR bid (in RA only)
Ibuprofen	Up to 400 mg tid	600 mg tid–qid	800 mg qid
Ketoprofen	25–50 mg tid	75 mg tid	IR = 300 mg/day (divide), SR = 200 mg/d
Naproxen	250 mg tid	500 mg bid	1250 mg/d (divided)
Naproxen sodium	275 mg tid	550 mg bid	1375 mg/d (divided)
Partially selective NSAIDs			
Meloxicam	7.5 mg/d		15 mg/d
Nabumetone	1000 mg/d		2000 mg/d (daily or divided bid)
Cox-2 inhibitors			
Celecoxib	200 mg/d		200 mg bid

COX, Cyclooxygenase; *IR,* immediate release; *NSAID,* nonsteroidal antiinflammatory drug; *RA,* rheumatoid arthritis; *SR,* sustained release
[a] This table does not represent exact or equivalent dosing conversions. It is based on U.S. Food and Drug Administration–approved dosing ranges and comparative doses from clinical trials.
From Agency for Healthcare Research and Quality. (n.d.). Analgesics for Osteoarthritis: An Update of the 2006 Comparative Effectiveness Review. Retrieved April 30, 2020 from https://www.ncbi.nlm.nih.gov/books/NBK65646/pdf/Bookshelf_NBK65646.pdf.

Table 10.5 | Parenteral Nonsteroidal Antiinflammatory Drugs

	Intravenous	Intramuscular
Ketorolac[a]		
<65 y	30 mg qid (max 120 mg/d)	30 mg qid (max 120 mg/d)
>65 y, renally impaired, weight <50 kg	15 mg qid (max 60 mg/d)	15 mg qid (max 60 mg/d)
Ibuprofen	400-800 mg IV every 6 h prn administered over 30 min	

max, Maximum. **(ref: ketorolac package insert, Caldolor package insert)**
[a] Use is limited to 5 days.

Topical Salicylates and NSAIDs

Salicylate-containing rubefacients cause irritation of the skin, and are thought to relieve pain in muscles, joints, and tendons and other musculoskeletal pain in the extremities by counter-irritation. Irritation of the sensory nerve endings alters or offsets pain in the underlying muscle or joints that are served by the same nerves (Moore, Derry, & McQuay, 2010). Methyl salicylate is an ester oil (wintergreen oil) that when applied topically induces skin redness and irritation, leading to analgesic effect. Methyl salicylate is converted to salicylate in the skin, salicylates are derivatives of salicylic acid related pharmacologically to aspirin and NSAIDs. Theoretically the conversion to salicylate may offer additional benefits; however, this has not been studied or proven. Additionally, only approximately 20% of topically applied methyl salicylate may be absorbed, leading to very low systemic levels of salicylate (Center for Drug Evaluation and Research 2008). A 2014 Cochrane meta-analysis was conducted to assess the efficacy and safety of topically applied salicylates in acute and chronic musculoskeletal pain in adults and found topically applied salicylates have very low relative risk and are very well tolerated by patients, but available evidence does not support their use for acute injuries or chronic musculoskeletal pain conditions (Derry, Matthews, & Wiffen, 2014).

Topical NSAIDs are used for a variety of acute and chronic pain conditions, including acute sprains and strains, chronic musculoskeletal pain, and various neuropathic conditions (Derry et al., 2017). Topical NSAIDs, like systemic NSAIDS, act to reversibly inhibit COX-mediating production of prostaglandins and TXA_2. Topical NSAIDs inhibit COX enzymes locally and peripherally with minimal systemic uptake (Derry et al., 2017). In general, with topical NSAIDs, plasma drug concentrations are far below (usually less than 5%) concentrations achieved after oral administration (Derry et al., 2017). In the United States the only FDA-approved topical NSAID is diclofenac, but in Europe there are numerous topical NSAIDS that have been used clinically (Peppin et al., 2015). Topical diclofenac is available as a patch for treatment of acute musculoskeletal pain, or as a gel or solution for management of pain related to osteoarthritis (Peppin et al., 2015).

Other NSAIDS are sometimes prepared as topicals by compounding pharmacies but have not been studied as extensively as diclofenac, nor are they FDA approved for topical use in the United States. Research using nanotechnology for the preparation of new topical NSAIDs is underway (Elkomy, Elmenshawe, Eid, & Ali, 2016). Despite significantly lower systemic exposure, topical diclofenac products still have the same boxed warnings for cardiovascular and GI risk as oral NSAIDS. Table 10.6 includes a summary of topical diclofenac preparations. Additional information related to topical analgesics is provided in Chapter 16.

Other NSAID Routes

Ophthalmic Route

Ophthalmic NSAIDs are approved for several indications, including management of pain, discomfort, and inflammation associated with a variety of ocular conditions (Chandra Sekhar, Pathapati, Varalakshmi, Harshita, & Patra, 2015). Ophthalmic NSAIDs such as diclofenac, ketorolac, flurbiprofen, bromfenac, and nepafenac are used to treat pain and inflammation associated with cataract surgery and pain associated with corneal refractive surgery (Wilson, Schutte, & Abel, 2015). Administration of these medications is often associated with discomfort and a burning sensation that lasts for several minutes (Chandra Sekhar et al., 2015).

Intranasal Route

The intranasal (IN) route is another option that may be used for NSAID administration. Ketorolac is the only available intranasal NSAID because it is highly water soluble (Vadivelu et al., 2015). Each spray of intranasal medication provides 15.75 mg of ketorolac; the recommended dose for patients younger than 65 years of age is one spray in each nostril every 6 to 8 hours as needed (maximum dose 126 mg/day), or for those 65 years of age or older, one spray in only one nostril every 6 to 8 hours as needed (maximum dose 63 mg/day). The total duration of ketorolac use (including all formulations) is limited to 5 days to reduce risks of adverse effects. Intranasal ketorolac has the advantage of rapid administration because of ease of access of the intranasal route. In a review of ketorolac routes and indications, intranasal

Table 10.6 | Topical Diclofenac Product Descriptions

Product	Patch 1.3% (10 × 14 cm)	Gel 1%		Solution 1.5% (Drops)	Solution 2% (Pump)
FDA approved indication	Acute pain resulting from minor strains, sprains, and contusions	Osteoarthritis pain of knee(s) or hand(s)		Osteoarthritis pain of knee(s)	Osteoarthritis pain of knee(s)
Active ingredient	180 mg diclofenac epolamine/patch	10 mg diclofenac sodium/g of gel		16.05 mg diclofenac sodium/mL	20 mg diclofenac sodium/mL
Notable inactive ingredient	Epolamine	—		Dimethyl sulfoxide (DMSO)	Dimethyl sulfoxide (DMSO)
	(180 mg diclofenac epolamine/patch)	(10 mg diclofenac sodium/g of gel)		19 mg diclofenac sodium/ 40 drops	20 mg diclofenac/ pump actuation
Dosage	1 patch to the most painful area 2 times daily	*Upper extremities:* 2 g to affected area 4 times daily	*Lower extremities:* 4 g to affected area 4 times daily	40 drops per knee 4 times a day	2 pump actuations per knee 2 times a day
		Max: 32 g/d for all affected joints			
Administration	Do not wear patch when bathing or showering Edges of the patch may be taped down or a breathable nonocclusive mesh netting sleeve may be used	Dosing card should be used for each application Avoid showering/bathing for at least 1 h after application Do not use gel concomitantly with other topical products Avoid wearing clothing or gloves for at least 10 min after applying gel		Dispense 10 drops at a time either directly onto the knee or first into the hand and then onto the knee Apply evenly around front, back, and sides of the knee Avoid showering/bathing for at least 30 min after the application Wait until the treated area is dry before applying other topical products or wearing clothing over the area	The pump must be primed (4 actuations) before first use

ketorolac spray provides analgesia similar to that of intramuscular and intravenous ketorolac administration (Vadivelu et al., 2015). In an RCT of intranasal ketorolac in a multimodal analgesic plan for 321 postoperative patients after major abdominal surgery, when used in a multimodal pain management plan, intranasal ketorolac provided statistically significant pain relief and reduced morphine requirements by 34% in the ketorolac group compared to the placebo group in the first 72 postoperative hours (Moodie, Brown, Bisley, Weber, & Bynum, 2008). In a nonblinded prospective trial of intranasal ketorolac in the treatment of 82 patients with renal colic who presented to the emergency department, intranasal ketorolac followed by controlled doses of intravenous fentaNYL compared to intravenous ketorolac with the same doses of intravenous fentaNYL provided similar pain relief without significant adverse effects (Etteri, Maj, Maino, & Valli, 2018).

Monitoring Patients Receiving NSAID Therapy

Because of the risks for development of adverse effects, patients on chronic NSAID therapy may benefit from monitoring for bleeding, GI adverse effects, and impaired kidney function through periodic measurement of complete blood count, serum creatinine, and electrolyte concentrations (Pisano, 2016). It is necessary to assess for the addition of concurrent medications, such as antiplatelet agents; anticoagulants; blood pressure medications, including ACE/ARBs and/or diuretics, to minimize risks for potential harm associated with drug-drug interactions (Dreischulte, Morales, Bell, & Guthrie, 2015; Lanas, et al. 2015; Moore, Pollack, & Butkerait, 2015; Prieto-García et al., 2016). Periodic blood pressure monitoring is recommended for those who regularly use NSAIDs, particularly when high doses are used (Floor-Schreudering et al., 2015). Because of the potential for adverse effects, the lowest effective dose of NSAIDs for the shortest amount of time is recommended (Pergolizzi, Raffa, Nalamachu, & Taylor, 2016; Scheiman, 2016). The benefit of NSAID therapy, particularly with concurrent use of medications that increase NSAID-related risks, is evaluated on a consistent basis to ensure benefit outweighs risk of therapy (Pisano, 2016).

Use in Special Populations

Older Adults

Beers Criteria is a list of potentially inappropriate medications for use in older adults which is compiled and published by the American Geriatrics Society (American Geriatrics Society, 2019). The Beers Criteria advise NSAIDs should be used with caution in older adults; as people age, their ability to tolerate NSAIDs decreases and the risk for GI bleeding and renal effects increases (American Geriatrics Society, 2019). More COX-2–selective NSAIDs are better tolerated, but they increase the risk for cardiac events, pulmonary embolism, stroke, and deep venous thrombosis (DVT), and many of these patients already have a history of underlying risk in these areas. If lack of alternative treatment options exists in the setting of severe inflammatory pain (i.e., arthritis), NSAIDs should be trialed with caution and increased monitoring. They should not be considered for continued use unless significant clinical benefit is demonstrated. In a review of 16 studies examining NSAID use and fall risk among older adults, older adults who used NSAIDs had a higher rate of falls than those who did not use NSAIDs (Findley & Bulloch, 2015). These data are supported by an earlier study of fall risk that reported a 10-fold increase in likelihood of fall in older adults who took NSAIDs (Walker, Alrawi, Mitchell, Regal, & Khanderia, 2005). Older adults have more illnesses and take more medications than younger patients; therefore, older adults who take NSAIDs may be at increased risk for drug-disease and drug-drug interactions (Gnjidic et al., 2014).

When considering NSAID use for older adults, the risks need to be weighed against the benefits to determine if NSAID use is appropriate. For example, the older adult with rheumatoid arthritis who cannot use his hands without the antiinflammatory benefit of an NSAID may opt to accept the risk associated with NSAID use. It is recommended to reevaluate older adults 2 weeks after the introduction of NSAID therapy to evaluate effectiveness of treatment and assess for GI side effects, monitor blood pressure, and test renal function (Reid, Eccleston, & Pillemer, 2015). As for all patients, NSAIDs should be used at the lowest effective dose for the shortest length of time possible (Pergolizzi et al., 2016).

Patients With End-Stage Renal Disease

In patients with end-stage renal disease (ESRD) on hemodialysis, the risk of NSAID use on residual renal function necessitates avoidance of NSAIDs, if possible, because they may negatively affect dialysis adequacy (Mathew, Bettinger, Wegrzyn, & Fudin, 2016). Use of NSAIDs in this patient population poses other risks. In a case-crossover study of patients on hemodialysis who had suffered stroke, results demonstrated NSAID use, especially parenteral nonselective NSAIDs such as ketorolac, increased the risk for stroke (Hsu et al., 2017). Patients with ESRD receiving hemodialysis are at increased risk for development of other NSAID-related adverse effects such as hypertension and GI bleeding (Heleniak et al., 2017). Although patients with ESRD often experience chronic pain, the use of NSAIDs in a multimodal analgesia plan for these patients requires careful evaluation of the benefits versus the risks associated with their use.

Surgical Patients

Patients are often instructed to discontinue use of NSAIDs 7 to 10 days before surgery, but this is based on aspirin's risk for bleeding and not applicable to all NSAIDs. There are no identified studies that specifically evaluate bleeding risk for traditional NSAIDs. In the absence of prospective randomized trials, the pharmacokinetics of each NSAID is the most reliable guide for discontinuation before surgery. The most useful method to determine when an NSAID should be stopped is to check the drug elimination half-life, which is available in the FDA package insert under pharmacokinetics. Half-life is the amount of time required to decrease an administered dose by 50% in the plasma. Terminal half-life, however, is the amount of time required for plasma concentration to decrease by 50% after steady-state concentration has been established (Waller & Sampson, 2018). After 5 half-lives, roughly 97% of the drug has been eliminated from the body and is the standard for drug clearance. In guidelines developed by the ASRA, European Society of Regional Anaesthesia and Pain Therapy, American Academy of Pain Medicine, International Neuromodulation Society, North American Neuromodulation Society, and World Institute of Pain (Narouze et al., 2015), it is recommended when the exact bleeding risk is unknown, 5 half-lives should be used as the criteria for withholding the individual NSAID before surgery. After surgery, NSAIDs generally can be restarted quickly and may even aid in recovery by reducing postoperative pain, but the risk for postoperative bleeding may be higher after certain surgeries, thus necessitating consideration of individual risk.

Patients Who Have Undergone Bariatric Surgery

It is often recommended to avoid use of NSAIDs after weight loss surgery because of the risk for marginal ulcer development. In "Clinical Practice Guidelines for the Perioperative Nutritional, Metabolic, and Nonsurgical Support of the Bariatric Surgery Patient" (Mechanick et al., 2013), it is recommended to completely refrain from the use of NSAIDs after bariatric surgery, if possible. The guidelines include this recommendation because NSAID use has been associated with development of ulcerations and perforations of the surgical anastomosis; the guidelines include a recommendation for alternative analgesics (Mechanick et al., 2013). A systematic review that included 41 studies with 16,987 patients examined the incidence of marginal ulcer development in patients who had undergone laparoscopic Roux-en-Y gastric bypass; NSAID use, the position and size of the pouch, and smoking were associated with marginal ulceration (Coblijn, Goucham, Lagarde, Kuiken, & van Wagensveld, 2014).

Although there are recommendations to avoid NSAID use after bariatric surgery, recent interest in Enhanced Recovery After Surgery (ERAS) protocols in laparoscopic bariatric surgeries have resulted in recommendations for the use of NSAIDs in multimodal analgesic plans for postoperative analgesia (Awad et al., 2014; Matłok et al., 2015; Thorell et al., 2016). In a meta analysis of 12 RCTS involving 3829 patients, which examined complications of perioperative NSAID use in bariatric surgery patients, NSAIDs, particularly nonselective ones, increased risks of anastomatic leaks (Peng et al., 2016). Although there are limited studies of possible adverse outcomes related to perioperative use of NSAIDs in this patient population, to avoid potential adverse outcomes, concomitant use of PPIs may be beneficial in reducing ulceration risk (Coblijn et al., 2014).

Orthopedic Patients

NSAIDs as single medications or when used in multimodal analgesic plans of care may provide effective analgesia in a variety of orthopedic conditions (Dunn, Durieux, & Nemergut, 2016; Halawi, Grant, & Bolognesi, 2015; Tosounidis, Sheikh, Stone, & Giannoudis, 2015; Vannucci, Fossi, Gronchi, & Brandi, 2017; Zhang & Zhou, 2017). Over the years there have been debates about the risk of NSAID use and delayed bone healing, and many orthopedic surgeons continue to advise patients to avoid NSAIDs. Although there is evidence in animal studies to support the theory that NSAIDs inhibit bone healing, high-quality clinical studies in humans have not supported this theory (Fader et al., 2018; Richards, Graf, & Mashru, 2017). Two early systematic reviews concluded there is no evidence that NSAIDs inhibit bone healing (Kurmis, Kurmis, O'Brien, & Dalen, 2012; Pountos, Georgouli, Calori, & Giannoudis, 2012).

In a systematic review of 12 clinical articles and 24 literature reviews, there was significant variability in the interpretation of the findings that addressed the impact of NSAIDs on bone-healing; however, the greater number of reviews reported no impact on bone healing. Evidence was not conclusive to support the safe use of NSAIDs on bone healing, but the researchers stated there is no evidence to justify the withholding of NSAIDs in patients who would benefit from these medications for pain management (Marquez-Lara, Hutchinson, Nuñez Jr., Smith, & Miller, 2016). The general agreement among researchers and clinicians is that a short

duration of NSAID therapy after a fracture may be safe in the absence of other nonunion risk factors, and that large, high-quality studies are needed (Richards, Graf, & Mashru, 2017).

Similar debate exists about the use of NSAIDs in patients who have undergone spinal fusion. However, in a systematic review of 138 studies examining the effect of NSAIDS on spinal fusion, studies published after 2005 did not demonstrate any delay in fusion when NSAIDs were used for less than 2 weeks; the researchers concluded it is not contraindicated to use low-dose NSAIDs for a short time after spinal fusion (Sivaganesan, Chotai, White-Dzuro, McGirt, & Devin, 2017).

Acetaminophen

History

Acetaminophen and phenacetin are structurally similar derivatives of aniline dye developed as analgesic and antipyretic agents in the 19th century (Hayward, Powell, Irvine, & Martin, 2016). Phenacetin was widely used in the 20th century until it was recognized that phenacetin was nephrotoxic, and in the 1950s, biochemists Brodie and Axelrod demonstrated that the efficacy of phenacetin was from its active hepatic metabolite, acetaminophen (Brune, Renner, & Tiegs, 2015). Acetaminophen became available in the United States 1955 and elsewhere in the world throughout the 1950s, but it did not gain widespread acceptance until the 1970s because of safety concerns (Bertolini et al., 2006; Brune et al., 2015; Smith, 2009).

Pharmacologic Effects

Acetaminophen is not considered an NSAID and is often categorized as a weak antiinflammatory agent used mainly for reducing pain and fever. Paracetamol is the recommended international nonproprietary name of acetaminophen (Smith, 2009), and it is also known as acetyl-*para*-aminophenol (APAP) from its chemical name, N-acetyl-p-aminophenol (Brenner & Stevens, 2018). Acetaminophen is widely used as a first-line option for acute and chronic pain management because of its relative safety and tolerability.

The mechanism of action of acetaminophen is not well understood but it is thought to have primarily central and some peripheral effects (Graham, Davies, Day, Mohamudally, & Scott, 2013; Smith, 2009). Proposed mechanisms of action are inhibition of PGE_2 synthesis within the central nervous system, activation of spinal serotonergic descending system, interaction with the brain opioid system, interference with nitric oxide generation, and activation of spinal TRPA1 channels by the acetaminophen metabolites (Klinger-Gratz et al., 2017). Over the years there have been attempts to explain the analgesic effects of acetaminophen because, although it has analgesic and antipyretic effects similar to those of aspirin and the other NSAIDs, it lacks significant antiinflammatory effects or antiplatelet effects (Brenner & Stevens, 2018).

It has been proposed that the antiinflammatory effects of acetaminophen may be blocked by peroxides in inflamed tissues (Brenner & Stevens, 2018). Another theory is that acetaminophen inhibits COX-3, a recently identified variant of COX-1 in the brains of dogs (Hazarika & Selvam, 2015; Smith, 2009). Other animal studies point to a role of the cannabinoid system in contributing to the analgesic effect of acetaminophen in acute pain and inflammatory hyperalgesia (Klinger-Gratz et al., 2018). Unlike NSAIDs, acetaminophen is regarded as safe for use in patients at risk for renal impairment and is not associated with cardiovascular, thrombotic, or GI risks (Graham et al., 2013).

Acetaminophen is a weak acid that is essentially neutral at physiologic pH, and the oral formulation is rapidly absorbed from the gut after administration; it has high oral bioavailability (88%) and reaches peak blood concentration in approximately 90 minutes after ingestion (Mazaleuskaya et al., 2015). Intravenous acetaminophen has a faster onset and higher peak concentration than oral administration, but overall exposure is similar to that with the same oral dose. Peak concentration is reached immediately after the 15-minute infusion and is approximately 70% higher than the maximum concentration obtained by oral delivery. It is unknown if the higher peak concentration obtained with intravenous versus oral administration has a clinical benefit, but some studies suggest that timing the infusion before surgical incision provides greater benefit than administration immediately before skin closure (Macario & Royal, 2011). In pharmacodynamic studies, single doses of intravenous acetaminophen up to 3000 mg and repeated doses of 1000 mg every 6 hours for 48 hours have not been shown to cause a significant effect on platelet aggregation and therefore may be a safer alternative to NSAIDs in the perioperative setting (Drugs@FDA: Ofirmev, 2010).

Acetaminophen has minimal binding to plasma proteins and is widely distributed throughout the body (Brenner & Stevens, 2018). Under normal conditions, the majority (~90%) of acetaminophen is conjugated by phase II metabolic pathways into glucuronidated and sulfated metabolites that are then renally eliminated (Brenner & Stevens, 2018; Mazaleuskaya et al., 2015). A small amount (~2%) of acetaminophen is excreted unchanged in the urine. Approximately 10% of acetaminophen is oxidized by hepatic phase I metabolism by CYP2E1, 1A2, and 3A4 enzymes to form the highly reactive toxic metabolite N-acetyl-*para*-benzo-quinone imine (NAPQI). NAPQI is rapidly conjugated by hepatic glutathione (GSH) to form nontoxic compounds, mercaptate and cysteine, that are renally excreted (Mazaleuskaya et al., 2015; McGill & Jaeschke, 2013).

Indications for Use

Acetaminophen is widely used as a first-line option for pain management because of its relative safety and tolerability despite lower efficacy and lack of antiinflammatory properties in comparison to NSAIDs. It is routinely used for management of acute pain. Acetaminophen is available OTC for temporary relief of minor aches and pains caused by the common cold, headache, backache, minor pain of arthritis, toothache, muscular aches, premenstrual and menstrual cramps, and temporary fever reduction.

Intravenous acetaminophen use has become increasingly common for postoperative pain management (Macario, 2011). Intravenous acetaminophen is FDA approved for the management of mild to moderate pain, management of moderate to severe pain with adjunctive opioid analgesics, and reduction of fever (Drugs@FDA: Ofirmev, 2010). An advantage of intravenous acetaminophen is that it can be administered intraoperatively when oral acetaminophen would not be a viable option or postoperatively in patients who are unable to take or absorb oral medications. Several studies have demonstrated intravenous acetaminophen use in the perioperative setting can improve pain control and reduce opioid consumption in the perioperative and ambulatory surgery settings (Macario & Royal, 2011). At the present time, cost is identified as an obstacle to its use (Politi, Davis, & Matrka, 2017); however, the availability of intravenous acetaminophen provides an opportunity for inclusion of acetaminophen in multimodal analgesia plans of care, especially for patients who are unable to use the enteral route.

In an RCT that included 97 patients with elective colorectal procedures during the first 48 postoperative hours, those who received intravenous acetaminophen and intravenous opioid patient-controlled analgesia (PCA) (n = 47) had less opioid use, shorter lengths of hospital stay, better pain control, more rapid return of bowel function, and less postoperative ileus than those who received placebo and intravenous opioid PCA (n = 50) (Aryaie et al., 2018). In a meta-analysis of four studies that included 865 postoperative patients who underwent knee and hip total joint arthroplasty, intravenous acetaminophen, compared to placebo, was associated with significant reductions in pain scores and opioid consumption, as well as nausea and vomiting; the researchers identified the need for more RCTs due to the limited quality of currently available evidence (Liang, Cai, Li, & Ma, 2017).

In a retrospective analysis of data from the Premier Database, a database that contains inpatient information from participating hospitals across the United States, patients who had undergone orthopedic surgery who received both intravenous acetaminophen and intravenous opioids for postoperative analgesia had shorter hospital stays (reduced by 0.51 days), lower hospital costs ($634.8 less), and less opioid use than those who received only intravenous opioids (Hansen, Pham, Strassels, Balaban, & Wan, 2016). Similar outcomes, including reduced adverse effects, decreased length of stay, and lowered hospital costs, were found in an earlier review of the Premier Database that included matched-pairs analysis of adult inpatients who underwent elective total hip arthroplasty or total knee arthroplasty (Apfel, Jahr, Kelly, Ang, & Oderda, 2015).

As addressed in the NSAID section, guidelines for the management of acute postoperative pain include strong recommendation with high-quality evidence for the inclusion of acetaminophen and/or NSAIDs (unless contraindicated) in a multimodal treatment plan (Chou et al., 2016). In general, acetaminophen, when used with other pain relievers, including NSAIDs and opioids, can have a synergistic and dose-sparing effect. A double-blind clinical trial of 90 patients who underwent cesarean section illustrates the synergistic effect of acetaminophen when used along with an NSAID; pain scores and opioid requirements were significantly lower in the group that received a combination of acetaminophen and diclofenac suppository than for those who received either medication as a single agent (Bakhsha, Niaki, Jafari, Yousefi, & Aryaie, 2016). In a study of 408 patients who underwent removal of at least two impacted third molars, pain relief was greater and more rapid during the first 48 hours after molar removal in the group who received a fixed-dose combination of acetaminophen and ibuprofen, than in groups who received acetaminophen, ibuprofen, or placebo as monotherapy (Daniels, Atkinson, Stanescu, & Frampton, 2018).

A systematic review of 5 RCTs that examined interventions to treat acute pain after oral surgery identified pain as significantly better controlled in those who received a combination of acetaminophen and NSAIDs, compared to either medication alone; side effects were less in the combination group than in the ibuprofen monotherapy group (Alexander, Hall, Eriksson, & Rohlin, 2014). In a systematic review with network meta-analysis of RCTs that compared outcomes of postoperative pain therapies, the combination of acetaminophen with NSAIDs or nefopam (a nonopioid, nonsteroidal drug not available in the United States) was superior to other analgesics used alone (traMADol, corticosteroids, and metamizole) in reducing morphine PCA requirements (Martinez et al., 2016).

Routes, Formulations, and Dosing

Acetaminophen is widely available OTC as single-ingredient and in combination products for a variety of ailments, including cold, cough, allergy, and pain. It is also combined with opioids such as HYDROcodone and oxyCODONE for synergistic analgesic effect; the addition of acetaminophen to these medications may limit opioid use because of the risk of hepatotoxicity associated with over-ingestion of the acetaminophen component. Acetaminophen is also available in many formulations, including oral, liquid, rectal, and intravenous routes.

Dosing of acetaminophen will vary based on the patient population (i.e., adult, pediatric, infant), specific product, and route of administration. In general, acetaminophen for adults is dosed every 4 to 6 hours and the dose for an adult (who does not have factors that require dose limitations) should not exceed 4000 mg/day. For frail older patients, it is recommended to limit acetaminophen to 3000 mg/day because of age-related decline

Table 10.7 | Acetaminophen Formulations and Strengths

Dosage Formulation	Strength(s)
Tablet	325, 500 mg
Tablet, dispersible	80, 160 mg
Tablet, chewable	80 mg
Tablet, extended-release	650 mg
Capsule	500 mg
Oral solution	80 mg/0.8 mL, 100 mg/mL, 160 mg/5 mL, 325 mg/5 mL, 500 mg/15 mL, 1000 mg/30 mL
Oral suspension	80 mg/0.8 mL, 160 mg/5 mL
Oral gel	160 mg/5 mL
Rectal suppository	80, 120, 325, 650 mg
Intravenous	10 mg/mL

Data from: Malotte, K., & McPherson, M. L. (2015). *Acetaminophen: Information that patients need to know about their medication.* Retrieved April 30, 2020 from https://www.practicalpainmanagement.com/sites/default/files/acetaminophen%20.pdf.

in liver function (Bartoszczyk & Herr, 2016; Cornelius, Herr, Gordon, & Kretzer, 2017; Herndon et al., 2016). See Table 10.7 for commonly used acetaminophen formulations and strengths.

Dosage of intravenous acetaminophen is the same as oral dosing. Adults and adolescents weighing 50 kg and over, may be administered 1000 mg every 6 hours or 650 mg every 4 hours to a maximum of 4000 mg/day; intravenous acetaminophen may be administered without further dilution as a single or repeated dose as a 15-minute intravenous infusion (Drugs@FDA: Ofirmev, 2010). If doses less than 1000 mg are used, the appropriate dose must be withdrawn from the vial and placed into a separate container before administration (Drugs@FDA: Ofirmev, 2010). Precautions for the use of intravenous acetaminophen are similar to warnings with use of oral acetaminophen. Patients with hepatic impairment or active hepatic disease, alcoholism, chronic malnutrition, severe hypovolemia, or severe renal impairment (creatinine clearance ≤ 30 mL/min) may not be ideal candidates for intravenous acetaminophen.

Adverse Effects

In a systematic review that examined the long-term observational evidence of adverse effects associated with acetaminophen, the authors reported a dose-response relationship between acetaminophen and risks for mortality, GI bleeding, and cardiovascular and renal adverse events similar to those associated with NSAIDs (Roberts et al., 2015). The investigators acknowledged the limitations of the data, particularly because all studies were observational, contained multiple sources of potential bias, and called for further meta-analyses. Roberts et al. (2015) recommended careful consideration of risk when the analgesic benefit is unclear, as in the case of low back, hip, and knee osteoarthritis-related pain, and advised increased awareness of adverse effects associated with higher doses. Battaggia et al. (2016), in a critical review of the publication by Roberts et al. (2015), cited study limitations, including multiple sources of bias, and endorsed the need for high quality studies to further examine the safety issues related to acetaminophen use.

Hepatotoxicity

Hepatotoxicity is caused by accumulation of the NAPQI metabolite of acetaminophen. At hepatotoxic doses of acetaminophen, the primary phase II metabolic pathways are saturated and metabolism to NAPQI becomes the major metabolic pathway. Hepatic GSH that normally functions to convert NAPQI to nontoxic compounds becomes depleted, and reactive NAPQI binds to hepatocytes, causing oxidative injury and hepatocellular necrosis (Yoon, Babar, Choudhary, Kutner, & Pyrsopoulos, 2016).

Dose and pattern of use (acute high doses) of acetaminophen are primary factors related to development of hepatotoxicity; patient-specific factors that increase the risk for acetaminophen-induced hepatotoxicity include advanced age, genetic factors, malnutrition, preexisting liver dysfunction, concurrent hepatically metabolized drugs and herbal supplements, and chronic alcohol consumption (Yoon et al., 2016).

Early identification of acetaminophen toxicity is imperative for early treatment to prevent morbidity and mortality. It is estimated that more than half of all hepatotoxic acetaminophen cases are unintentional, and a large number of these cases result from ingestion of acetaminophen combination products, including acetaminophen with opioids (Serper et al., 2016). Research is needed to determine whether ingestion from single acetaminophen products results in a different pattern of hepatotoxicity from ingestion of combination acetaminophen products. It is essential to ensure patient education related to maximum acetaminophen doses, and ensure patients are aware of the need to read labels and avoid concurrent use of multiple OTC and prescription acetaminophen-containing products to reduce toxicity risks.

Clinical manifestations of acetaminophen overdose can be described by four sequential stages:

- Stage I occurs within 24 hours of overdose and is characterized by nonspecific symptoms of malaise, nausea, vomiting, and diaphoresis, with normal or elevated liver enzymes depending on the magnitude of the overdose.
- Stage II is generally within 24 to 72 hours of overdose and is also known as the latent period because of an improvement in symptoms but is characterized by elevations of aspartate aminotransferase (AST) and alanine aminotransferase (ALT).
- Stage III occurs between 72 and 96 hours of overdose and has the highest risk for mortality because of multiorgan failure. Stage III is characterized by a return of stage I symptoms, marked liver enzyme elevation, coagulopathy, jaundice, encephalopathy, and lactic acidosis.
- Stage IV is the recovery phase, which typically lasts 1 to 2 weeks, but duration can be prolonged based on the severity of the overdose (Yoon et al., 2016).

Treatment of Hepatotoxicity

The management of acute overingestion of acetaminophen depends on how quickly a patient presents for treatment. If medical attention is sought promptly, typically within 4 hours of ingestion, physical prevention of acetaminophen absorption may be an effective method to prevent toxicity. In a Cochrane Review of studies that examined interventions for acetaminophen overdose, reduction of acetaminophen absorption through administration of activated charcoal had a better risk-to-benefit ratio than gastric lavage or induced emesis (Chiew, Gluud, Brok, & Buckley, 2018). Patients at high risk for development of acetaminophen-induced hepatotoxicity, those in whom treatment was delayed more than 4 hours after ingestion, or those with established hepatotoxicity are usually treated with N-acetylcysteine; administration replenishes cellular GSH stores and can repair oxidative damage if it is administered within 8 to 10 hours of acetaminophen ingestion (Bateman, 2016). In cases of severe irreversible liver failure, liver transplantation can be considered as a life-saving measure (Lancaster, Hiatt, & Zarrinpar, 2015).

FDA Warnings

Overdose of acetaminophen is the most common cause of acute liver failure in the United States because of both intentional and nonintentional overdose (Yoon et al., 2016). The risk for hepatotoxicity is low, with doses up to 4000 mg/day per the FDA. Beginning in 2011 the FDA requested drug manufacturers to limit the amount of acetaminophen to 325 mg per dosage unit in combination with prescription medications, primarily opioid medications, including oxyCODONE, HYDROcodone, and codeine. The FDA also mandated the inclusion of a boxed warning highlighting the potential for severe liver injury (FDA Drug Safety, 2011). Although not required by the FDA, the maker of brand name acetaminophen products, McNeil-PPC, Inc., began revising OTC labels for products containing acetaminophen to limit daily doses to 3000 mg/day in an attempt to reduce the risk for accidental overdose (McNeil Consumer Healthcare, 2011). In 2013 the FDA released a safety announcement regarding the risk for developing Stevens-Johnson syndrome, a rare but serious skin reaction that may occur with acetaminophen or acetaminophen-containing products (FDA Drug Safety, 2013). The FDA requires all prescription drug products containing acetaminophen and all new OTC products to include a warning of skin reactions on the product label (FDA Drug Safety, 2013).

Monitoring of Patients

It is important to obtain a history of all medications that a patient is taking, OTC and prescribed, to identify possible multiple sources of acetaminophen use. The total daily dose and duration of acetaminophen therapy should be monitored. In situations of chronic ingestion, monitoring of hepatic function may be appropriate, especially in patients at high risk for hepatotoxicity, such as those with advanced age and those who chronically abuse alcohol. Effective relief of symptoms also should be evaluated.

Use in Special Populations

Older Adults
Acetaminophen has been considered a first-line analgesic for older patients with acute and chronic mild to moderate pain, particularly with musculoskeletal pain (Abdulla et al., 2013). Although the use of acetaminophen has been recommended to improve physical function, including activities of daily living participation and sleep (Dentino, Medina, & Steinberg, 2017), recent evidence demonstrates uncertain effectiveness and increased risks (Marcum, Duncan, & Makris, 2016). In a systematic review examining the efficacy and safety of acetaminophen (paracetamol) compared to placebo in those with spine, hip, and knee pain related to osteoarthritis, acetaminophen was not effective in improving pain, disability, or quality of life in those with low back pain and provided a small, but not clinically significant, improvement in pain and disability for those with hip and knee osteoarthritis (Machado et al., 2015). This review was limited to the short-term effects of acetaminophen use. Participants who took acetaminophen were more likely to have elevations in their liver function tests (compared to placebo), but the significance of the elevation was unclear (Machado et al., 2015).

Patients With Liver Disease
Acetaminophen may be used in patients with cirrhosis in reduced doses of 2 to 3 g/day (Hayward, Powell, Irvine, & Martin, 2016; Hong et al., 2016; Imani, Motavaf, Safari, & Alavian, 2014). However, in a summary of existing literature related to the use of analgesics in patients with cirrhosis, a dose limitation of 2 g/day is recommended (Rakoski et al., 2018). In a review of analgesic use in those with liver cirrhosis, acetaminophen at reduced doses of 2 to 3 g/day was found to be safe for long-term use (in excess of 14 days) (Imani et al., 2014). When used at recommended doses, acetaminophen is the preferred analgesic in those with liver disease, including cirrhosis, because of its lack of renal toxicity and absence of sedating effects (Imani et al., 2014). Cautious dosing and monitoring of the response to

acetaminophen is needed, particularly in patients with viral hepatitis or who are actively using alcohol or are malnourished or underweight (Imani et al., 2014).

Patients With Impaired Renal Function
Acetaminophen used at the recommended dosing has not been associated with acute nephrotoxicity (Hiragi et al., 2018). In a review of extrahepatic effects of acetaminophen, Kennon-McGill and McGill (2018) noted acetaminophen overdose has been demonstrated with renal toxicity, although the mechanisms are unknown. No evidence was identified to suggest acetaminophen-related extrahepatic toxicity with recommended doses.

Multimodal Use of Nonopioid Analgesics

Acetaminophen and NSAIDs, including celecoxib, are nonopioid analgesics that provide relief of mild to moderate pain when used as single agents. In recent years, researchers have examined effects of acetaminophen, NSAIDs, and COX-2 inhibitors use as single agents, or in combination with each other, and in combination with other coanalgesic medications in multimodal analgesic plans. End-points in these studies included opioid-sparing effects, analgesia, adverse effects, and patient satisfaction. In a randomized, multicenter, noninferiority study of patients with acute musculoskeletal trauma, combined treatment with diclofenac (an NSAID), and acetaminophen provided better analgesia than either medication alone, but acetaminophen as monotherapy was not found to provide inferior relief to the combined medications or diclofenac (Ridderikhof et al., 2018). In a scientific review of intravenous acetaminophen and ibuprofen for perioperative and postoperative pain management, both were found to be safe and effective when used as recommended, and when used as monotherapy or in combination, were found to reduce pain, fever, and opioid use (Koh, Nguyen, & Jahr, 2015).

The American Society of Anesthesiologists Task Force on Acute Pain Management (2012), in their guidelines for the perioperative management of acute pain, recommended, unless contraindicated, patients should receive an around-the-clock regimen of acetaminophen, NSAIDs, or COX-2 inhibitor. Similarly, in a clinical practice guideline developed through a joint effort by the APS, the American Society of Regional Anesthesia and Pain Management, the American Society of Anesthesiologists' Committee on Regional Anesthesia, and others, a preoperative dose of celecoxib was recommended, unless contraindicated. The use of acetaminophen, NSAIDs, or both, unless contraindicated, is also recommended as multimodal analgesia in patients with postoperative pain (Chou et al., 2016).

Acetaminophen and NSAIDs are associated with adverse effects, described earlier in this chapter. During the use of these medications in a multimodal plan of care, dosing precautions are required to prevent adverse effects; patient assessment for adverse effects and prompt treatment are necessary. Box 10.2 summarizes adverse effects of nonopioid analgesics and preventive and treatment measures.

Key Points

- Nonopioid analgesics, including NSAIDs and acetaminophen, may provide effective analgesia as single agents or when used in combination with other analgesic modalities in a multimodal analgesic plan.
- NSAIDs and acetaminophen are available OTC and in combination with other products, including prescription opioids, and patient education is essential to avoid toxicity related to overdose.
- Unless contraindicated, an NSAID and acetaminophen should be scheduled around the clock in the management of acute postoperative pain.
- Availability of NSAIDs and acetaminophen in a variety of formulations provide options for inclusion of these medications in multimodal analgesic plans for patients with a variety of medical conditions.
- Aspirin and NSAIDs reduce pain, inflammation, and fever by inhibition of prostaglandin synthesis.
- Aspirin and NSAIDs, through inhibition of prostaglandin synthesis, inhibit COX -1 and COX-2 enzymes. COX-2 inhibition is responsible for the antiinflammatory and analgesic effect of these medications.
- Aspirin and NSAIDs are associated with a number of risk factors, and their use in a multimodal analgesic plan must include consideration of risk versus benefit.
- When aspirin is used for cardiac protection, and a nonaspirin NSAID is used for other indications, the aspirin should be taken at least 30 minutes before the nonaspirin NSAID.
- Different NSAID preparations provide varying degrees of COX-1 and COX-2 inhibition. Inhibitory effects of the different medications should be considered in NSAID selection and dosing to reduce adverse effects.
  - COX-1 inhibition is responsible for inhibition of platelet function and may increase bleeding risks, particularly GI bleeding. GI bleeding risk is also increased because COX-1 plays a role in gastric epithelial cytoprotection, and NSAIDs are weak acids. Patients on nonselective NSAIDS who are at higher risk for GI bleeding (i.e., high doses, older patients, long-term therapy) may benefit from coadministration of gastroprotective agents such as proton pump inhibitors.
  - COX-2 inhibitors (celecoxib) are not associated with the same degree of GI bleeding risk as nonselective agents, but if used in combination with aspirin, gastroprotection is recommended.

- NSAIDs, particularly COX-2 inhibitors (celecoxib) pose increased cardiovascular risks, including hypertension, in those with cardiovascular risk factors.
- NSAIDs can cause adverse renal effects, such as acute renal injury, and risk is increased in those who are dehydrated or are on ACE or ARB medications, or on diuretics. Older patients, those with diabetes, renal insufficiency, ascites, or heart failure may be at increased risk.
- Nanotechnology and topical NSAIDs may improve NSAID-related safety.
- Acetaminophen is not an NSAID and is regarded as an analgesic agent and weak antiinflammatory drug.
  - Acetaminophen is recommended as a first-line analgesic for acute and chronic pain management because of its relative safety and tolerability.
  - Acetaminophen is available OTC as a single agent and in combination with other OTC and prescription medications, including opioids, thus increasing risks for acetaminophen toxicity. Acetaminophen toxicity is the major cause of acute liver failure.
- Acetaminophen dosing should be reduced in older patients and in those with liver disease. It is necessary to carefully consider individual patient characteristics and weigh the risks versus the benefits of acetaminophen use.

Case Scenario

Robert L., 76 years old, is transferred to a surgical floor after an open cholecystectomy and is reporting severe surgical site pain that increases with cough and movement. He has intravenous HYDROmorphone prescribed as needed *(prn)* for pain and is experiencing nausea and pruritus with use of HYDROmorphone. The surgical team members are trying to minimize Robert's opioid intake because they are concerned about adverse effects.

1. What other assessment information is needed to use nonopioid analgesics in developing a multimodal pain management plan?
2. What are the possible patient-specific barriers to use of nonopioid analgesics in the multimodal analgesic plan? Include indications and contraindications for use of acetaminophen and/or NSAIDs.
3. What are the possible organizational barriers to use of nonopioid analgesics in the multimodal analgesic plan, and what strategies can you use to address them?
4. Robert L. may report that acetaminophen will not work for him because it never works when he has a headache. How can you respond?
5. How might the multimodal analgesic plan be adjusted if Robert L. has a history of nonalcoholic cirrhosis?

References

Abdulla, A., Adams, N., Bone, M., Elliott, A. M., Gaffin, J., Jones, D., et al. (2013). Guidance on the management of pain in older people. *Age and Ageing, 42,* i1–i57.

Alexander, L., Hall, E., Eriksson, L., & Rohlin, M. (2014). The combination of non-selective NSAID 400 mg and paracetamol 1000 mg is more effective than each drug alone for treatment of acute pain. A systematic review. *Swedish Dental Journal, 38*(1), 1–14.

AlHajri, L. (2017). Enteric-Coated, extended-release and sustained-release formulations of NSAIDs: Do they reduce GI risks? *Annals of Pharmacotherapy, 51*(4), 354–356.

Altman, R., Bosch, B., Brune, K., Patrignani, P., & Young, C. (2015). Advances in NSAID development: evolution of diclofenac products using pharmaceutical technology. *Drugs, 75*(8), 859–877.

2019 American Geriatrics Society Beers Criteria® Update Expert Panel, Fick, D. M., Semla, T. P., Steinman, M., Beizer, J., Brandt, N., … Flanagan, N. (2019). American Geriatrics Society 2019 updated AGS Beers Criteria® for potentially inappropriate medication use in older adults. *Journal of the American Geriatrics Society, 67*(4), 674–694.

American Society of Anesthesiologists Task Force on Acute Pain Management. (2012). Practice guidelines for acute pain management in the perioperative setting: an updated report by the American Society of Anesthesiologists Task Force on Acute Pain Management. *Anesthesiology, 116,* 248–273.

Anwar, A., Anwar, I. J., & Delafontaine, P. (2015). Elevation of cardiovascular risk by non-steroidal anti-inflammatory drugs. *Trends in Cardiovascular Medicine, 25*(8), 726–735.

Apfel, C., Jahr, J. R., Kelly, C. L., Ang, R. Y., & Oderda, G. M. (2015). Effect of IV acetaminophen on total hip or knee replacement surgery: a case-matched evaluation of a national patient database. *American Journal of Health-System Pharmacy, 72*(22), 1961–1968.

Aryaie, A. H., Lalezari, S., Sergent, W. K., Puckett, Y., Juergens, C., Ratermann, C., et al. (2018). Decreased opioid consumption and enhance recovery with the addition of IV Acetaminophen in colorectal patients: a prospective, multi-institutional, randomized, double-blinded, placebo-controlled study (DOCIVA study). *Surgical Endoscopy, 38*(8), 3432–3438.

Auriel, E., Regev, K., & Korczyn, A. D. (2014). Nonsteroidal anti-inflammatory drugs exposure and the central nervous system. *Handbook of Clinical Neurology: Vol. 119* (pp. 577–584). St. Louis: Elsevier.

Awad, S., Carter, S., Purkayastha, S., Hakky, S., Moorthy, K., Cousins, J., et al. (2014). Enhanced recovery after bariatric surgery (ERABS): clinical outcomes from a tertiary referral bariatric centre. *Obesity Surgery, 24*(5), 753–758.

Bakhsha, F., Niaki, A. S., Jafari, S. Y., Yousefi, Z., & Aryaie, M. (2016). The effects of diclofenac suppository and intravenous acetaminophen and their combination on the severity of postoperative pain in patients undergoing spinal anaesthesia during cesarean section. *Journal of Clinical and Diagnostic Research: JCDR, 10*(7), UC09.

Bannuru, R. R., Schmid, C. H., Kent, D. M., Vaysbrot, E. E., Wong, J. B., & McAlindon, T. E. (2015). Comparative effectiveness of pharmacologic interventions for knee osteoarthritis: a systematic review and network meta-analysis. *Annals of Internal Medicine, 162*(1), 46–54.

Bartoszczyk, D. A., & Herr, K. A. (2016). Managing pain in frail elders. *American Nurse Today, 11*(4).

Bateman, D. N. (2016). Acetaminophen (paracetamol). *Critical Care Toxicology,* 1–25.

Battaggia, A., Aprile, P. L., Cricelli, I., Fornasari, D., Fanelli, A., Cricelli, C., et al. (2016). Paracetamol: A probably still safe drug. *Annals of the Rheumatic Diseases,* https://doi.org/10.1136/annrheumdis-2016-209713.

Bello, A. E., Kent, J. D., Grahn, A. Y., Ball, J., & Holt, R. J. (2015). One-year open-label safety evaluation of the fixed combination of ibuprofen and famotidine with a prospective analysis of dyspepsia. *Current Medical Research and Opinion, 31*(3), 397–405.

Bertolini, A., Ferrari, A., Ottani, A., Guerzoni, S., Tacchi, R., & Leone, S. (2006). Paracetamol: New vistas of an old drug. *CNS Drug Reviews, 12*(3-4), 250–275.

Brenner, G. M., & Stevens, C. W. (2018). *Drugs for pain, inflammation, and arthritic disorders.* In *Brenner & Stevens' Pharmacology* (5th Edition, p. 30): Elsevier. 343-356.

Brune, K., & Patrignani, P. (2015). New insights into the use of currently available non-steroidal anti-inflammatory drugs. *Journal of Pain Research, 8,* 105.118.

Brune, K., Renner, B., & Tiegs, G. (2015). Acetaminophen/paracetamol: A history of errors, failures and false decisions. *European Journal of Pain, 19*(7), 953–965.

Burke, M., R Pabbidi, M., Farley, J., & J Roman, R. (2014). Molecular mechanisms of renal blood flow autoregulation. *Current Vascular Pharmacology, 12*(6), 845–858.

Center for Drug Evaluation and Research. (2008). *Application 02-029 [SALONPAS patch (l-menthol 3%/methyl salicylate 10%)].* FDA Medical Review, Summary Review. Retrieved June 10, 2017 from https://www.accessdata.fda.gov/drugsatfda_docs/nda/2008/022029s000sumr.pdf.

Chandra Sekhar, G., Pathapati, R. M., Varalakshmi, U., Harshita, S. S., & Patra, R. (2015). Head-to-head comparison of tolerability and acceptability of single dose of four topical NSAIDS in patients undergoing cataract surgery: A randomized open label parallel group study. *Journal of Evidence based Medicine and Healthcare, 2*(31), 4568–4573.

Chiew, A. L., Gluud, C., Brok, J., & Buckley, N. A. (2018). Interventions for paracetamol (acetaminophen) overdose. *Cochrane Database of Systematic Reviews, 2,* CD003328.

Chou, R., Gordon, D. B., de Leon-Casasola, O. A., Rosenberg, J. M., Bickler, S., Brennan, T., … Griffith, S. (2016). Management of postoperative pain: A clinical practice guideline from the American Pain Society, the American Society of Regional Anesthesia and Committee on Regional Anesthesia, Executive Committee, and Administrative Council. *The Journal of Pain, 17*(2), 131–157.

Coblijn, U. K., Goucham, A. B., Lagarde, S. M., Kuiken, S. D., & van Wagensveld, B. A. (2014). Development of ulcer disease after Roux-en-Y gastric bypass, incidence, risk factors, and patient presentation: A systematic review. *Obesity Surgery, 24*(2), 299–309.

Cornelius, R., Herr, K. A., Gordon, D. B., & Kretzer, K. (2017). Acute Pain Management in Older Adults. *Journal of Gerontological Nursing, 43*(2), 18–27.

Daniels, S. E., Atkinson, H. C., Stanescu, I., & Frampton, C. (2018). Analgesic efficacy of an acetaminophen/ibuprofen fixed-dose combination in moderate to severe postoperative dental pain: A randomized, double-blind, parallel-group, placebo-controlled trial. *Clinical Therapeutics, 40*(10), 1765–1776.

Deardorff, W. J., & Grossberg, G. T. (2017). Targeting neuroinflammation in Alzheimer's disease: evidence for NSAIDs and novel therapeutics. *Expert Review of Neurotherapeutics, 17*(1), 17–32.

Dentino, A., Medina, R., & Steinberg, E. (2017). Pain in the elderly: Identification, evaluation, and management of older adults with pain complaints and pain-related symptoms. *Primary Care, 44*(3), 519–528.

Derry, S., Matthews, P. R., Wiffen, P. J., & Moore, R. A. (2014). Salicylate-containing rubefacients for acute and chronic musculoskeletal pain in adults. *The Cochrane Library,* (11), CD007403.

Derry, S., Wiffen, P. J., Kalso, E. A., Bell, R. F., Aldington, D., Phillips, T., et al. (2017). Topical analgesics for acute and chronic pain in adults-an overview of Cochrane Reviews. *Cochrane Database of Systematic Reviews,* (5), CD008609.

Desborough, M. J., & Keeling, D. M. (2017). The aspirin story: from willow to wonder drug. *British Journal of Haematology, 177*(5), 674–683.

Dowell, D., Haegerich, T. M., & Chou, R. (2016). CDC guideline for prescribing opioids for chronic pain—United States, 2016. *Journal of the American Medical Association, 315*(15), 1624–1645.

Dreischulte, T., Morales, D. R., Bell, S., & Guthrie, B. (2015). Combined use of nonsteroidal anti-inflammatory drugs with diuretics and/or renin–angiotensin system inhibitors in the community increases the risk of acute kidney injury. *Kidney International, 88*(2), 396–403.

Drugs@FDA. Caldolor® (ibuprofen) [Package Insert]. April 2016a. Retrieved July 27, 2017, from https://www.accessdata.fda.gov/drugsatfda_docs/label/2016/022348s010lbl.pdf.

Drugs@FDA. Cytotec® (misoprostol) [Package Insert]. December 2016b. Retrieved January 25, 2018a, from https://www.accessdata.fda.gov/drugsatfda_docs/label/2016/019268Orig1s049lbl.pdf.

Drugs@FDA. Indocin® (Indomethacin) [Package Insert]. June 10, 1965. Retrieved June 19, 2019 from: https://www.accessdata.fda.gov/drugsatfda_docs/label/2006/018332s029_017814s039_016059s096lbl.pdf.

Drugs@FDA. Ofirmev™ (Acetaminophen Injection) [Package Insert]. November 2010. Retrieved January 25, 2018b, from https://www.accessdata.fda.gov/drugsatfda_docs/label/2010/022450lbl.pdf.

Drugs@FDA. Toradol® (Ketorolac Tromethamine) [Package Insert]. March, 2014. Retrieved April 27, 2020 from https://www.accessdata.fda.gov/drugsatfda_docs/label/2014/074802s038lbl.pdf.

Dunn, L. K., Durieux, M. E., & Nemergut, E. C. (2016). Nonopioid analgesics: Novel approaches to perioperative analgesia for major spine surgery. *Best Practice & Research Clinical Anaesthesiology, 30*(1), 79–89.

Elkomy, M. H., Elmenshawe, S. F., Eid, H. M., & Ali, A. M. (2016). Topical ketoprofen nanogel: Artificial neural network optimization, clustered bootstrap validation, and in vivo activity evaluation based on longitudinal dose response modeling. *Drug Delivery, 23*(9), 3294–3306.

Etteri, M., Maj, M., Maino, C., & Valli, R. (2018). Intranasal ketorolac and opioid in treatment of acute renal colic. *Emergency Care Journal, 14*(1).

Fader, L., Whitaker, J., Lopez, M., Vivace, B., Parra, M., Carlson, J., et al. (2018). Tibia fractures and NSAIDs. Does it make a difference? A multicenter retrospective study. *Injury, 49*(12), 2290–2294.

Fanelli, A., Ghisi, D., Aprile, P. L., & Lapi, F. (2017). Cardiovascular and cerebrovascular risk with nonsteroidal anti-inflammatory drugs and cyclooxygenase 2 inhibitors: Latest evidence and clinical implications. *Therapeutic Advances in Drug Safety, 8*(6), 173–182.

Farber, H. R., Yiengst, M. J., & Shock, N. W. (1949). The effect of therapeutic doses of aspirin on the acid-base balance of the blood in normal adults. *The American Journal of the Medical Sciences, 217*(3), 256–262.

Findley, L. R., & Bulloch, M. N. (2015). Relationship between nonsteroidal anti-inflammatory drugs and fall risk in older adults. *The Consultant Pharmacist, 30*(6), 346–351.

Floor-Schreudering, A., Smet, P. A. D., Buurma, H., Kramers, C., Tromp, P. C., Belitser, S. V., et al. (2015). NSAID–antihypertensive drug interactions: Which outpatients are at risk for a rise in systolic blood pressure? *European Journal of Preventive Cardiology, 22*(1), 91–99.

Furst, D. E. (1994). Are there differences among nonsteroidal anti-inflammatory drugs? *Arthritis & Rheumatology, 37*(1), 1–9.

Gnjidic, D., Blyth, F. M., Le Couteur, D. G., Cumming, R. G., McLachlan, A. J., Handelsman, D. J., et al. (2014). Nonsteroidal anti-inflammatory drugs (NSAIDs) in older people: Prescribing patterns according to pain prevalence and adherence to clinical guidelines. *PAIN, 155*(9), 1814–1820.

Goldstein, J. L., & Cryer, B. (2015). Gastrointestinal injury associated with NSAID use: A case study and review of risk factors and preventative strategies. *Drug, Healthcare and Patient Safety, 7,* 31.

Goodwin, J. S., & Regan, M. (1982). Cognitive dysfunction associated with naproxen and ibuprofen in the elderly. *Arthritis & Rheumatism, 25*(8), 1013–1015.

Graham, G. G., Davies, M. J., Day, R. O., Mohamudally, A., & Scott, K. F. (2013). The modern pharmacology of paracetamol: therapeutic actions, mechanism of action, metabolism, toxicity and recent pharmacological findings. *Inflammopharmacology, 21*(3), 201–232.

Halawi, M. J., Grant, S. A., & Bolognesi, M. P. (2015). Multimodal analgesia for total joint arthroplasty. *Orthopedics, 38*(7), e616–e625.

Hansen, R. N., Pham, A., Strassels, S. A., Balaban, S., & Wan, G. J. (2016). Comparative analysis of length of stay and inpatient costs for orthopedic surgery patients treated with IV acetaminophen and IV opioids vs. IV opioids alone for post-operative pain. *Advances in Therapy, 33*(9), 1635–1645.

Hayward, K. L., Powell, E. E., Irvine, K. M., & Martin, J. H. (2016). Can paracetamol (acetaminophen) be administered to patients with liver impairment? *British Journal of Clinical Pharmacology, 81*(2), 210–222.

Hazarika, I., & Selvam, P. (2015). Cyclooxygenase 3 inhibition: A probable mechanism of acetaminophen in human-A Review. *Research & Reviews, 6*(3), 23–29. 2015.

Heleniak, Z., Cieplińska, M., Szychliński, T., Rychter, D., Jagodzińska, K., Kłos, A., et al. (2017). Nonsteroidal anti-inflammatory drug use in patients with chronic kidney disease. *Journal of Nephrology, 30*(6), 781–786.

Henry, D., Lim, L. L., Rodriguez, L. A. G., Gutthann, S. P., Carson, J. L., Griffin, M., ... Hill, S. (1996). Variability in risk of gastrointestinal complications with individual non-steroidal anti-inflammatory drugs: results of a collaborative meta-analysis. *British Medical Journal, 312*(7046), 1563–1566.

Herndon, C. M., Arnstein, P., Darnall, B., Hartrick, C., Hecht, K., Lyons, M., et al. (2016). *Principles of Analgesic Use.* Chicago, Ill: American Pain Society.

Hiragi, S., Yamada, H., Tsukamoto, T., Yoshida, K., Kondo, N., Matsubara, et al. (2018). Acetaminophen administration and the risk of acute kidney injury: A self-controlled case series study. *Clinical Epidemiology, 10*, 265–276.

Hochberg, M. C., Altman, R. D., April, K. T., Benkhalti, M., Guyatt, G., McGowan, J., et al. (2012). American College of Rheumatology 2012 Recommendations for the Use of Nonpharmacologic and Pharmacologic Therapies for in Osteoarthritis of the Hand, Hip, and Knee. *Arthritis Care & Research, 64*(4), 465–474.

Hong, Y. M., Yoon, K. T., Heo, J., Woo, H. Y., Lim, W., An, D. S., et al. (2016). The prescription pattern of acetaminophen and non-steroidal anti-inflammatory drugs in patients with liver cirrhosis. *Journal of Korean Medical Science, 31*(10), 1604–1610.

Hsu, C. C., Chang, Y. K., Hsu, Y. H., Lo, Y. R., Liu, J. S., Hsiung, C. A., & Tsai, H. J. (2017). Association of non-steroidal anti-inflammatory drug use with stroke among dialysis patients. *Kidney International Reports, 2*(3), 400–409.

Imani, F., Motavaf, M., Safari, S., & Alavian, S. M. (2014). The therapeutic use of analgesics in patients with liver cirrhosis: a literature review and evidence-based recommendations. *Hepatitis Monthly, 14*(10).

Jain, K., Mehra, N. K., & Jain, N. K. (2014). Potentials and emerging trends in nanopharmacology. *Current Opinion in Pharmacology, 15*, 97–106.

Joint Commission. (2012). *Sentinel event alert issue 49: Safe use of opioids in hospitals (August 8, 2012).*

Joint Commission, (2017) Pain assessment and management standards for hospitals. *R3 Report; Requirement, Rationale, Reference, Issue 11.* Retrieved 4 July 2019 from https://jntcm.ae-admin.com/assets/1/6/R3_Report_Issue_11_Pain_Assessment_2_11_19_REV.pdf.

Jungquist, C. R., Quinlan-Colwell, A., Vallerand, A., Carlisle, H. L., Cooney, M., Dempsey, S. J., ... Sawyer, J. (2020). American Society for Pain Management Nursing Guidelines on Monitoring for Opioid-Induced Advancing Sedation and Respiratory Depression: Revisions. *Pain Management Nursing, 21*(1), 7–25.

Kennon-McGill, S., & McGill, M. R. (2018). Extrahepatic toxicity of acetaminophen: Critical evaluation of the evidence and proposed mechanisms. *Journal of Clinical and Translational Research, 3*(3), 297–310.

Khan, S., Loi, V., & Rosner, M. H. (2017). Drug-induced kidney injury in the elderly. *Drugs & Aging, 34*(10), 729–741.

Klinge, M., Coppler, T., Liebschutz, J. M., Dugum, M., Wassan, A., DiMartini, A., et al. (2018). The assessment and management of pain in cirrhosis. *Current Hepatology Reports, 17*(1), 42–51.

Klinger-Gratz, P. P., Ralvenius, W. T., Neumann, E., Kato, A., Nyilas, R., Lele, Z., ... Zeilhofer, H. U. (2018). Acetaminophen relieves inflammatory pain through CB1 cannabinoid receptors in the rostral ventromedial medulla. *Journal of Neuroscience, 38*(2), 322–334.

Koh, W., Nguyen, K. P., & Jahr, J. S. (2015). Intravenous non-opioid analgesia for peri-and postoperative pain management: A scientific review of intravenous acetaminophen and ibuprofen. *Korean Journal of Anesthesiology, 68*(1), 3–12.

Kurmis, A. P., Kurmis, T. P., O'Brien, J. X., & Dalen, T. (2012). The effect of nonsteroidal anti-inflammatory drug administration on acute phrase fracture-healing: A review. *Journal of Bone and Joint Surgery, 94*(9), 815–823.

Lanas, Á., Carrera-Lasfuentes, P., Arguedas, Y., García, S., Bujanda, L., Calvet, X., et al. (2015). Risk of upper and lower gastrointestinal bleeding in patients taking nonsteroidal anti-inflammatory drugs, antiplatelet agents, or anticoagulants. *Clinical Gastroenterology and Hepatology, 13*(5), 906–912.

Lancaster, E. M., Hiatt, J. R., & Zarrinpar, A. (2015). Acetaminophen hepatotoxicity: An updated review. *Archives of Toxicology, 89*(2), 193–199.

Lewis, S. C., Langman, M. J. S., Laporte, J. R., Matthews, J. N., Rawlins, M. D., & Wiholm, B. E. (2002). Dose–response relationships between individual nonaspirin nonsteroidal anti-inflammatory drugs (NANSAIDs) and serious upper gastrointestinal bleeding: A meta-analysis based on individual patient data. *British Journal of Clinical Pharmacology, 54*(3), 320–326.

Liang, L., Cai, Y., Li, A., & Ma, C. (2017). The efficiency of intravenous acetaminophen for pain control following total knee and hip arthroplasty: a systematic review and meta-analysis. *Medicine, 96*(46).

Lovell, A. R., & Ernst, M. E. (2017). Drug-Induced Hypertension: Focus on Mechanisms and Management. *Current Hypertension Reports, 19*(5), 39.

Loy, V. (2017). Health Maintenance in Liver Disease and Cirrhosis. In *Liver Disorders* (pp. 89–98). Cham, Switzerland: Springer.

Macario, A., & Royal, M. A. (2011). A literature review of randomized clinical trials of intravenous acetaminophen (paracetamol) for acute postoperative pain. *Pain Practice, 11*(3), 290–296.

Machado, G. C., Maher, C. G., Ferreira, P. H., Day, R. O., Pinheiro, M. B., & Ferreira, M. L. (2017). Non-steroidal anti-inflammatory drugs for spinal pain: a systematic review and meta-analysis. *Annals of the Rheumatic Diseases, 76*(7), 1269–1278.

Machado, G. C., Maher, C. G., Ferreira, P. H., Pinheiro, M. B., Lin, C. W. C., Day, R. O., et al. (2015). Efficacy and safety of paracetamol for spinal pain and osteoarthritis: Systematic review and meta-analysis of randomised placebo controlled trials. *British Medical Journal, 350*, h1225.

Marcum, Z. A., Duncan, N. A., & Makris, U. E. (2016). Pharmacotherapies in geriatric chronic pain management. *Clinics in Geriatric Medicine, 32*(4), 705–724.

Maniar, K. H., Jones, I. A., Gopalakrishna, R., Vangsness, J. R., & T, C. (2017). Lowering side effects of NSAID usage in osteoarthritis: Recent attempts at minimizing dosage. *Expert Opinion on Pharmacotherapy, 19*(2), 93–102.

Manvelian, G., Daniels, S., & Gibofsky, A. (2012). The pharmacokinetic parameters of a single dose of a novel nano–formulated, lower dose oral diclofenac. *Postgraduate Medicine, 124*(1), 117–123.

Marquez-Lara, A., Hutchinson, I. D., Nuñez, F., Jr., Smith, T. L., & Miller, A. N. (2016). Nonsteroidal anti-inflammatory drugs and bone-healing: A systematic review of research quality. *JBJS Reviews, 4*(3).

Martinez, V., Beloeil, H., Marret, E., Fletcher, D., Ravaud, P., & Trinquart, L. (2016). Non-opioid analgesics in adults after major surgery: Systematic review with network meta-analysis of randomized trials. *British Journal of Anaesthesia, 118*(1), 22–31.

Mathew, R. O., Bettinger, J. J., Wegrzyn, E. L., & Fudin, J. (2016). Pharmacotherapeutic considerations for chronic pain in chronic kidney and end-stage renal disease. *Journal of Pain Research, 9*, 1191.

Matłok, M., Pędziwiatr, M., Major, P., Kłęk, S., Budzyński, P., & Małczak, P. (2015). One hundred seventy-nine consecutive bariatric operations after introduction of protocol inspired by the principles of enhanced recovery after surgery (ERAS®) in bariatric surgery. *Medical Science Monitor: International Medical Journal of Experimental and Clinical Research, 21*, 791–797.

Mazaleuskaya, L. L., Sangkuhl, K., Thorn, C. F., FitzGerald, G. A., Altman, R. B., & Klein, T. E. (2015). PharmGKB summary: Pathways of acetaminophen metabolism at the therapeutic versus toxic doses. *Pharmacogenetics and Genomics, 25*(8), 416–426.

McAlindon, T. E., Bannuru, R., Sullivan, M. C., Arden, N. K., Berenbaum, F., Bierma-Zeinstra, S. M., et al. (2014). OARSI guidelines for the non-surgical management of knee osteoarthritis. *Osteoarthritis and Cartilage, 22*(3), 363–388.

McGettigan, P., & Olsen, A. M. S. (2017). NSAIDs for high-risk patients: none, celecoxib, or naproxen? *The Lancet, 389*(10087), 2351–2352.

McGill, M. R., & Jaeschke, H. (2013). Metabolism and disposition of acetaminophen: Recent advances in relation to hepatotoxicity and diagnosis. *Pharmaceutical Research, 30*(9), 2174–2187.

McNeil Consumer Healthcare Announces Plans for New Dosing Instructions for Tylenol® Products | Johnson & Johnson. (2011, July 28). Retrieved May 31, 2017, from https://www.jnj.com/media-center/press-releases/mcneil-consumer-healthcare-announces-plans-for-new-dosing-instructions-for-tylenol-products.

Mechanick, J. I., Youdim, A., Jones, D. B., Garvey, W. T., Hurley, D. L., McMahon, M. M., … Dixon, J. B. (2013). Clinical practice guidelines for the perioperative nutritional, metabolic, and nonsurgical support of the bariatric surgery patient—2013 update: Cosponsored by American Association of Clinical Endocrinologists, the Obesity Society, and American Society for Metabolic & Bariatric Surgery. *Obesity, 21*(S1), S1–S27.

Mekaj, Y. H., Daci, F. T., & Mekaj, A. Y. (2015). New insights into the mechanisms of action of aspirin and its use in the prevention and treatment of arterial and venous thromboembolism. *Therapeutics and Clinical Risk Management, 11*, 1449–1456.

Mitchell, J. A., Larkin, S., & Williams, T. J. (1995). Cyclooxygenase-2: regulation and relevance in inflammation. *Biochemical Pharmacology, 50*(10), 1535–1542.

Moodie, J. E., Brown, C. R., Bisley, E. J., Weber, H. U., & Bynum, L. (2008). The safety and analgesic efficacy of intranasal ketorolac in patients with postoperative pain. *Anesthesia & Analgesia, 107*(6), 2025–2031.

Moore, N., Pollack, C., & Butkerait, P. (2015). Adverse drug reactions and drug–drug interactions with over-the-counter NSAIDs. *Therapeutics and Clinical Risk Management, 11*, 1061.

Moore, R. A., Derry, S., & McQuay, H. J. (2010). Topical analgesics for acute and chronic pain in adults. *The Cochrane Library*. Retrieved July 6, 2019 from https://www.ncbi.nlm.nih.gov/pmc/articles/PMC4234085/.

Morís, G., & García-Moncó, J. C. (2018). Drug-induced aseptic meningitis and other mimics. In *CNS Infections* (pp. 275–300). Cham: Springer.

Narouze, S., Benzon, H. T., Provenzano, D. A., Buvanendran, A., De Andres, J., Deer, T. R., et al. (2015). Interventional spine and pain procedures in patients on antiplatelet and anticoagulant medications: Guidelines from the American Society of Regional Anesthesia and Pain Medicine, the European Society of Regional Anaesthesia and Pain Therapy, the American Academy of Pain Medicine, the International Neuromodulation Society, the North American Neuromodulation Society, and the World Institute of Pain. *Regional Anesthesia and Pain Medicine, 40*(3), 182–212.

Negm, A. A., & Furst, D. E. (2017). Nonsteroidal Anti-Inflammatory Drugs, Disease-Modifying Antirheumatic Drugs, Nonopioid Analgesics, & Drugs Used in Gout. In B. G. Katzung (Ed.), *Basic & Clinical Pharmacology, 14e*. New York, NY: McGraw-Hill. Retrieved September 24, 2018 from http://accessmedicine.mhmedical.com.lproxy.nymc.edu/content.aspx?bookid=2249&sectionid=175221264.

Nissen, S. E., Yeomans, N. D., Solomon, D. H., Lüscher, T. F., Libby, P., Husni, M. E., et al. (2016). Cardiovascular safety of celecoxib, naproxen, or ibuprofen for arthritis. *New England Journal of Medicine, 375*, 2519–2529.

Ofman, J. J., Maclean, C. H., Straus, W. L., et al. (2002). A meta-analysis of severe upper gastrointestinal complications of nonsteroidal anti-inflammatory drugs. *Journal of Rheumatology, 29*, 804–812.

Pasero, C. & McCaffery, M. (2011). Nonopioid analgesics. In *Pain Assessment and Pharmacologic Management.* (pp. 6, 180, 182, 186, 192, 198). St. Louis: Mosby.

Pathan, S. A., Mitra, B., & Cameron, P. A. (2018). A systematic review and meta-analysis comparing the efficacy of nonsteroidal anti-inflammatory drugs, opioids, and paracetamol in the treatment of acute renal colic. *European Urology, 73*(4), 583–595.

Patrono, C. (2016). Cardiovascular effects of cyclooxygenase-2 inhibitors: A mechanistic and clinical perspective. *British Journal of Clinical Pharmacology, 82*(4), 957–964.

Patrono, C., & Baigent, C. (2017). Coxibs, Traditional NSAIDs, and cardiovascular safety post-PRECISION: What we thought we knew then and what we think we know now. *Clinical Pharmacology & Therapeutics, 102*(2), 238–245.

Peck, K. R., Roland, M. M., & Smitherman, T. A. (2018). Factors associated with medication-overuse headache in patients seeking treatment for primary headache. *Headache: The Journal of Head and Face Pain, 58*(5), 648–660.

Pelletier, J. P., Martel-Pelletier, J., Rannou, F., & Cooper, C. (2016). Efficacy and safety of oral NSAIDs and analgesics in the management of osteoarthritis: Evidence from real-life setting trials and surveys. *Seminars in Arthritis and Rheumatism, 45*(4), S22–S27.

Peng, F., Liu, S., Hu, Y., Yu, M., Chen, J., & Liu, C. (2016). Influence of perioperative nonsteroidal anti-inflammatory drugs on complications after gastrointestinal surgery: a meta-analysis. *Acta Anaesthesiologica Taiwanica, 54*(4), 121–128.

Pepine, C. J., & Gurbel, P. A. (2017). Cardiovascular safety of NSAIDs: Additional insights after PRECISION and point of view. *Clinical Cardiology, 40*(12), 1352–1356.

Peppin, J. F., Albrecht, P. J., Argoff, C., Gustorff, B., Pappagallo, M., Rice, F. L., et al. (2015). Skin matters: A review of topical treatments for chronic pain. Part two: Treatments and applications. *Pain and Therapy, 4*(1), 33–50.

Pergolizzi, J. V., Jr., Raffa, R. B., Nalamachu, S., & Taylor, R., Jr. (2016). Evolution to low-dose NSAID therapy. *Pain Management, 6*(2), 175–189.

Pinals, R. S., & Frank, S. (1967). Relative efficacy of indomethacin and acetylsalicylic acid in rheumatoid arthritis. *New England Journal of Medicine, 276*(9), 512–514.

Pisano, M. (2016). NSAIDs: Balancing the risks and benefits. *US Pharm, 41*(3), 24–26.

Politi, J. R., Davis, R. L., II, & Matrka, A. K. (2017). Randomized prospective trial comparing the use of intravenous versus oral acetaminophen in total joint arthroplasty. *The Journal of Arthroplasty, 32*(4), 1125–1127.

Pountos, I., Georgouli, T., Calori, G. M., & Giannoudis, P. V. (2012). Do nonsteroidal anti-inflammatory drugs affect bone healing? A critical analysis. *Scientific World-Journal, 2012,* 606404.

Prieto-García, L., Pericacho, M., Sancho-Martínez, S. M., Sánchez, Á., Martínez-Salgado, C., López-Novoa, J. M., et al. (2016). Mechanisms of triple whammy acute kidney injury. *Pharmacology & Therapeutics, 167,* 132–145.

Rakoski, M., Goyal, P., Spencer-Safier, M., Weissman, J., Mohr, G., & Volk, M. (2018). Pain management in patients with cirrhosis. *Clinical Liver Disease, 11*(6), 135.

Reid, M. C., Eccleston, C., & Pillemer, K. (2015). Management of chronic pain in older adults. *British Medical Journal, 350*(7995), 1–10.

Richards, C. J., Graf, K. W., & Mashru, R. P. (2017). The effect of opioids, alcohol, and nonsteroidal anti-inflammatory drugs on fracture union. *Orthopedic Clinics, 48*(4), 433–443.

Richy, F., Bruyère, O., Ethgen, O., Rabenda, V., Bouvenot, G., Audran, M., et al. (2004). Time dependent risk of gastrointestinal complications induced by non-steroidal anti-inflammatory drug use: A consensus statement using a meta-analytic approach. *Annals of the Rheumatic Diseases, 63*(7), 759–766.

Ridderikhof, M. L., Lirk, P., Goddijn, H., Vandewalle, E., Schinkel, E., Van Dieren, S., et al. (2018). Acetaminophen or nonsteroidal anti-inflammatory drugs in acute musculoskeletal trauma: A multicenter, double-blind, randomized, clinical trial. *Annals of Emergency Medicine, 71*(3), 357–368.

Roberts, E., Nunes, V. D., Buckner, S., Latchem, S., Constanti, M., Miller, P., et al. (2015). Paracetamol: Not as safe as we thought? A systematic literature review of observational studies. *Annals of the Rheumatic Diseases, 75*(3), 552–559.

Rostom, A., Muir, K., Dube, C., Lanas, A., Jolicoeur, E., & Tugwell, P. (2009). Prevention of NSAID-related upper gastrointestinal toxicity: A meta-analysis of traditional NSAIDs with gastroprotection and COX-2 inhibitors. *Drug, Healthcare and Patient Safety, 1,* 47.

Scheiman, J. M. (2016). NSAID-induced Gastrointestinal Injury. *Journal of Clinical Gastroenterology, 50*(1), 5–10.

Schmeltzer, P. A., Kosinski, A. S., Kleiner, D. E., Hoofnagle, J. H., Stolz, A., Fontana, R. J., et al. Drug-Induced Liver Injury Network (DILIN) (2016). Liver injury from nonsteroidal anti-inflammatory drugs in the United States. *Liver International, 36*(4), 603–609.

Schrör, K., & Voelker, M. (2016). *NSAIDS and aspirin: Recent advances and implications for clinical management.* In *NSAIDs and Aspirin* (pp. 107-122). Cham, Switzerland: Springer.

Serper, M., Wolf, M. S., Parikh, N. A., Tillman, H., Lee, W. M., & Ganger, D. R. (2016). Risk factors, clinical presentation, and outcomes in overdose with acetaminophen alone or with combination products: Results from the Acute Liver Failure Study Group. *Journal of Clinical Gastroenterology, 50*(1), 85–91.

Sivaganesan, A., Chotai, S., White-Dzuro, G., McGirt, M. J., & Devin, C. J. (2017). The effect of NSAIDs on spinal fusion: A cross-disciplinary review of biochemical, animal, and human studies. *European Spine Journal, 26*(11), 2719–2728.

Smith, H. S. (2009). Potential analgesic mechanisms of acetaminophen. *Pain Physician, 12*(1), 269–280.

Sostres, C., & Lanas, Á. (2016). Appropriate prescription, adherence and safety of non-steroidal anti-inflammatory drugs. *Medicina Clínica (English Edition), 146*(6), 267–272.

Tegner, W. S. (1939). The treatment of the rheumatic diseases in the United States and the continent of Europe. *Annals of the Rheumatic Diseases, 1*(4), 249.

Thorell, A., MacCormick, A. D., Awad, S., Reynolds, N., Roulin, D., Demartines, N., et al. (2016). Guidelines for perioperative care in bariatric surgery: Enhanced Recovery After Surgery (ERAS) society recommendations. *World Journal of Surgery, 40*(9), 2065–2083.

Tosounidis, T. H., Sheikh, H., Stone, M. H., & Giannoudis, P. V. (2015). Pain relief management following proximal femoral fractures: Options, issues and controversies. *Injury, 46,* S52–S58.

Ugurlucan, M., Caglar, I. M., Caglar, F. N., Ziyade, S., Karatepe, O., Yildiz, Y., et al. (2012). Aspirin: from a historical perspective. *Recent Patents on Cardiovascular Drug Discovery, 7*(1), 71–76.

Ungprasert, P., Cheungpasitporn, W., Crowson, C. S., & Matteson, E. L. (2015). Individual non-steroidal anti-inflammatory drugs and risk of acute kidney injury: A systematic review and meta-analysis of observational studies. *European Journal of Internal Medicine, 26*(4), 285–291.

U.S. Food and Drug Administration (FDA) (April 7, 2005). Postmarket drug safety information for patients and providers.COX-2 selective (includes Bextra, Celebrex, and Vioxx) and non-selective non-steroidal anti-inflammatory drugs (NSAIDs). Retrieved June 19, 2019, from https://www.fda.gov/drugs/postmarket-drug-safety-information-patients-and-providers/cox-2-selective-includes-bextra-celebrex-and-vioxx-and-non-selective-non-steroidal-anti-inflammatory

U.S. Food and Drug Administration (FDA) Drug Safety Communication: FDA warns of rare but serious skin reactions with the pain reliever/fever reducer acetaminophen (2013, Aug 1). Retrieved July 27, 2017, from https://www.fda.gov/Drugs/DrugSafety/ucm363041.htm.

U.S. Food and Drug Administration (FDA) FDA Drug Safety Communication: Prescription acetaminophen products to be limited to 325 mg per dosage unit; Boxed warning will highlight potential for severe liver failure. (2011, Jan 11). Retrieved May 31, 2017 from https://www.fda.gov/Drugs/Drug Safety/ucm239821.htm.

U.S. Food and Drug Administration (FDA) (7-9 2015). FDA Drug Safety Communication: FDA strengthens warning that non-aspirin nonsteroidal anti-inflammatory drugs (NSAIDs) can cause heart attacks or strokes. Retrieved June 19, 2019 from https://www.fda.gov/Drugs/DrugSafety/ucm451800.htm.

U.S. Food and Drug Administration (FDA). (2018). *Orange book: Approved drug products with therapeutic equivalence evaluations.* Retrieved June 19, 2019 from https://www. accessdata.fda.gov/scripts/cder/ob/search_product.cfm.

Vadivelu, N., Gowda, A. M., Urman, R. D., Jolly, S., Kodumudi, V., Maria, M., et al. (2015). Ketorolac tromethamine–routes and clinical implications. *Pain Practice, 15*(2), 175–193.

Vaezi, M. F., Yang, Y. X., & Howden, C. W. (2017). Complications of proton pump inhibitor therapy. *Gastroenterology, 153*(1), 35–48.

Vannucci, L., Fossi, C., Gronchi, G., & Brandi, M. L. (2017). Low-dose diclofenac in patients with fragility fractures. *Clinical Cases in Mineral and Bone Metabolism, 14*(1), 15–17.

Walker, P. C., Alrawi, A., Mitchell, J. F., Regal, R. E., & Khanderia, U. (2005). Medication use as a risk factor for falls among hospitalized elderly patients. *American Journal of Health-System Pharmacy, 62*(23), 2495–2499.

Waller, D. G., & Sampson, A. P. (2018). In Waller D. G., Sampson A. P. (Eds.), 29 - *Nonsteroidal Antiinflammatory Drugs* Elsevier. https://doi-org.lproxy.nymc.edu/10.1016/ B978-0-7020-7167-6.00029-4.

Weersink, R. A., Bouma, M., Burger, D. M., Drenth, J. P., Harkes-Idzinga, S. F., Hunfeld, N. G., et al. (2018). Evidence-based recommendations to improve the safe use of drugs in patients with liver cirrhosis. *Drug Safety,* 1–11.

Wilson, D. J., Schutte, S. M., & Abel, S. R. (2015). Comparing the efficacy of ophthalmic NSAIDs in common indications: A literature review to support cost-effective prescribing. *Annals of Pharmacotherapy, 49*(6), 727–734.

Wysenbeek, A. J., Klein, Z., Nakar, S., & Mane, R. (1988). Assessment of cognitive function in elderly patients treated with naproxen. A prospective study. *Clinical and Experimental Rheumatology, 6*(4), 399–400.

Yang, M., He, M., Zhao, M., Zou, B., Liu, J., Luo, L. M., et al. (2017). Proton pump inhibitors for preventing non-steroidal anti-inflammatory drug induced gastrointestinal toxicity: A systematic review. *Current Medical Research and Opinion, 33*(6), 973–980.

Yoon, E., Babar, A., Choudhary, M., Kutner, M., & Pyrsopoulos, N. (2016). Acetaminophen-induced hepatotoxicity: A comprehensive update. *Journal of Clinical and Translational Hepatology, 4*(2), 131–142.

Yuan, J. Q., Tsoi, K. K. F., Yang, M., Wang, J. Y., Threapleton, D. E., Yang, Z. Y., et al. (2016). Systematic review with network meta-analysis: Comparative effectiveness and safety of strategies for preventing NSAID-associated gastrointestinal toxicity. *Alimentary Pharmacology & Therapeutics, 43*(12), 1262–1275.

Zhang, C. H., & Zhou, X. P. (2017). Effectiveness of various non-steroidal anti-inflammatory drugs in pain management of patients with vertebral fracture: A comparative clinical study. *Tropical Journal of Pharmaceutical Research, 16*(9), 2275–2279.

Zhang, W., Nuki, G., Moskowitz, R. W., Abramson, S., Altman, R. D., Arden, N. K., et al. (2010). OARSI recommendations for the management of hip and knee osteoarthritis: part III: Changes in evidence following systematic cumulative update of research published through January 2009. *Osteoarthritis and Cartilage, 18*(4), 476–499.

Zhou, Y., Boudreau, D. M., & Freedman, A. N. (2014). Trends in the use of aspirin and nonsteroidal anti-inflammatory drugs in the general US population. *Pharmacoepidemiology and Drug Safety, 23*(1), 43–50.

Chapter 11 Opioid Analgesics

Maureen F. Cooney

CHAPTER OUTLINE

Section 1, pg. 223

Opioid Pharmacology, pg. 223

Background, pg. 223

Opioid Receptors, pg. 224

Discovery, pg. 225

Nomenclature, pg. 226

Opioid Receptor Signaling, pg. 226

Factors Affecting Drug Response, pg. 226

Pharmacodynamics, pg. 226

Pharmacokinetics, pg. 227

Pharmacogenomics, pg. 230

Opioid Classes, pg. 232

Phenanthrenes, pg. 232

Phenylpiperadines, pg. 233

Diphenylheptane, pg. 234

Phenylpropylamines, pg. 235

Benzomorphans, pg. 235

Key Points, pg. 236

Section 2, pg. 236

Opioid Selection, pg. 236

Indications and Use of Opioids, pg. 236

Morphine, pg. 238

Codeine, pg. 242

FentaNYL, pg. 243

HYDROcodone, pg. 247

HYDROmorphone, pg. 248

Meperidine, pg. 249

Methadone, pg. 249

Levorphanol, pg. 255

OxyCODONE, pg. 256

OxyMORphone, pg. 258

Other Mu Opioid Analgesics, pg. 259

Dual Mechanism Analgesics, pg. 261

Partial Mu Agonist, pg. 264

Mixed Agonist-Antagonist Opioids, pg. 266

Opioid Antagonists, pg. 267

Key Points, pg. 269

Section 3, pg. 269

Opioid Dosing Practices, pg. 269

Initiation of Opioid Therapy, pg. 270

Titration of Short-Acting Opioid Dose, pg. 270

Use of Modified-Release Opioids, pg. 272

Titration of Modified-Release Opioid, pg. 272

Continuous Intravenous Opioid Infusions, pg. 273

Opioid Rotation or Switch, pg. 273

Rotating From Other Opioids to Methadone, pg. 280

Buprenorphine, pg. 286

Tapering and Discontinuing Opioid Therapy, pg. 287

Opioid Safety in the Community, pg. 288

Key Points, pg. 289

Case Scenario, pg. 289

References, pg. 291

OPIOIDS are effective analgesics and often included in the treatment of moderate to severe pain; they may be appropriately used in multimodal treatment plans, especially in the settings of acute nonsurgical pain, postoperative pain, and cancer pain. Opioid use in patients with chronic noncancer pain has increasingly been challenged because of a lack of evidence to support the effectiveness and safety of this therapy (Herndon et al., 2016). In recent years, awareness of the prevalence of opioid use disorder and its complications has contributed to the controversy related to opioid use and led to more conservative opioid prescribing and monitoring practices. There are legitimate concerns about the use of opioids and opioid-related adverse outcomes. However, it is also important to recognize that opioids are effective analgesics and have an important role in multimodal pain management in carefully selected and closely monitored patients, including those who have not responded to nonopioid and/or nonpharmacologic approaches (Herndon, et al., 2016). Opioid-related risks can be reduced by appropriate patient selection, dosing, and monitoring. Risks can be mitigated by the use of multimodal analgesia (MMA) plans that include opioids in combination with non-opioid analgesics, coanalgesics, and nonpharmacologic therapies. To ensure effective, appropriate, and safe use of opioids, it is necessary for clinicians involved in the prescription and/or administration of opioids to be well informed about these medications. The three sections of this chapter address opioid pharmacology, opioid selection, and opioid dosing practices.

Section 1 | Opioid Pharmacology

Mena Raouf, Jeffrey J. Bettinger, Erica L. Wegrzyn, Jeffrey Fudin

Background

Opioids have been used for thousands of years for treatment of pain and are among the oldest medications used by humans. The use of opium dates back to 3400 BCE by Sumerians, Babylonians, and Egyptians (Atkinson, Coleman, & Fudin, 2018). To exemplify their utility, they are commercially available for virtually every route of administration, including oral (PO), rectal (PR), topical, sublingual (SL), buccal, transmucosal (TM), intranasal (IN), intravenous (IV), intramuscular (IM), subcutaneous (subcut), epidural, intrathecal (IT), and extemporaneously compounded as topical.

Opium is the dried latex derived from the opium poppy *(Papaver somniferum)*. In 1804 morphine was isolated from the opium poppy, becoming the first pharmaceutical extracted from a natural product. In addition to morphine, the opium latex contains the opiates codeine and thebaine and nonanalgesic alkaloids such as papaverine and noscapine. Therefore the terms *natural opioids* and *opiates* refers to morphine, codeine, and thebaine (Vallejo, Barkin, & Wang, 2011). Semisynthetic opioids are derived from natural opioids through chemical modification of functional groups, such as oxyCODONE, HYDROcodone, and HYDROmorphone, because they are all phenanthrenes by chemical structure (more on this later). Synthetic opioids such as fentaNYL, meperidine (Demcrol), and methadone (Dolophine) are completely human-made in a laboratory. Classification of opioids by chemical class is listed in Table 11.1.

Table 11.1 | Chemical Classes of Opioids

Phenanthrenes	Benzomorphans	Phenylpiperidines	Diphenylheptanes	Phenylpropyl Amines
Morphine	**Pentazocine**	**Meperidine**	**Methadone**	**TraMADol**
Buprenorphine[*,b]	Diphenoxylate	Alfentanil	Methadone	Tapentadol
Butorphanol[*,b]	Loperamide	FentaNYL	Propoxyphene	TraMADol
Codeine[a]	Pentazocine	Meperidine		
Dextromethorphan[*,b]		Remifentanil		
Heroin		SUFentanil		
(diacetyl-morphine)[b]				
Morphine[a]				
HYDROcodone[*,b]				
HYDROmorphone[*,b]				

Table 11.1 | Chemical Classes of Opioids—Cont'd

Morphine	Pentazocine	Meperidine	Methadone	TraMADol
Levorphanol[*,b]				
Methylnaltrexone[†,b,c]				
Morphine (opium, concentrate)[a]				
Nalbuphine[*,b]				
Naloxone[*,b]				
Naloxegol[*,b,c]				
Naltrexone[†,b]				
OxyCODONE[*,b]				
OxyMORphone[*,b]				
Cross-Sensitivity Risk				
Probable	Possible	Low risk	Low risk	Low risk

[*] Agents lacking the 6-OH group of morphine, possibly decreases cross-tolerability within the phenanthrene group
[†] Six position is substituted with a ketone group and tolerability is similar to hydroxylation
[a] Naturally occurring.
[b] Semisynthetic.
[c] PAMORA (peripherally acting mu opioid receptor antagonists) for prevention of opioid-induced constipation)

With permission from Dr. Jeffrey Fudin. Revised from Chemical Classes of Opioids (Fudin 2016), http://paindr.com/wp-content/uploads/2016/11/Opioid-Structural-Classes_edited-November-2016.pdf

Opioid Receptors

Opioid receptors are expressed in pain transmission and modulation pathways, including afferent neurons, spinal cord, limbic system, midbrain, and thalamus, as described in Chapter 3 (Vallejo et al., 2011; Waldhoer, Bartlett, & Whistler, 2004). Opioid receptors are particularly abundant in the periaqueductal gray, dorsal horn of the spinal cord, brainstem, thalamus, and cortex. They are also present in other areas of the body such as gastrointestinal (GI) tract, skin, hypothalamus, pituitary gland, and immune cells, where they perform nonanalgesic functions.

To date, four opioid receptors have been identified: mu (μ), delta (δ), kappa (κ), and opioid receptor like-1 (ORL1) (Hoffman et al., 2015; Vallejo et al., 2011; Waldhoer et al., 2004). Some receptors are further divided into subunits that are responsible for different effects. Clinical effects related to opioid receptor activation are listed in Table 11.2. Opioid effect results from the binding of the opioid (agonist) to its receptor (Fig. 11.1). Most opioids are mu agonists that also have varying activity at the kappa receptor. There are no commercially available delta or ORL1 receptor agonists to date.

Table 11.2 | Clinical Effects of Opioid Receptor Activation

1996 Conventional Name	IUPHAR Name	Clinical Effect	Examples of Opioids With Mu Affinity
$\mu1$ (Mu1)	MOP	Supraspinal analgesia	Morphine
		Peripheral analgesia	Codeine
		Sedation	HYDROmorphone
		Euphoria	FentaNYL
		Prolactin release	SUFentanil
$\mu2$ (Mu2)		Spinal analgesia	Alfentanil
		Respiratory depression	OxyCODONE
		Physical dependence	OxyMORphone
		Gastrointestinal dysmotility	Methadone

Table 11.2 | Clinical Effects of Opioid Receptor Activation—Cont'd

1996 Conventional Name	IUPHAR Name	Clinical Effect	Examples of Opioids With Mu Affinity
		Pruritus	Levorphanol
		Bradycardia	
		Growth hormone release	
κ1 (Kappa1)	KOP	Spinal analgesia	*Examples of opioids with κ affinity*
		Miosis	Butorphanol
		Diuresis	Nalbuphine
κ2 (Kappa2)		Psychotomimesis	Pentazocine
		Dysphoria	Buprenorphine
κ3 (Kappa3)		Supraspinal analgesia	Weak affinity: methadone, SUFentanil
Δ (Delta)	DOP	Spinal and supraspinal analgesia	*Examples of opioids with Δ affinity*
		Modulation of μ-receptor function	Levorphanol
		Inhibit release of dopamine	Weak affinity: SUFentanil, morphine, methadone, oxyMORphone
Nociceptin/orphanin FQ	NOP	Anxiolysis	
		Analgesia	

IUPHAR, International Union of Basic and Clinical Pharmacology.

From Nelson, L. S., & Olsen, D. Opioids. In: R. S. Hoffman, M. Howland, N. A. Lewin, L. S. Nelson, & L. R. Goldfrank (Eds.). *Goldfrank's toxicologic emergencies* (10th ed.). New York: McGraw-Hill; 2015.

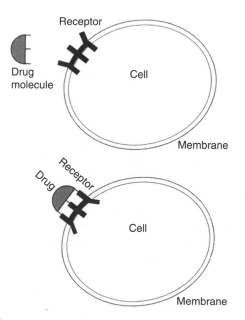

Fig. 11.1 | Medication and Receptor Activation. (From Spencer, R. T. [1993]. Pharmacodynamics and pharmacokinetics. In Nichols, L. W., Spencer, R. T., Bergan, F. W., & Eisenhauer, L. A. *Clinical pharmacology and nursing management* [4th ed.]. Philadelphia: Lippincott Williams & Wilkins.) As appears in Pasero, C., & McCaffery, M. *Pain assessment and pharmacologic management* [p. 284]. St. Louis, MO: Mosby. May be duplicated for use in clinical practice.

Discovery

Despite the long-standing history of their use, the presence of opioid receptors was not proposed until the mid-20th century. Studies on antagonism of morphine by nalorphine suggested the presence of more than one receptor and more than one binding site on a receptor (Martin, Eades, Thompson, Huppler, & Gilbert, 1976). Such binding sites were discovered in 1973 (Pert & Snyder, 1973). The reason behind the presence of these receptors that combine with opioids remained unclear and drove research to identify the endogenous (naturally occurring) ligands for these receptors. Of note, ligands are molecules that signal a separate protein by binding to that target protein. The presence of endogenous ligands was uncovered in 1975 with the discovery of met-enkephalin and leu-enkephalin, followed by the discovery of β-endorphin and dynorphin (Akil, 1984; Hughes et al., 1976). These endogenous ligands for opioid receptors were named *endorphins* (endogenous morphine). Endorphins are located throughout the peripheral and central nervous systems, and although they are recognized as endogenous opioids, they are also associated with other effects such as mood, learning and memory, and social bonding (Ballantyne & Sullivan, 2017).

Nomenclature

In older literature, opioid receptors were identified by the Greek symbol that represents them: δ, μ, or κ. However, the International Union of Pharmacology (IUPHAR) Committee on Receptor Nomenclature and Drug Classification has twice recommended nomenclature change from Greek symbols to make the names of opioid receptors consistent with those of other neurotransmitters (Dhawan, Cesselin, & Raghubir, 1996; Waldhoer et al., 2004). In the first proposal, receptors were named by their opioid peptide (OP) with a subscript representing the chronologic order of discovery. The δ receptor was discovered first and therefore renamed OP_1, the κ receptor was renamed OP_2, and the μ receptor, the third identified opioid receptor, was renamed OP_3. The currently proposed nomenclature recommends adding a single letter before the OP designation. The δ receptor is represented as DOP (delta opioid peptide), the κ receptor is represented as KOP (kappa opioid peptide), and the μ receptor is represented as MOP (mu opioid peptide). This classification eliminated grouped variants of opioid receptor under one nomenclature. For example, μ1 and μ2 receptors are identified as MOP. Throughout this book, the terms mu opioid and mu opioid agonists are often used to refer to MOP.

Opioid Receptor Signaling

Opioid receptors are made up of seven transmembrane-spanning proteins coupled to inhibitory G-proteins (G_i), which on activation decrease adenyl cyclase production of the secondary messenger cyclic adenosine monophosphate (cAMP) (Al-Hasani & Bruchas, 2011). This is important because normally neurotransmitter release from neurons requires depolarization of the nerve terminal and calcium influx into the synaptic terminal through voltage-gated calcium channels, causing neurotransmitter-vesicle fusion with the plasma membrane, leading to its subsequent release. Thus the reduction in cAMP production caused by activation of opioid receptors inhibits influx of calcium and hyperpolarizes the cell through activation of potassium channels. The end result is an inhibition of neuronal signaling, which in turn inhibits spinal cord pain transmission (Al-Hasani & Bruchas, 2011; Vallejo et al., 2011).

Factors Affecting Drug Response

Individual variability in drug response can be explained by multiple parameters, including age, gender, weight, disease severity, comorbidities, pharmacokinetics, and pharmacogenetics. These factors and the corresponding impact are discussed throughout this chapter.

Pharmacodynamics

Pharmacodynamics is the study of how the drug affects the body through interaction with the receptor. The pharmacodynamics of a drug help predict its clinical effects, including efficacy and adverse effects.

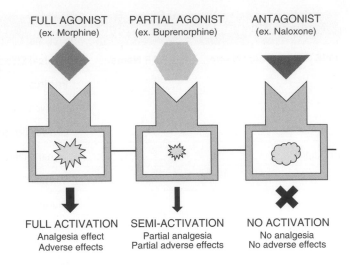

Fig. 11.2 | **Opioid Binding and Receptor Activation.** (Created and printed with permission by Dr. Thien C. Pham.)

Opioids are classified into full agonist, partial agonist, antagonist, or agonist/antagonist (Vallejo et al., 2011). The corresponding effects of agonists, partial agonist, and agonist/antagonist are illustrated in Fig. 11.2.

- *Full agonists* bind to the receptor tightly and undergo a significant conformational change that produces maximal effect after receptor activation. Examples of full agonists are morphine, oxyCODONE, HYDROcodone, codeine, methadone, heroin (diacetyl morphine) and fentaNYL.

- *Partial agonists,* such as butorphanol and traMADol, cause less conformational change and receptor activation than full agonists. At lower doses, full agonists and partial agonists may provide similar efficacy. As the dose of a full opioid agonist increases, there is a corresponding increase in analgesia and respiratory depression. However, as the dose of a partial agonist increases, the activity will eventually plateau, or reach a ceiling effect, and further dose increases will not provide additional efficacy but could incur additional side effects. The partial agonist may have the same affinity for the receptor as the full agonist, and in some cases, the partial agonist may even have stronger affinity for the receptor than the full agonist, but the partial agonist will cause less receptor activation and effect.

- *Antagonists,* such as naloxone and naltrexone, bind to the receptor but do not result in receptor activation. The major effect of the antagonist is prevention of agonists from activating the receptor. Because naloxone and naltrexone usually have a higher affinity toward the receptor than the full agonist, they will bump the full agonist off the receptor and cause reversal of the opioid effects.

- *Agonists/antagonists,* including pentazocine, nalbuphine, buprenorphine, and butorphanol,

Table 11.3 | Receptor Effects of Opioid Agonists/Antagonists

Opioid	Mu	Kappa	Delta
Buprenorphine	Partial agonists	Antagonist	Antagonist (weak)
Butorphanol	Antagonist	Agonist	—
Nalbuphine	Antagonist	Agonist	—
Pentazocine	Partial agonist	Agonist	—

exhibit agonist activity at some opioid receptors and antagonist activity at other opioid receptor(s). For example, nalbuphine binds to the MOP receptor and does not activate it (a MOP antagonist); however, it binds to and activates the KOP receptor (a KOP agonist). The receptor-specific effects of opioid agonists/antagonists are included in Table 11.3.

In addition to the opioid activity that results once a medication binds to the receptor, there are factors that affect how a medication reaches and binds to a receptor. Two important concepts are affinity and binding capacity. Affinity is the pull a drug has toward the receptor. High affinity means a low concentration of a drug is adequate to maximally occupy the receptor binding site, whereas low affinity means that a higher concentration of the drug is needed to occupy the receptor binding site. Binding capacity is the ability of the drug to hold on to the receptor and form intermolecular forces. High binding capacity means that the drug is strongly bound to the receptor and is hard to displace by another ligand. One way to think of binding capacity is that strongly bound drugs are comparable to a strong magnet whereas weakly bound opioids are similar to a weak magnet.

Pharmacokinetics

Pharmacokinetics is the study of how the body acts on drugs, compared to the aforementioned pharmacodynamics (how the drug acts on the body). More specifically, pharmacokinetics involves ADME, which is an accepted acronym for *a*bsorption, *d*istribution, *m*etabolism, and *e*xcretion. These characteristics may vary greatly among various opioids, and a complete understanding of these pharmacokinetic parameters is paramount in guiding optimal treatment selection and providing safe dosing when starting opioids, adding one or more opioid(s) to another, or rotating opioids.

Absorption

The majority of opioids are available as oral formulations because most are adequately absorbed within the GI tract. Others, mainly buprenorphine and fentaNYL, are available only as transdermal, sublingual, submucosal, buccal, or injectable formulations because of their extremely low oral bioavailability and high hepatic first-pass metabolism

(Drewes et al., 2013). In other words, buprenorphine or fentaNYL would not provide adequate analgesia if administered orally because serum concentrations would not be high enough to cause an effect.

One major problem for orally available opioids is that some are substrates for efflux-transport proteins in the intestinal lumen. These proteins normally serve as a protective mechanism that binds certain substances (including some opioids) and pulls them back into the gut lumen, thus protecting the body by preventing absorption of certain drugs or toxins. Presence of these proteins when certain opioids are used could reduce their overall absorption and systemic concentration, although most of the time it can be overcome by increasing the oral dose. One example of this property is that 10 mg of intravenous morphine is approximately equivalent to 30 mg of oral morphine. This disparity is due to p-glycoprotein (P-gp) transporters preventing oral morphine absorption and affecting first-pass metabolism through the liver before reaching the bloodstream.

Other examples of substrate binding include natural proteins that bind together with drugs. This is common with drug metabolism and may be necessary for the medication to have an effect. For example, cytochrome 2D6 (CYP2D6) enzymes combine with codeine, and as a result codeine is metabolized to morphine. The efficacy and safety of codeine largely depend on CYP2D6 activity. In this case, codeine is the drug and CYP2D6 is the substrate.

The most common transporter protein for opioids belongs to the adenosine triphosphate (ATP) binding cassette efflux transport system, and specifically are P-gp transporters, as noted earlier with morphine (Drewes et al., 2013; Somogyi, Barratt, & Coller, 2007). P-gp transporters are mainly expressed along apical epithelial cell membranes throughout the GI tract and in the blood-brain barrier (BBB) and act by binding to substrates and transporting them back out of the cell in the direction from which they came (Drewes et al., 2013; Somogyi et al., 2007). This prevents drug absorption in the GI tract and/or reduces penetration to the central nervous system (CNS) in the BBB so that the desired analgesic effect will not be possible. Notable opioid P-gp substrates include fentaNYL, morphine, and methadone. If these medications are given along with drugs that may induce (increase) or inhibit P-gp expression or given to patients with P-gp pharmacogenomic variability that might enhance or promote absorption across the GI membrane to the systemic circulation or peripheral blood into the CNS, the effect of these medications may be greater or less than expected (Drewes et al., 2013; Somogyi et al., 2007). Specific drugs that inhibit or induce P-gp are beyond the scope of this chapter, but lists are readily available, regularly updated, and retrievable by most medical and scientific electronic search platforms.

Distribution

After drugs are absorbed, they are distributed systemically throughout the body to various tissues. For opioids, the goal is generally to reach the CNS, where they combine with various opioid receptors, the target of which is usually the mu opioid receptor, to elicit analgesia. As mentioned earlier, P-gp plays a major role in preventing certain opioids from crossing the BBB; however, the amount of serum protein binding and volume of distribution (Vd) will also have an impact. Vd is defined as the amount a certain drug is distributed throughout the body, mainly in tissues. The extent to which an opioid binds to circulating plasma proteins and its Vd are both important characteristics to consider because individual variations in these parameters will affect overall efficacy and toxicity. In short, if the drug is bound too tightly to proteins or trapped within an organ, it will not be available to cross the BBB and therefore cannot elicit a response within the CNS.

Metabolism

Metabolism is the process of transforming substances into chemically different compounds, also known as metabolites, by enzymatic reactions so they may be more easily excreted from the body. Although these reactions can occur anywhere in the body, the primary site of these enzymatic reactions is within the liver. In general, the liver functions to convert medications to a more water-soluble form to set the stage for excretion through the kidney. There are generally two forms of metabolism that dictate metabolite generation: phase I and phase II metabolism. Phase I metabolism involves oxidation or hydrolysis reactions with the major goal of modifying substances to be further metabolized. Phase I is mainly carried out by the CYP450 enzyme system (Sekhri & Cooney, 2017). Phase II metabolism involves conjugating substances into more hydrophilic compounds through glucuronidation and sulfation-type reactions, so they can be renally excreted. To further detail, glucuronidation is the process by which a glucose molecule is chemically attached to the parent drug or a metabolite of that drug, which enhances the water solubility of the drug.

Usually phase I precedes phase II reactions; however, some medications do not require phase I reactions and go directly to phase II. It is also important to note that drugs can be metabolized into active or inactive metabolites or both, with active meaning they have some type of action on their therapeutic target, leading to new or additional efficacy and/or toxicity. Therefore drug metabolism can have a significant impact on a patient's response to medications.

More than 50% of all medications, including many opioids, are metabolized by CYP3A4, subjecting them to a high risk for drug-drug interactions (Deer et al., 2013). Other important CYP isoenzymes that contribute to opioid metabolism include 2D6, 2C9, 2C19, and 2B6. Drug-drug interactions commonly occur because many drugs either inhibit or induce the expression of hepatic CYP enzymes, and these enzymes are subject to a high degree of pharmacogenetic variability (further explained in the next section). Hepatic CYP enzymes may have significant effects on serum concentrations of opioids and many other drugs and their metabolites.

Drug-Drug Interactions: Phase I Metabolism

CYP450 inhibitors are medications (or foods) that inhibit (reduce) production of specific enzymes that play an important role in the metabolism of some other medications, including opioids. Hepatic inhibition (reduction) of the specific enzymes by a drug (or food) happens within 48 hours of starting the new drug. When an inhibitor of an enzyme is given along with a parent medication that is metabolized into inactive metabolites by that same enzyme, the result would be increased serum concentrations of the parent drug, leading to toxicity and/or overdose. However, if the parent compound (an opioid) has limited or no pharmacologic activity and relies on its active metabolite(s) to yield its effect, inhibiting conversion to the active metabolite reduces or eliminates efficacy. In the case of an opioid, such a circumstance could not only limit and reduce its analgesic effect but could also put the patient at increased risk for withdrawal. Clinical application of concepts related to CYP450 inhibition is provided in Box 11.1.

CYP450 inducers are drugs (or foods) that induce (increase) production of certain enzymes, and therefore enhance the liver's output of those enzymes, increasing their availability to metabolize the affected drug. However, in the case of induction, increased enzyme production (or induction) is not seen for up to 3 weeks. For example, if metabolism of an opioid results in production of an inactive metabolite, an inducer may reduce the amount of available active opioid by speeding up its metabolism into an inactive metabolite, resulting in a decrease in the analgesic effect of the opioid and an increased risk of possible withdrawal. If the parent compound (opioid) has no or limited pharmacologic activity and relies on its active metabolite(s)

Box 11.1 | Clinical Application of Cytochrome P450 Inhibition

- Codeine is a relatively weak mu agonist and is primarily metabolized by CYP2D6 into its pharmacologically active metabolite morphine (Smith, 2009; Deer et al., 2013). If this metabolism does not occur, the patient will not receive the analgesic effect that would be expected.
- If codeine were to be given with the antiarrhythmic drug amiodarone, a medication that strongly inhibits the CYP2D6 isoenzyme, the patient would experience much less efficacy and possibly undergo withdrawal because codeine would not be activated into its morphine metabolite.
- Many antidepressants, such as venlafaxine, buPROPion, and DULoxetine, commonly prescribed for patients with pain syndromes, are CYP2D6 inhibitors and may also reduce the effectiveness of codeine.
- FentaNYL, a strong mu agonist, is primarily metabolized via CYP3A4 into norfentanyl, an inactive metabolite (Smith, 2009). If amiodarone, which also inhibits CYP3A4, were given concomitantly with fentaNYL, there would be less metabolism of fentaNYL into its inactive

metabolite, and higher serum concentrations of fentaNYL would be expected, increasing the risk for toxicity and overdose.
- A complex interaction occurs between omeprazole and HYDROcodone. Omeprazole inhibits CYP3A4 and CYP2D6, which are the same enzymes responsible for metabolizing HYDROcodone. HYDROcodone is an active compound that is metabolized to inactive forms of norhydrocodone by CYP3A4; it is also metabolized to the more potent HYDROmorphone by CYP2D6 and eventually glucuronidated to an inactive form of HYDROmorphone. When the CYP enzymes are inhibited by omeprazole, the active HYDROcodone parent compound may remain available longer, thus resulting in increased opioid-related risks.
- Another complex example is the conversion of oxyCODONE (an active drug) by CYP3A4 to noroxycodone (inactive) and by CYP2D6 to oxyMORphone (active, and perhaps twice as potent as oxyCODONE).

Box 11.2 | Clinical Application of Cytochrome P450 Induction

- If rifAMPin, a CYP2D6 inducer, was newly introduced to a patient who had been regularly receiving codeine, after about 3 weeks there would be increased metabolism of codeine into morphine. Thus increased concentrations of morphine would be expected, increasing the risk for toxicity and/or overdose (Smith, 2009).
- If carBAMazepine, a potent CYP3A4 inducer, was given to a patient who had been receiving fentaNYL, increased concentrations of norfentanyl (an inactive metabolite) would be expected, resulting in reduced analgesia and possible development of withdrawal.

to yield its effect, an inducer may increase the patient's risk for toxicity and/or overdose. Clinical application of concepts related to CYP450 induction is provided in Box 11.2.

For medications that undergo phase I metabolism by multiple isoenzymes, drug-drug interactions may become much more complex and variable. Some drugs may either inhibit or induce multiple isoenzymes, which will increase the complexity of the patient case and may more greatly affect overall outcomes. For example,

amiodarone is an inhibitor of both CYP2D6 and CYP3A4 and when used with an opioid, varied interactions are possible.

Drug-Drug Interactions: Phase II Metabolism

The risk for drug-drug interactions with phase II metabolism is much less than with phase I metabolism because there are very few drugs that inhibit or induce phase II enzymes. The primary enzyme mediators of phase II metabolism are the uridine diphosphate glucuronosyltransferase (UGT) enzymes. This is the phase in which a glucose molecule becomes attached to the parent drug and/or its metabolite(s). Opioids that primarily undergo phase II metabolism include morphine, oxyMORphone, HYDROmorphone, tapentadol, and levorphanol. These opioids may be preferred over others if patients intermittently require medications that interact with phase I enzymes, because there will be much less variability in metabolism of these medications, resulting in more consistent analgesia and improved safety. Notwithstanding, even these medications may be affected by drug-drug interactions or genetic variability because of enhanced or diminished absorption, which depends on P-gp, as noted earlier.

Clearance

Clearance is the final major concept in regard to pharmacokinetics. Drugs are normally cleared by renal, fecal, skin, or lung elimination or a combination of these routes.

Clearance has the biggest impact on half-life ($T_{(1/2)}$), which is the time required for a drug to decrease to 50% of its final concentration. To illustrate, if the blood level of a specific drug is 100 ng/mL and 4 hours later it decreases to 50 ng/mL, its half-life would be 4 hours. Half-life varies from medication to medication. For example, the half-life of morphine is 2 to 4 hours, whereas the half-life of methadone is variable and ranges from 8 to 90 hours (McPherson, Costantino, & McPherson, 2018).

Renal Excretion

The degree to which opioids and their metabolites are renally eliminated can dictate overall treatment selection and dosing. This pharmacokinetic characteristic is extremely important to consider in those with chronic kidney disease and the elderly, who often have diminished renal function. These populations have decreased elimination of opioids, which rely on renal excretion, resulting in increased risks for opioid accumulation, toxicity, and overdose. Analysis of creatinine clearance is often used to measure kidney function, and a high creatinine level may indicate reduced renal function. Normal serum creatinine and creatinine clearance values vary with age, gender, and weight. Box 11.3 provides values for all age groups and one of the formulas used for calculating creatinine clearance.

FentaNYL, oxyCODONE, HYDROcodone, and tapentadol are opioids that are at least 50% renally excreted and should be avoided or used cautiously in those with diminished renal function (Atkinson, Wegrzyn, & Bettinger, 2014). It is noteworthy that morphine also should be avoided in these populations. Whereas morphine is metabolized in the liver through phase II metabolism, its 3- and 6-glucoronide metabolites accumulate with reduced renal clearance. These metabolites are commonly known as morphine-3-glucuronide (M3G) and morphine-6-glucuronide (M6G) and are further described in a later section. Recognizing all of these key differences aids in optimal treatment selection and minimizes the potential for adverse event occurrence.

Pharmacogenomics

Pharmacogenomics is the study of how medication actions and reactions vary because of the patient's individual genetic makeup (Ting & Schug, 2016). This relatively new field combines pharmacology (the science of drugs) and genomics (the study of genes and their functions) to develop effective, safe medications and doses that will be tailored to a person's genetic makeup. Although interindividual genetic variations can lead to differences in both pharmacodynamic characteristics (i.e., receptor expression and signal transduction elements) and pharmacokinetic characteristics (i.e., expression of metabolizing enzymes and transporters), when it comes to opioids, there is generally a far greater emphasis on the pharmacokinetic implications of pharmacogenomic variability.

BOX 11.3 Creatinine Values and Clearance Calculations

SERUM CREATININE

- Newborns: 0.3–1.0 mg/dL
- Infants: 0.2–0.4 mg/dL
- Children: 0.3–0.7 mg/dL
- Adolescents: 0.5–1.0 mg/dL
- Adult males: 0.6–1.5 mg/dL
- Adult females: 0.5–1.2 mg/dL
- Elderly: May be normal, but creatinine clearance may be decreased

CREATININE CLEARANCE

- Newborns: 40–65 mL/min
- Males younger than 40 years: 97–137 mL/min
- Females younger than 40 years: 88–128 mL/min
- Adult males: 85–125 mL/min
- Adult females: 75–115 mL/min
- Elderly: Decreased

Creatinine clearance can be easily estimated using the following formula[a]:

Creatinine clearance (mL/min) = (140 − age) × (Weight in kg) ÷ (Serum creatinine [mg/dL] × 72)

[a] For women, multiply this amount by 0.85.
From Pasero, C., & McCaffery, M. *Pain assessment and pharmacologic management* (p. 290). St. Louis, MO: Mosby. © 2011, Pasero, C. & McCaffery, M. May be duplicated for use in clinical practice.

Genotype is the specific DNA sequence of an individual's genetic makeup that codes for specific physical characteristics or the phenotype of that individual (Wright & Fessele, 2017). Variable gene makeup can grossly affect reactions, efficacy, and side effects of drugs, which are especially dependent on polymorphic differences in CYP enzymes and P-gp expression, but also other phenotypes that are outside the scope of this chapter. Some important variable phenotypes for opioid response and/or toxicity include *OPMR-1, ABC1* genes, *COMT, MTHFR*, and others.

Depending on phenotype, a patient of the same gender, similar weight, and same overall health with the same diagnosis and on the same medications could have variable responses to their newly prescribed drug, including efficacy and toxicity, no efficacy and no toxicity, efficacy and no toxicity, and no efficacy and toxicity. It is for these reasons that individualized medication therapy and employment of pharmacogenetic testing will likely be the new standard in the future.

As outlined earlier in this chapter, P-gp reuptake transporters play a very important role when it comes to overall GI absorption and penetration of opioids across the BBB.

The *ABCB1* gene encodes the phenotypic expression of P-gp and is known to be highly polymorphic (Somogyi et al., 2007). Although it is known that mutations to this gene can affect P-gp expression, the clinical relevance when it comes to opioid efficacy remains controversial and contradictory.

Polymorphisms are alterations or mutations within certain sections of the genome that change the phenotypic expression of proteins, causing variations among individuals (Argoff, 2014). Genetic polymorphisms to alleles (alternative forms of the same gene arising from mutations) encoding for enzyme systems responsible for metabolizing opioids do have a significant clinical impact on opioid therapeutics. Both the CYP and UGT enzyme systems are affected by these polymorphisms, which produce enzymes with varying rates of metabolism. The CYP2D6 enzyme serves as a good example. Four different allelic combinations have been shown to produce four different CYP2D6 phenotypes with differing rates of metabolism (Deer et al., 2013; Somogyi et al., 2007). Two nonfunctional alleles produce poor metabolizers, at least one reduced functional allele produces intermediate metabolizers, at least one functional allele produces intermediate metabolizers, and multiple functional alleles and/or promoter mutations to the *CYP2D6* gene produce ultrarapid metabolizers or poor metabolizers (Deer et al., 2013). CYP2D6 poor metabolizers have the lowest rates of metabolism, followed by intermediate metabolizers, then extensive metabolizers (considered the norm), and finally ultrarapid metabolizers have the highest rates of metabolism. These variants are extremely important when it comes to predicting opioid response and toxicity. Because this applies to each CYP gene (2D6, 3A4, 1A3, 2C9, etc.), it is easy to see how different populations can have a vastly different response to medications.

If a patient is taking codeine and is a poor metabolizer of CYP2D6, production of its active metabolite morphine will be greatly reduced; thus it is likely the patient would experience little to no pain relief. If a patient is taking codeine and is an ultrarapid metabolizer of CYP2D6, production of its active metabolite morphine would be greatly enhanced; thus the patient is at greater risk for toxicity and overdose. This genetic variation is the reason codeine now has a black box warning for mothers who are nursing their infants and for children receiving codeine-containing cough products, as well as other child-related warnings, because infant and child deaths have been reported.

CYP2D6 is just one example; other enzymes are susceptible to genetic variation. CYP enzymes 3A4 and 2C9, as well as UGT enzyme 2B7 (notable for metabolizing buprenorphine, dihydrocodeine, dihydromorphine, HYDROmorphone, naloxone, naltrexone, and oxyMORphone) have been shown to have different genetic polymorphisms leading to variations in metabolism rates (Somogyi et al., 2007; Wirz, Wartenberg, & Nadstawek 2007).

CYP variations are not unique to opioid analgesics or any analgesics, because about 25% of all medications rely on the CYP system for metabolism. Examples of other medications that rely on the CYP system for metabolism include celecoxib (CYP2C9), carisoprodol and citalopram (CYP2C19), acetaminophen (CYP2E1, 1A2, 2A6, 3A4), and most antidepressants commonly used to treat neuropathic pain (Janicki, 2013). It is important to be aware of these variations because patients requiring analgesics may be taking a combination of medications that rely on the CYP system. Table 11.4 summarizes some potential drug interactions for CYP3A4 and CYP2D6. Many on-line

Table 11.4 | Potential Drug Interactions From Major Cytochrome P450 Enzymes CYP3A4 and CYP2D6

Enzyme	Substrates	Inhibitors	Inducers
CYP3A4	ALPRAZolam, amitriptyline, buPROPion, dexamethasone, dextromethorphan, diazePAM, fentaNYL, FLUoxetine, ketamine, lidocaine, meperidine, methadone, predniSONE, sertraline, venlafaxine	FLUoxetine, PARoxetine, propoxyphene, venlafaxine	CarBAMazepine, dexamethasone, phenytoin, rifAMPin
CYP2D6	Amitriptyline, buPROPion, codeine, desipramine, dextromethorphan, doxepin, FLUoxetine, haloperidol, HYDROcodone, methadone, morphine, nortriptyline, oxyCODONE, PARoxetine, sertraline, traMADol, venlafazine	Celecoxib, buPROPion, desipramine, haloperidol, metoclopramide, PARoxetine, venlafaxine	CarBAMazepine, dexamethasone, phenytoin, rifAMpin

From Pasero, C., & McCaffery, M. *Pain assessment and pharmacologic management* (p. 289). St. Louis, MO: Mosby. Data from Clinical Pharmacology Online. Gold Standard, Inc. Retrieved from http://clinicalpharmacology.com; Cytochrome P450 Interactions ©GlobalRPh Inc. Retrieved from http://www.globalrph.com/cytochrome.htm; Cytochrome P450 and drug interactions (drugs that induce or inhibit various cytochrome P-450 systems). Retrieved from http://www.edhayes.com/CYP450-3.html. © 2011, Pasero, C., & McCaffery, M. May be duplicated for use in clinical practice.

interactive websites such as http://www.globalrph.com/cytochrome.htm and http://www.medscape.com/druginfo/druginterchecker provide information related to CYP450 enzyme interactions.

Opioid Classes

Phenanthrenes

As outlined in Table 11.1, the phenanthrene class is the largest of all the classes and contains the prototypical opiate, morphine. Also included here are semisynthetic opioids HYDROcodone, oxyCODONE, and several others. The term *opiate* refers to drugs that come from natural sources. *Opioid* includes semisynthetic and synthetic agents. Of note, although opium has traditionally been considered the only naturally occurring opiate from the poppy plant, we know that kratom, from *Mitragyna speciosa,* a tree indigenous to Southeast Asia, provides opiate activity too. For the purposes of this chapter, we will collectively refer to these medications as opioids.

Phenanthrenes are divided into two subcategories, hydroxylated phenanthrenes and dehydroxylated phenanthrenes, the latter of which lacks a hydroxyl group at the sixth position and are indicated by an asterisk. The absence of this hydroxyl group is associated with improved GI tolerability compared to hydroxylated phenanthrenes (Wirz et al., 2007). Indications for the use of opioids include moderate to severe pain not resolved by nonopioid therapies, exercise, physical therapy, various physical modalities, and where nonopioid medications have failed or are contraindicated. Naloxone, a mu receptor antagonist indicated for reversal of opioid-induced respiratory depression (OIRD), is included in this category but does not provide analgesic activity; however, in very low doses it has been shown to ameliorate opioid side effects and promote analgesia (Elzey, Fudin, & Edwards, 2016; Gan et al., 1997).

Many of the dehydroxylated phenanthrenes are available in extended-release, long-acting, and immediate-release formulations. Extended-release formulations are generally reserved for opioid-tolerant patients in need of around-the-clock (ATC) analgesia, with the exception of extended-release tapentadol, which can be started in opioid-naïve patients at 50 mg bid (approximately every 12 hours) according to the package insert (Drugs@FDA: Nucynta ER, 2016). In 2013 the U.S. Food and Drug Administration (FDA) updated the indication for all extended-release and long-acting opioids such that their indication is "for the management of pain severe enough to require daily, around-the-clock, long-term opioid treatment and for which alternative treatment options are inadequate" (FDA, 2013, p. 8). It is important to note that tolerance is developed over time with any opioid regardless of subclass and therefore it is important to start low and titrate

carefully to avoid opioid-induced respiratory depression or withdrawal. Adult dosing of commonly prescribed phenanthrenes for the treatment of pain is listed in Table 11.5.

As described earlier, morphine is metabolized to M3G and M6G through phase II glucuronidation. The M6G metabolite is more potent than the parent drug and has a longer half-life. It is an active opioid metabolite with potent analgesic effects and a long half-life (longer than the parent morphine) (Klimas & Mikus, 2014). Repeated dosing in patients with reduced renal function can cause the active metabolite M6G to accumulate and result in improved analgesia but also increased sedation and respiratory depression. The M3G metabolite lacks analgesic activity but with reduced renal function, it can accumulate and lead to neurotoxicity. Neurotoxicity can also occur at high doses of intravenous morphine because of the preservatives in multidose vials (i.e., phenols, formaldehyde, bisulfate, or parabens). The use of preservative-free or single-use morphine vials for high-dose intravenous morphine is an alternative to avoid this potential adverse effect.

The dehydroxylated phenanthrene opioid group also includes the partial agonist/antagonists buprenorphine, butorphanol, and nalbuphine, outlined in Table 11.5. Buprenorphine is a semisynthetic partial agonist/antagonist, similar in chemical structure to HYDROcodone, oxyCODONE, levorphanol, HYDROmorphone, oxy-MORphone, naloxone, and butorphanol (Lutfy & Cowan, 2004). Buprenorphine has different indications depending on the product. In some formulations it is approved in the United States to treat moderate to severe pain; in others it is used to treat opioid use disorder. Doses used for pain are much lower than doses used for opioid use disorder. Buprenorphine formulations that are FDA approved for pain indications include Buprenex (injection), Butrans (transdermal), and Belbuca (buccal) (Indivor, 2016; Purdue Pharma, 2017; Endo Pharmaceuticals, 2016). The buccal and transdermal formulations are indicated for the management of pain severe enough to require daily, ATC, long-term opioid treatment. Buprenorphine in opioid use disorder is addressed in Chapter 14. Buprenorphine products that are FDA approved for treatment of opioid dependence include Probuphine (implant), Subutex (sublingual), Suboxone (sublingual, film), Bunavail (buccal), and Zubsolv (sublingual), the latter three of which are coformulated with naloxone (Braeburn Pharmaceuticals, Inc., 2018; Drugs@FDA: Bunavail, 2014; Orexo US, Inc., 2018; Reckitt Benckiser Pharmaceuticals, 2018; Roxane Laboratories, 2015). A monthly subcutaneous extended-release buprenorphine injection is now also available for treatment of moderate to severe opioid use disorder (Drugs@FDA: Sublocade™).

Buprenorphine has a unique pharmacologic profile that distinguishes it from its dehydroxylated phenanthrene counterparts (Lutfy & Cowan, 2004; Pillarisetti &

Table 11.5 | Adult Dosing of Common Phenanthrenes for the Treatment of Pain[a]

Medication	Common Starting Doses: Suggest starting at lowest end of dosing range and titrating based on patient response
HYDROcodone	IR: 5–10 mg PO q4–6h. Commonly prescribed as a combination product with acetaminophen or ibuprofen; not available as a single agent ER 12-h formulation: 10 mg PO every 12 hours ER 24-h formulation: 20 mg PO/day
OxyCODONE	IR: 5–10 mg PO q4–6h. Commonly prescribed as a combination product with acetaminophen or ibuprofen; also available as a single agent ER/LA: 10–20 mg PO every 12 hours
Morphine	IR: 10–30 mg PO q4–6h SR: 15 mg–30 mg PO q8–12h ER: 15 mg–30 mg PO q12–24h IV: 5–10 mg q4h
HYDROmorphone	IR: 2–4 mg PO q4h ER: 8 mg–12 mg PO q24h IV: 0.5–2 mg q4h
OxyMORphone	IR: 5–10 mg PO q4–6h ER: 5 mg PO q12h IV: 1 mg q3–4h
Buprenorphine	TDS: 5 mcg/h–20 mcg/h Buccal: 75 mcg, 150 mcg, 300 mcg, 450 mcg, 600 mcg, 750 mcg, 900 mcg every twelve hours IV: 0.3 mg q6–8h

ER, extended release; *IR*, immediate release, *IV*, intravenous; *LA*, long-acting; *PO*, orally; *SR*, sustained release.

[a] *Notes:*
1. Use only the lowest effective dose
2. Use in multimodal analgesia plan to minimize opioid dose and optimize analgesia
3. Lower doses may be appropriate for those at increased risk for opioid-related adverse effects.
4. IV and IR formulations are usually administered as prn medications, especially in opioid-naïve patients.
5. Modified-release medications (ER and SR) are scheduled medications.
6. Ensure assessment of effectiveness and adverse effects.

Khanna, 2015). Buprenorphine is a partial agonist at the mu opioid receptor and an antagonist at the kappa receptor, as mentioned previously. It has a strong affinity and high binding capacity, slow and incomplete dissociation from the mu receptor, and a long elimination half-life. Because of its partial agonist effect at the mu receptor, it provides similar opioid effects (e.g., analgesia, euphoria, respiratory depression) to full agonists. Theoretically, buprenorphine's maximal opioid effects are less than those of full agonists, although studies have shown similar efficacy between morphine and buprenorphine (White et al., 2017). Buprenorphine also has been thought to have a ceiling effect on respiratory depression because of its partial agonist activity, making it a safer option for patients at increased risk for respiratory depression (Dahan, 2006). However, recent studies have raised doubts about these claims (White et al., 2017). Its ability to cause euphoria has a ceiling effect, making it a better option for pain management in patients with high risk for abuse or misuse. As with full opioid agonists, buprenorphine also works on peripheral opioid receptors, including those in the gut. Therefore constipation can be a side effect of buprenorphine therapy; however, it may be less than the constipation associated with the traditional mu opioid agonists.

Phenylpiperadines

The most commonly prescribed phenylpiperadine is fentaNYL. Remifentanil, SUFentanil, and alfentanil are extremely potent phenylpiperadines reserved for surgical procedures under the direction of an anesthesiologist and/or collaborating nurse anesthetist. Additionally, there have been several illegally manufactured potent fentaNYL derivatives such as carfentanil, which have made their way to the streets and are responsible for many of the unintentional deaths among substance abusers (Drug Enforcement Administration, 2016).

FentaNYL is used intravenously or intramuscularly (although intramuscular injections should be avoided, if possible) in the inpatient setting for the treatment of acute pain and is available as a transmucosal immediate-release fentaNYL (TIRF) product indicated for breakthrough pain in patients with cancer. TIRFs are restricted by the federal Risk Evaluation Mitigation Strategy (REMS) program, requiring clinicians and pharmacists to register before prescribing or dispensing. FentaNYL is also available in a transdermal patch, which is indicated for patients who are opioid tolerant requiring chronic 24-hour analgesia. Because the fentaNYL patch is indicated only for patients who are opioid tolerant, the patient's previous opioid dose should be considered when determining an appropriate fentaNYL starting dose.

Diphenylheptane

The only available diphenylheptane on the United States market is methadone.

Methadone

Methadone is a nontraditional synthetic opioid and offers a unique, attractive, and inexpensive treatment option for multimodal pain management. Its multimodal activity is due to its unique mechanism; in addition to mu opioid agonism, methadone also acts as a kappa antagonist and N-methyl-D-aspartate (NMDA) antagonist. It also has noradrenergic activity, which includes reuptake blockade of norepinephrine and serotonin. Norepinephrine activity specifically provides synergistic activity in pain reduction similar to the analgesic activity of serotonin-norepinephrine reuptake inhibiting antidepressants and most tricyclic antidepressants mentioned in Chapter 15. This results in benefits for neuropathic pain that are not seen with pure mu opioid agonists (Aiyer, Mehta, Gungor, & Gulati, 2018; Pham, Fudin, & Raffa, 2015; Zorn & Fudin, 2011). Methadone's unique combination of receptor sites can provide analgesic benefit in patients intolerant to other traditional opioids.

The pharmacokinetics of methadone are important to consider. It is characterized by a long and variable half-life that can range from 15 to 60 hours and could even extend up to 150 hours in some patients with a genetic polymorphism. It is also prone to CYP450 enzyme drug-drug interactions and risk for QTc prolongation, which can lead to torsades de pointes and sudden cardiac death (Pham et al., 2015). Box 11.4 highlights medications that can prolong QTc and require caution and careful monitoring when used in combination with methadone. The QTc prolongation risk requires patients on chronic methadone to have electrocardiogram (ECG) monitoring. Because the major metabolism of methadone is through CYP3A4 and CYP2B6, care is needed to avoid use with inhibitors or inducers of either enzyme. Reduced CYP2B6 activity, as determined by pharmacogenetic testing or by concomitant use of another medication that is a CYP2B6 inhibitor, must be assessed carefully because decreased CYP2B6 metabolism of methadone can lead to an increased risk for torsades de pointes and sudden death.

Box 11.4	Common QTc Prolonging Drugs

- Atypical antipsychotics
- Amiodarone
- Buprenorphine (in higher than FDA-approved doses for pain)
- ChlorproMAZINE
- Citalopram
- Dofetelide
- Haloperidol
- Itraconazole/ketoconazole
- Macrolide antibiotics
- Methadone
- Ondansetron/dolasetron
- Quinolone antibiotics
- Sertraline
- Sotalol
- Venlafaxine

Initial methadone dosing should start low and be increased slowly (no more frequently than 7 days between titrations). A recommended initial starting dose is 2.5 mg bid. The dose should be titrated slowly to three or four times daily when used for analgesia (as distinct from the once-daily dose used in the treatment of opioid use disorder). Although the half-life of methadone is long, the analgesic properties last for only 6 to 8 hours (Herndon et al., 2016; Rajan & Scott-Warren, 2015). Methadone therefore should not be dosed once a day when used for analgesia. Both tablet and liquid formulations are available for use for the treatment of pain; however, the dispersible disks, also known as *diskets,* are available in the outpatient setting only for use in methadone maintenance clinics and detoxification centers.

Of note, levorphanol, which belongs to the phenanthrene chemical class of medications, has mechanisms nearly identical to those of methadone. This allows for unique benefits in the treatment of neuropathic pain, in addition to nociceptive pain. Levorphanol, however, has almost no serotonin activity, so it is better tolerated and has reduced risk for serotonin syndrome when given with drugs that have serotonergic properties. The half-life of levorphanol is also long but is more predictable and less variable at 16 hours compared to methadone (Pham et al., 2015). Levorphanol is metabolized by phase II and avoids the CYP450 interactions outlined earlier. Further, there is no risk for QTc prolongation with levorphanol. This allows for benefits similar to those of methadone, with an improved safety profile. Levorphanol is available in 2-mg tablets, which can be split for ease of dosing and titration, similar to methadone. Unfortunately, the use of levorphanol has been largely limited in recent years because of costs.

Table 11.6 | Adult Dosing of Phenylpropylamines

Drug	Common Dosing	Special Considerations
TraMADol	50–100 mg PO q4–6h; MDD 400mg ER: 100–200 mg PO daily; MDD 300mg	Commonly prescribed as a combination product with acetaminophen, but also available as single agent Avoid concomitant use of other serotonergic drugs
Tapentadol	IR: 50–100 mg PO q4–6h ER: 50–250 mg PO bid	Phase II metabolism Minimal serotonergic activity compared to traMADol IR MDD: 700mg for first 3 days, then 600 mg ER MDD: 500 mg

ER, Extended release; *IR,* immediate release; PO, orally.

Phenylpropylamines

Phenylpropylamines comprise two nontraditional opioids, traMADol and tapentadol. Both have benefits for neuropathic and nociceptive pain because of noradrenergic activity. TraMADol also has serotonergic activity. TraMADol and tapentadol are structurally similar; and although tapentadol does carry a warning for serotonin syndrome, it in fact has limited, if any, serotonin activity (Raouf, Glogowski, Bettinger, & Fudin, 2017). Adult dosing for the phenylpropylamines, traMADol and tapentadol, is listed in Table 11.6.

TraMADol

TraMADol exhibits extremely weak opioid activity, having 6000 times less affinity for the mu opioid receptor than morphine. This likens its opioid effect to that of dextromethorophan, which has similar binding affinity. TraMADol can be beneficial in the treatment of neuropathic pain because of its noradrenergic activity; however, it is important to always consider serotonergic effects, particularly when combined with other serotonergic drugs such as selective serotonin reuptake inhibitors (SSRIs) (Raffa et al., 1992). The use of several concomitant serotonin-acting agents can increase the risk for serotonin syndrome. Cyclobenzaprine, a tricyclic skeletal muscle relaxant that is sometimes prescribed along with traMADol, is an inhibitor of serotonin reuptake, and the combination of these medications may further increase risks for serotonin syndrome (Beakley, Kaye, & Kaye, 2015). TraMADol use with antidepressants that block reuptake of serotonin, such as FLUoxetine and other serotonin reuptake inhibitors, tertiary tricyclic antidepressants such as amitriptyline, serotonin-norepinephrine reuptake inhibitors such as DULoxetine, some antipsychotics such as QUEtiapine and many others not listed here, increase the potential for serotonin syndrome. TraMADol may decrease the seizure threshold, increasing the risk for seizure activity even in individuals with no history of seizures (Labate,

Newton, & Vernon, 2005). Abrupt discontinuation of traMADol may increase risks for opioid and serotonin and norepinephrine reuptake inhibitor withdrawal symptoms (Miotto et al., 2017).

TraMADol is a prodrug and relies on metabolism by CYP2D6 and CYP3A4 to its active metabolite O-desmethyltramadol (M1) to provide analgesic benefits. It has five metabolites in total and is therefore highly vulnerable to altered metabolism because of genetic polymorphism and CYP450 drug interactions.

Tapentadol

Tapentadol has significantly greater mu opioid activity than traMADol, demonstrating only 18 times less the affinity for the mu receptor compared to morphine. As noted earlier, significant serotonin effects have not been observed with tapentadol. Additionally, it undergoes phase II metabolism, avoiding concerns associated with traMADol and the CYP450 system. This allows for fewer drug-drug interactions and decreased risk for altered metabolism resulting from genetic polymorphisms.

Benzomorphans

The use of benzomorphans, particularly by someone who is not a pain specialist, is very limited. This opioid class is seldom used in clinical practice. Pentazocine, a benzomorphan, is typically considered a last-line option for pain management because of risks for accumulation, with even mildly hepatic or renal impairment, which can lead to neurotoxicity. Additionally, its activity as a partial agonist/antagonist (similar to buprenorphine) results in a plateau effect on analgesic activity. Although diphenoxylate and loperamide are included in this chemical class, neither are used clinically for pain management. In recent years, over-the-counter (OTC) loperamide has gained popularity as a drug of abuse when taken in high doses (Miller, Panahi, Tapia, Tran, & Bowman, 2017). This presents a very high risk for torsades de pointes, ventricular tachycardia, and death.

Key Points

- Opioids are effective analgesics that may be used in MMA plans to treat moderate to severe pain.
- Careful patient selection and monitoring for effectiveness and unintended effects are important to safe and effective opioid use.
- Opioids activate natural receptors within the CNS known as opiate receptors and thereby inhibit neuronal signaling involved in transmission of pain signals.

- Opioid analgesics provide symptomatic pain relief, but the underlying disease remains.
- Two patients receiving the same opioid at the same dose may have different analgesic and nonanalgesic effects. It is important to understand this variability exists and why it exists when initiating, titrating, and rotating opioids to individualize therapy.

This article is the sole work of the authors, and stated opinions or assertions do not reflect the opinions of employers, employee affiliates, or any pharmaceutical companies listed. It was not prepared as part of the authors' duties as federal employees.

Section 2 | Opioid Selection

Maureen F. Cooney

MANY factors are considered when determining the appropriate opioid, route, and dose to treat the patient with pain. These include the unique characteristics of the various opioids and patient characteristics, such as pain intensity, age, coexisting disease, current drug regimen, potential drug interactions, prior treatment outcomes, and patient preference (Box 11.5). It is important to use a multimodal approach to pain treatment that, whenever possible, includes nonopioid analgesics, coanalgesics, and nonpharmacologic interventions to minimize opioid requirements and optimize pain relief. The characteristics of opioid analgesics vary widely. There have been few randomized controlled trials that have compared one opioid directly with another. Wide variations exist in patient response to all opioids. Therefore no opioid can be said to be clinically superior to all others in providing analgesia. Understanding the unique characteristics of each opioid helps determine the optimal opioid analgesic for the individual patient.

As described earlier, a number of different classes of opioids are used in the management of pain. The purpose of this section is to elaborate on those classes and provide more detail related to the use of selected mu agonists, dual-mechanism analgesics, mixed agonist-antagonist action medications, and opioid antagonists in clinical practice, beginning with morphine (the prototypic full mu opioid agonist), followed by other full mu opioid agonists in alphabetical order. The section concludes with discussion of other medications that act on opioid receptors. Many of the currently used opioids have been available for decades, and much of the research related to individual opioids was conducted years ago, thus limiting the availability of more recent references.

Indications and Use of Opioids

Opioids are effective analgesics for many different pain conditions and, when used, should be incorporated into multimodal treatment plans. They are often indicated for the management of moderate to severe nociceptive pain, but also may be effective in some neuropathic conditions (Finnerup et al., 2015). Opioids are used in acute pain and cancer pain and, when necessary, are included in multimodal treatment plans for carefully selected patients with chronic noncancer pain. Full mu opioid agonists may be formulated in combination with a nonopioid (usually acetaminophen or a nonsteroidal antiinflammatory drug [NSAID]) and are used for moderate pain. Examples of these combination products are oxyCODONE with acetaminophen and HYDROcodone with ibuprofen. Although these medications are sometimes referred to as weak opioids, the dose-limiting factor is the nonopioid in the combination. Other medications referred to as weak opioids and used for moderate pain include the partial agonists and mixed agonist-antagonists. All full mu agonists are capable of producing comparable analgesia if an equianalgesic (equivalent) dose is provided and therefore may be used to treat moderate to severe pain depending on dose selection. Equianalgesic dose selection is described in detail in Section 3 of this chapter. See Table 11.7 for information on selected mu opioid analgesics.

Box 11.5 | Use of Opioids

- Perform a comprehensive assessment that addresses pain, all comorbidities, and functional status.
- Develop an individualized treatment plan that includes specific goals related to pain intensity, activities (function), and adverse effects (e.g., pain rating of 3 on a scale of 0–10 to ambulate or walk the dog accompanied by minimal or no sedation, and other adverse effects are tolerable and manageable).
- Use multimodal analgesia (i.e., this should be the regular practice for treatment of most types of pain).
- Assess for presence preoperatively of underlying persistent pain in surgical patients and optimize its treatment.
- Consider the potential for development of persistent postsurgical pain associated with type of surgery in surgical patients and provide multimodal analgesia.

Consider introduction of multimodal therapies before surgery for all patients (e.g., provide nonopioid analgesics preemptively, intraoperatively, or as soon as a patient is admitted to the pediatric intensive care unit). Often included in Enhanced Recovery After Surgery Society protocols.

- Provide analgesics before painful procedures.
- Medication selection
  - Consider diagnosis, condition, or surgical procedure, current or expected pain intensity, age, whether major organ failure is present (especially renal, hepatic, or respiratory), and presence of coexisting disease.
  - Consider pharmacologic issues (e.g., accumulation of metabolites and effects of concurrent drugs, including over-the-counter drugs, and possible interactions).
  - Consider individual differences (note prior treatment outcomes) and patient preference.
  - Be aware of available routes of administration (e.g., oral, transdermal, rectal, intravenous, subcutaneous, perineural, intraspinal) and formulation (e.g., short-acting or modified-release).
  - Be aware of cost differences.
- Route selection
  - Use least invasive route possible.
  - Consider convenience and patient's ability to adhere to the regimen (ease of use).
  - Consider staff's (or family's, patient's) ability to monitor and provide care required (e.g., parenteral and intraspinal routes in the home setting).
- Dosing and dose titration
  - Consider previous dosing requirement and relative analgesic potencies when initiating therapy.

- Use pain intensity and equianalgesic chart to determine starting dose with consideration of patient's current status (e.g., sedation and respiratory status) and comorbidities (e.g., medical frailty), and then titrate until adequate analgesia is achieved or dose-limiting adverse effects are encountered (see Chapter 12).
- Use appropriate dosing schedule (i.e., around the clock or as needed).
- When a dose is safe but additional analgesia is desired, titrate upward by 25% for slight increase, 50% for moderate increase, and 100% for considerable increase in analgesia.
- Provide supplemental doses for breakthrough pain.
- Consider patient-controlled analgesia (see Chapter 17).
- Recognize that for persistent cancer or noncancer pain, tolerance is rarely the "driving force" for dose escalation; consider disease progression when increasing dose requirements occur.
- Trials of alternative opioids
  - Trial of another opioid should be done only after the first opioid has been titrated upward to determine whether adequate analgesia can be obtained without significant adverse effects.
  - Be aware of incomplete cross-tolerance, and start the new opioid at about 50% of the estimated equianalgesic dose (see later in this chapter).
- Treatment of adverse effects (see Chapters 12 and 13)
  - Be aware of the prevalence and impact of opioid adverse effects.
  - Remember that most opioid adverse effects are dose dependent; always consider decreasing the opioid dose as a method of treating or eliminating an adverse effect; adding nonopioid analgesics for additive analgesia facilitates this approach.
  - Use a preventive approach in the management of constipation, including for patients receiving short-term opioid treatment (e.g., postoperative patients).
  - Use a preventive, multimodal antiemetic approach for patients with moderate to high risk for postoperative nausea and vomiting.
  - Prevent respiratory depression by monitoring sedation levels in opioid-naïve patients and decreasing the opioid dose as soon as increased sedation is detected.
  - Advise patient/family which adverse effects are likely to subside with long-term opioid treatment (e.g., nausea, cognitive effects).
  - Consider changing the opioid if adverse effects overshadow efficacy.

Continued

Box 11.5   Use of Opioids—cont'd

- Monitoring
  - Continually and consistently evaluate the treatment plan on the basis of the specific goals identified at the outset and assess pain intensity, adverse effects, and activity levels. Focus on functional improvement and clinically meaningful pain relief.
  - Make necessary modifications to treatment plan.
- Tapering and cessation of treatment
  - If a decrease in dose or cessation of treatment is appropriate, do so in accordance with an assessment of pain and after evaluation of functional outcomes.
  - Be aware of potential for withdrawal syndrome and need for tapering schedule in patients who have been receiving opioid therapy for more than a few days.

- Use equianalgesic dosing to determine appropriate decreases in doses (see discussion in text).

Modified from Pasero, C., & McCaffery, M. *Pain assessment and pharmacologic management* (pp. 324–325). St. Louis, MO: Mosby. Data from Argoff, C. E., Abrecht, P., Irving, G., & Rice, F. (2009). Multimodal analgesia for chronic pain: Rationale and future directions. *Pain Medicine, 10* (Suppl 2), S53–S66; Coyle, N., Cherny, N., & Portenoy, R. K. (1995). Pharmacologic management of cancer pain. In D. McGuire, C. H. Yarbro, & B. R. Ferrell (Eds.), *Cancer pain management* (2nd ed.). Boston: Jones and Bartlett; Fine, P. G., Mahajan, G., & McPherson, M. L. (2009). Long-acting opioids and short-acting opioids: Appropriate use in chronic pain management. *Pain Medicine, 10* (Suppl 2), S79–S88. © 2011, Pasero, C. & McCaffery, M. May be duplicated for use in clinical practice.

Formulations

The terms *short-acting, immediate release,* and *normal release* are used interchangeably to describe oral opioids that have an onset of action of approximately 30 minutes and a relatively short duration of 3 to 4 hours. It should be noted that although the term *immediate release* is often used, it may be misleading because most of the oral opioid analgesics do not have an immediate release or onset of analgesia. The term *rapid onset* may be accurately applied to opioids such as TIRF formulations because of their significantly faster onset of action compared with other short-acting opioids (TIRF REMS Access [n.d.]). The terms *modified release, extended release, sustained release, controlled release,* and *prolonged release* are used to describe opioids formulated to release over a prolonged period. Most often, the terms are applied to oral or transdermal formulations.

Opioid-Related Labeling and Safety Practices

Some of the generic and brand name opioid formulations have sound-alike/look-alike name similarities (e.g., HYDROmorphone and morphine, HYDROmorphone and HYDROcodone, OxyCONTIN and MS Contin, Roxanol and Roxicodone), which have been cited as a cause of medication errors (Institute for Safe Medication Practices [ISMP], 2016). Some ways to avoid confusion when prescribing opioids are to use Tall Man Letters (e.g., HYDROmorphone, OxyCONTIN, oxyCODONE), never express doses of liquid opioids in milliliters alone (include milligram amount), and write out opioid name modifiers (e.g., *extended release* rather than *ER* or *immediate release* rather than *IR*) (ISMP, 2016). In a systematic review of 16 studies, of which 13 were carried out in laboratory settings, tall-man lettering was found to improve

readability of medication container labels (Larmené-Beld, Alting, & Taxis, 2018).

Adverse Effects

All opioids have similar opioid-related adverse effects. See Chapters 12 and 13 for further details. If an individual opioid is associated with unique adverse effects, it is described in the following paragraphs.

Assessment and Monitoring of Patients on Opioid Therapy

Similar assessment and monitoring for effect and adverse effects is needed for all opioid medications. See Chapters 6 and 7 for details related to pain assessment and reassessment, and Chapter 13 for further detail related to monitoring for adverse effects. If an individual opioid requires specific monitoring, it is described in the following paragraphs. Some opioids are problematic for patients with acute or chronic kidney failure and require dose adjustments and opioid rotation in some situations. See Table 11.8 for information related to the use of selected mu opioid agonists in patients with renal failure or undergoing dialysis.

Morphine

Indications and Uses

Morphine has been extensively researched and widely used in many patient populations and clinical scenarios. Morphine plays a large role in the worldwide treatment of cancer pain and has a long history in the management of other types of pain. Most research related to the use of morphine and other mu opioid agonists was conducted over 10 years ago, whereas more recent research efforts

Table 11.7 | Overview of Selected Mu Opioid Agonist Medications

Mu Opioid Agonist Drug	Routes Administered	Comments
Morphine	PO (short-acting and modified-release), SL, R, IV, (IM), subcut, E, IT, IA	Standard for comparison. Multiple routes of administration. Several modified-release formulations available, but they are not therapeutically equivalent. Begin with lower doses in older adults. Active metabolite M6G can accumulate with repeated dosing in renal failure. Oral bioavailability is 20% to 30%. **IM administration of any opioid is to be avoided.**
Codeine	PO, (IM), subcut	Limited usefulness. Codeine is a prodrug and requires CYP2D6 metabolism to convert into morphine. Usually compounded with nonopioid. FDA restriction against use of codeine to treat pain or cough in children under 12 years of age, or in those under 18 years of age who have had a tonsillectomy/adenoidectomy and FDA recommends avoidance in obese children, and those with increased respiratory-related risks aged 12–18 years. FDA advises against use of codeine by nursing mothers because of potential harm to infants. Used orally for mild to moderate pain, but analgesia is inferior to that of ibuprofen. IV route not recommended, subcut route rarely used. **IM administration of any opioid is to be avoided.**
FentaNYL	OT, B, IV, (IM), TD, E, IT, IN	Fast-acting; short half-life (except TD). At steady state, slow elimination from tissues can lead to a prolonged half-life (up to 12 h). TD fentaNYL is indicated for management of pain severe enough to require an opioid analgesic and for which alternative treatments are inadequate. It is not approved for use in opioid-naïve patients and is not appropriate for acute pain management. OTFC and buccal fentaNYL are approved for management of breakthrough pain in opioid-tolerant individuals.
HYDROcodone	PO	Used for moderate to moderately severe pain; available in nonopioid combination only.
HYDROmorphone	PO (short-acting and modified-release), R, IV, (IM), subcut, E, IT	Useful alternative to morphine. Metabolite may accumulate with long-term, high-dose administration. Available in high-potency parenteral formulation (10 mg/mL) useful for subcut infusion; oral modified-release formulation available. **IM administration of any opioid is to be avoided.**
Levorphanol	PO, IV, (IM), subcut	Long half-life can lead to accumulation within 2–3 days of repetitive dosing. **IM administration of any opioid is to be avoided.**
Meperidine		No longer recommended for the management of any type of pain because of potential toxicity from accumulation of metabolite, normeperidine.
Methadone	PO, SL, R, IV, subcut, (IM), E, IT	Long half-life can lead to delayed toxicity from accumulation. See text for information on methadone. **IM administration of any opioid is to be avoided.**
OxyCODONE	PO (short-acting and modified-release), R	Used for pain severe enough to require an opioid analgesic and for which alternative treatments are inadequate (used for moderate pain when combined with a nonopioi acetaminophen or ibuprofen). Rectal and parenteral formulation not available in the United States. Oral formulation can be administered rectally. **IM administration of any opioid is to be avoided.**

Continued

Table 11.7 | Overview of Selected Mu Opioid Agonist Medications—Cont'd

Mu Opioid Agonist Drug	Routes Administered	Comments
OxyMORphone	PO (short-acting and modified-release) IV, (IM), subcut, R	Used for pain severe enough to require an opioid analgesic and for which alternative treatments are inadequate. Available in 5-mg rectal suppositories. **IM administration of any opioid is to be avoided.**

B, Buccal; *CYP2D6*, cytochrome 2D6; *E*, epidural analgesia; *FDA*, U.S. Food and Drug Administration; *IA*, intraarticular; *IM*, intramuscular; *IT*, intrathecal analgesia; *IN*, intranasal; *IV*, intravenous; *M6G*, morphine-6-glucuronide; *NR*, not recommended; *OT*, oral transdermal; *OTFC*, oral transmucosal fentaNYL citrate; *PO*, oral; *R*, rectal; *subcut*, subcutaneous; *SL*, sublingual; *TD*, transdermal.

Modified From Pasero, C., & McCaffery, M. *Pain assessment and pharmacologic management* (pp. 326–327). St. Louis, MO: Mosby.; Burnham, R., McNeil, S., Hegedus, C., & Gray, D. S. (2006). Fibrous myopathy as a complication of repeated intramuscular injection for chronic headache. *Pain Research and Management, 11*(4), 249–252; Chamberlin, K. W., Cottle, M., Neville, R., & Tan, J. (2007). Oral oxymorphone for pain management. *Annals of Pharmacotherapy, 41*(7), 1144–1152; Coda, B. A. (2006). Opioids. In P. G. Barash, B. F. Cullen, & R. K. Stoelting (Eds.). *Clinical anesthesia* (5th ed.). Philadelphia: Lippincott, Williams & Wilkins; Dale, O., Hjortkjær, R., & Kharasch, E. D. (2002). Nasal administration of opioids for pain management in adults. *Acta Anaesthesiology Scandinavia, 46*(7), 759–770; Davis, M. P., Varga, J., Dickerson, D., Walsh, D., LeGrand, S. B., & Lagman, R. (2003). Normal-release and controlled-release oxycodone: Pharmacokinetics, pharmacodynamics, and controversy. *Supportive Care in Cancer, 11*(2), 84–92; De Pinto, M., Dunbar, P. J., & Edwards, W. T. (2006). Pain management. *Anesthesiology Clinics of North America, 24*(1), 19–37; Du Pen, S., Du Pen, A., & Hillyer, J. (2006). Intrathecal hydromorphone for intractable nonmalignant pain: A retrospective study. *Pain Medicine, 7*(1), 10–15; Fick, D. M., Cooper, J. W., Wade, W. E., Waller, J. L., Maclean, J. R., & Beers, B. H. (2003). Updating the Beers criteria for potentially inappropriate medication use in older adults: Results of a US consensus panel of experts. *Archives of Internal Medicine, 163*(22), 2716–2724; Fong, H. K., Sands, L. P., & Leung, J. M. (2006). The role of postoperative analgesia in delirium and cognitive decline in elderly patients: A systematic review. *Anesthesia and Analgesia, 102*(4), 1255–1266; Fukuda, K. (2005). Intravenous opioid anesthetics. (2005). In R. D. Miller (Ed.), *Miller's anesthesia* (6th ed.). St. Louis, MO: Churchill Livingstone; Furlan, A. D., Sandoval, J. A., Mailis-Gagnon, A., & Tunks, E. (2006). Opioids for chronic noncancer: Pain a meta-analysis of effectiveness and side effects. *Canadian Medical Association Journal, 174*(11), 1589–1594; Gupta, S., & Sathyan, G. (2007). Providing constant analgesia with OROS hydromorphone. *Journal of Pain Symptom Management, 33*(2S), S19–S24; Gutstein, H., & Akil, H. (2006). Opioid analgesics. In L. L. Brunton (Ed.), *Goodman & Gilman's the pharmacological basis of therapeutics* (11th ed). New York: McGraw-Hill; Hagen, N. A., & Babul, N. (1997). Comparative clinical efficacy and safety of a novel controlled-release oxycodone formulation and controlled-release hydromorphone in the treatment of cancer pain. *Cancer, 79*, 1428–1437; Hale, M. E., Ahdieh, H., Ma, T., & Rauk R. (2007). Efficacy and safety of OPANA ER (oxymorphone extended release) for relief of moderate to severe chronic low back pain in opioid-experienced patients: A 12-week, randomized, double-blind, placebo-controlled study. *Journal of Pain, 8*(2), 175–184; Hanks, G., Cherny, N. I., & Fallon, M. (2004). Opioid analgesics. In D. Doyle, G. Hanks, & N. I. Cherny (Eds.), *Oxford textbook of palliative medicine* (3rd ed.). New York: Oxford University Press; Kalso, E. (2005). Oxycodone. *Journal of Pain Symptom Management, 29*(Suppl. 5), S47–S56; Kumar, M. G., & Lin, S. (2007). Hydromorphone in the management of cancer-related pain: An update on routes of administration and dosage forms. *Journal of Pharmacological Science, 10*(4), 504–518; Latta, K. S., Ginsberg, B., & Barkin, R. L. (2002). Meperidine: A critical review. *American Journal of Therapeutics, 9* (1), 53–68; Lugo, R. A., & Kern, S. E. (2004). The pharmacokinetics of oxycodone. *Journal of Pain and Palliative Care Pharmacotherapy, 18*(4), 17–30; McIlwain, H., & Ahdieh, H. (2005). Safety, tolerability, and effectiveness of oxymorphone extended release for moderate to severe osteoarthritis pain. A one year study. *American Journal of Therapeutics, 12*(2), 105–112; Miller, M. G., McCarthy, N., O'Boyle, C. A., & Kearney, M. (1999). Continuous subcutaneous infusion of morphine vs. hydromorphone: A controlled trial. *Journal of Pain Symptom Management, 18*(1), 9–16; Mitchell, A., van Zanten, S. V., Inglis, K., & Porter, G. (2008). A randomized controlled trial comparing acetaminophen plus ibuprofen versus acetaminophen plus codeine plus caffeine after outpatient general surgery. *Journal of the American College of Surgeons, 206*(3), 472–479; Murray, A., & Hagen, N. A. Hydromorphone. (2005). *Journal of Pain Symptom Management, 29*(Suppl. 5), S57–S66; Prommer, E. (2006). Oxymorphone: A review. *Supportive Care in Cancer, 14*(2), 109–115; Prommer, E. (2007). Levorphanol: The forgotten opioid. *Supportive Care in Cancer, 15*, 259–264; Prommer, E. E. (2007). Levorphanol revisited. *Journal of Palliative Medicine, 10*(6), 1228–1230; Quigley, C. (2002). Hydromorphone for acute and chronic pain. *Cochrane Database of Systematic Reviews*, (1):CD003447; Quigley, C., & Wiffen, P. (2003). A systematic review of hydromorphone in acute and chronic pain. *Journal of Pain Symptom Management, 5*(2), 169–178; Riley, J., Eisenberg, E., Müller-Schwefe, G., Drewes, A. M., & Arendt-Nielsen, L. (2008). Oxycodone: A review of its use in the management of pain. *Current Medical Research and Opinion, 24*(1), 175–192; Sarhill, N., Walsh, D., & Nelson, K. A. (2001). Hydromorphone: Pharmacology and clinical applications in cancer patients. *Supportive Care in Cancer, 9*(2), 84–96; Susce, M. T., Murray-Carmichael, E., & de Leon, J. (2006). Response to hydrocodone, codeine and oxycodone in a CYP2D6 poor metabolizer. *Progress in Neuro-Psychopharmacology and Biological Psychiatry, 30*(7), 1356–1358; Wright, A. W., Mather, L. E., & Smith, M. T. (2001). Hydromorphone-3-glucuronide: A more potent neuro-excitant than its structural analogue, morphine-3-glucuronide. *Life Science, 69*(4), 409–420. © 2011, Pasero, C., & McCaffery, M. May be duplicated for use in clinical practice.

Table 11.8 | Opioid Use During Renal Failure and Dialysis

Opioid	Comments About Use During Renal Failure	Comments About Use During Dialysis
Morphine	Avoid use. Metabolites can accumulate, and adverse effects can be prolonged.	Choose another opioid if possible. Parent drug and metabolites are removed by dialysis, but "rebound" accumulation can occur between dialysis sessions as drug and metabolites reequilibrate between CNS and plasma.
Codeine	Do not use. Metabolites can accumulate and cause serious adverse effects.	Do not use. Parent drug and metabolites can accumulate and cause serious adverse effects.
FentaNYL[a,b]	Use cautiously. Appears safe, particularly for short-term use. Metabolites are inactive, but accumulation of parent drug may occur. Cautious use and careful monitoring of adverse effects is advised with long-term use and continuous intravenous or intraspinal infusion.	Not removed by dialysis. Appears safe, particularly for short-term use. Metabolites are inactive, and no adverse effects have been reported during dialysis. In most cases, no dose adjustments are necessary, but use caution during and after titration. FentaNYL may absorb onto one type of filter in which changing the filter is recommended.
HYDROcodone	Use cautiously, monitor adverse effects closely, and adjust dose as needed. Metabolite can accumulate causing neuroexcitation.	Parent drug can be removed, but metabolite can accumulate and may pose risk.

Table 11.8 | Opioid Use During Renal Failure and Dialysis—Cont'd

Opioid	Comments About Use During Renal Failure	Comments About Use During Dialysis
HYDROmorphone	Use cautiously, carefully monitor for adverse effects, and adjust dose as needed. Metabolite can accumulate, causing neuroexcitation, but the drug has been used safely in patients with renal failure. May be an option in patients with ESRD who are unable to tolerate other opioids.	Parent drug can be removed, but metabolite can accumulate and may pose a risk. Use cautiously and monitor patient closely during dialysis.
Meperidine	Do not use. Metabolite accumulation increases adverse effects.	Do not use. No data on drug or metabolites during dialysis, but risk for adverse effects is plausible.
Methadone[a]	Use with caution as methadone is associated with increased risks in all patient populations. No clear increased risk in ESRD as it is eliminated primarily by hepatic metabolism, but more research regarding its excretion is needed. Parent drug and metabolites are excreted into the gut, and renal excretion varies widely.	Metabolites are inactive, but use with caution because parent drug is not removed by dialysis.
OxyCODONE	Further research is needed to make conclusive recommendations. Parent drug and metabolite (oxyMORphone) can accumulate. If used, administer with great caution and carefully monitor adverse effects.	Monitor closely for adverse effects as there is insufficient research to provide conclusive evidence of safety. In a small study (n = 20), a limited amount of oxycodone and noroxycodone were dialyzed (Samolsky Dekel et al., 2017).

CNS, Central nervous system; ESRD, end-stage renal disease.

[a] Not dialyzed; considered "safe," but cautious titration and close monitoring for a protracted period are recommended in patients with renal failure or undergoing dialysis (Dean, 2004).

[b] The other fentaNYLs (i.e., remifentanil, SUFentanil, and alfentanil) have been designated as safe for use in patients with renal impairment (Wellington & Chia, 2009), but further research and clinical experience with their use in these patients is warranted.

From Pasero, C., & McCaffery, M. (2011). *Pain assessment and pharmacologic management* (p. 364). St. Louis, MO: Mosby. Data from Dean, M. (2004). Opioids in renal failure and dialysis patients. *Journal of Pain Symptom Management, 28*(5), 497–504; Johnson, S. J. (June, 2007). Opioid safety in patients with renal or hepatic dysfunction. *Pain Treatment Topics.* Retrieved February 2, 2009 from http://www.pain-topics.org; Kurella, M., Bennett, W. M., & Chertow, G. M. (2003). Analgesia in patients with ESRD: A review of available evidence. *American Journal of Kidney Disease, 42*(2), 217–228; Wellington, J., & Chia Y. Y. (2009). Patient variables influencing acute pain management. In R. S. Sinatra, O.A. de Leon-Casasola, B. Ginsberg, E. R. Viscusi (Eds.), *Acute Pain Management,* Cambridge, New York: Cambridge University Press. © 2011, Pasero, C., & McCaffery, M. May be duplicated for use in clinical practice.

have involved the use of nonopioids in multimodal treatment plans. Older studies demonstrated efficacy for the use of morphine as a primary drug for acute postoperative pain management (McCartney & Niazi, 2006) and a wide range of other painful conditions, including severe angina pectoris (Mouallem, Schwartz, & Farfel, 2000), and prehospital admission trauma and medical conditions (Ricard-Hibon et al., 2008). As part of a standard anesthetic regimen, intravenous morphine, but not intravenous fentaNYL, suppressed several components of the inflammatory response to cardiopulmonary bypass in patients undergoing coronary artery bypass graft surgery (Murphy, Szokol, Marymont, Avram, & Vender, 2007). More recently, morphine use in this scenario has decreased, with emphasis on the use of fast-track early extubation protocols and increased use of adjuvant sedation and nonopioids to provide analgesia during cardiopulmonary bypass (Barry, Chaney, & London, 2015).

Improvement in neuropathic pain has been reported when morphine was used in combination with first-line adjuvant analgesics such as the gabapentinoids (i.e., gabapentin and pregabalin) and the coanalgesic antidepressants (Gilron, Tu, Holden, Jackson, & DuMerton-Shore, 2015; Wang, Yang, Shen, & Luo, 2017). Opioids are not first-line analgesics for neuropathic pain, and a Cochrane review concluded there is insufficient evidence to support or negate the usefulness of morphine in the treatment of neuropathic pain (Cooper et al., 2017).

Routes and Formulations

Morphine is available in a variety of formulations for multiple routes of administration. A Cochrane Collaboration review of 62 studies of oral morphine for cancer pain concluded well-controlled research with large numbers of patients is lacking, but studies confirm morphine is effective and oral morphine continues to be the preferred analgesic for moderate or severe cancer pain (Wiffen, Wee, & Moore, 2016).

Morphine may be administered by several routes: oral, intravenous, subcutaneous, intramuscular, intraspinal (epidural and intrathecal), intranasal, sublingual/buccal, intrapulmonary, rectal, intraarticular, vaginal, and topical (Brokjær et al., 2015; Herndon et al., 2016; Kestenbaum et al., 2014; Webster et al., 2018). Poor lipid solubility precludes transdermal absorption and also complicates reliable delivery through mucous membranes, such as the sublingual/buccal route (Coluzzi, 1998; Garg & Saini, 2015; Reisfield & Wilson, 2007). In a review of the use of sublingual opioids in palliative medicine, Reisfield and Wilson (2007) noted wide variations in the pharmacokinetics of sublingual morphine and concluded that highly hydrophilic opioids, such as morphine, have limited bioavailability. Highly concentrated morphine liquid (morphine sulfate in a 20-mg/1-mL preparation) is used as a sublingual medication in end-of-life situations in which oral and parenteral routes are not available and may provide analgesia when titrated to drug effect (Coluzzi, 1998). Some of the effect may be related to a degree of GI absorption from swallowed medication (Reisfield & Wilson, 2007). The evidence for vaginal administration of morphine is limited to case reports (Ostrop, Lamb, & Reid, 1998). Topical application of morphine is reported for painful wounds, in which case it is presumed to have a primary local action; there is a dearth of systematic research on this use, and it should not be considered an approach for systemic analgesic therapy (Paice et al., 2008; Zeppetella, Porzio, Aielli, 2007). Nebulized morphine was studied in a randomized controlled trial of 300 patients with severe traumatic pain. Titrated boluses of nebulized morphine 10 mg provided pain relief similar to that of titrated morphine 2 mg IV doses and resulted in fewer side effects. Nebulized 20-mg doses provided better analgesia without an increase in side effects (Grissa et al., 2015).

Morphine's effectiveness as an analgesic is therefore established for specific systemic routes of administration—oral and parenteral—and intraspinal routes. Intramuscular administration is not recommended for morphine or any other analgesic because of the painful injection and unreliable absorption (Herndon et al., 2016). The oral formulations of morphine are available in liquids, tablets, and capsules and in both short-acting and modified-release preparations.

Pharmacologic Considerations

As described earlier, morphine and its metabolites, M3G and M6G, are renally excreted. In patients with renal insufficiency there is an increased risk of morphine toxicity because of accumulation of morphine and its metabolites. M3G has been associated with neurotoxic effects, and metabolite accumulation in chronic kidney disease may contribute to sedation, altered mental states, myoclonus, and respiratory depression (Herndon et al., 2016). It is important to consider the need to reduce morphine doses in patients with renal insufficiency, the elderly, or use alternative opioids to minimize these risks (Sverrisdóttir et al., 2015).

Morphine is hydrophilic (soluble in an aqueous solution), which contributes to its delayed ability to cross the BBB, slower onset, and longer duration of action compared to those of the more lipophilic (soluble in fatty tissue) opioid medications, such as fentaNYL and SUFentanil. The length of time it takes for morphine to reach its analgesic site of action and to be eliminated must be considered when determining indications for its use and timing of subsequent doses. For example, morphine, with a half-life of 2 to 4 hours and an analgesic effect of 4 to 5 hours (Sheth, Holtsman, & Mahajan, 2018) would not be preferred over a lipophilic opioid such as fentaNYL when the goal is to have a rapid onset for procedural analgesia and elimination of opioid effect soon after the procedure is completed.

Codeine

Indications and Uses

Codeine is the prototypical "weak" opioid used primarily for short-term acute pain. It is usually prescribed as an oral combination product that also contains aspirin or acetaminophen. Codeine combination products also may include caffeine or a muscle relaxant. Combination preparations that include codeine are not appropriate for moderate to severe or escalating pain because of the dosing limitations inherent in the nonopioid constituent.

Routes and Formulations

Single-product codeine formulation is not FDA-approved for use in children (FDA, 2018) or used in clinical practice for adults, and combination codeine products are not dosed higher than 60 mg of codeine per dose because higher doses are not as effective as other opioids. When studied as a single-product entity, doses above 65 mg provided diminishing incremental analgesia but increasing adverse effects (Miaskowski et al., 2005).

Pharmacologic Considerations

Codeine is a prodrug, and, when absorbed, 10% of codeine is metabolized in the liver to morphine, its active form (Mercadante, 2015), which probably provides the bulk of its analgesic effect. The metabolism of codeine to morphine depends on the presence of the enzyme CYP450 2D6 (Mercadante, 2015) (see earlier for a detailed discussion of this enzyme system). Genetic polymorphisms that effect 2D6 metabolism may result in variability in codeine metabolism and potential for inadequate pain relief and serious life-threatening respiratory depression. The risk for altered metabolism has resulted in avoidance of codeine when other alternatives are possible.

Adverse Effects

Genetic polymorphisms may alter codeine metabolism and result in potential inadequate pain relief or serious life-threatening respiratory depression. Recognizing these risks, the FDA (2018) issued a contraindication for the use of codeine to treat pain or cough in children under 12 years of age and warns against the use of codeine in those aged 12 to 18 years who are obese or who have increased respiratory-related risks (obstructive sleep apnea or severe lung disease). The FDA also warns against the use of codeine for mothers who are nursing their infants, because of the potential for ultrarapid metabolizers to secrete high levels of codeine in their breast milk. Other codeine-related adverse effects include the adverse effects associated with all opioid medications. See Chapter 12 for further detail.

FentaNYL

FentaNYL is the prototype in a subset of mu agonists that includes SUFentanil, alfentanil, and remifentanil. Indications for fentaNYL vary depending on the route of administration. Pharmacology, adverse effects, and monitoring implications are also affected by the fentaNYL formulation and administration route, and therefore content related to fentaNYL is organized according to route.

Parenteral FentaNYL

Indications and Uses

Parenteral fentaNYL is administered for the management of acute pain as a bolus and as a continuous infusion. FentaNYL, like morphine and HYDROmorphone, may be used for postoperative pain management by intravenous patient-controlled analgesia (PCA). (See Chapter 17 for details related to PCA.) Earlier studies have shown that parenteral fentaNYL can be administered by subcutaneous infusion (Anderson & Shreve, 2004). Its rapid onset and short duration in the non–steady state situation make fentaNYL the most commonly used opioid in combination with benzodiazepines for procedural analgesia and sedation.

There have been no recent randomized controlled trials (RCTs) comparing intravenous fentaNYL, morphine, and HYDROmorphone. In an older retrospective analysis of medical records, adverse effects associated with morphine (N = 93), HYDROmorphone (N = 89), and fentaNYL (N = 72) by postoperative intravenous PCA were compared and lower mean rates of nausea, pruritus, urinary retention, and sedation were found with fentaNYL; there were no differences among the opioids in incidence of respiratory depression, headache, agitation, confusion, and hallucinations (Hutchison et al., 2006). In an RCT involving 50 patients who had undergone general or gynecologic surgery who received either morphine or fentaNYL by intravenous PCA, no difference was found between the medications in terms of efficacy, side effects, or patient satisfaction (Hong, Flood, & Diaz, 2008). However, well-controlled research is needed to draw conclusions regarding differences.

Pharmacologic Considerations

FentaNYL differs in many ways from morphine. Its lipophilicity provides wide and rapid distribution after intravenous administration, as well as ready passage through the BBB. When given as a single IV bolus, fentaNYL's onset (within 1–5 minutes) is faster and its duration (sometimes < 1 hour) is shorter than those of morphine because the drug moves from the blood to the lungs, muscle, and fat (Stanley, 2014). It also is approximately 100 times more potent than morphine, so a single intravenous bolus of 100 mcg produces roughly the same analgesia as intravenous morphine 10 mg (Sheth et al., 2018); however, caution is recommended when converting to and from fentaNYL because studies demonstrate considerable variability in conversion ratios.

When fentaNYL or some other very lipophilic drug is administered to the patient who is not receiving regular dosing, the blood levels decline quickly as the drug redistributes into fatty tissue. This redistribution, or alpha phase, is associated with a short half-life and a brief duration of clinical effects. With fentaNYL, it is typically only minutes long. Although fentaNYL is a rapid and short-acting medication, regular dosing of fentaNYL or any lipophilic drug eventually leads to a steady state in which there is equilibrium between the blood and fatty tissues. A bolus injection in this setting still has a redistribution phase, but most of the elimination time, the beta phase, results from metabolism and redistribution of drug from fat back into blood. As a result, in this setting, the half-life, and the duration of effect after the bolus, is much longer. The so-called *terminal elimination half-life* is the half-life that is obtained after the redistribution has taken place. Given these kinetics, reports of the half-life of fentaNYL vary in the literature depending on whether the study measured the decline in concentration in a steady-state situation.

An understanding of fentaNYL pharmacokinetics in the critical care setting is important in understanding the duration of the effect of this medication. A continuous infusion of intravenous fentaNYL has variable pharmacokinetics, influenced by the length of time the patient has received the infusion. Elimination half-time is the time it takes for a drug to be decreased by 50% of its steady-state concentration. Another term, *context-sensitive half-time*, takes into account the duration of the infusion (Whiteley & Hardman, 2017). The context-sensitive half-time is a better predictor of the duration of the effect of a medication such as fentaNYL than elimination half-life because it considers the time required for drug concentration to decrease to half of its concentration after a specific infusion duration. When the infusion duration of fentaNYL is increased from 1 to 8 hours, the context-sensitive half-time increases 10-fold (Whiteley & Hardman, 2017).

FentaNYL's lipophilicity and storage in fatty tissue has significant implications for obese patients in the perioperative setting. If perioperative dosing is based on body weight alone, obese patients are likely to receive too high of a dose. Dosing based on a calculated "pharmacokinetic mass" (i.e., for patients weighing 140–200 kg, dosing weights of 100–108 kg are projected) has been shown in two clinical studies to provide safe and effective intraoperative and postoperative analgesia at lower doses than would be predicted by actual weight (Shibutani, Inchiosa, Sawada, & Bairamian, 2004, 2005). This is a result of a nonlinear relationship between total body weight and fentaNYL clearance. These results are supported by a study of fentaNYL pharmacokinetics in critically ill medical and surgical patients in which body weight was found to have a significant effect on fentaNYL clearance and distribution in peripheral compartments, with overestimation of fentaNYL requirements in obese patients and very lean patients when fentaNYL is dosed by usual body weight calculations (Choi et al., 2016). Clinical application of this information necessitates awareness that fentaNYL doses in obese and very lean patients should be more conservative than usual weight-based calculations.

FentaNYL is metabolized in the liver primarily by CYP3A4, has no active metabolites, and produces minimal hemodynamic effects (Stanley, 2014; Suzuki & El-Haddad, 2017). These characteristics have made fentaNYL among the favored opioids for use in the critically ill, including critically ill older adults and those who are hemodynamically unstable (Barr et al., 2013; Choi et al., 2016). There is minimal concern about the effects of fentaNYL in patients with renal failure and liver failure when individual doses of the medication are administered. In the previously described study of the pharmacokinetics of fentaNYL infusions in the critically ill, a history of severe liver disease or congestive heart failure, but not age or renal failure, were shown to affect fentaNYL clearance and distribution into the peripheral compartments. Study results support earlier reports that individual doses of fentaNYL in liver and renal failure are not problematic, but patients receiving continuous infusions may have prolonged and increased opioid effects (Dean, 2004).

Other Considerations

Specific pharmacologic effects must be considered in parenteral fentaNYL administration. With rapid intravenous administration of high doses, fentaNYL can produce chest wall rigidity and subsequent difficult ventilation (Stanley, 2014). The mechanism of fentaNYL-induced cough (also reported with SUFentanil) is not well understood but may be histamine related. Interventions to reduce fentaNYL-induced cough during anesthesia induction include preinduction incentive spirometry, accupressure and a variety of medications, including magnesium sulfate, dezocine, and oxyCODONE (Goyal, Bhargava, & Baj, 2017; Huang, Wang, Xu, & Li, 2015; Liu, An, Su, Zhang, & Gui, 2015; Liu, Zhou, Wei, & Ma, 2015; Solanki, Doctor, Kapila, Gehdoo, & Divatia, 2016).

Another consideration related to parenteral fentaNYL is the impact of its lipophilicity on the pharmacokinetics of subcutaneous fentaNYL infusions. In a study of the pharmacokinetics of continuous subcutaneous fentaNYL infusions compared to transdermal fentaNYL in a cohort of patients with cancer, slow absorption with significant interindividual variation was noted with subcutaneous

administration. It was also noted that plasma levels fall more slowly after subcutaneous infusion than what is reported with intravenous infusion, thus necessitating caution and more conservative dosing when rotating from a subcutaneous infusion to a transdermal patch than with intravenous to transdermal rotation practices (Oosten et al., 2016).

Transmucosal FentaNYL

Indications and Uses

TIRF products are indicated for relief of breakthrough cancer pain in opioid-tolerant patients and are restricted by the federal REMS program. TIRF products are used for the treatment of breakthrough cancer pain (BTCP) in patients who are receiving modified-release opioids such as the fentaNYL transdermal patch. They are not approved for use in patients who are opioid naïve or who have acute postoperative pain (Herndon et al., 2016).

Pharmacologic Considerations

Breakthrough cancer pain is associated with a rapid onset, peak intensity within several minutes, and short duration of approximately 30 minutes (Bhatnagar et al., 2014). TIRF products have a rapid onset of action to address breakthrough cancer pain and have greater bioavailabilty than oral products because of minimal first-pass effect (Chang, Roeland, Atayee, Revta, & Ma, 2015). In a systematic review of 44 studies, TIRF products were shown to be effective in the management of breakthrough cancer pain and had stronger evidence for use than oral opioids (Brant, Rodgers, Gallagher, & Sundaramurthi, 2017). There is some variability in absorption of transmucosal fentaNYL because it is affected by how long and how closely the product is in contact with the mucosa. Individual titration, usually beginning with the lowest dose, is necessary. The fentaNYL pectin-based nasal spray product has been shown to be effective in the treatment of breakthrough cancer pain in patients with head and neck cancer and treatment-associated mucositis (Mazzola et al., 2017). A benefit of these products is that they afford patients with cancer an alternative route to intravenous administration for rapid relief of breakthrough cancer pain.

Other Considerations

TIRF products are available in sublingual tablet and spray, buccal tablet and soluble film, oral transmucosal product, and fentaNYL pectin nasal spray formulations (Chang A. et al., 2015). Dosing of transmucosal fentaNYL products is determined by titration of doses to achieve optimal relief without significant adverse effects. Dosing is not determined based on dose of the modified-release opioid or the dose of short-acting opioids that have been used. Dose adjustment on the basis of age alone is not required (Gordon, 2006; Kharasch, Hoffer, & Whittington, 2004), although elimination in older adults is prolonged (Gordon, 2006). The TIRF transmucosal products differ in formulation and are not bioequivalent to each other, so caution is necessary when changing from one product to another (Chang A. et al., 2015). Clinicians are advised to refer to the specific product information for the selected TIRF for dosing and administration guidelines.

Transdermal FentaNYL

Indications and Uses

The lipophilicity and potency of fentaNYL make it an excellent opioid for use as a transdermal medication. The transdermal fentaNYL patch is indicated for the treatment of chronic pain in opioid-tolerant individuals. Transdermal fentaNYL has been shown to be effective for persistent cancer-related pain and various types of noncancer pain. Numerous research studies conducted before 2011 demonstrated the efficacy of transdermal fentaNYL in the treatment of persistent cancer pain, acute exacerbations of cancer pain, AIDS-related pain, persistent postsurgical pain, persistent musculoskeletal pain, and other pain conditions (Pasero & McCaffrey, 2011). In a meta-analysis of 35 studies involving 3406 patients comparing transdermal fentaNYL to oral morphine in the treatment of cancer pain, similar efficacy was shown between the opioids (Wang, Ma, Zhu, & Peng, 2018). Although efficacy is well supported by older studies, there have been few recent studies related to the efficacy of transdermal fentaNYL.

Approval in the United States for the use of the transdermal fentaNYL patch is limited to the treatment of persistent, moderate to severe chronic pain in patients who are opioid tolerant when a continuous ATC opioid medication is necessary for an extended period and pain cannot be adequately managed by other medications (Drugs@FDA: Duragesic CII, 2016). The use of transdermal fentaNYL and other modified-release opioids requires careful patient selection, and the FDA cautions these products should be reserved as second-line approaches when alternative options have been ineffective, not tolerated, or not adequate. Safety concerns related to accidental overdose and death and risks associated with misuse, abuse, and opioid use disorder have resulted in several FDA safety announcements and changes in labeling requirements over recent years.

Pharmacologic Considerations

The transdermal patch is designed to release fentaNYL continuously over 3 days when applied to intact skin (Drugs@FDA: Duragesic CII, 2016; Lane, 2013). The transdermal system provides analgesia by passive diffusion of the fentaNYL across the skin and into the systemic circulation. A lipid-rich intracellular pathway permits passive diffusion of highly lipophilic drugs through this and other layers. With patch application, a subcutaneous depot or reservoir of fentaNYL is established in the skin near the patch, but after systemic uptake, the drug also redistributes into fat and muscle. At steady state, the level of drug in the blood represents the end result of absorption from the patch, movement into and out of these storage sites in various tissues, and drug elimination processes (Drugs@FDA: Duragesic CII, 2016; Lane, 2013). Despite changes in aging skin as a result of decreased water and lipid content, absorption of transdermal fentaNYL is not dramatically affected by age; however, older adults are more likely to experience skin irritation (Drugs@FDA: Duragesic CII, 2016).

Transdermal fentaNYL has been manufactured in reservoir and matrix delivery systems. The initial formulation was the reservoir patch, which contained a fentaNYL-gel reservoir that diffuses through a membrane to the skin. This formulation was at greater risk for accidental leakage and abuse (Schug & Ting, 2017). The newer matrix system contains fentaNYL dissolved in an inert polymer matrix that controls drug release and eliminates leakage risks (Lane, 2013; Pastore, Kalia, Horstmann, & Roberts, 2015; Schug & Ting, 2017). A number of newer patch delivery systems are under development, with some designed to reduce tampering risks. Patients should be monitored closely when switching from one patch formulation to another to ensure ease of use, satisfactory analgesia, and tolerable and manageable adverse effects.

FentaNYL patches are available in 12, 25, 50, and 100 mcg/h doses. The lowest available dose of transdermal delivery system, 12.5 mcg/h of fentaNYL, is prescribed as a 12-mcg/h patch to avoid decimal place error. Initial fentaNYL patch doses vary according to daily oral morphine equivalent requirements. For example, the fentaNYL product information suggests a 25-mcg/h fentaNYL patch as the initial starting dose for patients with a morphine equivalent daily dose (MEDD) of 60 to 134 mg/day (Drugs@FDA: Duragesic CII, 2016). When initiating transdermal fentaNYL, serum levels will rapidly increase over the first 3 days, continuing to increase to a lesser extent on days 4 through 6. It is advised that after the initial dose application, the dose should not be increased for at least 3 days, and subsequent increases should be based on assessment after at least two 3-day applications (Drugs@FDA: Duragesic CII, 2016), to ensure the patient is at a steady-state serum fentaNYL concentration before increasing the dose. After steady state is achieved using transdermal fentaNYL, half-life is affected by continued absorption from the skin depot under the patch; the half-life is therefore typically over 24 hours (Drugs@FDA: Duragesic CII, 2016).

The typical dosing interval for transdermal fentaNYL is to change the transdermal patch every 72 hours; however, for unclear reasons, some patients may report decreased efficacy, or end-of-dose failure, on the third day of patch application. These patients may experience improved efficacy with an adjustment in the frequency of patch changes to every 48 hours (Arnet, Schacher, Balmer, Koeberle, & Hersberger, 2016). A once-daily fentaNYL patch is available in Japan to address the problem of end-of-dose failure (Koike et al., 2016).

Other Considerations

Transdermal fentaNYL is associated with adverse effects similar to those of other full mu opioid agonists (see Chapters 12 and 13) but has been associated with less constipation, nausea and vomiting, drowsiness, and urinary retention than oral morphine (Wang et al., 2018). In a systematic review of transdermal fentaNYL in the treatment of cancer pain that included nine studies with 1244 patients, most participants had no worse than mild pain with treatment, and transdermal fentaNYL was associated with less constipation (28%) than oral morphine (46%) (Hadley, Derry, Moore, & Wiffen, 2012). Although recent studies are lacking, earlier research indicates side effect reduction, and significant improvements in many of the indicators of quality of life (e.g., sleep, mood) may be primary reasons patients frequently express a preference for transdermal fentaNYL over other modified-release formulations (Allan et al., 2001; Berliner, Giesecke, Bornhövd, 2007; Kornick, Santiago-Palma, Moryl, Payne, & Obbens, 2003).

If respiratory depression occurs with use of transdermal fentaNYL, despite reversal of respiratory depression with an opioid antagonist such as naloxone, the patient must be monitored closely after discontinuation of the patch because transdermal fentaNYL has a half-life of 20 to 27 hours, significantly longer than naloxone's half-life. The FDA (Drugs@FDA: Duragesic CII, 2016) recommends monitoring for at least 72 to 96 hours beyond the overdose. If naloxone is necessary, higher doses than those used for reversal of respiratory depression with other opioids may be required, and treatment may necessitate use of a naloxone infusion (Suzuki & El-Haddad, 2017).

Clinicians often express concern that transdermal fentaNYL will not be effective in cachectic patients because they lack subcutaneous fat. A small number of studies have examined the effects of body mass index on absorption of fentaNYL with a transdermal patch. Only one study showed a significant difference in serum fentaNYL levels (Heiskanen et al., 2009). In a study comparing plasma fentaNYL concentrations at 48 hours and 72 hours after application of a fentaNYL patch to 10 patients with normal weight and 10 patients with cachexia, serum fentaNYL was twice as low in patients with cachexia as it was in patients with normal body mass index (Heiskanen et al., 2009). The researchers pointed out that absorption of transdermal fentaNYL is governed by skin permeability and local blood flow, not by the amount of subcutaneous adipose tissue a patient has and that other factors, such as xerosis (abnormal dryness of the skin), may have been the cause. Others note serum albumin levels were not compared by Heiskanen et al. and suggest the lower serum fentaNYL levels in patients with cachexia may have been related to hypoalbuminemia (Kuip, Zandvliet, Koolen, Mathijssen, & Rijt, 2017). Transdermal fentaNYL efficacy must be carefully assessed when initiating this route of opioid therapy in a patient with cachexia, and pain control must be closely monitored in patients who are already using transdermal fentaNYL and develop cachexia. If analgesia is inadequate, doses may be increased or the patient switched to another opioid formulation.

Box 11.6 describes important educational content for clinicians, patients, and care providers.

Box 11.6 FentaNYL Transdermal Patch Instructions

- Appropriate application site should be considered when applying transdermal fentaNYL patches. Intact, flat skin surface is necessary to optimize patch adherence. Excess hair may be clipped, not shaven, and inflamed or irradiated skin should be avoided.
- Patients and caregivers should wash hands after applying transdermal fentaNYL patches to avoid inadvertent fentaNYL absorption.
- Application site should be rotated to minimize skin irritation.
- Patches should not be cut as a means of reducing medication dose; instead, lower dose patches should be prescribed.
- Patches can become loosened and may accidentally dislodge, posing a safety risk to others, particularly children. Fatalities related to inadvertent ingestion and inappropriate patch adherence and heating have occurred, and children are at increased risks. To prevent accidental dislodgement, loosened edges of patches should be taped or an adhesive film cover should be placed over the patch.
- Heat may increase the rate of absorption of fentaNYL from the patch, thus increasing risks for opioid-related respiratory depression. Patients and caregivers should be educated not to expose the transdermal application site to heat, including a heating pad application, electric blankets, submersion in hot water, or other sources of sustained heat, because this can dangerously increase absorption (Drugs@FDA: Duragesic CII, 2016).
- Patients with fever should be assessed for signs of excessive sedation and respiratory depression because fever may increase transdermal fentaNYL absorption (Drugs@FDA: Duragesic CII, 2016; Weaver, 2014).
- Proper patch disposal is important to reduce risks for misuse of the medication, diversion, and environmental contamination, especially because significant amounts of fentaNYL remain in the patch after 3 days of use. Used, unused, and discontinued patches should be folded in half, sticky side in, and returned to a drug take-back program or facility, but when not available, the FDA and manufacturers recommend flushing the product down the toilet (Drugs@FDA: Duragesic CII, 2016).

It is important to ensure adequate hand-off communication about the use of the fentaNYL patch. All clinicians need to be informed about the location and dose of the patch to prevent adverse patient outcomes. It is important for clinicians to inspect patients for the presence of fentaNYL patches on admission, especially when patients are unable to provide an accurate medication history. It is also necessary to ensure that prescribed patches remain adherent, because they can be inadvertently dislodged or, in some cases, purposefully diverted.

HYDROcodone

Indications and Uses

HYDROcodone is available in several different short-acting, fixed-dose combinations with nonopioids and in single-entity extended-release preparations for the treatment of pain. HYDROcodone in combination products is useful for the management of moderate to moderately severe pain (Greenwood, Clements, & Alper, 2017). The dose of nonopioid constituent in the combination product places a ceiling limit on the daily amount of the combination product that can be taken. In 2012, HYDROcodone bitartrate in combination products was the most commonly used medication for acute and chronic pain in the United States (Manchikanti, Alturi, Kaye, & Kaye, 2015). The FDA (2014a), in approval of two different single-entity, extended-release HYDROcodone analgesics, cautions the use of these medications should be reserved to treat pain severe enough to require daily, ATC, long-term opioids for which alternative treatments (e.g., nonopioid analgesics or immediate-release opioids) have been found to be inadequate.

Most of the research supporting the efficacy of short-acting HYDROcodone combination preparations for the treatment of acute pain was conducted over two decades ago. However, in a 2015 RCT of 240 adults presenting to the emergency department with acute extremity pain related to sprains, strains, and fractures, HYDROcodone with acetaminophen and oxyCODONE with acetaminophen resulted in similar efficacy; side effects of nausea and dizziness were significantly more frequent in the oxyCODONE with acetaminophen group (Chang, Bijur, Holden, & Gallagher, 2015).

More recent HYDROcodone research efforts have been directed toward the use of the extended-release products. In a study of 391 opioid-tolerant patients with moderate to severe pain for more than 3 months who received individualized single-entity, extended-release HYDROcodone doses of 20 to 300 mg bid for up to 48 months, 59% reported a moderate or substantial ($\geq 30\%$) reduction in pain scores (Argoff et al., 2015). Secondary functional outcomes demonstrated significant improvements ($P < .001$) in the Oswestry Disability Inventory, all pain interference outcomes, and Subject Global Assessment of Medication. The most commonly reported adverse events were constipation (12.5%), back pain (11.1%), nausea (9.9%), vomiting (9.7%), and arthralgia (7.8%).

A post-hoc analysis of two phase III trials of once-daily, single-entity, extended-release HYDROcodone included a 12-week placebo RCT and an open-label, 52-week trial of participants whose primary pretrial analgesic was HYDROcodone with acetaminophen combination tablets (Bartoli, Michna, He, & Wen, 2015). In both trials, an initial dose-titration period with the extended-release HYDROcodone was conducted. The RCT involved a fixed-dose, double-blind trial, and the open-label trial used flexible-dose maintenance treatment. Results of the 12-week RCT demonstrated better pain relief with the HYDROcodone than with placebo during double-blind treatment. Of the participants in the open-label flexible-dose 52-week trial, 57% completed the 1-year maintenance period. The average pretrial pain score was 6.3 (on a scale of 0–10), and during the maintenance period the mean pain scores ranged between 3.6 and 4.1. Participants had access to supplemental pain medication during the trial, and use of the supplemental medication decreased or was unchanged during the year-long maintenance treatment. The authors reported safety and tolerability of the once-daily, single-entity HYDROcodone product as similar to those of other opioids.

Routes and Formulations

HYDROcodone is available as a short-acting opioid in combination with nonopioid analgesics, including acetaminophen and ibuprofen. HYDROcodone is also available in single-entity, modified (extended)-release formulations. Most HYDROcodone combination products are available in tablet form, and some are available in capsule or liquid form. Combination medications containing HYDROcodone and a nonopioid drug illustrate MMA because the combination can provide more effective relief than either drug alone. Ibuprofen combined with a variety of HYDROcodone doses was shown to increase the effectiveness of HYDROcodone seven-fold in animal research (Kolesnikov, Wilson, & Pasternak, 2003).

The extended-release HYDROcodone 12-hour and 24-hour products, available in capsule and tablet forms, were approved by the FDA in recent years. At least one of these products has FDA-approved labeling describing the product's abuse-deterrent properties (Drugs@FDA, Hysingla ER, 2016). The abuse-deterrent properties result from physicochemical formulations that make them difficult to physically alter, which is expected to deter intranasal, intravenous, and oral abuse.

Pharmacologic Considerations

HYDROcodone is an active metabolite of benzhydrocodone. It has weak mu opioid receptor affinity, and its metabolite, HYDROmorphone, has strong affinity, but it is unclear whether the analgesic efficacy is related to HYDROcodone or its metabolite (Singla & Sloan, 2013). Short-acting HYDROcodone reaches peak serum levels by 60 minutes and peak effect by 120 minutes; it has a plasma half-life of approximately 4.5 hours (Drugs@ FDA: Vicoprofen, 2016). Like codeine, HYDROcodone is metabolized by the CYP2D6 enzyme, and polymorphisms of CYP2D6 may result in rapid and poor metabolizers of this medication (Singla & Sloan, 2013).

Other Considerations

The adverse effects of HYDROcodone are comparable to those of other opioids. To ensure safety, it should be specifically noted that the name HYDROcodone is similar in appearance and sound to oxyCODONE, oxyMORphone, and HYDROmorphone. An increased level of alertness is required to prevent medication errors with these opioids.

With rising awareness of national opioid abuse and opioid use disorder crisis, the FDA, in an effort to curtail availability and abuse of this opioid, rescheduled HYDROcodone products from Schedule III of the Controlled Substances Act to Schedule II in 2014 (Greenwood et al., 2017). As a result of the classification of HYDROcodone as a Schedule II opioid, tighter controls have been placed on the prescribing of HYDROcodone products and it is no longer possible to refill HYDROcodone prescriptions (Jones, Lurie, & Throckmorton, 2016). In the first year after the reclassification of HYDROcodone, Jones et al. (2016) reported that compared to the 12 months before reclassification, HYDROcodone prescriptions decreased by 22.0% and the amount of dispensed HYDROcodone combination product tablets decreased by 16.0%. The marked decline was in large part the result of the elimination of refills (73.7%). Of note, in the 12 months after the reclassification of HYDROcodone, prescriptions for non–HYDROcodone combination product opioid analgesics increased by 4.9%, with an increase in dispensed tablets by 1.2%. Along with the reclassification of HYDROcodone, the FDA placed a limit of 325 mg on the dose of acetaminophen that could be combined with each unit of HYDROcodone (and other medications) in recognition of the risks for hepatotoxicity associated with overuse and abuse of opioid-acetaminophen combination products (FDA, 2014b). Although the amount of acetaminophen in a single dose unit of HYDROcodone is limited, it is still necessary to avoid prescribing or administering medications that would permit amounts of nonopioids to exceed the daily maximum dose for acetaminophen, aspirin, or ibuprofen. It is critical to ensure patients are educated and understand the dangers of exceeding these amounts.

Benzhydrocodone

A short-acting opioid that was approved in 2018 is included in this section on HYDROcodone because the product contains benzhydrocodone and acetaminophen. Benzhydrocodone, the prodrug for HYDROcodone, must be metabolized by enzymes in the intestinal tract to enable its pharmacologic effects. Because the pharmacologic effects of benzhydrocodone rely on intestinal enzyme activity, its potential for intravenous or intranasal misuse may be reduced (Guenther et al., 2018).

According to the FDA (2018) full prescribing information, benzhydrocodone with acetaminophen is available in an immediate-release tablet form that contains 6.12 mg of benzhydrocodone and 325 mg acetaminophen. The HYDROcodone content of one tablet of benzhydrocodone is 7.5 mg of HYDROcodone bitartrate (Drugs@FDA: Apadaz, 2018). Dosing, actions, side effects, and warnings are similar to those for HYDROcodone products.

HYDROmorphone

Indications and Uses

HYDROmorphone is a full mu opioid agonist often used as an alternative to morphine, especially for acute pain. HYDROmorphone, like morphine and other single-entity full mu opioid agonists, is used for the treatment of acute pain, postoperative pain, and cancer pain and in carefully selected patients with chronic, nonmalignant pain.

In a review that compared the analgesic efficacy of HYDROmorphone to oxyCODONE or morphine in 504 participants with moderate to severe cancer pain, there was little difference in analgesic efficacy or side effects between HYDROmorphone and the other opioids (Bao et al., 2016). In a meta-analysis in which the analgesic benefits and side effects of HYDROmorphone (494 patients) and morphine (510 patients) were compared, HYDROmorphone was slightly more effective ($P = .012$) than morphine and side effects were similar (Felden et al., 2011). There is some limited evidence that HYDROmorphone may offer some benefits because it has been associated with less nausea, vomiting, pruritus, and sedation (Sheth et al., 2018). HYDROmorphone is often recommended as the first alternative for opioid rotation when morphine toxicity symptoms develop. Some clinicians will use HYDROmorphone in older adults as a first-line opioid instead of morphine because of the theoretically improved tolerance in the presence of decreased renal function; however, this practice has not been studied and has not been recommended in published guidelines. Well-designed studies are needed to draw conclusions regarding differences among the various opioids.

Routes and Formulations

Like morphine, HYDROmorphone is available in several formulations for use in different routes. Oral short-acting HYDROmorphone is available in tablets and an oral solution. Parenteral formulations of HYDROmorphone are used for bolus injections and infusions, with the intravenous route being the preferred parenteral route. The availability of HYDROmorphone in a concentrated parenteral formulation (10 mg/mL) also makes it a viable option for use in subcutaneous injections or infusions. In a longitudinal study of patients with cancer in an inpatient palliative care setting who received medications by the subcutaneous route, HYDROmorphone was the most frequently administered medication (59% of all subcutaneous administrations) (Bartz et al., 2014). The epidural and intrathecal routes have been used for acute and persistent cancer and noncancer pain (Bujedo, 2014; Galica et al., 2018; Shah, Baqai-Stern, A., & Gulati, 2015). A HYDROmorphone 3-mg suppository may be administered rectally and provides a treatment option when other routes are unavailable (Ripamonti & Bosco, 2015).

Pharmacologic Considerations

Oral short-acting HYDROmorphone is approximately 60% bioavailable, with an onset of action of 30 minutes (Sheth et al., 2018), a half-life of 2 to 3 hours, and a duration of approximately 3 to 4 hours (Drugs@FDA: Dilaudid, 2016). The extended-release oral formulation of HYDROmorphone, after a single dose, has a gradual increase in plasma concentration over 6 to 8 hours, with sustained concentrations for 18 to 24 hours; and after two or three consecutive daily doses, a steady state is reached (Drugs@FDA: Exalgo, 2013). The 3-mg HYDROmorphone rectal suppository has low bioavailability (~36%), and absorption is varied based on factors described in Chapter 9.

HYDROmorphone, like morphine, is hydrophilic, but it is 10 times more lipid soluble than morphine, reflected in the fact that it has a faster intravenous onset of action than morphine (intravenous bolus onset in 5 minutes and peak in 8–20 minutes), and its duration is approximately 4 hours (Sheth et al., 2018).

HYDROmorphone is metabolized in the liver and eliminated via the kidneys (Sheth et al., 2018). It undergoes extensive first-pass metabolism and is metabolized primarily in the liver by glucuronidation to HYDROmorphone-3-glucuronide. It is not significantly metabolized by CYP450 activity (Mercadante, 2015). HYDROmorphone-3-glucuronide (H3G) is a neuroexcitatory metabolite which is also renally excreted and may account for neurotoxicity at high doses. However, H3G is usually produced in small quantities, and therefore, even with renal insufficiency, neurotoxicity seldom develops (Sheth et al., 2018). Patients with mild to moderate renal failure who are receiving high doses of HYDROmorphone for extended periods should be monitored for signs of neurotoxicity (Lee, Ganta, Horton, & Chai, 2016).

The equianalgesic dose conversion between morphine and HYDROmorphone is unclear and may vary with the administration route (Sheth et al., 2018) and length of time a patient has taken one medication or the other. Published equianalgesic tables typically show oral HYDROmorphone to be five times more potent than oral morphine and four times more potent than oxyCODONE (Mercadante & Bruera, 2016); intravenous HYDROmorphone may be seven times more potent than intravenous morphine (Sheth et al., 2018). It is essential to recognize the potency of HYDROmorphone compared to morphine and other opioids to prevent inadvertent opioid overdose.

Meperidine

Indications and Uses

Meperidine was once the most widely used opioid analgesic. Its popularity as an analgesic was associated with the misconception that its anticholinergic effects resulted in less biliary spasm or renal colic. In recent years, use of meperidine has markedly declined (Piper, Shah, Simoyan, McCall, & Nichols, 2018) and it has been either removed from or severely restricted on hospital formularies, the result of concerted efforts to improve patient safety during opioid use (Friesen, Falk, & Bugden, 2015; Gordon, Jones, Goshman, Foley, & Bland, 2000; Raymo, Camejo, & Fudin, 2007).

Meperidine's use as an analgesic has been mostly abandoned, but low doses (12.5–25 mg IV) are sometimes used to treat shivering in patients who have received general or spinal anesthesia, transfusion, or medications, such as amphotericin (Fadeyi & Pomper, 2016; Lin et al., 2017).

Adverse Effects

The FDA-required product information for meperidine contains multiple black box warnings. The metabolite of meperidine, normeperidine, is associated with serotonergic properties and CNS toxicity. Accumulation of normeperidine may lead to anxiety, tremors, myoclonus, and generalized seizures, which are not reversed with naloxone (Herndon et al., 2016).

Oral meperidine is associated with greater risks than the intravenous formulation because it undergoes extensive first-pass metabolism, resulting in greater amounts of toxic metabolite formation (Herndon et al., 2016). Patients with renal or CNS disease are at particularly high risk. The Beers Criteria of inappropriate medication use in older individuals lists meperidine as an agent that should be avoided because of its anticholinergic effects and the risk for accumulation of neurotoxic metabolites (2019 American Geriatrics Society Beers Criteria® Update Expert Panel, 2019).

Methadone

Indications and Uses

Methadone is a unique opioid analgesic that may have advantages over other opioids in carefully selected and closely monitored patients. Methadone is used in the treatment of cancer pain and chronic noncancer pain (Chow & Issa, 2017). Methadone acts as a multimodal agent because it is a mu opioid agonist, a kappa antagonist, and an NMDA antagonist and also has noradrenergic activity. Based on extensive preclinical science, it is thought that NMDA receptor antagonism has the potential to produce analgesic effects independent of the opioid effect, at least in some neuropathic pain states; it has been shown in animal models to reduce opioid tolerance (Posa, Accarie, Noble, & Marie, 2016). Although methadone is often used in the treatment of neuropathic pain, clinical studies to support the use of methadone in neuropathic conditions have yielded conflicting results (Aiyer et al., 2018; McNicol, Ferguson, & Schumann, 2017).

Methadone's efficacy, high oral bioavailability, rapid analgesic onset, long half-life, low rate of tolerance, and low cost may make it a viable first-line treatment option for cancer pain (Mercadante & Bruera, 2018). Methadone is synthetic and structurally unrelated to other opioids, and for this reason it may be an alternative for the rare patient with a true allergy to another opioid.

See Table 11.9 for a summary of advantages and disadvantages related to methadone use.

Mercadante and Bruera (2018), in a systematic review of the use of methadone as a first-line analgesic for cancer pain, found that although available data were not adequate to draw conclusions, methadone provided analgesia and side effect profiles similar to the other opioids but offered the additional benefits of stable dosing with limited tendency to increase the dose. It was also successfully used as a first-line agent in opioid-naïve patients. The authors noted that the use of methadone as a first-line

Table 11.9 | Methadone Advantages and Disadvantages

Advantages	Disadvantages
Multiple mechanisms of action	Very wide interindividual pharmacokinetic and pharmacodynamic variability. A complex medication requiring prescribers who are knowledgeable about the unique pharmacological properties of this medication.
Agonist at mu, delta, and kappa opioid receptors	Long half-life and wide distribution may cause accumulation and potential toxicity with improper prescribing and/or inadequate monitoring. Monitor carefully.
NMDA receptor antagonist	Large number of drug-drug interactions because of metabolism by multiple CYP450 pathways
Serotonin and norepinephrine reuptake inhibitor	Variable dose ratio when converting from other opioids
May be helpful for neuropathic as well as nociceptive pain	No consensus on best procedure for switching from another opioid; requires specific expertise or consultation with expert
Onset of action comparable to morphine (30–60 minutes). Peak plasma concentration in 2.5 to 4 hours.	Not appropriate for use in pain emergency
Prolonged analgesia (usually 8–12 hours, but for some patients only 6 hours) once steady state is reached	Requires patient/family who can remain adherent to prescribed regimen
Increased effectiveness with long-term dosing	Requires close monitoring, especially during titration phase
Excellent option when rotating from other opioids because of ineffectiveness or adverse effects	Tablets are available only in 5- and 10-mg strengths[a]
Oral bioavailability may be as high as 80%–85%	Potential for QTc prolongation and torsades de pointes
No neurotoxic metabolites	Reluctance to prescribe and use because of perceived stigma of a drug used to treat opioid use disorder
May be used in most patients with renal insufficiency	
May be used in most patients with hepatic insufficiency	
Relative potency of methadone increases with rising dose of other opioid (dose ratio decreases as prior opioid dose increases)	
Relatively inexpensive	
Multiple routes of administration[a]	
May be alternative when patient is allergic to other opioids (is structurally unrelated to other opioids)	

Continued

Table 11.9	Methadone Advantages and Disadvantages—cont'd
Advantages	**Disadvantages**
Constipation develops more slowly and may be less than with morphine and HYDROmorphone	
Available in tablet, parenteral, and liquid formulations; may be compounded for rectal administration[a]	

[a] Available dose forms/strengths may vary in different countries.
CYP450, Cytochrome P450; *NMDA*, N-methyl-D-aspartate.

Modified from Pasero, C., & McCaffery, M. (2011). *Pain assessment and pharmacologic management* (p. 340). St. Louis, MO: Mosby. Data from Daeninck, P. J., & Bruera, E. (1999). Reduction in constipation and laxative requirements following opioid rotation to methadone: A report of four cases. *Journal of Pain Symptom Management, 18*(4), 303–309; Davis, M. P., & Walsh, D. (2001). Methadone for relief of cancer pain: A review of pharmacokinetics, pharmacodynamics, drug interactions and protocols of administration. *Supportive Care in Cancer, 9*(2), 73–83; Krantz, M. J., Martin, J., Stimmel, B., et al. (2009). QTc interval screening in methadone treatment. *Ann Intern Med, 150*(6), 387–395; Lynch, M. E. (2005). A review of the use of methadone for the treatment of chronic noncancer pain. *Pain Research and Management, 10*(3), 133–144; Mannino, R., Coyne, P., Swainey, C., Hansen, L. A., & Lyckholm L. (2006). Methadone for cancer-related neuropathic pain: A review of the literature. *Journal of Opioid Management, 2*(5), 269–276; Rajan, J., & Scott-Warren, J. (2015). The clinical use of methadone in cancer and chronic pain medicine. *BJA Education, 16*(3), 102–106; Weschules, D. J., & Bain, K. T. (2008). A systematic review of opioid conversion ratios used with methadone for the treatment of pain. *Pain Medicine, 9*(5), 595–612. © 2011, Pasero, C., & McCaffery, M. May be duplicated for use in clinical practice.

opioid may be preferred and less problematic to its use as a second-line agent because use as the first-line agent does not involve the challenging and potentially dangerous dose conversions associated with rotation from another opioid to methadone (Mercadante & Bruera, 2018).

Methadone is often considered an alternative agent when the efficacy of the original opioid, availability, side effects, or other factors necessitate a rotation. Up to 44% of patients with cancer pain will require opioid rotation during the course of pain treatment (McLean & Twomey, 2015). In a prospective, open-label study, the efficacy and safety of a rotation to methadone from another opioid was examined in 145 patients in an outpatient cancer clinic (Porta-Sales, Garzón-Rodríguez, Villavicencio-Chávez, Llorens-Torromé, & González-Barboteo, 2016). Efficacy was shown because by day 28 the median worst and average pain scores were significantly reduced from baseline ($P < 0.0001$) and there was no increase in opioid toxicity during the study.

Methadone has been used for chronic noncancer pain and some types of neuropathic pain (Rajan & Scott-Warren, 2015). Methadone (and other opioids) use in the treatment of these conditions may decline as a result of more recent attention to the potential for adverse effects associated with the use of opioids in the treatment of chronic noncancer pain (Els et al., 2017), the conflicting evidence to support methadone use in the treatment of neuropathic pain (McNicol et al., 2017), the rising awareness of prescription methadone–related unintentional deaths (Lev et al., 2015), and clinical practice guidelines that cite the lack of evidence to support opioid use in chronic noncancer pain treatment (Dowell, Haegerich, & Chou, 2016).

Methadone has been investigated for breakthrough pain via both oral and sublingual routes. In general, methadone is not used for both baseline and breakthrough pain relief because of risks for accumulation and adverse events. In methadone safety guidelines published by the American Pain Society (APS) and College on Problems of Drug Dependence in collaboration with

the Heart Rhythm Society (hereafter referred to as the APS methadone safety guidelines), the use of methadone for breakthrough pain is not recommended (Chou et al., 2014). However, case reports, particularly in end-of-life situations, have been published that report the efficacy of use of sublingual and rectal aqueous methadone for breakthrough cancer pain when other medications are poorly tolerated (Hagen, Fisher, & Stiles, 2007; Hawley, Wing, & Nayar, 2015).

Routes and Formulations

Although methadone is usually administered orally (tablets and liquid are available), it can be given intravenously, intramuscularly, subcutaneously, sublingually, rectally, and topically. A guideline for the use of parenteral methadone in pain and palliative care has been published (Shaiova et al., 2008). Most published reports on continuous subcutaneous administration indicate that local irritation is a problem (Nicholson, Watson, Derry, & Wiffen, 2017); flushing of the access site with normal saline has been reported to minimize irritation so sites can be maintained for prolonged periods without the need for dose limitation or medications added to prevent irritation (Hum, Fainsinger, & Bielech, 2007). Although a commercial product is not available, rectal administration of a compounded methadone preparation is very effective. The oral-to-rectal dose ratio for aqueous methadone is 1:1, with rapid absorption because rectal bioavailability is approximately 80% (Hawley, Wing, & Nayar, 2015). Because of its lipophilicity, the bioequivalence of buccal methadone is comparable to that of oral methadone (Hawley et al., 2015).

Pharmacologic Considerations

The pharmacology of methadone has been addressed earlier, but to highlight its clinical usefulness, after an oral dose, methadone has an onset of analgesia comparable to that of morphine (30–60 minutes). Plasma concentrations peak at approximately 2 to 4 hours after oral administration

(Nicholson et al., 2017; Rajan & Scott-Warren, 2015). Its oral bioavailability is 80% to 85%, which is significantly higher than that of morphine. The commonly used conversion ratio of parenteral-to-oral methadone dose is 1:2 but more specific conversion guidelines are provided later in this chapter. In a study of parenteral to oral methadone conversion in patients with cancer pain, Gonzalez-Barboteo et al. (2016) reported similar analgesia but lower toxicity when a more conservative 1:1.2 dosing ratio was used. The elimination half-life of methadone is long and highly variable. Elimination of methadone is primarily via feces.

The duration of analgesia after an oral dose of methadone is approximately 6 hours or less, particularly in those who have not been receiving regular doses, but may be prolonged with repeated dosing because peripheral tissues act as a reservoir and maintain plasma levels (Herndon et al., 2016; Rajan & Scott-Warren, 2015). The half-life, as noted previously, is usually 15 to 60 hours but may be longer (Herndon et al., 2016) and is typically approximated at about 24 hours (McPherson et al., 2018). These characteristics have an impact on clinical management, especially during the initial titration phase. After dosing begins or is increased, accumulation may occur for many days, or even weeks, before a steady state is approached. Methadone does not have neurotoxic metabolites, unlike morphine and HYDROmorphone. See Box 11.7 for highlights related to methadone pharmacokinetics and Box 11.8 for a summary of clinically important methadone characteristics.

Other Considerations

Methadone is a complex analgesic associated with multiple safety concerns. To be used optimally and safely, a clinician well versed in its characteristics should be involved in care planning and implementation. Patient selection and close monitoring during the titration phase are critical elements in pain management with this drug. See Box 11.9 for recommendations for patient selection for outpatient initiation of methadone for pain management.

The APS methadone safety guidelines were developed to promote safer methadone prescribing for substance use disorder and chronic pain (Chou et al., 2014). The guidelines include dosing recommendations for initiation of methadone in patients with chronic pain who are opioid naïve, those who are rotating to methadone from relatively low doses of other opioids, and those who are rotating to methadone from higher doses of another opioid. For patients who are considered by the APS to be opioid naïve (taking less than 60 mg/day of oral morphine), initial starting doses of 2.5 mg every 8 hours are recommended. Subsequent dose increases should not exceed 5 mg/day, and increases should not be made more frequently than every 5 to 7 days (Chou et al., 2014). Hospice and palliative care experts recommend similar dosing practices (McPherson et al., 2018). Rotation practices involving methadone are addressed later in this chapter. See Box 11.10, adapted from the APS guidelines, for recommendations related to initiation and dosing of methadone for analgesia.

Box 11.7	Highlights of Methadone's Unique Pharmacokinetics

- Methadone has several unique pharmacokinetic idiosyncrasies that make it difficult to titrate when initiating or discontinuing therapy, and therefore both must be done carefully and slowly over a prolonged period to ensure safety.
- Methadone has an extremely high volume of distribution (Vd) and is highly lipid soluble, which causes it to be rapidly transferred to tissues after oral absorption (Ferrari, Coccia, Bertolini, & Sternieri, 2004).
  - Methadone is associated with significant interindividual variability. In general, a larger patient with more body fat will most likely require a higher dose after reaching steady state than a cachectic patient lacking body fat.
    - This is because higher concentrations of methadone will be taken up into the available tissue in larger patients, because they have a larger volume of tissue to sequester the methadone (Ferrari et al., 2004). Therefore

higher doses are needed to ensure that sufficient drug concentration is available in systemic circulation to cross the blood-brain barrier and bind to mu opioid receptors in the central nervous system (CNS).
- Methadone has a very long and variable half-life (Cohen, 2015) and must be carefully dosed with assessment of individual characteristics and responses.
  - Methadone is rapidly transferred to tissues, then slowly released back into systemic circulation over prolonged and variable spans of time. The variability in release back into systemic circulation affects ultimate delivery to the CNS.
- Methadone's analgesic efficacy lasts 4 to 8 hours, and it must therefore be dosed 3 or 4 times daily irrespective of its long half-life and Vd.
- This is due to dissociation of the drug from the binding site but high volume of distribution, which results in tissue accumulation.

Box 11.8 | Summary of Clinically Important Methadone Characteristics

- Highly lipophilic
  - Oral bioavailability 80% to 85%
  - Wide distribution
  - Readily crosses blood-brain barrier
- Highly protein bound
- Wide distribution as a result of lipophilicity and protein binding
  - Slow elimination
  - Long but highly variable half-life
  - Accumulation and potential resultant toxicity
- Short duration of action (4–6 hours) with initial dosing; longer duration (8–12 hours) with accumulation
- When switching from another opioid (e.g., morphine), the morphine-to-methadone dose ratio varies with the morphine dose; methadone potency increases significantly as the morphine dose increases; published dose ratios vary from 4:1 (<90 mg morphine/day) to 20:1 (>1000 mg morphine/day)
- Multiple analgesic mechanisms of action
  - Active at mu, kappa, and delta opioid receptors
  - N-Methyl-D-aspartate receptor antagonist
- Effective in neuropathic pain states
- Potential decreased level of physiologic tolerance
  - Serotonin and norepinephrine reuptake inhibitor
- Elimination mostly via nonrenal routes; dose adjustment not normally necessary for renal insufficiency
  - Urine pH affects excretion: Urine pH less than six increases urinary excretion of methadone
  - Metabolizes in intestines as well as liver; dose adjustment not normally required in hepatic failure

- Wide interindividual variability in pharmacokinetics and response
- Large number of drug-drug interactions mediated by cytochrome (CY) P450 system (primarily via CYPC4A, but also CYP2D6 and CYP1A2; other CYP450 enzymes may have a smaller role in metabolism)
- Potential for cardiac arrhythmia, especially at methadone doses more than 100 mg/day (extended QTc interval with potential to induce torsades de pointes)
- No active metabolites

From Pasero, C., & McCaffery, M. (2011). *Pain assessment and pharmacologic management* (p. 342). St. Louis, MO: Mosby. Data from Davis, M. P., & Walsh, D. (2001). Methadone for relief of cancer pain: A review of pharmacokinetics, pharmacodynamics, drug interactions and protocols of administration. *Supportive Care in Cancer, 9*(2), 73–83; Fredheim, O. M., Moksnes, K., Borchgrevink, P. C., Kaasa, S., & Dale, O. (2008). Clinical pharmacology of methadone for pain. *Acta Anaesthesiology Scandinavia, 52*(7), 879–889; Krantz, M. J., Martin, J., Stimmel, B., Mehta, D., & Haigney, M. C. (2009). QTc interval screening in methadone treatment. *Annals of Internal Medicine, 150*(6), 387–395; Lynch, M. E. (2005). A review of the use of methadone for the treatment of chronic noncancer pain. *Pain Research and Management, 10*(3), 133–144; Mannino, R., Coyne, P., Swainey, C., Hansen, L. A., & Lyckholm, L. (2006). Methadone for cancer-related neuropathic pain: A review of the literature. *Journal of Opioid Management, 2*(5), 269–276; Mercadante, S., & Bruera, E. (2006). Opioid switching: A systematic and critical review. *Cancer Treatment Reviews, 32*(4), 304–315; Weschules, D. J., & Bain, K. T. (2008). A systematic review of opioid conversion ratios used with methadone for the treatment of pain. *Pain Medicine, 9*(5), 595–612. © 2011, Pasero, C., & McCaffery, M. May be duplicated for use in clinical practice.

Box 11.9 | Patient Selection for Outpatient Initiation of Methadone for Pain

1. Patients who live alone are generally not good candidates for methadone initiation. If the patient lives alone, strong consideration to how monitoring and reporting will occur is necessary.
2. Is the patient reliable? Able to follow instructions? Willing to have daily monitoring by phone?
3. Does the patient have a reliable family member who can monitor and communicate with the clinician? Make sure current contact information is available.
4. Is there a personal or family cardiac history? Consider baseline electrocardiogram.
5. Review all current medications for potential drug-drug interactions.
6. Give written instructions and a written schedule of doses and times, contact information during office hours, and when the practice is closed.
7. Confirm the patient's phone number(s), which may be different from what is in the records. The clinician needs to make sure contact information is available for at least one family member.

Box 11.10 | Recommendations for Use and Dosing of Methadone for Analgesia

1. Consult with a pain management expert who is competent in methadone management. Familiarity with methadone and individualization of care are essential to safe management.
2. Determine the patient's appropriateness for methadone (including assessment of medical and behavioral risks).
3. Educate patients about the risks and adverse effects of methadone (using informed consent).
4. Ensure an acceptable QTc on a baseline electrocardiogram (ECG) (generally ≤450 ms).
5. Calculate previous morphine equivalent daily dose (MEDD) and stop other opioids.
6. Starting dose of methadone.
   a. If on a low MEDD (40–60 mg) (or if opioid naïve), start methadone at 2.5 mg PO bid or tid;
   b. If opioid tolerant and on higher MEDD, refer to methods for rotation from another opioid to methadone in Boxes 11.16, 11.17, and 11.18 and Table 11.11.
   c. Initial doses should never exceed 30 to 40 mg/day.

7. Titrate based on effect no more frequently every 5 to 7 days, with conservative increases in daily dose (not to exceed 5 mg in opioid naïve or 10 mg in opioid tolerant).
8. Close assessment for adverse effects:
   a. Expect maximum adverse effects to occur 5 to 7 days after dose change.
   b. Treat adverse effects.
   c. Check ECG 2 to 4 weeks after methadone initiation, when dose exceeds 30 mg, and again if dose exceeds 100 mg, and when other risks for QTc interval prolongation develop.

From Chou, R., Cruciani, R. A., Fiellin, D. A., Compton, P., Farrar, J. T., Haigney, M. C., . . . & Mehta, D. (2014). Methadone safety: A clinical practice guideline from the American Pain Society and College on Problems of Drug Dependence, in collaboration with the Heart Rhythm Society. *The Journal of Pain, 15*(4), 321–337; Herndon, C. M., Arnstein, P., Darnall, B., Hartrick, C., Hecht, K., Lyons, M., & Sehgal, N. (2016). *Principles of analgesic use.* Chicago: American Pain Society; McPherson, M. L., Costantino, R. C., & McPherson, A. L. (2018). Methadone: Maximizing safety and efficacy for pain control in patients with cancer. *Hematology/Oncology Clinics of North America, 32*(32), 3, 405–415.

Unlike morphine and HYDROmorphone, there are no methadone toxic metabolites to accumulate in renal failure, and dose adjustment in the presence of renal insufficiency is generally not necessary (Elefritz, Murphy, Papadimos, & Lyaker, 2016). However, as with other opioids, initial doses for older adults should be lower and dosing intervals longer than for healthy younger adults (McPherson et al., 2018; Nicholson et al., 2017); the half-life in older adults is likely to be relatively longer than in younger patients (Gallagher, 2009; Sunilkumar & Lockman, 2018). Some methadone metabolism occurs in the intestine rather than the liver. There are no specific recommendations for methadone dose reductions in cirrhosis or stable chronic liver disease, but because CYP450 enzymes are involved in methadone metabolism, it is appropriate to use low doses with cautious dose titration and observation for adverse effects (Elefritz et al., 2016). Methadone may be less likely to cause severe constipation than other opioids, but this has not been confirmed (Rajan & Scott-Warren, 2015).

Drug-Drug Interactions

Major safety and clinical management limitations of methadone are related to multiple pharmacodynamic and pharmacokinetic drug-drug interactions associated with its use (McPherson et al., 2018). Limited evidence exists related to the degree of harm associated with these interactions, but some may result in alterations in methadone blood levels, increased sedative or respiratory depressant risks, and/or

prolonged QT intervals (Chou et al., 2014). The increased drug-drug interaction potential is related to methadone's reliance on the CYP450 enzymes for metabolism. It is important to review patients' medication histories to identify risks for drug-drug interactions that may necessitate closer monitoring, elimination or replacement of methadone or other medications, or dose reductions. Patients should be educated to inform prescribers of all medications they are taking, including OTC medications, to identify potential drug-drug interactions (McPherson et al., 2018).

Like all opioids, methadone is a CNS depressant, and therefore its use in patients who are taking other CNS depressants such as the benzodiazepines, increases risks for advancing sedation and respiratory depression (McPherson et al., 2018). To illustrate this point, methadone and benzodiazepines both cause sedation and a high number of cases of methadone-related overdose have been associated with the concomitant use of these medications (Leece et al., 2015). Therefore, it is recommended that in general the combination of these medications should be avoided, or, if used, careful risk-benefit assessment should be conducted (Chou et al., 2014).

As addressed earlier, a potential drug-drug interaction that may involve methadone is the risk for prolongation of the QTc interval seen on ECG. A critically prolonged QTc interval—one greater than 500 ms—may lead to torsades de pointes, a potentially fatal cardiac arrhythmia (Chou et al., 2014). Methadone as a single agent may increase QTc in some patients, and there is cumulative risk when methadone is used with other medications that also increase the QTc (McPherson et al., 2018). See Box 11.4 for a list of medications associated with QTc prolongation. Other risk factors include structural heart disease, electrolyte abnormalities, advanced age, female gender, genetic polymorphisms, bradycardia, and a history of QTc prolongation (McPherson et al., 2018).

Although there is no consensus among experts related to ECG monitoring for QTc prolongation, the APS methadone safety guidelines have been published (see Box 11.11).

Methadone is a serotonin reuptake inhibitor, and therefore caution must be exercised when used along with other serotonergic agents, such as the monoamine oxidase inhibitors (MAOIs), selective serotonin reuptake inhibitors (SSRIs), serotonin-norepinephrine reuptake inhibitors (SNRIs), and tricyclic antidepressants because of the potential for serotonin syndrome (Baldo, 2018). Methadone also poses risks for other nondrug interactions. A known food interaction (grapefruit juice inhibits gut-wall CYP3A4) and herb interaction (St. John's wort induces CYP3A4 metabolism) (Chou et al., 2014) further underscores the complexity of methadone and reinforces the need for thorough history taking and patient teaching. A drug interaction should be suspected whenever a new drug or remedy is introduced and there is a sudden increase in pain or increase in sedation when the methadone dose is stable.

Renal excretion of methadone is affected by urine pH. Methadone renal clearance is markedly increased in a low pH environment (Chong & Johnson, 2017). Although decreased renal function is not generally a concern with methadone use, drug-drug interactions may interfere with methadone pharmacokinetics. Medications that lower urine pH, such as furosemide, and drugs that increase urine pH, such as sodium bicarbonate and acetaZOLAMIDE, must therefore be used with caution.

The risk for methadone accumulation during initial treatment and dose titration necessitates caution and assessment for adverse effects. It is important to frequently assess the inpatient who is receiving methadone during initial dose titration for signs of progressing sedation and respiratory depression. It is also important to provide reassessment of outpatients during dose titration and educate patients and their significant others about signs of opioid-related adverse effects. The APS methadone safety guidelines recommend face to face or phone assessment of patients for adverse effects, especially for signs and symptoms of excessive sedation, respiratory depression, and cardiac arrhythmia within 3 to 5 days of methadone initiation or upward dose titration (Chou et al., 2014).

Clinicians and patients may be more familiar with the use of methadone as maintenance therapy in the treatment of opioid use disorder than its use in pain management. Despite significantly increased use of methadone as an analgesic, some patients are reluctant to take it or other opioids because of fears of opioid use disorder and the perceived stigma of taking a medication that is used in its treatment (Fishman, Wilsey, Mahajan, & Molina, 2002; Gunnarsdottir et al., 2017; Valeberg, Miaskowski, Paul, & Rustøen, 2016). In a survey of physicians in outpatient pain practices, 5 of 13 physicians who did not prescribe methadone cited concerns about social stigma as the reason for not prescribing it (Shah & Diwan, 2010). It is important to elicit patient and family concerns and provide clarification. The indication should be written on the prescription to avoid misunderstanding among patients, family members, and clinicians.

When using methadone to treat pain, as with other opioids, consideration should be given for the use of nonopioids and nonpharmacologic approaches in a multimodal plan of care. Although methadone is associated with a number of potential drug-drug interactions, there are nonopioids that do not present risks for dangerous interactions. For example, in a small trial (N = 22) involving patients who required multilevel spinal surgery, patients who received an intraoperative and postoperative ketamine infusion in addition to methadone PCA required 70% less methadone in the first 24 hours compared to those who received methadone PCA and placebo (Pacreu, Candil, Moltó, Carazo, & Galinski, 2012).

Box 11.11 | Methadone EKG QTc Monitoring Recommendations

- Consider doing a baseline ECG if one was done in previous year and QTc was less than 450 ms and there were no new risk factors.
- Baseline ECG is unnecessary if one was done in preceding 3 months and QTc was less than 450 ms.
- Baseline ECG before methadone therapy is initiated if patient is at risk for QTc prolongation:
  - Prior ECG with QTc greater than 450 ms
  - History suggestive of ventricular arrhythmia
- Avoid methadone if QTc is greater than 500 ms.
- Consider alternatives to methadone if QTc is more than 450 ms and less than 500 ms.
- If risk factors for prolonged QTc, prior QTc greater than 450 ms, or a history of syncope exist, repeat ECG 2 to 4 weeks after starting methadone and after significantly increasing doses.
- If started on lower doses, repeat the ECG when methadone doses are increased to 30 to 40 mg/day and again at 100 mg/day (Chou et al., 2014).

Levorphanol

Indications and Uses

Levorphanol (Levo-Dromoran) is a synthetic opioid with activity at the mu, kappa, and delta opioid receptor sites, and, like methadone, it also is an NMDA antagonist. In addition, it is an inhibitor of serotonin and norepinephrine reuptake (Reddy, Ng, Mallipeddi, & Bruera, 2018), which may contribute to its efficacy in neuropathic pain conditions. It has not been widely used clinically since newer formulations of other opioids have become available. Many clinicians are unfamiliar with its pharmacology because it has not received widespread marketing, is more expensive, and is less commercially available than methadone and other opioids (Gudin, Fudin, & Nalamachu, 2016). It is seldom mentioned in the literature, and few recent studies of levorphanol have been published. Levorphanol may be difficult for patients to obtain because of limited Drug Enforcement Agency (DEA) production quotas (Herndon et al., 2016).

Levorphanol, because of its activity at multiple receptor sites, may be an effective first-line analgesic in cancer pain and in pain conditions such as neuropathic and central pain that have not been controlled by more commonly used opioids (Gudin et al., 2016). Levorphanol is used as a long-acting medication, so a short-acting or immediate-release opioid and/or nonopioid analgesic would be required for breakthrough or acute pain.

A study using levorphanol at two dose levels established that neuropathic pain is responsive to opioid treatment (Rowbotham et al., 2003). In fact, all types of neuropathic pain responded to levorphanol except central poststroke pain in the study. In the higher dose arm (mean was ~9 mg/day) apparent CNS toxicity occurred (i.e., irritability, mood changes, confusion, weakness). The reasons and risk factors for these changes were unknown. Close monitoring and dose and interval changes are indicated for older adults and those with impaired renal function.

McNulty et al. (2007) published a small study of the use of levorphanol in patients who had been previously treated with methadone for refractory chronic noncancer pain and in hospice patients with primarily cancer pain. Of those with chronic noncancer pain who had been switched from methadone to levorphanol because of poor pain control, 40% reported excellent relief and 35% experienced fair relief (N = 20). Of 11 hospice patients with cancer, 55% reported excellent relief and 18% reported fair relief. Levorphanol was well tolerated.

Routes and Formulations

Levorphanol is available in the United States orally only in 2-mg tablets, which can make titration difficult. A levorphanol dose of 4 mg is proposed to be equivalent to 30 mg of oral morphine. The recommended starting dose of levorphanol is 1 mg PO, every 6 to 8 hours with weekly upward titration by 25% depending on the patient's response (Pham et al., 2015).

Pharmacologic Considerations

Levorphanol metabolism is similar to morphine metabolism. It undergoes glucuronidation in the liver and is renally excreted. Because it does not undergo phase I liver metabolism, it is not affected by the CYP450 system and therefore poses fewer potential drug-drug interactions than methadone. Compared to methadone, levorphanol has more reliable pharmacokinetics and does not pose a risk of QTc prolongation (Gudin et al., 2016). Levorphanol's duration of analgesia ranges from 6 to 15 hours (Pham et al., 2015). Levorphanol has a half-life of 12 to 16 hours, which is shorter than the half-life of methadone, but the half-life of levorphanol may be increased to 90 to 120 hours with continued dosing (Herndon et al., 2016). The discrepancy between analgesic duration and half-life can predispose levorphanol to accumulation.

OxyCODONE

Indications and Uses

OxyCODONE is used in the management of acute pain, cancer pain, and some noncancer chronic pain conditions. The controlled-release formulation is approved by the FDA for the treatment of pain that is severe enough to necessitate the use of daily, ATC, chronic opioid therapy when alternatives to opioids have not been effective (Drugs@FDA: OxyContin®, 2018). However, earlier published studies have reported efficacy in the use of the controlled-release formulation in the treatment of acute postsurgical pain after different surgeries, including orthopedic and breast surgery (de Beer et al., 2005; Kampe et al., 2004; Sunshine et al., 1996). Of note, these studies examined controlled-release oxyCODONE before its reformulation with abuse-deterrent properties in 2010.

OxyCODONE is often used in the treatment of acute postsurgical pain because it provides advantages over other opioids. The greater oral bioavailability of oxyCODONE compared to oral morphine may offer better pain relief. It has been shown to provide greater efficacy in reducing visceral pain and is associated with less nausea and pruritus and fewer hallucinations than morphine (Cheung, Ching Wong, Qiu, & Wang, 2017). In a review of 26 trials of oxyCODONE (including immediate-release and sustained-release formulations), for the treatment of acute pain in a variety of surgical conditions, Cheung et al. (2017) reported superior efficacy over placebo, and greater or similar efficacy compared to intravenous opioids in those who underwent knee arthroplasty, spine surgery, caesarean section, laparoscopic colorectal surgery, and cardiac surgery.

Immediate-release and controlled-release oxycodone have been extensively studied in patients with cancer pain. In a Cochrane review that included 26 studies with 2648 participants, oxyCODONE was found to provide pain relief similar to that of morphine and other strong opioids and was associated with similar adverse effects (Schmidt-Hansen, Bennett, Arnold, Bromham, & Hilgart, 2017). Both oxyCODONE and morphine were reported as appropriate first-line opioids for the treatment of cancer pain.

Routes and Formulations

OxyCODONE is available in single-entity oral formulations and in a variety of fixed combinations with acetaminophen, aspirin, and ibuprofen. Like HYDROcodone combination products, the use of oxyCODONE in combination products offers the benefit of an MMA approach in a single product. However, the dose of nonopioid constituent in the combination product places a ceiling limit on the daily amount of the combination product that can be taken.

As a single agent, oxyCODONE is available as a tablet, capsule, and elixir, and in a controlled-release or modified-release (every 12 hours) formulation. Newer combination oxyCODONE-naloxone products have been developed for their abuse deterrent properties and benefits of reduced peripheral opioid side effects. Sustained-release oxyCODONE-naloxone combination products are associated with less constipation than single-product, sustained-release oxyCODONE (Davis & Goforth, 2016). In a study of 69 patients with severe pain who had opioid-induced constipation refractory to laxatives, a significant reduction in constipation ($P < .001$) was demonstrated when patients were treated with sustained-release oxyCODONE-naloxone compared to sustained-release oxyCODONE, and pain relief and quality of life were also improved (Poelaert et al., 2015).

In 2016, a new extended-release, abuse-deterrent formulation of oxycodone (oxycodone DETERx™) was approved by the FDA (Drugs@FDA: Xtampza ER). Like other modified-release products, this medication is indicated for management of pain severe enough to require daily, around-the-clock, long-term use of opioids for which alternative treatments have not been effective.

Oxycodone DETERx™ is available in capsules that contain microspheres with an oxycodone base and an inactive ingredient to make the product more difficult to tamper with or alter for abuse purposes (Kopecky, Fleming, Levy-Cooperman, O'Connor, & Sellers, 2017). Capsules are available in oxycodone base formulations of 9, 13.5, 18, 27, or 36mg, which are equivalent to oxycodone HCL of 10, 15, 20, 30, or 40mg, respectively (Drugs@FDA: Xtampza ER). This medication can be prescribed to opioid-naive patients, if appropriate, with initial doses of 9mg orally every 12 hours. Patients should be instructed to take the medication with food. Recommended doses for rotation from another oxycodone product or other opioid to Oxycodone DETERx™ are provided in the product information (Drugs@FDA: Xtampza ER). One of the benefits of this oxycodone product is that it is a capsule containing microspheres. For patients who cannot swallow the capsule or who require medication administration via a feeding tube, the capsule can be opened and the the microspheres can be sprinkled onto a small amount of soft food for swallowing or poured directly into the feeding tube and flushed with water through the tube.

OxyCODONE is not available in the United States in suppository form for rectal administration; however, oral preparations may be administered rectally when other enteral routes are not possible. Absorption and peak blood levels by the rectal route appear to be comparable to those of the oral route, but maximum blood concentration is prolonged. In a review of alternative routes of opioid administration in palliative care, onset of analgesia was found to be slower with rectal administration of oxyCODONE than with intravenous administration but duration of action was longer (Kestenbaum et al., 2014). An intravenous formulation of oxyCODONE is available in other countries but not in the United States.

Pharmacologic Considerations

OxyCODONE binds to the mu opioid receptor, but in contrast to morphine and HYDROmorphone, oxyCODONE also binds to the kappa receptor (Sheth et al., 2018). Kappa and mu opioid receptors are found in the both the central and peripheral nervous systems. This dual action and interaction between receptor types theoretically may provide clinical advantages of oxycodone in some pain states. Kappa receptor activity in the abdominal organs is believed to account for the greater efficacy of oxycodone in relieving visceral pain than morphine (Ruan, Mancuso, & Kaye, 2017). In animal studies, topical oxyCODONE provided an analgesic response that was thought to be related to the presence of kappa receptors located on peripheral nerve endings (Smith et al., 2015).

OxyCODONE is metabolized in the liver primarily by the CYP450 2D6 enzyme and also by CYP450 3A4, and excreted by the kidneys. It is recommended to reduce the starting dose of oxyCODONE in advanced liver disease by 30% to 50%, and the dosing interval may need to be increased (Soleimanpour, Safari, Nia, Sanaie, & Alavian, 2016). Dose reductions and longer dosing intervals are also recommended in renal insufficiency and failure (Koncicki, Brennan, Vinen, & Davison, 2015). OxyMORphone is a potent metabolite of oxyCODONE, but it does not account for oxyCODONE's analgesic effect because it is not produced in significant amounts (Sheth et al., 2018). Unchanged oxyCODONE and multiple metabolites produced by other pathways appear to produce oxyCODONE's pharmacodynamic effects, although the role of the metabolites has not been well described (Ruan et al., 2017).

Approximately 10% of the population have genetically low levels of the CYP450 2D6 enzyme, resulting in lower concentrations of oxymorphone. Although oxycodone's analgesic effect is not usually related to oxymorphone, in a small number of patients, this may result in the need for higher than usual doses of oxyCODONE to obtain adequate pain relief. Similarly, analgesia may also be reduced in those with concurrent use of medications that inhibit the CYP450 2D6 enzyme. Analgesia may be enhanced by the concurrent use of medications that inhibit the CYP450 3A4 enzymes (Sheth et al., 2018).

Other Considerations

There are only a few head-to-head studies comparing oxyCODONE with other analgesics. Compared with morphine, oxyCODONE is more potent, has greater oral bioavailability (55%–64% versus 24%–40% for morphine), comparable onset of action (30 to 60 minutes) and half-life (3 to 4 hours), and a similar adverse effect profile (Sheth et al., 2018).

A meta-analysis identified four RCTs that compared oral oxyCODONE with either oral morphine (N = 3) or oral HYDROmorphone (N = 1) and concluded there were no significant differences in efficacy and tolerability between the opioids (Reid, Martin, Sterne, Davies, & Hanks, 2006). A Cochrane Collaboration review concluded single oxyCODONE doses higher than 5 mg are effective for postoperative pain and two to three times stronger than codeine (Gaskell, Derry, Moore, & McQuay, 2009). Efficacy was increased when oxyCODONE was combined with acetaminophen. OxyCODONE 10 mg plus acetaminophen (650 mg) provided good analgesia to half of those treated, comparable to NSAIDs but with a longer duration of action.

When taken in fixed combination with a nonopioid, it is critical for patient safety and treatment efficacy to establish exactly what dose of the nonopioid the patient is taking. Care should be taken to avoid prescribing or administering amounts that would exceed the daily maximum dose for acetaminophen, aspirin, or ibuprofen. Patients also should be educated to avoid taking additional nonopioids that could result in excess dosing (see discussion related to HYDROcodone).

In a narrative review of clinical trials that examined the use of oxyCODONE in the management of acute postoperative pain, studies were identified that examined the use of oxyCODONE in an MMA plan. Six studies demonstrated oxyCODONE in a multimodal plan was associated with analgesia comparable to that of intravenous PCA opioid, and reduced adverse effects, reduced opioid consumption, earlier analgesic discontinuation, shortened hospitalization, and reduced cost were also reported (Cheung et al., 2017).

OxyMORphone

Indications and Uses

OxyMORphone is a semisynthetic mu opioid agonist used in the treatment of moderate to severe acute pain (Endo Pharmaceuticals, 2010; Vadivelu et al., 2013). At equianalgesic dosing, oxyMORphone provides analgesia comparable to that of oxyCODONE (Mayyas, Fayers, Kaasa, & Dale, 2010).

Routes and Formulations

OxyMORphone is available in short-acting 5- or 10-mg oral tablets and a parenteral formulation (1 mg/mL). The modified-release (extended-release) formulation, originally approved for use in the treatment of chronic pain, was voluntarily withdrawn by the manufacturer in 2017 (Endo Pharmaceuticals, 2017) because of FDA concerns that the abuse deterrent properties were not as effective as intended (FDA, 2017).

Pharmacologic Considerations

OxyMORphone is an oxyCODONE metabolite. The oral bioavailability of oxyMORphone is only 10%, which is lower than the oral bioavailability of morphine or oxyCODONE. However, oxyMORphone is more lipid soluble than either morphine or oxyCODONE (Mercadante, Porzio, & Gebbia, 2014). Its greater lipid solubility facilitates greater movement across the BBB, resulting in a slightly faster onset of action than morphine and a mean time to maximum plasma concentration of 30 minutes compared to 1.2 hours for morphine (Vadivelu et al., 2013; Sheth et al., 2018). OxyMORphone undergoes extensive phase II metabolism in the liver; therefore there is little risk for CYP450 drug-drug interactions; the primary metabolites, oxyMORphone-3-glucuronide and 6-hydroxymorphone have not been well studied, but oxyMORphone-3-glucuronide may provide some analgesia (Vadivelu et al., 2013). OxyMORphone is excreted via the kidneys and produces clinically inert metabolites. Reduced doses are required with impaired hepatic or renal function, and it is contraindicated in those with moderate to severe liver impairment.

Other Considerations

The analgesic potency of oral oxyMORphone is twice that of oral oxyCODONE and 3 times that of oral morphine (Endo Pharmaceuticals., 2010). Parenterally, oxyMORphone is 10 times more potent than intravenous morphine (Vadivelu et al., 2017). When given intravenously it has a quick onset (5–10 minutes). Its peak time is 15 minutes, and its duration is 3 to 6 hours. The oral formulation provides analgesia in 30 to 45 minutes (Vadivelu, 2013). In a review of studies that included immediate-release and extended-release oxyMORphone, two RCTs demonstrated rapid and effective analgesia of immediate-release oxyMORphone in patients with moderate to severe postoperative pain; six RCTs and three open-label studies of extended-release oxyMORphone for chronic cancer or noncancer pain demonstrated comparable pain relief and side effects to modified-release morphine and oxyCODONE preparations (Sloan & Barkin, 2008). OxyMORphone was shown to not induce histamine release after intravenous administration (Hermens, Ebertz, Hanifin, & Hirshman, 1985).

The safety, efficacy, and adverse effect profiles of oral oxyMORphone are similar to those of other mu agonist opioids (Vadivelu et al., 2013). Precautions must be taken related to the timing of oral oxyMORphone administration. Food, particularly food with a high fat content, has been found to increase the plasma concentration of oral oxyMORphone by as much as 38%, so the drug should be taken on an empty stomach (1 hour before or 2 hours after a meal) (Drugs@FDA: Opana, 2018). This is an important consideration when selecting an opioid because oral oxyMORphone would not be an appropriate medication for patients who are unable to follow these limitations related to the timing of food consumption. Like other opioids, alcohol should not be used along with oxyMORphone to reduce the risk for excessive sedation and respiratory depression.

It should be noted that the name oxyMORphone is similar in appearance and sound to oxyCODONE, HYDROcodone, and HYDROmorphone. An increased level of awareness is required to prevent medication errors with these opioids.

Other Mu Opioid Analgesics

Some mu opioid analgesics are primarily used in the anesthesia setting, but may offer analgesic options in limited situations for select patients. A brief overview of alfentanil, remifentanil, and SUFentanil is provided.

Alfentanil

Indications and Uses
Alfentanil is approved for use in general anesthesia and monitored anesthesia care. It is rarely used for pain management outside of the anesthesia setting because it has an extremely short half-life. It was studied for use in procedural sedation in the ED, and although it provided effective analgesia, it was associated with respiratory risks similar to those associated with propofol (Miner et al., 2011).

Routes and Formulations
Alfentanil is usually administered as an intravenous infusion, but there are limited reports of subcutaneous infusions of alfentanil in palliative care settings (Dickman et al., 2015). There are no advantages to epidural use of alfentanil. When studied as an epidural agent, epidural alfentanil provided similar analgesia and was associated with adverse effects similar to those of intravenous alfentanil (Coda, Brown, Risler, Syrjala, & Shen, 1999).

Pharmacologic Considerations
Alfentanil is the least potent of the fentanyl products but it is highly lipophilic. Alfentanil has an onset of action in 20 seconds, peaks within 90 seconds of injection, and has a very short duration of action (7–15 minutes) (Fontaine, Latarjet, Payre, Poupelin, & Ravat, 2017). It is widely distributed in the body, like fentaNYL, and is rapidly cleared from the CNS. Alfentanil is metabolized in the liver and has no clinically significant metabolites but requires lowered doses with liver failure and can be safely used for patients with end-stage renal disease (Findlay & Isles, 2015; Fontaine et al., 2017; Soleimanpour et al., 2016).

Other Considerations
Alfentanil is associated with fewer cardiovascular complications than fentaNYL and remifentanil (Soleimanpour, Safari, Nia, Sanaie, & Alavian, 2016). It is not used for postoperative analgesia because of its short half-life and availability of fentaNYL and other opioid analgesics.

Remifentanil

Indications and Uses
Remifentanil is approved for the induction and maintenance of general anesthesia (Drugs@FDA: Ultiva, 2001). Remifentanil's characteristics allow easy titration for intraoperative sedation and analgesia; it is also used for procedural sedation because its short half-life affords rapid recovery from sedation. Remifentanil has been studied in combination with propofol and other sedatives (ketamine) in patient-controlled sedation; it has demonstrated safety and efficacy for GI procedures (including outpatient colonoscopies) (Sultan, 2014) and gynecologic procedures (oocyte retrieval for in-vitro fertilization) (Morue et al., 2018). It has also been used as a target-controlled intravenous infusion (titrated according to respiratory rate). The drug is capable of providing extremely rapid and intense analgesia with minimal effect on cognition, making it suitable for procedures during which patient response to instruction is required, such as fiberoptic intubation (Liu et al., 2015). Remifentanil has been found to be safe and effective for analgesia and sedation during extracorporeal shock-wave lithotripsy (ESWL). In a study comparing the safety and efficacy of target-controlled remifentanil infusion to target-controlled SUFentanil infusion, SUFentanil PCA, and morphine PCA in patients undergoing ESWL, remifentanil provided more effective analgesia with no increase in adverse effects (Fouladi & Soleimani, 2017).

Remifentanil is approved as an anesthetic agent, but outside of the operating room it has been used off-label, especially in the obstetric field. It has been used in PCA in the management of labor pain and during anesthesia for cesarean delivery. In a review of the use of remifentanil for labor analgesia, it was found to have less effect on the fetus than other opioids, but was associated with a significantly higher rate of excessive sedation and respiratory depression than that provided by epidural analgesia (Van De Velde & Carvalho, 2016). Epidural analgesia also provided more effective and reliable pain relief. The authors recommended that remifentanil use in labor should be limited to patients who are not candidates for epidural analgesia, and, if remifentanil is used, patients require higher levels of monitoring (Van De Velde & Carvalho, 2016).

Remifentanil has been used as a continuous intravenous infusion for analgesia and sedation in critically ill patients. In a systematic review that included 23 RCTs and 1905 patients, remifentanil provided efficacy and safety similar to those of other opioids and was associated with shorter duration of mechanical ventilation, faster time to extubation after sedation was stopped, and reduced intensive care unit (ICU) length of stay (Zhu, Wang, Du, & Xi,

2017). It has also shown efficacy and safety in studies of critically ill patients who have undergone cardiothoracic surgery and neurosurgical procedures.

Routes and Formulations

Remifentanil is available only for intravenous use. Because remifentanil is formulated in glycine, it is not recommended for spinal or epidural administration (Thompson & Rowbotham, 1996).

Pharmacologic Considerations

Remifentanil has pharmacodynamics similar to those of fentaNYL. It has unique pharmacokinetics. After the administration of an intravenous dose over 60 seconds, it has a rapid distribution half-life of 1 minute, a slower distribution half-life of 6 minutes, and a terminal elimination half-life of 10 to 20 minutes. The effective biological half-life of remifentanil is 3 to 10 minutes, with a similar half-life after discontinuation of prolonged infusions (Drugs@FDA: Ultiva, 2001). The pharmacokinetics of remifentanil are unaffected by the presence of renal or hepatic impairment.

Other Considerations

The nonlabeled use of remifentanil for postoperative pain management is often restricted to monitored settings, such as the postanesthesia care unit (PACU) or ICU, because of the need for close monitoring, risks for life-threatening adverse effects, and ready access to anesthesia clinicians.

The short duration of action of remifentanil after a dose or after discontinuation of an infusion makes it an inappropriate choice for intermittent administration in the management of acute postoperative pain. In these situations, the use of MMA, including regional anesthesia, nonopioid analgesics, and a longer acting opioid may be necessary. Like other mu opioids, remifentanil produces dose-related analgesia and adverse effects; nausea and pruritus are common. It is associated with a high incidence of adverse respiratory events, including respiratory depression (Anderson, 2017), necessitating close monitoring of sedation level and respiratory status, as detailed in Chapter 13. Like the other fentaNYL products, muscle rigidity, in particular chest wall rigidity requiring resuscitation, can occur (Anderson, 2017).

Another concern with remifentanil use is the association of remifentanil with the development of acute opioid tolerance and opioid-induced hyperalgesia. Chapter 12 provides a more detailed discussion of opioid-induced hyperalgesia. Although remifentanil has been identified with these conditions in many studies, systematic reviews have not shown consistent results. In a review of acute opioid tolerance and opioid-induced hyperalgesia related to the perioperative use of remifentanil, Kim, Stoicea, Soghomonyan, and Bergese (2015) reported that remifentanil intravenous infusions at rates of 0.1 mcg/kg/min or more, either alone or with inhalation anesthetics, may be associated with acute opioid tolerance and opioid-induced hyperalgesia, but it is unclear whether the use of other medications factored into the development of these conditions. They found no evidence to suggest the need for remifentanil dose reductions. In a systematic review by Fletcher and Martinez (2014), hyperalgesia was noted in more patients in the first 24 hours postoperatively who received high intraoperative doses of remifentanil compared with those who did not, as evidenced by a slight increase in pain at rest and a moderate increase in postoperative morphine use. However, the authors noted that the evidence was not robust and no adverse outcomes resulted from the hyperalgesic state; therefore they did not recommend any change in the use of intraoperative remifentanil.

SUFentanil

Indications and Uses

SUFentanil is another very potent, lipophilic mu agonist opioid analgesic usually used in perioperative or procedural settings. SUFentanil's rapid onset, high efficacy, and lack of active metabolites make it an option for treatment of acute postoperative pain and a promising opioid for the treatment of breakthrough pain.

It is sometimes used for the management of acute pain in intravenous PCA. In a small study comparing efficacy and safety of SUFentanil intravenous PCA to morphine intravenous PCA in 42 postoperative patients after lumbar fusions, the medications provided similar pain relief (Do Keun Kim, Kim Oh, Jung, & Kim, 2017). The incidence of nausea and vomiting was significantly less in the SUFentanil group ($P = .04$). The authors suggested SUFentanil should be considered an option for postoperative pain management in patients who have GI problems with fentaNYL.

In another study, 72 patients were randomized to receive either HYDROmorphone intravenous PCA or SUFentanil intravenous PCA after elective laparoscopic or open radical surgery for colorectal cancer (Yang et al., 2018). Results demonstrated no significant difference in analgesic effect between the medications, but HYDROmorphone was associated with greater improvement in mood and SUFentanil was associated with more nausea and pruritus.

Sublingual SUFentanil is indicated for the management of acute pain severe enough to require an opioid for which alternative treatments are inadequate. Sublingual SUFentanil may only be administered by health care providers in certified medical facilities such as hospitals, surgical centers, and emergency departments for a maximum of three days (Drugs@FDA: DSUVIA® 2018).

Routes and Formulations

SUFentanil is usually administered as an intravenous infusion or PCA, epidural, or intrathecal infusion, but other routes may be used. SUFentanil is sometimes combined with a local anesthetic and administered via the epidural route (Youssef et al., 2014). Few studies have compared efficacy of SUFentanil when administered through different routes. In a 2005 study comparing intrathecal to intravenous administration of SUFentanil, those who received intrathecal administration had significantly faster pain relief and required less rescue medication than those who received intravenous SUFentanil (Fournier, Weber, & Gamulin, 2005). In a study of 60 participants who underwent elective lower limb surgery with epidural local anesthetic, postoperative pain was better controlled, and there was less effect on blood pressure and fewer side effects in those who received epidural SUFentanil in the recovery room than in those who received the medication by intrathecal or intravenous routes (Dwivedi & Agarwal, 2015). The results of this small study are perplexing because it could be posited that the epidural intravenous route would be the least effective as the lipophilicity of SUFentanil would cause the medication to be absorbed into the epidural fat, thereby reducing its effectiveness.

Properties such as SUFentanil's high lipophilicity and lack of active metabolites have attracted investigators and clinicians to consider the use of SUFentanil in alternative routes that require high potency and low volume, such as sublingual transmucosal delivery for acute postoperative pain (Fisher, Chang, Wada, Dahan, & Palmer, 2018; Porela-Tiihonen, Kokki, & Kokki, 2017). These properties make the medication suitable for breakthrough pain. A 30-mcg sublingual tablet formulation of SUFentil was approved by the FDA in 2018 for administration to patients by a health care provider in a certified medically supervised health care setting (Drugs@FDA: DSUVIA®, 2018). A disposable single-dose applicator is provided with each tablet to assist health care providers to place the 30-mcg tablet under the patient's tongue. Doses may be repeated no more often than every 60 minutes, if needed, for a maximum of 12 doses in a 24-hour period (Drugs@FDA: DSUVIA® 2018).

The efficacy and safety of the single-dose health care provider administered SUFentanil 30-mcg sublingual tablet was studied in a randomized, double-blind, placebo-controlled trial of 161 patients (age 18 to 69 years) with acute postoperative pain after abdominal surgery (Drugs@FDA: DSUVIA®, 2018). Patients received a SUFentanil 30-mcg sublingual tablet or placebo as needed with a minimum of 60 minutes between doses. Morphine 1 mg IV was available as a rescue dose. The patients who received the sublingual SUFentanil experienced significantly better pain relief than those who received placebo. The time to meaningful pain relief was 54 minutes for the sublingual SUFentanil group compared to 84 minutes for the placebo group; 22% of those in the sublingual SUFentanil group compared to 65% of those in the placebo group took rescue medication within the first 12 hours of the study.

A study in Europe, where a sublingual SUFentanil patient-administered opioid system is approved, compared sublingual SUFentanil to morphine intravenous PCA in postoperative patients (Frampton, 2016). In a head-to-head comparison the sublingual SUFentanil was associated with a faster onset of analgesia and greater efficacy as determined by patient and health care professional global assessments of the method of pain control. Ease of use and overall satisfaction was higher with the SUFentanil system. Adverse effects of the sublingual SUFentanil system were similar to those associated with other opioids.

Pharmacologic Considerations

SUFentanil is the most lipid-soluble opioid (twice that of fentaNYL) and is approximately 12 times more potent than fentaNYL and 400 times more potent than morphine (van de Donk, Ward, Langford, & Dahan, 2018). SUFentanil is metabolized by CYP3A4, but its metabolites are inactive, making it one of the safer opioids for use in patients with chronic liver and renal failure (Herndon et al., 2016; Soleimanpour et al., 2016). Like other highly lipophilic drugs, SUFentanil is fast-acting (intravenous peak analgesic effect is ~ 3 minutes) and has a short duration of action (< 1 hour) because it moves rapidly from plasma to opioid receptor action sites (van de Donk et al., 2018; Sheth et al., 2018).

As with fentaNYL, SUFentanil has a wide volume of distribution, but clearance is much faster.

Other Considerations

As with other opioids, whenever possible, an MMA plan of care incorporating nonopioids and nonpharmacologic interventions should be included when SUFentanil is used. For example, in an RCT that included 60 patients who underwent a lung resection for lung cancer, those who were treated with music therapy before and after surgery had lower pain scores, blood pressure, heart rate, and anxiety in the first 24 hours postoperatively ($P < 0.01$) and used less SUFentanil PCA ($P < .01$) than those treated with PCA alone (Wang et al., 2015).

Dual-Mechanism Analgesics

Some mu opioid receptor agonists are unique because they have an additional mechanism of action that involves their ability to inhibit neurotransmitter reuptake (Herndon et al., 2016). Two of the more frequently used dual-mechanism analgesics in clinical practice are traMADol and tapentadol.

TraMADol

Indications and Uses

TraMADol is a synthetic atypical opioid analgesic indicated for moderate to moderately severe pain. Earlier studies examined the analgesic benefits of traMADol compared to other opioids, but no recent research has been identified. A study comparing traMADol with acetaminophen to HYDROcodone with acetaminophen and placebo in adults with partial ankle ligament tear showed

1 to 2 capsules of 37.5 mg traMADol/325 mg acetaminophen provided equivalent analgesia and comparable adverse effects to 7.5 mg HYDROcodone/650 mg acetaminophen (Hewitt et al., 2007). In another study, the efficacy and tolerability of traMADol and HYDROcodone with acetaminophen was compared in a double-blind RCT of 118 patients with chronic cancer pain (Rodriguez et al., 2008). No statistically significant difference was shown between these medications with initial doses of traMADol 200 mg/day and HYDROcodone/acetaminophen 25 mg/2500 mg/day and doubled daily doses of each medication. TraMADol was associated with more mild side effects (i.e., nausea, vomiting, appetite loss, and weakness) than HYDROcodone/acetaminophen.

TraMADol has been used in the treatment of a variety of pain states, including postoperative pain, minor musculoskeletal trauma, migraine/headache, cancer-related pain, and pain from rheumatoid arthritis and osteoarthritis (OA). Recent reviews have examined the use of oral traMADol in various pain states. A Cochrane review from 2016 compared the efficacy of a single dose of traMADol 75 mg against placebo, and traMADol 75 mg combined with dexketoprofen 25 mg (an NSAID, not available in the United States) in the management of acute postoperative pain of 1853 patients after hip replacement, hysterectomy, and surgical removal of wisdom teeth (Derry, Cooper, & Phillips, 2016). As a single agent, traMADol provided at least 50% pain relief in 45% of patients compared to 53% of those who received only the NSAID. When traMADol was combined with an NSAID, over 66% of participants had efficacy of greater than 50% compared to placebo with efficacy of 32%. The authors concluded traMADol combined with the NSAID provided good levels of pain relief with long duration of action to most participants compared to either agent alone or to placebo (Derry et al., 2016). A 2017 Cochrane review cites limited, low-quality evidence for use of traMADol in the treatment of cancer pain in adults (Wiffen, Derry, & Moore, 2017). It is regarded as a second-line analgesic with weak evidence in guidelines for neuropathic pain (Finnerup et al., 2015). In a systematic review of the use of traMADol in treating neuropathic pain, although over 50% of studies showed pain reduction of 50% or more from baseline, small study size and pooled data sets resulted in a determination of insufficient quality data to provide evidence of traMADol's efficacy in relieving neuropathic pain (Duehmke et al., 2017). MacLean & Schwartz (2015) conducted a review of the use of traMADol in the treatment of pain associated with fibromyalgia and found fair evidence to support its use as a second-line medication.

TraMADol has been used as a treatment option for older adults with nociceptive pain not adequately managed with acetaminophen (Makris, Abrams, Gurland, & Reid, 2014; Reid, Eccleston, & Pillemer, 2015). Short-acting traMADol, in reduced doses, is listed as an option for persistent pain in older adults, but it is recommended to avoid the extended-release product, especially in older patients with reduced renal function (2019 American Geriatrics Society Beers Criteria® Update Expert Panel, 2019). In an older study that stratified patients by age (younger than 65, 65, younger than 75, 75 or older), the drug was well tolerated and effective for moderate to severe cancer and noncancer pain, and there were no significant differences in tolerability and effectiveness across age groups (Likar et al., 2006). A Cochrane review and a later systematic review and meta-analysis by the same researchers concluded that the analgesic and functional outcome benefits are small and adverse events are reversible and not life-threatening but are often a cause of treatment cessation for osteoarthritis (Cepeda, Camargo, Zea, & Valencia, 2006, 2007).

In the United States, traMADol is available in oral short-acting and modified-release tablets and in a combination tablet with acetaminophen. Short-acting traMADol is available in 50-mg tablets. Modified-release traMADol (100, 200, and 300 mg) is effective for 24 hours. Different formulations, including parenteral and rectal suppositories are available in other areas of the world (Miotto et al., 2017).

Pharmacologic Considerations

As mentioned previously, traMADol binds to the mu opioid receptor site and also inhibits serotonin and norepinephrine reuptake, resulting in inhibition in pain transmission in the spinal cord (Vazzana et al., 2015). TraMADol has 70% oral bioavailability, is subject to first-pass effect, and is metabolized via the CYP2D6 pathway. Both traMADol and its active metabolite, M1, are excreted by the kidneys. TraMADol is a very weak mu receptor agonist, and its mu receptor activity is mostly related to the M1 metabolite. M1 has 200 times stronger affinity for the mu receptor, is two to four times more potent, and has a longer half-life than traMADol (Miotto et al., 2017; Vazzana et al., 2015). The peak effect of the short-acting traMADol formulation occurs in 3 hours, and its duration is approximately 6 hours (Miotto et al., 2017).

TraMADol is estimated to be eight times less potent than morphine in its ability to bind to the mu opioid receptor, but because of its dual activity, its analgesic potency is estimated to be two to three times less than that of morphine (Fudin, Raouf, & Wegrzyn, 2017). It is difficult to compare the potency of traMADol to that of other mu receptor agonists because traMADol's efficacy results from its dual mechanisms of action.

Other Considerations

TraMADol, despite its widespread use and reports of abuse, was not a controlled substance until 2014, when it was identified as a Schedule IV controlled substance under the Controlled Substances Act in the United States (Drug Enforcement Administration, 2014). Acetaminophen combined with traMADol appears to enhance effectiveness beyond the degree expected, demonstrating a "supra-additive effect" (Filitz et al., 2008), thus supporting the benefits of MMA. The combination traMADol-acetaminophen product contains 25% less tra-MADol (37.5 mg) than the usual initial dose single product (50 mg), and the combination product was found to have a faster onset of analgesia (17 minutes) than traMADol as a single agent (51 minutes) (Sawaddiruk, 2011).

The maximum recommended dose of short-acting traMADol is 400 mg/day, and the dose limit for the modified-release preparation is 300 mg/day (Miotto et al., 2017). The dosing limit in older adults is 300 mg/day (Malec & Shega, 2015). Lower doses are advised in patients who are taking other serotonergic medications and in those with impaired renal or liver function (Hassamal, Miotto, Dale, & Danovitch, 2018).

The most common adverse effects of traMADol are nausea and vomiting, dizziness, drowsiness, and constipation (Vazzana et al., 2015). The risk for respiratory depression is lower than with pure mu agonist opioids but may occur, particularly with coingestion of other respiratory depressant medications, such as benzodiazepines and medications with serotonergic effects (Vazzano et al., 2015). Because traMADol is largely dependent on the CYP2D6 metabolic pathway for analgesic activation, individual genetic polymorphisms and drug interactions must be taken into consideration. Individuals who are ultra-rapid CYP2D6 metabolizers may have increased amounts of the active metabolite, M1, leading to higher than usual levels of analgesia with traMADol, but also experience more side effects such as miosis and nausea (Miotto et al., 2017). Like single ingredient codeine, traMADol is not FDA-approved for use in children, and the FDA warns against the use of tramadol for mothers who are nursing their infants, because of the potential for harm to their infants (FDA, 2018).

Two major adverse effects, serotonin syndrome and seizures, may be associated with traMADol use (Vazzana et al., 2015). The SSRIs (e.g., FLUoxetine, PARoxetine) may inhibit hepatic metabolism of traMADol via the CYP2D6 enzyme system, leaving more parent compound form of traMADol, thereby increasing the risk for serotonin syndrome (Miotto et al., 2017). Serotonin syndrome may manifest as shivering, nausea, low-grade fever, sweating, mental confusion, and delirium. TraMADol is also contraindicated in patients who are receiving MAOIs, because MAOIs inhibit serotonin metabolism (Miotto et al., 2017). TraMADol has been associated with seizure development possibly because of a lowering of the seizure threshold (Miotto et al., 2017) or inhibition of γ-aminobutyric acid (GABA) receptors (Vazzana et al., 2015). When traMADol was compared to tapentadol, a review of case reports showed a significantly higher rate of seizures and vomiting among those taking traMADol (Tsutaoka, Ho, Fung, & Kearney, 2015). Seizures may occur in the first 24 hours of therapy and have been identified in patients with and without seizure histories (Miotto et al., 2017). To reduce seizure risk, it is recommended traMADol be taken within the recommended dose range and avoided in seizure-prone patients. Monitoring for seizure occurrence and cautious use is advised in those who are concurrently taking SSRIs and other drugs that can lower the seizure threshold (Miotto et al., 2017). It is also suggested to gradually reduce traMADol doses to prevent withdrawal seizures if the drug is to be discontinued.

Tapentadol

Indications and Uses
Tapentadol is a Schedule II drug indicated for moderate to severe pain. In a systematic review and meta-analysis of nine RCTs with 3961 participants, the safety and efficacy of immediate-release tapentadol for moderate to severe pain was compared to placebo or immediate-release oxyCODONE 10 mg (Xiao, Li, Feng, Ye, & Wang, 2017). Tapentadol doses of 50, 75, and 100 mg were reported to provide efficacy similar to that of immediate-release oxyCODONE 10 mg. Tapentadol 75 mg provided significantly better pain relief than tapentadol 50 mg. Tapentadol 50- and 75-mg doses were associated with fewer total side effects than oxyCODONE 10 mg, and nausea and constipation were significantly less with both tapentadol doses ($P < 0.05$). The authors concluded the 75-mg dose might be the best dose to provide relief of moderate to severe acute pain with fewer side effects.

In a systematic and critical review of tapentadol in the treatment of cancer pain in opioid-tolerant patients, Mercadante (2017) reported tapentadol was well tolerated and provided effective pain relief while being associated with a low incidence of GI side effects. However, observational studies had a small sample size and controlled studies did not show superiority of tapentadol over other opioids. Mercadante (2017) cited the need for additional studies of tapentadol in the management of patients who need strong opioids to address cancer pain.

In a Cochrane review of the efficacy, safety, and tolerability of tapentadol in the treatment of chronic musculoskeletal pain, four studies involving 4094 patients were examined in which tapentadol was compared to placebo or oxyCODONE (Santos, Alarcão, Fareleira, Vaz-Carneiro, & Costa, 2015). Moderate-quality evidence showed 30% of those treated with tapentadol had at least 50% reduction in pain compared to 20% of those treated with placebo or oxyCODONE. Moderate-quality evidence showed that 20% of those treated with tapentadol withdrew because of side effects, compared to withdrawal rates of 10% in those who received placebo or 30% in those treated with oxyCODONE. GI side effects (i.e., constipation, nausea, and vomiting) and pruritus (i.e., itching) were less with tapentadol than with oxyCODONE. The incidence of fatigue, insomnia, somnolence, and headache was similar in the tapentadol and oxyCODONE groups.

Routes and Formulations
A short-acting formulation of tapentadol is available in 50-, 75-, and 100-mg tablets (Drugs@FDA: Nucynta, 2009). A modified-release formulation of tapentadol

(extended release) is also available for the management of pain severe enough to necessitate the use of daily, continuous opioid treatment in pain that is responsive to opioid therapy and has not responded to other treatment options (Drugs@FDA: Nucynta ER, 2016).

Pharmacologic Considerations

Tapentadol is a centrally acting analgesic with a dual mechanism of action, binding as an agonist to the mu opioid receptor site and also blocking the reuptake of norepinephrine. Tapentadol binds to mu opioid receptors in the presynapses and postsynapses, which results in inhibition of the pain impulses in ascending pathways. As a result of binding to the presynaptic receptors, tapentadol inhibits glutamate and release of substance P, thereby reducing activation of the ascending pathways. As a result of inhibition of the norepinephrine reuptake transported, tapentadol blocks norepinephrine reuptake and increases the inhibitory effect of the descending pathways (Zajączkowska et al., 2018). It is metabolized in the liver via phase II glucuronidation to nonactive metabolites and is not metabolized through the CYP450 system.

Tapentadol reaches maximum serum concentration in approximately 1.25 hours and has a terminal half-life of 4 hours (Drugs@FDA: Nucynta, 2009).

Other Considerations

In a review comparing the pharmacology and toxicology of tapentadol to those of traMADol, the reviewers noted tapentadol has a number of advantages because it does not rely on metabolic activation via the CYP450 system, has strong opioid activity, and works through norepinephrine reuptake inhibition (Faria et al., 2018). As a result, the reviewers reported tapentadol is associated with fewer risks for serotonergic effects, less dependence and abuse risks, more linear pharmacokinetics, fewer GI side effects, and greater applicability to the treatment of chronic and neuropathic pain.

Tapentadol differs from traMADol in that it does not directly block the reuptake of serotonin. However, it is difficult to conclude that the risk for serotonin syndrome is absent with tapentadol because there is a paucity of evidence to support such a claim. Although Gressler, Hammon, and Painter (2017) found no studies that identified the development of serotonin syndrome in patients taking tapentadol, they noted nausea, diarrhea, constipation, fatigue, vomiting, and somnolence were frequently reported adverse effects. It was not possible for the reviewers to draw conclusions related to risk for tapentadol-associated serotonin syndrome because none of the examined studies differentiated between the adverse events in those patients who took serotonergic drugs and those who did not.

In a systematic review of 24 peer-reviewed papers that examined the development of serious adverse effects associated with tapentadol, Channell and Schug (2018) reported tapentadol has been associated with serious effects. Respiratory depression, confusion, coma, hallucinations/delusions, seizures, tachycardia, hypertension, and agitation are included among the noted adverse effects. However, tapentadol was found to be unlikely to cause serotonin syndrome. When compared to pure mu agonist opioids, tapentadol was associated with significantly less toxicity.

Tapentadol is a relatively new analgesic that may offer significant advantages over pure mu opioid agonists and traMADol, but cost and accessibility may limit its use. Although more experience has been acquired in the use of tapentadol, and an increased number of studies have been published that point to the low risk for serotonin syndrome in patients taking tapentadol, the evidence remains inconclusive. For this reason, it is necessary to exercise the same precautions for tapentadol as one would apply to traMADol (i.e., avoid combining tapentadol with other drugs that increase serotonin level, such as traMADol and SSRIs). Tapentadol should not be administered with MAOIs. As with other opioids, additive toxicity may occur with concurrent use of CNS depressants.

Partial Mu Agonist

Buprenorphine

Indications and Uses

Buprenorphine is used in the treatment of acute pain, cancer pain, chronic noncancer pain, and as medication-assisted therapy in the treatment of opioid use disorder (Davis, Pasternak, & Behm, 2018). Buprenorphine, because of its unique pharmacology, is of research interest because of its potential to cause less tolerance and hyperalgesia than full mu opioid agonists, and for its efficacy in the treatment of neuropathic pain.

In a systematic review that included studies in which transdermal buprenorphine was compared to transdermal fentaNYL in patients with cancer pain, the medications provided similar pain relief, but transdermal buprenorphine required less upward dose titration over time (Ahn et al., 2017). Transdermal buprenorphine was preferred over transdermal fentaNYL in patients with cancer with renal impairment because no dose adjustments were necessary (Ahn et al., 2017).

In a review of clinical trials involving transdermal buprenorphine, the patch was found to be well tolerated and provided good background pain relief in patients with chronic noncancer pain such as osteoarthritis, chronic back pain, and other chronic conditions of moderate pain intensity (Pergolizzi et al., 2015). Functional improvements have been noted in those with chronic noncancer pain with use of the transdermal formulation (Miller et al., 2014; Yarlas et al., 2015). Within 4 weeks of treatment with transdermal buprenorphine, patients with chronic noncancer pain were noted to have improvements in sleep and sleep quality (Yarlas et al., 2016).

In a multicenter, randomized, double-blind, placebo-controlled, parallel-group trial study of 183 patients with moderate to severe diabetic peripheral neuropathy, transdermal buprenorphine with doses ranging from 5 mcg/h to 40 mcg/h, was found to be effective (defined as a 30% decrease in average pain intensity at the end of the 12th week compared with baseline) (Simpson & Wlodarczyk, 2016). However, a number of patients in the treatment group (37/93) withdrew because of side effects (untreated nausea and vomiting). Although a few studies demonstrated efficacy in specific neuropathic pain conditions, more research is needed. Wiffen et al. (2015) in a Cochrane review were unable to refute or support its use in neuropathic pain conditions because of the lack of large, robust randomized trials with patient-centered outcomes.

The use of buprenorphine for acute pain may be less familiar to many clinicians than its use in chronic pain. Both sublingual and parenteral formulations have been used to treat acute pain.

A number of studies, including parenteral (intravenous or intramuscular) and sublingual buprenorphine formulations, have examined its use for acute pain management in the ED and in postoperative settings (White et al., 2017). In a systematic review of nine RCTs with 826 patients, sublingual buprenorphine (in doses ranging from 0.4–2 mg) was compared to intravenous or intramuscular morphine in four ED studies and five postoperative studies. Sublingual buprenorphine provided pain relief similar to that with intravenous morphine during the first hour after administration and after another hour, buprenorphine had a greater analgesic effect than morphine, probably because of its slower elimination pharmacokinetics (Vlok, An, Binks, Melhuish, & White, 2018). In a study of patients with renal colic in the ED, sublingual buprenorphine and intravenous morphine provided similar time to the first experience of pain relief (Hosseininejad et al., 2016). In a systematic review of 28 RCTs with 2210 patients, intravenous and sublingual buprenorphine preparations were compared to morphine in the treatment of acute pain in hospitalized patients (White et al., 2017). Similar analgesia and side effects were found between the two medications in patients in the ED and in those who had undergone surgery.

Routes and Formulations

Buprenorphine, for the treatment of pain, is currently available in three approved formulations: transdermal, buccal, and parenteral. Although published studies have included the use of sublingual buprenorphine for pain, sublingual formulations in the United States are only FDA approved for the treatment of opioid use disorder, and are not approved for pain management. A transdermal formulation is available in 5-, 10-, and 20-mcg/h strengths (in the United States) and is reapplied every 7 days. Because the highest available transdermal dose is 20 mcg/h, use of the transdermal formulation is limited to those requiring less than 80 MEDDs, and higher doses are considered off-label use (Foster, Twycross, Mihalyo, & Wilcock,

2013). In a systematic review of various buprenorphine formulations in the treatment of chronic pain conditions, the transdermal formulation was effective in treating chronic pain because it significantly reduced pain against a comparator in 10 out of 15 studies (Aiyer et al., 2018).

The more recently released buccal formulation is a film that dissolves within 30 minutes of placement on the buccal tissue. The buccal film was noted to reach therapeutic plasma concentrations more rapidly than the transdermal formulation (Bai, Xiang, & Finn, 2016). It was studied in patients who were previously receiving up to 160 mg MEDD for chronic pain treatment and was found to have efficacy and tolerability over a 48-week period with dose titration up to 900 mcg twice daily (Hale, Urdaneta, Kirby, Xiang, & Rauck, 2017). In a phase III randomized withdrawal study of opioid-naïve patients with chronic low back pain, buprenorphine buccal film (doses ranging from 150–450 mcg every 12 hours), demonstrated 30% or greater pain relief and tolerability compared to placebo (Rauck, Potts, Xiang, Tzanis, & Finn, 2016). In a phase III multicenter, double-blind, placebo-controlled randomized withdrawal study of opioid-tolerant patients with moderate to severe chronic low back pain who used ATC opioids (up to 160 mg MEDD), the buccal film (doses ranging from 150–900 mcg every 12 hours) provided clinically significant pain control compared to placebo over a 12- week period (Gimbel et al., 2016). The side effect profile of the buccal formulation was similar to that of other opioids and transdermal buprenorphine (Rauck et al., 2016; Gimbel et al., 2016).

The parenteral formulation of buprenorphine is generally reserved for acute pain and has been used in continuous infusions in end-of-life situations (Foster et al., 2013). Parenteral buprenorphine is available in a 0.3-mg/mL formulation, and 0.3 mg is estimated to have an analgesic and respiratory depressant effect similar to parenteral morphine 10 mg (Jonan, Kaye, & Urman, 2018; Reckitt Benckiser Pharmaceuticals, 2016). The intravenous formulation is administered over at least 2 minutes, and the dose of intravenous (and intramuscular) buprenorphine is 300 mcg every 6 or 8 hours prn (Foster et al., 2013). If pain is not relieved after 30 to 60 minutes, the dose may be repeated once (Reckitt Benckiser Pharmaceuticals, 2016).

Pharmacologic Considerations

As described earlier, buprenorphine is referred to as a partial agonist at the mu opioid receptor and an antagonist at the kappa opioid receptor, with some weak activity at the delta opioid receptor (Davis et al., 2018; Jonan et al., 2018). Buprenorphine has a long and variable half-life, which may be related to its high lipophilicity and slow dissociation from the mu opioid receptor (Jonan et al., 2018). Buprenorphine has greater affinity for the mu opioid receptor than morphine and most other mu-opioid agonists. It is approximately 50 times more potent than morphine (White et al., 2017) and, in addition to its analgesic properties, is used in medication-assisted treatment for opioid use disorder (described in Chapter 14). Because it is eliminated by nonrenal pathways, buprenorphine is safely used in patients with renal failure and is a preferred analgesic for older patients (Davis et al., 2018; Pergolizzi et al., 2015). In analgesic doses, it has not been associated with prolongation of the QTc and risk for cardiac dysrhythmias, and, although buprenorphine and its metabolite are metabolized by CYP3A4, at therapeutic doses, there is little risk for drug-drug interactions (Khanna & Pillarisetti, 2015).

Other Considerations

Buprenorphine's high affinity for mu opioid receptors may result in dose- and concentration-dependent inhibition or displacement of other mu opioid receptor agonists (Silverman, Raffa, Cataldo, Kwarcinski, & Ripa, 2017). This potential has resulted in concerns that patients receiving buprenorphine for analgesia would be unable to receive adequate relief of breakthrough pain with the use of immediate-release opioids. However, it has been shown that buprenorphine's analgesic effect occurs with only 5% to 10% of the mu opioid receptor sites being occupied (Davis et al., 2018), and therefore other receptor sites are available for binding with other opioids (Davis et al., 2018; Pergolizzi et al., 2010). As a result, other opioids can provide effective breakthrough pain relief when administered to patients who are receiving analgesic doses of buprenorphine.

Breakthrough pain may be treated with nonopioid analgesics, although full mu agonist opioids have also been used to provide relief. For breakthrough pain in patients with the transdermal product, oral morphine in doses up to 10 mg for the 20-mcg/h patch may be effective for breakthrough pain (Foster et al., 2013). Silverman et al. (2017), in a post hoc analysis of the use of immediate-release opioids for supplemental analgesia in patients receiving transdermal buprenorphine for moderate to severe pain, reported patients who received immediate-release opioids along with the use of the transdermal buprenorphine had lower pain scores and pain interference than those who did not receive immediate-release opioids. Silverman et al. (2017) also reported an extensive literature review that yielded many studies supporting the concomitant use of immediate-release opioids and transdermal buprenorphine, even with higher transdermal buprenorphine doses than are used in the United States.

In early publications, because of its partial mu opioid agonism, buprenorphine was reported to have an analgesic ceiling effect with doses beyond 32 mg. However, in more recent studies, the analgesic ceiling effect has been disputed because it has been noted in clinical practice that there is no bell-shaped dose-response curve or plateau on the dose-response curve (Khanna & Pillarisetti, 2015). In other words, as the dose of buprenorphine is increased the analgesic effect is also increased. Similarly, as the dose of buprenorphine increases, there may also be a risk for respiratory depression. In systematic reviews of buprenorphine in the treatment of acute pain, buprenorphine compared to morphine was found to provide comparable analgesia and was associated with the same risk for adverse effects, including respiratory depression (Vlok et al., 2018; White et al., 2017). It is unclear whether the respiratory depressant effect was due to buprenorphine alone or if it was as the result of other medications used in the MMA plan.

Adverse effects associated with buprenorphine may include respiratory depression, although reviews show conflicting results (Khanna & Pillarisetti, 2015; White et al., 2017). However, despite the unclear effect, in vulnerable patients, particularly the elderly and those with underlying ventilatory impairment, the risk for respiratory depression should be considered. Buprenorphine's high affinity for the mu opioid receptor may result in resistance to reversal with naloxone (Jonan et al., 2018). In vulnerable patients in the acute care setting, close monitoring is suggested, and escalation to a higher level of care is recommended if signs of respiratory depression develop (White et al., 2017).

Other side effects associated with buprenorphine are similar to those of the full mu opioid agonists, but the intensity of the effects may be less. In a review by White et al. (2017), sedation, nausea, vomiting, dizziness, and hypotension were similar in patients who received morphine or buprenorphine but buprenorphine was associated with less pruritus (White et al., 2017). Buprenorphine may cause less constipation than full mu opioid agonists (Khanna & Pillarisetti, 2015), and the buccal formulation may be less constipating than the sublingual form (Webster, Camilleri, & Finn, 2016).

Mixed Agonist-Antagonist Opioids

Mixed alpha antagonist opioids are analgesics that provide pain relief by binding to the kappa opioid receptor while antagonizing or blocking the mu opioid receptor. These medications have an analgesic dose ceiling level, limiting the ability to titrate them to higher doses when pain is not relieved at a lower dose. Because they are not active at the mu opioid receptor, they may pose less risk for respiratory depression and other side effects associated with pure mu opioid agonists. The pharmacology of the mixed agonist-antagonists (butorphanol, nalbuphine, and pentazocine) are addressed earlier in this chapter. There is a lack of strong evidence to support the use of these medications in the management of acute and cancer pain over full mu opioid agonists that can be titrated (Herndon et al., 2016); therefore further details about their use is limited to the information discussed earlier in this chapter. Chapter 12 provides a description of the use of nalbuphine, a mixed agonist-antagonist, in the prevention of opioid-induced pruritus.

Opioid Antagonists

Indications and Uses

Opioid antagonists are used to reverse the effects of opioid agonists. The commonly used opioid antagonists include naloxone and naltrexone. A third agent, nalmefene, was withdrawn from the U.S. market over a decade ago because of low sales but is approved in some countries outside the United States for the treatment of alcohol use disorder (Skolnick, 2018). Naloxone is the primary antagonist used to reverse opioid-induced respiratory depression. Naltrexone is primarily used for opioid detoxification and in medication-assisted treatment of opioid use disorder (see Chapter 14). Other antagonists, including methylnaltrexone and alvimopan, are used for their potential to block the peripheral mu receptors while sparing the mu receptors in the CNS and are used in the treatment of opioid-induced constipation. These peripherally acting mu opioid receptor antagonists are further described in Chapter 12.

Routes and Formulations

The route and formulation of opioid antagonists depend on the specific product and indication. Information related to naloxone follows in subsequent paragraphs. Information related to naltrexone is provided in Chapter 14, and information related to use of the peripherally acting opioid receptor antagonists is provided in Chapter 12.

Pharmacologic Considerations

Opioid antagonists are medications that bind to the opioid receptors but produce no analgesia. When an antagonist is present, it competes with the opioid agonist molecules for binding sites on the receptors and blocks the analgesic and other opioid effects. These medications antagonize mu, kappa, and delta opioid receptors.

Other Considerations

When using an opioid antagonist, it is important to ensure that the use is appropriate. Before the use of an antagonist to reverse opioid-induced respiratory depression, the patient should be carefully assessed to determine that reversal is necessary. If the patient is exhibiting confusion or is difficult to arouse, the mental status changes may not be opioid related but may be related to a metabolic problem, disease progression, or another cause. In general, if the patient has acceptable oxygenation and respiratory rate and depth, an opioid antagonist is unlikely to be beneficial and may be problematic.

Naloxone

Indications and Uses

As discussed earlier, naloxone is an opioid antagonist that binds tightly to the mu opioid receptor, causing the dissociation of mu opioid agonists. It is combined in some newer opioid formulations to act as an abuse deterrent.

Routes and Formulations

In the event of opioid-induced respiratory depression, naloxone can be administered intravenously, intramuscularly, or by intranasal spray to reverse opioid effects. In emergency situations where intravenous access is not available, it can be administered (off-label) via endotracheal or intraosseous routes. In severe cases it can be given as a continuous intravenous infusion in a critical care setting. When administered intravenously, naloxone has a very rapid onset of action (2 minutes), a peak concentration in 10 minutes, and a half-life of approximately 60 minutes (Pani, Dongare, & Mishra, 2015).

Two FDA-approved naloxone products designed for layperson administration include the Evzio Auto Injector and Narcan Intranasal (Elzey et al., 2016). Evzio has audible directions to assist the person administering the medication in an emergency overdose setting. Narcan was the original branded injectable product containing naloxone decades ago. Although a branded Narcan injectable is no longer available, the intranasal FDA-approved formulation does in fact have rights to the name Narcan and is marketed as such in the intranasal formulation. An important counseling point is that when administered intranasally, naloxone is absorbed through the mucosal lining of the nares and does not require the patient to breathe in the medication. Notwithstanding, it is important to note that there can be reduced exposure to the intranasal vessels and decreased systemic absorption in patients with intermittent or chronic sinusitis and/or a deviated septum because of diminished circulation from intranasal substance abuse. Naloxone products specifically FDA approved by the injectable route (intravenous or intramuscular) are frequently used off-label by attaching an atomizer to the syringe tip and spraying half the dose into one nostril and half into the other. This is an off-label use but has become an inexpensive in-home option, popularized and supported by third-party insurance payers for economic reasons.

Pharmacologic Considerations

Naloxone binds to opioid receptors but produces no analgesia. When naloxone is present, it competes with the opioid agonist molecules for binding sites on the receptors and blocks the analgesic and other opioid effects. The extent and duration of the reversal of opioid effects varies depending on a number of factors, including the specific opioid used, the opioid dose, concurrent medications, and route of opioid and naloxone administration.

Other Considerations

Because of the short half-life of naloxone, those who require naloxone for reversal of opioid-induced respiratory depression require close monitoring for recurrence of respiratory depression, and may need repeated doses or continuous infusions of naloxone because the half-life of naloxone may be shorter than the half-life of the opioid. When naloxone is needed to reverse the effect of

Box 11.12 Naloxone Administration in Adults

1. Patients who require naloxone (Narcan) usually meet all of the following criteria[a]:
   - Minimal or no response to physical stimulation
   - Shallow respirations or respiratory rate less than 8 breaths/min
   - Pinpoint pupils
2. Stop the administration of the opioid and any other sedative drugs. If given intravenously, maintain intravenous access.
3. Summon help. Call rapid response team if indicated by patient status, and ask a coworker to prepare naloxone (see No. 4) and bring it to you. Remain with the patient, continue to attempt to vigorously arouse him or her, and support respirations as indicated by patient status.
4. Ask coworker to mix 0.4 mg (1 ampule) of naloxone and 10 mL of normal saline in a syringe for intravenous administration.[b,c]
5. Administer the dilute naloxone solution IV very slowly (0.5 mL over 2 minutes)[c–e] while you observe the patient's response (titrate to effect).
6. The patient should open his or her eyes and talk to you within 1 to 2 minutes. If not, continue intravenous naloxone at the same rate up to a total of 0.8 mg or 20 mL of dilute naloxone. If no response, begin looking for other causes of sedation and respiratory depression.
7. Discontinue the naloxone administration as soon as the patient is responsive to physical stimulation and able to take deep breaths when told to do so. Keep the syringe nearby. Another dose of naloxone may be needed as early as 30 minutes after the first dose because the duration of naloxone is shorter than the duration of most opioids.
8. Assign a staff member to monitor sedation and respiratory status and to remind the patient to deep breathe every 1 to 2 minutes until the patient becomes more alert.
9. Notify the primary prescribing clinician and pain service. Document your actions.
10. Provide a nonopioid for pain relief.
11. Resume opioid administration at half the original dose when the patient is easily aroused and respiratory rate is more than 9 breaths/min.
12. Monitor sedation and respiratory status in accordance with the pharmacokinetics of the opioid administered.[e]

---

[a] Orders for opioids should include the administration of naloxone according to the American Pain Society (APS) recommendations, or a protocol incorporating the APS recommendations can be adopted for use by any nurse who suspects a patient is experiencing clinically significant opioid-induced respiratory depression.

[b] If naloxone is available only in a prefilled syringe, 10 mL of saline can be drawn into a 12-mL syringe, leaving enough room to accept the transfer of naloxone from the prefilled syringe. This procedure would ensure correct dilution.[c]

[c] If the intravenous route is inaccessible, administer undiluted naloxone 0.4 mg, subcutaneously or intramuscularly. The patient should respond within 5 minutes. If not, repeat dose up to a total of 2 mg. Intranasal naloxone (2 mg) has been shown to be as safe and effective as intramuscular and intravenous naloxone in the treatment of opioid overdose with a favorable response within 10 minutes; however, an additional dose of naloxone was more likely when given intranasally (see text for discussion and references). More well-controlled research is needed to recommend this route of administration for naloxone.

[d] This is the recommended amount and rate for administering naloxone to reverse opioid-induced respiratory depression. Administering a larger amount in a shorter period than this risks reversing more than opioid-induced respiratory depression (e.g., analgesia).

[e] If sedation and respiratory depression occur during administration of transdermal fentaNYL, remove the patch; if naloxone is necessary, treatment will be needed for a prolonged period after initial resuscitation, and the typical approach involves a naloxone infusion (see text). Patient must be closely monitored for at least 24 hours after discontinuation of the transdermal fentaNYL.

From Pasero, C., & McCaffery, M. (2011). *Pain assessment and pharmacologic management* (p. 521). St. Louis, MO: Mosby. Data from American Pain Society. (2003). *Principles of analgesic use in the treatment of acute and cancer pain* (5th ed.). Glenview, IL, Author.

NOTE: This box provides the recommended titrate-to-effect procedure for administering naloxone (Narcan) to reverse clinically significant respiratory depression. Giving too much naloxone or giving it too fast can precipitate severe pain, which is extremely difficult to control, and increase sympathetic activity, leading to hypertension, tachycardia, ventricular dysrhythmias, pulmonary edema, and cardiac arrest. In physically dependent patients, withdrawal syndrome can be precipitated; patients who have been receiving opioids for more than 1 week may be exquisitely sensitive to antagonists.
© 2011, Pasero, C. May be duplicated for use in clinical practice.

---

a long-acting opioid, it may be necessary to administer a continuous naloxone infusion in a critical care setting so the patient's response can be closely monitored until the duration of effect of the long-acting opioid has passed.

When using naloxone to reverse respiratory depression in the clinical setting, careful dose titration is necessary to ensure adequate reversal of the opioid effect without causing naloxone-related adverse effects. The recommended procedure for administration and titration of naloxone is described in Box 11.12. Naloxone has been shown to increase respiratory rate in patients with opioid-induced respiratory depression within 1 to 2 minutes of intravenous administration. If the initial dose is ineffective, repeated doses are given until the desired effect is obtained. Patients who have received opioids for more than a week and require naloxone to reverse somnolence or respiratory depression may be extremely sensitive to naloxone's effects (Herndon et al., 2016). Excessive naloxone dosing can precipitate severe pain associated with sudden opioid withdrawal. Small doses should be given slowly to prevent loss of pain control and withdrawal symptoms. Excessive dosing or too rapid administration of naloxone can result in increased sympathetic activity leading to tachycardia, hypertension, ventricular tachycardia, pulmonary edema, and cardiac arrest (Pani et al., 2015).

Key Points

- When an opioid is necessary, it should be used as one component of an MMA pain management plan.
- The decision to include an opioid in the pain management plan of care should be based on assessment of an individual's condition, comorbidities, pain, goals for treatment, consideration of treatment options, and assessment of opioid-related risks and benefits.
- Many factors are included in selection of an appropriate opioid, including:
  o Diagnosis, condition, surgical procedure, current or anticipated pain intensity, age, organ failure (renal, hepatic, or respiratory), presence of coexisting disease, prior treatment outcomes, patient preference, prior experience
  o Unique characteristics of the various opioids, opioid availability, ease of administration, route availability, frequency of dosing, cost, medication regimen, potential medication interactions, risk for metabolite accumulation
- Full mu opioid agonists such as morphine, HYDROmorphone, oxyCODONE, and fentaNYL are usually considered first-line opioids when it

is determined that opioid therapy is appropriate. Although these medications have similar mechanisms of action, a number of factors, including pharmacogenetics, affect the individual's response to the specific medication.
- If a full mu opioid agonist is not providing adequate pain relief despite dose titration and the patient is developing side effects, including sedation, a different full mu opioid agonist may provide improved analgesia with fewer side effects.
- Methadone is a full mu agonist that has unique pharmacodynamics and pharmacokinetics that make it an important treatment option in chronic pain.
- Dual-mechanism medications such as traMADol and tapentadol act on the mu opioid receptor and also inhibit neurotransmitter reuptake.
- Buprenorphine, a partial mu agonist, provides an important treatment option for some patients who may not require or who cannot tolerate full mu opioid agonists. Buprenorphine is associated with less tolerance and hyperalgesia than full mu opioid agonists and may be effective for the treatment of neuropathic pain.
- Mu opioid agonists are associated with a risk for dangerous adverse effects such as advancing sedation and respiratory depression.
- Naloxone is an opioid antagonist with a short half-life that binds tightly to the mu opioid receptor and causes displacement of the mu opioid agonist, thereby reversing the mu opioid effect.

Maureen F. Cooney of Section 2 acknowledges contributions of Mena Raouf, Jeffrey J. Bettinger, Erica L. Wegrzyn, and Jeffrey Fudin to this section.

Section 3 | Opioid Dosing Practices

Maureen F. Cooney

THIS section provides information related to selection of opioid formulations, dosing, and opioid rotation (switching). As addressed throughout this book, whenever possible, if opioid therapy is necessary, it should be included as a component of an MMA plan of care. It is necessary to weigh the benefits and risks of opioid therapy and use opioids only for pain that is opioid-responsive. Opioids are generally reserved for moderate to severe acute pain and cancer pain that is inadequately relieved with nonopioid analgesics and/or coanalgesics. When

possible, patients and clinicians need to discuss and agree on the goals of opioid therapy, the plan for assessment and reassessment of opioid therapy goals, and plan for the next steps if goals of opioid therapy are not achieved. It is important to recognize that opioid therapy is only expected to provide partial relief of pain and therefore requires realistic goal setting and use of nonopioid and nonpharmacologic approaches. Evidence is lacking to support the safety and efficacy of long-term opioid use to treat chronic noncancer pain.

Initiation of Opioid Therapy

When it is determined that opioids are necessary, it is important to select the medication based on each individual's unique characteristics and condition. Chapter 9 describes many of the variables involved in selection of opioid, route, and dose, including age, condition, previous opioid exposure, and pain intensity. If a patient has received an opioid in the past, it may be beneficial to provide a medication that was previously effective and well tolerated. When opioids are necessary, the oral formulation is preferred. Intravenous opioids are generally reserved for patients with very severe acute pain, and parenteral (intravenous or subcutaneous) opioids are used for those who cannot swallow or absorb oral medications.

Opioid therapy is usually initiated with a short-acting (immediate-release) oral opioid administered by one administration route. This allows for simpler identification of medication effects and adverse responses and may lower the risk for adverse events. In acute pain situations, it may be necessary to offer a second route (or medication) for the treatment of severe or breakthrough pain. For example, a patient who is taking oxyCODONE every 4 hours for acute postoperative pain may require a dose of intravenous morphine or HYDROmorphone if a dressing change or procedure is immediately required or if pain suddenly escalates after a physical therapy session. With appropriate monitoring (see Chapter 13), the concomitant administration of a parenteral or transmucosal opioid may ensure very rapid relief while the baseline medication is administered orally.

The initial dose of a short-acting opioid is usually based on specific product dosing information and consideration of the patient's pain intensity and other factors, such as age, opioid tolerance, comorbidities, sedation level, drug-drug interactions, and other risk factors for opioid-related respiratory depression (see Chapter 13). A patient is considered opioid tolerant if the patient has taken the equivalent of 60 mg or more of oral morphine for at least a week (FDA, 2015). Pain intensity is never the only factor used to determine opioid use or dose (see Chapter 9). Considerable individual variation exists in the opioid dose required for comfort (De Gregori et al., 2016; Herndon et al., 2016). For example, research has established that specific genetic variants have been shown to affect pain and opioid requirements among patients during the postoperative period (Lu, 2015). This wide variability reinforces the need for close assessment and prompt and individualized attention to unrelieved pain. In general, for opioid-naïve adults older than 70 years, it is recommended to reduce the starting dose of short-acting opioids by 25% to 50% of the usual initial dose and titrate up (or down) depending on response and side effects (Herndon et al., 2016). Many opioid dose tables include a starting opioid dose, but these tables must

be used with caution, and starting doses must be individualized. Some pain management guidelines, such as those published by the National Cancer Comprehensive Network (NCCN) (Swarm et al., 2018), offer similar recommendations for individualization and suggest initial oral morphine doses of 5 to 15 mg or initial intravenous morphine doses of 2 to 5 mg or their equivalent doses of other opioids.

Titration of Short-Acting Opioid Dose

Titration of the opioid dose is often necessary at the beginning of therapy and repeatedly during the course of treatment. Patients with acute pain, particularly postoperative pain, may require upward dose titration to establish effective pain relief and eventual taper downward as pain resolves, while patients with cancer pain may require upward titration during the course of the disease. Titration of opioid dose is based on assessment of pain and the patient's response to opioid administration.

Valuable information is obtained by asking patients to describe the patterns of pain they are experiencing. For example, patients commonly take more breakthrough doses during the times when they are active than when they are resting. Many patients would prefer a rescue dose during these periods of activity rather than risk increased sedation that can accompany an increase in the usual opioid dose. Some patients prefer less than complete pain relief rather than risk nausea or other adverse effects with an increased dose.

Provided an MMA plan is implemented, inadequate pain relief is addressed by increases in the short-acting opioid dose until adequate analgesia is reported or until intolerable and unmanageable adverse effects occur. The goal of titration is to use the smallest dose that provides satisfactory pain relief with the fewest adverse effects. Titration is an important tool in providing effective pain relief while minimizing potential harm. Serious adverse effects, including respiratory depression and cardiac arrest, have been associated with aggressive opioid dosing and inadequate assessments of responses. The use of fixed, rigid protocols in which patients receive the same initial doses and fixed (often weight-based) titration doses increases risks for harm. Safer dosing requires assessment of the analgesic, sedation, and respiratory response to each dose, particularly as doses accumulate. For patients receiving oral short-acting opioids, a second dose of the oral short-acting opioid may be taken if pain is not adequately relieved and at least 2 hours has passed since the previous dose (Herndon et al., 2016). The NCCN (Swarm et al., 2018) recommends that in patients with moderate to severe cancer pain, if pain is unchanged or increased 1 hour after the initial dose of an oral opioid, the dose may be increased by 50% to 100%. The key principles in dose titration include the need for assessment of opioid effectiveness and for signs of serious adverse effects at the peak time of opioid effect and dose adjustments based on responses.

The first sign that an increase in opioid dose is needed is most commonly a decrease in the duration of analgesia for a given opioid dose (Pasero & McCaffery, 2011). For example, patients receiving intravenous PCA may repeatedly attempt to self-administer PCA doses before the programmed lockout (delay) interval elapses, or those receiving oral opioids may report increased pain before the end of the dosing interval. When an increase in the opioid dose is necessary, it may be done by percentages. When a slight improvement in analgesia is needed, a 25% increase in the total daily opioid dose may be sufficient; for a moderate effect, a 50% increase, and for a strong effect, such as for the treatment of severe pain, a 100% increase may be indicated. The time at which the dose should be increased is typically determined by considering the onset or peak effect of the opioid. For example, titration of intravenous opioid doses may occur as often as every 5 to 15 minutes (depending on the lipid solubility of the drug), whereas titration of oral modified-release opioids may occur every 24 to 48 hours (Pasero & McCaffery, 2011).

Titration of Short-Acting Opioids in Patients With Severe Acute Pain

Providing effective pain control while minimizing opioid-induced adverse effects presents special challenges for clinicians who work in outpatient surgery settings, PACUs, and ICUs, because they also must deal with the additional CNS depression caused by the sedative and anesthetic agents that are administered intraoperatively and sometimes throughout care in the ICU. Similarly, clinicians working with patients in the ED with severe trauma-related pain or severe acute pain associated with other conditions must also consider the effects of other medications and interventions on patient responses to opioids. Pain may be very severe, and the need for rapid analgesia may add to the challenges of ensuring safety in patients who may be hemodynamically unstable. Furthermore, many of these patients are opioid naïve, which places them at greater risk for adverse opioid-induced effects, particularly excessive sedation and respiratory depression. Many specialty organizations have developed guidelines for the management of acute pain in special patient populations. For example, guidelines are available for the management of acute pain in postoperative patients (Chou et al., 2016), in critically ill patients (Devlin et al., 2018), and in patients with blunt trauma (Galvagno et al., 2016).

It is necessary to ensure use of multimodal medications, nonpharmacological approaches, and interventional techniques to optimize comfort and improve pain relief. The use of intravenous nonopioid analgesics and local anesthetics may reduce opioid requirements while optimizing pain relief. Before a patient who has experienced trauma or has undergone surgery becomes sufficiently recovered to provide self-reports of pain, the nurse should assume that pain

is present by the fact that sufficient noxious stimuli are present (see Chapter 7). If needed, an intravenous bolus of an opioid can be administered and then repeated after the bolus reaches peak effect, based on assessment of the patient's response. It is important to administer an initial dose that will provide significant relief but not result in serious adverse effects. Although weight is usually not considered in adult opioid dosing, some protocols use weight to guide initial doses. In a review of opioid use in acute trauma protocols, MacKenzie, Zed, and Ensom (2016) noted the use of morphine 0.1 mg/kg IV followed by additional boluses of morphine 0.05 mg/kg every 5 minutes as needed achieved pain control in 40% of patients at 10 minutes and 76% at 60 minutes. In the review, one study was identified that used fentaNYL 0.1 mcg/kg IV every 5 minutes until analgesia was obtained. The authors concluded one opioid is not superior over another because all could be titrated to desired effect. They reported that morphine and HYDROmorphone can be titrated intravenously every 5 minutes until adequate pain control and absence of significant adverse effects and fentaNYL can be titrated every 3 minutes.

The mu agonist opioids—morphine, HYDROmorphone, and fentaNYL—are most commonly used for initial titration in patients with severe acute pain. Although no opioid is more appropriate than another, important patient characteristics such as organ function and hemodynamic stability deserve consideration when selecting an opioid for titration. For example, fentaNYL is favored in patients with any type of end-organ failure. It also produces minimal hemodynamic effects, which adds to its appeal for patients with unstable blood pressure.

In addition to patient characteristics, the pharmacokinetics of the opioids and the goals of treatment are considered when deciding which opioid is best for titration in particular patients. As discussed, morphine is hydrophilic and requires several minutes to cross the BBB and yield peak effects after intravenous administration; the more lipophilic opioids such as fentaNYL cross the blood-brain barrier very quickly and produce peak effects almost immediately when given intravenously. HYDROmorphone is less hydrophilic than morphine, so it has an intermediate effect. These pharmacokinetics help explain why fentaNYL is often selected when the goal is to control severe, rapidly escalating pain quickly (e.g., severe pain on admission to the ED or PACU). Although intravenous fentaNYL's short duration is an advantage when short patient stays are expected, it can be a drawback when pain is expected to be continuous. For example, fentaNYL tends to be a first-choice opioid for procedural pain and is a logical selection in an ambulatory surgery PACU or ED where the goal is to transition patients quickly to the oral analgesic that the patients will take after discharge. However, morphine or HYDROmorphone may be a more appropriate opioid selection when an intravenous opioid is needed for ongoing continuous pain. For example, a short lockout (delay) interval is prescribed when fentaNYL is used for intravenous PCA, whereas longer lockout intervals are used with morphine and HYDROmorphone PCA (see Chapter 17).

For patients who have undergone major surgery, many receive intraoperative fentaNYL and additional doses may be given in the PACU but are usually followed by either HYDROmorphone or morphine for longer lasting analgesia. However, caution is needed and close assessment is required when different opioids are combined, because peak times and half-lives vary; if adverse effects occur, it is difficult to interpret which one opioid might be responsible. Therefore a general principle of initial opioid titration in patients with acute pain is to consider the plan for continued postoperative pain management. As an example, for the patient who is admitted to the PACU after major abdominal surgery and is unable to take oral medications, if HYDROmorphone intravenous PCA is prescribed for the first 24 hours postoperatively, as well as scheduled intravenous nonopioids, HYDROmorphone loading doses are preferred over fentaNYL, unless the patient has severe, rapidly escalating pain on admission to the PACU. Use of the same medication for bolus dose titration and PCA allows assessment of effect and side effects in a closely monitored setting. When repeating bolus opioid doses, it is important to wait until the previous dose has reached its peak effect and allow enough time for it to be effective before administering a subsequent dose.

When titrating opioids to treat severe acute pain, patients must be observed closely for adverse effects, particularly sedation and respiratory depression (see Chapter 13). Particularly with intravenous opioids, adverse effects such as development of chest wall rigidity related to the speed of opioid injection can be reduced by following recommended injection rates and closely assessing for adverse effects (see Chapter 9). It is important to remember that sedation can occur before pain is completely relieved and sleep during opioid titration is usually not normal sleep but primarily the result of the sedative effects of the opioid. This type of rapid dosing always carries the risk for excessive sedation and respiratory depression (see Chapter 13); these parameters must be carefully assessed during titration and for at least 3 hours after the peak of the last dose administered (Herndon et al., 2016).

Use of Modified-Release Opioids

As noted in the earlier individual opioid descriptions, most modified-release opioids are approved by the FDA for the treatment of pain that is severe enough to necessitate the use of daily, ATC, chronic opioid therapy when alternatives to opioids have not been effective (FDA, 2013). Modified-release opioids, including sustained-release (SR), extended-release (ER), and controlled-release (CR), may be added to the pain management plan when the patient meets the FDA criteria and the short-acting opioid has been titrated to an effective level. Modified-release

opioids have been used in some patients with acute postoperative pain, but as the pain levels and opioid requirements vary with acute postoperative pain, this practice is not recommended and potentially dangerous. For patients with cancer and carefully selected patients with noncancer chronic pain requiring daily, ATC, chronic opioids as part of an MMA plan, modified-release opioids (oral or transdermal) of the same or similar short-acting opioid may be added to the pain management plan.

One approach to the introduction of a modified-release opioid is to determine the average daily dose of the short-acting opioid and, if planning to use a modified-release product that is the same as the short-acting one, start the modified-release opioid daily dose at the average daily short-acting dose (divided over the day according to dosing recommendations); Reduce the short-acting opioid to a dose that is 5% to 15% of the 24-hour dose of the modified-release opioid to be taken every 4 hours as needed (Herndon et al., 2016). McPherson (2018) recommends a similar approach, to calculation of the modified-release opioid dose, but suggests the short-acting dose, when used as a rescue medication, may be 10% to 20% of the 24-hour dose of the modified-release opioid, available as often as every 1 to 2 hours. The modified-release medication is used as a scheduled medication, never as an as-needed medication (Herndon et al., 2016).

If a selected modified-release medication is different from the short-acting opioid, the daily dose of the short-acting opioid is used to calculate an equianalgesic daily dose of the modified-release medication, and then the calculated modified-release dose is reduced by 30% to account for incomplete cross-tolerance; the daily dose of the modified-release medication is divided over the day according to dosing recommendations (Herndon et al., 2016). More conservative dose reductions (up to 50%) to account for incomplete cross-tolerance may be appropriate, provided the patient has access to short-acting opioids to address periods of inadequate pain relief. As mentioned previously, incomplete cross-tolerance means that a patient who has developed tolerance to one opioid analgesic may not be equally tolerant to another.

If a decision is made to use methadone as a long-acting opioid rather than one of the modified-release agents, to optimize efficacy and patient safety, consultation with a professional who is knowledgeable about methadone's unique pharmacology is advised. The intricacies of methadone dose selection are described later in this chapter.

Titration of Modified-Release Opioid

When an increase in the modified-release opioid is needed, it may be indicated by a patient report of breakthrough pain occurring toward the end of the continuous analgesic dosing interval (referred to as end-of-dose failure), such as in the 11th hour of a 12-hour dosing schedule or 48 hours after placement of a fentaNYL patch. Patients with cancer pain may report the need for an increased number of breakthrough doses. As a rule of thumb, two or more breakthrough doses during a 12-hour period (four to six daily) should alert the clinician that the opioid regimen needs to be reevaluated. Repeated doses of a short-acting opioid necessitate assessment of the dose of the modified-release medications. Re-evaluation for an increase in dose necessitates a thorough assessment, as described in Chapter 5, including assessment for changes in the pain condition, new sources of pain, tolerance, function, and adverse effects and for development of aberrant behaviors.

The modified-release opioid dose may be increased according to assessment of analgesia, side effects, and calculation of the daily amount of short-acting opioid that has been required. Further increases in modified-release doses may be necessary as disease progresses or tolerance develops. When an increase in the opioid dose is necessary, it can be done by percentages. As in titration of short-acting opioids for acute pain, when a slight improvement in analgesia is needed, a 25% increase in the total daily opioid dose may be sufficient; for a moderate effect, a 50% increase, and for a strong effect, such as for the treatment of severe pain, a 100% increase may be indicated. The time at which the dose should be increased is typically determined by considering the onset or peak effect of the opioid. An oral modified-release opioid may be titrated every 24 to 48 hours. Increases in the modified-release opioid may need to be accompanied by proportional increases in the breakthrough dose, so that the size of breakthrough doses remains an effective percentage of the fixed dose. Whenever the dose of the baseline opioid is increased, the efficacy of the breakthrough pain dose should be reevaluated and adjusted as needed.

Titrations and conversions of short-acting and modified-release opioids addressed in the previous paragraphs do not apply to the dosing of the transmucosal fentaNYL and other TIRFs.

Continuous Intravenous Opioid Infusions

In patients with severe pain who require intravenous opioid therapy in the critical care or closely monitored setting, a continuous parenteral opioid infusion may be necessary after initial pain control with parenteral boluses. Continuous infusions are usually avoided, especially in opioid-naïve patients, or in acute pain, because of risks for adverse effects (Herndon et al., 2016). Other patients, including those who are opioid tolerant with severe pain, patients with severe cancer pain, and patients at the end of life, may require continuous parenteral opioid infusions outside the critical care setting (including hospice and home care) after assessment of benefits and risks.

Intravenous bolus loading doses are administered and titrated to achieve adequate pain relief. Various methods are used to calculate the dose of the continuous infusion. To maintain analgesia, the continuous opioid infusion may be initiated at one-fourth of the total of intravenous bolus loading doses (Herndon et al., 2016). The full effect of the continuous infusion will not be experienced until five elimination half-lives have passed, which, for morphine or HYDROmorphone may be in the range of 10 to 12 hours. Once the steady state of the continuous infusion has been achieved, the hourly dose may be titrated up or down based on patient response. Close monitoring and assessment of effect and adverse effects is necessary during this time, because patients may develop advancing sedation and respiratory depression (see Chapter 13).

Additional bolus doses (breakthrough, rescue, or supplemental doses) of the parenteral opioid may be needed to titrate the initial infusion dose to an effective level or to address breakthrough pain associated with cancer pain or pain related to procedures or activities. It is important to assess for possible causes of inadequate pain control, including an infiltrated intravenous access, kinked tubing, tubing disconnection, or mechanical device failure. When it has been determined an additional dose is necessary, it is usually calculated as 5% to 15% of the 24-hour dose (Herndon et al., 2016) or 25% to 50% of the hourly dose (Pasero & McCaffery, 2011). Administration of bolus doses requires preassessment and postassessment of pain, sedation level, and respiratory status. The frequency of repeated dosing depends on the onset of action and timing of peak effect of the medication. For example, lipophilic medications such as fentaNYL rapidly cross the BBB (in 1–5 minutes) and may be bolused more frequently than morphine, which takes 15 to 30 minutes to cross the BBB (Herndon et al., 2016). If the patient requires bolus doses totaling the hourly infusion rate or more or if frequent boluses are needed, the hourly infusion rate may require an increase.

Opioid Rotation or Switch

Opioid rotation or switch from one opioid to another may be necessary for a number of reasons. If rotation is considered to be the result of inadequate pain relief, before considering a rotation or switch to a different opioid, it may be possible to improve pain relief through optimization of an MMA plan and opioid dose adjustments. Inadequate pain relief or side effects may not be appropriate reasons to rotate (switch) to a different opioid. With few exceptions, the effectiveness and adverse effects associated with opioids are related to the opioid dose rather than the particular medication or route. If opioid-related adverse drug effects are present, they can often be resolved by opioid dose reduction along with use of nonopioid MMA measures to optimize pain relief.

Opioid rotation is sometimes necessitated by the development of tolerance to a particular opioid. As described in Chapter 12, tolerance is a state of adaptation in which higher doses of a medication are required over time to obtain the original effectiveness of a medication (Herndon et al., 2016). As it relates to opioids, tolerance means that over time the opioid will not have the same effects as it had when introduced and higher doses or rotation to a different opioid may be necessary to achieve the same degree of analgesia previously provided by the original, lower dose of an opioid.

Opioid rotation or change in administration route may become necessary because of changes in the patient's condition, including comorbidities and drug-drug interactions or availability of a route (McPherson, 2018). Some opioids are not available in every route, so the need for a change in route may necessitate the use of an alternative opioid. For example, a patient who was taking oral oxyCODONE and is now unable to take oral medication may require rotation to a new parenteral opioid. For other reasons, including pharmacogenetics, interindividual variability, and interactions of coadministered medications, even opioids of the same class can have different effects in individuals. If dose titration does not result in the desired effect, rotation from one opioid to a different one may be necessary because of lack of efficacy, tolerance to the opioid analgesic effect, side effects, and hyperalgesia (Rennick et al., 2015). Other reasons for opioid rotation include medication shortages and lack of supply, the need to accommodate a patient's need for a reduction in frequency of dosing or number of pills per dose, or in response to cost and accessibility of particular opioids (McPherson, 2018).

Opioids are often compared to each other in terms of their analgesic effect, and their oral morphine equivalanet daily dose (MEDD) (McPherson, 2018; Rennick et al., 2015; Schatman, Fudin, & Cleary, 2016). Often termed *opioid equivalence,* equating opioid overall MEDD helps characterize opioid potency, estimates overall respiratory depression risk, and allows practitioners to more easily transition from one opioid to the next (opioid rotation). Although there are several potential advantages when equating opioids in terms of dose, equianalgesic conversion still requires awareness of individual responses to medications, a high level of expertise, and an extensive knowledge of the physiochemical, pharmacodynamic, and pharmacokinetic characteristics of opioids.

Determination of opioid equivalence is the first and perhaps most significant challenge involved in opioid rotation. Differences in potency, receptor binding ability, volume of distribution, lipophilicity, route of administration, absorption, and individual patient factors are important variables that must be considered during the rotation process; for these reasons, any dose calculation should only be considered an estimate. Equianalgesic dose tables (charts), including online opioid conversion calculators, are an attempt to estimate the equivalent analgesic effect of one opioid dose compared to another. Table 11.10 is an example of a frequently published equianalgesic table that presents estimated equianalgesic doses and pharmacokinetic information available for commonly used opioids. McPherson (2018) published an updated equianalgesic opioid dosing table that is slightly different from other published tables and conversion calculator applications and is "based on the equianalgesic doses used by most health care practitioners and the best available evidence" (McPherson, 2018, p. 6). For example, the updated equianalgesic dosing table by McPherson (2018) approximates parenteral morphine 10 mg to morphine 25 mg orally. Morphine 25 mg orally is approximately equivalent to oxycodone 20 mg orally. Parenteral morphine 10 mg is approximately equianalgesic to hydromorphone 2 mg parenterally or 5 mg orally (McPherson, 2018).

Table 11.10 | Frequently Published Equianalgesic Dose Chart With Opioid Pharmacokinetic Information

A Guide to Using Equianalgesic Dose Charts[a]

- *Equianalgesic* means approximately the same pain relief.

- The equianalgesic chart is a guideline for selecting doses for opioid-naïve patients. Doses and intervals between doses are titrated according to individuals' responses.

- The equianalgesic chart is helpful when switching from one drug to another or switching from one route of administration to another.[b]

- Doses in this equianalgesic chart suggest a ratio for comparing the analgesic effects of one drug to those of another.

- The longer a patient has been receiving an opioid, the more conservative the starting dose of a new opioid should be.

Opioid	Oral (PO) (Over ~4 h) Traditional	Parenteral (IV/subq/IM[c]) (Over ~4 h)	Onset (min)	Peak (min)	Duration (h)[d]	Half-Life (h)
Mu Agonists						
Morphine	30 mg	10 mg	30–60 (PO) 30–60 (MR)[e]	60–90 (PO) 90–180 (MR)[e]	3–6 (PO) 8–24 (MR)[e]	2–4

Table 11.10 | Frequently Published Equianalgesic Dose Chart With Opioid Pharmacokinetic Information—cont'd

Drug						
			30–60 (R) 5–10 (IV) 10–20 (subq)	60–90 (R) 15–30 (IV) 30–60 (subq)	4–5 (R) 3–4 (IV)[d,f] 3–4 (subq)	
Codeine	200 mg NR	130 mg	30–60 (PO) 10–20 (subq)	60–90 (PO) ND (subq)	3–4 (PO) 3–4 (subq)	2–4
FentaNYL		100 mcg IV 1 mcg/h of TD fentaNYL is approximately equal to 2 mg/24 h of oral morphine[i]	5 (OT)[g] 5 (B)[g] 3–5 (IV) 12–16 h (TD)	15 (OT)[g] 15 (B)[g] 15–30 (IV) 24 h (TD)	2–5 (OT)[g] 2–5 (B)[g] 2 (IV)[d,f] 48–72(TD)	3–4[h] > 24 (TD)
HYDROcodone	30 mg[j] NR	—	30–60 (PO)	60–90 (PO)	4–6 (PO)	4
HYDROmorphone	7.5 mg	1.5 mg[k]	15–30 (PO) 15–30 (R) 5 (IV) 10–20 (subq)	30–90 (PO) 30–90 (R) 10–20 (IV) 30–90 (subq)	3–4 (PO) 3–4 (R) 3–4 (IV)[d,f] 3–4 (subq)	2–3
Levorphanol	4 mg	2 mg	30–60 (PO) 10 (IV) 10–20 (subq)	60–90 (PO 15–30 (IV) 4–6 (IV)[b,e] 4–6 (IV) 60–90 (subq) 4–6 (IV) 4–6 (IV)	4–6 (PO) 4–6 (subq)	12–15
Meperidine Not Recommended for analgesic purposes: Information provided to rotate off meperidine to another opioid	300 mg NR	75 mg	30–60 (PO) 5–10 (IV) 10–20 (subq)	60–90 (PO) 10–15 (IV) 15–30 (subq)	2–4 (PO) 2–4 (IV)[d,f] 2–4 (subq)	2–3
Methadone	(See Boxes 11.17 to 11.19 and Table 11.11)					
OxyCODONE	20 mg	—	30–60 (PO) 30–60 (MR)[l] 30–60 (R)	60–90 (PO) 90–180 (MR)[l] 30–60 (R)	3–4 (PO) 8–12 (MR)[l] 3–6 (R)	2–3 (short acting) 4.5 (MR)[l]
OxyMORphone	10 mg (10 mg R)	1 mg	30–45 (PO) 15–30 (R) 5–10 (IV) 10–20 (subq)	30–90 (PO) 60 (MR)[m] 120 (R) 15–30 (IV) ND (subq)	4–6 (PO) 12 (MR)[m] 3–6 (R) 3–4 (IV)[d,f] 3–6 (subq)	7–11 (PO 2 (parenteral)

[a] This table provides equianalgesic doses and pharmacokinetic information about selected opioid drugs. Characteristics and comments about selected mu opioid agonist drugs can be found in Table 11.7.

[b] An expert panel was convened for the purpose of establishing a new guideline for opioid rotation and recently proposed a two-step approach (Fine, P. G., & Portenoy, R. K. (2009). Ad Hoc Expert Panel on Evidence Review and Guidelines for Opioid Rotation. Establishing "best practices" for opioid rotation: conclusions of an expert panel. *Journal of Pain & Symptom Management, 38*(3), 418–425.). The approach presented in the text for calculating the dose of a new opioid can be conceptualized as the panel's Step One, which directs clinicians to calculate the equianalgesic dose of the new opioid based on the equianalgesic table. Step Two suggests that clinicians perform a second assessment of patients to evaluate the current pain severity (perhaps suggesting that the calculated dose be increased or decreased) and to develop strategies for assessing and titrating the dose and to determine the need for breakthrough doses and calculate those doses.

[c] The intramuscular route for opioid administration should be avoided and information is therefore omitted.

Table 11.10 | Frequently Published Equianalgesic Dose Chart With Opioid Pharmacokinetic Information—cont'd

^d Duration of analgesia is dose dependent; the higher the dose, usually the longer the duration.

^e As in, for example, morphine modified-release products. Some products have duration of 8 hours, others are 12–24 hours. Refer to the product information for specific medications.

^f The intravenous route produces the highest peak concentration of the drug, and the peak concentration is associated with the highest level of toxicity (e.g., sedation). To decrease the peak effect and lower the level of toxicity, intravenous boluses may be administered more slowly (e.g., morphine 5 mg over a 15-min period); or smaller doses may be administered more often (e.g., morphine 2 mg every 1–1.5 hours).

^g The delivery system for transmucosal fentaNYL influences potency (e.g., buccal fentaNYL is approximately twice as potent as oral transmucosal fentaNYL).

^h At steady state, slow release of fentaNYL from storage in tissues can result in a prolonged half-life (e.g., 4–5 times longer).

ⁱ This is the ratio that is used clinically.

^j Equianalgesic data are not available.

^k The recommendation that 1.5 mg of parenteral HYDROmorphone is approximately equal to 10 mg of parenteral morphine is based on single-dose studies. With repeated dosing of HYDROmorphone (as during patient-controlled analgesia), it is more likely that 2–3 mg of parenteral HYDROmorphone is equal to 10 mg of parenteral morphine.

^l As in, for example, modified-release oxyCODONE.

^m As in modified-release oxyMORphone.

ⁿ Used in combination with mu agonist opioids, this drug may reverse analgesia and precipitate withdrawal in opioid-dependent patients.

^o In opioid-naïve patients who are taking occasional mu agonist opioids, such as HYDROcodone or oxyCODONE, the addition of butorphanol nasal spray may provide additive analgesia. However, in opioid-tolerant patients such as those receiving ATC morphine, the addition of butorphanol nasal spray should be avoided because it may reverse analgesia and precipitate withdrawal.

ATC, Around-the-clock; *B,* buccal; *IM,* intramuscular; *IV,* intravenous; *MR,* oral modified-release; *ND,* no data; *NR,* not recommended; *OT,* oral transmucosal; *PO,* oral; *R,* rectal; *subq,* subcutaneous; *TD,* transdermal.

Modified from Pasero, C., & McCaffery, M. *Pain assessment and pharmacologic management* (pp. 444–446). St. Louis, MO: Mosby. Data from American Pain Society. (2003). *Principles of analgesic use in the treatment of acute pain and chronic cancer pain.* Glenview, IL, Author; Breitbart, W., Chandler, S., Eagel, B., Ellison, N., Enck, R. E., Lefkowitz, M., & Payne, R. (2000). An alternative algorithm for dosing transdermal fentanyl for cancer-related pain. *Oncology, 14*(5), 695–705 (see discussion in same issue, pp. 705, 709–710, 712, 17; Coda, B. A., Tanaka, A., Jacobson, R. C., Donaldson, G., & Chapman, C. R. (1997). Hydromorphone analgesia after intravenous bolus administration. *Pain, 71*(1), 41–48; Donner, B., Zenz, M., Tryba, M., & Strumpf, M. (1996). Direct conversion from oral morphine to transdermal fentanyl: A multicenter study in patients with cancer pain. *Pain, 64*(3), 527–534; Dunbar, P. J., Chapman, C. R., Buckley, F. P., & Gavin, J. R. (1996). Clinical analgesic equivalence for morphine and hydromorphone with prolonged PCA. *Pain, 68,* 226–270; Fine, P. G., Portenoy, R. K., & Ad Hoc Expert Panel on Evidence Review and Guidelines for Opioid Rotation. (2009). Establishing best practices for opioid rotation: Conclusions of an expert panel. *Journal of Pain Symptom Management, 38*(3), 418–425; Gutstein, H. B., & Akil, H. (2006). Opioid analgesics. In L. L. Brunton, J. S. Lazo, & K. L. Parker (Eds.), *Goodman & Gilman's The pharmacological basis of therapeutics* (11th ed.). New York: McGraw-Hill; Hanks, G., Cherny, N. I., & Fallon, M. (2004). Opioid analgesic therapy. In D. Doyle, G. Hanks, N. I. Cherny, & K. Calman, (Eds.), *Oxford textbook of palliative medicine* (3rd ed.)., New York: Oxford Press; Johnson, R. E., Fudala, P. J., & Payne, R. (2005). Buprenorphine: Considerations for pain management. *Journal of Pain Symptom Management, 29*(3), 297–326; Kaiko, R. F., Lacouture, P., Hopf, K., Brown, J., & Goldenheim, P.. (1996). Analgesic onset and potency of oral controlled release (CR) oxycodone CR and morphine. *Clinical Pharmacology & Therapeutics, 59*(2), 130–133; Knotkova, H., Fine, P. G., & Portenoy, R. K. (2009). Opioid rotation: The science and limitations of the equianalgesic dose table. *Journal of Pain Symptom Management, 38*(3), 426–439; Lawlor, P., Turner, K., Hanson, J., & Bruera, E. (1997). Dose ratio between morphine and hydromorphone in patients with cancer pain: A retrospective study. *Pain, 72*(1, 2), 79–85; Manfredi, P. L., Borsook, D., Chandler, S. W., & Payne, R. (1997). Intravenous methadone for cancer pain unrelieved by morphine and hydromorphone: Clinical observations. *Pain, 70,* 99–101; Portenoy, R. K. (1996). Opioid analgesics. In R. K. Portenoy, & R. M. Kanner (Eds.), *Pain management: Theory and practice.* Philadelphia, FA Davis; Sittl, R., Likar, R., & Nautrup, B. P. (2005). Equipotent doses of transdermal fentanyl and transdermal buprenorphine in patients with cancer and noncancer pain: Results of a retrospective cohort study. *Clinical Therapeutics, 27*(2), 225–237; Skaer, T. L. (2004). Practice guidelines for transdermal opioids in malignant pain. *Drugs, 64*(23), 2629–2638; Skaer, T. L. (2006). Transdermal opioids for cancer pain. *Health and Quality of Life Outcomes, 4,* 24; Vogelsang, J., & Hayes, S. R. (1991). Butorphanol tartrate (Stadol): A review. *Journal of Post Anesthesia Nursing, 6*(2), 129–135; Weinberg, D. S., Inturrisi, C. E., Reidenberg, B., Moulin, D. E., Nip, T. J., Wallenstein, S., . . . Foley, K. M. (1988). Sublingual absorption of selected opioid analgesics. *Clinical Pharmacology & Therapeutics, 44,* 335–342; Wilson, J. M., Cohen, R. I., Kezer, E. A., Schange, S. J., & Smith, E. R. (1995). Single and multiple-dose pharmacokinetics of dezocine in patients with acute and chronic pain. *Journal of Clinical Pharmacology, 35,* 395–403. © 2011, Pasero, C., & McCaffery, M. May be duplicated for use in clinical practice.

It is necessary to recognize the limitations of equianalgesic dosing tables. Dose conversion ratios may vary from table to table, and many are not well supported by research. Webster and Fine (2012b) identified many potential problems associated with the tables and studies used to develop the dose conversion ratios:

1. Some studies used to develop the dose conversion ratios used a single dose or small dose ranges to calculate the equianalgesic dose.
2. These ratios may not apply to those who are receiving chronic opioid therapy.
3. Studies did not account for responses based on ethnicity, advanced age, concomitant medication use, or comorbidities.
4. For several opioids, potency may vary depending on the direction of the rotation (switch) and tables may not indicate this.
5. Studies did not account for major interindividual differences in opioid responsiveness, as little was known about genetic polymorphisms.

The many limitations of equianalgesic conversion tables, charts, or online calculators, and lack of consensus related to rotation guidelines require that when rotating opioids, it is necessary to be conservative and carefully assess the patient's response as one opioid is changed to another, or when an alternative route of an opioid is selected. Incorporating all of the potential individual patient variabilities into a simple equation to help guide dose conversion is not only challenging but also leaves room for extensive inconsistency among different calculators and large room for error. As a result of inaccurate conversions, there are risks that may result in undertreatment of pain or significant adverse effects.

Although many health professionals prescribe opioids and rotate patients from one opioid route to another or from one opioid to another, there are concerns about the accuracy and ability of clinicians to perform these conversions. Rennick et al. (2015) described the variability in clinicians' calculations of a MEDD, irrespective of genetic variation, in a survey in which physicians, pharmacists, and nurse practitioners were requested to convert doses of several opioids into their MEDD. The clinicians were charged with calculating the oral MEDD of HYDROcodone 80 mg, transdermal fentaNYL patches 75 mcg/h, methadone 40 mg, oxyCO-DONE 120 mg, and HYDROmorphone 48 mg (Rennick et al., 2015). The results, in mean MEDD (± standard deviation) included 88 (±42) mg for HYDROcodone, 183 (±136) mg for fentaNYL, 188 (±122) mg for methadone, 176 (±38) mg for oxyCODONE, and 192 (±55) mg for HYDROmorphone. Although the wide range of results is very problematic, the large variation in standard deviation values for fentaNYL (±136 mg) and methadone (±122 mg) are of particular concern (Rennick et al., 2015). Using the lower end of the standard deviation value could result in inadequate pain relief and possible withdrawal, whereas the upper end could easily result in increased frequency of side effects, opioid-induced respiratory depression, and increased morbidity and mortality. To reduce the risk for either outcome, clinicians need to be aware of techniques for opioid rotation.

One technique used for opioid rotation is to stop the original opioid and, using the opioid dose conversion ratio on an equianalgesic chart, select the equianalgesic dose of the new opioid based on the dose of the original opioid (Brooks, Kominek, Pham, & Fudin, 2016). For patients who are opioid naïve and require a relatively quick transition to the new opioid, this method may be appropriate. For example, a patient who has received 10 mg of oxyCODONE four times daily over the past 5 days for severe pain associated with an orthopedic injury may require rotation to parenteral morphine postoperatively because of severe postoperative nausea. In this situation, 5 mg of intravenous morphine, an equianalgesic dose, may be appropriate.

However, when rotating an opioid-tolerant patient to an alternative opioid drug, it is important to assume cross-tolerance will be incomplete (Brooks et al., 2016). This means a patient who has developed tolerance to one opioid analgesic may not be equally tolerant to another and may experience serious opioid-related adverse effects if an equivalent dose of the new opioid is used. To address incomplete cross-tolerance, some experts recommend a 25% to 50% reduction of the equianalgesic dose of the new opioid with the availability of additional medication for inadequate relief (Herndon et al., 2016). For patients on high doses of the initial opioid, or for older adults, medically fragile patients, or nonwhite patients, it is prudent to reduce the dose of the new opioid to 50% of the equianalgesic dose of the original opioid (Smith & Peppin, 2014). Assessment of the patient's response to opioid rotation is necessary because even with careful attention to dose conversions, some patients will experience inadequate pain relief and others will experience side effects because of individual variability in responses. MMA plans are important as they may reduce opioid requirements and risks for adverse effects.

Another approach to opioid rotation involves the gradual reduction and discontinuation of the original opioid with introduction of the new opioid at its lowest available dose and gradual up-titration of the new opioid based on effect (Webster & Fine, 2012a). This technique is more appropriate for use in situations in which a gradual rotation can be tolerated by the patient because it may take 3 to 4 weeks for the rotation to be completed. A major benefit of this technique is that it allows rotation without reliance on a potentially flawed equianalgesic dosing chart. Webster and Fine (2012a) recommend the following:

1. Reduce the current total daily dose of the original opioid by 10% to 30% while starting the new opioid at a dose normally used for the opioid-naïve patient (or lowest available dose in the desired formulation).
2. Continue to reduce the total daily dose of the original opioid by 10% to 25% per week while increasing the dose of the new opioid by 10% to 20% based on the patient's response (efficacy and safety) until the original opioid is discontinued.
3. Use a short-acting opioid (and multimodal nonopioid interventions) throughout the process to ensure pain relief and prevent withdrawal.

With either opioid rotation technique, it is important to ensure patients are carefully assessed to determine whether pain is adequately relieved and if the opioid rotation is resulting in potentially dangerous adverse effects. In acute care settings, patients who are undergoing opioid rotation require frequent screening for pain and pain assessments and assessments of sedation levels and respiratory status as presented in Chapter 13. When rotation is necessary for outpatients, patients and their caregivers require education about the potential for inadequate analgesia and adverse effects and instructions to address either concern. The optimization of MMA techniques is particularly important during opioid rotation, to ensure adequate pain control. Box 11.13 provides an example of an opioid conversion.

Opioid rotation from another opioid to transdermal fentaNYL is sometimes confusing to clinicians. The manufacturer of the transdermal fentaNYL patch has published a table of conversion values from oral morphine to transdermal fentaNYL patch strengths, but the morphine values include a fairly wide range at each dosing interval. The manufacturer recommended conversions may be conservative and may increase the patient's risk for increased pain, withdrawal, and lengthy duration of titration to an effective dose (McPherson, 2018). A more straightforward conversion approach introduced by Breitbart et al. (2000) and used by many clinicians is the use of morphine 2 mg/day PO to 1 mcg transdermal fentaNYL patch per hour conversion. This approach is described in Box 11.14 and an example of rotation from morphine to a fentaNYL patch is provided in Box 11.15.

Box 11.13 | Example of Opioid Conversion: OxyCODONE to Morphine

SCENARIO

A patient has been receiving oxyCODONE controlled-release (CR) 20 mg PO every 12 hours for a year and HYDROcodone/acetaminophen 10 mg/325 mg PO every 4 hours prn (usually takes 1 or 2 tablets per day).

It is necessary to convert the oxyCODONE CR to extended-release (ER) morphine because the patient's insurance will no longer cover the oxyCODONE CR.

1. Calculate the total daily dose of oxyCODONE:

Total daily dose of oxyCODONE: 40 mg (20 mg + 20 mg)

2. Convert 40 mg oxyCODONE to equivalent morphine dose:

OxyCODONE to morphine conversion ratio: 20 mg PO oxyCODONE = 30 mg PO morphine (using the equianalgesic dosing in Table 11.10)

If 20 mg oxyCODONE = 30 mg morphine, then 40 mg oxyCODONE = 60 mg oral morphine

3. To account for incomplete cross-tolerance, the morphine ER dose needs to be reduced by 25% to 50%. Therefore the daily dose of morphine ER (with a 50% reduction) may be 30 mg.
4. Stop the oxyCODONE CR and start morphine ER 15 mg every 12 hours.
5. The HYDROcodone/acetaminophen would be continued as prescribed.

Box 11.14 | Rotation From Morphine Equivalent Daily Dose to Transdermal FentaNYL

1. Calculate the morphine equivalent daily dose (MEDD) that has been used to control the patient's pain.
2. Use a conversion of 2 mg PO **MEDD** (2 mg PO morphine equivalent daily dose) to 1 **mcg/h** transdermal fentaNYL to calculate the dose of the transdermal patch.
   NOTE: It is extremely important to ensure that the morphine equivalent daily dose is calculated as mg/d and is converted to a transdermal fentanyl dose of μg/h.
3. The patch dose is then rounded up or down based on the transdermal patch strengths that are available from the manufacturer (12 mcg/h, 25mcg/h, 50 mcg/h, 75 mcg/hr, or 100 mcg/h). The patient's pain and general condition are considered in the decision to round up or down.
   a. If pain has been stable and adequately controlled on the initial MEDD used for the conversion, consider rounding down to the next patch strength.
   b. If pain has not been well controlled on the initial MEDD used for the conversion, and there are no signs of opioid-induced respiratory depression, consider rounding up to the next patch strength.

Data from Breitbart, W., Chandler, S., Eagel, B., et al. (2000). An alternative algorithm for dosing transdermal fentanyl for cancer-related pain. *Oncology (Williston Park)*, 14(5), 695-717. Breitbart, W., Chandler, S., Ellison, N., Enck, R. E., Lefkowitz, M., & Payne, R. (2000). An alternative algorithm for dosing transdermal fentanyl for cancer-related pain. Retrieved August 8, 2020 from https://www.cancernetwork.com/view/jun-j-mao-md-msce-on-next-steps-in-acupuncture-for-managing-pain-in-cancer-survivors. McPherson, M. L., & McPherson, M. L. (2019). *Demystifying opioid conversion calculations* (2nd ed.). Bethesda, MD: American Society of Health-System Pharmacists.

Similarly, confusion may arise if it becomes necessary to rotate a patient from a fentaNYL transdermal patch to another opioid. After fentaNYL patch removal, it may take 17 hours or more to reduce the serum fentaNYL concentration by 50% and up to 68 hours after patch removal to eliminate nearly all the fentaNYL from the serum (McPherson, 2018). Individual patients may have variations in the rate of elimination. Because of the slow elimination of fentaNYL after patch removal, a gradual introduction of the replacement opioid is needed. The conversion from transdermal fentaNYL to another opioid often considers 1 mcg/h transdermal fentaNYL to be equivalent to 2 mg MEDD. However, Reddy et al. (2016), in a study to determine the opioid rotation ratio of patients with cancer from transdermal fentaNYL to other opioids, noted a 1 mcg/h transdermal fentaNYL to 2.4 mg MEDD ratio. To rotate from the transdermal fentanyl patch to another modified-release opioid,

Box 11.15 | Conversion From Oral Morphine to Transdermal FentaNYL: Application

To convert a modified-release oral morphine dose to a starting transdermal fentaNYL dose, consider morphine 2 mg/24 h orally to be approximately equianalgesic to fentaNYL 1 mcg/h transdermally.[a]

SELECTING A STARTING DOSE

1. Calculate the patient's current 24-hour morphine dose.

Example: If the patient is receiving 60 mg PO of modified-release morphine every 12 hours, the total 24-hour dose of morphine is 60 mg × 2 (doses per day) = 120 mg.

2. Determine the initial dose of transdermal fentaNYL by dividing the 24-hour morphine dose by 2 (morphine-to-fentaNYL conversion ratio of 2:1).

Example: 120 mg of morphine ÷ 2 = 60 mcg/h of transdermal fentaNYL

3. Round up or down to the available fentaNYL patch strength based on the clinical status of the patient. There are four available patch strengths that provide options for starting transdermal fentaNYL therapy in this patient example: 12 mcg/h, 25 mcg/h, 50 mcg/h, and 75 mcg/h.
   a. If the patient has adequate pain relief from the current morphine dose, it is possible to start with a 12-mcg/h patch plus a 50-mcg/h patch (62 mcg/h).
   b. If a more conservative starting dose is desired (e.g., in the frail older patient or a patient with a chronic pulmonary condition), start with the lower nearest patch strength (50 mcg/h).
   c. If the current morphine dose is not providing sufficient analgesia, start with the higher nearest patch strength (75 mcg/h).
4. Apply the fentaNYL patch at the time the patient takes the last dose of modified-release morphine.
5. Monitor the patient for adequacy of pain relief and development of adverse effects.

TREATMENT OF BREAKTHROUGH PAIN DURING CONVERSION

1. The minimum amount of each rescue dose should be 25% of the total dose of the previous opioid the patient received in the past 24 hours.

Example: Using oral morphine for breakthrough pain
   a. 120 mg of morphine was taken in the past 24 hours
   b. 120 mg × 0.25 (25%) = 30 mg

2. Provide as-needed (prn) rescue doses in the amount of 30 mg every 3 to 4 hours prn for breakthrough pain.

TITRATION

1. Constant serum levels are achieved in 16 to 20 hours; steady state is attained at 72 hours of transdermal patch application.
2. After 24 to 30 hours (and always by 72 hours), determine if the patch dose is sufficient based on ongoing evaluation of pain relief and the requirement for breakthrough doses.
3. If breakthrough pain is persistent and frequent, no adverse effects are present, and nonopioid analgesic approaches are optimized, it may be necessary to increase the dose of transdermal fentaNYL.
4. The dose of transdermal fentaNYL may be increased by 25% to 50%. At low doses, such as in the example, the dose of the patch may be conservatively increased by 12 mcg/h.
5. In a small group of patients, adjustment of the dosing interval may be necessary. Patches should be changed every 48 hours in patients who have well-controlled pain for only 48 hours and require more breakthrough doses on the third day of a 72-hour interval.
6. The number of patches that may be applied is limited only by dose requirement and body surface on which to apply and rotate the patches.

---

[a] When studies that clarify equianalgesic dosing are lacking, such as is the case with fentaNYL, various conversion formulas evolve. These formulas, and even the ones used in this text, are not necessarily comparable; different formulas lead to different answers. This conversion formula may be used to convert the patient from oral morphine to transdermal fentaNYL and vice versa. The current recommendation by the manufacturer may be used only to convert from oral morphine to transdermal fentaNYL, but not vice versa, and the clinician should expect that approximately 50% of the patients will require additional analgesia.

From Pasero, C., & McCaffery, M. (2011). *Pain assessment and pharmacologic management* (p. 393). St. Louis, MO: Mosby. Data from Breitbart, W., Chandler, S., Eagel, B., Ellison, N., Enck, R. E., Lefkowitz, M., & Payne, R. (2000). An alternative algorithm for dosing transdermal fentanyl for cancer-related pain. *Oncology (Williston Park), 14*(5), 695–705; Carr, D. B., & Goudas, L. C. (2000). The Brietbart et al article reviewed. *Oncology, 14*(5), 712, 717; Donner, B., Zenz, M., Tryba, M., Strumpf, M. (1996). Direct conversion from oral morphine to transdermal fentanyl: A multicenter study in patients with cancer pain. *Pain, 64,* 527–534; Hewitt, D. J. (2000). The Brietbart et al article reviewed. *Oncology, 14*(5), 705, 709–710. © 2011, Pasero, C., & McCaffery, M. May be duplicated for use in clinical practice.

calculate the 24-hour dose of the new opioid that will be required to replace the dose of the fentanyl patch using the 1 mcg/h transdermal fentanyl dose to 2 mg of oral morphine equivalent dose (or a 1 mcg/h transdermal fentanyl dose to 2.4 mg oral morphine equivalent dose). Then remove the patch, and for the first 12 hours after patch removal, provide the usual breakthrough opioid doses. Twelve hours after patch removal, administer 50% of the new opioid dose and continue availability of the breakthrough opioid doses. Twenty-four hours after the patch has been removed, start the regular dosing schedule for the new opioid along with the usual breakthrough opioid doses (McPherson, 2018). Of note, when switching an opioid-tolerant person from another opioid to transdermal fentaNYL or vice versa, it is not necessary to consider an incomplete cross-tolerance dose reduction of the transdermal fentaNYL because the incomplete cross-tolerance factor has already been considered (McPherson, 2018).

Certain opioids, particularly methadone and buprenorphine, must be converted to and from with even more care and caution because of their physiochemical, pharmacologic, and pharmacokinetic characteristics. For this reason, it is often recommended that rotations involving methadone and buprenorphine be guided by clinicians who are knowledgeable about the unique characteristics of these medications and conversions involving these medications.

Rotating From Other Opioids to Methadone

Safely rotating a patient from another opioid to methadone is a clinical challenge, particularly because of methadone's complex pharmacokinetic and pharmacodynamic characteristics (McLean & Twomey, 2015; McPherson, 2018; McPherson, Costantino, & McPherson, 2018). Box 11.16 describes methadone characteristics that should be considered when determining methadone dosing. Methadone offers several advantages over other opioids, but particularly with cancer pain, methadone offers superior benefits because of its long half-life, lack of active metabolites, availability in multiple dose forms, and low cost (McPherson et al., 2018). On the other hand, barriers to methadone use include its variable and unpredictable dose conversion ratio, complex pharmacology, risk for genetic polymorphisms, CYP450 metabolism with potential drug-drug interaction, risks for accumulation, and potential for QT prolongation (Mercadante & Bruera, 2018).

It is widely agreed among pain specialists that published equianalgesic dose tables do not adequately reflect the complex pharmacology of methadone and the clinical reality of patient management (Chou et al., 2014; Karimian, Atayee, Ajayi, & Edmonds. 2017; McLean & Twomey, 2015; McPherson et al., 2018; Rajan & Scott-Warren, 2015). Over the years, attempts have been made to determine

| **Box 11.16** | Factors to Consider With Methadone Dosing |

1. Onset of action is comparable to that of other oral opioids, about 30 to 60 minutes.
2. Duration of analgesia with acute dosing (e.g., the beginning of the titration period) is 4 to 6 hours.
3. Duration of analgesia with long-term dosing may be 8 to 12 hours or longer.
4. Peak effect is at about 2.5 hours.
5. Steady state will not be reached for several days; in occasional patients who experience longer methadone half-life, this may take as long as several weeks.
6. Drug accumulation occurs during initial titration when the concentration in the blood continues to increase above the effective analgesic level and into the toxic range as a result of the relatively prolonged period required to approach steady state.
7. Do not increase the methadone dose for at least 5 days (significant toxicity from accumulation becomes evident on days 3–5); may decrease the dose by 50% for excess sedation (consider also skipping a dose; consider increasing the interval to 12 hours).
8. Use a short-acting opioid for breakthrough pain.
9. Monitor patient closely. If an outpatient, contact daily by phone. Assess for pain level, use of breakthrough analgesic, sedation, and any other symptoms.
10. Continue to monitor closely until pain and methadone dose are stable for 5 days after the last dose or increment adjustment.

the equianalgesic dose ratio of other opioids, principally morphine, to methadone (Chou et al., 2014; Mercadante & Bruera, 2016). It is now recognized that the conversion ratio from another opioid to methadone is not fixed. The relative potency of methadone rises in comparison to that of other opioids in those who are receiving high doses of other opioids (McLean & Twomey, 2015; Mercadante & Bruera, 2016). For example, for patients taking a MEDD less than 100 mg, one suggestion is that the morphine to methadone ratio is 3:1 (Chou et al., 2014). As the daily morphine dose rises, the ratio of morphine to methadone increases to as much as 15:1 in those taking more than 1000 mg of MEDD (Chou et al., 2014; Herndon et al., 2016). Research-derived tables that match morphine dose ranges to ratios of morphine to methadone are intended to guide selection of a safe starting dose, but these tables are not identical, as illustrated in Table 11.11. Box 11.17 provides examples and application of the use of the different morphine-to-methadone ratios to obtain a methadone starting dose. Weschules and Bain (2008) conclude that the actual dose ratio used to

Table 11.11 | Comparison of Selected Methods of Converting Oral Morphine to Methadone

	Bruera & Sweeney, 2002	Morley & Makin, 1998	Mercadante et al., 2001	Ayonrinde & Bridge, 2000	Ripamonti et al., 1998	Blackburn et al., 2002	Indelicato & Portenoy, 2002
Conversion ratio (morphine sulfate [MS] to methadone) (all doses are PO in mg)	1:1 (MS dose <100)	10:1	4:1 (MS dose <90)	3:1 (MS dose <100)	4:1 (MS dose <90)	10:1	1.5:1 (oral) 1:1 (parenteral)
	10:1 (MS dose >500)		8:1 (MS dose 90–300)	5:1 (MS dose 101–300)	8:1 (MS dose 90–300)		
			12:1 (MS dose >300)	10:1 (MS dose 301–600)	12:1 (MS dose >300)		
				12:1 (MS dose 601–800)			
				15:1 (MS dose 801–1000)			
				20:1 (MS dose >1001)			
Starting dose	10% of daily PO MS dose × 0.33 or 0.5	10% of daily PO MS dose	As above + additional 20%–30% as priming dose on day 1 or 2	As above + additional 25%–50% as loading dose × 2 days	10% of daily PO MS dose × 0.33	Loading dose of 1/10 of the total morphine equivalent dose of previous 24 h; additional loading dose may be given at 12 h for severe pain. Subsequent doses are 1/2 of loading dose	Reduce calculated dose by 75%–90%
Starting dose limit	None	30 mg/dose	None	None	None	30 mg/dose	None
Dosing interval	8 h	q3h prn × 6 days; then every 12 hours fixed dose based on previous 48-h total dose	8 h	6 h increasing to 8–12 h over several days	8 h	12 h	
Breakthrough interval		As above	Up to 3 doses per day			"Ideally" 3 h, but may be decreased if necessary or incorporated in the 12-h dose	
Breakthrough drug	Use short-acting drug initially, then 10% of daily methadone	Methadone	Methadone: 1/6 of daily dose	Short-acting opioid	Use short-acting opioid initially, then 10% of daily methadone	Methadone: 1/8 of loading dose	None

Continued

Table 11.11 | Comparison of Selected Methods of Converting Morphine to Methadone—cont'd

	Bruera & Sweeney, 2002	Morley & Makin, 1998	Mercadante et al., 2001	Ayonrinde & Bridge, 2000	Ripamonti et al., 1998	Blackburn et al., 2002	Indelicato & Portenoy, 2002
Gradual substitution versus acute conversion	1/3–1/2 reduction in MS each day for 2–3 days; only increase methadone dose on day 2 or 3 if pain is moderate to severe	Stop previous opioid	Stop previous opioid	Regular doses of previous opioid stopped, but short-acting opioids (morphine or oxyCODONE) used for breakthrough pain	1/3 reduction in MS each day for 3 days; only increase methadone dose on day 2 or 3 if pain is moderate to severe	Stop previous opioid	
Additional reduction after conversion calculation							Reduce calculated dose by 75%–90%
Planned conversion period	3 days	6 days	4 days	"Several days"		5+ days; regular 12-h doses should not be increased for 5 days, but may be decreased for toxicity	
Route	Oral or rectal	Oral	Oral				
Study method	Review	Prospective N = 146	Prospective N = 50	Prospective N = 14	Prospective N = 49	Prospective N = 9	Review

MS, Morphine sulfate; *N*, Number; *PO*, oral.

From Pasero, C., & McCaffery, M. (2011). *Pain assessment and pharmacologic management* (pp. 346–347). St. Louis, MO: Mosby. Data from Ayonrinde, O. T., & Bridge, D. T. (2000). The rediscovery of methadone for cancer pain management. *Medical Journal of Australia, 173*(10), 536–540; Blackburn, D., Somerville, E., & Squire, J. (2002). Methadone: An alternative conversion regime. *European Journal of Palliative Care, 9*(3), 92–96; Bruera, E., & Sweeney, C. (2002). Methadone use in cancer patients with pain: A review. *Journal of Palliative Medicine, 5*(1), 127–138; Indelicato, R. A., & Portenoy, R. K. (2002). Opioid rotation in the management of refractory cancer pain. *Journal of Clinical Oncology, 20*(1), 348–352; Mercadante, S., Casuccio, A., Fulfaro, F., Groff, L., Boffi, R., Villari, P., . . . Ripamonti, C. (2001). Switching from morphine to methadone to improve analgesia and tolerability in cancer patients: A prospective study. *Journal of Clinical Oncology, 19*(11), 2898–2904; Morley, J. S., & Makin, M. K. (1997). Comments on Ripamonti et al. *Pain, 73*(1), 114; Ripamonti, C., Groff, L., Brunelli, C., Polastri, D., Stavrakis, A., & De Conno, F. (1998). Switching from morphine to oral methadone in treating cancer pain: What is the equianalgesic dose ratio? *Journal of Clinical Oncology, 16*(10), 3216–3221. © 2011, Pasero, C., & McCaffery, M. May be duplicated for use in clinical practice.

determine the starting dose of methadone is probably less important than careful patient selection and close systematic monitoring of the patient during the titration period.

Once the initial starting dose of methadone is selected, it is then necessary to determine how the conversion will be implemented. Different techniques have been developed to rotate other opioids to methadone. McLean and Twomey (2015), in a systematic review of studies that examined methods of methadone rotation, identified five different rotation strategies (Table 11.12). Box 11.18 illustrates the application of one of these strategies, the rapid conversion stop and go method. Low-quality evidence was available to recommend one rotation technique over another, but the authors stressed the importance of close monitoring of patients during the initial days after rotation to

methadone. Given the potential risks associated with methadone rotation, patients should be hospitalized for rotation if adequate supervision during the conversion is not possible in a community setting.

The factors outlined earlier strongly highlight the need for a systematic procedure and the assistance of a clinician experienced in the use of methadone when rotating between another opioid and methadone. See Box 11.19 for an example of a switch from another opioid to methadone. Those caring for patients during rotation and titration involving methadone must be skilled in the assessment of patients for adverse effects and use of MMA to address inadequate pain control. In addition, patients and families require education about the safe use of methadone, its benefits, potential side effects, and need for monitoring and follow-up.

Box 11.17 | Switching to Methadone From Another Opioid

EXAMPLES OF METHODS TO DETERMINE STARTING DOSE

1. Complete thorough assessment of patient's pain and response to opioid therapy (including opioid risk assessment for adverse effects). Consider drug-drug interactions and reduce calculated methadone dose if patient is taking an enzyme-inhibiting medication.
2. Convert all current opioid(s) (short-acting and modified-release) to oral morphine equivalents using a standard equianalgesic table and determine 24-hour morphine equivalent daily dose (MEDD) in the previous 24 hours (NOTE: if there has been rapid dose escalation in the past few days, consider using the 24-hour dose from the most recent stable day).
3. Match the 24-hour morphine dose to a morphine-to-methadone dose ratio table to approximate the equianalgesic dose of methadone, as shown in the following examples:

EXAMPLE 1: AYONRINDE AND BRIDGE CONVERSION

Morphine Dose Range (24 Hours)	Morphine-to-Methadone Ratio
≤ 100 mg	3:1
101–300 mg	5:1
301–600 mg	10:1
601–800 mg	12:1
801–1000 mg	15:1
> 1000 mg	20:1

From Ayonrinde, O. T., & Bridge, D. T. (2000). The rediscovery of methadone for cancer pain management. *Medical Journal of Australia, 173* (10), 536–540.

APPLICATION

If a patient was receiving the equivalent of 120 mg oral morphine daily (morphine 30 mg PO qid), the daily methadone dose, using the 5:1 morphine-to-methadone Ayonrinde and Bridge Conversion, would be 24 mg, which, if dosed three times daily, would be rounded down to 5 mg PO tablets every 8 hours based on the conversion table above. (NOTE: Methadone is available as 5-mg tablets, therefore requiring rounding down. If using methadone liquid, it would be possible to measure out 8 mg liquid for each dose.)

EXAMPLE 2: MERCADANTE ET AL. CONVERSION (2001)

Morphine Dose Range (24 Hours)	Morphine-to-Methadone Ratio
< 90 mg	4:1
90–300 mg	8:1
> 300 mg	12:1

From Mercadante, S., Casuccio, A., Fulfaro, F., Groff, L., Boffi, R., Villari, P., . . . Ripamonti, C. (2001). Switching from morphine to methadone to improve analgesia and tolerability in cancer patients: A prospective study. *Journal of Clinical Oncology, 19*(11), 2898–2904. https://doi.org/10.1200/jco.2001.19.11.2898

APPLICATION

If a patient was receiving the equivalent of 120 mg PO morphine daily (morphine 30 mg PO qid), the daily methadone dose using the 8:1 morphine-to-methadone Mercadante et al. conversion ratio would be 15 mg, which, if dosed three times daily, would be 5 mg PO tid based on the table presented earlier.

EXAMPLE 3: RIPAMONTI ET AL. CONVERSION (1998)

Morphine Dose Range (24 Hours)	Morphine-to-Methadone Ratio
< 90 mg	4:1
90–300 mg	6:1
> 300 mg	8:1

From Ripamonti, C., Groff, L., Brunelli, C., Polastri, D., Stavrakis, A., & Conno, F. D. (1998). Switching from morphine to oral methadone in treating cancer pain: What is the equianalgesic dose ratio? *Journal of Clinical Oncology, 16*(10), 3216–3221. https://doi.org/10.1200/jco.1998.16.10.3216

Continued

Box 11.17 Switching to Methadone From Another Opioid—cont'd

APPLICATION

If a patient was receiving the equivalent of oral morphine 120 mg/day (morphine 30 mg PO qid), the daily methadone dose, using the 6:1 morphine-to-methadone Ripamonti et al. Conversion, would be 20 mg, which, if dosed three times daily, would be rounded down to 5 mg PO tid based on the conversion table presented earlier. (*Note:* Methadone is available as 5- and 10-mg tablets, therefore requiring rounding down.)

EXAMPLE 4: AMERICAN PAIN SOCIETY CONVERSION (HERNDON ET AL., 2016)

Morphine Dose Range (24 Hours)	Morphine-to-Methadone Ratio
<100 mg	3:1
100–300 mg	5:1
300–600 mg	8:1
600–1000 mg	10:1
>1000 mg	15:1

From Herndon, C. M., Arnstein, P., Darnall, B., Hartrick, K., Lyons, M., & Sehgal, N. (2016). *Principles of analgesic use.* Chicago: American Pain Society.

APPLICATION

If a patient was receiving the equivalent of 120 mg oral morphine daily (morphine 30 mg PO qid), the daily methadone dose, using the 5:1 morphine-to-methadone American Pain Society Conversion, would be 24 mg, which, if dosed three times daily, would be rounded down to 5-mg PO tablets tid based on the conversion table presented previously. (*Note:* Methadone is available as 5- or 10-mg tablets, therefore requiring rounding down. If using methadone liquid, it would be possible to measure out 8 mg liquid for each dose.)

EXAMPLE 5: FUDIN FACTOR

The Fudin Factor is a mathematical equation for morphine-to-methadone conversion that is based on Ripamonti's conversion schematic that also relied on similar conversion schematics by Ayonrinde and Bridge and Mercadante (Ayonrinde & Bridge, 2000; Brennan, Fudin & Perkins, 2012; Ripamonti et al., 1998; Mercadante & Bruera, 2016). An on-line methadone conversion calculator using the Fudin Factor equation is available on the Practical Pain Management website at https://opioidcalculator.practicalpainmanagement.com/conversion.php. (*Note:* On-line conversion calculations should be double-checked against traditional methods for methadone conversion.)

APPLICATION

If a patient was receiving the equivalent of 120 mg oral morphine daily (morphine 30 mg PO qid), the daily methadone dose, using the Fudin Factor equation in the on-line opioid calculator described above, would be 18.6 mg if it is determined to not consider incomplete cross-tolerance (Opioid Calculator, 2017). If dosed three times daily, it would be rounded down to 5-mg PO tablets tid. (*Note:* Methadone is available as 5- or 10-mg tablets, therefore requiring rounding down.)

The Practical Pain Management Opioid Calculator provides an option for modification of the new opioid dose based on consideration of incomplete cross-tolerance.

If incomplete cross-tolerance in this example was considered, and a 50% reduction was selected, the starting dose of methadone would be a daily dose of 9.3 mg.

Table 11.12 | Main Methods of Rotation to Methadone

Rotation Method	Description
3DS (3 Day Switch Method)	Day 1—30% of original opioid replaced with an equianalgesic dose of methadone given in three daily divided doses. Days 2 and 3—dose of methadone is increased by 30% and dose of original opioid reduced by 30% each day.
RC stop and go (Rapid Conversion stop and go)	Original opioid is discontinued. Daily methadone dose is calculated according to evidence-based conversion ratios and given in three regular divided daily doses. Regular methadone dose titrated to achieve effective analgesia. It has been argued that a higher priming dose of methadone (20%–30% higher than as calculated using published conversion ratios) may be required initially.
AL stop and go (ad libitum method)	Original opioid is discontinued. A fixed dose of methadone that is one-tenth of the actual or calculated morphine equivalent oral daily dose up to a maximum of 30 mg is calculated. The fixed dose is taken orally as required but not more frequently than every 3 hours. Day 6—The methadone requirement of the previous 2 days is noted and converted into a regular every 12-hour regimen.
German model	Original opioid is discontinued. Methadone is prescribed at a dose of 5–10 mg PO q4h and every 1 hour as needed. Days 2 and 3—The dose of methadone is titrated up by 30% until analgesia is achieved. After 72 hours, methadone dosing is changed to an every 8 hours and every 3 hours as-needed regimen at the same dose as prescribed on Days 2 and 3. The methadone dose is titrated up until analgesia is achieved.
Outpatient titration	Original opioid continued at same dose. Methadone commenced at 5 mg PO q4h and increased by 5 mg/dose every 3 days until improved analgesia is noted. Original opioid then reduced by one-third, and the methadone dose increased according to breakthrough requirements. The original opioid dose is reduced, and the methadone dose increased accordingly over a variable period.

3DS, Three-day switch; *AL,* ad libitum; *RC,* rapid conversion.

From McLean, S. & Twomey, F. (2015). Methods of rotation from another strong opioid to methadone for the management of cancer pain: A systematic review of the available evidence. *Journal of Pain Symptom Management, 50*(2), 248–259, Table 1.

Box 11.18 | Application of the Methadone Rapid Conversion Stop and Go Method

SCENARIO

Patient has been receiving morphine 30 mg PO qid for several months, and a decision is made to switch to methadone.
1. Stop the previous scheduled opioid.
2. Using the Mercadante et al. conversion ratio, the calculated daily methadone dose would be 15 mg.
3. Methadone will be started at the time the next morphine dose was due.
4. Start methadone in three regular divided daily doses of 5 mg PO.
5. Titrate the methadone dose carefully to achieve effective pain relief.

From McLean, S., & Twomey, F. (2015). Methods of rotation from another strong opioid to methadone for the management of cancer pain: A systematic review of the available evidence. *Journal of Pain and Symptom Management, 50*(2), 248–259; McPherson, M. L., Costantino, R. C., & McPherson, A. L. (2018). Methadone: Maximizing safety and efficacy for pain control in patients with cancer. *Hematology/Oncology Clinics of North America, 32*(32), 3, 405–415; Pasero, C., & McCaffery, M. (2011). *Pain assessment and pharmacologic management* (p. 345). St. Louis, MO: Mosby.

Box 11.19   Patient Example of Switch to Methadone From Another Opioid

PATIENT EXAMPLE: METHADONE

Mr. A. is a 48-year-old man with cancer metastatic to liver and bone in several locations. In addition, he has severe chemotherapy-induced peripheral neuropathy. His analgesics include gabapentin and short-acting oxyCODONE. He takes oxyCODONE modified-release 30 mg every 12 hours and oxyCODONE 10 mg approximately three times daily for breakthrough pain. His pain is continuous. His insurance does not cover any modified-release opioids, and, in addition, the insurance limits the number of tablets that can be dispensed at any one time, requiring frequent prescriptions. A decision is made to convert his oxyCODONE modified-release to methadone. Because his current medication pattern includes oxyCODONE prn, it will be continued for breakthrough pain.

Using a standard equianalgesic table (see Table 11.10), 20 mg PO oxyCODONE is equivalent to 30 mg PO morphine, so the 60 mg of oxyCODONE is changed to PO morphine equivalents (90 mg/day).

Using a dose-range table (see Table 11.11), 90 mg morphine per day yields a morphine-to-methadone dose ratio of 3:1 if the American Pain Society conversion ratio is used.

In this case, the daily methadone starting dose will be 30 mg.

Methadone comes in 5- and 10-mg tablets. It would be convenient to use a schedule of 10 mg every 8 hours.

The nurse calls Mr. A. daily at about the same time. After the first four doses, Mr. A. reports reduction in pain and less use of oxyCODONE; however, he also reports falling asleep watching television, which is unusual for him. At the patient's request, the dose is reduced to 5 mg every 8 hours.

On day 4, the patient continues to report improved pain and the sedation has resolved.

Buprenorphine

Buprenorphine, described in greater detail in Chapter 14, is unique because it is a partial mu receptor agonist, with extremely high binding affinity toward the mu receptor and a relatively slow dissociation rate from that receptor. Because of these characteristics, rotating to and from buprenorphine poses clinical challenges. When converting to buprenorphine from a pure opioid agonist such as morphine, it is necessary to recognize that buprenorphine, like naloxone, may displace the pure agonist from the opioid receptor and may result in opioid withdrawal. When rotating opioid-tolerant patients with pain to buprenorphine from other opioids, it is necessary to avoid withdrawal and minimize loss of analgesia. The manufacturer of a buprenorphine buccal film (indicated for severe pain) recommends discontinuing all ATC opioids when starting the buprenorphine and suggests patients be tapered to 30 mg MEDD or less before starting the buprenorphine product (Drugs@ FDA: Belbuca, 2018). Once buprenorphine has been initiated, dose adjustments, according to the individual buprenorphine formulation's product information recommendations, can be made. Buprenorphine initiation in medication-assisted treatment of opioid use disorder is a separate topic and is described in Chapter 14.

Webster et al. (2016) conducted a study to determine whether opioid-tolerant patients with chronic pain who were receiving daily morphine or oxyCODONE with a MEDD dose of at least 80 mg could be safely rotated to buccal buprenorphine without the need for complete cessation of the full mu opioid agonist. The researchers, in a randomized, double-blind, double-dummy, active-controlled, two-period crossover study, found patients with chronic pain receiving ATC morphine or oxyCODONE could be rotated to buccal buprenorphine at approximately 50% of the full mu opioid agonist dose (using a 100:1 morphine-to-buprenorphine dose conversion ratio) without an increased risk for opioid withdrawal or loss of analgesia.

Caution is also necessary when converting from buprenorphine to another opioid. It is recommended to titrate the dose of buprenorphine as low as possible before initiating the new opioid. This is necessary because the new opioid is unlikely to displace buprenorphine from the mu receptor, because buprenorphine has a higher binding affinity than all other prescription opioid agonists, including naloxone. If buprenorphine has been stopped or is being titrated down while another opioid is titrated up, analgesia from the new opioid may be limited until buprenorphine no longer occupies the mu opioid receptors. It is difficult to determine how effective the new opioid will be until the buprenorphine effect is extinguished. This is particularly important to consider in patients who have stopped buprenorphine just before surgery, because postoperative pain may not be adequately relieved by usual doses of short-acting mu opioid agonists, such as morphine, HYDROmorphone, or oxycodone, until buprenorphine is no longer occupying the mu opioid receptors (see Chapter 14). When buprenorphine no longer occupies the receptor, all of the new opioid may then occupy available mu opioid receptors, potentially increasing the risk for adverse effects, including opioid-induced respiratory depression.

As stated earlier, multimodal pain management approaches may aid in addressing analgesic requirements, and, if needed, full mu opioid agonists may be administered for breakthrough pain during the rotation period, although cautious dosing and close assessment is recommended.

Tapering and Discontinuing Opioid Therapy

Physical dependence on opioids is an adaptive response to the use of opioids over a period that results in symptoms of withdrawal if opioids are reversed, rapidly decreased, or abruptly discontinued (Jamison & Mao, 2015). The exact dose and duration of opioid use expected to result in physical dependence is unknown. There is little agreement about the optimal method of tapering and discontinuing opioids, and there is a paucity of research, particularly related to the tapering of opioids used in the treatment of acute pain.

It is possible for patients with declining acute pain, including postoperative pain, to experience symptoms of withdrawal, although opioids may not have been used for a prolonged period. Symptoms may develop if opioids are rapidly decreased or abruptly discontinued. Although severe surgical pain is expected to abate over several days, postoperative pain severe enough to require opioids may persist for weeks to months (Chou et al., 2016). The APS, American Society of Regional Anesthesia and Pain Medicine, and American Society of Anesthesiologists, in guidelines for management of acute postoperative pain, recommended that patients who were opioid naïve before surgery and received opioids for 1 to 2 weeks postoperatively should be advised to gradually reduce opioid doses to prevent significant withdrawal signs and symptoms; reductions in doses by 20% to 25% of the discharge dose every 1 to 2 days is suggested (Chou et al., 2016). An MMA plan of care is useful throughout the postoperative period to reduce postoperative opioid use and facilitate adequate pain control during opioid tapering and discontinuation. Transitions in care, especially when postoperative patients require continued opioid therapy after leaving the acute care setting, may pose challenges to effective analgesia and appropriate opioid tapering. In many U.S. states, limits have been placed on the number of days for which a prescriber may provide opioids for patients on discharge from the hospital. If additional opioids are needed, the patients may need to follow up with their surgeons or primary care providers. Some hospitals have developed transitional pain management care teams to provide support to patients and primary care providers to improve pain management, reduce withdrawal risks, and reduce risks for chronic opioid use (Clarke et al., 2018; Friedman, Arzola, Postonogova, Malavade, & Siddiqui, 2017; Hollmann, Rathmell, & Lirk, 2019).

For chronic pain, the goal of tapering may be to reduce opioids to a level that safely and effectively achieves goals of opioid therapy or the goal may be to ultimately discontinue opioid therapy. Opioid tapers should be planned to take place over a long enough time to prevent signs and symptoms of opioid withdrawal. Tapering schedules require consideration of individual patient needs; for example, pregnant patients may require a very conservative taper to avoid withdrawal that may jeopardize the patient or fetus (Dowell et al., 2016). Others may require more rapid tapers, particularly if there are concerns related to medical comorbidities or for potential overdose.

The Centers for Disease Control and Prevention (CDC) and other professional organizations have developed guidelines for the management of patients with chronic pain that include recommendations for tapering (reducing or weaning) opioid doses in patients who require higher doses of opioids and receive long-term opioid therapy. In guidelines for chronic pain management, the CDC recommends that if patients do not experience improvements in pain and function at MEDD of 90 mg/day or more, if escalating doses are necessary, or if patients have been receiving MEDD of 90 mg/day or more for an extended period, a plan should be made to taper opioid doses to a lower dose or discontinuation if possible (Dowell et al., 2016). The CDC recommends tapering the opioid dosage by approximately 10% per week, although a slower taper, such as 10% per month, for patients who have taken opioids for a very prolonged period may be necessary (Dowell et al., 2016). Guidelines for opioid therapy in the treatment of chronic pain published by the U.S. Department of Veterans Affairs (VA) and U.S. Department of Defense advise an opioid taper if the risks for long-term opioid therapy outweigh the benefits (Rosenberg, Bilka, Wilson, & Spevak, 2017). These guidelines suggest a taper by 5% to 20% of the original dose each week and a gradual taper of 5% to 20% every 4 weeks for higher opioid doses and those who have received prolonged opioid therapy (Rosenberg et al., 2017). Follow-up for reassessment is recommended within 1 week to 1 month after any opioid dosage adjustment, and patients should be educated about self-management strategies and opioid-related risks (Rosenberg et al., 2017).

In addition to the previous guidelines, other practices are used in opioid tapering. When patients have been receiving long-acting opioids, a suggestion is to change the long-acting medication to its lowest dosage form and then taper the number of tablets (capsules, pills, patches) according to a schedule (Berna, Kulich, & Rathmell, 2015). For example, a patient who has been prescribed controlled-release oxyCODONE 80-mg tablets bid could be prescribed controlled-release oxyCODONE 10-mg tablets and then directed to gradually reduce the number of tablets taken every 12 hours over an extended period. When the smallest dose has been reached, the duration between doses can be prolonged and the medication can be stopped when it is taken less than daily (Berna et al., 2015; Jancin, 2017). A tapering plan used in a study by Sullivan et al. (2017) implemented a schedule in which the opioid dose was reduced by 10% of the original opioid dose on a weekly basis until the patient received 30% of the original dose; at this dose, the taper was recalculated, and this dose became the basis for continued reductions of 10% each week until the opioid was discontinued.

Multimodal pharmacologic and nonpharmacologic pain management strategies are important in ensuring adequate analgesia during an opioid taper. Psychological support and nonpharmacologic interventions to promote comfort and anxiety reduction are major considerations in opioid tapering. Interdisciplinary chronic pain management programs and strategies such as cognitive-behavioral therapies have been used in supporting opioid tapering efforts (Berna et al., 2015; Clarke et al., 2018; Guildford, Daly-Eichenhardt, Hill, Sanderson, & McCracken, 2018; Rosenberg et al., 2017; Sullivan et al., 2017). Resources to assist in opioid tapers have been developed by the CDC and the VA. A pocket tool developed by the CDC is available at https://www.cdc.gov/drugoverdose/pdf/clinical_pocket_guide_tapering-a.pdf. The VA tool to guide decisions related to chronic opioid therapy opioid tapering is available at https://www.pbm.va.gov/PBM/AcademicDetailingService/Documents/Academic_Detailing_Educational_Material_Catalog/52_Pain_Opioid_Taper_Tool_IB_10_939_P96820.pdf#.

Opioid Safety in the Community

Prescribers have a responsibility to be well informed about appropriate pain management strategies including the importance of multimodal analgesia, and principles of safe opioid prescribing. The National Pain Strategy describes gaps in education of health care providers related to pain and pain care and identifies strategies and resources to optimize the competencies of health professionals in providing pain care, including specific strategies on safe opioid prescribing practices (IPRCC, 2015, P.42). The U.S. Department of Health and Human Services (DHHS) has developed resource material for medical professionals to promote responsible and effective opioid prescribing in the treatment of pain (DHHS, 2019). In 2016, the CDC published "A Guideline for Prescribing Opioids for Chronic Pain" to assist primary care providers to prescribe opioids appropriately in the treatment of chronic noncancer pain (Dowell, Haegerich, & Chou, 2016). In addition to guidance regarding patient assessment, opioid prescribing, initiation, and dosing strategies, risk assessment and mitigation, the guideline recommends that clinicians offer naloxone prescriptions to patients at increased risk for overdose, including those taking opioid doses of 50 mg MEDD or higher. Some of the content

in the CDC guidelines has been criticized and misinterpreted by various parties. In 2020, the American Medical Association (AMA) urged the CDC to review and revise the 2016 guidelines to assure protection of patients with pain and address the unintended consequences and misapplication of the guidelines (AMA, 2020).

Increased opioid misuse and abuse evolved into a public health crisis during the first two decades of the 21st century (Volkow & Collins, 2017). Many factors have contributed to this crisis. The over-prescription of opioids following various procedures, and storage of unused opioids by individuals when they were no longer required are factors that contribute to the excessive amount of unused opioid medications available in communities (Hasak et al., 2018; Linnaus et al., 2019; Vadivelu, Kai, Kodumudi, Sramcik, & Kaye, 2018). Availability of unused supplies of opioids increases risks of diversion and distribution into the community where they may be illegally sold and consumed for nonmedical opioid use, thus contributing to the opioid crisis. According to a 2015 national survey, nearly half of those who misused opioids obtained them from a friend or family member (Han et al, 2017).

Efforts have been made to reduce the amount of unused prescription opioids in communities. Researchers have published studies of opioid prescribing practices; they have studied the quantities of opioids prescribed upon hospital discharge after specific procedures and the amounts of opioids reported by patients as unused. In a study by Fujii et al. (2018), researchers analyzed the quantity of opioids prescribed and used for general, urology, and orthopedic surgery patients, and examined the proportion of patients who received instructions on opioid disposal and nonopioid pain management strategies. They found the median opioid use after surgery was 27% of the quantity prescribed, and only 18% of patients received disposal instructions. Awareness of the quantity of unused opioids in communities has led to development of State and system-level policies to reduce the quantities of leftover opioids by placing limitations on the dose and/or number of days that opioids may be prescribed following patients' hospitalizations (Davis, Lieberman, Hernandez-Delgado, & Suba, 2019).

All clinicians, including prescribers, nurses, and pharmacists, have the responsibility to educate patients and their family members about the risks associated with opioid use, safety, storage, and disposal to reduce opioid misuse and the supply of leftover opioids in communities. Nurses, because they are often involved in providing discharge instructions when patients leave health care settings, need to be well informed about the information that should be provided to patients related to opioid safety. Costello and Thompson (2015) surveyed 133 nurses to explore their knowledge and attitudes related to opioid use. Their study revealed a significant knowledge gap and lack of sufficient information about opioids that the authors concluded may affect the nurses' ability to provide effective medication instructions to their patients. In a study of 1632 perianesthesia nurses' knowledge and promotion of safe opioid use, storage and disposal, Odom-Forren and Brady (2019) reported that although perianesthesia nurses were generally knowledgeable about opioids and 82% discussed opioid side effects with patients, fewer nurses promoted safe opioid use (27%), storage (23%), and disposal (18%). Similar studies have been conducted in other practice settings, including emergency departments, where inadequacies were found in clinicians' knowledge or interventions related to patient education about opioid use and safety practices.

In efforts to optimize safe use, storage, and disposal of opioids in the community, the DHHS has compiled resources for patients and health care providers readily available on the internet (DHHS, 2018). Similarly, the CDC has numerous resources and factsheets available for clinicians and patients to provide education about opioid risks, adverse effects, options to opioid therapy, safe opioid use, storage, and disposal (CDC, 2016). Resources for clinicians and patients related to opioid misuse, overdose prevention, and treatment are also available with links to additional HHS material (CDC, 2020). Many organizations have standardized patient education plans to guide clinicians on the content that should be provided to patients related to opioid safety at the time of discharge. It is important for all clinicians involved in the care of patients receiving opioids to be knowledgeable about opioids and inform patients and their family members about available resources and the safe use of these medications to optimize pain relief and mitigate risks of harm to patients and the communities in which they live.

Key Points

- When opioids are necessary for adequate pain management, it is important to select the medication based on each individual's unique characteristics and condition.
- Opioid therapy is expected to provide only partial relief of pain; realistic goal setting and use of nonopioid and nonpharmacologic approaches are necessary for safe and effective analgesia.
- There is a lack of evidence to support the long-term safety and efficacy of chronic opioid use to treat chronic noncancer pain.
- Opioid therapy is usually initiated with a short-acting (immediate-release) oral opioid administered by one administration route; when rapid relief of severe pain is needed, the intravenous route is the route of choice.
- Many factors are considered in the selection of an initial opioid dose; specific medication dosing information provides only an estimate for starting doses; patient characteristics, including age, comorbidities, and opioid tolerance are considered in dose selection.
- Selection of an opioid dose based on pain intensity is potentially dangerous.
- Modified-release (sustained-release or long-acting) opioids are reserved for the treatment of pain that is severe enough to necessitate the use of daily, ATC, chronic opioid therapy when alternatives to opioids have not been effective (FDA, 2013). They are not indicated for the management of acute pain.
- It is sometimes necessary for patients to be rotated or switched from one opioid to another.
- Opioid rotation may be necessary for reasons such as change in patient condition, development of comorbidities, development of tolerance or side effects from one opioid, or to address pill burden, cost, or opioid availability.
- Opioids are often compared to each other in terms of their analgesic effect and their oral MEDD.
- Equianalgesic dose tables (charts) are used to estimate the equivalent analgesic effect of one opioid to another; the tables provide only estimates, and individual patient effects may vary.
- When a patient is tolerant to one opioid, when switching to another opioid, it is necessary to reduce the equianalgesic dose of the new opioid by 25% to 50% to account for incomplete cross-tolerance.
- The duration of opioid use that results in opioid dependence and tolerance is variable; opioid-naïve patients who have used opioids for 1 to 2 weeks should reduce opioid use gradually (once pain has been reduced) by 20% to 25% of the discharge dose every 1 to 2 days to prevent opioid withdrawal.
- Patients who have taken opioids for a prolonged period may require a weekly taper of 10% of the opioid dose, and for some a slower taper of 10% per month is necessary to prevent withdrawal symptoms.
- Multimodal pharmacologic and nonpharmacologic approaches are useful in limiting opioid requirements and providing adequate pain relief during opioid rotations and tapering.
- Clinicians have a responsibility to be informed and educate patients about safe opioid use, storage, and disposal, especially when prescriptions are written for opioid use in the outpatient setting.

Maureen F. Cooney of Section 3 acknowledges contributions of Mena Raouf, Jeffrey J. Bettinger, Erica L. Wegrzyn, and Jeffrey Fudin to this section.

Case Scenario

Ms. J. is a 58-year-old opioid-naïve woman in the trauma intensive care unit after a motor vehicle collision. She denies any allergies and has a negative medical history; her only prior surgery was for cholecystectomy 10 years ago. As a result of the crash, Ms. J. sustained a number of significant injuries, including a sternal fracture, multiple rib fractures, pulmonary contusions, a large liver laceration, and several transverse process fractures. A central line and two chest tubes were placed last evening. She had a hypotensive episode 24 hours ago and was placed on vasopressors, which were recently discontinued, and her vital signs have stabilized. Of note, her serum creatinine has increased to 1.8 mg/dL since arrival at the hospital. Despite the around-the-clock use of intravenous acetaminophen, Ms. J.'s pain remains severe and the clinicians are considering the use of opioids to optimize her analgesia.

1. What opioids might be most beneficial and least likely to affect Ms. J.'s blood pressure and kidney function at this time? What is your rationale for suggesting these opioids?
2. Ms. J.'s liver enzymes have markedly increased in the past 24 hours. Acetaminophen was discontinued. What impact may her altered liver function have on opioid selection?
3. What opioids might be least appropriate? Provide a rationale for avoidance of these medications.
4. What route of opioid administration would be suggested and why?
5. How will you address Ms. J.'s question about opioid side effects and her request to have the opioid with the least constipating effect?

Ms. J.'s condition gradually improves, and she is transferred to the trauma floor. She continues to have severe pain, particularly when attempting to turn in bed or transfer with assistance to a chair for short periods. Her chest tubes are still in place. She is eating a regular diet and is beginning to participate in physical therapy.

6. What modifications to the analgesic plan of care may be considered at this time?
7. What are some possible reasons why Ms. J.'s pain may not be adequately controlled with her current opioid regimen?
8. Ms. J. reports the opioid she is currently receiving is causing her to have nausea and pruritus. What strategies can be used to address these side effects?

Ms. J. has remained in the hospital for 3 weeks because she developed a pulmonary embolus despite prophylactic anticoagulation during her hospitalization. Over the course of the 3 weeks, she was rotated from intravenous HYDROmorphone to oral HYDROmorphone. She is currently taking oral HYDROmorphone 4 mg every 4 hours around the clock but finds that the HYDROmorphone continues to be associated with pruritus. She will be transferred to an acute rehabilitation setting, and it is anticipated that she will continue to require opioids, at an even higher dose, because of the escalation in physical therapy she will be undergoing. She requests a change in her opioid therapy to a different opioid and one that will

---

Box 11.20   Driving While Taking Opioids

- It is generally recommended to avoid driving while receiving any sedating medications.
- There is precedent for driving when on continuous long-term opioid therapy at regular doses (Byas-Smith, Chapman, Reed, & Cotsonis, 2005; Fishbain et al., 2002, 2003; Gaertner et al., 2006; Galski, Williams, & Ehle, 2000; Menefee et al., 2004; Sabatowski et al., 2003).
  - In a study of 20 patients with chronic noncancer pain who were receiving stable doses of chronic opioid therapy, no significant differences in driving performance were found when compared to performance of healthy controls (Schumacher et al., 2017). The researchers recommended that an individual patient assessment be performed to determine fitness to drive.
  - In a systematic review that included three studies of patients on chronic opioids with stable doses, no impairment of simulated driving was found, and, in one study, more severe pain was associated with poorer driving performance (Ferreira, Boland, Phillips, Lam, & Currow, 2018). The authors identified the need for prospective studies to address the safety of driving and chronic opioid use.

- Clinicians do not generally support driving while on opioid therapy, but there may be unique circumstances that the prescribing clinician and the patient must discuss and evaluate, with consideration of local, state, and federal regulation.
- When combining opioids with other sedating medications, this can be problematic. Prescribers and patients need to discuss what medications, prescribed and over-the-counter (OTC), are being taken to determine whether combinations of medications place the patient and others at increased risk for harm when driving.
  - Certain OTC drugs (and prescribed drugs), such as omeprazole for gastrointestinal symptoms, could actually inhibit the metabolism of HYDROcodone if taken within 48 hours. This could result in a longer availability of the active HYDROcodone parent compound.
- Although it is important for patients with chronic pain to be functional, which may include driving, the benefits and liability must be balanced against risks.

give her more continuous relief, with the availability of a rescue dose for physical therapy.

9. Describe opioids that may be beneficial for Ms. J. as she transitions to the acute rehabilitation setting.
10. Calculate an appropriate dose of a modified-release opioid and an opioid for a rescue dose if pain is severe after therapy.

After 2 weeks in the acute rehabilitation setting, Ms. J. is ready for discharge home. Her pain has significantly improved, and she is not requiring any short-acting opioids. She has been taking her modified-release opioid, controlled-release oxyCODONE 30 mg PO bid.

11. Describe an appropriate pain management plan of care for Ms. J. at this time.
12. Ms. J. is concerned that she may experience opioid withdrawal. How can the risk for withdrawal be minimized?
13. Ms. J.'s spouse is concerned that Ms. J. may need to take opioids for an extended period because she will continue to receive outpatient therapies her father has offered to drive June to outpatient physical therapy but he has been taking extended-release morphine 30 mg bid for chronic back pain for several years. Ms. J.'s spouse asks if it is safe for Ms. J.'s father to drive while receiving opioid therapy. Refer to Box 11.20 for information related to driving while receiving opioid therapy.

References

Ahn, J. S., Lin, J., Ogawa, S., Yuan, C., O'Brien, T., Le, B. H., … Ganapathi, A. (2017). Transdermal buprenorphine and fentanyl patches in cancer pain: a network systematic review. *Journal of Pain Research, 10*, 1963.

Aiyer, R., Mehta, N., Gungor, S., & Gulati, A. (2018). A systematic review of NMDA receptor antagonists for treatment of neuropathic pain in clinical practice. *The Clinical Journal of Pain, 34*(5), 450–467.

Akil, H. (1984). Endogenous Opioids: Biology and Function. *Annual Review of Neuroscience, 7*(1), 223–255. https://doi.org/10.1146/annurev.neuro.7.1.223.

Al-Hasani, R., & Bruchas, M. R. (2011). Molecular Mechanisms of Opioid Receptor-dependent Signaling and Behavior. *Anesthesiology, 115*(6), 1363–1381. https://doi.org/10.1097/aln.0b013e318238bba6.

Allan, L., Hays, H., Jensen, N. H., de Waroux, B. L. P., Bolt, M., Donald, R., & Kalso, E. (2001). Randomised crossover trial of transdermal fentanyl and sustained release oral morphine for treating chronic non-cancer pain. *British Medical Journal, 322*(7295), 1154.

2019 American Geriatrics Society Beers Criteria® Update Expert Panel, Fick, D. M., Semla, T. P., Steinman, M., Beizer, J., Brandt, N., … Flanagan, N. (2019). American Geriatrics Society 2019 updated AGS Beers Criteria® for potentially inappropriate medication use in older adults. *Journal of the American Geriatrics Society, 67*(4), 674–694.

American Medical Association. (2020). *Letter to the U.S. Centers for Disease Control and Prevention Re: Docket No. CDC-2020-0029.* Retrieved Sept. 6, 2020 from https://searchlf.ama-assn.org/undefined/documentDownload?uri=%2Funstructured%2Fbinary%2Fletter%2FLETTERS%2F2020-6-16-Letter-to-Dowell-re-Opioid-Rx-Guideline.pdf.

Anderson, B. (2017). The use of remifentanil as the primary agent for analgesia in parturients. *Critical Care Nursing Clinics, 29*(4), 495–517.

Anderson, S. L., & Shreve, S. T. (2004). Continuous subcutaneous infusion of opiates at end-of-life. *Annals of Pharmacotherapy, 38*(6), 1015–1023.

Argoff, C. E. (2014). An Introduction to Pharmacogenetics in Pain Management: Knowledge of How Pharmacogenomics May Affect Clinical Care. In H. T. Benzon, J. P. Rathmell, C. L. Wu, D. C. Turk, C. E. Argoff, & R. W. Hurley (Eds.), *Practical Management of Pain* (5th Ed., pp. 132–138). Philadelphia, PA: Mosby.

Argoff, C., Arnstein, P., Stanos, S., Robinson, C. Y., Galer, B. S., & Gould, E. (2015). Relationship between change in pain intensity and functional outcomes in patients with chronic pain receiving twice daily extended-release hydrocodone bitartrate. *Journal of Opioid Management, 11*(5), 417–424.

Arnet, I., Schacher, S., Balmer, E., Koeberle, D., & Hersberger, K. E. (2016). Poor adhesion of fentanyl transdermal patches may mimic end-of-dosage failure after 48 hours and prompt early patch replacement in hospitalized cancer pain patients. *Journal of Pain Research, 9*, 993–999.

Atkinson, T., Coleman, J. J., & Fudin, J. (2018). Opioid medications, old wine in new bottles. In J. F. Peppin, J. J. Coleman, K. K. Dineen, & A. J. Ruggles (Eds.), *Prescription Drug Diversion and Pain: History, Policy, and Treatment* (p. 1). New York: Oxford University Press.

Atkinson, T. J., Wegrzyn, E. L., & Bettinger, J. J. (2014). Dialysis, Opioids, and Pain Management: Where's the Evidence? *Practical Pain Management, 14*(8), 49–57.

Ayonrinde, O. T., & Bridge, D. T. (2000). The rediscovery of methadone for cancer pain management. *Medical Journal of Australia, 173*(10), 536–540.

Bai, S. A., Xiang, Q., & Finn, A. (2016). Evaluation of the pharmacokinetics of single- and multiple-dose buprenorphine buccal film in healthy volunteers. *Clinical Therapeutics, 38*(2), 358–369.

Baldo, B. A. (2018). Opioid analgesic drugs and serotonin toxicity (syndrome): mechanisms, animal models, and links to clinical effects. *Archives of toxicology, 92*(8), 2457–2473.

Ballantyne, J. C., & Sullivan, M. D. (2017). Discovery of endogenous opioid systems: what it has meant for the clinician's understanding of pain and its treatment. *Pain, 158*(12), 2290–2300.

Bao, Y. J., Hou, W., Kong, X. Y., Yang, L., Xia, J., Hua, B. J., & Knaggs, R. (2016). Hydromorphone for cancer pain. *Cochrane Database of Systematic Reviews, 10*, CD011108.

Barr, J., Fraser, G. L., Puntillo, K., Ely, E. W., Gélinas, C., Dasta, J. F., … Coursin, D. B. (2013). American College of Critical Care Medicine Clinical practice guidelines for the management of pain, agitation, and delirium in adult patients in the intensive care unit. *Critical Care Medicine, 41*(1), 263–306.

Barry, A. E., Chaney, M. A., & London, M. J. (2015). Anesthetic management during cardiopulmonary bypass: a systematic review. *Anesthesia & Analgesia*, 120(4), 749–769.

Bartoli, A., Michna, E., He, E., & Wen, W. (2015). Efficacy and safety of once-daily, extended-release hydrocodone in individuals previously receiving hydrocodone/acetaminophen combination therapy for chronic pain. *Postgraduate Medicine*, 127(1), 5–12.

Bartz, L., Klein, C., Seifert, A., Herget, I., Ostgathe, C., & Stiel, S. (2014). Subcutaneous administration of drugs in palliative care: results of a systematic observational study. *Journal of Pain and Symptom Management*, 48(4), 540–547.

Beakley, B. D., Kaye, A. M., & Kaye, A. D. (2015). Tramadol, Pharmacology, Side Effects, and Serotonin Syndrome: A Review. *Pain Physician*, 18(4), 395–400.

Berliner, M. N., Giesecke, T., & Bornhövd, K. D. (2007). Impact of transdermal fentanyl on quality of life in rheumatoid arthritis. *The Clinical Journal of Pain*, 23(6), 530–534.

Berna, C., Kulich, R. J., & Rathmell, J. P. (2015, June). Tapering long-term opioid therapy in chronic noncancer pain: evidence and recommendations for everyday practice. In *Mayo Clinic Proceedings* (Vol. 90, No. 6, pp. 828–842): Elsevier.

Bhatnagar, S., Saraswathi Devi, N. K., Jain, P. N., Durgaprasad, G., Maroo, S. H., & Patel, K. R. (2014). Safety and efficacy of oral transmucosal fentanyl citrate compared to morphine sulphate immediate release tablet in management of breakthrough cancer pain. *Indian Journal of Palliative Care*, 20(3), 182.

Braeburn Pharmaceuticals, Inc. (2018). *Package Insert*. NJ: Princeton.

Brant, J. M., Rodgers, B. B., Gallagher, E., & Sundaramurthi, T. (2017). Breakthrough cancer pain: A systematic review of pharmacologic management. *Clinical Journal of Oncology Nursing*, 21(3), 71–80. Supplement.

Breitbart, W., Chandler, S., Eagel, B., Ellison, N., Enck, R. E., Lefkowitz, M., & Payne, R. (2000). An alternative algorithm for dosing transdermal fentanyl for cancer-related pain. *Oncology*, 14(5), 695–705.

Brennan, M. J., Fudin, J., & Perkins, R. J. (2012). PPM launches online opioid calculator. *Pract Pain Manage*, 13(2), 81–85.

Brokjær, A., Kreilgaard, M., Olesen, A. E., Simonsson, U. S., Christrup, L. L., Dahan, A., & Drewes, A. M. (2015). Population pharmacokinetics of morphine and morphine-6-glucuronide following rectal administration–A dose escalation study. *European Journal of Pharmaceutical Sciences*, 68, 78–86.

Brooks, A., Kominek, C., Pham, T. C., & Fudin, J. (2016). Exploring the use of chronic opioid therapy for chronic pain: when, how, and for whom? *Medical Clinics*, 100(1), 81–102.

Bujedo, B. M. (2014). Spinal opioid bioavailability in postoperative pain. *Pain Practice*, 14(4), 350–364.

Byas-Smith, M. G., Chapman, S. L., Reed, B., & Cotsonis, G. (2005). The Effect of Opioids on Driving and Psychomotor Performance in Patients With Chronic Pain. *The Clinical Journal of Pain*, 21(4), 345–352. https://doi.org/10.1097/01.ajp.0000125244.29279.c1.

Centers for Disease Control and Prevention (CDC). (2016). Prescription opioids: What you need to know. Retrieved June 1, 2020 from http://www.cifsf.org/uploads/3/2/0/9/32099267/opioid_fact_sheet_cdc.pdf.

Centers for Disease Control and Prevention (CDC). (2020). Opioid overdose. Retrieved June 1, 2020 from https://www.cdc.gov/drugoverdose/index.html.

Cepeda, M. S., Camargo, F., Zea, C., & Valencia, L. (2006). Tramadol for osteoarthritis. *The Cochrane Library*, 3, CD005522.

Cepeda, M. S., Camargo, F., Zea, C., & Valencia, L. (2007). Tramadol for osteoarthritis: a systematic review and meta-analysis. *The Journal of Rheumatology*, 34(3), 543–555.

Chang, A., Roeland, E. J., Atayee, R. S., Revta, C., & Ma, J. D. (2015). Transmucosal immediate-release fentanyl for breakthrough cancer pain: opportunities and challenges for use in palliative care. *Journal of Pain & Palliative Care Pharmacotherapy*, 29(3), 247–260.

Chang, A. K., Bijur, P. E., Holden, L., & Gallagher, E. J. (2015). Comparative Analgesic Efficacy of Oxycodone/Acetaminophen Versus Hydrocodone/Acetaminophen for Short-term Pain Management in Adults Following ED Discharge. *Academic Emergency Medicine*, 22(11), 1254–1260.

Channell, J. S., & Schug, S. (2018). Toxicity of tapentadol: a systematic review. *Pain Management*, 8(5), 327–329.

Cheung, C. W., Ching Wong, S. S., Qiu, Q., & Wang, X. (2017). Oral oxycodone for acute postoperative pain: a review of clinical trials. *Pain Physician*, 20, SE33–SE52.

Choi, L., Ferrell, B. A., Vasilevskis, E. E., Pandharipande, P. P., Heltsley, R., Ely, E. W., … Girard, T. D. (2016). Population pharmacokinetics of fentanyl in the critically ill. *Critical Care Medicine*, 44(1), 64.

Chong, W. S., & Johnson, D. S. (2017). Update on opioid pharmacology. *Update in Anaesthesia*, 32(n/a), 28–32.

Chou, R., Cruciani, R. A., Fiellin, D. A., Compton, P., Farrar, J. T., Haigney, M. C., … Mehta, D. (2014). Methadone safety: a clinical practice guideline from the American Pain Society and College on Problems of Drug Dependence, in collaboration with the Heart Rhythm Society. *The Journal of Pain*, 15(4), 321–337.

Chou, R., Gordon, D. B., de Leon-Casasola, O. A., Rosenberg, J. M., Bickler, S., Brennan, T., … Griffith, S. (2016). Management of Postoperative Pain: a clinical practice guideline from the American Pain Society, the American Society of Regional Anesthesia and Pain Medicine, and the American Society of Anesthesiologists' committee on regional anesthesia, executive committee, and administrative council. *The Journal of Pain*, 17(2), 131–157.

Chow, R. M., & Issa, M. (2017). Methadone. In R. J. Young, M. Nguyen, E. Nelson, & R. D. Urman (Eds.), *Pain Medicine, An Essential Review* (pp. 157–158). Cham, Switzerland: Springer International Publishing.

Clarke, H., Azargive, S., Montbriand, J., Nicholls, J., Sutherland, A., Valeeva, L., … Katznelson, R. (2018). Opioid weaning and pain management in postsurgical patients at the Toronto General Hospital Transitional Pain Service. *Canadian Journal of Pain*, 2(1), 236–247.

Coda, B. A., Brown, M. C., Risler, L. B., Syrjala, K., & Shen, D. D. (1999). Equivalent analgesia and side effects during epidural and pharmacokinetically tailored intravenous infusion with matching plasma alfentanil concentration. *Anesthesiology: The Journal of the American Society of Anesthesiologists*, 90(1), 98–108.

Cohen, H. (2015). *Casebook in Clinical Pharmacokinetics and Drug Dosing*. New York: McGraw-Hill.

Coluzzi, P. H. (1998). Sublingual morphine: efficacy reviewed. *Journal of Pain and Symptom Management*, 16(3), 184–192.

Cooper, T. E., Chen, J., Wiffen, P. J., Derry, S., Carr, D. B., Aldington, D., … Moore, R. A. (2017). Morphine for chronic neuropathic pain in adults. *The Cochrane Library*, 5, CD011669.

Costello, M., & Thompson, S. (2015). Preventing opioid misuse and potential abuse: The nurse's role in patient education. *Pain Management Nursing*, 16(4), 515–519.

Dahan, A. (2006). Opioid-induced respiratory effects: New data on buprenorphine. *Palliative Medicine*, 20(1), 3–8. https://doi.org/10.1191/0269216306pm1126oa.

Davis, M. P., & Goforth, H. W. (2016). Oxycodone with an opioid receptor antagonist: a review. *Journal of Opioid Management*, 12(1), 67–85.

Davis, C. S., Lieberman, A. J., Hernandez-Delgado, H., & Suba, C. (2019). Laws limiting the prescribing or dispensing of opioids for acute pain in the United States: A national systematic legal review. *Drug and alcohol dependence*, 194, 166–172.

Davis, M. P., Pasternak, G., & Behm, B. (2018). Treating Chronic Pain: An Overview of Clinical Studies Centered on the Buprenorphine Option. *Drugs*, 78(12), 1211–1228.

Dean, M. (2004). Opioids in renal failure and dialysis patients. *Journal of Pain and Symptom Management*, 28(5), 497–504.

de Beer, J. D. V., Winemaker, M. J., Donnelly, G. A., Miceli, P. C., Reiz, J. L., Harsanyi, Z., ... Darke, A. C. (2005). Efficacy and safety of controlled-release oxycodone and standard therapies for postoperative pain after knee or hip replacement. *Canadian Journal of Surgery*, 48(4), 277.

Deer, T. R., Leong, M. S., Buvanendran, A., Gordin, V., Kim, P. S., Panchal, S. J., & Ray, A. L. (2013). *Comprehensive Treatment of Chronic Pain by Medical, Interventional, and Integrative Approaches. The American Academy Of Pain Medicine Textbook on Patient Management*. New York: Springer.

De Gregori, M., Diatchenko, L., Ingelmo, P. M., Napolioni, V., Klepstad, P., Belfer, I., ... Normanno, M. (2016). Human genetic variability contributes to postoperative morphine consumption. *The Journal of Pain*, 17(5), 628–636.

Derry, S., Cooper, T. E., & Phillips, T. (2016). Single fixed-dose oral dexketoprofen plus tramadol for acute postoperative pain in adults. *Cochrane Database Syst Rev*, 9, CD012232.

Devlin, J. W., Skrobik, Y., Gélinas, C., Needham, D. M., Slooter, A. J., Pandharipande, P. P., ... Balas, M. C. (2018). Executive Summary: Clinical Practice Guidelines for the Prevention and Management of Pain, Agitation/Sedation, Delirium, Immobility, and Sleep Disruption in Adult Patients in the ICU. *Critical Care Medicine*, 46(9), 1532–1548.

Dhawan, B. N., Cesselin, F., & Raghubir, R. (1996). International Union of Pharmacology. XII: Classification of receptors. *Pharmacological Reviews*, 48, 567–592. https://doi.org/10.1124/pr.54.2.161.

Dickman, A., Roberts, E., Bickerstaff, M., Jackson, R., Weir, P., & Ellershaw, J. (2015). Chemical Compatibility/Stability of Alfentanil with Commonly Used Supportive Drug Combinations Administered by Continuous Subcutaneous Infusions for End of Life Care. *BMJ Supportive & Palliative Care*, 5(1), 103.

Do Keun Kim, S. H. Y., Kim, J. Y., Oh, C. H., Jung, J. K., & Kim, J. (2017). Comparison of the effects of sufentanil and fentanyl intravenous patient controlled analgesia after lumbar fusion. *Journal of Korean Neurosurgical Society*, 60(1), 54.

Dowell, D., Haegerich, T. M., & Chou, R. (2016). CDC Guideline for Prescribing Opioids for Chronic Pain—United States, 2016. *JAMA*, 315(15), 1624. https://doi.org/10.1001/jama.2016.1464.

Drewes, A. M., Jensen, R. D., Nielsen, L. M., Droney, J., Christrup, L. L., Arendt-Nielsen, L., ... Dahan, A. (2013). Differences between opioids: pharmacological, experimental, clinical and economical perspectives. *British Journal of Clinical Pharmacology*, 75(1), 60–78. https://doi.org/10.1111/j.1365-2125.2012.04317.x.

Drug Enforcement Administration. (2014). 21 CFR Part 1308 [Docket No. DEA-351] Schedule of controlled substances: placement of tramadol into schedule IV. In *U.S. Department of Justice Drug Enforcement Administration Diversion Control Division Rules*. Retrieved June 30, 2019, from https://www.deadiversion.usdoj.gov/fed_regs/rules/2014/fr0702.htm.

Drug Enforcement Administration (2016). DEA Releases 2016 Drug Threat Assessment: Fentanyl-related overdose deaths rising at an alarming rate. (2016, December 06). Retrieved August 01, 2017, from https://www.dea.gov/divisions/hq/2016/hq120616.shtml.

Drugs@FDA. Apadaz™ (Benzhydrocodone and acetaminophen) [Package Insert]. (2018). Retrieved June 21, 2019, from https://www.accessdata.fda.gov/drugsatfda_docs/label/2018/208653s000lbl.pdf.

Drugs@FDA. Belbuca™ (Buprenorphine) [Package Insert]. (2018). Retrieved June 28, 2019, https://www.accessdata.fda.gov/drugsatfda_docs/label/2015/207932s000lbl.pdf.

Drugs@FDA. Bunavail® (Buprenorphine and naloxone) buccal film [Package Insert]. (2014). Retrieved April 1, 2020, https://www.accessdata.fda.gov/drugsatfda_docs/label/2014/205637s000lbl.pdf.

Drugs@FDA. DSUVIA® (Sufentanil) [Package Insert]. (2018). Retrieved March 28, 2020, https://www.accessdata.fda.gov/drugsatfda_docs/label/2018/209128s000lbl.pdf.

Drugs@FDA. Duragesic® CII (Fentanyl Transdermal System [Package Insert]. (2016). Retrieved June 21, 2019, from https://www.accessdata.fda.gov/drugsatfda_docs/label/2016/019813s069lbl.pdf.

Drugs@FDA. Exalgo® (Hydromorphone Extended-Release Tablets) [Package Insert]. (2013). Retrieved June 21, 2019, from https://www.accessdata.fda.gov/drugsatfda_docs/label/2013/021217s005lbl.pdf.

Drugs@FDA. Dilaudid® Oral Liquid and Dilaudid® Tablets (hydromorphone hydrochloride) CS-II [Package Insert]. (2016). Retrieved June 21, 2019, from https://www.accessdata.fda.gov/drugsatfda_docs/label/2007/019892s015lbl.pdf.

Drugs@FDA: XTAMPZA ER (oxycodone extended-release capsules). [Package Insert]. (2016). Retrieved September 3, 2020 from https://www.accessdata.fda.gov/drugsatfda_docs/label/2016/208090s000lbl.pdf.

Drugs@FDA. Hysingla™ ER (Hydrocodone Bitartrate) [Package Insert]. (2016). Retrieved June 21, 2019, from https://www.accessdata.fda.gov/drugsatfda_docs/label/2016/206627s004lbl.pdf.

Drugs@FDA. Nucynta® (Tapentadol) [Package Insert]. (2009). Retrieved June 21, 2019, from https://www.accessdata.fda.gov/drugsatfda_docs/label/2010/022304s003lbl.pdf.

Drugs@FDA. Nucynta® ER (Tapentadol) extended-release tablets. [Package Insert]. (2016). Retrieved June 29, 2019, from https://www.accessdata.fda.gov/drugsatfda_docs/label/2016/200533s014lbl.pdf.

Drugs@FDA. Opana® (Oxymorphone hydrochloride) [Package Insert]. (2018). Retrieved June 28, 2019, from https://www.accessdata.fda.gov/drugsatfda_docs/label/2018/021611s013s015lbl.pdf.

Drugs@FDA. OxyContin® (Oxycodone hydrochloride) extended-release tablets [Package Insert]. (2018). Retrieved June 22, 2019, from https://www.accessdata.fda.gov/drugsatfda_docs/label/2018/022272s039lbl.pdf.

Drugs@FDA. Sublocade™ (buprenorphine extended-release) injection for subcutaneous use [Package Insert]. (2017). Retrieved Sept. 3, 2020 from https://www.accessdata.fda.gov/drugsatfda_docs/label/2017/209819s000lbl.pdf.

Drugs@FDA. Ultiva® (Remifentanil) [Package Insert]. (2001). Retrieved June 21, 2019, from https://www.accessdata.fda.gov/drugsatfda_docs/label/2004/20630se5-005_ultiva_lbl.pdf.

Drugs@FDA. Vicoprofen® 7.5mg/200mg (Hydrocodone Bitartrate and Ibuprofen Tablets) [Package Insert]. (2016). Retrieved June 21, 2019, from https://www.accessdata.fda.gov/drugsatfda_docs/label/2016/020716s012s013s014s015s016lbl.pdf.

Duehmke, R. M., Derry, S., Wiffen, P. J., Bell, R. F., Aldington, D., & Moore, R. A. (2017). Tramadol for neuropathic pain in adults. *Cochrane Database of Systematic Reviews*, 6, CD003726.

Dwivedi, S., & Agarwal, S. K. (2015). Comparative evaluation of intrathecal, epidural and intravenous bolus sufentanil for post operative analgesia in lower limb surgery. *Journal of Evolution of Medical and Dental Sciences*, 4(48), 8288–8293.

Elefritz, J. L., Murphy, C. V., Papadimos, T. J., & Lyaker, M. R. (2016). Methadone analgesia in the critically ill. *Journal of Critical Care*, 34, 84–88.

Els, C., Jackson, T. D., Kunyk, D., Lappi, V. G., Sonnenberg, B., Hagtvedt, R., ... Straube, S. (2017). Adverse events associated with medium-and long-term use of opioids for chronic non-cancer pain: an overview of Cochrane Reviews. *Cochrane Database Syst Rev*, 10, CD012509.

Elzey, M. J., Fudin, J., & Edwards, E. S. (2016). Take-home naloxone treatment for opioid emergencies: A comparison of routes of administration and associated delivery systems. *Expert Opinion on Drug Delivery*, 14(9), 1045–1058. https://doi.org/10.1080/17425247.2017.1230097.

Endo Pharmaceuticals. (2010). Opana® ER (oxymorphone hydrochloride) extended-release tablets: Full prescribing information. Retrieved June 29, 2019, from http://www.opana.com.

Endo Pharmaceuticals. (2016). *Belbuca*. Malvern, PA: Package Insert.

Endo Pharmaceuticals (2017). Endo provides update on Opana® Er. Available at http://investor.endo.com/news-releases/news-release-details/endo-provides-update-opanar-er.

Fadeyi, E. A., & Pomper, G. J. (2016). Febrile, allergic, and non-immune transfusion reactions. In T. L. Simon, J. McCullough, F. I. Snyder, B. G. Solheim, & R. G. Strauss (Eds.), *Rossi's Principles of Transfusion Medicine* (5th Ed., pp. 652–666). Hoboken, NJ: John Wiley & Sons, Ltd.

Faria, J., Barbosa, J., Moreira, R., Queirós, O., Carvalho, F., & Dinis-Oliveira, R. J. (2018). Comparative pharmacology and toxicology of tramadol and tapentadol. *European Journal of Pain*, 22(5), 827–844.

Felden, L., Walter, C., Harder, S., Treede, R. D., Kayser, H., Drover, D., ... Lötsch, J. (2011). Comparative clinical effects of hydromorphone and morphine: a meta-analysis. *British Journal of Anaesthesia*, 107(3), 319–328.

Ferrari, A., Coccia, C., Bertolini, A., & Sternieri, E. (2004). Methadone—metabolism, pharmacokinetics and interactions. *Pharmacological Research*, 50(6), 551–559. https://doi.org/10.1016/j.phrs.2004.05.002.

Ferreira, D. H., Boland, J. W., Phillips, J. L., Lam, L., & Currow, D. C. (2018). The impact of therapeutic opioid agonists on driving-related psychomotor skills assessed by a driving simulator or an on-road driving task: A systematic review. *Palliative Medicine*, 32(4), 786–803.

Filitz, J., Ihmsen, H., Günther, W., Tröster, A., Schwilden, H., Schüttler, J., & Koppert, W. (2008). Supra-additive effects of tramadol and acetaminophen in a human pain model. *Pain*, 136(3), 262–270.

Findlay, M., & Isles, C. (2015). The challenges of renal replacement therapy in the elderly. In *Clinical Companion in Nephrology* (pp. 229–233). Cham, Switzerland: Springer International.

Finnerup, N. B., Attal, N., Haroutounian, S., McNicol, E., Baron, R., Dworkin, R. H., ... Kamerman, P. R. (2015). Pharmacotherapy for neuropathic pain in adults: a systematic review and meta-analysis. *The Lancet Neurology*, 14(2), 162–173.

Fishbain, D. A., Cutler, R. B., Rosomoff, H. L., & Rosomoff, R. S. (2002). Can Patients Taking Opioids Drive Safely? A structured evidenced-based review. *Journal of Pain & Palliative Care Pharmacotherapy*, 16(1), 9–28. https://doi.org/10.1080/j354v16n01_03.

Fishbain, D. A., Cutler, R., Rosomoff, H. L., & Rosomoff, R. S. (2003). Are Opioid-Dependent/Tolerant Patients Impaired in Driving-Related Skills? A Structured Evidence-Based Review. *Journal of Pain and Symptom Management*, 25(6), 559–577. https://doi.org/10.1016/s0885-3924(03)00176-3.

Fisher, D. M., Chang, P., Wada, D. R., Dahan, A., & Palmer, P. P. (2018). Pharmacokinetic Properties of a Sufentanil Sublingual Tablet Intended to Treat Acute Pain. *Anesthesiology: The Journal of the American Society of Anesthesiologists*, 128(5), 943–952.

Fishman, S. M., Wilsey, B., Mahajan, G., & Molina, P. (2002). Methadone reincarnated: novel clinical applications with related concerns. *Pain Medicine*, 3(4), 339–348.

Fletcher, D., & Martinez, V. (2014). Opioid-induced hyperalgesia in patients after surgery: a systematic review and a meta-analysis. *British Journal of Anaesthesia*, 112(6), 991–1004.

Fontaine, M., Latarjet, J., Payre, J., Poupelin, J. C., & Ravat, F. (2017). Feasibility of monomodal analgesia with IV alfentanil during burn dressing changes at bedside (in spontaneously breathing non-intubated patients). *Burns*, 43(2), 337–342.

Foster, B., Twycross, R., Mihalyo, M., & Wilcock, A. (2013). Buprenorphine. *Journal of Pain and Symptom Management*, 45(5), 939–949.

Fouladi, A., & Soleimani, A. (2017). Comparison of different analgesic techniques for pain relief during extracorporeal shock wave lithotripsy: a double-blind, randomized clinical trial. *Acta Informatica Medica*, 25(2), 94.

Fournier, R., Weber, A., & Gamulin, Z. (2005). Intrathecal sufentanil is more potent than intravenous for postoperative analgesia after total-hip replacement. *Regional Anesthesia and Pain Medicine*, 30(3), 249–254.

Frampton, J. E. (2016). Sublingual sufentanil: a review in acute postoperative pain. *Drugs*, 76(6), 719–729.

Friedman, Z., Arzola, C., Postonogova, T., Malavade, A., & Siddiqui, N. T. (2017). Physician and Patient Survey of Taper Schedule and Family Physician Letters Following Discharge from the Acute Pain Service. *Pain Practice*, 17(3), 366–370.

Friesen, K. J., Falk, J., & Bugden, S. (2015). Voluntary warnings and the limits of good prescribing behavior: the case for de-adoption of meperidine. *Journal of Pain Research*, 8, 879.

Fudin, J., Raouf, M., & Wegrzyn, E. L. (2017). *Opioid Dosing Policy: Pharmacological Considerations Regarding Equianalgesic Dosing*. Lenexa, KS: American Academy of Integrative Pain Management.

Fujii, M. H., Hodges, A. C., Russell, R. L., Roensch, K., Beynnon, B., Ahern, T. P., ... MacLean, C. D. (2018). Post-discharge opioid prescribing and use after common surgical procedure. *Journal of the American College of Surgeons, 226*(6), 1004–1012.

Gaertner, J., Radbruch, L., Giesecke, T., Gerbershagen, H., Petzke, F., Ostgathe, C., ... Sabatowski, R. (2006). Assessing cognition and psychomotor function under long-term treatment with controlled release oxycodone in non-cancer pain patients. *Acta Anaesthesiologica Scandinavica, 50*(6), 664–672. https://doi.org/10.1111/j.1399-6576.2006.01027.x.

Galica, R. J., Hayek, S. M., Veizi, E., McEwan, M. T., Katta, S., Ali, O., ... Sondhi, N. (2018). Intrathecal Trialing of Continuous Infusion Combination Therapy with Hydromorphone and Bupivacaine in Failed Back Surgery Patients. *Neuromodulation: Technology at the Neural Interface, 21*(7), 648–654.

Gallagher, R. (2009). Methadone: an effective, safe drug of first choice for pain management in frail older adults. *Pain Medicine, 10*(2), 319–326.

Galski, T., Williams, J., & Ehle, H. T. (2000). Effects of Opioids on Driving Ability. *Journal of Pain and Symptom Management, 19*(3), 200–208. https://doi.org/10.1016/s0885-3924(99)00158-x.

Galvagno, S. M., Jr., Smith, C. E., Varon, A. J., Hasenboehler, E. A., Sultan, S., Shaefer, G., ... Joseph, B. A. (2016). Pain management for blunt thoracic trauma: a joint practice management guideline from the Eastern Association for the Surgery of Trauma and Trauma Anesthesiology Society. *Journal of Trauma and Acute Care Surgery, 81*(5), 936–951.

Gan, T. J., Ginsberg, B., Glass, P. S., Fortney, J., Jhaveri, R., & Perno, R. (1997). Opioid-sparing Effects of a Low-dose Infusion of Naloxone in Patient-administered Morphine Sulfate. *Anesthesiology, 87*(5), 1075–1081. https://doi.org/10.1097/00000542-199711000-00011.

Garg, R., & Saini, S. (2015). Sublingual Route During Perioperative and Chronic Pain Management. *Journal of Anesthesia and Critical Care Open Access, 3*(2), 00085.

Gaskell, H., Derry, S., Moore, R. A., & McQuay, H. J. (2009). Single dose oral oxycodone and oxycodone plus paracetamol (acetaminophen) for acute postoperative pain in adults. *The Cochrane Database of Systematic Reviews, 3*, CD002763.

Gilron, I., Tu, D., Holden, R. R., Jackson, A. C., & DuMerton-Shore, D. (2015). Combination of morphine with nortriptyline for neuropathic pain. *Pain, 156*(8), 1440–1448.

Gimbel, J., Spierings, E. L., Katz, N., Xiang, Q., Tzanis, E., & Finn, A. (2016). Efficacy and tolerability of buccal buprenorphine in opioid-experienced patients with moderate to severe chronic low back pain: results of a phase 3, enriched enrollment, randomized withdrawal study. *Pain, 157*(11), 2517.

Gonzalez-Barboteo, J., Porta-Sales, J., Nabal-Vicuña, M., Diez-Porres, L., Canal, J., Alonso-Babarro, A., ... Bruera, E. (2016). A randomized controlled trial (RCT) of 2 dose ratios for conversion from parenteral to oral methadone in patients with cancer pain. *Journal of Clinical Oncology, 34*(26), 206.

Gordon, D. B. (2006). Oral transmucosal fentanyl citrate for cancer breakthrough pain: a review. *Oncology Nursing Forum, 33*(2), 257.

Gordon, D. B., Jones, H. D., Goshman, L. M., Foley, D. K., & Bland, S. E. (2000). A quality improvement approach to reducing use of meperidine. *The Joint Commission Journal on Quality Improvement, 26*(12), 686–699.

Goyal, V. K., Bhargava, S. K., & Baj, B. (2017). Effect of preoperative incentive spirometry on fentanyl-induced cough: a prospective, randomized, controlled study. *Korean Journal of Anesthesiology, 70*(5), 550–554.

Greenwood, B. C., Clements, K., & Alper, C. J. (2017). The Effect of a Federal Controlled Substance Act Schedule Change on Hydrocodone Combination Products Claims in a Medicaid Population. *Journal of Managed Care & Specialized Pharmacy, 23*(5), 532–539.

Gressler, L. E., Hammond, D. A., & Painter, J. T. (2017). Serotonin syndrome in tapentadol literature: systematic review of original research. *Journal of Pain & Palliative Care Pharmacotherapy, 31*(3-4), 228–236.

Grissa, M. H., Boubaker, H., Zorgati, A., Beltaïef, K., Zhani, W., Msolli, M. A., ... Nouira, S. (2015). Efficacy and safety of nebulized morphine given at 2 different doses compared to IV titrated morphine in trauma pain. *The American Journal of Emergency Medicine, 33*(11), 1557–1561.

Gudin, J., Fudin, J., & Nalamachu, S. (2016). Levorphanol use: past, present and future. *Postgraduate Medicine, 128*(1), 46–53.

Guildford, B. J., Daly-Eichenhardt, A., Hill, B., Sanderson, K., & McCracken, L. M. (2018). Analgesic reduction during an interdisciplinary pain management programme: treatment effects and processes of change. *British Journal of Pain, 12*(2), 72–86.

Guenther, S. M., Mickle, T. C., Barrett, A. C., Roupe, K. A., Zhou, J., & Lam, V. (2018). Relative bioavailability, intranasal abuse potential, and safety of benzhydrocodone/acetaminophen compared with hydrocodone bitartrate/acetaminophen in recreational drug abusers. *Pain Medicine, 19*(5), 955–966.

Gunnarsdottir, S., Sigurdardottir, V., Kloke, M., Radbruch, L., Sabatowski, R., Kaasa, S., & Klepstad, P. (2017). A multicenter study of attitudinal barriers to cancer pain management. *Supportive Care in Cancer, 25*(11), 3595–3602.

Gutstein, H. B., & Akil, H. (2006). Opioid Analgesics. Opioid agonist/antagonist and partial agonists. In L. L. Brunton (Ed.), *Goodman & Gilman's the pharmacological basis of therapeutics* (11th Ed, pp. 574–576). Toronto: McGraw-Hill, Medical Publishing Division.

Hadley, G., Derry, S., Moore, R. A., & Wiffen, P. J. (2012). Transdermal fentanyl for cancer pain. *Cochrane Database of Systematic Reviews, 12*.

Hagen, N. A., Fisher, K., & Stiles, C. (2007). Sublingual methadone for the management of cancer-related breakthrough pain: a pilot study. *Journal of Palliative Medicine, 10*(2), 331–337.

Hale, M., Urdaneta, V., Kirby, M. T., Xiang, Q., & Rauck, R. (2017). Long-term safety and analgesic efficacy of buprenorphine buccal film in patients with moderate-to-severe chronic pain requiring around-the-clock opioids. *Journal of Pain Research, 10*, 233.

Han, B., Compton, W. M., Blanco, C., Crane, E., Lee, J., & Jones, C. M. (2017). Prescription opioid use, misuse, and use disorders in US adults: 2015 National Survey on Drug Use and Health. *Annals of Internal Medicine, 167*(5), 293–301.

Hasak, J. M., Bettlach, C. L. R., Santosa, K. B., Larson, E. L., Stroud, J., & Mackinnon, S. E. (2018). Empowering post-surgical patients to improve opioid disposal: a before and after quality improvement study. *Journal of the American College of Surgeons*, 226(3), 235–240.

Hassamal, S., Miotto, K., Dale, W., & Danovitch, I. (2018). Tramadol: understanding the risk of serotonin syndrome and seizures. *The American Journal of Medicine*, 131(11), 1382-e1.

Hawley, P., Wing, P., & Nayar, S. (2015). Methadone for pain: What to do when the oral route is not available. *Journal of Pain and Symptom Management*, 49(6), e4–e6.

Heiskanen, T., Mätzke, S., Haakana, S., Gergov, M., Vuori, E., & Kalso, E. (2009). Transdermal fentanyl in cachectic cancer patients. *PAIN®*, 144(1-2), 218–222.

Hermens, J. M., Ebertz, J. M., Hanifin, J. M., & Hirshman, C. A. (1985). Comparison of histamine release in human skin mast cells induced by morphine, fentanyl, and oxymorphone. *Anesthesiology*, 62(2), 124–129.

Herndon, C. M., Arnstein, P., Darnall, B., Hartrick, C., Hecht, K., Lyons, M., & Seghal, N. (2016). *Principles of Analgesic Use*. Chicago: American Pain Society.

Hewitt, D. J., Todd, K. H., Xiang, J., Jordan, D. M., Rosenthal, N. R., & CAPSS-216 Study Investigators. (2007). Tramadol/acetaminophen or hydrocodone/acetaminophen for the treatment of ankle sprain: a randomized, placebo-controlled trial. *Annals of Emergency Medicine*, 49(4), 468–480.

Hoffman, R. S., Howland, M. A., Lewin, N. A., Nelson, L., Goldfrank, L. R., & Flomenbaum, N. (2015). *Goldfranks toxicologic emergencies*. New York: McGraw-Hill Education.

Hollmann, M. W., Rathmell, J. P., & Lirk, P. (2019). Optimal postoperative pain management: redefining the role for opioids. *The Lancet*, 393(10180), 1483–1485.

Hong, D., Flood, P., & Diaz, G. (2008). The side effects of morphine and hydromorphone patient-controlled analgesia. *Anesthesia & Analgesia*, 107(4), 1384–1389.

Hosseininejad, S. M., Samakous, A. K., Montaze, S. H., Khati, I., Jahania, F., & Ahidasht, H. (2016). Comparing the Effects of Sublingual Buprenorphine and Intravenous Morphine on Acute Renal Colic Pain. *Journal of Mazandaran University of Medical Sciences*, 26(143), 1–10.

Huang, M., Wang, H., Xu, J., & Li, P. (2015). Comparison of oxycodone and dezocine for prevention of fentanyl-induced cough during anesthesia induction. *Chinese Journal of Anesthesiology*, 35(7), 787–789.

Hughes, J., Smith, T. W., Kosterlitz, H. W., Fothergill, L. A., Morgan, B. A., & Morris, H. R. (1976). Pharmacology identification of two related pentapeptides from the brain with potent opiate agonist activity. *Pain*, 2(3), 329. https://doi.org/10.1016/0304-3959(76)90018-x.

Hum, A., Fainsinger, R. L., & Bielech, M. (2007). Subcutaneous methadone—an issue revisited. *Journal of Pain and Symptom Management*, 34(6), 573–575.

Hutchison, R. W., Chon, E. H., Tucker, W. F., Jr., Gilder, R., Moss, J., & Daniel, P. (2006). A comparison of a fentanyl, morphine, and hydromorphone patient-controlled intravenous delivery for acute postoperative analgesia: a multicenter study of opioid-induced adverse reactions. *Hospital Pharmacy*, 41(7), 659–663.

Indivor. (2016). *Buprenex*. Richmond, VA: Package Insert.

Institute for Safe Medication Practices. (Nov. 20, 2016). Look-Alike Drug Names with Recommended Tall Man Letters.

Available at https://www.ismp.org/recommendations/tall-man-letters-list.

Interagency Pain Research Coordinating Committee. (2015). *National Pain Strategy: a comprehensive population health-level strategy for pain*. Washington, DC: Department of Health and Human Services. Retrieved June 1, 2020 from https://iprcc.nih.gov/sites/default/files/HHSNational_Pain_Strategy_508C.pdf.

Jamison, R. N., & Mao, J. (2015, July). Opioid analgesics. In *Mayo Clinic Proceedings* (Vol. 90, No. 7, pp. 957–968): Elsevier.

Jancin, B. (2017). Helpful schedules ease task of tapering opioids. In *Internal Medicine News, Health Reference Center Academic*. Retrieved June 30, 2019, from http://link.galegroup.com/apps/doc/A519252542/HRCA?u=nysl_me_nymcv&sid=HRCA&xid=885a5c47.

Janicki, P. K. (2013). Pharmacogenomics of Pain Management. In T. R. Deer, M. S. Leong, A. Buvanendran, V. Gordin, P. S. Kim, S. J. Panchal, & A. L. Ray (Eds.), *Comprehensive Treatment of Chronic Pain by Medical, Interventional, and Integrative Approaches: The American Academy of Pain Medicine Textbook on Patient Management* (pp. 23–33). New York: Springer.

Jonan, A. B., Kaye, A. D., & Urman, R. D. (2018). Buprenorphine formulations: clinical best practice strategies recommendations for perioperative management of patients undergoing surgical or interventional pain procedures. *Pain Physician*, 21, E1–E12.

Jones, C. M., Lurie, P. G., & Throckmorton, D. C. (2016). Effect of US Drug Enforcement Administration's rescheduling of hydrocodone combination analgesic products on opioid analgesic prescribing. *JAMA Internal Medicine*, 176(3), 399–402.

Kampe, S., Warm, M., Kaufmann, J., Hundegger, S., Mellinghoff, H., & Kiencke, P. (2004). Clinical efficacy of controlled-release oxycodone 20 mg administered on a 12-h dosing schedule on the management of postoperative pain after breast surgery for cancer. *Current Medical Research and Opinion*, 20(2), 199–202.

Karimian, P., Atayee, R. S., Ajayi, T. A., & Edmonds, K. P. (2017). Methadone dose selection for treatment of pain compared with consensus recommendations. *Journal of Palliative Medicine*, 20(12), 1385–1388.

Kestenbaum, M. G., Vilches, A. O., Messersmith, S., Connor, S. R., Fine, P. G., Murphy, B., ... Muir, J. C. (2014). Alternative routes to oral opioid administration in palliative care: a review and clinical summary. *Pain Medicine*, 15(7), 1129–1153.

Khanna, I. K., & Pillarisetti, S. (2015). Buprenorphine–an attractive opioid with underutilized potential in treatment of chronic pain. *Journal of Pain Research*, 8, 859.

Kharasch, E. D., Hoffer, C., & Whittington, D. (2004). Influence of age on the pharmacokinetics and pharmacodynamics of oral transmucosal fentanyl citrate. *Anesthesiology: The Journal of the American Society of Anesthesiologists*, 101(3), 738–743.

Kim, S. H., Stoicea, N., Soghomonyan, S., & Bergese, S. D. (2015). Remifentanil—Acute Opioid Tolerance and Opioid-Induced Hyperalgesia: A Systematic Review. *American Journal of Therapeutics*, 22(3), e62–e74.

Klimas, R., & Mikus, G. (2014). Morphine-6-glucuronide is responsible for the analgesic effect after morphine administration: a quantitative review of morphine, morphine-6-glucuronide, and morphine-3-glucuronide. *British Journal of Anaesthesia*, 113(6), 935–944.

Koike, K., Terui, T., Nagasako, T., Horiuchi, I., Machino, T., Kusakabe, T., ... Nishisato, T. (2016). A new once-a-day fentanyl citrate patch (Fentos® Tape) could be a new treatment option in patients with end-of-dose failure using a 72-h transdermal fentanyl matrix patch. *Supportive Care in Cancer*, 24(3), 1053–1059.

Kolesnikov, Y. A., Wilson, R. S., & Pasternak, G. W. (2003). The synergistic analgesic interactions between hydrocodone and ibuprofen. *Anesthesia & Analgesia*, 97(6), 1721–1723.

Koncicki, H. M., Brennan, F., Vinen, K., & Davison, S. N. (2015). An approach to pain management in end stage renal disease: Considerations for general management and intradialytic symptoms. *Seminars in Dialysis*, 28(4), 384–391.

Kopecky, E. A., Fleming, A. B., Levy-Cooperman, N., O'Connor, M., & Sellers, E. (2017). Oral human abuse potential of oxycodone DETERx®(Xtampza® ER). *The Journal of Clinical Pharmacology*, 57(4), 500–512.

Kornick, C. A., Santiago-Palma, J., Moryl, N., Payne, R., & Obbens, E. A. (2003). Benefit-risk assessment of transdermal fentanyl for the treatment of chronic pain. *Drug Safety*, 26(13), 951–973.

Kuip, E. J., Zandvliet, M. L., Koolen, S. L., Mathijssen, R. H., & Rijt, C. C. (2017). A review of factors explaining variability in fentanyl pharmacokinetics; focus on implications for cancer patients. *British Journal of Clinical Pharmacology*, 83(2), 294–313.

Labate, A., Newton, M. R., & Vernon, G. M. (2005). Tramadol and new-onset seizures. *The Medical Journal of Australia*, 182(1), 42–43.

Lane, M. E. (2013). The transdermal delivery of fentanyl. *European Journal of Pharmaceutics and Biopharmaceutics*, 84(3), 449–455.

Larmené-Beld, K. H., Alting, E. K., & Taxis, K. (2018). A systematic literature review on strategies to avoid look-alike errors of labels. *European Journal of Clinical Pharmacology*, 74(8), 985–993.

Lee, K. A., Ganta, N., Horton, J. R., & Chai, E. (2016). Evidence for neurotoxicity due to morphine or hydromorphone use in renal impairment: a systematic review. *Journal of Palliative Medicine*, 19(11), 1179–1187.

Leece, P., Cavacuiti, C., Macdonald, E. M., Gomes, T., Kahan, M., Srivastava, A., ... Canadian Drug Safety and Effectiveness Research Network. (2015). Predictors of opioid-related death during methadone therapy. *Journal of Substance Abuse Treatment*, 57, 30–35.

Lev, R., Petro, S., Lee, A., Lee, O., Lucas, J., Castillo, E. M., ... Vilke, G. M. (2015). Methadone related deaths compared to all prescription related deaths. *Forensic Science International*, 257, 347–352.

Likar, R., Wittels, M., Molnar, M., Kager, I., Ziervogel, G., & Sittl, R. (2006). Pharmacokinetic and pharmacodynamic properties of tramadol IR and SR in elderly patients: a prospective, age-group-controlled study. *Clinical Therapeutics*, 28(12), 2022–2039.

Lin, Y. C., Chen, C. Y., Liao, Y. M., Liao, A. H. W., Lin, P. C., & Chang, C. C. (2017). Preventing shivering with adjuvant low dose intrathecal meperidine: A meta-analysis of randomized controlled trials with trial sequential analysis. *Scientific Reports*, 7(1), 15323.

Linnaus, M. E., Sheaffer, W. W., Ali-Mucheru, M. N., Velazco, C. S., Neville, M., & Gray, R. J. (2019). The opioid crisis and surgeons: national survey of prescribing patterns and the influence of motivators, experience, and gender. *The American Journal of Surgery*, 217(6), 1116–1120.

Liu, H. H., Zhou, T., Wei, J. Q., & Ma, W. H. (2015). Comparison between remifentanil and dexmedetomidine for sedation during modified awake fiberoptic intubation. *Experimental and Therapeutic Medicine*, 9(4), 1259–1264.

Liu, H. L., An, L. J., Su, Z., Zhang, Y., & Gui, B. (2015). Magnesium sulphate suppresses fentanyl-induced cough during general anesthesia induction: a double-blind, randomized, and placebo-controlled study. *International Journal of Clinical and Experimental Medicine*, 8(7), 11332.

Lu, L. (2015). The impact of genetic variation on sensitivity to opioid analgesics in patients with postoperative pain: a systematic review and meta-analysis. *Pain Physician*, 18, 131–152.

Lutfy, K., & Cowan, A. (2004). Buprenorphine: A Unique Drug with Complex Pharmacology. *Current Neuropharmacology*, 2(4), 395–402. https://doi.org/10.2174/1570159043359477.

MacKenzie, M., Zed, P. J., & Ensom, M. H. (2016). Opioid pharmacokinetics-pharmacodynamics: clinical implications in acute pain management in trauma. *Annals of Pharmacotherapy*, 50(3), 209–218.

MacLean, A. J., & Schwartz, T. L. (2015). Tramadol for the treatment of fibromyalgia. *Expert Review of Neurotherapeutics*, 15(5), 469–475.

Malec, M., & Shega, J. W. (2015). Pain management in the elderly. *Medical Clinics*, 99(2), 337–350.

Makris, U. E., Abrams, R. C., Gurland, B., & Reid, M. C. (2014). Management of persistent pain in the older patient: a clinical review. *JAMA*, 312(8), 825–837.

Manchikanti, L., Alturi, S., Kaye, A. M., & Kaye, A. D. (2015). Hydrocodone bitartrate for chronic pain. *Drugs of Today*, 51(7), 415–427.

Martin, W. R., Eades, C. G., Thompson, J. A., Huppler, R. F., & Gilbert, P. E. (1976). The effects of morphine- and nalorphine-like drugs in the nondependent and morphine-dependent chronic spinal dog. *Journal of Pharmacology and Experimental Therapeutics*, 197(3), 517–532.

Mayyas, F., Fayers, P., Kaasa, S., & Dale, O. (2010). A systematic review of oxymorphone in the management of chronic pain. *Journal of Pain and Symptom Management*, 39(2), 296–308.

Mazzola, R., Ricchetti, F., Fiorentino, A., Giaj-Levra, N., Fersino, S., Tebano, U., ... Alongi, F. (2017). Fentanyl pectin nasal spray for painful mucositis in head and neck cancers during intensity-modulated radiation therapy with or without chemotherapy. *Clinical and Translational Oncology*, 19(5), 593–598.

McCartney, C. J., & Niazi, A. (2006). Use of opioid analgesics in the perioperative period. In G. Shorten, D. Carr, D. Harmon, M. Puig, & J. Browne (Eds.), *Postoperative Pain Management* (pp. 137–147):WB Saunders.

McLean, S., & Twomey, F. (2015). Methods of rotation from another strong opioid to methadone for the management of cancer pain: a systematic review of the available evidence. *Journal of Pain and Symptom Management*, 50(2), 248–259.

McNicol, E. D., Ferguson, M. C., & Schumann, R. (2017). Methadone for neuropathic pain in adults. *Cochrane Database Syst Rev*, 5, CD012499.

McNulty, J. P. (2007). Can levorphanol be used like methadone for intractable refractory pain? *Journal of Palliative Medicine*, 10(2), 293–296.

McPherson, M. L. (2018). *Demystifying opioid conversion calculations: a guide for effective dosing*. Bethesda, MD: American Society of Health-System Pharmacists.

McPherson, M. L., Costantino, R. C., & McPherson, A. L. (2018). Methadone: Maximizing Safety and Efficacy for

Pain Control in Patients with Cancer. *Hematology/Oncology Clinics of North America*, 32(3), 405–415.

Menefee, L. A., Frank, E. D., Crerand, C., Jalali, S., Park, J., Sanschagrin, K., & Besser, M. (2004). The Effects of Transdermal Fentanyl on Driving, Cognitive Performance, and Balance in Patients with Chronic Nonmalignant Pain Conditions. *Pain Medicine*, 5(1), 42–49. https://doi.org/10.1111/j.1526-4637.2004.04005.x.

Mercadante, S. (2015). Opioid metabolism and clinical aspects. *European Journal of Pharmacology*, 769, 71–78.

Mercadante, S. (2017). The role of tapentadol as a strong opioid in cancer pain management: a systematic and critical review. *Current Medical Research and Opinion*, 33(11), 1965–1969.

Mercadante, S., & Bruera, E. (2016). Opioid switching in cancer pain: From the beginning to nowadays. *Critical Reviews in Oncology/Hematology*, 99, 241–248.

Mercadante, S., & Bruera, E. (2018). Methadone as first line opioid in cancer pain management: a systematic review. *Journal of Pain and Symptom Management*, 55(3), 998–1003.

Mercadante, S., Porzio, G., & Gebbia, V. (2014). New opioids. *Journal of Clinical Oncology*, 32(16), 1671–1676.

Miaskowski, C., Cleary, J., Burney, R., Coyne, P., Finley, R., Foster, R., ... Weisman, S. J. (2005). *Guideline for the management of cancer pain in adults and children* (p. 3). Glenview, IL: American Pain Society.

Miller, H., Panahi, L., Tapia, D., Tran, A., & Bowman, J. D. (2017). Loperamide misuse and abuse. *Journal of the American Pharmacists Association*, 57(2), S45–S50. https://doi.org/10.1016/j.japh.2016.12.079.

Miller, K., Yarlas, A., Wen, W., Dain, B., Lynch, S. Y., Ripa, S. R., ... Raffa, R. (2014). The impact of buprenorphine transdermal delivery system on activities of daily living among patients with chronic low back pain: an application of the International Classification of Functioning, Disability and Health. *The Clinical Journal of Pain*, 30(12), 1015–1022.

Miner, J. R., Gray, R., Delavari, P., Patel, S., Patel, R., & Plummer, D. (2011). Alfentanil for procedural sedation in the emergency department. *Annals of Emergency Medicine*, 57(2), 117–121.

Miotto, K., Cho, A. K., Khalil, M. A., Blanco, K., Sasaki, J. D., & Rawson, R. (2017). Trends in tramadol: pharmacology, metabolism, and misuse. *Anesthesia & Analgesia*, 124(1), 44–51.

Morue, H. I., Raj-Lawrence, S., Saxena, S., Delbaere, A., Engelman, E., & Barvais, L. A. (2018). Placebo versus low-dose ketamine infusion in addition to remifentanil target-controlled infusion for conscious sedation during oocyte retrieval: A double-blinded, randomised controlled trial. *European Journal of Anaesthesiology*, 35(9), 667–674.

Mouallem, M., Schwartz, E., & Farfel, Z. (2000). Prolonged oral morphine therapy for severe angina pectoris. *Journal of Pain and Symptom Management*, 19(5), 393–397.

Murphy, G. S., Szokol, J. W., Marymont, J. H., Avram, M. J., & Vender, J. S. (2007). The effects of morphine and fentanyl on the inflammatory response to cardiopulmonary bypass in patients undergoing elective coronary artery bypass graft surgery. *Anesthesia & Analgesia*, 104(6), 1334–1342.

Nicholson, A. B., Watson, G. R., Derry, S., & Wiffen, P. J. (2017). Methadone for cancer pain. *The Cochrane Library.*, 2, CD003971.

Odom-Forren, J., Brady, J., Rayens, M. K., & Sloan, P. (2019). Perianesthesia nurses' knowledge and promotion of safe use, storage, and disposal of opioids. *Journal of PeriAnesthesia Nursing*, 34(6), 1156–1168.

Oosten, A. W., Abrantes, J. A., Jönsson, S., de Bruijn, P., Kuip, E. J., Falcão, A., ... Mathijssen, R. H. (2016). Treatment with subcutaneous and transdermal fentanyl: results from a population pharmacokinetic study in cancer patients. *European Journal of Clinical Pharmacology*, 72(4), 459–467.

Opioid Calculator. (2017, August 01). Retrieved from https://opioidcalculator.practicalpainmanagement.com/.

Orexo US, Inc. (2018). *Zubsolv*. Morristown, NJ: Package Insert.

Ostrop, N. J., Lamb, J., & Reid, G. (1998). Intravaginal morphine: an alternative route of administration. *Pharmacotherapy: The Journal of Human Pharmacology and Drug Therapy*, 18(4), 863–865.

Pacreu, S., Candil, J. F., Moltó, L., Carazo, J., & Galinski, S. F. (2012). The perioperative combination of methadone and ketamine reduces post-operative opioid usage compared with methadone alone. *Acta Anaesthesiologica Scandinavica*, 56(10), 1250–1256.

Paice, J. A., Von Roenn, J. H., Hudgins, J. C., Luong, L., Krejcie, T. C., & Avram, M. J. (2008). Morphine bioavailability from a topical gel formulation in volunteers. *Journal of Pain and Symptom Management*, 35(3), 314–320.

Pani, N., Dongare, P. A., & Mishra, R. K. (2015). Reversal agents in anaesthesia and critical care. *Indian Journal of Anaesthesia*, 59(10), 664.

Pasero, C., & McCaffery, M. (2011). Guidelines for selection of routes of opioid administration (Chapter 13). In C. Pasero, & M. McCaffery (Eds.), *Pain Assessment and Pharmacologic Management*. St. Louis, MO: Mosby.

Pastore, M. N., Kalia, Y. N., Horstmann, M., & Roberts, M. S. (2015). Transdermal patches: history, development and pharmacology. *British Journal of Pharmacology*, 172(9), 2179–2209.

Pergolizzi, J., Aloisi, A. M., Dahan, A., Filitz, J., Langford, R., Likar, R., ... Sacerdote, P. (2010). Current knowledge of buprenorphine and its unique pharmacological profile. *Pain Practice*, 10(5), 428–450.

Pergolizzi, J. V., Jr., Scholten, W., Smith, K. J., Leighton-Scott, J., Willis, J. C., & Henningfield, J. E. (2015). The unique role of transdermal buprenorphine in the global chronic pain epidemic. *Acta Anaesthesiologica Taiwanica*, 53(2), 71–76.

Pert, C. B., & Snyder, S. H. (1973). Opiate Receptor: Demonstration in Nervous Tissue. *Science*, 179(4077), 1011–1014. https://doi.org/10.1126/science.179.4077.1011.

Pham, T. C., Fudin, J., & Raffa, R. B. (2015). Is levorphanol a better option than methadone? *Pain Medicine*, 16(9), 1673–1679. https://doi.org/10.1111/pme.12795.

Pillarisetti, S., & Khanna, I. (2015). Buprenorphine – an attractive opioid with underutilized potential in treatment of chronic pain. *Journal of Pain Research*, 859. https://doi.org/10.2147/jpr.s85951.

Piper, B. J., Shah, D. T., Simoyan, O. M., McCall, K. L., & Nichols, S. D. (2018). Trends in Medical Use of Opioids in the US, 2006–2016. *American Journal of Preventive Medicine*, 54(5), 652–660.

Poelaert, J., Koopmans-Klein, G., Dioh, A., Louis, F., Gorissen, M., Logé, D., & van Megen, Y. J. (2015). Treatment with prolonged-release oxycodone/naloxone improves pain relief and opioid-induced constipation compared with prolonged-release oxycodone in patients with chronic severe pain and laxative-refractory constipation. *Clinical Therapeutics*, 37(4), 784–792.

Porela-Tiihonen, S., Kokki, M., & Kokki, H. (2017). Sufentanil sublingual formulation for the treatment of acute, moderate to severe postoperative pain in adult patients. *Expert Review of Neurotherapeutics*, 17(2), 101–111.

Porta-Sales, J., Garzón-Rodríguez, C., Villavicencio-Chávez, C., Llorens-Torromé, S., & González-Barboteo, J. (2016). Efficacy and safety of methadone as a second-line opioid for cancer pain in an outpatient clinic: a prospective open-label study. *The Oncologist*, 21(8), 981–987.

Posa, L., Accarie, A., Noble, F., & Marie, N. (2016). Methadone reverses analgesic tolerance induced by morphine pretreatment. *International Journal of Neuropsychopharmacology*, 19(7), pyv108.

Purdue Pharma. (2017). *Butrans*. Stamford, CT: Package Insert.

Raffa, R. B., Friderichs, E., Reimann, W., Shank, R. P., Codd, E. E., & Vaught, J. L. (1992). Opioid and nonopioid components independently contribute to the mechanism of action of tramadol, an 'atypical' opioid analgesic. *Journal of Pharmacology and Experimental Therapeutics*, 260(1), 275–285.

Rajan, J., & Scott-Warren, J. (2015). The clinical use of methadone in cancer and chronic pain medicine. *BJA Education*, 16(3), 102–106.

Raouf, M., Glogowski, A. J., Bettinger, J. J., & Fudin, J. (2017). Serotonin-norepinephrine reuptake inhibitors and the influence of binding affinity (Ki) on analgesia. *Journal of Clinical Pharmacy and Therapeutics*, 42(4), 513–517. https://doi.org/10.1111/jcpt.12534.

Rauck, R. L., Potts, J., Xiang, Q., Tzanis, E., & Finn, A. (2016). Efficacy and tolerability of buccal buprenorphine in opioid-naive patients with moderate to severe chronic low back pain. *Postgraduate Medicine*, 128(1), 1–11.

Raymo, L. L., Camejo, M., & Fudin, J. (2007). Eradicating analgesic use of meperidine in a hospital. *American Journal of Health-System Pharmacy*, 64(11), 1148–1152.

Reckitt Benckiser Pharmaceuticals. (2016). Prescription Drug Information: Buprenex. Retrieved June 30, 2019, from https://rxdruglabels.com/lib/rx/rx-meds/buprenex-2/.

Reckitt Benckiser Pharmaceuticals. (2018). *Suboxone*. Richmond, VA: Package Insert.

Reddy, A., Ng, A., Mallipeddi, T., & Bruera, E. (2018). Levorphanol for Treatment of Intractable Neuropathic Pain in Cancer Patients. *Journal of Palliative Medicine*, 21(3), 399–402.

Reddy, A., Yennurajalingam, S., Reddy, S., Wu, J., Liu, D., Dev, R., & Bruera, E. (2016). The opioid rotation ratio from transdermal fentanyl to "strong" opioids in patients with cancer pain. *Journal of Pain and Symptom Management*, 51(6), 1040–1045.

Reid, C. M., Martin, R. M., Sterne, J. A., Davies, A. N., & Hanks, G. W. (2006). Oxycodone for cancer-related pain: meta-analysis of randomized controlled trials. *Archives of Internal Medicine*, 166(8), 837–843.

Reid, M. C., Eccleston, C., & Pillemer, K. (2015). Management of chronic pain in older adults. *BMJ*, 350(7995), 1–10.

Reisfield, G. M., & Wilson, G. R. (2007). Rational use of sublingual opioids in palliative medicine. *Journal of Palliative Medicine*, 10(2), 465–475.

Rennick, A., Atkinson, T., Cimino, N. M., Strassels, S. A., McPherson, M. L., & Fudin, J. (2015). Variability in Opioid Equivalence Calculations. *Pain Medicine.*, 17(5), 892–898. https://doi.org/10.1111/pme.12920.

Ricard-Hibon, A., Belpomme, V., Chollet, C., Devaud, M. L., Adnet, F., Borron, S., ... Marty, J. (2008). Compliance with a morphine protocol and effect on pain relief in out-of-hospital patients. *The Journal of Emergency Medicine*, 34(3), 305–310.

Ripamonti, C., Groff, L., Brunelli, C., Polastri, D., Stavrakis, A., & Conno, F. D. (1998). Switching from morphine to oral methadone in treating cancer pain: What is the equianalgesic dose ratio? *Journal of Clinical Oncology*, 16(10), 3216–3221. https://doi.org/10.1200/jco.1998.16.10.3216.

Ripamonti, C. I., & Bosco, M. (2015). Alternative routes for systemic opioid delivery. In E. Bruera, I. Higginson, & C. F. von Gunten (Eds.), *Textbook of Palliative Medicine and Supportive Care* (2nd Ed., p. 431). Boca Raton, FL: CRC Press.

Rodriguez, R. F., Castillo, J. M., Castillo, M. P., Montoya, O., Daza, P., Rodríguez, M. F., ... Angel, A. M. (2008). Hydrocodone/acetaminophen and tramadol chlorhydrate combination tablets for the management of chronic cancer pain: a double-blind comparative trial. *The Clinical Journal of Pain*, 24(1), 1–4.

Rosenberg, J. M., Bilka, B. M., Wilson, S. M., & Spevak, C. (2017). Opioid therapy for chronic pain: Overview of the 2017 US Department of Veterans Affairs and US Department of Defense clinical practice guideline. *Pain Medicine*, 19(5), 928–941.

Rowbotham, M. C., Twilling, L., Davies, P. S., Reisner, L., Taylor, K., & Mohr, D. (2003). Oral opioid therapy for chronic peripheral and central neuropathic pain. *New England Journal of Medicine*, 348(13), 1223–1232.

Roxane Laboratories. (2015). *Subutex*. Columbus, OH: Package Insert.

Ruan, X., Mancuso, K. F., & Kaye, A. D. (2017). Revisiting Oxycodone Analgesia: A Review and Hypothesis. *Anesthesiology Clinics*, 35(2), e163–e174.

Sabatowski, R., Schwalen, S., Rettig, K., Herberg, K. W., Kasper, S. M., & Radbruch, L. (2003). Driving Ability Under Long-Term Treatment with Transdermal Fentanyl. *Journal of Pain and Symptom Management*, 25(1), 38–47. https://doi.org/10.1016/s0885-3924(02)00539-0.

Samolsky Dekel, B. G., Donati, G., Vasarri, A., Croci Chiocchini, A. L., Gori, A., Cavallari, G., ... Melotti, R. M. (2017). Dialyzability of oxycodone and its metabolites in chronic noncancer pain patients with end-stage renal disease. *Pain Practice*, 17(5), 604–615.

Santos, J., Alarcão, J., Fareleira, F., Vaz-Carneiro, A., & Costa, J. (2015). Tapentadol for chronic musculoskeletal pain in adults. *Cochrane Database Syst. Rev*, 5, CD009923.

Sawaddiruk, P. (2011). Tramadol hydrochloride/acetaminophen combination for the relief of acute pain. *Drugs of Today (Barcelona, Spain: 1998)*, 47(10), 763–772.

Schatman, M. E., Fudin, J., & Cleary, J. P. (2016). The MEDD myth: The impact of pseudoscience on pain research and prescribing-guideline development. *Journal of Pain Research*, 153. https://doi.org/10.2147/jpr.s107794.

Schmidt-Hansen, M., Bennett, M. I., Arnold, S., Bromham, N., & Hilgart, J. S. (2017). Oxycodone for cancer-related pain. *The Cochrane Library*, 8, CD003870.

Schug, S. A., & Ting, S. (2017). Fentanyl formulations in the management of pain: an update. *Drugs*, 77(7), 747–763.

Schumacher, M. B., Jongen, S., Knoche, A., Petzke, F., Vuurman, E. F., Vollrath, M., & Ramaekers, J. G. (2017). Effect of chronic opioid therapy on actual driving performance in non-cancer pain patients. *Psychopharmacology*, 234(6), 989–999.

Sekhri, N. K., & Cooney, M. F. (2017). Opioid Metabolism and Pharmacogenetics: Clinical Implications. *Journal of PeriAnesthesia Nursing*, 32(5), 497–505.

Shah, R., Baqai-Stern, A., & Gulati, A. (2015). Managing intrathecal drug delivery (ITDD) in cancer patients. *Current Pain and Headache Reports*, 19(6), 20.

Shah, S., & Diwan, S. (2010). Methadone: does stigma play a role as a barrier to treatment of chronic pain. *Pain Physician*, 13(3), 289–293.

Shaiova, L., Berger, A., Blinderman, C. D., Bruera, E., Davis, M. P., Derby, S., ... Perlov, E. (2008). Consensus guideline on parenteral methadone use in pain and palliative care. *Palliative & Supportive Care*, 6(2), 165–176.

Sheth, S., Holtsman, M., & Mahajan, G. (2018). Major Opioids in Pain Management. In H. T. Benzon, S. N. Raja, S. S. Liu, S. M. Fishman, & S. P. Cohen (Eds.), *Essentials of Pain Medicine* (4th Ed., pp. 373–384), Elsevier.

Shibutani, K., Inchiosa, M. A., Sawada, K., & Bairamian, M. (2004). Accuracy of Pharmacokinetic Models for Predicting Plasma Fentanyl Concentrations in Lean and Obese Surgical Patients Derivation of Dosing Weight ("Pharmacokinetic Mass"). *Anesthesiology: The Journal of the American Society of Anesthesiologists*, 101(3), 603–613.

Shibutani, K., Inchiosa, M. A., Jr., Sawada, K., & Bairamian, M. (2005). Pharmacokinetic mass of fentanyl for postoperative analgesia in lean and obese patients. *British Journal of Anaesthesia*, 95(3), 377–383.

Singla, A., & Sloan, P. (2013). Pharmacokinetic evaluation of hydrocodone/acetaminophen for pain management. *Journal of Opioid Management*, 9(1), 71–80.

Silverman, S., Raffa, R. B., Cataldo, M. J., Kwarcinski, M., & Ripa, S. R. (2017). Use of immediate-release opioids as supplemental analgesia during management of moderate-to-severe chronic pain with buprenorphine transdermal system. *Journal of Pain Research*, 10, 1255.

Simpson, R. W., & Wlodarczyk, J. H. (2016). Transdermal buprenorphine relieves neuropathic pain: a randomized, double-blind, parallel-group, placebo-controlled trial in diabetic peripheral neuropathic pain. *Diabetes Care*, 39(9), 1493–1500.

Skolnick, P. (2018). On the front lines of the opioid epidemic: rescue by naloxone. *European Journal of Pharmacology*, 835(n/a), 147–153.

Sloan, P. A., & Barkin, R. L. (2008). Oxymorphone and oxymorphone extended release: a pharmacotherapeutic review. *Journal of Opioid Management*, 4(3), 131–144.

Smith, H. S. (2009). Opioid Metabolism. *Mayo Clinic Proceedings*, 84(7), 613–624. https://doi.org/10.1016/s0025-6196(11)60750-7.

Smith, H. S., & Peppin, J. F. (2014). Toward a systematic approach to opioid rotation. *Journal of Pain Research*, 7, 589–608.

Smith, M. T., Wyse, B. D., Edwards, S. R., El-Tamimy, M., Gaetano, G., & Gavin, P. (2015). Topical application of a novel oxycodone gel formulation (tocopheryl phosphate mixture) in a rat model of peripheral inflammatory pain produces localized pain relief without significant systemic exposure. *Journal of Pharmaceutical Sciences*, 104(7), 2388–2396.

Solanki, S. L., Doctor, J. R., Kapila, S. J., Gehdoo, R. P., & Divatia, J. V. (2016). Acupressure versus dilution of fentanyl to reduce incidence of fentanyl-induced cough in female cancer patients: a prospective randomized controlled study. *Korean Journal of Anesthesiology*, 69(3), 234–238.

Soleimanpour, H., Safari, S., Nia, K. S., Sanaie, S., & Alavian, S. M. (2016). Opioid drugs in patients with liver disease: a systematic review. *Hepatitis Monthly*, 16(4), e32636. https://doi.org/10.5812/hepatmon.32636omogyi.

Somogyi, A. A., Barratt, D. T., & Coller, J. K. (2007). Pharmacogenetics of Opioids. *Clinical Pharmacology & Therapeutics*, 81(3), 429–444. https://doi.org/10.1038/sj.clpt.6100095.

Stanley, T. H. (2014). The fentanyl story. *The Journal of Pain*, 15(12), 1215–1226.

Sullivan, M. D., Turner, J. A., DiLodovico, C., D'Appollonio, A., Stephens, K., & Chan, Y. F. (2017). Prescription opioid taper support for outpatients with chronic pain: a randomized controlled trial. *The Journal of Pain*, 18(3), 308–318.

Sultan, S. S. (2014). Patient-controlled sedation with propofol/remifentanil versus propofol/alfentanil for patients undergoing outpatient colonoscopy, a randomized, controlled double-blind study. *Saudi Journal of Anaesthesia*, 8(Suppl 1), S36.

Sunilkumar, M. M., & Lockman, K. (2018). Practical pharmacology of methadone: A long-acting opioid. *Indian Journal of Palliative Care*, 24(Suppl 1), S10.

Sunshine, A., Olson, N. Z., Colon, A., Rivera, J., Kaiko, R. F., Fitzmartin, R. D., ... Goldenheim, P. D. (1996). Analgesic efficacy of controlled-release oxycodone in postoperative pain. *The Journal of Clinical Pharmacology*, 36(7), 595–603.

Suzuki, J., & El-Haddad, S. (2017). A review: fentanyl and non-pharmaceutical fentanyls. *Drug & Alcohol Dependence*, 171, 107–116.

Sverrisdóttir, E., Lund, T. M., Olesen, A. E., Drewes, A. M., Christrup, L. L., & Kreilgaard, M. (2015). A review of morphine and morphine-6-glucuronide's pharmacokinetic–pharmacodynamic relationships in experimental and clinical pain. *European Journal of Pharmaceutical Sciences*, 74(n/a), 45–62.

Swarm, R.A., Paice, J. A., Anghelescu, D. L., Are, M., Bruce, J. Y., Buga, S, ...Gurski, L. A. (2018). NCCN Clinical Practice Guidelines in Oncology (NCCN Guidelines®). Retrieved August, 2018, from https://www.nccn.org/professionals/physician_gls/pdf/pain.pdf.

Thompson, J. P., & Rowbotham, D. J. (1996). Remifentanil-an opioid for the 21st century. *British Journal of Anaesthesia*, 76(3), 341–343.

Ting, S., & Schug, S. (2016). The pharmacogenomics of pain management: Prospects for personalized medicine. *Journal of Pain Research*, 9, 49–56. https://doi.org/10.2147/JPR.S55595.

TIRF REMS Access. (n.d.). Retrieved August 01, 2017, from http://www.TIRFREMSaccess.com/.

Tsutaoka, B. T., Ho, R. Y., Fung, S. M., & Kearney, T. E. (2015). Comparative toxicity of tapentadol and tramadol utilizing data reported to the national poison data system. *Annals of Pharmacotherapy*, 49(12), 1311–1316.

U.S. Department of Health and Human Services, (2018). Prevent Opioid Abuse and Addiction. Retrieved June 3, 2020 from https://www.hhs.gov/opioids/prevention/index.html.

U.S. Department of Health and Human Services, (2019). Safe Opioid Prescribing. Retrieved June 3, 2020 from https://www.hhs.gov/opioids/prevention/safe-opioid-prescribing/index.html.

U.S. Food and Drug Administration. (2014a). Information Page: FDA approves extended-release, single-entity hydrocodone product with abuse-deterrent properties. Retrieved June 21, 2019, from https://www.fda.gov/Drugs/DrugSafety/PostmarketDrugSafetyInformationforPatientsandProviders/ucm420978.htm.

U.S. Food and Drug Administration. (2013). ER/LA Opioid Analgesic Class Labeling Changes and Postmarket Requirements Letter to ER/LA opioid application holders. (n.d.). Retrieved August 01, 2017 from https://www.fda.gov/downloads/Drugs/DrugSafety/InformationbyDrugClass/UCM367697.pdf.

U.S. Food and Drug Administration. (2014b). Information by drug class: *All manufacturers of prescription combination drug products with more than 325 mg of acetaminophen have discontinued marketing* https://www.fda.gov/Drugs/DrugSafety/InformationbyDrugClass/ucm390509.htm.

U.S. Food and Drug Administration. (2015). Extended-release (ER) and long-acting (LA) opioid analgesics Risk Evaluation and Mitigation Strategy (REMS). Retrieved August 22, 2018, from http://www.fda.gov/downloads/drugs/drugsafety/postmarket-drugsafetyinformationforpatientsandproviders/ucm311290.pdf.

U.S. Food and Drug Administration. (2017). FDA requests removal of Opana ER for risks related to abuse. Rockville, MD; 2017 Jun 8. Retrieved June 29, 2019 , from https://www.fda.gov/newsevents/newsroom/pressannouncements/ucm562401.htm.

U.S. Food and Drug Administration. (2018). Drug Safety Communication: FDA restricts use of prescription codeine pain and cough medicines and tramadol pain medicines in children; recommends against use in breastfeeding women. Retrieved June 29, 2019, from https://www.fda.gov/Drugs/DrugSafety/ucm549679.htm.

Vadivelu, N., Chang, D., Helander, E. M., Bordelon, G. J., Kai, A., Kaye, A. D., ... Julka, I. (2017). Ketorolac, oxymorphone, tapentadol, and tramadol: a comprehensive review. *Anesthesiology Clinics, 35*(2), e1–e20.

Vadivelu, N., Kai, A. M., Kodumudi, V., Sramcik, J., & Kaye, A. D. (2018). The opioid crisis: a comprehensive overview. *Current Pain and Headache Reports, 22*(3), 16.

Vadivelu, N., Maria, M., Jolly, S., Rosenbloom, J., Prasad, A., & Kaye, A. D. (2013). Clinical applications of oxymorphone. *Journal of Opioid Management, 9*(6), 439–452.

Valeberg, B. T., Miaskowski, C., Paul, S. M., & Rustøen, T. (2016). Comparison of oncology patients' and their family caregivers' attitudes and concerns toward pain and pain management. *Cancer Nursing, 39*(4), 328–334.

Vallejo, R., Barkin, R. L., & Wang, V. C. (2011). Pharmacology of opioids in the treatment of chronic pain syndromes. *Pain Physician, 14*(4), 343–360.

van de Donk, T., Ward, S., Langford, R., & Dahan, A. (2018). Pharmacokinetics and pharmacodynamics of sublingual sufentanil for postoperative pain management. *Anaesthesia, 73*(2), 231–237.

Van De Velde, M., & Carvalho, B. (2016). Remifentanil for labor analgesia: an evidence-based narrative review. *International Journal of Obstetric Anesthesia, 25*, 66–74.

Vazzana, M., Andreani, T., Fangueiro, J., Faggio, C., Silva, C., Santini, A., ... Souto, E. B. (2015). Tramadol hydrochloride: pharmacokinetics, pharmacodynamics, adverse side effects, co-administration of drugs and new drug delivery systems. *Biomedicine & Pharmacotherapy, 70*, 234–238.

Vlok, R., An, G. H., Binks, M., Melhuish, T., & White, L. (2018). Sublingual buprenorphine versus intravenous or intramuscular morphine in acute pain: A systematic review and meta-analysis of randomized control trials. *The American Journal of Emergency Medicine, 37*(3), 381–386.

Volkow, N. D., & Collins, F. S. (2017). The role of science in addressing the opioid crisis. *New England Journal of Medicine, 377*(4), 391–394.

Waldhoer, M., Bartlett, S. E., & Whistler, J. L. (2004). Opioid Receptors. *Annual Review of Biochemistry, 73*, 953–990. https://doi.org/10.1146/annurev.biochem.73.011303.073940.

Wang, D. D., Ma, T. T., Zhu, H. D., & Peng, C. B. (2018). Transdermal fentanyl for cancer pain: Trial sequential analysis of 3406 patients from 35 randomized controlled trials. *Journal of Cancer Research and Therapeutics, 14*(8), 14.

Wang, Y., Yang, H., Shen, C., & Luo, J. (2017). Morphine and pregabalin in the treatment of neuropathic pain. *Experimental and Therapeutic Medicine, 13*(4), 1393–1397.

Wang, Y., Tang, H., Guo, Q., Liu, J., Liu, X., Luo, J., & Yang, W. (2015). Effects of intravenous patient-controlled sufentanil analgesia and music therapy on pain and hemodynamics after surgery for lung cancer: a randomized parallel study. *The Journal of Alternative and Complementary Medicine, 21*(11), 667–672.

Weaver, J. M. (2014). Multiple risks for patients using the transdermal fentanyl patch. *Anesthesia Progress, 61*(1), 1.

Webster, L. R., & Fine, P. G. (2012a). Overdose Deaths Demand a New Paradigm for Opioid Rotation: Table 1. *Pain Medicine, 13*(4), 571–574. https://doi.org/10.1111/j.1526-4637.2012.01356.x.

Webster, L. R., & Fine, P. G. (2012b). Review and critique of opioid rotation practices and associated risks of toxicity. *Pain Medicine, 13*(4), 562–570.

Webster, L. R., Camilleri, M., & Finn, A. (2016). Opioid-induced constipation: rationale for the role of norbuprenorphine in buprenorphine-treated individuals. *Substance Abuse and Rehabilitation, 7*, 81–86.

Webster, L. R., Gruener, D., Kirby, T., Xiang, Q., Tzanis, E., & Finn, A. (2016). Evaluation of the tolerability of switching patients on chronic full μ-opioid agonist therapy to buccal buprenorphine. *Pain Medicine, 17*(5), 899–907.

Webster, L. R., Pantaleon, C., Iverson, M., Smith, M. D., Kinzler, E. R., & Aigner, S. (2018). Intranasal Pharmacokinetics of Morphine ARER, a Novel Abuse-Deterrent Formulation: Results from a Randomized, Double-Blind, Four-Way Crossover Study in Nondependent, Opioid-Experienced Subjects. *Pain Research and Management, 18*, 7276021.

Wellington, C. (2009). Patient variables influencing acute pain management. Chapter 3. In R. S. Sinatra, O. deLeon-Casasola, B. Ginsberg, & E. Viscusi (Eds.), *Acute Pain Management* (p. 38). Cambridge University Press.

Weschules, D. J., & Bain, K. T. (2008). A systematic review of opioid conversion ratios used with methadone for the treatment of pain. *Pain Medicine, 9*(5), 595–612.

White, L. D., Hodge, A., Vlok, R., Hurtado, G., Eastern, K., & Melhuish, T. M. (2017). The efficacy and adverse effects of buprenorphine in acute pain management: a systematic review and meta-analysis of randomised controlled trials. *British Journal of Anaesthesia, 120*(4), 668–678.

Whiteley, W. J., & Hardman, J. G. (2017). Pharmacokinetic analysis. *Anaesthesia & Intensive Care Medicine, 18*(9). 455–457.

Wiffen, P. J., Derry, S., & Moore, R. A. (2017). Tramadol with or without paracetamol (acetaminophen) for cancer pain. *Cochrane Database Systematic Reviews, 5*, CD012508.

Wiffen, P. J., Wee, B., & Moore, R. J. (2016). Oral morphine for cancer pain. *Cochrane Database Syst Rev. 2016 Apr 22*, (4). https://doi.org/10.1002/14651858.CD003868.pub4.

Wiffen, P. J., Derry, S., Moore, R. A., Stannard, C., Aldington, D., Cole, P., & Knaggs, R. (2015). Buprenorphine for neuropathic pain in adults. *Cochrane Database of Systematic Reviews, 9*, CD011603.

Wirz, S., Wartenberg, H. C., & Nadstawek, J. (2007). Less nausea, emesis, and constipation comparing hydromorphone and morphine? A prospective open-labeled investigation on cancer pain. *Supportive Care in Cancer, 16*(9), 999–1009.

Wright, F., & Fessele, K. (2017). Primer in genetics and genomics, article 5—Further defining the concepts of genotype and phenotype and exploring genotype–phenotype associations. *Biological Research for Nursing, 19*(5), 576–585.

Xiao, J. P., Li, A. L., Feng, B. M., Ye, Y., & Wang, G. J. (2017). Efficacy and safety of tapentadol immediate release assessment in treatment of moderate to severe pain: a systematic review and meta-analysis. *Pain Medicine, 18*(1), 14–24.

Yang, Y., Wu, J., Li, H., Ye, S., Xu, X., Cheng, L., … Feng, Z. (2018). Prospective investigation of intravenous patient-controlled analgesia with hydromorphone or sufentanil: impact on mood, opioid adverse effects, and recovery. *BMC Anesthesiology, 18*(1), 37.

Yarlas, A., Miller, K., Wen, W., Lynch, S. Y., Munera, C., Pergolizzi, J. V., Jr., … Ripa, S. R. (2015). Buprenorphine transdermal system compared with placebo reduces interference in functioning for chronic low back pain. *Postgraduate Medicine, 127*(1), 38–45.

Yarlas, A., Miller, K., Wen, W., Lynch, S. Y., Ripa, S. R., Pergolizzi, J. V., & Raffa, R. B. (2016). Buprenorphine Transdermal System Improves Sleep Quality and Reduces Sleep Disturbance in Patients with Moderate-to-Severe Chronic Low Back Pain: Results from Two Randomized Controlled Trials. *Pain Practice, 16*(3), 345–358.

Youssef, N., Orlov, D., Alie, T., Chong, M., Cheng, J., Thabane, L., & Paul, J. (2014). What epidural opioid results in the best analgesia outcomes and fewest side effects after surgery?: a meta-analysis of randomized controlled trials. *Anesthesia & Analgesia, 119*(4), 965–977.

Zajączkowska, R., Przewłocka, B., Kocot-Kępska, M., Mika, J., Leppert, W., & Wordliczek, J. (2018). Tapentadol–a representative of a new class of MOR-NRI analgesics. *Pharmacological Reports., 70*(4), 812–820.

Zeppetella, G., Porzio, G., & Aielli, F. (2007). Opioids applied topically to painful cutaneous malignant ulcers in a palliative care setting. *Journal of Opioid Management, 3*(3), 161–166.

Zhu, Y., Wang, Y., Du, B., & Xi, X. (2017). Could remifentanil reduce duration of mechanical ventilation in comparison with other opioids for mechanically ventilated patients? A systematic review and meta-analysis. *Critical Care, 21*(1), 206.

Zorn, K. E., & Fudin, J. (2011). Treatment of Neuropathic Pain: The Role of Unique Opioid Agents. *Practical Pain Management, 11*(4), 26–33.

Chapter 12 Common Unintended Effects of Opioids

Ann Quinlan-Colwell, Maureen F. Cooney

CHAPTER OUTLINE

Constipation, pg. 306

    Assessment of Opioid-Induced Constipation, pg. 307

    Prevention and Management of Opioid-Induced Constipation, pg. 307

    Pharmacologic Management, pg. 307

    Nonpharmacologic Management, pg. 310

Xerostomia (Dry Mouth), pg. 311

    Assessment, pg. 311

    Prevention and Management, pg. 311

Opioid-Induced Nausea and Vomiting, pg. 312

    Assessment, pg. 312

    Prevention and Management, pg. 312

Pruritus, pg. 314

    Assessment, pg. 315

    Prevention and Management of Opioid-Induced Pruritus, pg. 316

Urinary Retention, pg. 319

    Assessment for Urinary Retention, pg. 320

    Prevention and Management of Opioid-Related Urinary Retention, pg. 320

Hypogonadism, pg. 321

    Assessment, pg. 322

    Prevention and Management of Opioid-Induced Hypogonadism, pg. 322

Sedation, pg. 323

    Assessment, pg. 324

    Prevention and Management, pg. 324

Myoclonus, pg. 325

    Assessment, pg. 325

    Prevention and Management, pg. 326

Opioid-Induced Hyperalgesia, pg. 326

    Prevention, pg. 327

Physical Dependence on Opioids, pg. 327

    Assessment, pg. 327

    Prevention and Management, pg. 328

Opioid Tolerance, pg. 328

Immune Suppressing Effect of Opioids, pg. 328

Key Points, pg. 329

Case Scenario, pg. 329

References, pg. 329

LIKE all medications, opioids have effects that are not intended. Pharmacokinetics (how medications move through the body), pharmacodynamics (the effect of medications on the body and mechanism of action), and an individual's genetic makeup are factors that may contribute to the development of unintended opioid effects of the medications (Oosten, Oldenmenger, Mathijssen, & van der Rijt, 2015). Risks for the development of unintended effects are multifactorial. Medication *and botanical related* factors, including dose, frequency, drug-drug interactions, and timing of administration, can lead to undesired effects.

Patient-related factors such as age, gender, genetic factors, and physical condition may contribute to the development of unintended effects. For example, with some medications, gender may contribute to unanticipated effects. When receiving similar doses of a medication, women, *compared to men,* may have larger volumes of distribution of lipophilic medications because they typically have greater percentages of body fat despite having lower total body weight. During menstrual cycles, there can be an increased risk of side effects related to changes in body fluid and renal filtration (Carter et al., 2014a). Some diseases may increase the risk for development of unintended effects, particularly if the diseases are not recognized. Patients with undiagnosed hypertension or diabetes, for example, may have reduced kidney function, which may lead to greater accumulation of medications and their metabolites. Social factors such as smoking and alcohol abuse can alter the metabolism of medications and cause unintended effects.

The unplanned effects of opioids range from nuisance (mild pruritis) to life threatening (respiratory depression and arrest) with wide variability of severity, intensity, and tolerability within the range. Often comfort and quality of life are compromised by these effects (He, Jiang, & Li, 2016; Oosten et al., 2015). As many as 80% of patients who receive opioids for pain control experience at least one undesirable effect, with drowsiness, constipation, and nausea most frequently reported (Gan et al., 2014a). See Table 12.1 for the major common unintended effects of opioids. These effects are often very distressing to patients and may interfere with pain management. In a two-part study in six Western European countries, the participants reported greater concern about enduring the adverse effects of opioids than about achieving relief from pain (Chancellor, Martin, Liedgens, Baker, & Müller-Schwefe, 2012). In that study, the participants concerns were inconsistent with their physicians' goals for treatment

Table 12.1 | Major Adverse Effects of Opioids

Classification	Drugs	Adverse Effects and Relative Risks
Phenanthrenes	Morphine	*Dermatologic:* Pruritus ($\leq$80%) *Gastrointestinal:* Constipation ($\geq$9%), nausea (oral, 7% and >10%; epidural or intrathecal, 15%–70%), vomiting (>10%) *Neurologic:* Dizziness (6%), headache (>10%), light-headedness, somnolence ($\geq$9%) *Renal:* Urinary retention (oral, <5%; epidural/intrathecal, 15%–70%)
	Codeine	*Cardiovascular:* Hypotension (1%–10%), tachycardia or bradycardia (1%–10%) *Dermatologic* (1%–10%): Pruritus (1%–10%), rash (1%–10%), urticaria (1%–10%) *Gastrointestinal:* Constipation (>10%), nausea (1%–10%), vomiting (1%–10%), anorexia (1%–10%), xerostomia (1%–10%) *Neurologic:* Drowsiness (>10%), dizziness (1%–10%), light-headedness (1%–10%), sedated, somnolence *Renal:* Urinary retention *Respiratory:* Dyspnea (1%–10%) *Ophthalmic:* Blurred vision (1%–10%), visual disturbances
	HYDROmorphone	*Dermatologic:* Flushing (extended-release, <2%), pruritus (extended-release, 1%–8%), sweating *Gastrointestinal:* Constipation (extended-release, 7%–31%), nausea (extended-release, 9%–28%), vomiting (extended-release, 6%–14%) *Neurologic:* Asthenia (extended-release, 1%–11%), dizziness (extended-release, 2%–11%), headache (extended-release, 5%–12%), light-headedness, sedated (extended-release, <2%), somnolence (extended-release, 1%–15%)
	OxyCODONE	*Dermatologic:* Pruritus (controlled-release, 13%; immediate-release, $\geq$3%), sweating (controlled-release, 5%; immediate-release, <3%) *Gastrointestinal:* Abdominal pain ($\leq$5%), constipation (controlled-release, 23%; immediate-release, $\geq$3%), nausea (controlled-release, 23%; immediate-release, $\geq$3%), vomiting (controlled-release, 12%; immediate-release, $\geq$3%), xerostomia (controlled-release, 6%; immediate-release, <3%) *Neurologic:* Asthenia (controlled-release, 6%; immediate-release, $\geq$3%), dizziness (controlled-release, 13%; immediate-release, $\geq$3%), headache (controlled-release, 7%; immediate-release, $\geq$3%), somnolence (controlled-release, 23%; immediate-release, $\geq$3%)
	Levorphanol	*Cardiovascular:* Hypotension (1%–10%) *Dermatologic:* Pruritus (>10%) *Gastrointestinal:* Constipation (1%–10%), nausea (>10%), vomiting (1%–10%) *Psychiatric:* Altered mental status (1%–10%), disturbance in mood (1%–10%)
	HYDROcodone[a]	*Dermatologic:* Pruritus, rash *Gastrointestinal:* Constipation, bowel obstruction, nausea, vomiting, pharyngeal dryness, xerostomia *Neurologic:* Confusion, dizziness, impaired cognition, lethargy, sedated, somnolence *Psychiatric:* Anxiety, dysphoric mood, euphoria, fear, mood swings *Renal:* Urinary retention, spasm of bladder, urethral spasm *Respiratory:* Depression, tight chest

Table 12.1 | Major Adverse Effects of Opioids—cont'd

Classification	Drugs	Adverse Effects and Relative Risks
	OxyMORphone	*Cardiovascular:* Hypotension (<10%) *Dermatologic:* Pruritus (≤15.2%), sweating (1% to <10%) *Gastrointestinal:* Abdominal pain (1% to <10%), constipation (4.1%–27.6%), nausea (2.9%–33.1%), vomiting (≤15.6%), xerostomia (1%–<10%) *Neurologic:* Confusion (≤10%), dizziness (≤17.8%), headache (2.9%–12.2%), somnolence (1.9%–19.1%) *Respiratory:* Dyspnea (1% to <10%), hypoxia (1%– <10%) *Other:* Fever (1%–14.2%)
	Buprenorphine	*Dermatologic:* Application-site erythema (5%–10%), application-site irritation (3%–5%), application-site rash (6%–9%), pruritus, application site (4%–15%) *Gastrointestinal:* Constipation (14%), nausea (23%), vomiting (11%), xerostomia (≥5%) *Neurologic:* Dizziness (16%), headache (16%), somnolence (14%)—does have ceiling dose for analgesia. Not recommended above 30 mg total daily dose. Buprenorphine is associated with less QTc prolongation than methadone, but this can occur at higher doses
	Butorphanol	*Gastrointestinal:* Nausea and vomiting (13%) *Neurologic:* Dizziness (19%–54%), insomnia (11%), sedated (30%–40%), somnolence (43%–88%) *Respiratory:* Nasal congestion (13%), long-term use of intranasal product (13%)
Phenylpiperidines	FentaNYL	*Dermatologic:* Application-site reaction (adults, ≥1%; pediatrics, 3%–10%), diaphoresis (adults: transdermal ≥10%, sublingual ≥1%; pediatrics: transdermal ≥1%), pruritus (transdermal, 3%–10%; sublingual, ≥1%) *Gastrointestinal:* Abdominal pain (transdermal, 3%–10%; sublingual, ≥1%), constipation (adults, ≥10%; pediatrics, 3%–10%), diarrhea (adults: transdermal 3%–10%, sublingual ≥1%; pediatrics: transdermal ≥1%), indigestion (transdermal, 3%–10%; sublingual, ≥1%), loss of appetite (transdermal, 3%–10%; sublingual, ≥1%), nausea (≥10%), vomiting (≥10%), xerostomia (adults: transdermal ≥10%, sublingual ≥1%; pediatrics: transdermal ≥1%) *Neurologic:* Asthenia (adults, ≥9.7%; pediatrics, 3%–10%), confusion (adults: transdermal ≥10%, sublingual ≥1%; pediatrics: transdermal ≥1%), dizziness (adults, 3%–10%; pediatrics, ≥1%), feeling nervous (3%–10%), headache (transdermal, 3%–10%; sublingual, ≥1%), insomnia (adults, ≥1%; pediatrics, 3%–10%), somnolence (adults, ≥9.5%; pediatrics, 3%–10%) *Psychiatric:* Anxiety (adults, 3%–10%; pediatrics, ≥1%), depression (adults: transdermal 3%–10%, sublingual ≥1%; pediatrics: transdermal ≥1%), euphoria (3%–10%), hallucinations (adults: transdermal 3%–10%, sublingual ≥1%; pediatrics: transdermal ≥1%) *Renal:* Urinary retention (adults: transdermal 3%–10%, sublingual <1%; pediatrics: transdermal ≥1%) *Respiratory:* Dyspnea (adults: transdermal 3%–10%, sublingual 10.4%; pediatrics: transdermal ≥1%), upper respiratory infection (3%–10%) *Other:* Fatigue (transdermal, 3%–10%; sublingual, ≥1%), influenza-like symptoms (3%–10%)
	Alfentanil	*Cardiovascular:* Bradyarrhythmia (14%), hypertension (18%), hypotension (10%), tachycardia (12%) *Gastrointestinal:* Nausea (28%), vomiting (18%)
	SUFentanil	*Cardiovascular:* Bradyarrhythmia (3%–9%), hypotension (3%–9%) *Dermatologic:* Pruritus (25%) *Gastrointestinal:* Nausea (3%–9%), vomiting (3%–9%) *Musculoskeletal:* Muscle rigidity, chest wall (3%–9%) *Neurologic:* Somnolence (3%–9%)
	Meperidine[b]	*Dermatologic:* Sweating, pruritus, rash, urticaria *Gastrointestinal:* Abdominal cramps, anorexia, biliary spasm, constipation, nausea, paralytic ileus, sphincter of Oddi spasm, vomiting, xerostomia *Neurologic:* Agitation, confusion, delirium, disorientation, dizziness, light-headedness, sedation *Neuromuscular and skeletal:* Muscle twitching, myoclonus, tremor, weakness *Ocular:* Visual disturbances

Continued

Table 12.1 | Major Adverse Effects of Opioids—cont'd

Classification	Drugs	Adverse Effects and Relative Risks
	Methadone[a]	*Cardiovascular:* Cardiac dysrhythmia, hypotension *Endocrine metabolic:* Diaphoresis *Gastrointestinal:* Constipation, nausea, vomiting *Neurologic:* Asthenia, dizziness, light-headedness, sedated
Other	Tapentadol	*Gastrointestinal:* Constipation (8%–17%), nausea (21%–30%), vomiting (8%–18%) *Neurologic:* Dizziness (17%–24%), headache (extended-release tablets, 10%–15%), somnolence (12%–15%); avoid combining with SNRI or SSRI
	TraMADol	*Dermatologic:* Flushing (8%–16%), pruritus (3%–11.9%) *Gastrointestinal:* Constipation (9%–46%), nausea (15%–40%), vomiting (5%–17%), dyspepsia (1%–13%) *Neurologic:* Dizziness (7%–28.2%), headache (3%–15.8%), insomnia (1%–10.9%), somnolence (4%–20.3%) *Neuromuscular and skeletal:* Weakness (4%–12%); avoid combining with SNRI or SSRI

SNRI, Serotonin-norepinephrine reuptake inhibitor; *SSRI,* selective serotonin reuptake inhibitor.
[a] Frequency of adverse effects not defined.
[b] Meperidine is not recommended for use as an analgesic medication.
From Carter, G. T., Duong, V., Ho, S., Ngo, K. C., Greer, C. L., & Weeks, D. yL. (2014). Side effects of commonly prescribed analgesic medications. *Physical Medicine and Rehabilitation Clinics, 25*(2), 457–470.

of pain. Interestingly, those concerns for adverse effects are consistent with the work done in the United States by Gan, Habib, Miller, White, & Apfelbaum (2014a).

The purpose of this chapter is to provide a review of common unintended effects of opioids and identify strategies to prevent, minimize, and, when necessary, treat them. Through the use of nonopioid medications, interventional techniques and nonpharmacologic therapies, multimodal analgesia (MMA) provides a basis for opioids to be used in lower doses that result in fewer side effects (Gan et al., 2014a; Youssef, et al, 2014).

Constipation

Constipation resulting from opioids is very common, but unlike other opioid-related side effects, tolerance to it does not commonly develop (Kumar, Barker, & Emmanuel, 2014; Mann & Chai, 2014). Opioid-induced constipation (OIC) is also different from functional constipation, which is constipation not related to the use of opioids. Functional constipation is characterized by difficulty passing stool; stool that may be hard or lumpy; inability to completely pass stool; fewer than three bowel movements per week; and/or needing to use aids to facilitate passing stool (Kumar et al., 2014; Willens, 2015).

OIC is part of the broader category of opioid-induced bowel dysfunction and is the most frequently reported gastrointestinal (GI) side effect of opioids, with prevalence reports ranging from 41% to greater than 90% (Camilleri et al., 2014; Doran, Lembo, & Cremonini, 2014). OIC is a bowel disorder that results from the activity of opioids in the GI tract and central nervous system (CNS) (Lacy

et al., 2016). OIC is defined as a change (either new or worsening symptoms) from baseline bowel habits and defecation patterns occurring after the start of opioid therapy. It is characterized by any or all of the following: reduction in the frequency of bowel movements (e.g., fewer than three bowel movements per week), increase in straining to pass stool, sense of incomplete evacuation after bowel movement, subjective perception of distress related to defecation, and harder stool consistency (Camilleri, Lembo, & Katzka, 2017; Lacy et al., 2016). See Box 12.1 for characteristics of OIC.

When exogenous opioids bind to mu receptors in the GI tract, several things occur. Peristalsis is repressed, and longitudinal muscles in both the small intestines and colon relax as a result of diminished release of acetylcholine. Movement through the small bowel slows. The exogenous opioids cause a decrease in intestinal secretions, which in turn results in reabsorption of fluids and electrolytes, resulting in dryer, harder stools that are more difficult to move. In addition, they cause increased tone of the anal sphincter causing a decrease in the sensation to trigger defecation (Levine & Shega, 2013). Because the underlying pathophysiologic effect (Box 12.2) on the mu receptors in the GI tract is so different, OIC often is not able to be managed with treatments commonly used for functional constipation (Camilleri et al., 2014).

OIC negatively affects quality of life, and patients may limit the use of opioids to relieve pain rather than experience the constipation (Kumar et al., 2014). However, the researchers of one study (n = 500) evaluated people from four countries (United States, Germany, Canada, United Kingdom) who were experiencing OIC while being treated with opioids for

Box 12.1	Diagnostic Criteria for Opioid-Induced Constipation

1. New, or worsening, symptoms of constipation when initiating, changing, or increasing opioid therapy that must include two or more of the following:
   a. Straining during more than one-fourth (25%) of defecations
   b. Lumpy or hard stools (Bristol Stool Form Scale 12) more than one-fourth (25%) of defecations
   c. Sensation of incomplete evacuation more than one-fourth (25%) of defecations
   d. Sensation of anorectal obstruction/blockage more than one-fourth (25%) of defecations
   e. Manual maneuvers to facilitate more than one-fourth (25%) of defecations (e.g., digital evacuation, support of the pelvic floor)
   f. Fewer than three spontaneous bowel movements per week
2. Loose stools are rarely present without the use of laxatives.

From Lacy, B. E., Mearin, F., Chang, L., Chey, W. D., Lembo, A. J., Simren, M., & Spiller, R. (2016). Bowel disorders. *Gastroenterology*, *150*(6), 1393–1407.

Box 12.2	Effects of Mu Opioid Receptors in the Gastrointestinal Tract

- Nonperistaltic esophageal contractions
- Reduced gastric motility and emptying
- Increase in tone of pyloric sphincter
- Reduced secretions (gastrointestinal, biliary, and pancreatic)
- Restraint of intestinal propulsion
- Enhanced water absorption from bowel
- Increased tone of anal sphincter
- Constriction of sphincter of Oddi
- Intensification of amplitude of nonpropulsive segmental contractions

From Camilleri, M., Drossman, D. A., Becker, G., Webster, L. R., Davies, A. N., & Mawe, G. M. (2014). Emerging treatments in neurogastroenterology: A multidisciplinary working group consensus statement on opioid-induced constipation. *Neurogastroenterology & Motility, 26*(10), 1386–1395.

noncancer pain (Coyne et al., 2014). In that study, the majority of respondents reported continuing to use opioids despite OIC interfering with work and quality of life while experiencing only slight pain relief. In addition to those issues, OIC is associated with hemorrhoid formation, accompanying pain, and serious consequences, including bowel obstruction with potential rupture and even death (Kumar et al., 2014). The goal of treatment is for the patient to ease defecation, which frequently means easily passing stool every day or every other day without straining (Levine & Shega, 2013).

Assessment of Opioid-Induced Constipation

Assessment of bowel function should be standard practice for patients receiving opioids, but it is not routinely done. Barriers to assessment for OIC include lack of knowledge about OIC by clinicians, embarrassment by patients, lack of assessment skill by clinicians, or no available assessment tool (Camilleri et al., 2014). The Bowel Function Index (Fig. 12.1) is an easy-to-use three-item questionnaire designed specifically to evaluate OIC. It is a useful tool to evaluate constipation and the effect on the quality of life of patients with and without cancer and using opioids to manage chronic pain (Abramowitz et al., 2013; Rentz, Yu, Müller-Lissner, & Leyendecker, 2009; Willens, 2015).

Prevention and Management of Opioid-Induced Constipation

Prevention of OIC is the optimal approach, but it is not without challenges. Selection of opioids reported to be less constipating is a prevention option, but that decision must be balanced with the effectiveness of analgesia, other medications prescribed, and comorbidities. In one report, OIC was reported to be significantly less likely to develop in patients receiving tapentadol compared to immediate-release oxyCODONE (Kwong et al., 2013). It is important to know that even when opioid medications may be considered less likely to cause OIC, they may still be constipating because they are involved in slower gastric emptying (Camilleri et al., 2017). More commonly, preventive efforts involve the prescription of laxatives along with prescription of opioids (Levine & Shega, 2013). From one study with patients living with cancer (n = 348) the researchers reported daily dosing of polyethylene glycol (13.81 g) and sodium picosulphate (10 mg) was more effective than lactulose and the participants had low incidence of OIC (Wirz, Nadstawek, Elsen, Junker, & Wartenberg, 2012). Because a multimodal approach for pain management facilitates using less of any one medication, including opioids, a multimodal approach is an important approach in preventing or minimizing OIC.

Pharmacologic Management

Pharmaceutical management options are extensive. There are several options for laxatives to prevent and alleviate OIC (Table 12.2). The actions of these agents are all different.

Bowel Function Index (BFI)
Please complete all items in this assessment.
1. Ease of defecation (NAS) during the last 7 days according to patient assessment: 0 = easy/no difficulty 100 = severe difficulty
Ask the subject: *"During the last 7 days, how would you rate your ease of defecation on a scale from 0 to 100, where 0 = easy or no difficulty and 100 = severe difficulty?"* ***If the subject requires clarification, ask:*** *"During the last 7 days, how easy or difficult was it to have a bowel movement on a scale from 0 to 100, where 0 = easy or no difficulty and 100 = severe difficulty?"*
2. Feeling of incomplete bowel evacuation (NAS) during the last 7 days according to patient assessment: 0 = not at all 100 = very strong
Ask the subject: *"During the last 7 days, how would you rate any feeling of incomplete bowel evacuation on a scale from 0 to 100, where 0 = no feeling of incomplete evacuation and 100 = a very strong feeling of incomplete evacuation?"* ***If the subject requires clarification, ask:*** *"During the last 7 days, how strongly did you feel that you did not empty your bowels completely? Please indicate how strong this feeling was on a scale from 0 to 100, where 0 = not at all and 100 = very strong"*
3. Personal judgement of patient (NAS) regarding constipation during the last 7 days: 0 = not at all 100 = very strong
Ask the subject; *"During the last 7 days, how would you rate your constipation on a scale from 0 to 100, where 0 = not at all and 100 = very strong"* ***If the subject requires clarification, ask:*** *"During the last 7 days, how would you rate how constipated you felt on a scale from 0 to 100, where 0 = not at all and 100 = very strong"*

Fig. 12.1 | **Bowel Function Index.** (From Meissner, W., Leyendecker, P., Mueller-Lissner, S., Nadstawek, J., Hopp, M., Ruckes, C., Wirz, S., Fleischer, W., … & Reimer, K. (2009). A randomised controlled trial with prolonged-release oral oxycodone and naloxone to prevent and reverse opioid-induced constipation. *Pain, 13*(1), 56–64.)

- *Stimulants* (e.g., senna, bisacodyl, cascara sagrada) are designed to encourage muscle contractions and are the first-line treatment.
- *Surfactants or stool softeners* (e.g., docusate sodium and mineral oil) are used to soften stools along with stimulants.
- *Bulking agents* (e.g., methylcellulose, psyllium) can be used to increase the bulk of the stool and keep fluids in the gut; however, it is imperative that adequate fluid is consumed or constipation can be intensified.
- *Osmotics* (e.g., polyethylene glycol, magnesium sulfate, magnesium hydroxide) are designed to bring water to the gut lumen of the colon and keep it there, promoting greater fluid in the small bowel. Some *osmotics* (e.g., magnesium salts) are intended to cause softer stools with easier passage because of triggering water being secreted into the intestinal lumen (Camilleri, 2017; Coyne et al., 2014; Levine & Shega, 2013; Sandoval & Witt, 2015).
- *Rectal laxatives or agents* include suppositories and enemas. They are usually only used when oral agents are not effective because they tend to be uncomfortable,

potentially embarrassing, and inconvenient. In addition, they may not be effective if stool is high in the colon or intestines (Levine & Shega, 2013).

Because there is no evidence that one medication is preferable, it is most likely a multimodal approach to bowel management will be most effective (Caraceni et al., 2012). To provide a guideline for selecting laxative therapies, Levine and Shega (2013) developed an easy-to-follow stepwise laxative regimen (Fig. 12.2).

Opioid receptor antagonist laxatives or peripherally acting mu opioid antagonists (PAMORAs) are specifically formulated to help manage OIC by blocking the opioid receptors found in the GI tract but not affecting the CNS receptors (Lacy et al., 2016).

- *Methylnaltrexone* is a selective PAMORA derivative of naltrexone. It antagonizes the effects of opioids in the GI tract and increases orocecal transit time (Camilleri et al., 2017; Lacy et al., 2016; Nalamachu et al., 2015). It is available in oral formulation (Rauck, Slatkin, Harper, & Israel, 2017). It has

Table 12.2 | Commonly Used Laxatives for Opioid-Induced Constipation

Group	Action	Agents	Latency	Side Effects and Cautions
Bulking agents	Increase fecal bulk, retain fluid in gut lumen	Psyllium seed, bran, methylcellulose	Days	Bloating, flatulence, abdominal pain Risk of exacerbating constipation if inadequate fluid intake Generally not recommended in patients with advanced illness
Osmotics	Draw and maintain water within gut lumen, increase fluid secretion in small bowel	Magnesium sulfate (e.g., Milk of Magnesia, magnesium citrate, Epsom salt)	1–3 h	Abdominal cramping, watery stools, dehydration, hypermagnesemia, hypocalcemia, hyperphosphatemia Not recommended in patient with cardiac and renal disease
		Lactulose	24–48 h	Bloating, flatulence, colic, sweet taste, hypokalemia, hypernatremia, lactic acidosis, acid-base disturbance
		Sorbitol	24–48 h	Abdominal cramping, bloating, flatulence, sweet taste
		Polyethylene glycol (e.g., Miralax)	0.5–1 h	Nausea, abdominal cramping, bloating, diarrhea, flatulence, fecal incontinence Aspiration into lungs can result in pulmonary edema
Stimulants	Alter intestinal permeability, stimulates myenteric plexus to induce peristalsis	Anthroquinones (e.g., senna, cascara)	6–12 h	Abdominal cramping, colic, melanosis, coli with chronic use
		Bisacodyl	6–12 h	Abdominal cramping, electrolyte imbalance
Surfactants	Detergents, lubricate and soften stools	Docusate sodium	12–72 h	Limited efficacy, not recommended as a solo agent
Suppositories	Reflex evacuation through direct stimulation	Glycerin	0.25–1 h	Rectal irritation, ineffective if feces located higher in colon
		Bisacodyl	0.25–1 h	Rectal irritation, ineffective if feces located higher in colon
Enemas	Draw water into lumen	Saline, sodium phosphate	0.5–1 h	Dehydration, hypocalcemia, hyperphosphatemia Not recommended in patients with renal disease
	Distention, facilitating peristalsis	Tap water, soapsuds, mineral oil	0.5–1 h	Repeated tap water enemas may lead to fluid and electrolyte abnormalities Soapsuds have been associated with chemical colitis
Opioid receptor antagonists	Competitive opioid antagonist	Naloxone	0.5–4 h	Opioid withdrawal; not indicated in most patients
	Selective peripheral opioid antagonist	Methylnaltrexone	0.5–4 h	Abdominal cramps, nausea, soft stools, diarrhea, flatulence, nausea Contraindicated in setting of bowel obstruction

From Levine, S. K. & Shega, J. W. (2013). What medications are effective in preventing and relieving constipation in the setting of opioid use? (pp. 129–134.) In: E. Goldstein, & R. S. Morrison. *Evidence-based practice of palliative medicine.* Philadelphia, PA: Saunders.

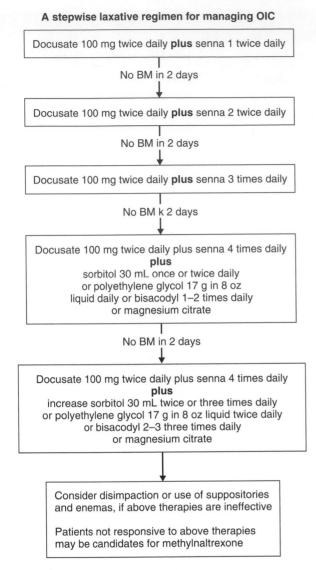

A stepwise laxative regimen for managing OIC

Docusate 100 mg twice daily **plus** senna 1 twice daily

No BM in 2 days

Docusate 100 mg twice daily **plus** senna 2 twice daily

No BM in 2 days

Docusate 100 mg twice daily **plus** senna 3 times daily

No BM k 2 days

Docusate 100 mg twice daily plus senna 4 times daily
plus
sorbitol 30 mL once or twice daily
or polyethylene glycol 17 g in 8 oz
liquid daily or bisacodyl 1–2 times daily
or magnesium citrate

No BM in 2 days

Docusate 100 mg twice daily plus senna 4 times daily
plus
increase sorbitol 30 mL twice or three times daily
or polyethylene glycol 17 g in 8 oz liquid twice daily
or bisacodyl 2–3 three times daily
or magnesium citrate

Consider disimpaction or use of suppositories
and enemas, if above therapies are ineffective

Patients not responsive to above therapies
may be candidates for methylnaltrexone

Fig. 12.2 | **Stepwise Laxative Regimen for Managing Opioid-Induced Constipation.** (From Levine, S. K., & Shega, J. W. [2013]. What medications are effective in preventing and relieving constipation in the setting of opioid use? (pp. 129–134.) In: E. Goldstein & R. S. Morrison. *Evidence-based practice of palliative medicine.* Philadelphia, PA: Saunders.)

also been shown to be effective when administered subcutaneously in patients with OIC and advanced illness (Nalamachu, 2015). A caution is the concern for gastric or intestinal perforation (Camilleri et al., 2017; Lacy et al., 2016).

- *Naloxegol* is an oral derivative of naloxone that was designed to act only outside the CNS, thus not having an effect on analgesia (Chey et al., 2014; Lacy et al., 2016). It acts locally in the GI tract and is reported to be effective, safe, and well-tolerated (Camilleri et al., 2017; Lacy et al., 2016; Webster et al., 2013). When taken daily during phase II trials with patients with OIC related to cancer and noncancer diagnoses, the frequency of spontaneous bowel movements was statistically significant (Webster et al., 2013).

Similar results were reported when used in phase III trials with patients with OIC related to noncancer diagnoses (Chey et al., 2014).

- *Naldemedine* is a PAMORA that was approved by the U.S. Food and Drug Administration (FDA) in 2017 as a treatment for OIC (Stern & Brenner, 2018). The authors of a phase II study reported that in a sample of 227 patients receiving opioids for cancer, naldemedine significantly reduced the symptoms of OIC and improved spontaneous bowel movements (Brower, 2017; Katakami et al., 2017).
- *Alvimopan* is another peripherally acting PAMORA. It is designed specifically to prevent or reduce postoperative ileus after resection of the bowel (Lacy et al., 2016) and enhance postoperative recovery (Simorov, Thompson, & Oleynikov, 2014). The results of a multicenter trial demonstrated that time in an intensive care unit, overall length of stay, and total hospital costs were reduced for patients who received alvimopan in conjunction with colonic segmental resections (Simorov et al., 2014). In that same study, length of stay was significantly reduced in patients who had alvimopan in conjunction with laparoscopic colectomies.

Nonpharmacologic Management

Patient education is important. Patients need to be taught the importance of basic nonpharmacologic lifestyle measures, including adequate fiber intake, ensuring adequate fluid intake, and regular daily physical exercise, which are all helpful in minimizing the severity of OIC (Kumar et al., 2014). Educating patients to detect and quickly respond to the physiologic impulse to evacuate (Dorn, Lembo, & Cremonini, 2014) can be helpful in minimizing the severity of OIC. When possible, it is desirable to condition the body to pass stool at a particular time each day (Levine & Shega, 2013). An important nonpharmacologic intervention is educating patients and families about the importance of optimizing these interventions and adhering to a prescribed medication regimen to promote regular passage of bowel movements and reporting any changes in function (Levine & Shega, 2013).

Acupuncture is an ancient Chinese medicine technique of inserting and then manipulating fine needles in specific predetermined points with the intention of achieving a certain effect (Anastasi, Capili, & Chang, 2017; Cheifetz, Gianotti, Luber, & Gibson, 2017; Chon & Lee, 2013). A recent review of systematic reviews and meta-analysis of studies using acupuncture to relieve chronic constipation concluded that it was effective with no clear undesirable effects (Wang & Yin, 2015). See Chapter 23 for further discussion about acupuncture.

Electroacupuncture is an intervention that uses acupuncture with electric current stimulation. It was used successfully in a clinical trial to shorten the duration of postoperative ileus (Ng, et al, 2013). The investigators of a large study (n = 1075) with people with chronic functional constipation concluded electroacupuncture seems to be a safe and effective intervention for people living with severe constipation resulting from ileus (Alper, Malone-Moses, & Manheimer, 2017). The authors acknowledged out-of-pocket and traveling costs could be prohibitive, particularly where electroacupuncture is not readily available. Although this study and the systematic review with acupuncture involved severe functional constipation that was not OIC, acupuncture or electroacupuncture may be helpful for patients with OIC. Certainly, clinical research is warranted to investigate the use among people living with OIC.

Reflexology is an ancient modality that involves using specific finger and hand movements applied to areas of the hands and feet that correspond to certain areas of the body with the intention of stimulating them to homeostasis and promote self-healing (Dahiya & Banerjee, 2016; Quinlan-Colwell, 2012). See Chapter 24 for further discussion of reflexology. Internationally it has been used as a treatment for constipation (Dahiya & Banerjee, 2016; Minagawa et al., 2016; Seyyedrassoli, 2016; Woodward, Norton, & Barriball, 2010). In a small study in the United Kingdom with women, foot reflexology was successful in relieving idiopathic constipation in 94% of the participants (Woodward et al., 2010). The authors of that study concluded although reflexology warrants further research, it is potentially beneficial for managing constipation. A study in Iran involving postoperative orthopedic patients (n = 60) also found reflexology beneficial in managing constipation. Those researchers noted it can be a clinically effective, cost-effective, and noninvasive nursing intervention (Seyyedrassoli, 2016). Although no studies were found that evaluated the benefit of foot reflexology specifically with OIC, one author (AQC) of this chapter has used it successfully for many years with patients suffering with OIC. Again, research in this area is needed.

Xerostomia (Dry Mouth)

Xerostomia, or dry mouth, which also can be a symptom of OIC, is a common side effect of opioid therapy (Drewes et al., 2016). The prevalence of xerostomia ranges from 1% to 94%, but with an overall rate of 48% or higher (Oosten et al., 2015). In addition to interfering with quality of life, dry mouth and hyposalivation can lead to infection of the oral cavity, dental caries, and halitosis (Scully, 2013). It is frequently reported with an intensity of moderate to severe, with the resulting stress considered to be "quite a bit" or greater (Oosten et al., 2015).

Assessment

Patients with xerostomia may report burning oral sensations, abnormal taste, dysarthria, dysphagia, dysgeusia, halitosis, and lack of retention of dentures. Health care providers may also note some of these signs during patient assessment. An examination of the mouth may reveal oral dryness, thickening of saliva, evidence of candidal infection (fissures on the corners of the mouth, white plaque on the mucosa, erythematous patches), and fissures of the tongue (Niklander et al., 2017).

Prevention and Management

Side effects are dose related, and a multimodal approach for pain management facilitates using less of any one medication, including opioids. Such a multimodal approach can be an important effort in preventing or minimizing the occurrence of dry mouth. Other interventions that address alleviating the symptom fall into two categories.

The first category involves avoiding things that may contribute to or intensify a dry mouth. Things to avoid include the following (Han, Suarez-Durall, & Mulligan, 2015; Mark, 2017; Scully, 2013):

- Dehydration
- Dry environments
- Dry, spicy, or salty foods
- Medications with anticholinergic or sympathomimetic effects
- Alcohol (including alcohol-based mouthwash)
- Smoking tobacco
- Caffeine
- Mouth breathing.

The second group of strategies involve improving moisture in the mouth. These include the following (Han et al., 2015; Mark, 2017; Scully, 2013; Villa, Connell, & Abati, 2015):

- Keeping the mouth wet by sucking on ice chips and frequent sips of water.
- Ensuring adequate hydration.
- Promoting salivation by chewing gum or sucking on hard candies.
- Using mucosal lubricants (e.g., olive oil).
- Keeping lips moist with lanolin-based lip balm.
- Using a humidifier while sleeping.
- Synthetic salivary substitutes are available commercially or can be made by adding 1/4 teaspoon of glycerin to 8 oz of water (Scully, 2013).
- Increasing humidity in the environment, particularly at night, is also helpful (Villa, Connell, & Abati, 2015).

Good oral hygiene by brushing with a soft-bristled brush and flossing along with regular dental evaluation and care are imperative (Mark, 2017; Plemons et al., 2014). When the situation is severe, and these measures are not effective, sialogogue medications (pilocarpine, cevimeline) can be prescribed to stimulate salivation (Plemons, Al-Hashimi, & Marek, 2014). Acupuncture, electrostimulation, laser therapy, and electric versus manual toothbrush have all been studied as interventions for dry mouth, but to date there is no evidence that they are effective (Furness, Bryan, McMillan, Birchenough, & Worthington, 2013).

Opioid-Induced Nausea and Vomiting

Nausea and vomiting in general occur as the result of stimulation of the GI tract, middle ear, or CNS (Harbord & Pomfret, 2013). They are considered repugnant symptoms (Horn & Yates, 2017), with patients reporting them as less desirable to tolerate than pain (Odom-Forren et al., 2013). Willingness of patients to endure some pain rather than experience nausea and vomiting was a finding in a study done by Gan et al. (2014a).

Nausea is a sensation indicating that vomiting will occur, although it may occur alone or in conjunction with actual vomiting (Pleuvry, 2015; Smith & Laufer, 2014). Nausea is generally an acute symptom when it is followed by vomiting (Harbord & Pomfret, 2013). Although there are a variety of reasons why nausea occurs, and the underlying mechanisms involved are not well understood, it is thought to involve the autonomic nervous system (Pleuvry, 2015). One reason for the lack of knowledge is the difficulty encountered when trying to get volunteers to consent to participate in research studies with nausea being induced as the phenomenon to be investigated. In the two-part Western European study, participants living with chronic pain ranked nausea as their primary concern and pain relief secondary to that (Chancellor et al., 2012).

Vomiting occurs as a reflexive action that is triggered within the medulla oblongata in response to communication from chemoreceptors or mechanoreceptors located in the upper GI tract, the chemoreceptor trigger zone (CTZ), or the vestibular system (Harbord & Pomfret, 2013). The act of vomiting involves a contraction and relaxation of the diaphragm and abdominal muscles concurrently, followed by a contraction that is constant and coordinated with muscles of the chest, pharynx, larynx, and intestinal muscles with closure of the glottis, elevation of the soft palate, and relaxation of the gastric fundus with expulsion of the gastric contents (Pleuvry, 2015).

Nausea and vomiting, like constipation, are common side effects of opioid therapy. They occur in 30% to 60% of people being treated with opioids, but there is wide variability in the occurrence, intensity, and tolerance that may develop among different people (Smith & Laufer, 2014). Opioid-induced nausea and vomiting (OINV) also negatively affect quality of life and often limits willingness to continue with opioid therapy (Marrett, Kwong, Frech, & Qian, 2016; Smith & Laufer, 2014). Although OINV are most commonly dose related and lessen during the first weeks of opioid therapy, some patients do not develop a tolerance even after years of opioid treatment (Smith & Laufer, 2014). Genetic factors, including polymorphisms, account for the extensive variations in both development and ability to modify the intensity of OINV (Smith & Laufer, 2014).

In addition to occurring solely in response to opioid treatment, OINV frequently occurs in conjunction with other responses, including chemotherapy (chemotherapy-induced nausea/vomiting [CINV]), radiation (radiation-induced emesis [RIE]), postoperatively (postoperative nausea/vomiting [PONV]) (Smith & Laufer, 2014), and postdischarge nausea and vomiting (PDNV) that occurs after ambulatory surgery (Odom-Forren et al., 2013). In addition, anticipatory nausea/vomiting (ANV) almost always results in actual vomiting and may result in persistent nausea/vomiting (PNV) (Kravits, 2015). As noted, because of the many different situations in which it occurs, combined with the loathsomeness of the experience, OINV has not frequently been researched as a separate entity so is not fully understood. It is thought that several factors contribute to OINV, including the following (Bashashati & McCallum, 2014; Smith & Laufer, 2014):

- Heightened sensitivity of the vestibular apparatus
- Result of stimulation of the mu opioid chemoreceptors in the CTZ
- Changes in esophageal function
- Delay in emptying of the GI tract
- Possible initiation of the vagovagal reflex pathway leading to reduction of gastric tone
- Morphine may cause some 5-HT_3 receptor constraint
- Role of delta and kappa receptors are not clear and may contribute to or modulate the response

Assessment

Assessment of nausea and vomiting should comprise all possible causes, including any possible underlying pathologic conditions, comorbidities, other newly introduced medications, and bowel function (Keeley, 2015). When assessment findings exclude other causes and lead to a diagnosis of OINV, the possible interventions are numerous.

Prevention and Management

Prevention of OINV involves avoidance, dose reductions, and opioid rotation. A multimodal approach for pain management facilitates using less of any one medication, including opioids; thus it is an important effort toward preventing or minimizing the development of OINV. Some other treatment measures discussed in this section also can be used for prevention when implemented before the development of OINV. Multimodal treatment of OINV can use pharmacologic and/or nonpharmacologic therapies.

Pharmacologic Management

Pharmacologic interventions for OINV range from adjusting the opioid prescription to a variety of medications that can treat OINV from a number of perspectives. As with OIC, reducing the dose or changing to another opioid to see if OINV resolves is an initial intervention (Bristow, Singh, & Ballantyne, 2014; Keeley, 2015). Tapentadol, which inhibits the reuptake of norepinephrine in addition to mu opioid receptor, is associated with less OINV than other oral opioids (Smith & Laufer, 2014).

PAMORAs are used to reverse the effect on the mu opioid receptors in the GI tract and chemoreceptor zone. Continuous infusions with low-dose naloxone, naltrexone, or nalmefene as well as subcutaneous administration of methylnaltrexone have all been effective in decreasing OINV (Bashashati & McCallum, 2014; Smith & Laufer, 2014). Alvimopan (described in detail in the earlier discussion of OIC) also decreases OINV postoperatively and enhances GI tract activity (Bashashati & McCallum, 2014).

Serotonin (5-HT₃) receptor antagonists include ondansetron, which is the most commonly used of the serotonin (5-HT$_3$) receptor antagonists. Other medications in this group include granisetron, dolasetron, tropisetron, and the newer second-generation palonosetron. The authors of a study comparing ondansetron with palonosetron reported significantly less PONV/OINV among those who received palonosetron (Moon, Joo, Kim, & Lee, 2012). The serotonin (5-HT$_3$) receptor antagonists have minimal side effects (e.g., headache and constipation) (Dronca & Loprinzi, 2012). Ondansetron now has an FDA black box warning after reports of prolongation of the QTc interval and other cardiac complications (Smith & Laufer, 2014).

Antidopaminergic or dopamine receptor antagonists include promethazine, prochlorperazine, and chlorproMAZINE are phenothiazine, dopamine D2 receptor (DRD2) antagonists that have established efficacy managing OINV (Andrews & Sanger, 2014; Bristow et al., 2014; Dronca & Loprinzi, 2012). The efficacy of prochlorperazine with OINV is the result of inhibition of DRD2 at the CTZ (Tsukuura et al., 2015). The phenothiazines also possess anticholinergic and antihistamine blocking properties (Dronca & Loprinzi, 2012).

Metoclopramide is a benzamide, DRD2 blocker. When used in higher doses it also blocks 5-HT$_3$ and serotonin receptors (Dronca & Loprinzi, 2012). Haloperidol and droperidol are butyrophenone, type 2 dopamine receptor antagonists. Despite the strong antiemetic effects (stronger than those of the phenothiazines), they are not frequently used because of the extrapyramidal, sedating, hypotensive, and cardiac side effects (QTc prolongation) (Dronca & Loprinzi, 2012). Droperidol has an FDA black box warning after reports of prolongation of the QTc interval and other cardiac complications (Smith & Laufer, 2014).

OLANZapine is an *atypical antipsychotic* and a *serotonin antagonist* that also blocks dopamine, histamine, and dopaminergic receptors (Bristow et al., 2014; Dronca & Loprinzi, 2012). It is effective as a treatment of nausea and vomiting by obstructing a number of neuronal receptors involved with nausea and vomiting and has been used effectively in patients with CINV and palliative care (Fonte, Fatigoni & Roila, 2015). As with the butyrophenones, use is limited by the side effects, which include anticholinergic and extrapyramidal effects, weight gain,

sedation, and, over time, an increased risk for developing diabetes (Dronca & Loprinzi, 2012).

Glucocorticosteroids include dexamethasone, which has more variability in prescribing and is more commonly used than methylPREDNISolone, which is the other corticosteroid used to treat nausea. Although the specific mechanism of action is not known, dexamethasone is used to prevent and treat CINV (Dronca & Loprinzi, 2012) and PONV. Use may be limited by the adverse effects, which include agitation, insomnia, alteration in mood, and GI disturbances (Dronca & Loprinzi, 2012).

Anticholinergic medications include scopolamine, which can be prescribed transdermally (Bristow et al., 2014). Effectiveness of the transdermal patch is presumed to be related to vestibular involvement in OINV (Smith & Laufer, 2014). It is FDA (2013) approved for both motion sickness and PONV and has typical anticholinergic side effects such as dry mouth, somnolence, dizziness, and agitation.

Tachykinin NK-1 receptor antagonists include aprepitant, which is an antiemetic medication that antagonizes the action of substance P. Although there are no studies to date in which they have been evaluated specifically with OINV, it is conceivable that they could be effective (Smith & Laufer, 2014).

Nonpharmacologic Management

Several nonpharmacologic interventions may be used to manage OINV. Acupuncture is an ancient traditional Chinese technique (see Chapter 23). Acupuncture of the P$_6$ acupoint is reported to be as effective as antiemetic medications to control PONV (Stoicea et al., 2015). In one systematic review, it was concluded that acupuncture was effective in reducing postoperative nausea (Holmér Pettersson & Wengström, 2012). The mechanism of action is thought to be activation of the release of endorphins, serotonin, and norepinephrine. This results in stimulation of both mu and delta opioid receptors (Lee & Warden, 2016). From work in both animal and human studies, it is thought that acupuncture is effective in controlling nausea because of the action on serotonin (Lee & Warden, 2016). It is reported to be effective in preventing or alleviating nausea in a variety of populations, including women with cancer (Rithirangsriroj, Manchana, & Akkayagorn, 2015), palliative care (Romeo et al., 2015), and PONV (Stott, 2016). See Chapter 23 for more discussion of acupuncture.

Acupressure for nausea and vomiting involves pressure being applied to the P$_6$ acupoint, which is located between the tendons of the carpi radialis and palmaris longus 4 cm proximal to the transverse crease of the hand. Like acupuncture, the mechanism of action is thought to be activation of an increase in beta-endorphin release from the hypothalamus in conjunction with tempering serotonin (Stoicea et al., 2015). In a study that used wristbands to apply pressure bilaterally to the P$_6$ acupoints, reduction of nausea was reported as statistically significant. However, another study found no benefit of acupressure compared to placebo (Stoicea et al., 2015). Yet, in a recent small study with patients who had undergone ambulatory surgery, the researchers concluded that acupressure was effective in preventing and treating PONV (Hofmann, Murray, Beck, & Homann, 2017). Additional research is needed on prevention or control of OINV with acupressure, which is cost effective and time efficient and has minimal adverse effects. See Chapter 23 for more discussion of acupressure.

Dietary modifications are imperative. It is important to ensure the diet is low in both fat and fiber as well as consisting of frequent but small servings. Recommendations are generally similar to those for patients with gastric emptying delay (Singh, Yoon, & Kuo, 2016). In one study it was observed that acute tryptophan depletion was related to an increase in nausea and vomiting (Rieber et al, 2010). That finding is interesting because acute tryptophan depletion is also observed with sluggish gastric emptying in women (Singh et al., 2016).

Ginger has a long history as a medicinal agent in India and other Eastern countries. It is ingested to prevent and treat nausea in a variety of conditions, including pregnancy (Ding, Leach, & Bradley, 2013), motion sickness (Kaur et al., 2015), and PONV (Singh et al., 2016). Information is inconsistent with CINV (Singh et al., 2016). Interestingly, although ginger was found to be effective in CINV with dogs, the results in humans with CINV have been variable (Kaur et al., 2015). See Chapter 26 for further discussion of ginger.

Aromatherapy in the form of isopropyl alcohol and peppermint oil have a relatively long history of use treating PONV. Although research studies have reported inconsistent results, a Cochrane Library review reported it as largely effective. In addition, in their 2006 guidelines, the American Society of PeriAnesthesia Nurses noted the benefit to be equal to the risks (Stoicea et al., 2015). Ginger is another substance used in an essential oil that was shown to be effective for a short time in preventing nausea but not vomiting in a small sample (n = 67) of women receiving chemotherapy (Lua, Salihah, & Mazlan, 2015). Ginger aromatherapy was also effective in controlling PONV in a study (n = 120) with nephrectomy patients (Adib-Hajbaghery & Hosseini, 2016). See Chapter 27 for further discussion of aromatherapy, including precautions and contraindications.

Hypnosis is used in a variety of types of nausea and vomiting. Hypnosis is an intervention with an identified "hypnosis induction" that begins with concentration approaches. This is followed by a "deepening" phase during which therapeutic suggestions by trained practitioners working with a patient generate desired changes in perception, thought, affect, conduct, performance, and sensation that both the patient and practitioner agree are desirable (Iserson, 2014; Kekecs, Nagy, & Varga, 2014; Kravits, 2015; Montgomery, Schnur, & Kravits, 2013; Stoicea et al., 2015). Therapeutic suggestions are designed to prevent, transform, or eliminate nausea and vomiting perceptions. A real benefit is that these suggestions can be designed to be effective after the actual hypnosis session (posthypnotic) so that the person can use the suggestion to prevent or manage any nausea and vomiting (Kravits, 2015). In addition, it is considered safe, time efficient, and low cost (Iserson, 2014).

Hypnosis is used to treat ANV (Kravits, 2015), CINV (Roila et al., 2016; Singh et al., 2016), and PONV (Kekecs et al., 2015; Stoicea et al., 2015). One meta-analysis of randomized control trials (RCTs) did not find hypnosis to be statistically significant in controlling PONV; however, the RCTs all had very small sample sizes (Kekecs et al., 2014). The 2016 Multinational Association of Supportive Care in Cancer and European Society of Medical Oncology rated hypnosis for CINV as grade II B (scale of I–V and A–D) (Roila et al., 2016). The strongest evidence for the effectiveness of medical hypnosis as treatment for nausea is involving ANV in patients preparing to undergo chemotherapy (Palsson, 2015). Additional research is needed to study the effectiveness of medical hypnosis with OINV and PONV. See Chapter 27 for more discussion on hypnosis.

Head-rest is a simple intervention that involves minimizing head movement to avoid OINV. It is based on the idea that stimulation of the vestibule-ocular reflex leads to OINV so by minimizing head movement, OINV is minimized or eliminated (Lehnen et al., 2015). Clearly, this is an intervention that could be effective for a short time, but not as a long-term intervention.

Pruritus

Pruritus is an unpleasant sensation and a very common unintended opioid effect (Benson, Campbell, & Phillips, 2015). Although opioid-induced itching is not a serious, life-threatening side effect, for many patients it is very disturbing and can result in the undertreatment of pain because the itch may be intolerable for some. The itching associated with opioid-induced pruritus (OIP) may range from mild to severe and may interfere with sleep, general comfort, and discontinuation of medication (Benson et al., 2015). Pruritus may be experienced all over the body but is usually localized to the face, neck, and upper thorax and seldom associated with a rash. When assessing patients, if a medication allergy to an opioid is reported, it is important to determine location of itching and presence or absence of rash, because patients often mistakenly report opioid-related pruritus as an allergic reaction. True opioid allergies (true immunoglobulin E [IgE]-mediated hypersensitivity reactions) are very rare, and many patients are inappropriately labeled as having an allergy to an opioid despite the lack of clinical evidence or diagnostic testing (Li, Ue, Wagner, Rutkowski, & Rutkowski, 2017).

The wide range in incidence of OIP is related to the route of administration, type of opioid, and dose.

Transdermal opioid administration, as with fentaNYL and buprenorphine patches, is associated with an incidence of 3% to 15%, but reactions are mostly localized to the site where the patch has been applied (Benson et al., 2015). Oral administration is associated with a 2% to 20% incidence, and the incidence increases to 10% to 50% after intravenous (IV) and 30% to 100% after epidural or spinal administration (Golembiewski, 2013). The highest risk (nearly 100%) occurs with intrathecal morphine administration, particularly to women in labor. The increased susceptibility in women in labor may be related to the interaction of estrogens with opioid receptors (Reich & Szepietowski, 2010). The epidural route has a lower incidence than the intrathecal route (Benson et al., 2015). The type and dose of opioid may also have some impact on the prevalence and severity of pruritus. Pruritus of less severity and shorter duration has been noted with the use of intrathecal fentaNYL and other more lipid-soluble opioids compared to intrathecal morphine (Kumar & Singh, 2013). In dosing studies, lower doses of intrathecal morphine and HYDROmorphone have been associated with less pruritus than with higher doses (Marroquin et al., 2017; Sultan, Halpern, Pushpanathan, Patel, & Carvalho, 2016). Long-acting oral opioids are associated with more pruritus than short-acting oral formulations (Benson et al., 2015).

The mechanism of OIP is not well understood, but studies have shown that central and peripheral mechanisms are involved. One proposed mechanism is that the sensation of itch is thought to be transmitted by unmyelinated C-fiber nociceptors from the periphery to the dorsal horn of the spinal cord, where they synapse and transmit via a distinct spinothalamic pathway (different from pain and temperature pathways) to the thalamus and somatosensory cortex (Ho & Gan, 2009). It has also been proposed that there is simultaneous activation of pain and itch C-fibers in response to noxious stimuli, but the perception of itch is inhibited in the brain by the perception of pain (Ho & Gan, 2009). However, when pain is alleviated with mu opioid agonists, the inhibition is diminished and itch is experienced. This proposed mechanism is less favored now because more evidence has accumulated related to the role of mu opioid receptors in OIP.

Evidence now points to a significant central mu opioid receptor–mediated mechanism in the development of OIP. The direct binding of mu opioids to these receptors in the brain and spinal cord, as well as changes in neurotransmission of these receptors, and interaction with other receptors, including 5-HT_3 and dopamine-2, are probable mechanisms of centrally-mediated pruritus (Benson et al., 2015; Golembiewski, 2013). The dorsal region of the spinal cord and the trigeminal nerve nucleus have high concentrations of mu opioid receptors as well as dopamine-2 receptors. The high density of receptors in these regions may account for the predominance of itching in the face, neck, and upper thorax, particularly with neuraxial opioids (Benson et al., 2015; Golembiewski, 2013). Experiments by Liu et al. (2011) identified that

a mu opioid receptor isoform, MOP1D, is required for intrathecal morphine-induced itch. Other opioid receptors, kappa and delta (see Chapter 11), are not associated with OIP, and kappa opioid receptors agonists have been found to block or inhibit OIP (Ko, 2015). Interactions between opioids and other mediators such as dopamine type 2 and prostaglandins may also contribute to pruritus. Growing awareness of the involvement of multiple receptors in the development of OIP is the subject of much research interest as new medications are sought to reduce unintended effects of opioid therapy.

Peripheral mechanisms, usually involving intravenous and oral opioid administration, have been found to have a minor role in OIP. Although there is a possible role of peripheral mu opioid receptors in itch, the more widely recognized peripheral mechanism that causes itch involves mast cell activation and histamine release. In studies that examined histamine release in response to opioids, morphine, codeine, and meperidine were noted to have this effect (Baldo & Pham, 2012). Similar results were reported in an older study comparing the effects of intradermal injections of opioids on histamine release from mast cells in which morphine, codeine, and meperidine increased histamine release, whereas fentaNYL, other fentaNYL-like opioids, and buprenorphine did not (Blunk et al., 2004). Methadone has also been shown to have a histamine-mediated pruritic effect that was not seen with oxyMORphone and fentaNYL (Benson et al., 2015). Although HYDROmorphone is a direct derivative of morphine with similar pharmacologic properties, it has not been shown to cause a significant histamine release (Ruan, Ma, Couch, Chen, & Bumgarner, 2015).

Assessment

In assessing patients for opioid-related unintended effects, it is useful to ask the patient to attempt to quantify the degree of pruritus so treatments can be initiated and responses can be determined. A number of self-report scales have been developed to facilitate assessment of pruritus. Similar to pain intensity ratings, measurements of itch intensity may be done using a visual analogue scale (VAS), numerical rating scale (NRS), verbal rating scale (VRS), and Verbal Numeric Rating Scale (VNRS). In a study of the horizontal and vertical VAS, NRS, and VRS, good reproducibility and correlation were found among the scales (Reich et al., 2012). A limitation of the VAS is that the patient must be able to use a writing implement to mark the itch intensity level on a line. The 4-point verbal rating scale (VRS-4) and an 11-point verbal numeric rating scale (VNRS-11) have been compared to each other, and good correlation has been shown (Reich et al., 2012). As a result of the strong correlation between the scales, each point on the VRS-4 could be substituted with a range on the VNRS so that 1 to 3 = mild itching, 4 to 7 = moderate itching, and 8 to 10 = severe itching (Jenkins, Spencer, Weissgerber, Osborne, &

Pellegrini, 2009). Similar cut-off points when comparing the VAS to a 5-point VRS were found, with the addition of a category for very severe itching with scores of 8 or 9 to 10 on the VAS (Kido-Nakahara et al., 2015). In a systematic review of patient-reported outcome measures in pruritus (although not specific to OIP), several scales were found to have the strong validity and reliability and are recommended for use in clinical research. The six scales are the Itch Severity Scale (ISS), Itchy Quality of Life (Itchy QoL), numerical rating scale-6 (NRS-6 on itch intensity), numerical rating scale-11 (NRS-11 on itch intensity), visual analogue scale horizontal (VAS horizontal on itch intensity), and verbal numerical scale (VNRS-4 on itch intensity) (Schoch, Sommer, Augustin, Ständer, & Blome, 2017).

Although clinicians may associate scratching or rubbing behaviors or skin scratch marks with signs of pruritus, similar to pain, the assessment of intensity requires a patient self-report. There is individual variation in behaviors associated with pruritus, and objective measurement of intensity is not possible. For the patient who is unable to self-report intensity of pruritus, observation of behaviors such as scratching, rubbing, and self-excoriation may provide indications of the presence of itch. Video recording of behaviors and a wrist activity monitor have been used to assess pruritus in other conditions associated with pruritus, but no literature is available to describe the use of similar instruments in OIP.

Prevention and Management of Opioid-Induced Pruritus

The identification of the association of 5-HT$_3$ receptors with OIP has led to studies into the use of 5-HT$_3$ antagonists in the prevention and treatment of OIP. The outcomes of these studies are inconclusive. In a systematic review, a decrease in the incidence and intensity of pruritus was noted in patients who received neuraxial opioids, including morphine, when a single intravenous dose of a 5-HT$_3$ antagonist (ondansetron, tropisetron, granisetron, or dolesetron) was given prophylactically (Bonnet, Marret, Josserand, & Mercier, 2008). In a more recent review, Ko (2015) cited conflicting evidence, noting that the administration of ondansetron reduced pruritus in patients who had received neuraxial morphine, fentaNYL, or a combination of mu opioid agonists, whereas in several other studies, ondansetron was ineffective in treating pruritus in patients who had received intrathecal fentaNYL or a combination of mu opioid agonists.

Because mu opioid receptors are highly implicated in the development of OIP, mu opioid antagonists such as naloxone and naltrexone have been considered as treatment options. In a meta-analysis of six RCTs that examined the effects of naloxone on opioid-induced side effects, naloxone was effective in preventing OIP (He et al., 2016). However, although these mu opioid antagonists may block the pruritic effect, the analgesic

effect may also be blocked. To prevent reversal of the analgesic effect, the dose of naloxone must be sufficient to reverse the itch, but low enough to prevent reversal of analgesia. Multiple studies, including a systematic review of obstetric patients who received intravenous naloxone (Kjellberg & Tramer 2001), demonstrated the effectiveness of mu opioid antagonists in treating the neuraxial OIP (Ko, 2015). A meta-analysis of six studies indicated that the occurrence rate of OIP was significantly lower in the naloxone-treated group than in the control group (He et al., 2016). Naloxone has a short duration of action (30–60 minutes depending on dose and route), and therefore it may be necessary to provide repeated naloxone dosing or, preferably, a low-dose continuous intravenous infusion (Benson et al., 2015). Although doses of up to 1 mcg/kg/h have been used, very low doses of intravenous naloxone infusions, 0.25 to 1 mcg/kg/h, are recommended (Benson et al., 2015; Golembiewski, 2013). Naltrexone, a longer acting mu opioid antagonist (4- to 5-hour half-life) that is twice as potent as naloxone, may provide some reversal of OIP with oral doses of 6 to 9 mg, but higher doses may block analgesia (Benson et al., 2015). Continuous intravenous naltrexone infusions may be effective at doses of 0.25 to 1 mcg/kg/h (Benson et al., 2015).

Nalbuphine, a mu opioid antagonist and kappa receptor agonist, at a 10-mg IV dose, is clinically indicated for moderate to severe pain because of its kappa agonist activity (Golembiewski, 2013). At lower doses, 3 to 5 mg IV, it has been used off-label for its mu antagonist effect in the prevention and treatment of OIP (Golembiewski, 2013). In a systematic review that included nine RCTs and one case study, Jannuzzi (2016) concluded that nalbuphine was superior to placebo, controls, diphenhydrAMINE, naloxone, or propofol in treating pruritus in patients who had undergone surgery and patients in childbirth who had received neuraxial opioids (Jannuzzi, 2016). Nalbuphine is also preferred over ondansetron because sedation is its only significant side effect (Benson et al., 2015). Nalbuphine may be preferred over mu opioid antagonists because it reverses pruritus and other mu opioid side effects without reversing analgesia (Benson et al., 2015). Jannuzzi (2015) noted that dose-finding studies are needed to optimize dosing, but Benson et al. (2015) recommend that a continuous intravenous infusion may be dosed at 2.5 mg/h. Butorphanol and pentazocine, other mixed agonist-antagonist opioids, have also shown efficacy in the treatment of opioid-induced itch (Kumar & Singh, 2013).

Droperidol, a potent dopamine-2 receptor antagonist with weak serotonin 5-HT$_3$ antagonist activity, has been extensively used for the treatment of PONV, but may also be considered as an alternative medication to treat OIP. Study results have been inconclusive, but in a study of 300 women who underwent cesarean sections and received spinal morphine, those in the droperidol group had less pruritus than those in placebo, propofol, alizapride, and promethazine groups (Horta et al., 2006). Another potent dopamine-2 receptor antagonist, metoclopromide, has been shown to be ineffective in reducing pruritus.

Propofol in subhypnotic doses (10-30 mg IV bolus over a 24-hour period) has been used for the prevention and treatment of OIP, although studies have provided inconclusive results (Kumar & Singh, 2013). The antipruritic properties of propofol are not well understood but may be related to its ability to inhibit posterior horn transmission in the spinal cord. In experiments on animals who received intrathecal morphine (Liu et al., 2014), propofol was found to inhibit scratching responses, and an increase in the expression of cannabinoid receptors was thought to contribute to the pruritus reduction (Liu et al., 2014).

Gabapentin, an anticonvulsant that is also used in the treatment of neuropathic pain, has shown efficacy in the treatment of intrathecal morphine-induced itch. When 1200 mg of gabapentin was preoperatively administered to 86 patients who received intrathecal morphine for limb surgery, there was significantly less (P = .01) pruritus in the gabapentin group (47.5%) compared to the placebo group (77.5%) (Sheen, Ho, Lee, Tsung, & Chang, 2008a). Similar reductions in pruritus were seen in a study of 80 patients who received 1200 mg of gabapentin before pilonidal cyst or unilateral inguinal hernia repair surgery with intrathecal morphine (Akhan et al., 2016). The antipruritic activity of gabapentin may be related to central reduction of itch perception, reduced excitability of spinal and supraspinal neurons, and the inhibition of spinal and supraspinal serotonergic circuits (Benson et al., 2015).

Mirtazapine, an antidepressant that has been studied for its ability to prevent intrathecal morphine pruritus, is a selective serotonin (5-HT$_2$/5-HT$_3$) inhibitor, an H1 receptor antagonist, and a kappa opioid agonist (Akhan et al., 2016; Benson et al., 2015). Both its antidepressant and antipruritic activity may be mediated centrally by its ability to activate kappa receptors (Kumar & Singh, 2013). Studies have shown that a preoperative 30-mg oral dose of mirtazapine can delay the time to onset and reduce the incidence, severity, and duration of intrathecal morphine-induced pruritus (Davis, Frandsen, Walsh, Andresen, & Taylor, 2003; Sheen, Ho, Lee, Tsung, & Chang, 2008b).

Clinicians may be familiar with the use of antihistamines, particularly diphenhydrAMINE and hydrOXYzine for the treatment of opioid-induced itch. Patients may be dissatisfied with the lack of relief and side effects (sedation) associated with antihistamines. Antihistamines are often ineffective treatment options for OIP because the cause of the pruritus may be centrally mediated rather than through mast cell activation and histamine release (Brennan, Josland, & Kelly, 2015). The histamine effect of many opioids is negligible or variable. It is possible for morphine and codeine to cause histamine release, but most OIP is related to central mu opioid effects. Reports of relief of OIP with antihistamines are more likely due to the sedating effect of the antihistamine that allows patients to sleep and interrupts the itch-scratch cycle than to any significant pharmacodynamic response (Ko, 2015; Kumar & Singh, 2013). Table 12.3 provides a summary of medications used in the prophylaxis and treatment of OIP.

Table 12.3 | Opioid-Induced Pruritus Prophylaxis/Treatment

Medication	Dose (refer to product information for dosing frequency)	Mechanism	Benefits	Warnings/Limitations
Naloxone	• Continuous IV infusion 0.25–1 mcg/kg/h	Mu opioid receptor antagonist	• Rapid onset	• Doses > 2 mcg/kg/h may reverse analgesia • Infusion needed because of short half-life (<1 h) • Not effective for intrathecal OIP
Naltrexone	• Oral: 9 mg • Epidural: Up to 0.3 mcg/kg/h • Continuous IV infusion: 0.25–1 mcg/kg/h	Mu opioid receptor antagonist	• Twice as potent as naloxone • Half-life 4–5 h	• 9-mg oral dose available from compounding pharmacies as smallest oral tablet is 25 mg • Oral doses more than 9 mg may reverse analgesia

Continued

Table 12.3 | Opioid-Induced Pruritus Prophylaxis/Treatment—cont'd

Medication	Dose (refer to product information for dosing frequency)	Mechanism	Benefits	Warnings/Limitations
Nalbuphine	• Continuous IV infusion: 2.5 mg/h • IV bolus: 2–3 mg • Epidural: 3–4 mg • IM: 1–5 mg	Mixed mu opioid agonist-antagonist	• Superior to propofol and ondansetron • Highly effective agent	• May cause sedation
Ondansetron	• IV bolus: 4 mg–8 mg	Serotonin (5-HT$_3$) receptor antagonist	• May be an effective prophylactic agent	• Mixed evidence for effectiveness as a treatment option • Potential for QTc prolongation
Droperidol	• IV bolus: 1.25–2.5 mg • Epidural: 1.25–5 mg	Dopamine (D2) receptor antagonist and weak 5-HT$_3$ antagonist	• Lacking strong evidence but may be superior to propofol as a prophylactic agent	• Less effective than mu opioid antagonists • Contraindicated in patients with QTc prolongation
Propofol	• IV bolus: 10–20 mg	May potentiate GABA-A receptor	• Possible prophylaxis for IT OIP • May relieve OIP associated with epidural morphine	• Limited evidence to support efficacy as a prophylactic or treatment option for OIP
Mirtazapine	• Oral: 30 mg	Presynaptic alpha$_2$ antagonist; 5-HT$_2$/5-HT$_3$ antagonist	• Central and peripherally acting • Longer duration than 5-HT$_3$ antagonists • Found to decrease incidence, duration, and severity of OIP after IT morphine	• Limited evidence to support efficacy as a prophylactic or treatment option for OIP
Gabapentin	• Oral: 1200 mg one time pre-op dose	Anticonvulsant and structural analog of GABA	• May reduce incidence, duration, and severity of OIP after IT morphine	• Limited evidence to support efficacy as a prophylactic or treatment option for OIP
Promethazine	• IV bolus: 50 mg	H1 antagonist (antihistamine), anticholinergic activity	• May reduce peripherally induced OIP	• Lacks evidence to support efficacy as a prophylactic or treatment option for neuraxial OIP • Boxed warning: Serious tissue injury, including gangrene
DiphenhydrAMINE	• Oral/IV bolus: 25–50 mg	H1 antagonist (antihistamine) with anticholinergic activity	• Sedating effect may decrease perception of OIP • Effective for peripherally induced OIP	• Ineffective for central (neuraxial) OIP • Increases sedation
HydrOXYzine	• Oral: 25–100 mg • IM: 25 mg (avoid this route if possible because of injection site pain and possible reaction)	H1 antagonist (antihistamine) with anticholinergic activity	• Sedating effect may decrease perception of OIP • Effective for peripherally induced OIP	• Ineffective for central (neuraxial) OIP • Increases sedation • Dose adjustment in renal impairment

GABA, γ-Aminobutyric acid; *H1*, histamine-1; *IM*, intramuscular; *IT*, intrathecal; *IV*, intravenous; *OIP*, opioid-induced pruritus.

Other Prevention and Management Considerations

Like many opioid-induced unintended effects, pruritus associated with opioids is best addressed by prevention, which is optimized by use of the lowest possible doses of the opioid that will provide effective relief of pain. The use of a multimodal analgesic plan for pain management is instrumental in achieving this goal. If OIP is present, strategies to reduce it include opioid rotation, dose reduction, administration route change, and nonpharmacologic comfort measures. Although dose reductions may be helpful, relief may not be adequate and it may be beneficial to change to an opioid or route that is less associated with pruritus. For example, if a patient is taking morphine and having pruritus, a rotation to HYDROmorphone, oxyMORphone, or fentaNYL, which have not been found to induce histamine release, may be helpful. If the patient with pruritus has been receiving an opioid with local anesthetic in an epidural solution, some pruritus relief may be possible if the opioid is removed from the epidural route and administered orally. Nonpharmacologic approaches, such as cool compresses or moisturizers, may be comforting, but there are no readily identified, evidence-based, nonpharmacologic approaches to OIP. If nonpharmacologic approaches and opioid adjustments mentioned at the beginning of this paragraph do not provide adequate relief, the use of pharmacologic interventions to prevent or treat OIP may be necessary. Table 12.4 summarizes the pharmacologic options for OIP that have been presented in this chapter.

Urinary Retention

Urinary retention is another unintended effect of opioid therapy. Pain, cystitis, and urinary tract infections are commonly recognized risks and complications of urinary retention, and other complications such as prolonged detrusor muscle impairments and chronic bladder problems may develop (Choi & Awad, 2013). Urinary retention can occur in any patients who receive opioids, but it is often seen and has been extensively studied in surgical patients because it often complicates the postoperative recovery period. The incidence of postoperative urinary retention may range from 2.1% to 36.6% (and higher), and the wide range may result from the lack of a single widely accepted definition of urinary retention (Choi & Awad, 2013; de Boer, Detriche, & Forget, 2017; Tischler et al., 2016). A summary of the mechanisms involved in micturition is provided in Box 12.3 and Fig. 12.3.

Although different mechanisms may be responsible for urinary retention, systemic opioids have been shown to exert a dose-dependent response. Opioids may cause a dose-dependent reduction in the sensation for urge to void, and although tolerance to urinary retention develops, the recovery of function varies based on the individual opioid's properties (Kowalik & Plante, 2016). The incidence of opioid-related urinary retention is affected by the type of opioid, route, dose, and duration of opioid administration. Mu receptor opioid agonists, particularly morphine, have been shown to have an antidiuretic effect and inhibit electrolyte excretion, while kappa receptor stimulation has a diuretic response without a direct electrolyte effect (Fukada, 2015). Opioids may inhibit the voiding reflex and increase the tone of the external sphincter (Bristow et al., 2014). Systemic opioids exert an effect on the spinal cord and block the parasympathetic effect of acetylcholine, which results in relaxation of the detrusor muscle and subsequent urinary retention (Choi & Awad, 2013). Spinal administration of short and long-acting opioids may also cause weakening of detrusor muscle contraction. Intrathecal morphine administration is associated with

---

Box 12.3 | Physiology: Micturition

Normal bladder function involves the storage and elimination of urine.

1. Bladder function is controlled by supraspinal and medullary centers via autonomic and somatic pathways.
2. Sympathetic nerves are involved in urinary collection by inhibiting micturition (voiding). The sympathetic activity of the hypogastric nerve prevents detrusor muscle contraction, which enables the bladder to fill.
3. Pudendal nerve activity is responsible for contraction of the bladder sphincters (S2-S4), thus preventing urine from flowing out of the bladder as urine collects.
4. Stretch receptors in the bladder wall (detrusor muscle) begin to signal the central nervous system via afferent nerves when about 150 mL of volume collects in the bladder. When the bladder fills to 300 to 400 mL, the voiding reflex can then be facilitated by centers in the pons to allow micturition. Neurotransmitters, including dopamine and serotonin.
5. For micturition to occur, the sympathetic activity of the pudendal nerve must be blocked to allow parasympathetic activity to relax the internal and external bladder sphincters.
6. Parasympathetic nerves (pelvic nerves S2–S4) facilitate activation of the detrusor muscle and relaxation of the urethral smooth muscle, thus permitting micturition to occur.

Modified from Kowalik, U., & Plante, M. K. (2016). Urinary retention in surgical patients. *Surgical Clinics of North America*, 96(3), 453–467; and Darrah, D. M., Griebling, T. L., & Silverstein, J. H. (2009). Postoperative urinary retention. *Anesthesiology Clinics*, 27(3), 465–484.

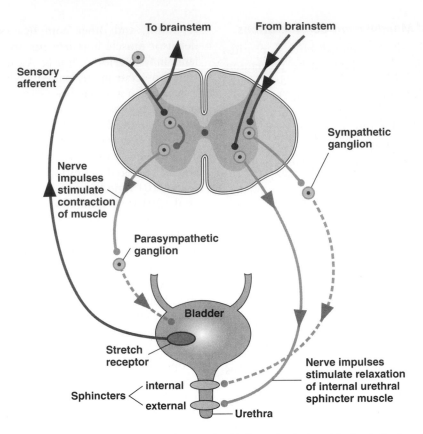

Fig. 12.3 | **Micturition Reflex Pathway.** (Courtesy McGill Molson Medical Informatics Project, Montreal, Quebec, Canada, with permission.)

a urinary retention incidence of 42% to 80% because of inhibition of parasympathetic activity and resulting relaxation of the detrusor muscle (de Boer et al., 2017). Although local anesthetics, which are often used in spinal anesthesia, are known to cause urinary retention, the incidence is increased when opioids are combined with local anesthetics. Longer acting neuraxial opioids such as epidural or intrathecal morphine have an increased incidence and longer duration of effect than shorter acting lipophilic opioids such as fentaNYL (Choi & Awad, 2013).

Assessment for Urinary Retention

The assessment of urinary retention related to opioid use is the same as the assessment for any other potential cause of retention. Awareness that the administration of opioids, especially in surgical patients, may contribute to the development of urinary retention necessitates monitoring of urinary output to ensure that output is sufficient, attention to complaints of bladder pain or discomfort, and examination for bladder distention, including bladder scanning. For postoperative patients, bladder ultrasound may be performed 4 hours after surgery or after Foley catheter removal. If the volume is more than 500 mL and the patient is unable to void, the bladder may be straight catheterized. Subsequent voiding attempts continue with ongoing assessment, scanning, and straight catheterization when residual volumes are more than 500 mL (Choi & Awad, 2013).

Prevention and Management of Opioid-Related Urinary Retention

Although indwelling urinary catheters are often used for the prevention of urinary retention in postoperative patients, particularly in those who have epidural catheters or have received spinal anesthesia, initiatives to reduce catheter-associated urinary tract infections have led to reductions in routine use of indwelling urinary catheters. Studies that examined the effect of early indwelling urinary catheter removal in patients with thoracic and lumbar epidural analgesia have demonstrated variable results.

Although epidural analgesia is associated with higher rates of urinary retention than systemic opioid administration, thoracic epidurals are associated with less urinary retention than lumbar epidurals. In a literature review of thoracic epidural analgesia for the management of postthoracotomy pain, the incidence of urinary retention in the 203 patients who had urinary catheters removed by the first day after surgery was 5.9%, almost five-fold lower than previously reported risks (Zaouter & Ouattara, 2015a). These results were not supported by another study, but the researchers noted the benefits of early removal on early mobilization and urinary tract infection reduction and suggest that early removal should be attempted (Hu et al., 2014). Others have recommended that in patients who have had thoracic surgery, the urinary catheter should be left in place until the epidural is removed, because significant urinary retention was noted with earlier removal and there was minimal risk for urinary tract infection if the urinary catheter was continued until the epidural was discontinued (Allen et al., 2016). Because lumbar spinal segments are involved in urinary tract function, it may be anticipated that the risk for urinary retention would be increased with lumbar epidural catheter infusion (Zaouter & Outtara, 2015b). Thus there may be more hesitation to remove urinary catheters soon after surgery for patients with lumbar epidurals, although if removed, trial voids and assessment for urinary retention may be attempted.

Many factors may contribute to the development of postoperative urinary retention, including opioid administration; therefore measures may be taken to reduce risks. These measures include, when possible, avoidance of other medications, such as anticholinergics, beta-blockers, and sympathomimetics, which contribute to retention, and avoidance of excessive administration of intravenous fluids (Umer, Ross-Richardson, & Ellner, 2015). Perioperative administration of larger volumes of intravenous fluids has been associated with an increased risk, but there is a lack of consensus as to the recommended limit (Kowalik & Plante, 2016). The most definitive recommendations for the prevention and reduction of opioid-related urinary retention are those that result in opioid reduction. To achieve this goal, while optimizing patient comfort, the implementation of multimodal analgesic measures is recommended. The addition of nonopioids, including acetaminophen, and use of opioid-sparing interventional techniques are recommended to facilitate less opioid use and lessen the unintended effect of urinary retention (de Boer et al., 2017).

Although many multimodal analgesic protocols include the use of nonsteroidal antiinflammatory drugs (NSAIDs), these medications have not been shown to reduce opioid-induced urinary retention and may increase the risk. NSAIDs are associated with a two-fold increase in the risk for urinary retention thought to be related to the inhibition of cyclooxygenase 2 (COX-2) and reduction in intravesical prostaglandin E_2 (PGE_2) levels (Darrah, Griebling, Silverstein, 2009). Other nonopioid analgesics, such as ketamine, have not been shown to contribute to urinary retention (Jouguelet-Lacoste, La Colla, Schilling, & Chelly, 2015). Other measures that may reduce opioid-related urinary retention include the use of regional anesthetic techniques, particularly techniques that do not include opioids, such as peripheral nerve blocks with local anesthetics. Epidural or intrathecal medications using lipophilic opioids such as fentaNYL, rather than morphine, are associated with less urinary retention and should be used when opioids are needed. The use of MMA and avoidance or early removal of urinary drainage catheters are measures that are strongly supported in many of

the Enhanced Recovery After Surgery (ERAS) protocols (Tan, Law, & Gan, 2015).

No recent published reviews have addressed the use of opioid antagonists in the prevention or treatment of opioid-related urinary retention. Although some literature points to a potential role for the use of peripherally acting opioid antagonists such as methylnaltrexone and alvimopam to address this unintended effect, there is a lack of evidence to support the use of these medications for this effect. A study of the use of methylnaltrexone in the prevention of opioid-related side effects in orthopedic patients who received intrathecal morphine did not show any reduction in the incidence of urinary retention (Zand, Amini, Asadi, & Farbood, 2015). Additional research to determine the role of peripheral opioid antagonists in the treatment of opioid-related urinary retention is needed. Although isolated studies have shown that opioid antagonists, such as naloxone, may reduce urinary retention (Gallo, DuRand, & Pshon, 2008), others (Wang, Pennefather, & Russell, 1998) have demonstrated that the central action of this intervention places the patient at risk for reversal of analgesia, and therefore this practice is not recommended.

Nonpharmacologic interventions, not specific for opioid-induced urinary retention, have been used to prevent and alleviate urinary retention. Having the patient void immediately before surgery may reduce the risk for postoperative urinary retention (Hansen, Søreide, Warland, & Nilsen, 2011). Practices such as lying flat and relaxing muscles, getting out of bed and standing in an upright position, relaxation techniques, taking a shower, applying ice, running water from a faucet, and tapping the groin are mentioned in the literature. A study by Afazel, Jalali, Sadat, and Mahmoodi (2014) of 126 men with postoperative urinary retention who were divided into three groups, compared the application of hot packs, gauze soaked in lukewarm water, and a control group of no intervention on the suprapubic regions of participants. Results indicated that retention was alleviated 71.4%, 59.5%, and 7.1% in the respective groups. The participants were heterogeneous for other risks for urinary retention, but most had received opioids.

Hypogonadism

Hypogonadism, or androgen deficiency, is a complication of chronic daily opioid use that can result in significant health problems. In a systematic review, although high-quality studies were lacking, there was fair evidence to associate hypogonadism with chronic opioid therapy (Birthi, Nagar, Nickerson, & Sloan, 2015). Hypogonadism may develop in both men and women, although there are few studies of opioid-induced hypogonadism in women. Hypogonadism develops as a result of reduction of gonadotropin-releasing hormone, which is responsible for the release of luteinizing hormone (LH) and follicle-stimulating hormone (FSH) from the pituitary gland (Ali, Raphael, Khan, Labib, & Duarte, 2016). Male hypogonadism is characterized by low testosterone levels, LH, and FSH, which account for symptoms of decreased libido, impotence, decreased body hair, decreased muscle strength, and fatigue. Female hypogonadism may result in decreased libido, irregular menstrual cycles, oligomenorrhea, amenorrhea, hot flashes, and inability to conceive (Ali, Raphael, Khan, Labib, & Duarte, 2016). Other consequences of hypogonadism include depression, osteoporosis, osteopenia, and reduced quality of life (Rubinstein & Carpenter, 2017). Opioid-induced hypogonadism is often undiagnosed because health providers may not ask about these symptoms and patients may be reluctant to report them.

In studies, the chronic use of long-acting opioids has shown an association with a higher risk of androgen deficiency than the chronic use of short-acting opioids (Rubinstein & Carpenter, 2014; Rubinstein, Carpenter, & Minkoff, 2013). Intrathecal opioid administration also has been associated with hypogonadism (Kim et al., 2014). The reason for the higher risk with long-acting opioids is proposed to be related to greater suppression of the hypothalamic-pituitary-gonadal axis as a result of constant, rather than variable, opioid levels. In a follow-up study, Rubinstein and Carpenter (2017) reported that methadone, oxyCODONE, and transdermal fentaNYL are associated with greater odds of developing androgen deficiency than HYDROcodone. They report that other factors contributing to hypogonadism include obesity, age 50 years or older, and at least two comorbidities (e.g., diabetes, hypertension, and hyperlipidemia).

Although chronic opioid use may lead to hypogonadism, it is interesting to note that low testosterone levels may affect endogenous opioid activity. Testosterone has a role in the binding of opioid receptors, dopamine activation, norepinephrine activity, and blood-brain barrier transport (Alyautdin, Khalin, Nafeeza, Haron, & Kuznetsov, 2014; Gudin, Laitman, & Nalamachu, 2015). Testosterone is involved in pain modulation, and low testosterone levels are associated with the development of fibromyalgia and other chronic pain conditions (White & Robinson, 2015). In a pilot study of the use of testosterone gel in 12 patients with fibromyalgia who had testosterone deficiency, it was shown that in addition to improvements in fatigue and libido, muscle pain and stiffness were significantly improved (White et al., 2015).

Assessment

Hypogonadism may be primary (the result of primary testicular or ovarian failure) or secondary (the result of secondary testicular or ovarian failure as a result of hypothalamic or pituitary malfunction). Opioid-induced

hypogonadism is a form of secondary hypogonadism. Diagnosis involves assessment of the patient's symptoms. For men, validated tools such as the Saint Louis University Androgen Deficiency in Aging Male (ADAM) with 97% sensitivity and 30% specificity, the Aging Male Survey (AMS) with 83% sensitivity and 39% specificity, and the Massachusetts Male Aging Study (MMAS) with 60% sensitivity and 59% specificity, have been developed as potential screening tools for hypogonadism in males (Morley, Perry, Kevorkian, & Patrick, 2006). Secondary hypogonadism in men is diagnosed by assessment of symptoms and laboratory values which show low serum testosterone and low LH and FSH. Women with secondary hypogonadism are also diagnosed by symptom assessment and the observation of low estrogen and FSH laboratory values. Physical findings of hypogonadism may include reduced facial and body hair, decreased muscle mass, weight gain, osteopenia, and osteoporosis (Raheem, Patel, Sisul, Furnish, & Hsieh, 2017). There is no consensus as to whether baseline laboratory testing or regular monitoring of androgen levels should be conducted for patients on chronic opioid therapy. Box 12.4 summarizes the criteria involved in the diagnosis of hypogonadism.

Prevention and Management of Opioid-Induced Hypogonadism

Prevention of opioid-induced hypogonadism can be facilitated by use of multimodal analgesic approaches to aid in the avoidance (if possible) and minimization of chronic opioid use. Hypogonadism risk appears to be increased with long-acting opioids; therefore pain management plans of care that include a foundation of nonopioid medications and interventions are preferred because it may be possible to limit opioids to short-acting formulations on an *as-needed* basis. If an opioid is necessary, HYDROcodone may result in less risk for hypogonadism than oxyCODONE, methadone, or transdermal fentaNYL (Rubinstein & Carpenter, 2017).

Although evidence is lacking, treatment of hypogonadism involves diet, exercise, opioid dose reduction, rotation, and, if possible, discontinuation of opioids (Brennan, 2013). In men, if opioid therapy cannot be discontinued, testosterone replacement therapy is initiated based on patient symptoms and serum levels. A number of clinical trials have been conducted to evaluate the use of testosterone replacement therapy in men with opioid-induced hypogonadism, although large, well-designed RCTs are lacking. In a study by Basaria et al. (2015), 84 men aged 18 to 64 who had opioid-induced hypogonadism participated in a trial in which 36 men were randomized to a group who received 12 weeks of testosterone replacement and 29 men who received placebo. After 12 weeks of treatment, those who received testosterone demonstrated improved pressure pain threshold, mechanical pain intensity, cold pressor pain, and mood compared to the placebo group. In another study, Raheem et al. (2016) followed 27 men with

Box 12.4	Diagnosis of Opioid-Induced Hypogonadism

- Clinical evaluation: Screen for the following symptoms:
  - Amenorrhea, irregular menses, galactorrhea
  - Decreased libido
  - Decreased muscle mass and strength
  - Depression and anxiety
  - Erectile dysfunction (men)
  - Hot flashes and night sweats
  - Infertility
  - Osteoporosis and fractures
  - Tiredness or fatigue
  - Decreased opioid effect
  - Pain
- Laboratory evaluation suggestions:
  - Dehydroepiandrosterone sulfate
  - Estradiol (women)
  - Free testosterone
  - Luteinizing hormone
  - Sex hormone–binding globulin

- Total testosterone
- Bone density (optional)
- Follicle-stimulating hormone
- Rule out other causes of central hypogonadism:
  - Alcoholism
  - Corticosteroid therapy
  - Hemochromatosis
  - Idiopathic gonadotropin or gonadotropin-releasing hormone deficiency
  - Pituitary-hypothalamic injury
- Tumors
- Trauma
- Radiation

Modified from Brennan, M. J. (2013). The effect of opioid therapy on endocrine function. *The American Journal of Medicine, 126*(3), S12–S18, Table 1.

opioid-induced hypogonadism for 18 months. Of the men, 11 received testosterone supplementation therapy and 16 patients were in the control group. Men in the treatment group reported significantly lower pain scores, had significant improvements in hypogonadal symptoms, and required significantly less opioid than those in the control group.

It is generally agreed that patients with serum total testosterone levels below 8.0 nmol/L will benefit from testosterone replacement (Ali et al., 2016). However, there is no consensus about the type of testosterone replacement therapy or dose that is optimal for the treatment of opioid-induced hypogonadism. Testosterone can be administered as a gel, patch, or depot injection, and the dose is determined by standard accepted guidelines, according to patient symptoms, baseline, and follow-up serum testosterone levels (Ali et al., 2016; O'Rourke & Wosnitzer, 2016).

Data to support the use of testosterone replacement therapy for women are limited. Testosterone replacement therapy is not approved for women by the FDA. However, when used off-label, it has been recommended that the starting doses be markedly less than those used for men. Dehydroepiandrosterone (DHEA) with a dose of 50 mg/day is another potential treatment for women with opioid-induced hypogonadism (Gudin et al., 2015). DHEA is available as a poorly regulated over-the-counter dietary supplement, thus having variable actual DHEA content.

Although testosterone replacement therapy may be beneficial in improving pain and symptoms of androgen insufficiency, long-term risks are not well known and there are a number of potential side effects identified in men, including hematologic abnormalities (polycythemia), lowered sperm counts, exacerbation of sleep-disordered breathing, infertility, prostatic hypertrophy, and cardiovascular risks (Brennan, 2013). There are concerns that testosterone therapy may increase the risks for development or progression of prostate cancer. Although risks are less well known in women, hormone therapy in women is associated with risks for cardiovascular disease and breast cancer (Brennan, 2013). In 2015 the FDA issued a safety announcement about the use of testosterone and noted that prescription testosterone products are approved only for certain medical conditions. Opioid-induced hypogonadism is not among the approved indications for use.

Sedation

Sedation and other cognitive changes are unintended consequences of opioid use. These changes may occur with acute and chronic opioid use and may range from impaired attention and concentration to delirium and sedation. Mu opioid receptor activation is often implicated in the cognitive changes seen with opioid therapy. Mu_2 receptor activation, in particular, has been associated with a number of opioid-related unintended effects, including the development of sedation (Wiffen, Wee, Derry, Bell, & Moore, 2017). However, some experts have postulated that the cholinergic system, because of its role in modulating cortical arousal and information processing, may contribute to the unintended effect of sedation (Dhingra, Ahmed, Shin, Scharaga, & Magun, 2015). Sedation is a particularly concerning unintended effect of opioid therapy because, in opioid-naïve patients as well as opioid-tolerant patients, it may precede respiratory depression, which is also associated with mu_2 activation.

The assessment of sedation in patients who are receiving opioids is an essential aspect of care because excessive sedation precedes the development of opioid-induced respiratory depression (Jungquist et al., 2016).

It is difficult to determine sedation prevalence because sedation lacks a widely accepted definition. Sedation occurs on a continuum ranging from mild drowsiness to unresponsiveness. Tools such as the Pasero Opioid Sedation Scale (POSS) have been developed to aid practitioners in identifying and intervening for advancing levels of opioid-induced sedation (Pasero, 2009). See Chapter 13 for discussion of the POSS. Although the Richmond Agitation Sedation Scale (RASS) is used to assess sedation, particularly in intensive care unit settings (Devlin et al., 2018), it is not specific to assessing sedation induced by opioids.

Recent data related to the prevalence of sedation in patients who receive opioids for acute postoperative pain are limited, but in drug safety studies, sedation is often cited as a common side effect of opioid administration. In a recent study of over 1100 emergency department patients who received morphine, drowsiness was identified in 8.9% of the patients within 6 hours of morphine administration (Bounes et al., 2017). In a review of opioid-related adverse events that developed in patients with cancer after starting opioid treatment, drowsiness was found to have a prevalence of approximately 20% and was reported as moderate to severe (Oosten et al., 2015). Sedation is often first noted on initial administration of an opioid and with increases in dose. Tolerance to the sedating effect of opioids has been shown to develop within a short period of opioid use if the dose remains stable (Trescot, 2016; Young-McCaughan & Maskowski, 2001).

Although there is less sedation with chronic use of opioids at stable doses, risk still exists. Cognitive effects and sedation also have been noted in patients who receive chronic opioid therapy. Memory deficits, sleep disturbances, fatigue, and somnolence have been reported as the most common unintended cognitive effects in 20% to 62% of this patient population (Dhingra et al., 2015). In systematic reviews, somnolence was reported in 23% of patients who received opioids for chronic cancer pain (Wiffen, Derry, & Moore, 2014) and 14% of adults with chronic noncancer pain (Moore & McQuay, 2005). Many of the studies and reviews published on unintended effects of chronic opioid therapy were done in the late 1990s and early 2000s. Results must be viewed carefully because study designs varied, terms were not well defined, and although studies of patients with chronic pain were used, the length of opioid treatment varied in some studies.

Assessment

The use of standardized monitoring tools and scales to facilitate assessment of sedation level is described in Chapter 13.

Prevention and Management

Opioid-induced sedation, like other opioid-related unintended effects, is best prevented or minimized through the use of MMA to minimize opioid administration while controlling pain. Another major consideration in the prevention or reduction of unintended sedation or other negative cognitive effects is to minimize drug-drug interactions that may contribute to these unintended effects. Concomitant use of opioids and benzodiazepines, antihistamines, or hypnotics increase risks for sedation and cognitive changes. Particularly with concomitant use of opioids and benzodiazepines, the risk for respiratory depression is increased.

The treatment of opioid-induced sedation for patients with acute pain is guided by the degree of sedation. Mild drowsiness in the first few days of opioid treatment is common and usually requires only patient reassurance that the drowsiness will resolve in a short time. More significant sedation may require more definitive interventions. The patient who is excessively sedated requires close monitoring for advancing sedation, which may precede the development of respiratory depression. In addition to frequent and skilled sedation assessment, patients who are more than slightly drowsy may require frequent stimulation to reduce the risk for hypoventilation. In the postanesthesia setting, nurses use a "stir up regimen" in which patients are verbally or tactilely stimulated to awaken, cough, deep breathe, and move to reduce the risks of anesthesia and opioid administration (Godden, 2018). In other settings, light verbal stimulation from staff members and visitors, as well as stimulation from procedures, may be adequate to address opioid-related sedation. If, however, sedation is more significant, opioid dose reduction and/or changes in dosing frequency (including patient-controlled analgesia) adjustment are necessary, because sedation, like many opioid-related unintended effects, is often dose dependent. If sedation advances and respiratory status is compromised (i.e., rate, depth, rhythm, carbon dioxide, or oxygenation levels), emergency measures, including naloxone administration and other rapid response interventions to support or restore adequate ventilation and oxygenation, are necessary.

Many patients with chronic pain who have been receiving chronic opioid therapy develop tolerance to the sedating effects of opioids when receiving a stable dose. However, some continue to experience sedation and, like the patient who receives opioids for acute pain, may benefit from dose reduction and/or opioid rotation. Reductions in opioid dose have been found to be particularly useful in reducing the cognitive unintended effects of opioids, including sedation and delirium (Rogers, Mehta, Shengelia, & Reid, 2013). If dose reductions are not effective in reducing unintended sedation or other cognitive effects or if dose reductions result in inadequate analgesia, rotation to another opioid may be helpful (Rogers et al., 2013; Smith & Peppin, 2014). Patients who have

Table 12.4 | Pharmacologic Approaches to Opioid-Induced Sedation

Medication	Dose and Route
Modafinil	100–200 mg/day PO
Methylphenidate	2.5–5 mg PO bid (morning and midday)
Dextroamphetamine	2.5–15 mg PO daily to bid
Caffeine	200 mg IV once daily or in caffeinated beverages as tolerated
Donepezil	2.5–15 mg PO once daily

IV, Intravenously; *PO*, orally.
From Dhingra, L., Ahmed, E., Shin, J., Scharaga, E., & Magun, M. (2015). Cognitive effects and sedation. *Pain Medicine, 16*(suppl_1), S37–S43.

experienced unintended effects of opioids in one class (e.g., morphine, oxyCODONE, or HYDROmorphone from the phenanthine class) may have a reduction in side effects if rotated to another class (e.g., fentaNYL from the phenylpiperidine class) (Rogers et al., 2013).

In limited situations, particularly in patients with cancer near the end of life, if the previously described measures do not adequately relieve opioid-induced sedation, CNS stimulants have been used to reduce sedation without adversely effecting analgesia. There is very limited data available to support this practice and this is an off-label use of these medications. The more commonly used and studied CNS stimulants are methylphenidate and modafinil (Dhingra et al., 2015). If these medications are not available or are poorly tolerated, other options include the use of psychostimulants such as caffeine or dextroamphetamine, although data to show effectiveness of these agents are limited (Dhingra et al., 2015). Donepezil, an acetylcholinesterase inhibitor, is another treatment option that, in limited studies, has demonstrated improved alertness without reducing analgesia (Bruera et al., 2003). The effects of the addition of the psychostimulant medications must be carefully monitored, because they can result in increased anxiety, insomnia, and loss of appetite (Ruddy, Barton, & Loprinzi, 2014). Monitoring is also indicated because of abuse and aberrant drug use behaviors associated with psychostimulant use (Dhingra et al., 2015). Table 12.4 provides a summary of medications that may be useful in the management of opioid-induced sedation.

Myoclonus

Opioids have been associated with several neuroexcitatory effects that may present as movement abnormalities. The cause of these abnormalities is poorly understood, and lim-ited research has been published regarding these conditions in recent years. Because myoclonic activity may arise from different causes, including medication-induced, further diagnostic evaluation may be necessary (Levy & Chen, 2016; Mills, & Mari, 2015). Myoclonus is a movement abnormality that may be associated with opioid use, regardless of administration route. Much of the research related to this unintended effect has occurred in patients with cancer, in whom opioids are often used in high doses over extended periods. The accumulation of opioid neuroexcitatory metabolites has been identified as a possible factor in the development of opioid-related myoclonus, although research is limited and results are conflicting (Lee, Ganta, Horton, & Chai, 2017). Morphine and HYDROmorphone have active neuroexcitatory metabolites that may accumulate, particularly with renal impairment. The morphine metabolite morphine-3-glucuronide (M3G), which has no analgesic effect, is a neuroexcitatory metabolite that contributes to myoclonus, hyperalgesia, allodynia, and seizures (Lee et al., 2017). HYDROmorphone-3-glucuronide (H3G) is the active HYDROmorphone metabolite, and although it has no analgesic effect, it has been shown, in rat studies, to cause dose-dependent myoclonus, agitation, and seizures (Lee et al., 2017).

The presence of neuroexcitatory metabolites is not sufficient to explain the development of myoclonus with opioid therapy. For example, neuroexcitatory changes have also been seen with fentaNYL and methadone, but these medications lack neuroexcitatory metabolites. Another proposed explanation for opioid-induced myoclonus is that neuroplastic changes from opioid use increase sensitivity to neuroexcitatory substances such as glutamate and N-methyl-D-aspartate (NMDA) (Lee, Silverman, Hansen, Patel, & Manchikanti, 2011). Alterations in serotonin metabolism and interactions with other neurotransmitters and dopamine uptake changes regulated by the glutaminergic system may also play a role (Mercadante, 1998). In some cases, preservatives used in parenteral opioid preparations and drug-drug interactions have been implicated in the development of myoclonus (Ahmedzai, 2017; Mercadante, 1998).

Assessment

When assessing patients on opioid therapy, especially during sleep, it is important to observe for abnormal movements and report these movements to ensure appropriate intervention. Known history of opioid use, especially opioids with neuroexcitatory metabolites in patients with decreased renal function, is useful in distinguishing opioid-induced myoclonus from other abnormal movement disorders. Myoclonus is evidenced by abnormal twitching and jerking of various muscle groups, usually involving the extremities (Mercadante, 1998). The frequency, duration, and intensity of the twitching and jerking movements vary among individuals.

Prevention and Management

Although the cause of myoclonus is not well understood, some measures can be taken to reduce risks for myoclonus development. The use of multimodal analgesic approaches and nonpharmacologic interventions may reduce opioid doses and duration of opioid therapy, thereby reducing the risks for myoclonus. Myoclonus is strongly associated with medications that have neuroexcitatory metabolites, such as morphine and HYDROmorphone. Therefore, in patients who require high doses of these agents and/or in patients with renal insufficiency, it is advisable to minimize or avoid use of these medications. Other medications, such as meperidine and traMADol, have proconvulsant metabolites that are associated with neuropsychiatric events and reduction in seizure threshold and therefore are avoided, particularly in renal insufficiency, especially when repeated doses are required (Lucyk & Nelson, 2016; Robottom, Shulman, & Weiner, 2012).

The treatment of opioid-induced myoclonus, in addition to the use of MMA, includes opioid dose reduction, if possible. If pain is not acceptable at lower doses of the same opioid, it may be necessary to rotate to an opioid that lacks neuroexcitatory metabolites such as fentaNYL or methadone (Mercadante, 1998). When possible, increased hydration may aid in elimination of toxic metabolites (Mercadante, 1998). If it is not possible to reduce the dose or rotate the opioid, coadministration of a benzodiazepine such as clonazePAM may reduce myoclonus; however, patients must be closely observed, because coadministration of an opioid and benzodiazepine increases risks for overdose, respiratory depression, and death (Hirschtritt, Delucchi, & Olfson, 2017).

Opioid-Induced Hyperalgesia

Hyperalgesia is the phenomenon in which pain is perceived as greatly intensified or exaggerated compared to what is expected to be perceived (Compton, Canamar, Hillhouse, & Ling, 2012). The International Association for the Study of Pain (IASP, 2014) specifies that the increase in hyperalgesia is in response to noxious stimuli that is expected to cause pain. Hyperalgesia may result from damage to tissue or nerves, from stress and particularly the stress related to illness, or as an unintended result of opioid administration (Jennings, Okine, Roche, & Finn, 2014; Mann & Chai, 2014).

Opioid-induced hyperalgesia (OIH) is defined as "a paradoxical condition where the intensity of the perceived pain increases rather than decreases in response to opioid administration" (Eisenberg, Suzan, & Pud, 2015, p. 632–633). An important distinction between OIH and opioid tolerance is that with OIH, opioids cause magnification of pain whereas with opioid tolerance, opioids still are used to alleviate pain (Mauermann et al., 2016). OIH is thought to occur when opioids intensify sensitivity

to unpleasant triggers (Fletcher & Martinez, 2014), and as a result the opioids actually increase the intensity of pain. Although the phenomenon has been observed since 1870 when the paradox was described by Albutt, there is still controversy as to whether it actually occurs as a separate entity, or, if instead, it is a misinterpretation of withdrawal, tolerance, or even substance use disorder (Eisenberg et al., 2015).

That it can occur with acute postoperative pain and with chronic pain and that the processes may be different at the different time frames complicate efforts in understanding OIH (Jamison & Mao, 2015; Lavand'homme & Steyaert, 2017). In addition, it is suggested that when postoperative OIH extends beyond areas of the actual surgical intervention, it is predictive of the acute postoperative pain evolving into chronic pain (Deumens et al., 2013). What does seem to be essential in the identification of OIH is that the paradox must occur while opioids are being taken and that it is a clinical syndrome (Lavand'homme & Steyaert, 2017).

In acute postoperative pain situations, remifentanil has been correlated with OIH (Wu, Huang, & Sun, 2015). A systematic review and meta-analysis of 27 studies suggested that acute pain intensity may increase postoperatively after high-dose remifentanil administration during surgery and that higher doses of morphine may be required in the immediate postoperative period (e.g., 24 hours) (Fletcher & Martinez, 2014). To date, research into OIH with acute pain is relatively new and there is little similarity among the samples, specifics, or results of the studies (Mauermann et al., 2016). Although postoperative OIH is most often associated with remifentanil and fentaNYL (Jamison & Mao, 2015; Lavand'homme & Steyaert, 2017; Raffa & Pergolizzi, 2013), researchers of a small Israeli study with 30 patients with chronic neuropathic lower back pain who were treated with oral HYDROmorphone for 1 month reported that OIH was induced by HYDROmorphone (Suzan, Eisenberg, Treister, Haddad, & Pud, 2013). Morphine has long been identified with OIH (Eisenberg et al., 2015). It is thought this is due, at least in part, to morphine causing an activation of excitatory receptors (e.g., NMDA receptor) (Raffa & Pergolizzi, 2013). The M3G metabolite of morphine also has been implicated in the development of hyperalgesia (Cortazzo, Copenhaver, & Fishman, 2014). In addition, OIH has been identified among people who are in medication-assisted therapy (methadone and buprenorphine) as treatment for substance use disorder (Compton et al., 2012) (see Chapter 14).

OIH may be treated pharmacologically. A basic option is to change the type of opioid used. Because there is incomplete cross-tolerance among opioids, when rotating from one opioid to another, the new opioid dose may provide adequate analgesia with a starting dose that is 25% to 50% less than the equianalgesic dose of the previous opioid. When this is done, not only is there a change in opioid but the lower dosing may be beneficial.

Rotation to methadone, which has a weak NMDA anta-goproperty, may be particularly beneficial (Pasero & McCaffery, 2012).

In subanesthetic doses, ketamine has been effective in minimizing (Allen & Ivester, 2017; Gristenko, Khelemsky, Kaye, Vadivelu, & Urman, 2014), treating, and in some cases reversing OIH (Pasero & McCaffery, 2012). Although there are few studies investigating the use of ketamine as a counter to OIH, it is considered an "anti-hyperalgesic medication" in some countries (Martinez et al., 2015). It is thought that this is the result of the action of ketamine in modulating proinflammatory cyto-kines (Kaye et al., 2017) by blocking NMDA receptors (Martinez, Derivaux, & Beloeil, 2015). Dosing and tim-ing of administration to counteract OIH are not currently established, but a general discussion of patient selection, dosing, and monitoring of ketamine can be found in Chapter 15.

Prevention

Preventing the development of OIH is often more reason-able than is treatment after it advances. MMA with an "opioid-sparing" approach is one effective intervention for preventing or at least minimizing the development of OIH (Weinbroum, 2012). This can be part of perioper-ative care beginning in the operating room with use of nonopioid medications, as well as regional and spinal anesthesia. An important component of this multimodal approach is inclusion of an NMDA receptor antagonist because studies have proposed that such agents can sig-nificantly decrease postoperative OIH (Wu et al., 2015). As noted, low-dose ketamine may be effective in minimiz-ing OIH (Allen & Ivester, 2017; Gristenko et al., 2014; Weinbroum, 2012). In addition, intravenously adminis-tered acetaminophen is used as an opioid-sparing medi-cation intraoperatively (Deumens et al., 2013; Pasero & McCaffery, 2012; Pasero & Stannard, 2012; Richebéet et al., 2011). Although it has not been researched specif-ically with prevention of OIH, it is reasonable for it to be used as a multimodal component for avoiding opioid monotherapy and reducing the doses of intraoperative opioids.

Magnesium sulfate, which physiologically blocks NMDA receptors, has been effective in treating postop-erative OIH by using magnesium sulfate bolus (30 mg/kg) at the beginning of surgery along with an intraoperative infusion (10 mg/kg/h) (Weinbroum, 2017). It has also been suggested that magnesium-rich foods (e.g., chocolate, avocados, pumpkin, banana, green leafy vegetables, and almonds) may be beneficial, especially in patients with OIH who have low levels of magnesium (Bell, Borzan, Kalso, & Simonnet, 2012). Postoperative OIH resulting from remifentanil was effectively diminished when mag-nesium was administered preoperatively at induction and continued postoperatively (Lavand'homme & Steyaert, 2017; Weinbroum, 2017).

A polyamine-deficient diet is suggested to be used as a preventive measure and as a potential treatment mea-sure. The basis for this diet being potentially effective is that polyamines, which result from food intake and bacterial metabolism in the GI tract, modulate the gluta-mate/NMDA receptor and counter NMDA upregulation activity. Studies done with rats have shown polyamine-deficient diets effective in reducing and/or preventing hyperalgesia (Bell et al., 2012; Le Roy, Laboureyras, Laulin, & Simonnet, 2013; Simonnet, Laboureyras, & Sergheraert, 2013). In humans, a polyamine light diet can be adopted by selecting foods to limit the intake of polyamines (Atiya Ali, Poortvliet, Strömberg, & Yngve, 2011; Büyükuslu, 2015; Simonnet et al., 2013). Cipolla, Havouis, and Moulinoux (2007) present a comprehensive discussion with a detailed listing of the polyamine con-tents in current food.

Physical Dependence on Opioids

Physical dependence is an expected adaptation to the exposure to medications of some classes that results in a withdrawal syndrome when the medication is abruptly stopped, doses are rapidly reduced, or an antagonist to the medication is given (O'Brien, 2011). This normal physiologic response occurs in patients who have been on long-term opioid therapy and does not imply opioid use disorder (addiction). There is individual variation in the duration of opioid use that will result in physi-cal dependence. The severity of withdrawal symptoms depends on several factors, including medication type, dosage, frequency of administration, and duration of treatment (Freynhagen et al., 2016). Chapters 11 and 14 also describe opioid dependence.

Assessment

The timing for the onset of opioid withdrawal, the severity, and the duration depend on the medication used and may be related to half-life. Opioid withdrawal is usually first experienced two to three half-lives after the last dose of an opioid (Gowing, Farrell, Ali, & White, 2016). For example, with a short-acting opioid such as morphine, withdrawal may develop in a range of 6 to 10 hours after the last dose, but may peak at 36 to 48 hours and then gradually sub-side (Katzung, Masters, & Trevor, 2012). Methadone has a longer and more variable half-life; therefore, it may take several days for withdrawal to peak and up to 2 weeks for signs and symptoms to subside (Katzung et al., 2012). Signs and symptoms of opioid withdrawal include anxiety, irritability, chills and hot flashes, yawning, nausea, vomit-ing, abdominal cramps, diarrhea, rhinorrhea, diaphoresis, and piloerection (Herndon et al., 2016). Scales such as the Clinical Opioid Withdrawal Scale (COWS), described in Chapters 6 and 14, may assist in the assessment of the patient who is experiencing opioid withdrawal.

Prevention and Management

The daily dose or duration of opioid use that may result in physical dependence is variable and not well known (Minozzi, Amato, & Davoli, 2013). Patients who require opioid therapy need to be advised of the potential for the development of physical dependence and the potential for the development of withdrawal or upon discontinuation of the opioids. Patients who receive opioids for acute postoperative pain or another acute pain condition, depending on dose and duration, and those on chronic opioid therapy may experience physical dependence. It is necessary to ensure that patients are educated about the difference between physical dependence and opioid use disorder and advised to discuss withdrawal symptoms and other concerns with health providers.

Withdrawal symptoms experienced by patients who are opioid dependent may be prevented or lessened by gradual dose reductions or tapering of the dose by 10% to 20% every 48 to 72 hours over a prolonged period; if abrupt cessation is necessary, cloNIDine 0.2 to 0.4 mg/day may be used to minimize discomfort for several days after the opioid has been discontinued (Cortazzo et al., 2013). TiZANidine, a skeletal muscle relaxant with alpha$_2$-adrenergic agonist properties, is another option to reduce the noradrenergic hyperactivity associated with opioid withdrawal (Gowing et al., 2016). Rotation off high-dose opioids to methadone, followed by a slow methadone taper is a technique that has been used to minimize withdrawal symptoms in patients who require an opioid taper. This technique has been used for opioid tapering because, although it requires a longer taper, methadone has a long half-life (24–36 hours and longer) and is associated with milder withdrawal symptoms than with other opioids (Gowing et al., 2016). Pregabalin is another medication used to reduce opioid withdrawal symptoms, but limited evidence exists to support its use (Freynhagen et al., 2016). An MMA plan and nonpharmacologic interventions may reduce opioid requirements and therefore physical dependence. Symptomatic approaches to withdrawal symptoms may be necessary. These approaches include pharmacologic and nonpharmacologic interventions, such as those identified earlier in this chapter, to provide symptomatic relief of nausea, diarrhea, and other withdrawal symptoms. Additional information is provided in Chapter 14.

Opioid Tolerance

Tolerance is a phenomenon in which higher doses of a medication are required over time to obtain the original extent of the medication effect. Tolerance is considered a state of adaptation that may result in decreased effectiveness or decreased duration of action of the medication (Herndon et al., 2016). As it relates to opioids, tolerance means that over time the opioid will not have the same effects as it had when introduced and higher doses may be necessary to achieve the same degree of analgesia that was achieved when the original, lower doses were used. With opioids, tolerance develops to both the analgesic effects (an undesirable effect) and many of the side effects (a desirable effect) (Bristow et al., 2014). This phenomenon is described in greater detail in Chapter 9.

The management of opioid tolerance traditionally involves increasing doses of opioid to effectively treat pain, provided other opioid-related side effects do not limit dose escalation. Although poorly understood, it is thought that the NMDA receptor plays a significant role in opioid tolerance. Medications that antagonize this receptor, such as ketamine, are sometimes used (particularly in the acute care setting and sometimes with cancer pain) to address the development of tolerance (Cortazzo et al., 2014). Another intervention to address opioid tolerance is opioid rotation.

Although opioid tolerance is an expected adaption to chronic opioid use, if a patient's pain increases, it is necessary to determine whether the loss of opioid effectiveness is related to disease progression, new pathologic condition, or some other factor (Herndon et al., 2016). Interventions to reduce opioid tolerance include limiting opioid doses and duration of opioid treatment. The use of a multimodal pain management approach may be helpful in ensuring adequate pain relief while reducing opioid use. Patient education is necessary to ensure that patients understand the development of opioid tolerance is a normal and anticipated response to continued opioid use, and interventions are available to address pain management concerns.

Immune Suppressing Effect of Opioids

Although an immunologic effect of opioids is not established as a common side effect, it is mentioned here in the interest of presenting a discussion of evolving awareness of other opioid-related unintended effects. Opioid-induced immunomodulation was first identified at the end of the 19th century in guinea pigs who were given morphine and subsequently noted to have immune suppression with less ability to fight bacteria (Benyamin et al., 2008). In other animal studies, morphine and fentaNYL have been implicated as contributing to weakened immune system function with effects on macrophage, T cells, and natural killer cells (Kim, 2018; Plein & Rittner, 2018) and immune response in bone cancer (Du et al., 2016). Current investigations regarding the immunosuppressive effect of opioids, possibly through altering gene expression of immunocytes on immune function, are focusing on the effects of different opioids, with postoperative infectious processes and with malignant tumor growth (Haroutounian, 2018).

The results of recent large studies are inconsistent. Those studies often involved patients diagnosed with immune system compromising conditions, which can be a significant confounder and limitation when evaluating the results of increased incidence of infection. In a large study (N = 1790) evaluating the relationship of opioid analgesic use with infection among people living with rheumatoid arthritis, a positive association between opioids and infection was reported (Wiese, Griffin, Stein, Mitchel, & Grijalva, 2016). In a different nested case-control matched study (N = 1233), an increased risk for developing invasive pneumococcal disease was associated with long-term use of opioids (Wiese et al., 2018). Another very large retrospective study (N = 36,486) evaluated a relationship of opioids and infection among recipients of renal transplants (Abbott et al., 2018). In that study the researchers reported an increased risk for morbidity and graft loss among the participants who reported long-term high-dose opioid use compared to recipients who did not use opioids or used them for only a brief time.

In contrast, the researchers of another large study (N = 4358) evaluated the effect of opioids on the recovery of CD4 cells among patients who were infected with human immunodeficiency virus (HIV) and had recently begun antiretroviral therapy (Edelman et al., 2016). In that study no effect on the CD4 counts were reported during a 2-year period. That is interesting because the participants in that study were receiving antiretroviral therapy. The effect of chronic opioid use on immune function was evaluated in a prospective study of Danish patients with breast cancer (N = 34,188) with no meaningful relationship found (Cronin-Fenton et al., 2015). These research efforts underscore that immunologic effect of opioids is an area in which additional rigorous research is needed. In a smaller, more recent study (N = 268) with patients who underwent surgery for oral cancer, the quantity of postoperative opioids was not considered predictive of recurrence-free survival; however, the researchers did find a small nonstatistically significant relationship with shorter overall survival (Patino et al., 2017). Although the results of research to date are inconsistent and inconclusive, the potential impact on the immune system is another important reason to use multimodal approaches to limit all potential adverse effects.

Key Points

- Most opioid-related unintended effects are dose related.
- Most opioid-related unintended effects, except constipation, resolve with continued use of the opioid.
- Opioid-naïve patients are at the greatest risk for the development of opioid-related unintended effects.
- Risk factors for the development of various opioid-related unintended effects, particularly dangerous effects such as respiratory depression, are considered and addressed when initiating opioid therapy. Chapter 13 more extensively addresses opioid-related respiratory depression.
- Opioid-related unintended effects can often be reduced or eliminated by dose reduction or opioid rotation.
- It is optimal to prevent opioid-related unintended effects through the use of multimodal analgesia, appropriate opioid dosing, and preventive nonpharmacologic and pharmacologic measures.
- There are many nonpharmacologic and pharmacologic approaches available to address opioid related unintended effects.
- The risk for unintended opioid-related effects such as dependence, tolerance, and hyperalgesia can be reduced by using the lowest effective doses of opioids for the briefest time possible.
- The development of dependence, tolerance, and hyperalgesia are unintended effects associated with opioid use over a period of time.
- When opioids are needed, the inclusion of nonpharmacologic and pharmacologic nonopioid analgesic approaches in a multimodal analgesic plan reduces opioid requirements and associated unintended effects.

Case Scenario

N. F. is an opioid-naïve, obese, otherwise healthy 54-year-old woman who had an open cholecystectomy yesterday under general anesthesia. She was started on morphine patient-controlled analgesia (PCA) after arriving on the floor to manage her incisional pain, which she is rating as 7 on a scale of 0 to 10. On rounds, you note that her PCA use has been minimal, yet she is drowsy and reporting severe nausea with more pain.

1. How will you assess N. F.'s pain and her inability to reduce it despite the availability of PCA?
2. What actual and potential unintended effects are interfering with N. F.'s pain relief?
3. What pharmacologic and nonpharmacologic measures can be implemented to reduce these unintended effects?
4. How can you anticipate and prevent some of the common unintended opioid effects?
5. How do you respond to N.F.'s concerns that she does not want to use the PCA because she is afraid she will become "addicted" to morphine?

References

Abbott, K. C., Fwu, C. W., Eggers, P. W., Eggers, A. W., Kline, P. P., & Kimmel, P. L. (2018). Opioid Prescription, Morbidity, and Mortality in US Transplant Recipients. *Transplantation*, 102(6), 994–1004.

Abramowitz, L., Béziaud, N., Caussé, C., Chuberre, B., Allaert, F. A., & Perrot, S. (2013). Further validation of the psychometric properties of the Bowel Function Index for evaluating opioid-induced constipation (OIC). *Journal of Medical Economics*, 16(12), 1434–1441.

Adib-Hajbaghery, M., & Hosseini, F. S. (2015). Investigating the effects of inhaling ginger essence on post-nephrectomy nausea and vomiting. *Complementary Therapies in Medicine*, 23(6), 827–831.

Afazel, M. R., Jalali, E., Sadat, Z., & Mahmoodi, H. (2014). Comparing the effects of hot pack and lukewarm-water-soaked gauze on postoperative urinary retention; a randomized controlled clinical trial. *Nursing and Midwifery Studies*, 3(4), E24606.

Ahmedzai, S. H. (2017). A fall from grace: exposing the neurotoxicities of morphine. *British Journal of Pain*, 11(1), 6–8.

Akhan, A., Subasi, F. D., Bosna, G., Ekinci, O., Pamuk, H., Batan, S., ... Turan, G. (2016). Comparison of mirtazapine, gabapentin and ondansetron to prevent intrathecal morphine-induced pruritus. *Northern Clinics of Istanbul*, 3(1), 53.

Ali, K., Raphael, J., Khan, S., Labib, M., & Duarte, R. (2016). The effects of opioids on the endocrine system: an overview. *Postgraduate Medical Journal*, 92(1093), 677–681.

Allen, C. A., & Ivester, J. R., Jr. (2017). Low-Dose Ketamine for Postoperative Pain Management. *Journal of PeriAnesthesia Nursing*, 33(4), 389–398.

Allen, M. S., Blackmon, S. H., Nichols, F. C., Cassivi, S. D., Harmsen, W. S., Lechtenberg, B., ... Shen, K. R. (2016). Optimal timing of urinary catheter removal after thoracic operations: a randomized controlled study. *The Annals of Thoracic Surgery*, 102(3), 925–930.

Alper, B. S., Malone-Moses, M., & Manheimer, E. W. (2017). Evidence for clinical practice: Point-of-care application of acupuncture for chronic severe functional constipation: A randomized controlled trial. *European Journal of Integrative Medicine*, 10, 57–58.

Alyautdin, R., Khalin, I., Nafeeza, M. I., Haron, M. H., & Kuznetsov, D. (2014). Nanoscale drug delivery systems and the blood–brain barrier. *International Journal of Nanomedicine*, 9(1), 795–811.

Anastasi, J. K., Capili, B., & Chang, M. (2017). Development of Acupuncture and Moxibustion Protocol in a Clinical Trial for Irritable Bowel Syndrome. *Journal of Acupuncture and Meridian Studies*, 10(1), 62–66.

Andrews, P. L., & Sanger, G. J. (2014). Nausea and the quest for the perfect anti-emetic. *European Journal of Pharmacology*, 722(1), 108–121.

Atiya Ali, M., Poortvliet, E., Strömberg, R., & Yngve, A. (2011). Polyamines in foods: development of a food database. *Food & Nutrition Research*, 55(1), 5572.

Baldini, G., Bagry, H., Aprikian, A., & Carli, F. (2009). Postoperative Urinary Retention Anesthetic and Perioperative Considerations. *Anesthesiology: The Journal of the American Society of Anesthesiologists*, 110(5), 1139–1157.

Baldo, B. A., & Pham, N. H. (2012). Histamine-releasing and allergenic properties of opioid analgesic drugs: resolving the two. *Anaesthesia and Intensive Care*, 40(2), 216.

Basaria, S., Travison, T. G., Alford, D., Knapp, P. E., Teeter, K., Cahalan, C., ... Martel, M. O. (2015). Effects of testosterone replacement in men with opioid-induced androgen deficiency: a randomized controlled trial. *Pain*, 156(2), 280.

Bashashati, M., & McCallum, R. W. (2014). Neurochemical mechanisms and pharmacologic strategies in managing nausea and vomiting related to cyclic vomiting syndrome and other gastrointestinal disorders. *European Journal of Pharmacology*, 722(1), 79–94.

Bell, R. F., Borzan, J., Kalso, E., & Simonnet, G. (2012). Food, pain, and drugs: Does it matter what pain patients eat? *Pain*, 153(10), 1993–1996.

Benson, J. L., Campbell, H. E., & Phillips, C. N. (2015). Opioid-induced pruritus. *The Consultant Pharmacist®*, 30(4), 221–227.

Benyamin, R., Trescot, A. M., Datta, S., Buenaventura, R., Adlaka, R., Sehgal, N., ... Vallejo, R. (2008). Opioid complications and side effects. *Pain Physician*, 11, S105–S120.

Birthi, P., Nagar, V. R., Nickerson, R., & Sloan, P. A. (2015). Hypogonadism associated with long-term opioid therapy: A systematic review. *Journal of Opioid Management*, 11(3), 255–278.

Blunk, J. A., Schmelz, M., Zeck, S., Skov, P., Likar, R., & Koppert, W. (2004). Opioid-induced mast cell activation and vascular responses is not mediated by μ-opioid receptors: an in vivo microdialysis study in human skin. *Anesthesia & Analgesia*, 98(2), 364–370.

Bonnet, M. P., Marret, E., Josserand, J., & Mercier, F. J. (2008). Effect of prophylactic 5-HT3 receptor antagonists on pruritus induced by neuraxial opioids: a quantitative systematic review. *British Journal of Anaesthesia*, 101(3), 311–319.

Bounes, V., Charriton-Dadone, B., Levraut, J., Delangue, C., Carpentier, F., Mary-Chalon, S., ... Ganetsky, M. (2017). Predicting morphine related side effects in the ED: An international cohort study. *The American Journal of Emergency Medicine*, 35(4), 531–535.

Brennan, M. J. (2013). The effect of opioid therapy on endocrine function. *The American Journal of Medicine*, 126(3), S12–S18.

Brennan, F. P., Josland, E., & Kelly, J. J. (2015). Chronic Pruritus: Histamine Is Not Always the Answer! *Journal of Pain and Symptom Management*, 50(4), 566–570.

Bristow, S., Singh, V., & Ballantyne, J. (2014). Opioids. In *Reference Module in Neuroscience and Biobehavioral Psychology Encyclopedia of the Neurological Sciences (2nd Ed)*. St. Louis, MO: Elsevier.

Brower, V. (2017). Naldemedine effective in treating opioid-induced constipation. *The Lancet Oncology*, 18(6), e306.

Bruera, E., Strasser, F., Shen, L., Palmer, J. L., Willey, J., Driver, L. C., & Burton, A. W. (2003). The effect of donepezil on sedation and other symptoms in patients receiving opioids for cancer pain: a pilot study. *Journal of Pain and Symptom Management*, 26(5), 1049–1054.

Büyükuslu, N. (2015). Dietary polyamines and diseases: reducing polyamine intake can be beneficial in cancer treatment. *Journal of Nutrients*, 2(2), 27–38.

Camilleri, M., Lembo, A., & Katzka, D. A. (2017). Opioids in gastroenterology: treating adverse effects and creating therapeutic benefits. *Clinical Gastroenterology and Hepatology*, 15(9), 1338–1349.

Camilleri, M., Drossman, D. A., Becker, G., Webster, L. R., Davies, A. N., & Mawe, G. M. (2014). Emerging treatments in neurogastroenterology: A multidisciplinary working group consensus statement on opioid-induced constipation. *Neurogastroenterology & Motility*, 26(10), 1386–1395.

Caraceni, A., Hanks, G., Kaasa, S., Bennett, M. I., Brunelli, C., Cherny, N., ... Haugen, D. F. (2012). Use of opioid analgesics in the treatment of cancer pain: Evidence-based recommendations from the EAPC. *The Lancet Oncology*, 13(2), e58–e68.

Carter, G. T., Duong, V., Ho, S., Ngo, K. C., Greer, C. L., & Weeks, D. L. (2014). Side effects of commonly prescribed analgesic medications. *Physical Medicine and Rehabilitation Clinics, 25*(2), 457–470.

Chancellor, J., Martin, M., Liedgens, H., Baker, M. G., & Müller-Schwefe, G. H. (2012). Stated preferences of physicians and chronic pain sufferers in the use of classic strong opioids. *Value in Health, 15*(1), 106–117.

Cheifetz, A. S., Gianotti, R., Luber, R., & Gibson, P. R. (2017). Complementary and alternative medicines used by patients with inflammatory bowel diseases. *Gastroenterology, 152*(2), 415–429.

Chey, W. D., Webster, L., Sostek, M., Lappalainen, J., Barker, P. N., & Tack, J. (2014). Naloxegol for opioid-induced constipation in patients with noncancer pain. *New England Journal of Medicine, 370*(25), 2387–2396.

Choi, S., & Awad, I. (2013). Maintaining micturition in the perioperative period: strategies to avoid urinary retention. *Current Opinion in Anesthesiology, 26*(3), 361–367.

Chon, T. Y., & Lee, M. C. (2013, October). Acupuncture. In *Mayo Clinic Proceedings: Vol. 88, No. 10* (pp. 1141–1146). Elsevier.

Cipolla, B. G., Havouis, R., & Moulinoux, J. P. (2007). Polyamine contents in current foods: a basis for polyamine reduced diet and a study of its long term observance and tolerance in prostate carcinoma patients. *Amino, 33*(2), 203–212.

Compton, P., Canamar, C. P., Hillhouse, M., & Ling, W. (2012). Hyperalgesia in heroin dependent patients and the effects of opioid substitution therapy. *The Journal of Pain, 13*(4), 401–409.

Cortazzo, M. H., Copenhaver, D., & Fishman, S. M. (2013). Major opioids and chronic opioid therapy. (pp. 495-508.e3). In H. Benzon, J. Rathmell, C. L. Wu, D. Turk, C. Argoff, & R. Hurley (Eds.), *Practical Management of Pain: Fifth Edition*. St. Louis, MO: Elsevier.

Coyne, K. S., LoCasale, R. J., Datto, C. J., Sexton, C. C., Yeomans, K., & Tack, J. (2014). Opioid-induced constipation in patients with chronic noncancer pain in the USA, Canada, Germany, and the UK: Descriptive analysis of baseline patient-reported outcomes and retrospective chart review. *ClinicoEconomics and Outcomes Research, 6*(5), 269–281.

Cronin-Fenton, D. P., Heide-Jørgensen, U., Ahern, T. P., Lash, T. L., Christiansen, P. M., Ejlertsen, B., … Sørensen, H. T. (2015). Opioids and breast cancer recurrence: A Danish population-based cohort study. *Cancer, 121*(19), 3507–3514.

Dabu-Bondoc, S., Franco, S. A., & Sinatra, R. S. (2009). Neuraxial analgesia with hydromorphone, morphine, and fentanyl: Dosing and safety guidelines. In R. S. Sinatra, O. A. de Leon-Cassola, B. Ginsbergm, & E. R. Viscusi (Eds.), *Acute Pain Management* (pp. 230-244). Cambridge, NY: Cambridge University Press.

Dahiya, S., & Banerjee, D. N. (2016). Complementary and alternative medicine: What is it good for? *Bulletin of Pharmaceutical Research, 6*(3), 83–92.

Darrah, D. M., Griebling, T. L., & Silverstein, J. H. (2009). Postoperative urinary retention. *Anesthesiology Clinics, 27*(3), 465–484.

Davis, M. P., Frandsen, J. L., Walsh, D., Andresen, S., & Taylor, S. (2003). Mirtazapine for pruritus. *Journal of Pain and Symptom Management, 25*(3), 288–291.

de Boer, H. D., Detriche, O., & Forget, P. (2017). Opioid related side effects: postoperative ileus, urinary retention, nausea and vomiting, and shivering. A review of the literature.

Best Practice & Research Clinical Anaesthesiology., 31(4), 499–504.

Deumens, R., Steyaert, A., Forget, P., Schubert, M., Lavand'homme, P., Hermans, E., & De Kock, M. (2013). Prevention of chronic postoperative pain: Cellular, molecular, and clinical insights for mechanism-based treatment approaches. *Progress in Neurobiology, 104*(1), 1–37.

Devlin, J. W., Skrobik, Y., Gélinas, C., Needham, D. M., Slooter, A. J., Pandharipande, P. P., … Balas, M. C. (2018). Clinical practice guidelines for the prevention and management of pain, agitation/sedation, delirium, immobility, and sleep disruption in adult patients in the ICU. *Critical Care Medicine, 46*(9), e825–e873.

Dhingra, L., Ahmed, E., Shin, J., Scharaga, E., & Magun, M. (2015). Cognitive effects and sedation. *Pain Medicine, 16*(suppl_1), S37–S43.

Ding, M., Leach, M., & Bradley, H. (2013). The effectiveness and safety of ginger for pregnancy-induced nausea and vomiting: a systematic review. *Women and Birth, 26*(1), e26–e30.

Dorn, S., Lembo, A., & Cremonini, F. (2014). Opioid-induced bowel dysfunction: Epidemiology, pathophysiology, diagnosis, and initial therapeutic approach. *The American Journal of Gastroenterology Supplements, 2*(1), 31–37.

Drewes, A. M., Munkholm, P., Simrén, M., Breivik, H., Kongsgaard, U. E., Hatlebakk, J. G., … Christrup, L. L. (2016). Definition, diagnosis and treatment strategies for opioid-induced bowel dysfunction—recommendations of the Nordic Working Group. *Scandinavian Journal of Pain, 11*(2), 111–122.

Dronca, R. S., & Loprinzi, C. (2012). Nausea and Vomiting. In *Management of Cancer in the Older Patient* (pp. 171–181). St. Louis: Elsevier.

Du, J. Y., Liang, Y., Fang, J. F., Jiang, Y. L., Shao, X. M., He, X. F., & Fang, J. Q. (2016). Effect of systemic injection of heterogenous and homogenous opioids on peripheral cellular immune response in rats with bone cancer pain: A comparative study. *Experimental and Therapeutic Medicine, 12*(4), 2568–2576.

Edelman, E. J., Gordon, K. S., Tate, J. P., Becker, W. C., Bryant, K., Crothers, K., … Rodriguez-Barradas, M. C. (2016). The impact of prescribed opioids on CD 4 cell count recovery among HIV-infected patients newly initiating antiretroviral therapy. *HIV Medicine, 17*(10), 728–739.

Eisenberg, E., Suzan, E., & Pud, D. (2015). Opioid-induced hyperalgesia (OIH): A real clinical problem or just an experimental phenomenon? *Journal of Pain and Symptom Management, 49*(3), 632–636.

Fletcher, D., & Martinez, V. (2014). Opioid-induced hyperalgesia in patients after surgery: A systematic review and a meta-analysis. *British Journal of Anaesthesia, 112*(6), 991–1004.

Fonte, C., Fatigoni, S., & Roila, F. (2015). A review of olanzapine as an antiemetic in chemotherapy-induced nausea and vomiting and in palliative care patients. *Critical Reviews in Oncology/Hematology, 95*(2), 214–221.

Freynhagen, R., Backonja, M., Schug, S., Lyndon, G., Parsons, B., Watt, S., & Behar, R. (2016). Pregabalin for the treatment of drug and alcohol withdrawal symptoms: a comprehensive review. *CNS Drugs, 30*(12), 1191–1200.

Fukada, K. (2015). Opioid analgesics. In R. Miller, L. Eriksson, L. Fleisher, J. Weiner-Kronish, N. Cohen, & W. Young (Eds.), *Miller's Anesthesia, Eighth Edition. Chapter 31* (pp. 864–914). Philadelphia: Saunders.

Furness, S., Bryan, G., McMillan, R., Birchenough, S., & Worthington, H. V. (2013). Interventions for the management of dry mouth: non-pharmacological interventions. *Cochrane Database Systematic Review*, (9), CD009603.

Gallo, S., DuRand, J., & Pshon, N. (2008). A study of naloxone effect on urinary retention in the patient receiving morphine Patient-controlled analgesia. *Orthopaedic Nursing*, 27(2), 111–115.

Gan, T. J., Habib, A. S., Miller, T. E., White, W., & Apfelbaum, J. L. (2014a). Incidence, patient satisfaction, and perceptions of post-surgical pain: Results from a US national survey. *Current Medical Research and Opinion*, 30(1), 149–160. https://doi.org/10.1185/03007995.2013.860019.

Gan, T. J., Diemunsch, P., Habib, A. S., Kovac, A., Kranke, P., Meyer, T. A., ... Bergese, S. D. (2014b). Consensus guidelines for the management of postoperative nausea and vomiting. *Anesthesia & Analgesia*, 118(1), 85–113.

Godden, B. (2018). Airway issues. In D. Stannard, & D. Krenzischeck (Eds.), *Perianesthesia Nursing Care: A Bedside Case for Safe Recovery* (2nd ed., pp. 23–31). Burlington, MA: Jones & Bartlett Learning.

Golembiewski, J. (2013). Opioid-induced pruritus. *Journal of PeriAnesthesia Nursing*, 28(4), 247–249.

Gowing, L., Farrell, M., Ali, R., & White, J. M. (2016). *Alpha2-adrenergic agonists for the management of opioid withdrawal*. The Cochrane Library.

Gristenko, K., Khelemsky, Y., Kaye, A. D., Vadivelu, N., & Urman, R. D. (2014). Multimodal therapy in perioperative analgesia. *Best Practice & Research Clinical Anesthesiology*, 28(1), 59–79.

Gudin, J. A., Laitman, A., & Nalamachu, S. (2015). Opioid related endocrinopathy. *Pain Medicine*, 16(suppl_1), S9–S15.

Han, P., Suarez-Durall, P., & Mulligan, R. (2015). Dry mouth: A critical topic for older adult patients. *Journal of Prosthodontic Research*, 59(1), 6–19.

Hansen, B. S., Søreide, E., Warland, A. M., & Nilsen, O. B. (2011). Risk factors of post-operative urinary retention in hospitalised patients. *Acta Anaesthesiologica Scandinavica*, 55(5), 545–548.

Hassan, I., & Haji, M. L. I. (2014). Understanding itch: an update on mediators and mechanisms of pruritus. *Indian Journal of Dermatology, Venereology, and Leprology*, 80(2), 106.

He, F., Jiang, Y., & Li, L. (2016). The effect of naloxone treatment on opioid-induced side effects: A meta-analysis of randomized and controlled trails. *Medicine*, 95(37), e4729. https://doi.org/10.1097?MD.0000000000004729.

Harbord, M., & Pomfret, S. (2013). Nausea and vomiting. *Medicine*, 41(2), 87–91.

Haroutounian, S. (2018). Postoperative opioids, endocrine changes, and immunosuppression. *Pain Reports*, 3(2), e640.

Herndon, C. M., Arnstein, P., Darnall, B., Hartrick, C., Hecht, K., Lyons, M., & Seghal, N. (2016). *Principles of Analgesic Use*. Chicago, Ill: American Pain Society.

Ho, K. Y., & Gan, T. J. (2009). Opioid-related adverse effects and treatment options. In *Acute pain management* (pp. 406–415). New York, NY: Cambridge University Press.

Hirschtritt, M. E., Delucchi, K. L., & Olfson, M. (2017). *Outpatient, combined use of opioid and benzodiazepine medications in the United States, 1993–2014*. Preventive Medicine Reports.

Hofmann, D., Murray, C., Beck, J., & Homann, R. (2017). Acupressure in management of postoperative nausea and vomiting in high-risk ambulatory surgical patients. *Journal of PeriAnesthesia Nursing*, 32(4), 271–278.

Holmér Pettersson, P., & Wengström, Y. (2012). Acupuncture prior to surgery to minimise postoperative nausea and vomiting: a systematic review. *Journal of Clinical Nursing*, 21(13-14), 1799–1805.

Horn, C. C., & Yates, B. J. (2017). Biology and control of nausea and vomiting 2015: Perspectives and overview of the conference. *Autonomic Neuroscience: Basic and Clinical*, 202(1), 3–4.

Horta, M. L., Morejon, L. C. L., Da Cruz, A. W., Dos Santos, G. R., Welling, L. C., Terhorst, L., ... Alam, R. U. Z. (2006). Study of the prophylactic effect of droperidol, alizapride, propofol and promethazine on spinal morphine-induced pruritus. *BJA: British Journal of Anaesthesia*, 96(6), 796–800.

Hu, Y., Craig, S. J., Rowlingson, J. C., Morton, S. P., Thomas, C. J., Persinger, M. B., ... Kozower, B. D. (2014). Early removal of urinary catheter after surgery requiring thoracic epidural: a prospective trial. *Journal of Cardiothoracic and Vascular Anesthesia*, 28(5), 1302–1306.

International Association for the Study of Pain (IASP). (2014). IASP Taxonomy. In *International Association for the Study of Pain*. Retrieved 06/22/17 https://www.iasp-pain.org/Education/Content.aspx?ItemNumber=1698.

Iserson, K. V. (2014). An hypnotic suggestion: review of hypnosis for clinical emergency care. *Journal of Emergency Medicine*, 46(4), 588–596.

Jamison, R. N., & Mao, J. (2015). Opioid analgesics. *Mayo Clinical Proceedings*, 90(7), 957–968.

Jannuzzi, R. G. (2016). Nalbuphine for treatment of opioid-induced pruritus: a systematic review of literature. *The Clinical Journal of Pain*, 32(1), 87–93.

Jenkins, H. H., Spencer, E. D., Weissgerber, A. J., Osborne, L. A., & Pellegrini, J. E. (2009). Correlating an 11-point verbal numeric rating scale to a 4-point verbal rating scale in the measurement of pruritus. *Journal of PeriAnesthesia Nursing*, 24(3), 152–155.

Jennings, E. M., Okine, B. N., Roche, M., & Finn, D. P. (2014). Stress-induced hyperalgesia. *Progress in Neurobiology*, 12(1), 1–18.

Jouguelet-Lacoste, J., La Colla, L., Schilling, D., & Chelly, J. E. (2015). The use of intravenous infusion or single dose of low-dose ketamine for postoperative analgesia: a review of the current literature. *Pain Medicine*, 16(2), 383–403.

Jungquist, C. R., Quinlan-Colwell, A., Vallerand, A., Carlisle, H. L., Cooney, M., Dempsey, S. J., ... Sawyer, J. (2020). American Society for Pain Management Nursing Guidelines on Monitoring for Opioid-Induced Advancing Sedation and Respiratory Depression: Revisions. *Pain Management Nursing*, 21(1), 7–25.

Jungquist, C. R., Correll, D. J., Fleisher, L. A., Gross, J., Gupta, R., Pasero, C., ... Polomano, R. (2016). Avoiding adverse events secondary to opioid-induced respiratory depression: Implications for nurse executives and patient safety. *Journal of Nursing Administration*, 46(2), 87–94.

Kandadai, P., Saini, J., Patterson, D., O'Dell, K., & Flynn, M. (2015). Urinary retention after hysterectomy and postoperative analgesic use. *Female Pelvic Medicine & Reconstructive Surgery*, 21(5), 257–262.

Katakami, N., Oda, K., Tauchi, K., Nakata, K., Shinozaki, K., Yokota, T., ... Boku, N. (2017). Phase IIb, randomized, double-blind, placebo-controlled study of naldemedine for the treatment of opioid-induced constipation in patients with cancer. *Journal of Clinical Oncology, 35*(17), 1921–1928.

Katzung, B. G., Masters, S. B., & Trevor, A. J. (2012). *Basic and clinical pharmacology twelfth edition.* International edition (pp. 636–650). McGraw-Hill.

Kaur, K., Saxena, A., Haniadka, R., Saldanha, E., D'Silva, P., Ponemone, V., ... Baliga, M. S. (2015). Medicinal benefits of ginger in various gastrointestinal ailments: Use in geriatric conditions. In *Foods and Dietary Supplements in the Prevention and Treatment of Disease in Older Adults* (pp. 51–61). St. Louis: Elsevier.

Kaye, A. D., Cornett, E. M., Helander, E., Menard, B., Hsu, E., Hart, B., & Brunk, A. (2017). An update on nonopioids: Intravenous or oral analgesics for perioperative pain management. *Anesthesiology Clinics, 35*(2), e55–e71.

Keeley, P. W. (2015). Nausea and vomiting. *Medicine, 43*(12), 709–711.

Kekecs, Z., Nagy, T., & Varga, K. (2014). The effectiveness of suggestive techniques in reducing postoperative side effects: A meta-analysis of randomized controlled trials. *Anesthesia & Analgesia, 119*(6), 1407–1419.

Kido-Nakahara, M., Katoh, N., Saeki, H., Mizutani, H., Hagihara, A., Takeuchi, S., ... Omoto, Y. (2015). Comparative cut-off value setting of pruritus intensity in visual analogue scale and verbal rating scale. *Acta Derm Venereol, 95*(3), 345–346.

Kim, C. H., Garcia, R., Stover, J., Ritchie, K., Whealton, T., & Ata, M. A. (2014). Androgen deficiency in long-term intrathecal opioid administration. *Pain Physician, 17*(4). E543-8.

Kim, R. (2018). Effects of surgery and anesthetic choice on immunosuppression and cancer recurrence. *Journal of Translational Medicine, 16*(1), 8.

Kjellberg, F., & Tramer, M. R. (2001). Pharmacological control of opioid-induced pruritus: a quantitative systematic review of randomized trials. *European Journal of Anaesthesiology, 18*(6), 346–357.

Ko, M. C. (2015). Neuraxial opioid-induced itch and its pharmacological antagonism. In *Pharmacology of Itch* (pp. 315-335). Berlin: Springer.

Kowalik, U., & Plante, M. K. (2016). Urinary retention in surgical patients. *Surgical Clinics of North America, 96*(3), 453–467.

Kravits, K. G. (2015). Hypnosis for the management of anticipatory nausea and vomiting. *Journal of the Advanced Practitioner in Oncology, 6*(3), 225–229.

Kumar, L., Barker, C., & Emmanuel, A. (2014). *Opioid-induced constipation: pathophysiology, clinical consequences, and management. Gastroenterology Research and Practice, 2014.* Article ID 141737, 6 pages https://doi.org/10.1155/2014/141737.

Kumar, K., & Singh, S. I. (2013). Neuraxial opioid-induced pruritus: an update. *Journal of Anaesthesiology Clinical Pharmacology, 29*(3), 303.

Kwong, W. J., Hammond, G., Upmalis, D., Okamoto, A., Yang, M., & Kavanagh, S. (2013). Bowel function after tapentadol and oxycodone immediate release (IR) treatment in patients with low back or osteoarthritis pain. *The Clinical Journal of Pain, 29*(8), 664–672.

Lacy, B. E., Mearin, F., Chang, L., Chey, W. D., Lembo, A. J., Simren, M., & Spiller, R. (2016). Bowel disorders. *Gastroenterology, 150*(6), 1393–1407.

Lavand'homme, P., & Steyaert, A. (2017). Opioid free anaesthesia. Opioid side effects: Tolerance and Hyperalgesia. *Best Practice & Research Clinical Anaesthesiology, 31*(4), 487–498.

Lee, E. J., & Warden, S. (2016). The effects of acupuncture on serotonin metabolism. *European Journal of Integrative Medicine, 8*(4), 355–367.

Lee, K., Ganta, N., Horton, J., & Chai, E. (2017). Evidence for Morphine or Hydromorphone-Induced Neurotoxicity in Renal Impairment: A Systematic Review (S705). *Journal of Pain and Symptom Management, 53*(2), 412.

Lee, M., Silverman, S., Hansen, H., Patel, V., & Manchikanti, L. (2011). A comprehensive review of opioid-induced hyperalgesia. *Pain Physician, 14*, 145–161.

Lehnen, N., Heuser, F., Sağlam, M., Schulz, C. M., Wagner, K. J., Taki, M., ... Schneider, E. (2015). Opioid-induced nausea involves a vestibular problem preventable by headrest. *PLoS ONE, 10*(8), e0135263.

Le Roy, C., Laboureyras, E., Laulin, J. P., & Simonnet, G. (2013). A polyamine-deficient diet opposes hyperalgesia, tolerance and the increased anxiety-like behaviour associated with heroin withdrawal in rats. *Pharmacology Biochemistry and Behavior, 103*(3), 510–519.

Levine, S. K., & Shega, J. W. (2013). What medications are effective in preventing and relieving constipation in the setting of opioid use? (pp. 129-134.). In E. Goldstein, & R. S. Morrison (Eds.), *Evidence-Based Practice of Palliative Medicine.* Philadelphia, PA: Saunders.

Levy, A., & Chen, R. (2016). Myoclonus: pathophysiology and treatment options. *Current Treatment Options in Neurology, 18*(5), 21.

Li, P. H., Ue, K. L., Wagner, A., Rutkowski, R., & Rutkowski, K. (2017). Opioid hypersensitivity: predictors of allergy and role of drug provocation testing. *The Journal of Allergy and Clinical Immunology: In Practice, 5*(6), 1601–1606.

Liu, X., Zhang, J., Zhao, H., Mei, H., Lian, Q., & Shangguan, W. (2014). The effect of propofol on intrathecal morphine-induced pruritus and its mechanism. *Anesthesia & Analgesia, 118*(2), 303–309.

Liu, X. Y., Liu, Z. C., Sun, Y. G., Ross, M., Kim, S., Tsai, F. F., ... Chen, Z. F. (2011). Unidirectional cross-activation of GRPR by MOR1D uncouples itch and analgesia induced by opioids. *Cell, 147*(2), 447–458.

Lua, P. L., Salihah, N., & Mazlan, N. (2015). Effects of inhaled ginger aromatherapy on chemotherapy-induced nausea and vomiting and health-related quality of life in women with breast cancer. *Complementary Therapies in Medicine, 23*(3), 396–404.

Lucyk, S., & Nelson, L. S. (2016). Opioids. Critical Care. *Toxicology,* 1–13.

Mann, M., & Chai, E. (2014). Opioid essentials. *Hospital Medicine Clinics, 3*(4), 567–581.

Mark, A. M. (2017). Limiting the effects of dry mouth. *The Journal of the American Dental Association, 148*(8), 626.

Marrett, E., Kwong, W. J., Frech, F., & Qian, C. (2016). Health Care Utilization and Costs Associated with Nausea and Vomiting in Patients Receiving Oral Immediate-Release Opioids for Outpatient Acute Pain Management. *Pain and Therapy, 5*(2), 215–226.

Marroquin, B., Feng, C., Balofsky, A., Edwards, K., Iqbal, A., Kanel, J., ... Wissler, R. (2017). Neuraxial opioids for post-cesarean delivery analgesia: can hydromorphone replace morphine? A retrospective study. *International Journal of Obstetric Anesthesia, 30*, 16–22.

Martinez, V., Derivaux, B., & Beloeil, H. (2015). Ketamine for pain management in France, an observational survey. *Anaesthesia Critical Care & Pain Medicine, 34*(6), 357–361.

Mauermann, E., Filitz, J., Dolder, P., Rentsch, K. M., Bandschapp, O., & Ruppen, W. (2016). Does fentanyl lead to opioid-induced hyperalgesia in healthy volunteers? A double-blind, randomized, crossover trial. *Anesthesiology: The Journal of the American Society of Anesthesiologists, 124*(2), 453–463.

Mercadante, S. (1998). Pathophysiology and treatment of opioid-related myoclonus in cancer patients. *Pain, 74*(1), 5–9.

Mills, K., & Mari, Z. (2015). An update and review of the treatment of myoclonus. *Current Neurology and Neuroscience Reports, 15*(1), 512.

Minagawa, T., Saitou, T., Suzuki, T., Domen, T., Yokoyama, H., Ishikawa, M., … Ishizuka, O. (2016). Impact of ao-dake-humi, Japanese traditional bamboo foot stimulator, on lower urinary tract symptoms, constipation and hypersensitivity to cold: A single-arm prospective pilot study. *BMC Complementary and Alternative Medicine, 16*(1), 513–521.

Minozzi, S., Amato, L., & Davoli, M. (2013). Development of dependence following treatment with opioid analgesics for pain relief: a systematic review. *Addiction, 108*(4), 688–698.

Montgomery, G. H., Schnur, J. B., & Kravits, K. (2013). Hypnosis for cancer care: Over 200 years young. *CA: A Cancer Journal for Clinicians, 63*(1), 31–44.

Moon, Y. E., Joo, J., Kim, J. E., & Lee, Y. (2012). Anti-emetic effect of ondansetron and palonosetron in thyroidectomy: a prospective, randomized, double-blind study. *British Journal of Anaesthesia, 108*(3), 417–422.

Moore, R. A., & McQuay, H. J. (2005). Prevalence of opioid adverse events in chronic non-malignant pain: systematic review of randomised trials of oral opioids. *Arthritis Research & Therapy, 7*(5), R1046.

Morley, J. E., Perry, H. M., Kevorkian, R. T., & Patrick, P. (2006). Comparison of screening questionnaires for the diagnosis of hypogonadism. *Maturitas, 53*(4), 424–429.

Nalamachu, S., Pergolizzi, J., Taylor, R., Slatkin, N., Barrett, C., & Forbes, W. P. (2015). Efficacy and tolerability of subcutaneous methylnaltrexone in patients with advanced illness and opioid-induced constipation: responder analysis of 2 randomized, placebo-controlled trials. *Pain Practice, 15*(6), 364–371.

Ng, S. S., Leung, W. W., Mak, T. W., Hon, S. S., Li, J. C. M., Wong, C. Y., … Lee, J. F. (2013). Electroacupuncture reduces duration of postoperative ileus after laparoscopic surgery for colorectal cancer. *Gastroenterology, 144*(2), 307–313.

Niklander, S., Veas, L., Barrera, C., Fuentes, F., Chiappini, G., & Marshall, M. (2017). Risk factors, hyposalivation and impact of xerostomia on oral health-related quality of life. *Brazilian Oral Research, 31*, e14.

O'Brien, C. (2011). Addiction and dependence in DSM-V. *Addiction, 106*(5), 866–867.

Odom-Forren, J., Jalota, L., Moser, D. K., Lennie, T. A., Hall, L. A., Holtman, J., … Apfel, C. C. (2013). Incidence and predictors of postdischarge nausea and vomiting in a 7-day population. *Journal of Clinical Anesthesia, 25*(7), 551–559.

Oosten, A. W., Oldenmenger, W. H., Mathijssen, R. H. J., & van der Rijt, C. C. D. (2015). A systematic review of prospective studies reporting adverse events of commonly used opioids for cancer-related pain: a call for the use of standardized outcome measures. *The Journal of Pain, 16*(1), 935–946.

O'Rourke, T. K., & Wosnitzer, M. S. (2016). Opioid-induced androgen deficiency (OPIAD): diagnosis, management, and literature review. *Current Urology Reports, 17*(10), 76.

Palsson, O. S. (2015). Hypnosis treatment of gastrointestinal disorders: a comprehensive review of the empirical evidence. *American Journal of Clinical Hypnosis, 58*(2), 134–158.

Pasero, C. (2009). Assessment of sedation during opioid administration for pain management. *Journal of Perianesthesia Nursing, 24*(3), 186–190. https://doi.org/10.1016/j.jopan.2009.03.005.

Pasero, C., & McCaffery, M. (2012). Opioid-induced hyperalgesia. *Journal of PeriAnesthesia Nursing, 27*(1), 46–50.

Pasero, C., & Stannard, D. (2012). The role of intravenous acetaminophen in acute pain management: a case-illustrated review. *Pain Management Nursing, 13*(2), 107–124.

Patino, M. A., Ramirez, R. E., Perez, C. A., Feng, L., Kataria, P., Myers, J., & Cata, J. P. (2017). The impact of intraoperative opioid use on survival after oral cancer surgery. *Oral Oncology, 74*, 1–7.

Plein, L. M., & Rittner, H. L. (2018). Opioids and the immune system–friend or foe. *British Journal of Pharmacology, 175*(14), 2717–2725.

Plemons, J. M., Al-Hashimi, I., & Marek, C. L. (2014). Managing xerostomia and salivary gland hypofunction: executive summary of a report from the American Dental Association Council on Scientific Affairs. *The Journal of the American Dental Association, 145*(8), 867–873.

Pleuvry, B. J. (2015). Physiology and pharmacology of nausea and vomiting. *Anesthesia and Intensive Care, 16*(9), 462–466.

Quinlan-Colwell, A. (2012). A review of pain assessment tools for use with the older adult patient. (pp 55-76). In *Compact Clinical Guide to Geriatric Pain Management*. NY: NY: Springer Publishing.

Raffa, R. B., & Pergolizzi, J. V. (2013). Opioid-induced hyperalgesia: is it clinically relevant for the treatment of pain patients? *Pain Management Nursing, 14*(3), e67–e83.

Raheem, O. A., Patel, S. H., Sisul, D., Furnish, T. J., & Hsieh, T. C. (2017). The Role of Testosterone Supplemental Therapy in Opioid-Induced Hypogonadism: A Retrospective Pilot Analysis. *American Journal of Men's Health, 11*(4), 1208–1213.

Rauck, R., Slatkin, N., Harper, J., & Israel, R. (2017). (220) Oral methylnaltrexone for adults with chronic noncancer pain and opioid-induced constipation (OIC): timing and characterization of clinical symptoms do not suggest opioid withdrawal with daily treatment. *The Journal of Pain, 18*(4), S31.

Reich, A., & Szepietowski, J. C. (2010). Opioid-induced pruritus: An update. *Clinical and Experimental Dermatology, 35*(1), 2–6.

Reich, A., Heisig, M., Phan, N. Q., Taneda, K., Takamori, K., Takeuchi, S., … Szepietowski, J. C. (2012). Visual analogue scale: evaluation of the instrument for the assessment of pruritus. *Acta Dermato-Venereologica, 92*(5), 497–501.

Rentz, A. M., Yu, R., Müller-Lissner, S., & Leyendecker, P. (2009). Validation of the Bowel Function Index to detect clinically meaningful changes in opioid-induced constipation. *Journal of Medical Economics, 12*(4), 371–383. https://doi.org/10.3111/13696990903430481.

Richebéet, P., Pouquet, O., Jelacic, S., Mehta, S., Calderon, J., & Janvier, G. (2011). Target-controlled dosing of remifentanil during cardiac surgery reduces postoperative hyperalgesia. *Journal of Cardiothoracic and Vascular Anesthesia, 25*(6), 917–926.

Rieber, N., Mischler, D., Schumacher, V., Muth, E., Bischoff, S., Klosterhalfen, S., … Enck, P. (2010). Acute tryptophan depletion increases experimental nausea but also induces hunger in healthy female subjects. *Neurogastroenterology & Motility, 22*(7), 752–e220.

Rithirangsriroj, K., Manchana, T., & Akkayagorn, L. (2015). Efficacy of acupuncture in prevention of delayed chemotherapy induced nausea and vomiting in gynecologic cancer patients. *Gynecologic Oncology*, 136(1), 82–86.

Robottom, B. J., Shulman, L. M., & Weiner, W. J. (2012). Drug-induced movement disorders: emergencies and management. *Neurologic Clinics*, 30(1), 309–320.

Rogers, E., Mehta, S., Shengelia, R., & Reid, M. C. (2013). Four strategies for managing opioid-induced side effects in older adults. *Clinical Geriatrics*, 21(4).

Roila, F., Molassiotis, A., Herrstedt, J., Aapro, M., Gralla, R. J., & Walsh, D. (2016). 2016 MASCC and ESMO guideline update for the prevention of chemotherapy- and radiotherapy-induced nausea and vomiting in advanced cancer patients. *Annals of Oncology*, 27(Suppl 5), v119–v133.

Romeo, M. J., Parton, B., Russo, R. A., Hays, L. S., & Conboy, L. (2015). Acupuncture to treat the symptoms of patients in a palliative care setting. *Explore: The Journal of Science and Healing*, 11(5), 357–362.

Rubinstein, A., & Carpenter, D. M. (2014). Elucidating risk factors for androgen deficiency associated with daily opioid use. *The American Journal of Medicine*, 127(12), 1195–1201.

Rubinstein, A. L., & Carpenter, D. M. (2017). Association Between Commonly Prescribed Opioids and Androgen Deficiency in Men: A Retrospective Cohort Analysis. *Pain Medicine*, 18(4), 637–644.

Rubinstein, A. L., Carpenter, D. M., & Minkoff, J. R. (2013). Hypogonadism in men with chronic pain linked to the use of long-acting rather than short-acting opioids. *The Clinical Journal of Pain*, 29(10), 840–845.

Ruan, X., Ma, L., Couch, J. P., Chen, T., & Bumgarner, G. W. (2015). Intractable pruritus during outpatient epidural hydromorphone infusion: a case report and a focused review of the literature. *Journal of Opioid Management*, 11(2), 184–190.

Ruddy, K. J., Barton, D., & Loprinzi, C. L. (2014). Laying to rest psychostimulants for cancer-related fatigue? *Journal of Clinical Oncology*, 32(18), 1865–1867. https://doi.org/10.1200/JCO.2014.55.8353.

Sandoval, K., & Witt, K. (2015). Gastrointestinal Drugs. In *Side Effects of Drugs Annual* (Vol. 37, pp. 433-459). Elsevier. https://doi.org/10.1016/bs.seda.2015.05.008.

Schoch, D., Sommer, R., Augustin, M., Ständer, S., & Blome, C. (2017). Patient-Reported Outcome Measures in Pruritus: A systematic review of measurement properties. *Journal of Investigative Dermatology*, 137(10), 2069–2077.

Scully, C. (2013). *Dry Mouth (xerostomia & hyposalivation) pp. 91-97* In: *Oral and Maxillofacial Medicine Third Edition*. St. Louis, MO: Elsevier.

Seyyedrassoli, A. (2016). Comparison of Effectiveness of Reflexology and Abdominal Massage on Constipation among Orthopedic Patients: A single-blind Randomized Controlled Trial. *International Journal of Medical Research and Health Sciences*, 5(10), 33–40.

Sheen, M. J., Ho, S. T., Lee, C. H., Tsung, Y. C., & Chang, F. L. (2008a). Preoperative gabapentin prevents intrathecal morphine-induced pruritus after orthopedic surgery. *Anesthesia & Analgesia*, 106(6), 1868–1872.

Sheen, M. J., Ho, S. T., Lee, C. H., Tsung, Y. C., Chang, F. L., & Huang, S. T. (2008b). Prophylactic mirtazapine reduces intrathecal morphine-induced pruritus. *British journal of Anaesthesia*, 101(5), 711–715.

Simonnet, G., Laboureyras, E., & Sergheraert, L. (2013). Polyamine deficient diet: A nutritional therapy for relieving abnormal and chronic pain. *PharmaNutrition*, 1(4), 137–140.

Simorov, A., Thompson, J., & Oleynikov, D. (2014). Alvimopan reduces length of stay and costs in patients undergoing segmental colonic resections: results from multicenter national administrative database. *The American Journal of Surgery*, 208(6), 919–925.

Singh, P., Yoon, S. S., & Kuo, B. (2016). Nausea: a review of pathophysiology and therapeutics. *Therapeutic Advances in Gastroenterology*, 9(1), 98–112.

Smith, H., & Laufer, A. (2014). Opioid induced nausea and vomiting. *European Journal of Pharmacology*, 722(1), 67–78.

Smith, H. S., & Peppin, J. F. (2014). Toward a systematic approach to opioid rotation. *Journal of Pain Research*, 7, 589.

Soergel, D. G., Subach, R. A., Burnham, N., Lark, M. W., James, I. E., Sadler, B. M., ... Webster, L. R. (2014). Biased agonism of the μ-opioid receptor by TRV130 increases analgesia and reduces on-target adverse effects versus morphine: a randomized, double-blind, placebo-controlled, crossover study in healthy volunteers. *PAIN*, 155(9), 1829–1835.

Stern, E. K., & Brenner, D. M. (2018). Spotlight on naldemedine in the treatment of opioid-induced constipation in adult patients with chronic noncancer pain: design, development, and place in therapy. *Journal of Pain Research*, 11, 195–199.

Stoicea, N., Gan, T. J., Joseph, N., Uribe, A., Pandya, J., Dalal, R., & Bergese, S. D. (2015). Alternative therapies for the prevention of postoperative nausea and vomiting. *Frontiers in Medicine*, 2(87). https://doi.org/10.3389/fmed.2015.00087.

Stott, A. (2016). Examining the efficacy of stimulating the PC6 wrist acupuncture point for preventing postoperative nausea and vomiting: A Cochrane review summary. *International Journal of Nursing Studies*, 64(1), 139–141.

Sultan, P., Halpern, S. H., Pushpanathan, E., Patel, S., & Carvalho, B. (2016). The effect of intrathecal morphine dose on outcomes after elective cesarean delivery: a meta-analysis. *Anesthesia & Analgesia*, 123(1), 154–164.

Suzan, E., Eisenberg, E., Treister, R., Haddad, M., & Pud, D. (2013). A negative correlation between hyperalgesia and analgesia in patients with chronic radicular pain: Is hydromorphone therapy a double-edged sword? *Pain Physician*, 16(1), 65–76.

Tan, M., Law, L. S. C., & Gan, T. J. (2015). Optimizing pain management to facilitate enhanced recovery after surgery pathways. *Canadian Journal of Anesthesia/Journal Canadien d'anesthésie*, 62(2), 203–218.

Tischler, E. H., Restrepo, C., Oh, J., Matthews, C. N., Chen, A. F., & Parvizi, J. (2016). Urinary retention is rare after total joint arthroplasty when using opioid-free regional anesthesia. *The Journal of Arthroplasty*, 31(2), 480–483.

Trescot, A. M. (2016). Opioid pharmacology and pharmacokinetics. In *Controlled substance management in chronic pain* (pp. 45–62). Springer.

Tsukuura, H., Ando, Y., Gyawali, B., Matsumoto, M., Sugishita, M., & Hasegawa, Y. (2015). Prophylactic use of antiemetics for prevention of opioid-induced nausea and vomiting: a questionnaire survey among Japanese physicians. *Journal of Palliative Medicine*, 18(11), 977–980.

Umer, A., Ross-Richardson, C., & Ellner, S. (2015). Incidence and risk factors for postoperative urinary retention: A retrospective, observational study with a literature review of preventive strategies. *Connecticut Medicine*, 79, 577–588.

U.S. Food and Drug Administration (FDA). (2013). *Highlights of Prescribing Information: Transdermal Scop (scopolamine).* https://www.accessdata.fda.gov/drugsatfda_docs/label/2013/017874s038lbl.pdf. Accessed 06/17/2017.

Villa, A., Connell, C. L., & Abati, S. (2015). Diagnosis and management of xerostomia & hyposalivation. *Therapeutics and Clinical Risk Management, 11*(12), 45–51. https://doi.org/10.2147/TCRM.S76282.

Wang, J., Pennefather, S., & Russell, G. (1998). Low-dose naloxone in the treatment of urinary retention during extradural fentanyl causes excessive reversal of analgesia. *British Journal of Anaesthesia, 80*(4), 565–566.

Wang, X., & Yin, J. (2015). Complementary and alternative therapies for chronic constipation. In *Evidence-Based Complementary and Alternative Medicine.* Article ID 396396. https://doi.org/10.1155/2015/396396.

Webster, L., Andrews, M., & Stoddard, G. (2003). Modafinil treatment of opioid-induced sedation. *Pain Medicine, 4*(2), 135–140.

Webster, L., Dhar, S., Eldon, M., Masuoka, L., Lappalainen, J., & Sostek, M. (2013). A phase 2, double-blind, randomized, placebo-controlled, dose-escalation study to evaluate the efficacy, safety, and tolerability of naloxegol in patients with opioid-induced constipation. *Pain, 154*(9), 1542–1550.

Weinbroum, A. A. (2012). Non-opioid IV adjuvants in the perioperative period: pharmacological and clinical aspects of ketamine and gabapentinoids. *Pharmacological Research, 65*(4), 411–429.

Weinbroum, A. A. (2017). Postoperative hyperalgesia: a clinically applicable narrative review. *Pharmacological Research, 120,* 188–205.

White, H. D., & Robinson, T. D. (2015). A novel use for testosterone to treat central sensitization of chronic pain in fibromyalgia patients. *International Immunopharmacology, 27*(2), 244–248.

White, H. D., Brown, L. A., Gyurik, R. J., Manganiello, P. D., Robinson, T. D., Hallock, L. S., ... Yeo, K. T. J. (2015). Treatment of pain in fibromyalgia patients with testosterone gel: Pharmacokinetics and clinical response. *International Immunopharmacology, 27*(2), 249–256.

Wiffen, P. J., Derry, S., & Moore, R. A. (2014). Impact of morphine, fentanyl, oxycodone or codeine on patient consciousness, appetite and thirst when used to treat cancer pain. *Cochrane Database Syst Rev, 5,* CD011056.

Willens, J. (2015). Understanding opioid-induced constipation. *Opioid-Induced Constipation, 1* (March 2015).

Wirz, S., Nadstawek, J., Elsen, C., Junker, U., & Wartenberg, H. C. (2012). Laxative management in ambulatory cancer patients on opioid therapy: a prospective, open-label investigation of polyethylene glycol, sodium picosulphate and lactulose. *European Journal of Cancer Care, 21*(1), 131–140.

Wiese, A. D., Griffin, M. R., Stein, C. M., Mitchel, E. F., Jr., & Grijalva, C. G. (2016). Opioid analgesics and the risk of serious infections among patients with rheumatoid arthritis: a self-controlled case series study. *Arthritis & Rheumatology, 68*(2), 323–331.

Wiese, A. D., Griffin, M. R., Schaffner, W., Stein, C. M., Greevy, R. A., Mitchel, E. F., & Grijalva, C. G. (2018). Opioid Analgesic Use and Risk for Invasive Pneumococcal Diseases: A Nested Case–Control Study. *Annals of Internal Medicine, 168*(6), 396–404.

Wiffen, P. J., Wee, B., Derry, S., Bell, R. F., & Moore, R. A. (2017). *Opioids for cancer pain-an overview of Cochrane reviews. Cochrane Database of Systematic Reviews.* Chichester, UK: John Wiley & Sons, Ltd.

Woodward, S., Norton, C., & Barriball, K. L. (2010). A pilot study of the effectiveness of reflexology in treating idiopathic constipation in women. *Complementary Therapies in Clinical Practice, 16*(1), 41–46.

Wu, L., Huang, X., & Sun, L. (2015). The efficacy of N-methyl-D-aspartate receptor antagonists on improving the postoperative pain intensity and satisfaction after remifentanil-based anesthesia in adults: a meta-analysis. *Journal of Clinical Anesthesia, 27*(4), 311–324.

Young-McCaughan, S., & Miaskowski, C. (2001). Definition of and mechanism for opioid-induced sedation. *Pain Management Nursing, 2*(3), 84–97.

Youssef, N., Orlov, D., Alie, T., Chong, M., Cheng, J., Thabane, L., & Paul, J. (2014). What epidural opioid results in the best analgesia outcomes and fewest side effects after surgery? A meta-analysis of randomized controlled trials. *Anesthesia & Analgesia, 119*(4), 965–977.

Zaouter, C., & Ouattara, A. (2015a). How long is a transurethral catheter necessary in patients undergoing thoracotomy and receiving thoracic epidural analgesia? Literature review. *Journal of Cardiothoracic and Vascular Anesthesia, 29*(2), 496–501.

Zaouter, C., & Ouattara, A. (2015b). Is Urinary drainage necessary in patients with thoracic epidural analgesia? A Prospective Analysis: Reply. *Journal of Cardiothoracic and Vascular Anesthesia, 29*(3), e31–e32.

Zand, F., Amini, A., Asadi, S., & Farbood, A. (2015). The effect of methylnaltrexone on the side effects of intrathecal morphine after orthopedic surgery under spinal anesthesia. *Pain Practice, 15*(4), 348–354.

Chapter 13 Preventing Opioid-Induced Advancing Sedation and Respiratory Depression

Carla R. Jungquist, Ann Quinlan-Colwell

CHAPTER OUTLINE

Opioids and Respiratory Function, pg. 338

Normal Respiratory Physiology and the Effect of Opioids, pg. 338

Advancing Sedation and Opioid-Induced Respiratory Depression, pg. 338

Incidence, pg. 338

Overview of Current Recommendations, pg. 339

Identification of the Risk Factors, pg. 339

Nonmodifiable Risk Factors, pg. 340

Risk Factors Associated With Naloxone Administration, pg. 340

Modifiable Risk Factors, pg. 341

Timing of Care and Assessments, pg. 342

Communication Within the Health Care Team, pg. 342

Health Care Team and Institutional Policies and Procedures, pg. 342

Associated Pharmacologic Factors, pg. 342

Formulations of Opioid Medications and Risks, pg. 342

Mechanisms of Delivery of Opioid Medications and Risks, pg. 345

Delivery Systems, pg. 346

Combining Classes of Medications and Their Synergistic Effects, pg. 346

Strategizing to Improve Safety for Patients at Risk, pg. 347

Assessing the Patient for Risk, pg. 347

Subjective Assessment of Risk, pg. 347

Objective Assessment of Risk, pg. 348

Detection Using Electronic Monitoring Devices, pg. 348

Monitoring the Patient, pg. 348

Procedures for Intermittent Nursing Assessment for All Patients on Opioids: Level of Sedation, pg. 348

Pasero Opioid Sedation Scale, pg. 349

Michigan Opioid Safety Score, pg. 349

Richmond Sedation Scale, pg. 350

Procedures for Intermittent Nursing Assessment for All Patients on Opioids: Respiratory Status, pg. 351

Continuous Electronic Monitoring, pg. 352

Pulse Oximetry, pg. 352

Respiratory Rate, pg. 352

Capnography, pg. 352

Minute Ventilation, pg. 352

Interventions After Assessment, pg. 353

Summary, pg. 353

Key Points, pg. 353

Case Scenario, pg. 354

Acknowledgments, pg. 354

References, pg. 354

PAIN management using opioids necessitates achieving a balance between adequate pain control and patient safety, including optimal respiratory function (Voscapoulos, Ladd, & George, 2015). Hospitalized patients who exhibit an opioid-related adverse event have 55% longer hospital stays, 47% higher costs associated with their care, a 36% increased risk for 30-day readmission, and a 3.4 times higher risk of inpatient mortality compared to those not having adverse drug events from opioids (Kessler, Shah, Gruschkus, & Raju, 2013). In a study of over 1.14 million nonsurgical admissions across 286 U.S. hospitals, about 50% of patients received opioid medications. In this study, 6 of every 1000 postoperative patients experienced a serious adverse event (defined by naloxone exposure or an opioid-related adverse drug event diagnostic code), including respiratory depression (Herzig, Rothberg, Cheung, Ngo, & Marcantonio, 2014).

Advancing sedation and opioid-induced respiratory depression (ASOIRD) can cause serious patient harm and have substantial financial consequences, costing hospitals an average of about $2.5 million per claim (Benumof, 2015; Fouladpour, Jesudoss, Bolden, Shaman, & Auckley, 2016; Lee et al., 2015; Svider et al., 2013). This chapter will present best nursing practices to ensure the safest and most effective pain management for the hospitalized patient. When using opioids, patient safety is the responsibility of the entire health care team and particularly the bedside nurse. Thus it is important for nurses to understand the (1) physiology of respiration, (2) influence opioids have on normal breathing and efficient ventilation of gas exchange, (3) risk factors for ASOIRD, and (4) best practices for individualizing monitoring of each patient.

Opioids and Respiratory Function

Normal Respiratory Physiology and the Effect of Opioids

The rate and depth of breath is mostly driven by carbon dioxide levels, although oxygen level does have a later influence. Central chemoreceptors in the medulla and peripheral receptors in carotid and aortic bodies regulate breathing by detecting rising carbon dioxide levels. Carbon dioxide crosses the blood-brain barrier, resulting in changes in the pH. Hydrogen ions maintain pH by increasing the respiratory rate, such as we see in the case of hypoventilation from opioids. ASOIRD occurs as the result of opioids suppressing the respiratory centers in the brain. Opioid medications blunt the normal respiratory rescue response to rising carbon dioxide and falling oxygen levels (Ladd et al., 2005; Sasaki, Meyer, & Eikermann, 2013). Additionally, opioids cause pharyngeal relaxation that enhances the normal sleep-induced airway relaxation. In patients with conditions such as obstructive sleep apnea (OSA), the addition of opioids can result in serious airway collapse, leading to hypoxemia, and blunted wakefulness response. This condition can lead to brain anoxia, hypoxia, ischemia, infarct, or even death (Lee et al., 2015).

Advancing Sedation and Opioid-Induced Respiratory Depression

In most cases, a patient experiencing opioid-induced advancing sedation and respiratory depression will exhibit a decrease in level of consciousness before signs of respiratory depression are displayed. The cause of decreased level of consciousness and respiratory depression from opioids is the result of their effect on the central nervous system (CNS). Nurses assess the level of sedation and the quality, rhythm, and rate of respirations to detect respiratory depression. Opioid-induced hypoventilation/respiratory compromise occurs when respiratory rate is less than 8 to 10 breaths/min and is accompanied by a decrease in oxygen saturation and level of responsiveness. Physiologically, respiratory depression or hypoventilation is the point when respiratory centers are no longer able to function in maintaining respiratory homeostasis by efficient gas exchange. Hypoventilation occurring from the influence of opioids results in rising carbon dioxide levels and then respiratory acidosis (Ladd et al., 2005).

Although not standard practice, one way to physiologically quantify a clinically relevant opioid-related respiratory event is to use the American Academy of Sleep Medicine criteria for sleep-disordered breathing. Sleep-disordered breathing is based on specific quantified criteria and diagnosed by a sleep study. Sleep studies are either in a laboratory and observed (polysomnography) by a technician or in home using a home sleep testing device. Both devices detect apneic events during sleep. The criterion used to identify a respiratory event is a pause in breath for more than 10 seconds with an oxygen desaturation of 3% (Kapur et al., 2017). A respiratory event could be either central or obstructive in origin. The following paragraphs will describe both types of respiratory events. Clinicians could use these criteria to identify an opioid-induced respiratory event using a bedside oximetry monitor as long as the patient is not on supplemental oxygen. Supplemental oxygen is known to blunt oxygen desaturation (Taenzer, Pyke, Herrick, Dodds, & McGrath, 2014).

Incidence

The incidence of ASOIRD is not well documented because most cases are not reported to governing agencies that collect data on sentinel and adverse events. According to a large meta-analysis, opioid-induced respiratory depression (OIRD) events are thought to be near 1.1% of all postsurgical patients receiving parenteral or epidural opioids (Cashman & Dolin, 2004). Many events are not reported as adverse events because the nurse intervenes by stimulating the patient or transferring the patient to the intensive care unit (ICU). Of reported serious ASOIRD events, 88% occurred within 24 hours of surgery and within 2 hours of the last nurse assessment of the patient (Benumof, 2015; Fouladpour et al., 2016; Lee et al., 2015; Svider et al., 2013). There is also evidence of rapid patient decline with patient harm within 15 minutes of a nursing assessment (Benumof, 2015; Fouladpour et al., 2016; Lee et al., 2015; Svider et al., 2013). Experts have deemed the majority of ASOIRD adverse events preventable with adequate monitoring.

Overview of Current Recommendations

The Joint Commission (TJC), the Institute for Healthcare Improvement (IHI), and Centers for Medicaid and Medicare Services (CMS) have issued alerts to draw attention to ASOIRD as a national problem. These alerts direct hospitals to take actions to prevent these occurrences with increased frequency of patient monitoring (Centers for Medicare and Medicaid Services (CMS), 2014; IHI, 2012; TJC, 2012). Professional organizations have developed evidence-based clinical practice guidelines (American Society of Anesthesiologists Task Force on Perioperative Management of Patients with Obstructive Sleep, 2014; Chou et al., 2016; Jarzyna et al., 2011). Along with guidelines for monitoring, there are guidelines that recommend opioid-sparing pain management interventions (Chou et al., 2016).

Unfortunately, there is very little evidence on which to base the monitoring guidelines, leaving the guidelines without specifics on timing or method of monitoring (e.g., continuous or intermittent pulse oximetry, capnography, or minute ventilation). Without adequate evidence to base clinical practices, some hospitals have elected to institute electronic monitoring of all patients on opioids. This has resulted in problems such as alarm fatigue, increased health care costs, work around behaviors (i.e., circumventing policies), and patient inconvenience from wearing electronic devices (Mitka, 2013; Pasero & von Baeyer, 2017; Sendelbach & Funk, 2013). Additionally, publications from hospitals that have instituted continuous monitoring have not documented consistent zero naloxone use, which needs to be a goal for safe and effective pain management. Current evidence on monitoring procedures and a review of factors that attribute to ASOIRD sentinel events has led most guidelines and quality monitoring organizations (TJC, IHI, and CMS) to recommend assessing the patient and environmental risk factors, institute systematic quality measures with tracking of events, and education of all members of the health care team. Quality measures may include the assessment of high-risk patients, implementation of an opioid-sparing multimodal analgesia (MMA) plan of care, and evaluation of the necessity and/or frequency of intermittent or continuous electronic system monitoring (Glowacki, 2015). When a patient is found to be at high risk, immediate implementation of opioid-sparing pain management as well as increasing the frequency of intermittent assessment or adding continuous monitoring using the appropriate electronic monitoring system is recommended.

Identification of the Risk Factors

The prevention of opioid-related adverse events is the responsibility of the facility as much as it is of individual clinicians. It is good practice for hospital administrators to initiate and support high-quality measures (see Chapter 28) that will allow the discovery and reporting of all opioid-related near-miss and events that cause patient harm. Instituting an action-oriented systematic process will allow facilities to recognize trends in adverse or near-miss events, and institute policies and procedures that will address the institutional risk factors for ASOIRD. Current best practices recommend the health care team assess all patients who will receive opioid medications for risk factors for ASOIRD (Box 13.1). Patient risk factors fall into the categories of modifiable and nonmodifiable. Nonmodifiable risk factors are unique factors of the patient that have an impact on the clinical plan of care. These factors cannot be changed (e.g., age, sex, genetics, comorbidities) (Box 13.1). Modifiable risk factors

---

| **Box 13.1** | Nonmodifiable Risk Factors |

Individual risks factors (if present indicate patient meets criteria for being at *higher* risk)
- Obesity hypoventilation syndrome
  - BMI $\geq$ 30 kg/m² *and*
  - ABG pCO$_2$ > 45 mm Hg (normal 35-45) *or* serum HCO$_3$ > 27 mmol/L (without other cause of metabolic alkalosis)
- Known or suspected sleep-disordered breathing
  - STOP-BANG total score > 3/8
  - Diagnosis of obstructive or central sleep apnea
- Comorbidities/ASA > 2
  - Cardiac and/or pulmonary (previous or current smoker and/or need for supplemental oxygen)
  - Renal (blood urea nitrogen > 30 mg/dL)
  - Hepatic (albumin level < 30 g/L)
- Obesity
- Substantive functional limitations
- Substance use disorder (tobacco, ETOH, opioid, illicit substances)
- Prior history or current (found observed in PACU) opioid-related sedation/respiratory event
- Prolonged (> 3 hours) surgery under general anesthesia
- Surgical site (head, neck, chest, upper abdominal)
- Requirement of higher than usual or frequently repeated doses of opioid medications
- First 24 hours after surgery or of starting opioids

ASA, American Society of Anesthesia; *BMI,* body mass index; *ETOH,* ethyl alcohol; *PACU,* postanesthesia care unit.

are hospital and clinical care issues that the health care team can modify or change (e.g., analgesic prescriptions, assessment parameters).

Nonmodifiable Risk Factors

It is well known that not all patients exhibit the same risk for ASOIRD. All patients administered opioids for acute pain are at some risk for developing ASOIRD, but some are at higher risk and require increased vigilance by the health care team. In recent years, some hospitals have started collecting data on patients who have required naloxone administration and/or initiation of the rapid response team for events thought to be ASOIRD. Publications from these root cause analyses and evidence developed during validation studies of new electronic monitoring devices have led to a better understanding of which patients are at higher risk. There is strong evidence that patients with signs and symptoms of or diagnosed OSA and obesity hypoventilation syndrome are at higher risk for ASOIRD.

Obstructive Sleep Apnea

OSA is consistently identified as a risk factor and a correlate of ASOIRD. In fact, respiratory arrest is considered the most common complication associated with OSA, with serious complications of anoxic brain injury and death seen increasingly as a primary contention in legal cases (Fouladpour et al., 2016). In a 24-month study of patients who required postoperative naloxone (n = 84,533), those with OSA were determined to be 2.45 times more likely to have OIRD or sedation related to opioids, and patients who had a respiratory adverse event in postoperative recovery unit (postanesthesia care unit [PACU]) were determined to be 5.11 times more likely to require naloxone to be administered (Weingarten et al., 2015). The authors of a large retrospective study analyzing postoperative respiratory complications (n = 108,479) concluded that when the Perioperative Sleep Apnea Prediction Assessment is used to identify OSA, there is an independent association between suspected OSA and the risk for having a postoperative respiratory complication (Ramachandran, Pandit, Devine, Tompson, & Shanks, 2017). OSA frequently coexists with obesity and morbid obesity (Peromaa-Haavisto et al., 2016). Despite this strong association, an extensive systematic review of respiratory distress among patients with OSA having bariatric surgery (n = 98,935) found no specific relationship between OSA and respiratory distress in this population (De Raaff, Coblijn, de Vries, & Van Wagensveld, 2016). The researchers of that study suggest the results may be due to improved monitoring and care of morbidly obese patients identified in a high-risk group. Use of a continuous positive airway pressure (CPAP) machine is most likely an important safety factor (Ireland, Chapman, Mathew, Herbison, & Zacharias, 2014). However, in a smaller study (n = 325) in patients with OSA who had undergone bariatric surgery,

the results were different. In that study, patients with OSA were significantly (P = .0002) more likely to experience respiratory complications if they did not use CPAP (14.9%) compared to those who did (2.95%) (Kong et al., 2016).

Screening for Obstructive Sleep Apnea

The STOP-BANG questionnaire (see Table 8.1) has been validated and is an effective screening tool for patients with OSA. Although a total score of greater than 3 of 8 is considered a positive screen for OSA, a total score of 5 or greater on the STOP-BANG instrument has been found to have 74% specificity and be 56% sensitive for the detection of OSA (Chung et al., 2008). The STOP-BANG questionnaire is being used more frequently by hospitals. In patients who have not been diagnosed with OSA, the practice of using overnight oximetry to screen for OSA occurs in some settings. If patients exhibit an average oxygen saturation level of less than 93% over the night, experience more than 29 desaturations per hour, or spend more than 7% of the night at an oxygen level less than 90%, they are 2.2 times more likely to experience a postoperative complication (Chung, Zhou, & Liao, 2014). See Chapter 8 for additional discussion of sleep and OSA.

Screening for Obesity Hypoventilation Syndrome

The diagnostic criteria for obesity hypoventilation syndrome (OHS) is body mass index (BMI) greater than 30 kg/m², hypoxemia (oxygen saturation [SpO_2] < 90% during sleep), and hypercapnia during the day. Compared with patients who have OSA alone, hospitalized patients with OHS are more likely to (1) be admitted to the ICU postoperatively, (2) require a tracheostomy, and (3) have increased lengths of hospital stay (Kaw et al., 2016).

The health care team can screen for OHS by assessing BMI greater than 30 kg/m², daytime oxygen level (<95%), partial pressure of carbon dioxide by arterial blood gas ($PaCO_2$) greater than 45 mm Hg, or serum bicarbonate (HCO_3) greater than 27 mmol/L (by admission chemistry profile) (Hart et al., 2014; Manuel, Hart, & Stradling, 2015).

Risk Factors Associated With Naloxone Administration

Naloxone is the rescue medication used to reverse the respiratory depressive effects of opioid medications. Hospitals have reviewed their naloxone use, reporting the characteristics of the patients who required naloxone administration for ASOIRD. Predictors were found to be (1) comorbid renal, cardiac, and respiratory disease; (2) history of smoking; (3) concurrent use of other sedating medications; (4) having undergone general anesthesia; (5) overweight (BMI ≥25); (6) older age (older than 60 years); (7) preoperative albumin less than 30 g/L; and (8) female sex (Khelemsky, Kothari, Campbell, & Farnad, 2015; Lee et al., 2015; Meisenberg, Ness, Rao, Rhule, & Ley, 2017; Rosenfeld et al., 2016; Story et al., 2009, 2010).

In one retrospective case-controlled study reviewing cases of naloxone used to reverse ASOIRD (n = 65), the investigators reported the patients who experienced ASOIRD had more risk factors (average of five risk factors) than the matched patients who did not experience ASOIRD (average of 3.3 risk factors). Consistent with other reports, the five patient characteristics significantly correlated with ASOIRD were coexisting renal disease, coexisting cardiac disease, coexisting respiratory disease, concurrent administration of medications sedating the CNS, and current smoker (Pawasauskas, Stevens, Youssef, & Kelley, 2014). There may be additional patient-specific risk factors. A randomized, double-blind and placebo-controlled adult twin study was done with 242 monozygotic and dizygotic twins who were administered either a steady-state infusion with the mu opioid agonist alfentanil or a placebo saline infusion (Angst et al., 2012). The researchers of that study reported that there were significant genetic effects or heritability of 30% of respiratory depression measured by respiratory rate and a familial aggregate effect (genetic and/or shared environmental effects) (Angst et al., 2012) of 31% measured by changes in transcutaneous carbon dioxide. In the same study, there was significant familial aggregate effect (29%) with sedation that was measured through a self-report on a visual analogue scale (VAS) (Angst et al., 2012). Clearly, additional research is needed to determine the relationships between patient-specific characteristics and the risk for ASOIRD. In studies of adverse events, reported risk factors were OSA, hypertension, coronary artery disease and dysrhythmias, diabetes, and congestive heart failure. Type of surgery is correlated with risk for ASOIRD. Surgery to repair aortic abdominal aneurysms, thoracic surgery, peripheral vascular procedures, upper abdominal surgery, neck surgery, bariatric surgery, and neurosurgery are associated with greater risk for respiratory complications compared to those undergoing spine, extremity, ear, nose, and throat surgery. Also, at greater risk are patients undergoing surgery with incisions going from above to below the umbilicus. The first 24 hours after surgery has been found to be the time when more patients will develop ASOIRD (Arozullah, Conde, & Lawrence, 2003; Lee et al., 2015; Ramachandran et al., 2011; Weingarten, 2015). Although in some studies age has been found to be a risk factor, other studies have shown that the presence for multiple morbidities is a stronger factor than age alone (Lee et al., 2015; Ramachandran et al., 2011; Weingarten et al., 2015).

Although there is not significant published evidence, clinically, experts report another category of patients at risk for ASOIRD (1) are those with chronic pain already on opioids before admission to the hospital, (2) those with a substance use disorder, and (3) patients who require multiple and higher than usual doses of opioids to control their acute pain. Multimodal pain management and the use of increased vigilance using continuous electronic monitoring (e.g., pulse oximetry or capnography) are recommended for patient safety (Chou et al., 2016).

Modifiable Risk Factors

Modifiable factors result from accidental or incidental influences from the environment or simply receiving care in the hospital setting. Modifiable risk factors for ASOIRD fall into the categories of (1) timing of care and nurse assessments, (2) health care team, (3) communication within the health care team, and (4) institutional policies and procedures. Using Embase, an extensive literature review identified no current information to support a correlation or relationship among patient discharge, environment, electronic medical record, handoff, hourly rounding, pain team presence, patient satisfaction, staffing, transfers, and staff turnover. There is a void of information regarding possible relationships, either correlational or causative, between OIRD and the various iatrogenic risk factors. Research among these factors and ASOIRD is needed. Although there is not published evidence, there is expert opinion that during hourly rounding nurses are doing a brief assessment of level of consciousness and noise from breathing, if sleeping, and other patient safety assessments and pain screen when the patient is awake.

Supplemental oxygen is often considered to be an intervention to provide safety when opioids are administered. However, in the 2016 American Society of Anesthesiologists (ASA) and American Society of Regional Anesthesia and Pain Medicine (ASRA) guidelines regarding respiratory depression and neuraxial opioids, it was noted that data were inadequate to conclude whether supplemental oxygen is beneficial to reduce hypoxia or hypoxemia in severity or frequency during administration of neuraxial opioids (ASA, 2016). In the same report, the authors noted that under certain circumstances (e.g., alteration in consciousness, respiratory depression, and hypoxemia [i.e. SpO_2 <90%]) supplemental oxygen is needed and that it should be available for patients if needed. Some concerns about using supplemental oxygen with patients receiving opioids are discussed in current literature. In a small proof of concept study (n = 20), it was noted that respiratory depression was more distinct in subjects who were inhaling hyperoxic gas compared to those inhaling normoxic gas mixtures, suggesting that ASOIRD can be intensified by the use of supplemental oxygen (Niesters, Mahajan, Aarts, & Dahan, 2013). This is reasonable because in the presence of supplemental oxygen, hypoxemia secondary to hypoventilation is delayed; supplemental oxygen can impair the accuracy and sensitivity of pulse oximetry and delay the ability to identify OIRD (Nagappa, Weingarten, Montandon, Sprung, & Chung, 2017).

Of all possible iatrogenic factors, the temporal relationship between starting opioids and ASOIRD is the strongest risk during the first 24 hours postoperatively (Weingarten, Warner, & Sprung, 2017). In a study done in a 268-bed tertiary teaching hospital, 61% of patients who required naloxone postoperatively (n = 251) did so within the first 24 hours of surgery (Rosenfeld et al., 2016).

Findings from a retrospective observational cohort study of a large database (n = 87,650) showed multiple patient-specific factors and most events occurring within 24 hours of initiation of opioid therapy. In that study, a critical respiratory event was reported for 34% of patients within the first 6 hours and for 81% of patients within the first day (Ramachandran et al., 2011). In another large retrospective cohort study (n = 84,533) that reviewed cases of patients hospitalized between 2008 and 2010, 58% of cases of OIRD occurred within 12 hours of discharge from anesthesia (Weingarten et al., 2015). Further, in that study, patients who had an adverse respiratory event while in the recovery room were more likely to also have an event during the post–recovery room period. This indicates there is an opportunity to identify ways to screen patients while in the postanesthesia unit who may be at higher risk for ASOIRD when they are transferred to other areas (Weingarten et al., 2015).

Timing of Care and Assessments

Patients are at the highest risk for OIRD during the 24 hours after a procedure (Khelemsky et al., 2015; Lee et al., 2015; Rosenfeld et al., 2016). There is evidence that patients who are assessed every 2 hours via intermittent pulse oximetry, sedation scale, and respiratory rate and quality are less likely to require naloxone intervention compared to patients assessed every 4 hours (Jungquist et al., 2016). Hourly rounding is a common procedure that nurses use to increase patient satisfaction with care and patient safety. Although there is no evidence that hourly rounding is a useful tool to prevent OIRD, there is evidence that hourly rounding improves pain management and decreases falls (Alaloul, Williams, Myers, Jones, & Logsdon, 2015; Kirk & Kane, 2016; Leone & Adams, 2016). Research to identify the possible effectiveness of hourly rounding to reduce the incidence of ASOIRD is needed.

Communication Within the Health Care Team

It is well known that inadequate or inaccurate communication is strongly associated with patient adverse events and negative outcomes (Lee, Allen, & Daly, 2012; Robinson, 2016) and sentinel events (Johnson, Logsdon, Fournier, & Fisher, 2016). Open and direct communication within the health care team is associated with safer patient care. Shift-to-shift handoff is an important communication strategy, but the benefits are mitigated when communication is not clear and complete (Matic, Davidson, & Salamonson, 2011). Hospitals have instituted standardized procedures for communication at patient handoff between levels of care or hospital units (Riesenberg, Leitzsch, & Cunningham, 2010). Unfortunately, there is a dearth of evidence on the effect of handoff communication on preventing ASOIRD. It is not clear how often respiratory status is discussed during even the most structured handoffs

(Johnson et al., 2016; Robinson, 2016). Research is needed, at a minimum, to identify barriers to effective communication and opportunities for improvement and to develop comprehensive tools and effective methods to educate staff members.

Health Care Team and Institutional Policies and Procedures

Although all nurses are considered to be pain management nurses, not all nurses have the expertise needed to address the needs of the patient with complex painful conditions. Additionally, novice nurses often lack the expertise needed to identify patients with early signs of respiratory compromise. For these reasons, it is important for hospitals to support the adaption of teams of experts to mentor nurses and provide a watchful eye on complex patients (Shelton et al., 2013; Story et al., 2013; Van den Heede, Clarke, Sermeus, Vleugels, & Aiken, 2007). The addition of a pain management team that has expertise in multimodal and opioid-sparing pain management is also considered helpful (Crawford, Boller, Jadalla, & Cuenca, 2016; Duncan et al., 2014; Hoda, Hamid, & Khan, 2007; McDonnell, Nicholl, & Read, 2003). The Institute for Safe Medication Practice (ISMP, 2013a) advised that hospitals establish policies and staff education based on established guidelines and standards of care. It is also important for hospitals to support the use of quality markers to track safe and effective pain management (Jungquist et al., 2014b).

Associated Pharmacologic Factors

All opioid medications have the potential to cause excessive sedation and respiratory depression. The difference among the opioids is their formulations and time to peak effect (see Box 13.2). Categories of pharmacologic risk factors include (1) formulations of opioid medications, (2) mechanisms of delivery, and (3) synergistic effects from coadministered medications.

Formulations of Opioid Medications and Risks

It is well known that patients who receive opioids are potentially at risk to have the serious side effect of OIRD. Earlier literature attributed ASOIRD to action of ventral medullary opioid receptors with opioids in the cerebrospinal fluid (CSF). The current explanation is that pre-Bötzinger complex neurons along with neurokinin-1 receptors are discriminately inhibited in the medulla (Green & Tay, 2016), leading to ASOIRD. Some opioids are considered to have less risk for OIRD. TraMADol is associated with less respiratory depression than other opioids (Green & Tay, 2016). Buprenorphine is reported to have a ceiling effect in avoiding respiratory depression when used appropriately (Wiegand, 2016); however, that

CHANGE THE WAY PAIN IS MANAGED

1. Promote a practice culture that views opioid-only pain treatment plans as unacceptable ("red flag").
2. Form a multidisciplinary task force (e.g., nurses from the perianesthesia setting and postoperative clinical units, pharmacists, surgeons, and anesthesia providers) to evaluate current pain management practices with a focus on those that increase the incidence of adverse events.
   a. Develop a process for identifying patients at the highest risk for opioid-induced adverse events preoperatively.
   b. Recognize the increased risk imposed by the coadministration of sedating adjuvant medications, such as benzodiazepines and antihistamines.
   c. Remember that opioid pain relief is usually dose related rather than opioid related. Rather than an "opioid laundry list" approach, establish PACU opioid titration protocols based on the goals of care and the pharmacokinetics and pharmacodynamics of the first-line opioids. For example, use fentaNYL in patients with severe pain on admission to the PACU and in those with an end-organ failure; otherwise, titrate using the opioid the patient is likely to receive after discharge from the PACU.
   d. Understand that many factors influence pain relief and there is no specific dose that will relieve pain of a specific intensity. Do not prescribe and administer opioid doses based on pain intensity ratings, for example, 2 mg intravenous (IV) morphine for pain ratings of 1 to 3 (on a scale of 0 to 10); 4 mg IV morphine for pain ratings of 4 to 6; and 6 mg IV morphine for pain ratings greater than 6. (Pasero, Quinn, Portenoy, McCaffery, & Rizos, 2011) Evaluate multiple factors, including sedation level, respiratory status, opioid tolerance, age, comorbidities, and pain intensity, when selecting an opioid dose.
   e. Do not establish PACU discharge criteria that require pain intensity be reduced to an arbitrary level (e.g., 4 on a scale of 0 to 10) before transfer to the clinical unit. Pain control is best viewed on a continuum and is the responsibility of every member of the health care team. Further titration after discharge from the PACU may be necessary and should be an accepted practice on the clinical units.
3. Review the relevant literature and develop multimodal pain treatment plans that have been shown to improve pain control while reducing opioid dose.
4. Expand the hospital formulary to provide reasonable options that will support MMA, for example, intravenous, oral, and rectal acetaminophen and NSAIDs.
   a. Although the cost of a drug is an important consideration, decisions about which analgesics will be available to the health care team should be based on the overarching goal of improving patient outcomes.
5. Include nonpharmacologic options in multimodal pain treatment plans.
   a. Implement creative approaches to increase the use of nonpharmacologic methods such as teaching pastoral care counselors and selected volunteers how to provide cognitive-behavioral approaches, including meditation, relaxation breathing, music therapy, and guided imagery, as well as when to suggest to the nursing staff the use of physical modalities, such as cold and heat therapy.
6. Optimize pain treatment in patients with preexisting chronic pain.
   a. Provide surgeons with information about which analgesics may be continued and which should be discontinued preoperatively in patients with preexisting pain.
   b. Establish a process for identifying patients with chronic pain preoperatively, so that their pain treatment can be optimized before the additional pain of surgery is inflicted.
   c. Contact the surgeon and/or anesthesiologist (preoperatively whenever possible) for analgesic orders in patients with poorly controlled chronic pain.
   d. Consider the preoperative administration of anticonvulsants to treat and prevent neuropathic pain.

ESTABLISH MONITORING PRACTICES THAT ENHANCE DECISION MAKING

1. Review current institutional monitoring practices for all opioid therapies and identify and correct those that may contribute to delayed detection of patient deterioration.
2. Review and apply evidence-based recommendations such as those presented in the American Society for Pain Management Nursing Evidence–based Guideline on Monitoring for Sedation and Respiratory Depression.
   a. Require systematic assessment of sedation and respiratory status in all patients receiving opioid therapy regardless of the type of opioid, dose, or route or method of administration.
      i. Expect nurses to reduce opioid dose as soon as increased sedation levels are detected.
   b. Consider risk factors to determine the need for mechanical monitoring. (See Box 13.3.)
      i. If mechanical monitoring is deemed necessary, provide it continuously rather than by intermittent spot checks.
      ii. If intermittent monitoring is implemented, be aware of its shortcomings and ensure proper sedation and respiratory assessments are conducted.
      iii. Systematically evaluate the need to add or discontinue mechanical monitoring based on the patient's condition.
      iv. Ensure that hospital protocol allows nurses to implement mechanical monitoring if and as soon as a patient's condition deteriorates.

Continued

v. If a patient's condition warrants closer monitoring than can be provided on the current clinical unit, the patient should be promptly moved to a more closely monitored setting.

3. Increase monitoring of sedation and respiratory status when other sedating medications, such as benzodiazepines and antihistamines, are coadministered with opioids.

4. Ensure that the hospital protocol supports the nurse's administration of diluted naloxone by titration-to-effect technique when clinically significant opioid-induced respiratory depression is detected. (See Box 13.3.)

PROVIDE COMPREHENSIVE EDUCATION

1. Educate primary care providers and staff on the compelling and urgent need for routine use of MMA.

2. Teach all nursing staff the importance and proper technique for assessment of respiratory status (depth, regularity, and rate obtained by watching the "rise and fall" of the patient's chest during respiration).

3. Reinforce that snoring is a respiratory obstruction and should be promptly evaluated.
   a. Teach ancillary staff and visitors to promptly report excessive sedation and snoring to nursing staff.

4. Teach nurses how to interpret and when to report the data obtained from respiratory assessment and mechanical monitoring, that is, recognition of trends that may indicate deterioration.

5. Talk with patients and families about pain (preoperatively whenever possible):
   a. Describe the purpose and the intention to use MMA and that opioids are just one analgesic that will likely (but not always) be used in the treatment plan.
   b. Establish comfort-function goals with patients by explaining that "zero" pain is unrealistic and rarely occurs after the surgery, but that the staff will accept their reports of pain and try to provide pain control that will help them accomplish their functional goals with relative ease.
   c. Remind patients that they may experience pain on awakening after the surgery and that medication will be provided with a focus on safely reducing the pain. Emphasize that safety always comes first!
   d. Reinforce practices that reduce patient risk for opioid-induced adverse events, such as patient-only use of patient-controlled analgesia.

EVALUATE PERSONAL PRACTICE

1. If nonopioid analgesics have not been prescribed, promptly contact the primary care provider for orders that ensure a nonopioid foundation for the treatment of postoperative pain for all patients undergoing surgery.

2. Implement multimodal pain treatment plans preoperatively whenever possible.

a. Remind primary care providers that many nonopioids have minimal or no effect on bleeding time and can be given preoperatively or intraoperatively.

3. Apply the principles of safe pain management.
   a. Appreciate the potency of the first-line opioids. By the IV route, 1 to 2 mg of morphine provides approximately the same analgesia as 0.1 to 0.2 mg of HYDROmorphone and 10 to 20 mcg of fentaNYL.
      i. Question the safety of a starting dose greater than 0.4 to 0.5 mg of HYDROmorphone in opioid-naïve patients.
   b. Reduce opioid dose in high-risk populations.
   c. Titrate opioids slowly and allow enough time to evaluate the patient response before administering subsequent doses.
   d. Recognize that "falling asleep" during an opioid titration indicates the patient is excessively sedated. Stop titration and allow the patient to "catch up."
   e. Do not administer a specific dose to achieve a specific pain intensity. The relationship between opioid dose and pain intensity is not linear. Consider multiple factors, including sedation level, respiratory status, and risk factors for opioid-induced respiratory depression, when determining whether to administer more opioid to a patient.
   f. View pain control on a continuum with the understanding that further titration maybe necessary after discharge from the PACU. Patient safety always comes first!
   g. Before the transfer to the clinical unit, obtain a baseline sedation level using the same sedation scale that is used to assess unwanted sedation on the clinical units. (See Box 13.3.)
   h. Patients are often sedated at discharge from the PACU as a result of anesthesia and other sedating medications given in the operating room and PACU. Inform the receiving nurse on the clinical unit whenever a patient has a sedation level of 3, so that opioid doses can be reduced or held and the patient watched closely until the sedation level improves.
   i. On transfer to the clinical unit, provide the receiving nurse with a comprehensive report of how pain was managed, including what medications and doses were administered, how well the medications were tolerated, and the patient's current pain intensity and sedation level. Inform the receiving nurse if the patient has any high-risk factors for an opioid-related sentinel event.

MMA, Multimodal anesthesia; *NSAID,* nonsteroidal antiinflammatory drug; *PACU,* postanesthesia care unit.
From Strategies to Prevent Opioid-Related Sentinel Events After Discharge from the PACU in Pasero (2013). The perianesthesia nurse's role in the prevention of opioid-related sentinel events. *Journal of PeriAnesthesia Nursing, 28*(1), 31–37.

effect is no longer present when other CNS depressants are ingested (Green & Tay, 2016). SUFentanil is reported to have a lower instance of OIRD and in a small study (n = 30) was found to have dramatically fewer instances of oxygen desaturation (3.4%) compared to morphine (23.3%) (Palmer, Royal, & Miller, 2014). The ASA Task Force (2016) concluded there was equivocal risk for administering hydrophilic opioids (e.g., morphine and HYDROmorphone) compared with lipophilic opioids (e.g., fentaNYL and SUFentanil) (see Chapter 11). The Task Force strongly advised that monitoring needs to be appropriate based on the pharmacodynamics and pharmacokinetics of the medication used; because of the longer duration of action, hydrophilic opioids are not appropriate to be administered neuraxially with patients undergoing outpatient surgery, and the lowest effective dose must always be administered. Patients receiving higher doses of opioids, including those who were using opioids on a regular basis before admission, were noted to be at higher risk for adverse respiratory events in one large study (Weingarten et al., 2015). Another group of patients at increased risk for respiratory events are those who receive systemic opioids in addition to neuraxial opioids (Green & Tay, 2016).

Mechanisms of Delivery of Opioid Medications and Risks

Precise data about the risk for OIRD and mechanism of delivery is difficult to identify because reports in the literature do not necessarily differentiate between patient-controlled analgesia (PCA) and epidural bolus delivery versus continuous infusion (Rosenfeld et al., 2016). Data are limited to compare neuraxial single-dose administration with other routes of administration (e.g., parenteral, oral, or transdermal); however, there seem to be fewer instances of ASOIRD when continuous epidural opioid infusions are compared with intravenous (IV) opioid infusions and no additional risk is noted with extended-release epidural morphine (ASA, 2016). Another confounding factor with delivery mechanisms is that epidural and intravenous PCA delivery are used more frequently after surgical procedures that are known to be more painful (Rosenfeld et al., 2016), making direct comparisons more difficult and less meaningful. Intravenous delivery of opioids primarily occurs in one of five ways (1) clinician-administered bolus doses as needed, (2) clinician-administered bolus doses scheduled on a regular basis, (3) continuous infusion, (4) PCA with bolus dose only, and (5) PCA with continuous infusion and bolus dose.

Clinician Boluses

When clinician-administered bolus doses are used, there is the advantage of the clinician being able to assess the patient before administration and after, when it is estimated for the opioid to take effect. A disadvantage to using clinician-administered intravenous bolus is that analgesia

benefit ebbs and flows with the peaks and troughs of the medication (Burwaiss & Comerford, 2013).

Continuous Intravenous Infusion

Continuous IV infusion of opioids have the benefit of providing more consistent analgesia once they achieve a steady plasma level. Because that necessitates 4 to 5 half-lives, ASOIRD may occur at a more variable time than can be seen with clinician-administered boluses (Burwaiss & Comerford, 2013). This is an important consideration when assessing patients for OIRD.

Intravenous Patient-Controlled Analgesia

Intravenous PCA (see Chapter 17) continues to be frequently used in hospitals, with the three most common opioids administered via PCA being morphine, HYDROmorphone and fentaNYL. The 2016 guideline from the American Pain Society (APS), the American Society of Regional Anesthesia and Pain Medicine (ASRA), and the ASA's Committee on Regional Anesthesia (ASA-CRA) strongly recommended that when parenteral opioids are needed postoperatively, intravenous PCA be used whenever the patient is appropriate for PCA use (Chou et al., 2016). The same guideline strongly recommends to not routinely use basal or continuous infusions with PCA in part because of the increased risk for OIRD and particularly because there is no evidence of improved analgesia (Chou et al., 2016). That recommendation is consistent with the safe practice recommendation from the Institute for Safe Medical Practice (ISMP, 2013b) that advised basal infusions on intravenous PCA only be used with patients who are opioid tolerant and that patients need to be monitored with continuous pulse oximetry or capnography (ISMP, 2009a, b).

Neuraxial Analgesia

Neuraxial analgesia denotes the administration of medications, single injection, continuous infusions, intermittent infusion, or patient-controlled administration into the epidural or spinal spaces (ASA, 2016). The APS, ASRA, and ASA-CRA guideline strongly recommended using neuraxial analgesia with "major thoracic and abdominal procedures, particularly in patients at risk for cardiac complications, pulmonary complications, or prolonged ileus" (Chou et al., 2016, p. 143). Although it is thought that there is less risk for OIRD with neuraxial analgesia, this may not be true with morphine. Since morphine is hydrophilic, it is more likely to result in rostral spread, which may account for the greater risk for ASOIRD with morphine compared to fentaNYL, which is lipophilic and more likely to be absorbed where it is injected (see Chapter 18) (Green & Tay, 2016; Palmer et al., 2014).

Epidural Analgesia

Epidural analgesia can be administered as bolus injections, continuous infusion, or patient-controlled epidural analgesia (PCEA) using opioids, local analgesia, or a combination of the two and the possible addition of cloNIDine

(Chou et al., 2016). A benefit to adding local analgesia or cloNIDine to the infusion or PCEA is that they are opioid sparing, thus reducing the amount of opioid needed to achieve adequate analgesia, further reducing the risk for ASOIRD (see Chapters 17 and 18).

Peripheral Regional Analgesia

Peripheral regional anesthesia is strongly recommended as an important component of postoperative MMA by the APS, ASRAPM, and ASA-CRA for surgical procedures, including those involving shoulders, lower extremities, hemorrhoids, thoracotomies, circumcisions, and cesarean sections (Chou et al., 2016). The same panel strongly recommended that whenever it is anticipated that pain control will require longer than a single-dose injection, a continuous infusion of local analgesia is needed (Chou et al., 2016) (see Chapter 18).

Wound Infiltration Analgesia

Wound infiltration analgesia is used at times as a component of MMA. A British study (n = 498) compared epidural analgesia with IV PCA and local analgesia infusion into the wound after liver resection. The researchers reported similar analgesia with lower opioid consumption and no serious adverse events, including no ASOIRD (Wong-Lun-Hing et al., 2014). Another study, done in Italy (n = 55), compared infusions of bupivacaine with infusion of saline in patients after thoracotomy who also had IV PCA with morphine. The researchers reported that the patients with bupivacaine infusions had lower pain scores both at rest and with movement and used less morphine, resulting in faster recovery of respiratory function (Fiorelli et al., 2015). Researchers in California theorized that pain could be reduced and be better controlled by infiltrating the total knee arthroplasty surgical wound with local anesthetics before implanting the knee component. In their retrospective case-controlled study (n = 76), the researchers reported significantly lower pain intensity scores and lower opioid consumption (Kuo & Grotkopp, 2017) (see Chapter 18).

Periarticular Injections

Periarticular injections are increasingly used as part of opioid-sparing MMA after total hip and total knee arthroplasties. These are effective when specific nociceptors within the joints are targeted (Ross, Greenwood, Sasser, & Jiranek, 2017). Medications used in the periarticular "cocktails" include local anesthetics, nonsteroidal anti-inflammatory drugs (NSAIDs), and corticosteroids with either an intravenous solution or a liposomal product (Bagsby, Ireland, & Meneghini, 2014; Ross et al., 2017). In one study (n = 103) patients who received liposomal injections did not have a statistical difference in analgesia or side effects, but they did have longer lengths of stay (Klug, Rivey, & Carter, 2016). The investigators of a study in Japan (n = 77) compared periarticular injections with and without a corticosteroid and concluded that patients who received a corticosteroid had significantly lower pain intensity scores early during the postoperative period with similar rates of adverse events (Tsukada, Wakui, & Hoshino, 2016). A 2015 study compared periarticular injections with local anesthetics with femoral and sciatic nerve blocks and found that whereas pain intensity scores were similar and length of stay was less, opioid use on the day of surgery was greater among the patients who received the periarticular injections (Spangehl et al., 2015) (see Chapter 18).

Delivery Systems

Clinicians need appropriate education, resources, and supervision when caring for patients receiving analgesia by these delivery routes (Chou et al., 2016). Whenever opioids are administered via equipment, it is important to remember that equipment can malfunction and lead to oversedation and respiratory sedation (Palmer et al., 2014). A particular concern is for excessive delivery of elastomeric pumps without alarms (Chou et al., 2016). Not only do patients need to be assessed and reassessed on a regular basis, but it is imperative the delivery system equipment is checked for proper function on a regular basis as well. Facilities need to have policies, procedures, education, and resources available for clinicians (Chou et al., 2016) (see Chapter 17).

Combining Classes of Medications and Their Synergistic Effects

MMA has been found to decrease opioid requirement. Unfortunately, medications such as gabanoids, which are commonly used in multimodal protocols, also have sedative properties. Although MMA is recommended, vigilance for ASOIRD continues to be necessary. In some patients, benzodiazepines and antihistamines are prescribed for comorbid conditions seen with both acute and chronic pain. The ASA Task Force (2016) advised caution when coadministering parenteral opioids and hypnotics when neuraxial opioids have been administered and that more intense and longer duration monitoring is needed when this is done and with coadministration of sedatives or magnesium. Patients who receive other sedating medications (e.g., benzodiazepines, anxiolytics, gabapentinoids, hypnotics, spasmolytics, antiepileptics, antipsychotics, anesthetics, and antihistamines) are at greater risk of having a serious adverse respiratory event (Lee et al., 2015; Pawasauskas et al., 2014; Sigmarsdottir, Gudmundsdottir, Zoëga, & Gunnarsson, 2017; Weingarten et al., 2015). A major concern is that opioids and other sedating medications interact with different receptors, which can result in a synergistic or enhanced risk for OIRD that is particularly great during sleep (Arora, Cao, & Javaheri, 2014). The results of a large (n = 8170) retrospective case-control Veterans Administration study included that the likelihood of experiencing ASOIRD was almost two times greater among patients using an antidepressant and 1.49 times greater among patients using a prescription benzodiazepine in addition to an opioid (Zedler et al., 2015). The researchers developed a tool to assess the risk for ASOIRD or overdose among veterans using prescription opioids for pain and concomitant use of antidepressants or benzodiazepines. The tool known as the Veterans Health Administration Risk for Overdose or Serious Opioid-induced Respiratory Depression (VA-RIOSORD) is reported to have excellent predictive accuracy among veterans and nonveterans and was considered valid through retrospective review, but still needs prospective validity testing in clinical situations (Zedler, Saunders, Joyce, Vick, & Murrelle, 2017). Respiratory depression is a major adverse drug event independently associated with benzodiazepines (Niedrig, Hoppe, Mächler, Russmann, & Russmann, 2016). The concomitant administration or use of opioids and benzodiazepines is known to increase risk for OIRD, but because benzodiazepines can also depress respiration, it is not clear whether that is due to a synergistic or additive effect (Jones, Mogali, & Comer, 2012; Niedrig et al., 2016). However, laboratory animal studies have shown that when there is a combination benzodiazepine and opioid, respiratory depression occurs more quickly and more intensely than when either is present alone (Jones, Mogali & Comer, 2012). An additional risk when benzodiazepines and opioids are used concomitantly is that naloxone is not as effective reversing respiratory depression, because benzodiazepines generally are reversed with flumazenil (Jones, Mogali, & Comer, 2012).

Fewer data are available regarding concomitant use of opioids with the other sedating medications. Although antihistamines are associated with ASOIRD (Cooney, 2015), other than acknowledging that they can be sedating and can also enhance the sedative effects of opioids (Anwari & Iqbal, 2003; Pasero, 2013), there is little information addressing this phenomenon in the literature (Jarzyna et al., 2011). A recent report of toxicology postmortem findings in a number of opioid deaths did report the presence of antihistamines in addition to opioids and other substances (Jones, 2017). Research is needed to explore the relationships when other sedating or potentiating medications are coadministered with opioids. This is consistent with the recommendations of authors of a systematic review noting gaps in research to support practice guidelines for management of acute postoperative pain. The authors of that review recommended well-designed research to fill the gaps and to use MMA, including nonopioid medications, nonpharmacologic interventions, and patient education (Gordon et al., 2016).

Strategizing to Improve Safety for Patients at Risk

Providing safe and effective pain management is an ethical responsibility of all health care clinicians. In the 2012 sentinel event alert issued by TJC (2012), this responsibility was stressed and brought to the attention of hospital administrators as well. The increased awareness of needing to balance patient safety with efficacious analgesia is critical to developing a strategy to achieve the balance. In many cases there needs to be a paradigm shift from pain-free analgesia to analgesia to control pain. An important component in this paradigm shift is to use MMA (Chou et al., 2016). It is imperative to understand and communicate that multimodal does not mean opioids are eliminated but rather that they are used judiciously in conjunction with nonopioid analgesic medications, coanalgesic medications, and nonpharmacologic interventions. The foundation of this effort must be the assessment of pain, function, and potential adverse events (see Chapters 5-8 and 12). Patients need to be assessed for risk for opioid-related adverse events before starting opioids and reassessed after administration of opioids (Glowacki, 2015).

Assessing the Patient for Risk

As mentioned previously, most patients will maintain their airway and metabolize opioid medications without clinically relevant signs of OIRD. However, predicting who will develop clinically relevant ASOIRD with 100% sensitivity and specificity is very difficult. There is some evidence that the current screening tools (STOP-BANG or Berlin questionnaire) that are validated to screen for OSA are not as sensitive to detect patients who experience ASOIRD (Nagappa et al., 2015). Although the STOP-BANG questionnaire total score of 8 of 8 has been found to be 99% specific for screening for moderate to severe OSA, it has not been found to have a high specificity for ASOIRD (Chung et al., 2008). In a study of postoperative patients, at least 18.3% of patients with non-sleep apnea developed moderate to severe sleep-disordered breathing after surgery (Chung et al., 2015). Currently, there are no validated screening tools to detect the patient at high risk for ASOIRD. See Box 13.1 for a list of risk factors for ASOIRD. Therefore it is important that assessment of ASOIRD of all patients receiving opioids be an ongoing and interactive process. It is important for clinicians to be vigilant and increase monitoring frequency or add continuous electronic monitoring when signs of ASOIRD may be present. The time of increased risk in all patients is during the first 24 hours after surgery or initiation of parenteral opioid medications.

Subjective Assessment of Risk

Current clinical practice guidelines recommend using the STOP-BANG questionnaire to screen all patients for ASOIRD. In addition to using the STOP-BANG questionnaire, all patients need to be screened according to nonmodifiable level of risk using the evidence presented in

Table 8.1 and Box 13.1. Additionally, it is important for clinicians to learn to use patient assessment and electronic monitoring data to detect ASOIRD.

Objective Assessment of Risk

Although clinicians are accustomed to using pulse oximetry to assess the patients' current oxygen saturation, nurses have not been trained to use trend monitoring to detect ASOIRD. Trend monitoring is a technique that captures patient baseline values (before surgery and/or opioid medications are started) and compares them to current readings. Current practice is for the nurse to measure oxygen saturation intermittently and then compare the reading to a threshold of concern (usually 90%) that is prescribed by a provider. Nursing interventions will then be based on whether the patient is above or below that threshold. The traditional threshold used to identify respiratory compromise via pulse oximetry is below 90% saturated. Unfortunately, in some cases, waiting until patients meet that threshold will be too late. When using trend monitoring, the nurse will be able to recognize respiratory compromise earlier in the declining trajectory.

Moving to trend monitoring will require a paradigm shift for nurses' critical thinking skills and for manufacturers of electronic monitoring devices. To date, data on defining a clinically relevant change in respiratory status before and after opioid administration are limited. Using the American Academy of Sleep Medicine definition, a 3% decrease in oxygen saturation from baseline is clinically relevant and meets the criteria for a respiratory event (Kapur et al., 2017). There is lack of evidence on the clinically relevant duration of the respiratory events after opioid administration. Some researchers have used the duration of 10 minutes of sustained hypoventilation (patient's respiratory status not returning to baseline or before opioid administration) to define clinically important OIRD (Galvagno, Brayanov, Williams, & George, 2017).

Detection Using Electronic Monitoring Devices

PACU nurses are in a good position to detect ASOIRD. Most PACUs use pulse oximetry to assess for respiratory compromise during recovery from anesthesia. Electronic monitoring devices currently used in most PACUs are cardiac and pulse oximetry. In patients receiving supplemental oxygen, pulse oximetry will not be a reliable measure of respiratory compromise (Liao et al., 2017). Using continuous capnography or minute ventilation in the PACU may allow nurses to identify OIRD, although evidence is still sparse in this area (Galvagno et al., 2017). Using the Academy of Sleep Medicine criteria for an apnea event, nurses could compare before and after opioid doses and identify the patient that has sustained (10 minutes) respiratory compromise after opioid administration. Another sign of OIRD is oxygen desaturation levels precipitously and repeatedly falling below 80% during sleep or deep sedation (Chung, Chan, & Liao, 2017) (see later section on capnography and minute ventilation).

Monitoring the Patient

As mentioned previously, the first 24 hours after surgery or initiation of parenteral opioids is the period when the patient is at most risk. It is good clinical care to monitor all patients closely (perhaps with continuous electronic monitoring or definitely with 2-hourly nursing assessment and hourly rounding checks) during that time. Patients found to be at higher risk definitely need to receive more vigilant and/or continuous electronic monitoring during the first 24 hours. It is good practice for all patients to be assessed every 2 hours in the first 24 hours using a validated sedation scale, intermittent pulse oximetry, and respiratory rate and quality (Jungquist et al., 2016).

Procedures for Intermittent Nursing Assessment for All Patients on Opioids: Level of Sedation

In a review of opioid-induced adverse events, somnolence was documented in 62% of the cases before the event was detected (Lee et al., 2015). This supports the need for ongoing sedation assessments and recognition by nurses that excessive sedation is a cardinal sign of impending respiratory depression. Additionally, anecdotal data from hospital surveillance of naloxone use indicate that patients who received oral opioids are as likely to receive naloxone as patients who received parenteral or neuraxial opioids. According to current practice guidelines, level of sedation is to be assessed and quantified using reliable and valid sedation scales (Jarzyna et al., 2011). Unfortunately, the use of validated sedation scales is not common practice in all hospitals (Jungquist et al., 2016). Two practice analysis surveys conducted in 2009 and 2013 by the American Society for Pain Management Nursing (ASPMN) revealed that 64% and 90%, respectively, of practicing nurses reported that their hospitals or units had sedation scales with numeric ratings for assessing opioid-induced sedation with opioid therapy (Jungquist, Willens, Dunwoody, Klingman, & Polomano, 2014a; Willens, Jungquist, Cohen, & Polomano, 2013). There are two types of validated scales used to assess level of sedation. An example of a commonly used sedation scale validated for intentional sedation is the Richmond Agitation and Sedation (RASS). An example of the second type of scale that was developed specifically to assess for opioid-related sedation is the Pasero Opioid Sedation Scale (POSS) (Box 13.3). According to ASPMN membership, the POSS and RASS were among the most commonly used (Pasero, 2009; Sessler et al., 2002).

| **Box 13.3** | Pasero Opioid-Induced Sedation Scale (POSS) With Interventions[a] |

S = Sleep, easy to arouse

Acceptable, no action necessary, may increase opioid dose if needed

1 = Awake and alert

Acceptable, no action necessary, may increase opioid dose if needed

2 = Slightly drowsy, easily aroused

Acceptable, no action necessary, may increase opioid dose if needed

3 = Frequently drowsy, arousable, drifts off to sleep during conversation

Unacceptable, monitor respiratory status and sedation level closely until sedation level is stable at less than 3 and respiratory status is satisfactory; decrease opioid dose 25% to 50%[b] or notify primary[c] or anesthesia provider for orders, consider administering a nonsedating, opioid-sparing nonopioid, such as acetaminophen or a nonsteroidal antiinflammatory drug, if not contraindicated; and ask patient to take deep breaths every 15 to 30 minutes.

4 = Somnolent, minimal or no response to verbal and physical stimulation

Unacceptable, stop opioid, consider administering naloxone,[d],[e] stay with the patient, stimulate, and support respiration as indicated by the patient status, *call rapid response team (code blue) if indicated, notify primary or anesthesia provider, monitor respiratory status and sedation level closely until sedation level is stable at less than 3 and respiratory status is satisfactory.*

From Pasero C. (2013). The perianesthesia nurse's role in the prevention of opioid-related sentinel events. *Journal of PeriAnesthesia Nursing, 28*(1), 31–37.

[a] Appropriate action is given in italics at each level of sedation.

[b] Opioid analgesic orders or a hospital protocol should include the expectation that a nurse will decrease the opioid dose if a patient is excessively sedated.

[c] For example, the physician, nurse practitioner, advanced practice nurse, or physician assistant responsible for the pain management prescription.

[d] For adults experiencing respiratory depression, mix 0.4 mg of naloxone and 10 mL of normal saline in syringe and administer this dilute solution very slowly (0.5 mL over 2 min) while observing the patient's response (titrate to effect). If sedation and respiratory depression occur during administration of transdermal fentaNYL, remove the patch; if naloxone is necessary, treatment will be needed for a prolonged period and the typical approach involves a naloxone infusion. Patient must be monitored closely for at least 24 hours after discontinuation of the transdermal fentaNYL.

e Hospital protocols should include the expectation that a nurse will administer naloxone to any patient suspected of having life-threatening opioid-induced sedation and respiratory depression.

Pasero Opioid Sedation Scale

The POSS is specifically designed to assess patients for sedation secondary to ASOIRD (Nisbet & Mooney-Cotter, 2009; Pasero, 2013; Quinlan-Colwell, 2013). Sedation occurs in advance of respiratory depression in most cases. It is important to use a sedation scale that is validated for the purpose for which it was designed. The researchers in a recent multisite retrospective study found that unintended sedation was likely assessed earlier by using the POSS and thus acted upon before the patient developed respiratory depression (Davis et al., 2017). The authors of that study suggest that in future research, POSS scores of 3 or 4 may be preferable to naloxone use as measures of OIRD (see Box 13.3).

POSS, when compared to the RASS, scored higher in ease of use, nursing confidence, and usefulness in clinical decision-making (Nisbet & Mooney-Cotter, 2009). The POSS is also easy to document in medical records (both paper and electronic) (Quinlan-Colwell, 2013). It provides clear information to share with patients and families regarding the importance of safe administration of opioids. For example, if a patient is assessed as above 3 (frequently drowsy, falls asleep midsentence) on the POSS, the nurse can share this information and educate that it is not safe to continue to administer opioids until the POSS score is 2 or lower. Because the patient descriptors on the POSS are standardized, communication among staff is more accurate and consistent, which contributes to improved patient safety (Quinlan-Colwell, Thear, Miller-Baldwin, & Smith, 2017). As discussed previously, accuracy of communication is an important component of improving patient safety and reducing adverse events. From a medicolegal perspective, the POSS documentation provides clear and standardized information about the sedation level of the patient when opioids were administered or held (Pasero, 2013; Quinlan-Colwell, 2013).

Michigan Opioid Safety Score

The Michigan Opioid Safety Score (MOSS) is another tool used to assess safety among patients receiving opioids (Fig. 13.1). Like the POSS, it was designed to standardize assessment and improve communication among clinicians. Thus it is used to guide opioid administration by combining a health risk, respiratory rate, and measurement of sedation (Soto & Yaldou, 2015). The developers reported excellent interrater reliability with the tool, but to date no validity has been established for it (Yaldou, Cooper, & Soto, 2017).

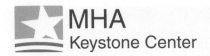

Michigan Opioid Safety Score (MOSS)

Roy Soto, M.D.

RISK STRATIFICATION

MOSS = Health Risk (maximum of 2 points) + RR Score +/- mPOSS STOP modifier (Possible score 0–4 with possible STOP modifier)		Circle point score if any criteria apply to patient	MOSS Score (Total Points)
A) Health Risk			
Group 1	• OSA • Snoring • BMI >40	1	
Group 2	• Abd/Thor surgery • Anesthesia time >3hr [within 24hr of assessment]	1	
Group 3	• Concomitant sedatives received within 2 hours	1	
Group 4	• Age >75 • Smoker	1	
If points total for this section is >2, enter "2" for MOSS Score here:			
B) Respiratory Rate			
Respiratory Rate ≥10		0	
Respiratory Rate <10		2	
Add points from this section to MOSS Score above and enter here:			
C) Modified Pasero Opioid-Induced Sedation Scale (mPoss): STOP Modifier			
Excessively sedated, drifts off to sleep, difficult to arouse or unarousable		STOP	
If STOP is circled for this section, enter "STOP" for MOSS Score and follow guidelines below			

MOSS INTERPRETATION

STOP	STOP	Stop all opioids Notify primary physician Institute increased levels of monitoring Consider anesthesia/pain consultation Ensure multimodal analgesia delivered Consider reversal agents (naloxone or flumazanil as appropriate)
4	CAUTION	Decrease opioid dose Increase levels of monitoring
3		Ensure multimodal analgesia delivered
2	CONCERN	Increase opioids as needed with special attention Consider increased levels of monitoring Ensure multimodal analgesia delivered
1	SAFE	Safe to proceed with further opioid dosing
0		Ensure multimodal analgesia delivered

Fig. 13.1 | Michigan Opioid Safety Score (MOSS). (From Soto, R., & Yaldou, B. (2015). The Michigan Opioid Safety Score (MOSS): a patient safety and nurse empowerment tool. *Journal of PeriAnesthesia Nursing, 30*(3), 196-200.

Richmond Sedation Scale

The RASS is an excellent tool with established validity and reliability for assessing sedation, particularly in the ICU (Barr et al., 2013). Although there is preliminary evidence the RASS can be used as a valid tool to assess seda-

tion and agitation with palliative sedation (Bush et al., 2014; Ely et al., 2003), there is no evidence that it can be used specifically to manage sedation related to opioid administration. Little evidence exists to support whether to use the POSS, MOSS, or RASS in an ICU setting. The best way to consider this is to think about the intention for the individual patient. If the patient is being administered opioids for analgesia and there is no intention for the person to be sedated, the POSS or MOSS is the appropriate tool for assessment of sedation. If the patient is being administered opioids for analgesia and receiving other medications for sedation or agitation, it is appropriate to use the RASS for assessing sedation and agitation.

Procedures for Intermittent Nursing Assessment for All Patients on Opioids: Respiratory Status

Observation of respiratory status requires more than just counting breaths per minute. Normal respiratory oxygenation and effective ventilation are both critical criteria when measuring the patient's respiratory assessment, not solely the rate. It is important to observe the depth, rhythm, and noise of the breaths. Normal respiratory rate ranges between 10 and 20 breaths/min (Jarvis, 2016). As mentioned previously, general consensus is that a respiratory rate less than 10 or greater than 18 breaths/min is a sign of respiratory distress. Opioids will result in a slowed rate and diminished volume initially. As the body compensates for the rising carbon dioxide levels, the respiratory rate will increase. A sign of respiratory compromise is when the respiratory rate continues to be greater than 18 breaths/min. Respiratory rhythm is usually even except when in rapid eye movement (REM) sleep when an irregular pattern is expected. Normal, nonobstructive breaths are audible and also at times with quiet snoring. Moderate to loud snoring, especially when accompanied by irregular breathing rhythm and gasps after a pause in breath, is a sign of an obstructed airway and OSA. Appropriate assessment of breathing occurs as the nurse approaches the bed, before waking the patient, remembering that respiration is most vulnerable during sleep and when sedated with medications (Box 13.4).

Most hospitals now have equipment available for clinicians to intermittently measure oxygen saturation. Although measuring oxygen saturation can be helpful, often the task is delegated to nursing assistants. Proper technique in effectively measuring oxygen saturation requires critical thinking and assessment skills. Because respiration is the most vulnerable during sleep and at peak effect of sedating medications, timing of the measurement is key. A pulse oximetry finger probe needs to be placed on the finger of the resting or sleeping patient and at the time of peak drug effect. It is important for assessment to occur without disturbing or arousing the patient, or breathing will not be observed at its most vulnerable time. Remember that most adverse events occur when the patient is sleeping. It is also important to make sure the finger probe is left in place for at least a full minute and the recorded data point is the lowest

| Box 13.4 | Clinical Application |

Mr. S. was admitted to the general care floor from the postoperative care unit at 1600. He had undergone an open cholecystectomy. His vitals were stable, and he was alert on arrival to the unit. Within an hour he was requesting pain medication for a pain level of 8 on a scale of 0 to 10 in the incisional area. The nurse medicated him with 1 mg IV HYDROmorphone after assessing his sedation level, respiratory rate and quality, and intermittent pulse oximetry. His pulse oximetry reading was 96% on room air, his respiratory rate was 20, and he was able to use his spirometry within normal range. He was alert. She returned for a 30-minute reassessment and found that he was sleeping. To assess the patient at his most vulnerable respiratory state, she walked quietly to the bedside and observed his breathing. His respiratory rate was 12 breaths/min and irregular, and he was snoring quietly. She gently placed the pulse oximeter on his finger and waited until the reading stabilized (about 30 seconds). The reading was moving between 90% and 92%. She then spoke his name quietly, and he opened his eyes quickly and spoke to her. She waited about a minute while speaking with him and then assessed his level of sedation. He was a level 2 (slightly drowsy, easily aroused) on the POSS. His pain was 3 on a scale of 0 to 10, which was an acceptable level according to him. Noticing that his oxygen level was dropping as low as 90%, she initiated continuous pulse oximetry monitoring. She also adjusted his next dose of HYDROmorphone to 0.5 mg IV, elected to give him acetaminophen with the HYDROmorphone, and applied ice to his incisional area.

observed reading. The most common obstacles to obtaining accurate oxygen saturation readings are (1) supplemental oxygen, (2) poor circulation in the finger, and (3) fingernail polish (Liao et al., 2017). Pulse oximetry is not as sensitive to assess for respiratory compromise in patients on supplemental oxygen. When only pulse oximetry is available for assessment, in patients on non–medically indicated supplemental oxygen, it makes better sense to remove the supplemental oxygen before measuring oxygen saturation. The consistent use of supplemental oxygen on all patients in the postoperative period is not evidence based and could be considered unnecessary and an impediment to accurate assessment for respiratory compromise. Capnography and minute ventilation are effective in assessing for respiratory compromise in patients on supplemental oxygen. Nurses have traditionally used the threshold of SpO_2 less than 90% saturated to determine respiratory compromise, but, as mentioned previously, research indicates that a change in paradigm is needed. To improve patient safety, nurses compare the current reading to the patient's baseline, and, if a 3%

decline has occurred, nurses reassess opioid dosing and identify opportunities to reduce opioid exposure and increase use of nonopioid strategies as part of an MMA plan of care. Another significant sign of OSA and OIRD is oxygen desaturation levels precipitously and repeatedly falling below 80% during sleep or deep sedation (Liao et al., 2017). When continuous monitoring is not available, the addition of hourly rounding with an observation of the patients' level of consciousness and breathing quality adds another safety procedure to 2-hourly assessment.

Continuous Electronic Monitoring

The safest method of detecting ASOIRD and preventing adverse events that may result in the need for naloxone administration and rapid response team activation is to use continuous electronic monitoring. Unfortunately, most hospitals do not have sufficient equipment and resources to provide this level of monitoring, and there is no evidence to support using continuous monitoring is superior to intermittent nurse assessment (sedation scale, pulse oximetry, respiration rate and quality). Timing of continuous monitoring could be most effective during the first 24 hours after anesthesia or initiation of opioid medications (Ramachandran et al., 2011). If the patient shows signs of ASOIRD, continuous monitoring is strongly advised to continue to the point at which parenteral opioids are no longer being used. Choosing the correct monitoring system requires full understanding of respiratory physiology, patient comorbid medical conditions, site of surgery, need for supplemental oxygen, and acceptability of the patient to wearing the device.

Pulse Oximetry

Pulse oximetry is a measure of the percent of hemoglobin binding sites in the bloodstream occupied by oxygen. Normal oxygen saturation is between 95% to 100%. During sleep, normal oxygen saturation can drop as low as 92% (Chung et al., 2014). Measuring pulse oximetry on a continuous basis allows nurses to observe changes over time as well as real-time trend assessment. Continuous oximetry also serves as patient observation when the nurse is unable to be continuously with the patient. Continuous electronic monitoring is never a replacement for 2- to 4-hourly nursing assessment of the patient. Pulse oximetry is generally acceptable to patients, because it is more comfortable than wearing a capnography cannula. As mentioned previously, supplemental oxygen can blunt the detection of respiratory compromise and is therefore not the best choice (Arakawa et al., 2013). There is evidence that capnography may be a more effective tool to assess for respiratory compromise with or without supplemental oxygen (Burton, Harrah, Germann, & Dillon, 2006; Jolley, Bell, Rafferty, Moxham, & Strang, 2015). Although instituting continuous pulse oximetry in all patients receiving opioids has been found to decrease

rescue events and transfer to an ICU, the increased number of alarms on the units have caused alarm fatigue (Durbin, 2016; Taenzer, Pyke, McGrath, & Blike, 2010). Research shows that only 36% of pulse oximetry alarms are clinically relevant (Voepel-Lewis et al., 2013). It is important that alarm settings are patient specific with consideration of the patient's baseline/pre-opioid oxygen saturation level.

Respiratory Rate

Continuous monitoring of just respiratory rate is an option but has not been validated for detection of OIRD. One device that measures respiratory rate acoustically has been found to be more comfortable and tolerated than capnography masks in patients being monitored in the emergency room for alcohol intoxication (Guechi et al., 2015). Although respiratory rate is one measure of respiratory status, unlike advance sedation, it is not thought to be sensitive for early detection of respiratory compromise.

Capnography

It is known that carbon dioxide levels increase before oxygen levels decrease in the setting of respiratory compromise. It makes physiologic sense to measure end-tidal carbon dioxide levels ($ETCO_2$) using capnography when monitoring for OIRD. Additionally, there is evidence supporting the effectiveness (McCarter, Shaik, Scarfo, & Thompson, 2008). Normal levels of exhaled carbon dioxide are considered to range between 33 and 43 mm Hg, just a bit lower than arterial levels that range from 35 to 45 mm Hg (Hinkelbein, Floss, Denz, & Krieter, 2008; Liu, Lee, & Bongard, 1992). Levels above 50 mm Hg are generally considered clinically dangerous. The use of capnography has increased over the past years because of knowledge that using supplemental oxygen can result in an inaccurate assessment of respiratory status with pulse oximetry. One of the issues for the patient using capnography is the discomfort of the cannula that is worn just under the nose. Displacing the capnography cannula because of this discomfort is a common cause of false alarms with capnography. Additionally, the cannula can impair a tight seal required for positive airway pressure (PAP) masks often used by patients with OSA during sleep.

Minute Ventilation

Minute ventilation is defined as the total amount of gas exhaled by the lungs per minute. The normal minute ventilation is 5 to 10 L/min. Minute ventilation has been measured on ventilated patients for years. Recently there has been development and validation of a newer technology that measures minute ventilation in the nonintubated patient. Using two chest (upper sternal and midaxillary) leads, the monitor detects tidal volume and respiratory rate. This device has been found to be more comfortable and as effective as capnography (Fleming, Voscopoulos, & George, 2015; Holley et al., 2016). The chest leads appear to be more comfortable than capnography cannulas for patients to wear. Clinicians are able to use a form of trend monitoring when using this device. The monitor displays real-time minute ventilation and activates an alarm when it drops below 40% of the patient's normal minute ventilation (Voscopoulos, Theos, Tillmann Hein, & George, 2017). This technology is new, and many clinicians are not familiar with measuring and interpreting minute ventilation. Education of clinicians will need to occur before this technology could be clinically applicable.

Interventions After Assessment

Assessment after the delivery of opioids is most effective at peak effect and at a minimum of at least every 2 hours for 24 hours and until the patient does not exhibit any signs of ASOIRD. Assessment is an ongoing and iterative process. Data from the assessment are used to adjust pain interventions to best meet the individual patients' functional needs in the safest manner. If a patient is assessed as not responsive to verbal or tactile stimuli and/or if the respiratory rate is less than 10 breaths/min, it is advised that the clinician first stop the administration of an opioid or other sedating medication, then engage the patient by stimulation by raising the head of the bed and verbally and tactically stimulating the patient as appropriate. The prescriber needs to be contacted, and administration of naloxone should be considered. Most hospitals now have rapid response teams that will assist the bedside nurse in assessment and intervention when a patient is considered at risk for decline. If naloxone is indicated, the recommended way to prepare and administer naloxone to adults experiencing OIRD is to "mix 0.4 mg of naloxone with 10 mL of normal saline in a syringe and administer this dilute solution very slowly (0.5 mL over 2 minutes) while observing the patient's response (titrate-to-effect)" (see Box 13.1) (Pasero, 2013, p. 35). If the formulation of opioid allows for a longer duration of action than the naloxone (e.g., transdermal fentaNYL), the naloxone may need to be repeated. Once the patient is out of immediate danger, opioid-sparing pain management strategies need to be put in place. Because the patient continues to be at higher risk through the following 24 hours, it is important for continuous electronic monitoring to be instituted.

Summary

Monitoring patients for advancing sedation and OIRD is an integral part of safe and effective pain care. Because most patients will tolerate opioid medications without adverse effects, some clinicians have not focused on this clinical problem. Recent evidence reveals that around 1% of hospitalized patients receiving opioid medications continue to experience adverse events as a result of the respiratory depressing effects of opioids. In deep dive analysis, it was discovered that certain patients are at higher risk than others. Hospitals attempting to institute continuous electronic monitoring to address the problem have found that alarm fatigue can contribute to negative patient outcomes (Mitka, 2013; Pasero & von Baeyer, 2017; Sendelbach & Funk, 2013). Continuous electronic monitoring is expensive, and there is not sufficient evidence that demonstrates that it is superior to intermittent nursing assessment per best practice. Current recommendations to promote safe and effective pain management are (1) applying opioid-sparing pain management techniques, (2) screening all patients for risk for ASOIRD, and (3) increasing vigilance of patients at higher risk. Increasing vigilance requires either continuous electronic monitoring or 2-hourly nursing assessments using a sedation scale, intermittent pulse oximetry, and assessment of respiratory rate and quality. The choice of the appropriate type of electronic monitor requires knowledge that supplemental oxygen will blunt the effectiveness of using pulse oximetry. It is important that the use of supplemental oxygen be clinically necessary and evidence based. Capnography or minute ventilation monitoring may be better choices for patients requiring supplemental oxygen therapy. The timing, nature, frequency, and intensity of monitoring for ASOIRD are informed by the ongoing comprehensive assessment of the following:

- Patient risk
- Type of opioid (especially if combined with other sedating medications)
- Presence of respiratory interventions (e.g., PAP therapy, supplemental oxygen)
- Patient responses to clinical care

Timing of nurse assessments and duration of increased vigilance and monitoring are most effective when based on the evidence that reveals that respiration is the most vulnerable during sleep, during the first 24 hours after surgery, or at initiation or increasing the dose of parenteral opioid therapy. Additionally, nursing education of the problem and the use of the appropriate monitoring system needs to be encouraged and used. Health care facilities are advised to have policies and procedures in place to surveil naloxone use, activate the rapid response team, and institute safe and effective opioid-sparing pain management. It is important for procedures to include the use of "trend" monitoring, providing nurses with readily available data on the patient's baseline readings for comparison purposes.

Key Points

- All patients receiving opioid analgesia are at risk for advancing sedation and opioid-induced respiratory depression (ASOIRD) and require increased vigilance within the first 24 hours of initiating opioid therapy.

- Increased vigilance is defined as nursing assessment, with monitoring at peak drug effect every 2.5 hours for the first 24 hours or the use of the appropriate continuous electronic monitor.
- Nursing assessment must include the rate and quality of respiration, oxygen saturation, and level of sedation.
- All patients must be assessed for risk for ASOIRD with intervention prescribed as soon as risk level is stratified.
- Assessment for ASOIRD is an ongoing process by which detection, increased vigilance, and opioid-sparing pain management are instituted as soon as higher risk is determined.
- Nurses need to appropriately use trend monitoring to recognize the signs of respiratory compromise. Nurses in the PACU are in a good position to identify OIRD using the appropriate electronic monitoring device.
- Hospitals must have policies and procedures in place to surveil and deep dive into adverse events such as naloxone administration. Identifying institutional risk factors must occur along continuous evaluation and modification of policies and procedures to improve patient safety when opioids are administered.
- Hospitals must have continuous electronic monitoring available, with policies in place that empower nurses to apply continuous electronic monitoring without a provider's order.

Case Scenario

The patient, 76-year-old Mr. B., underwent an emergent open cholecystectomy for listhesis. He was admitted to the general care unit at 9 p.m. from the emergency room after receiving three doses of HYDROmorphone 0.5 mg IV for pain and one dose of ondansetron 4 mg IV to control vomiting. He was febrile at 38 degrees Celsius. His pain was well controlled, he had no nausea, but he was drowsy. His medical history includes well-controlled hypertension and 10- to 20 cigarettes per day smoker for the past 50 years. Admission vital signs were B/P 138/78, P 52, RR 18, T 38 C. Pulse oximeter value was 96% on room air. Satisfied that the patient was resting quietly for now, the nurse went to admit her next patient. At 10 p.m. during her hourly rounding, she noticed that he was sitting up in pain and complaining of severe nausea. She reassessed his vital signs and medicated him again with 0.5 mg HYDROmorphone and 4 mg of ondansetron. At 10:30 p.m. she went back in to check him and noticed that he was snoring lightly and appeared to be sleeping. She decided to let him sleep. At 11 p.m. the nursing tech went in to perform routine vital signs and found that he woke when touched but was very drowsy. His vital signs were B/P 110/70, P 70, RR 22, T 38.6 C. Pulse oximeter reading was 92%. The tech reported the patient's status to the nurse, expressing some concern about his drowsiness.

The nurse performed an assessment and decided that he was experiencing advancing sedation and opioid-induced respiratory depression. She called the hospitalist, who ordered one dose of ketorolac 15 mg IV and rectal acetaminophen for temperature, instituting opioid-sparing pain management. The nurse initiated continuous pulse oximetry monitoring as well as the use of a sedation scale assessment every 2 hours.

In this case, the nurse and the nursing assistant were vigilant, but did not follow best practices. If best practices were employed, the patient would have been assessed for risk for advancing sedation and opioid-induced respiratory depression (ASOIRD) at admission. They would have found that he was a current smoker of more than 20 years and therefore at higher risk for ASOIRD. Additionally, he was experiencing drowsiness, which was a sign of ASOIRD. If the nursing assistant had not gone into the room at that time, the ASOIRD could have advanced to an adverse event. Best practices would have instituted the use of a sedation scale such as the POSS or the MOSS that would have guided care. Additionally, if available, continuous electronic monitoring was indicated.

Acknowledgments

The authors would like to acknowledge fellow members of the American Society for Pain Management Nursing workgroup who are revising the clinical practice guidelines for monitoring patients for ASOIRD. The members are: Heather Carlisle, Maureen Cooney, Susan Dempsey, Danielle Dunwoody, Angelika Maly, Kathy Meloche, Rosemary Polomano, Jason Sawyer, Navdeep Singh, Denise Sullivan Ashley Sweet, April Vallerand, Chris Watson. The members have contributed to the review of the literature and development of best practice recommendations.

References

Alaloul, F., Williams, K., Myers, J., Jones, K. D., & Logsdon, M. C. (2015). Impact of a Script-based Communication Intervention on Patient Satisfaction with Pain Management. *Pain Management Nursing*, 16(3), 321–327. https://doi.org/10.1016/j.pmn.2014.08.008.

American Society of Anesthesiologists Task Force on Neuraxial Opioids and the American Society of Regional Anesthesia and Pain Medicine. (2016). Practice guidelines for the prevention, detection, and management of respiratory depression associated with neuraxial opioid administration. *Anesthesiology*, 124(3), 535–552.

American Society of Anesthesiologists Task Force on Perioperative Management of patients with obstructive sleep. (2014). Practice guidelines for the perioperative management of patients with obstructive sleep apnea: an updated report by the American Society of Anesthesiologists Task Force on Perioperative Management of patients with obstructive sleep apnea. *Anesthesiology, 120*(2), 268–286. https://doi.org/10.1097/ALN.0000000000000053.

Angst, M. S., Lazzeroni, L. C., Phillips, N. G., Drover, D. R., Tingle, M., Ray, A., ... Clark, J. D. (2012). Aversive and Reinforcing Opioid Effects: A Pharmacogenomic Twin Study. *Anesthesiology: The Journal of the American Society of Anesthesiologists, 117*(1), 22–37.

Anwari, J. S., & Iqbal, S. (2003). Antihistamines and potentiation of opioid induced sedation and respiratory depression. *Anaesthesia, 58*(5), 494–495.

Arakawa, H., Kaise, M., Sumiyama, K., Saito, S., Suzuki, T., & Tajiri, H. (2013). Does pulse oximetry accurately monitor a patient's ventilation during sedated endoscopy under oxygen supplementation? *Singapore Medicine Journal, 54*(4), 212–215.

Arora, N., Cao, M., & Javaheri, S. (2014). Opioids, sedatives, and sleep hypoventilation. *Sleep Medicine Clinics, 9*(3), 391–398.

Arozullah, A. M., Conde, M. V., & Lawrence, V. A. (2003). Preoperative evaluation for postoperative pulmonary complications. *The Medical Clinics of North America, 87*(1), 153–173.

Bagsby, D. T., Ireland, P. H., & Meneghini, R. M. (2014). Liposomal bupivacaine versus traditional periarticular injection for pain control after total knee arthroplasty. *The Journal of Arthroplasty, 29*(8), 1687–1690.

Barr, J., Fraser, G. L., Puntillo, K., Ely, E. W., Gélinas, C., Dasta, J. F., ... Coursin, D. B. (2013). Clinical practice guidelines for the management of pain, agitation, and delirium in adult patients in the intensive care unit. *Critical Care Medicine, 41*(1), 263–306.

Benumof, J. L. (2015). Mismanagement of obstructive sleep apnea may result in finding these patients dead in bed. *Canadian Journal of Anaesthesia.* https://doi.org/10.1007/s12630-015-0513-x.

Burton, J. H., Harrah, J. D., Germann, C. A., & Dillon, D. C. (2006). Does end-tidal carbon dioxide monitoring detect respiratory events prior to current sedation monitoring practices? *Acad Emergency Medicine, 13*(5), 500–504. https://doi.org/10.1197/j.aem.2005.12.017.

Burwaiss, M., & Comerford, D. (2013). Techniques of opioid administration. *Anaesthesia & Intensive Care Medicine, 14*(11), 491–495.

Bush, S. H., Grassau, P. A., Yarmo, M. N., Zhang, T., Zinkie, S. J., & Pereira, J. L. (2014). The Richmond Agitation-Sedation Scale modified for palliative care inpatients (RASS-PAL): a pilot study exploring validity and feasibility in clinical practice. *BMC Palliative Care, 13*(1), 17.

Cashman, J. N., & Dolin, S. J. (2004). Respiratory and haemodynamic effects of acute postoperative pain management: evidence from published data. *British Journal of Anaesthesia, 93*(2), 212–223. https://doi.org/10.1093/bja/aeh180.

Centers for Medicare and Medicaid Services (CMS). (2014). *Requirements for Hospital Medication Administration, Particularly Intravenous (IV) Medications and Post-Operative Care of Patients Receiving IV Opioids.* Baltimore, MD: Department of Health and Human Services.

Chou, R., Gordon, D. B., de Leon-Casasola, O. A., Rosenberg, J. M., Bickler, S., Brennan, T., ... Wu, C. L. (2016). Management of Postoperative Pain: A Clinical Practice Guideline From the American Pain Society, the American Society of Regional Anesthesia and Pain Medicine, and the American Society of Anesthesiologists' Committee on Regional Anesthesia, Executive Committee, and Administrative Council. *Journal of Pain, 17*(2), 131–157. https://doi.org/10.1016/j.jpain.2015.12.008.

Chung, F., Chan, M. T., & Liao, P. (2017). Perioperative nocturnal hypoxemia matters in surgical patients with obstructive sleep apnea. *Canadian Journal of Anaesthesia, 64*(1), 109–110. https://doi.org/10.1007/s12630-016-0755-2.

Chung, F., Zhou, L., & Liao, P. (2014). Parameters from preoperative overnight oximetry predict postoperative adverse events. *Minerva Anestesiol, 80*(10), 1084–1095.

Chung, F., Liao, P., Yang, Y., Andrawes, M., Kang, W., Mokhlesi, B., & Shapiro, C. M. (2015). Postoperative sleep-disordered breathing in patients without preoperative sleep apnea. *Anesthesia & Analgesia, 120*(6), 1214–1224. https://doi.org/10.1213/ANE.0000000000000774.

Chung, F., Yegneswaran, B., Liao, P., Chung, S. A., Vairavanathan, S., Islam, S., ... Shapiro, C. M. (2008). STOP questionnaire: a tool to screen patients for obstructive sleep apnea. *Anesthesiology, 108*(5), 812–821. https://doi.org/10.1097/ALN.0b013e31816d83e4.

Cooney, M. F. (2015). Management of postoperative pain in opioid-tolerant patients. *Journal of PeriAnesthesia Nursing, 30*(5), 436–443.

Crawford, C. L., Boller, J., Jadalla, A., & Cuenca, E. (2016). An Integrative Review of Pain Resource Nurse Programs. *Critical Care Nursing Quarterly, 39*(1), 64–82. https://doi.org/10.1097/CNQ.0000000000000101.

Davis, C., Geik, C., Arthur, K., Fuller, J., Johnston, E., Levitt, F., ... Walroth, T. (2017). A Multisite Retrospective Study Evaluating the Implementation of the Pasero Opioid-Induced Sedation Scale (POSS) and Its Effect on Patient Safety Outcomes. *Pain Management Nursing, 18*(4), 193–201. https://doi.org/10.1016/j.pmn.2017.03.006.

De Raaff, C. A., Coblijn, U. K., de Vries, N., & Van Wagensveld, B. A. (2016). Is fear for postoperative cardiopulmonary complications after bariatric surgery in patients with obstructive sleep apnea justified? A systematic review. *The American Journal of Surgery, 211*(4), 793–801.

Duncan, F., Day, R., Haigh, C., Gill, S., Nightingale, J., O'Neill, O., ... Group, N. (2014). First steps toward understanding the variability in acute pain service provision and the quality of pain relief in everyday practice across the United Kingdom. *Pain Medicine, 15*(1), 142–153. https://doi.org/10.1111/pme.12284.

Durbin, C. G., Jr. (2016). Physiologic Monitoring: Improving Safety or Increasing Risk? *Respiratory Care, 61*(8), 1110–1121. https://doi.org/10.4187/respcare.04931.

Ely, E. W., Truman, B., Shintani, A., Thomason, J. W., Wheeler, A. P., Gordon, S., ... Sessler, C. N. (2003). Monitoring sedation status over time in ICU patients: reliability and validity of the Richmond Agitation-Sedation Scale (RASS). *JAMA, 289*(22), 2983–2991.

Fiorelli, A., Izzo, A. C., Frongillo, E. M., Del Prete, A., Liguori, G., Di Costanzo, E., ... Santini, M. (2015). Efficacy of wound analgesia for controlling post-thoracotomy pain: a randomized double-blind study. *European Journal of Cardio-Thoracic Surgery, 49*(1), 339–347.

Fleming, E., Voscopoulos, C., & George, E. (2015). Non-invasive respiratory volume monitoring identifies opioid-induced respiratory depression in an orthopedic surgery patient with diagnosed obstructive sleep apnea: a case report. *Journal of Medical Case Reports*, 9, 94. https://doi.org/10.1186/s13256-015-0577-9.

Fouladpour, N., Jesudoss, R., Bolden, N., Shaman, Z., & Auckley, D. (2016). Perioperative Complications in Obstructive Sleep Apnea Patients Undergoing Surgery: A Review of the Legal Literature. *Anesthesia and Analgesia.*, 122(1), 145–151. https://doi.org/10.1213/ANE.0000000000000841.

Galvagno, S. M., Jr., Brayanov, J., Williams, G., & George, E. E. (2017). Anesthesia and Postoperative Respiratory Compromise Following Major Lower Extremity Surgery: Implications for Combat Casualties. *Mil Med*, 182(S1), 78–86. https://doi.org/10.7205/MILMED-D-16-00048.

Glowacki, D. (2015). Effective pain management and improvements in patients' outcomes and satisfaction. *Critical Care Nurse*, 35(3), 33–41.

Gordon, D. B., de Leon-Casasola, O. A., Wu, C. L., Sluka, K. A., Brennan, T. J., & Chou, R. (2016). Research gaps in practice guidelines for acute postoperative pain management in adults: findings from a review of the evidence for an American Pain Society Clinical Practice Guideline. *The Journal of Pain*, 17(2), 158–166.

Green, C. J. G., & Tay, Y. C. (2016). Techniques of opioid administration. *Anesthesia and Intensive Care Medicine*, 17(9), 454–459.

Guechi, Y., Pichot, A., Frasca, D., Rayeh-Pelardy, F., Lardeur, J. Y., & Mimoz, O. (2015). Assessment of noninvasive acoustic respiration rate monitoring in patients admitted to an Emergency Department for drug or alcoholic poisoning. *Journal of Clinical Monit Comput*, 29(6), 721–726. https://doi.org/10.1007/s10877-015-9658-y.

Hart, N., Mandal, S., Manuel, A., Mokhlesi, B., Pepin, J. L., Piper, A., & Stradling, J. R. (2014). Obesity hypoventilation syndrome: does the current definition need revisiting? *Thorax*, 69(1), 83–84. https://doi.org/10.1136/thoraxjnl-2013-204298.

Herzig, S. J., Rothberg, M. B., Cheung, M., Ngo, L. H., & Marcantonio, E. R. (2014). Opioid utilization and opioid-related adverse events in nonsurgical patients in US hospitals. *Journal of Hospital Medicine*, 9(2), 73–81. https://doi.org/10.1002/jhm.2102.

Hinkelbein, J., Floss, F., Denz, C., & Krieter, H. (2008). Accuracy and precision of three different methods to determine Pco2 (Paco2 vs. Petco2 vs. Ptcco2) during interhospital ground transport of critically ill and ventilated adults. *Journal of Trauma*, 65(1), 10–18. https://doi.org/10.1097/TA.0b013e31815eba83.

Hoda, M. Q., Hamid, M., & Khan, F. A. (2007). Audit of an acute pain service in a tertiary care hospital in a developing country. *Journal of the Pakistan Medical Association*, 57(11), 560–562.

Holley, K., MacNabb, C. M., Georgiadis, P., Minasyan, H., Shukla, A., & Mathews, D. (2016). Monitoring minute ventilation versus respiratory rate to measure the adequacy of ventilation in patients undergoing upper endoscopic procedures. *J Clin Monit Comput*, 30(1), 33–39. https://doi.org/10.1007/s10877-015-9674-y.

Institute for Healthcare Improvement. (2012). *How-to Guide: Prevent Harm from High-Alert Medications*. Cambridge, MA: Institute for Healthcare Improvement.

Institute for Safe Medical Practice (ISMP). (2009a). Beware of basal opioid infusions with PCA therapy. *ISMP Medication Safety Alert-Acute Care, March 12, 2009*. https://www.ismp.org/newsletters/acutecare/showarticle.aspx?id=50.

Institute for Safe Medical Practice (ISMP). (2009b). Beware of basal opioid infusions with PCA therapy. *ISMP Medication Safety Alert- Nurse Advise-ERR. Acute Care, October, 2009, Vol 7*(10), 1–2.

Institute for Safe Medical Practice (ISMP). (2013a). Drawn curtains, muted alarms, and diverted attention lead to tragedy in the Postanesthesia Care Unit. *ISMP Medication Safety Alert - Acute Care, March 21, 2013*. https://www.ismp.org/newsletters/acutecare/showarticle.aspx?id=44. Accessed 7/19/2020.

Institute for Safe Medical Practice (ISMP). (2013b). Fatal PCA adverse events continue to happen... Better patient monitoring is essential to prevent harm. *ISMP Medication Safety Alert - Acute Care, May 30, 2013*.

Ireland, C. J., Chapman, T. M., Mathew, S. F., Herbison, G. P., & Zacharias, M. (2014). Continuous positive airway pressure (CPAP) during the postoperative period for prevention of postoperative morbidity and mortality following major abdominal surgery (Review). *Cochrane Database of Systematic Reviews*, 2014(8), 1–57. https://doi.org/10.1002/14651858.CD008930.pub2.

Jarvis, C. (2016). *Physical Examination & Health Assessment* (7th ed., p. 136). St. Louis, MO: Elsevier.

Jarzyna, D., Jungquist, C. R., Pasero, C., Willens, J. S., Nisbet, A., Oakes, L., ... Polomano, R. C. (2011). American Society for Pain Management Nursing guidelines on monitoring for opioid-induced sedation and respiratory depression. *Pain Management Nursing*, 12(3), 118–145. e110 https://doi.org/10.1016/j.pmn.2011.06.008.

Johnson, F., Logsdon, P., Fournier, K., & Fisher, S. (2016). SWITCH for safety: Perioperative hand-off tools. *AORN Journal*, 98(5), 494–507.

Jolley, C. J., Bell, J., Rafferty, G. F., Moxham, J., & Strang, J. (2015). Understanding Heroin Overdose: A Study of the Acute Respiratory Depressant Effects of Injected Pharmaceutical Heroin. *PLoS One*, 10(10). https://doi.org/10.1371/journal.pone.0140995.

Jones, A. W. (2017). Postmortem toxicology findings from medicolegal investigations of drug-related deaths among the rich and famous. *Toxicologie Analytique et Clinique*, 29(3), 298–308.

Jones, J. D., Mogali, S., & Comer, S. D. (2012). Polydrug abuse: a review of opioid and benzodiazepine combination use. *Drug and Alcohol Dependence*, 125(1), 8–18.

Jungquist, C. R., Willens, J. S., Dunwoody, D. R., Klingman, K. J., & Polomano, R. C. (2014a). Monitoring for opioid-induced advancing sedation and respiratory depression: ASPMN membership survey of current practice. *Pain Management Nursing*, 15(3), 682–693. https://doi.org/10.1016/j.pmn.2013.12.001.

Jungquist, C. R., Pasero, C., Tripoli, N. M., Gorodetsky, R., Metersky, M., & Polomano, R. C. (2014b). Instituting best practice for monitoring for opioid-induced advancing sedation in hospitalized patients. *Worldviews Evidence Based Nursing*, 11(6), 350–360. https://doi.org/10.1111/wvn.12061.

Jungquist, C. R., Correll, D. J., Fleisher, L. A., Gross, J., Gupta, R., Pasero, C., ... Polomano, R. (2016). Avoiding Adverse Events Secondary to Opioid-Induced Respiratory Depression: Implications for Nurse Executives and Patient Safety. *Journal of Nursing Administration*, 46(2), 87–94. https://doi.org/10.1097/NNA.0000000000000301.

Kapur, V. K., Auckley, D. H., Chowdhuri, S., Kuhlmann, D. C., Mehra, R., Ramar, K., & Harrod, C. G. (2017). Clinical Practice Guideline for Diagnostic Testing for Adult Obstructive Sleep Apnea: An American Academy of Sleep Medicine Clinical Practice Guideline. *Journal of Clinical Sleep Medicine*, *13*(3), 479–504. https://doi.org/10.5664/jcsm.6506.

Kaw, R., Bhateja, P., Paz, Y. M. H., Hernandez, A. V., Ramaswamy, A., Deshpande, A., & Aboussouan, L. S. (2016). Postoperative Complications in Patients With Unrecognized Obesity Hypoventilation Syndrome Undergoing Elective Noncardiac Surgery. *Chest*, *149*(1), 84–91. https://doi.org/10.1378/chest.14-3216.

Kessler, E. R., Shah, M., Gruschkus, S. K., & Raju, A. (2013). Cost and quality implications of opioid-based postsurgical pain control using administrative claims data from a large health system: opioid-related adverse events and their impact on clinical and economic outcomes. *Pharmacotherapy*, *33*(4), 383–391. https://doi.org/10.1002/phar.1223.

Khelemsky, Y., Kothari, R., Campbell, N., & Farnad, S. (2015). Incidence and Demographics of Post-Operative Naloxone Administration: A 13-Year Experience at a Major Tertiary Teaching Institution. *Pain Physician*, *18*(5), E827-829.

Kirk, K., & Kane, R. (2016). A qualitative exploration of intentional nursing round models in the emergency department setting: investigating the barriers to their use and success. *Journal of Clinical Nursing*, *25*(9-10), 1262–1272. https://doi.org/10.1111/jocn.13150.

Klug, M. J., Rivey, M. P., & Carter, J. T. (2016). Comparison of intraoperative periarticular injections versus liposomal bupivacaine as part of a multimodal approach to pain management in total knee arthroplasty. *Hospital Pharmacy*, *51*(4), 305–311.

Kong, W. T., Chopra, S., Kopf, M., Morales, C., Khan, S., Zuccala, K., ... Chronakos, J. (2016). Perioperative risks of untreated obstructive sleep apnea in the bariatric surgery patient: a retrospective study. *Obesity Surgery*, *26*(12), 2886–2890.

Kuo, A. C., & Grotkopp, E. (2017). A Simple Method Associated with Reduced Opioid Consumption After Total Knee Arthroplasty. *The Journal of Arthroplasty*, *32*(10), 3034–3037.

Ladd, L. A., Kam, P. C., Williams, D. B., Wright, A. W., Smith, M. T., & Mather, L. E. (2005). Ventilatory responses of healthy subjects to intravenous combinations of morphine and oxycodone under imposed hypercapnic and hypoxaemic conditions. *British Journal of Clinical Pharmacology*, *59*(5), 524–535. https://doi.org/10.1111/j.1365-2125.2005.02368.x.

Lee, L. A., Caplan, R. A., Stephens, L. S., Posner, K. L., Terman, G. W., Voepel-Lewis, T., & Domino, K. B. (2015). Postoperative opioid-induced respiratory depression: a closed claims analysis. *Anesthesiology*, *122*(3), 659–665. https://doi.org/10.1097/ALN.0000000000000564.

Lee, P., Allen, K., & Daly, M. (2012). A 'communication and patient safety' training programme for all healthcare staff: Can it make a difference? *BMJ Quality & Safety*, *21*(1), 84–88.

Leone, R. M., & Adams, R. J. (2016). Safety Standards: Implementing Fall Prevention Interventions and Sustaining Lower Fall Rates by Promoting the Culture of Safety on an Inpatient Rehabilitation Unit. *Rehabiltation Nursing*, *41*(1), 26–32. https://doi.org/10.1002/rnj.250.

Liao, P., Wong, J., Singh, M., Wong, D. T., Islam, S., Andrawes, M., ... Chung, F. (2017). Postoperative Oxygen Therapy in Patients With OSA: A Randomized Controlled Trial. *Chest*, *151*(3), 597–611. https://doi.org/10.1016/j.chest.2016.12.005.

Liu, S. Y., Lee, T. S., & Bongard, F. (1992). Accuracy of capnography in nonintubated surgical patients. *Chest*, *102*(5), 1512–1515.

Manuel, A. R. G., Hart, N., & Stradling, J. R. (2015). Is a raised bicarbonate, without hypercapnia, part of the physiologic spectrum of obesity-related hypoventilation? *Chest*, *147*(2), 362–368. https://doi.org/10.1378/chest.14-1279.

Matic, M., Davidson, P. M., & Salamonson, Y. (2011). Review: Bringing patient safety to the forefront through structured computerisation during clinical handover. *Journal of Clinical Nursing*, *20*(1-2), 184–189.

McCarter, T., Shaik, Z., Scarfo, K., & Thompson, L. J. (2008). Capnography monitoring enhances safety of postoperative patient-controlled analgesia. *American Health Drug Benefits*, *1*(5), 28–35.

McDonnell, A., Nicholl, J., & Read, S. M. (2003). Acute pain teams and the management of postoperative pain: a systematic review and meta-analysis. *Journal of Advanced Nursing*, *41*(3), 261–273.

Meisenberg, B., Ness, J., Rao, S., Rhule, J., & Ley, C. (2017). Implementation of solutions to reduce opioid-induced oversedation and respiratory depression. *American Journal of Health System Pharmacy*, *74*(3), 162–169. https://doi.org/10.2146/ajhp160208.

Mitka, M. (2013). Joint Commission warns of alarm fatigue: multitude of alarms from monitoring devices problematic. *JAMA*, *309*(22), 2315–2316. https://doi.org/10.1001/jama.2013.6032.

Nagappa, M., Weingarten, T. N., Montandon, G., Sprung, J., & Chung, F. (2017). Opioids, respiratory depression and sleep-disordered breathing. *Best Practice & Research Clinical Anaesthesiology*, *31*(4), 469–485.

Nagappa, M., Liao, P., Wong, J., Auckley, D., Ramachandran, S. K., Memtsoudis, S., ... Chung, F. (2015). Validation of the STOP-Bang Questionnaire as a Screening Tool for Obstructive Sleep Apnea among Different Populations: A Systematic Review and Meta-Analysis. *PLoS One*, *10*(12). https://doi.org/10.1371/journal.pone.0143697.

Niedrig, D. F., Hoppe, L., Mächler, S., Russmann, H., & Russmann, S. (2016). Benzodiazepine Use During Hospitalization: Automated Identification of Potential Medication Errors and Systematic Assessment of Preventable Adverse Events. *PloS ONE*, *11*(10), e0163224.

Niesters, M., Mahajan, R. P., Aarts, L., & Dahan, A. (2013). High-inspired oxygen concentration further impairs opioid-induced respiratory depression. *British Journal of Anaesthesia*, *110*(5), 837–841.

Nisbet, A. T., & Mooney-Cotter, F. (2009). Comparison of selected sedation scales for reporting opioid-induced sedation assessment. *Pain Management Nursing*, *10*(3), 154–164. https://doi.org/10.1016/j.pmn.2009.03.001.

Palmer, P. P., Royal, M., & Miller, R. D. (2014). Novel delivery systems for postoperative analgesia. *Best Practice & Research Clinical Anaesthesiology*, *28*(1), 81–90.

Pasero, C. (2009). Assessment of sedation during opioid administration for pain management. *J Perianesth Nurs*, *24*(3), 186–190. https://doi.org/10.1016/j.jopan.2009.03.005.

Pasero, C., Quinn, T. E., Portenoy, R. K., McCaffery, M., & Rizos, A. (2011). Opioid analgesics. In C. Pasero, & M. McCaffery (Eds.), *Pain Assessment and Pharmacologic Management* (pp. 277–622). Mosby/Elsevier: St. Louis, MO.

Pasero, C. (2013). The perianesthesia nurse's role in the prevention of opioid-related sentinel events. *Journal of PeriAnesthesia Nursing, 28*(1), 31–37.

Pasero, C., & von Baeyer, C. L. (2017). Guest Editorial: What nurses' work-arounds tell us about pain assessment. *International Journal of Nursing Studies, 67*(2), A1–A2.

Pawasauskas, J., Stevens, B., Youssef, R., & Kelley, M. (2014). Predictors of naloxone use for respiratory depression and oversedation in hospitalized adults. *American Journal of Health-System Pharmacy, 71*(9).

Peromaa-Haavisto, P., Tuomilehto, H., Kössi, J., Virtanen, J., Luostarinen, M., Pihlajamäki, J., ... Victorzon, M. (2016). Prevalence of obstructive sleep apnoea among patients admitted for bariatric surgery. A prospective multicentre trial. *Obesity Surgery, 26*(7), 1384–1390.

Quinlan-Colwell, A. (2013, April). A tool to assess sedation and so much more. *SPS News, 1*(8).

Quinlan-Colwell, A., Thear, G., Miller-Baldwin, E., & Smith, A. (2017). Use of the Pasero Opioid-induced Sedation Scale (POSS) in pediatric patients. *Journal of Pediatric Nursing, 33*(1), 83–87.

Ramachandran, S. K., Pandit, J. D., Devine, S., Tompson, A., & Shanks, A. (2017). Postoperative respiratory complications in patients at risk for obstructive sleep apnea: A single-institution cohort study. *Anesthesia & Analgesia, 125*(1), 272–279.

Ramachandran, S. K., Haider, N., Saran, K. A., Mathis, M., Kim, J., Morris, M., & O'Reilly, M. (2011). Life-threatening critical respiratory events: a retrospective study of postoperative patients found unresponsive during analgesic therapy. *Journal of Clinical Anesthesia, 23*(3), 207–213. https://doi.org/10.1016/j.jclinane.2010.09.003.

Riesenberg, L. A., Leitzsch, J., & Cunningham, J. M. (2010). Nursing handoffs: a systematic review of the literature. *American Journal of Nursing, 110*(4), 24–34. quiz 35-26 https://doi.org/10.1097/01.NAJ.0000370154.79857.09.

Robinson, N. L. (2016). Promoting patient safety with perioperative hand-off communication. *Journal of PeriAnesthesia Nursing, 31*(3), 245–253.

Rosenfeld, D. M., Betcher, J. A., Shah, R. A., Chang, Y. H., Cheng, M. R., Cubillo, E. I., ... Trentman, T. L. (2016). Findings of a Naloxone Database and its Utilization to Improve Safety and Education in a Tertiary Care Medical Center. *Pain Practitioner, 16*(3), 327–333. https://doi.org/10.1111/papr.12277.

Ross, J. A., Greenwood, A. C., Sasser, P., & Jiranck, W. A. (2017). Periarticular Injections in Knee and Hip Arthroplasty: Where and What to Inject. *The Journal of Arthroplasty, 32,* S77–S80.

Sasaki, N., Meyer, M. J., & Eikermann, M. (2013). Postoperative respiratory muscle dysfunction: pathophysiology and preventive strategies. *Anesthesiology, 118*(4), 961–978. https://doi.org/10.1097/ALN.0b013e318288834f.

Sendelbach, S., & Funk, M. (2013). Alarm fatigue: a patient safety concern. *AACN Advances in Critical Care, 24*(4), 378–386. quiz 387-378 https://doi.org/10.1097/NCI.0b013e3182a903f9.

Sessler, C. N., Gosnell, M. S., Grap, M. J., Brophy, G. M., O'Neal, P. V., Keane, K. A., ... Elswick, R. K. (2002). The Richmond Agitation-Sedation Scale: validity and reliability in adult intensive care unit patients. *American Journal of Respiratory & Critical Care Medicine, 166*(10), 1338–1344. https://doi.org/10.1164/rccm.2107138.

Shelton, A., Jones, D., Story, D. A., Heland, M., Bellomo, R., & Austin Health Post-Operative Surveillance Team, I. (2013). Survey of attitudes of nurses and junior doctors to co-management of high risk surgical patients. *Contemporary Nurse, 44*(2), 189–195. https://doi.org/10.5172/conu.2013.44.2.189.

Sigmarsdottir, B. D., Gudmundsdottir, Th. K., Zoëga, S., & Gunnarsson, P. S. (2017). Drugs that can cause respiratory depression with concomitant use of opioids. *Scandinavian Journal of Pain, 16*(1), 186.

Soto, R., & Yaldou, B. (2015). The Michigan Opioid Safety Score (MOSS): a patient safety and nurse empowerment tool. *Journal of PeriAnesthesia Nursing, 30*(3), 196–200.

Spangehl, M. J., Clarke, H. D., Hentz, J. G., Misra, L., Blocher, J. L., & Seamans, D. P. (2015). The Chitranjan Ranawat Award: periarticular injections and femoral & sciatic blocks provide similar pain relief after TKA: a randomized clinical trial. *Clinical Orthopaedics and Related Research®, 473*(1), 45–53.

Story, D. A., Fink, M., Leslie, K., Myles, P. S., Yap, S. J., Beavis, V., ... McNicol, P. L. (2009). Perioperative mortality risk score using pre- and postoperative risk factors in older patients. *Anaesth Intensive Care, 37*(3), 392–398.

Story, D. A., Shelton, A., Jones, D., Heland, M., Belomo, R., & Austin Health Post-Operative Surveillance Team, I. (2013). Audit of co-management and critical care outreach for high risk postoperative patients (The POST audit). *Anaesth Intensive Care, 41*(6), 793–798.

Story, D. A., Leslie, K., Myles, P. S., Fink, M., Poustie, S. J., Forbes, A., ... New Zealand College of Anaesthetists Trials, G. (2010). Complications and mortality in older surgical patients in Australia and New Zealand (the REASON study): a multicentre, prospective, observational study. *Anaesthesia, 65*(10), 1022–1030. https://doi.org/10.1111/j.1365-2044.2010.06478.x.

Svider, P. F., Pashkova, A. A., Folbe, A. J., Eloy, J. D., Setzen, M., Baredes, S., & Eloy, J. A. (2013). Obstructive sleep apnea: strategies for minimizing liability and enhancing patient safety. *Otolaryngol Head Neck Surgery, 149*(6), 947–953. https://doi.org/10.1177/0194599813504074.

Taenzer, A. H., Pyke, J. B., McGrath, S. P., & Blike, G. T. (2010). Impact of pulse oximetry surveillance on rescue events and intensive care unit transfers: a before-and-after concurrence study. *Anesthesiology, 112*(2), 282–287. https://doi.org/10.1097/ALN.0b013e3181ca7a9b.

Taenzer, A. H., Pyke, J., Herrick, M. D., Dodds, T. M., & McGrath, S. P. (2014). A comparison of oxygen saturation data in inpatients with low oxygen saturation using automated continuous monitoring and intermittent manual data charting. *Anesthesia & Analgesia, 118*(2), 326–331. https://doi.org/10.1213/ANE.0000000000000049.

The Joint Commission. (2012). *Sentinel Event Alert: safe use of opioids in hospitals.* Retrieved from Washington, DC http://www.jointcommission.org/sea_issue_49/. Accessed 8/13/2017.

Tsukada, S., Wakui, M., & Hoshino, A. (2016). The impact of including corticosteroid in a periarticular injection for pain control after total knee arthroplasty: a double-blind randomised controlled trial. *The Bone & Joint Journal, 98*(2), 194.

Van den Heede, K., Clarke, S. P., Sermeus, W., Vleugels, A., & Aiken, L. H. (2007). International experts' perspectives on the state of the nurse staffing and patient outcomes literature. *Journal of Nursing Scholarship, 39*(4), 290–297. https://doi.org/10.1111/j.1547-5069.2007.00183.x.

Voepel-Lewis, T., Parker, M. L., Burke, C. N., Hemberg, J., Perlin, L., Kai, S., & Ramachandran, S. K. (2013). Pulse oximetry desaturation alarms on a general postoperative adult unit: a prospective observational study of nurse response time. *International Journal of Nursing Studies, 50*(10), 1351–1358. https://doi.org/10.1016/j.ijnurstu.2013.02.006.

Voscapoulos, C., Ladd, D., & George, E. (2015). (129) The use of a non-invasive respiratory volume monitor to identify patients at high-risk for opioid-induced respiratory depression for a low-dose opioid regimen in the PACU. *The Journal of Pain, 16*(4, S), s8.

Voscopoulos, C., Theos, K., Tillmann Hein, H. A., & George, E. (2017). A risk stratification algorithm using non-invasive respiratory volume monitoring to improve safety when using post-operative opioids in the PACU. *J Clin Monit Comput, 31*(2), 417–426. https://doi.org/10.1007/s10877-016-9841-9.

Wiegand, T. J. (2016, March). The New Kid on the Block—Incorporating Buprenorphine into a Medical Toxicology Practice. *Journal of Medical Toxicology, Vol. 12*(1), 6470.

Weingarten, T. N., Warner, L. L., & Sprung, J. (2017). Timing of postoperative respiratory emergencies: when do they really occur? *Current Opinion in Anesthesiology, 30*(1), 156–162.

Weingarten, T. N., Herasevich, V., McGlinch, M. C., Beatty, N. C., Christensen, E. D., Hannifan, S. K., ... Schroeder, D. R. (2015). Predictors of delayed postoperative respiratory depression assessed from naloxone administration. *Anesthesia and Analgesia, 121*(2), 422.

Willens, J. S., Jungquist, C. R., Cohen, A., & Polomano, R. (2013). ASPMN survey—nurses' practice patterns related to monitoring and preventing respiratory depression. *Pain Management Nursing, 14*(1), 60–65. https://doi.org/10.1016/j.pmn.2013.01.002.

Wong-Lun-Hing, E. M., Dam, R. M., Welsh, F. K., Wells, J. K., John, T. G., Cresswell, A. B., & Rees, M. (2014). Postoperative pain control using continuous im bupivacaine infusion plus patient-controlled analgesia compared with epidural analgesia after major hepatectomy. *HPB, 16*(7), 601–609.

Yaldou, B., Cooper, M., & Soto, R. (2017). Inter-Rater Reliability and Reception of the Michigan Opioid Safety Score. *Journal of PeriAnesthesia Nursing, 33*(4), 412–419.

Zedler, B., Xie, L., Wang, L., Joyce, A., Vick, C., Brigham, J., ... Murrelle, L. (2015). Development of a risk index for serious prescription opioid-induced respiratory depression or overdose in Veterans' Health Administration patients. *Pain Medicine, 16*(8), 1566–1579.

Zedler, B. K., Saunders, W. B., Joyce, A. R., Vick, C. C., & Murrelle, E. L. (2017). Validation of a screening risk index for serious prescription opioid-induced respiratory depression or overdose in a US commercial health plan claims database. *Pain Medicine, 19*(1), 68–78.

Chapter 14 Opioid Use Disorder

Ann Quinlan-Colwell, Maureen F. Cooney

CHAPTER OUTLINE

Substance Use Disorder and Opioid Use Disorder, pg. 361

Pathophysiology of Substance Use Disorder, pg. 361

Terminology Related to Substance Use Disorder, pg. 361

Ethical Challenges in the Treatment of Pain in Patients With Comorbid Opioid Use Disorder, pg. 363

Caring for Patients With Pain and Opioid Use Disorder, pg. 363

Clinical Challenges of Treating Pain With Comorbid Opioid Use Disorder, pg. 363

Risk Factors for Development of Opioid Use Disorder, pg. 364

Treatment of Opioid Use Disorder, pg. 365

Pain and Opioid Use Disorder: Acute Care Setting, pg. 369

Screening for Opioid Use Disorder in the Acute Care Setting, pg. 369

Acute Pain Management of the Patient With Active Opioid Use Disorder Who Is Not in Active Treatment, pg. 369

Acute Pain Management for Patients on Medication-Assisted Treatment, pg. 370

Acute Pain Management for Patients With Opioid Use Disorder in Recovery Without Medication-Assisted Treatment, pg. 373

Acute Pain Management: Special Considerations, pg. 373

Discharge Planning for Patients With Opioid Use Disorder, pg. 374

Chronic Pain Management in Patients With Opioid Use Disorder, pg. 374

Chronic Pain Management for Patients With Opioid Use Disorder on Medication-Assisted Treatment: Special Considerations, pg. 375

Chronic Pain Management for Patients in Recovery Without the Use of Medication-Assisted Treatment, pg. 375

Chronic Pain Management for Patients With Active Opioid Use Disorder Who Are Not in Recovery, pg. 375

Strategies to Reduce Risk, pg. 376

Universal Precautions, pg. 376

Opioid Selection, pg. 376

Designing a Safe Treatment Plan, pg. 376

Overdose Prevention, pg. 377

Additional Considerations, pg. 377

Key Points, pg. 377

Case Scenario, pg. 379

References, pg. 379

THE multimodal analgesia (MMA) approach toward pain management is particularly important when working with patients who live with substance use disorder (SUD) (either active use or in recovery). Many health care providers, in a variety of settings, are called on to help patients with SUD manage pain. Age, gender, ethnicity, and socioeconomic status of such patients are diverse. The 24-year-old woman who began using opioids while in an abusive relationship now needs a cardiac valve replacement after developing endocarditis as a complication of intravenous use of heroin and will need help with postoperative pain. The 51-year-old executive who became dependent on opioids after a sports injury will need pain management following orthopedic surgery. The 65-year-old grandmother who was prescribed opioids for chronic back pain, then obtained opioids from several physicians and began using heroin after being dismissed by prescribers, now needs help managing pain from the epidural abscess that developed as a result of using heroin.

In each of these, and numerous similar situations, a person needs appropriate pain management along with caring intervention for SUD. Clinicians are called on to compassionately use evidence informed knowledge when caring for patients with complex needs related to the dual diagnoses of pain and SUD. When doing so, it is of paramount importance for clinicians to recognize their own knowledge deficits, biases, and fears so they can view people with SUD as people who need safe and effective pain management. The purpose of this chapter is to provide clinicians with evidence informed information about SUD, effective therapies for treating SUD, and appropriate use of MMA to most effectively care for patients with SUD who experience acute and/or chronic pain.

Substance Use Disorder and Opioid Use Disorder

In recent years, the term *addiction* has been replaced with the phrase *substance use disorder* (SUD), which involves the problematic use of substances classified in 10 categories (e.g., alcohol, sedative, stimulants, opioids, etc.) (American Psychiatric Association [APA], 2013). The criteria for diagnosis of SUD is further subdivided into groupings related to impaired control, social impairment, hazardous use, and pharmacologic criteria related to the substance. The severity of SUD is determined by the total number of criteria identified, ranging on a continuum from mild (2 or 3 items), to moderate (4 or 5 items), to severe (6–11 items) (APA, 2013). A full description of the criteria for opioid use disorder can be accessed in the APA, 2013 reference. Regardless of severity, SUD is chronic and like many chronic illnesses is associated with periods of exacerbation and remission.

During the first two decades of the 21st century, increased opioid misuse and abuse evolved into a public health crisis (Volkow & Collins, 2017). The import of this was clear when data from 2015 showed 1 in 10 Americans older than 12 years (>27 million) reported using an illicit substance during the previous month; nonmedical opioids followed marijuana as the second most common illegally used substance (Center for Behavioral Health Statistics and Quality, 2016); opioid overdose deaths tripled from the year 2000 to more than 15,000; and deaths from heroin overdose totaled 13,000, representing a four-fold increase from 2010 (Centers for Disease Control and Prevention, 2017). Also in 2015, more than 2 million individuals sought treatment for an SUD (Center for Behavioral Health Statistics and Quality, 2016). Although 2 million is an extremely large number, these individuals represent a fraction of the people who could benefit from treatment. Many people do not have access to treatment for a variety of reasons, including the lack of available treatment programs and the lack of access to available programs (U.S. Department of Health and Human Services [DHHS], 2013).

Opioid use disorder (OUD) is a subcategory of SUD. Although the criteria for OUD are similar to those in the general category of SUD, they are specific to the class of opioids. Criteria include the continued use of an opioid for longer than intended, strong desire to continue to use despite harm, inability to control use or stop use, excess time spent involved with use, interference with obligations, continued use despite harmful results, need for increased doses (when not used for legitimate medical need), and continued use to prevent withdrawal (APA, 2013). Similar to other SUDs such as alcohol use disorder, OUD exists on a continuum. In addition, some individuals who have OUD may also use other substances and thus have co-occurring SUD disorders (Kampman & Jarvis, 2015).

Pathophysiology of Substance Use Disorder

The vulnerability of some people to SUD is influenced by physical, social, environmental (e.g., exposure, access), psychological, and genetic factors, many of which continue not to be well understood (Sharma, Bruner, Barnett, & Fishman, 2016; Turton & Lingford-Hughes, 2016). Over the years, numerous theories, arising from a variety of clinical specialties, have been developed to explain the phenomena of SUD. There is general acceptance among the theories that three recurring processes are involved: *reward, withdrawal,* and *preoccupation* or *craving,* which intensify over time and may lead to physiologic changes in the reward, stress, and executive function systems of the brain (Koob & Volkow, 2016). Significant work in the field of neurobiology has resulted in findings that improved understanding of SUD and stimulated continued research into areas of prevention and treatment.

The neurobiology of opioid abuse is extremely complex and related to opioids binding at various sites within the brain, resulting in different physiologic effects. A basic explanation of the neurobiology of OUD involves the binding of opioids to the mu opioid receptors throughout the brain, especially in the ventral tegmental area, which releases dopamine into the nucleus accumbens, thus activating *reward* sensations. Although multiple neurotransmitters, receptors, and pathways are involved in reward and SUD, dopamine plays a major role in the reward pathways (Koob & Volkow, 2016). Cerebral (hippocampal area) processing of particular past experiences and the emotional (amygdala) status of the person contribute to how the opioid is experienced. The integration of this information influences behavior and use of the substance. The neurobiologic response to stress affects the hypothalamic-pituitary-adrenal (HPA) axis and can also affect substance use, craving, and risk for relapse (Kreek et al., 2012). Susceptible individuals who no longer have access to the substance of abuse may experience depression in mood, preoccupation with the substance, and craving that are relieved by taking the substance of abuse again (Nestler, 2015). With opioid use, changes in the dopaminergic and endogenous opioid system underlie some of the predisposition to OUD and explain the relapsing nature of the disease. Genetics is thought to play a role in the development of SUDs, and emerging research has identified multiple genetic variants that can contribute to increased risk for opioid misuse (Mistry, Bawor, Desai, Marsh, & Samaan, 2014). Although the specific genes related to SUD have not been identified, it is estimated that 40% to 60% of the risk for SUD is genetic (Volkow & Warren, 2014).

Terminology Related to Substance Use Disorder

Clinicians sometimes use terminology that labels patients and can negatively affect appropriate care. In the past, there was a lack of universally accepted definitions to explain opioid-related effects and there were inconsistencies in the use of these terms (Kaye et al., 2017a). In the *Diagnostic and Statistical Manual of Mental Disorders,* fifth edition (DSM-5) (APA, 2013), some of the definitions and criteria for SUD were revised, redefined, and further clarified. During assessment and care of patients with SUD and OUD, appropriate terminology should be used to the fullest extent possible (Box 14.1).

Opioid tolerance is a complex phenomenon that develops with repeated opioid exposure, resulting in a decrease in the analgesic effect of the opioid, thus necessitating an increase in dose to achieve the same level of adequate pain relief (Stromer, Michaeli, & Sandner-Kiesling, 2013). Although it is not completely understood, individuals are considered to be opioid tolerant if they received the equivalent of a minimum of 60 mg of oral morphine daily for 1 week or longer (U.S. Food and Drug Administration, 2015a). For example, a patient who has been taking oxyCODONE 10 mg five times daily for the past 7 days would be considered opioid tolerant. When an individual develops opioid tolerance, the person may also develop tolerance to some side effects (e.g., nausea and pruritus) that are often experienced during initiation of opioid therapy.

Physical dependence is an expected physiologic response to repeated opioid administration that is caused by a type of "counter-adaptation" that occurs in opioid receptors and in the physiologic process of transduction and transmission (Volkow & McLellan, 2016, p. 1255). When physical dependence has developed and the opioids are abruptly stopped, the person may experience withdrawal symptoms (APA, 2013). However, when the opioid is discontinued in the absence of addiction, dependency resolves over time commensurate with the length of time the opioid was used (Volkow & McLellan, 2016). Physical dependence alone does not constitute SUD. *Withdrawal* symptoms will occur when there is abrupt cessation or too rapid of a reduction in opioid use regardless of the underlying reason for using the opioid (e.g., either chronic pain or OUD) as soon as 1 week after starting use of opioids. Physical dependence also can occur with other medications such as glucocorticoids, in which a patient would require a dose taper after taking the medication for a time. A simplistic example of dependence is the withdrawal headache that develops when a person who drinks coffee on a regular basis abruptly stops all caffeine intake. See Chapter 12 for additional discussion on physical dependence.

Box 14.1 | Terminology

Addiction: Primary, chronic neurobiologic disease with genetic, psychosocial, and environmental factors influencing its development and manifestation. Characterized by behaviors that include one or more of the following: impaired control over drug use, compulsive use, continued use despite harm, and craving (has been replaced by terms *substance use disorder* or *opioid use disorder* by the American Psychiatric Association (2013)

Opioid-induced hyperalgesia: Phenomenon in which escalating doses of opioids usually in those treated for a period with opioids results in less effective pain relief and may actually cause more pain (still controversial)

Opioid use disorder (OUD): Use of opiates for nonmedical purposes and can range on a continuum from mild to severe

Substance use disorder: Use of substances divided into 10 classes for nonmedical purposes and can range on a continuum from mild to severe. The criteria for a diagnosis of substance use disorder (SUD) are subdivided into groupings related to impaired control, social impairment, hazardous use, and pharmacologic criteria related to the substance of abuse

Physical dependence: State of adaptation that is manifested by a drug class in which an abrupt cessation, dose reduction, or decreasing blood levels can cause uncomfortable symptoms (*example*: withdrawal syndrome related to opioids and may range in severity from mild to severe)

Tolerance: Diminution of one or more of the substance's effects or side effects over time; state of adaptation in which the exposure to a drug induces changes that result in a decrease of the medication side effects such as nausea, pruritus, and respiratory depression, such as in the case of opioid tolerance

Withdrawal state: Cluster of symptoms related to cessation of use or reduction in dose of a psychoactive substance such as opioids. Measurement of opioid withdrawal severity can be done through use of the Clinical Opioid Withdrawal Scale

American Psychiatric Association. (2013). *Diagnostic and statistical manual of mental disorders* (5th ed.). Arlington, VA: American Psychiatric Association; Wilford, B. B. (2014). Appendix 1: ASAM addiction terminology. In: R. K. Ries, D. A. Fiellin, S. C. Miller, & R. Saitz (Eds.), *The ASAM principles of addiction medicine* (5th ed). Philadelphia, PA: Wolters Kluwer; Wesson, D. R., & Ling W. (2003). The Clinical Opiate Withdrawal Scale (COWS). *Journal of Psychoactive Drugs, 35,* 253–259; Ling, W. (2012). Buprenorphine implant for opioid addiction. *Pain Management, 2,* 345–350; and Liu, Y., Lin, D., Wu, B., & Zhou, W. (2016). Ketamine abuse potential and use disorder. *Brain Research Bulletin, 126,* 68–73.

Opioid withdrawal consists of a constellation of symptoms both physical (e.g., nausea, mydriasis, piloerection) and psychological (e.g., anxiety, agitation, mood change), that occur when opioids are abruptly discontinued (Chou et al., 2015). Opioid withdrawal alone is not diagnostic of OUD. Withdrawal is also discussed in Chapter 12.

The duration of opioid withdrawal depends on the half-life of the medication. For example, it may start as early as 4 hours after the last dose of heroin or may not start until 36 hours after the last dose of methadone. For medications with short half-lives the withdrawal period can continue up to 5 days, but in the case of methadone the acute phase may be less severe or the withdrawal may last up to 14 days because of the longer half-life. There is a concept of prolonged withdrawal that can persist for months; however, it continues to be a controversial subject (Tetrault & O'Connor, 2014). Measurement of the severity of opioid withdrawal is done using validated tools including the Objective Opioid Withdrawal Scale (OOWS), the Subjective Opioid Withdrawal Scale (SOWS), or the Clinical Opioid Withdrawal Scale (COWS) (Kampman & Jarvis, 2015). Withdrawal is also briefly discussed in Chapter 12.

Opioid-induced hyperalgesia is another potential effect of opioids that has been defined as an abnormal sensitivity to pain and has been thought to be associated with long-term use of opioids (Kim et al., 2014). In the case of opioid-induced hyperalgesia, with escalating doses of opioids pain intensifies instead of lessening (Eisenberg, Suzan, & Pud, 2015). This phenomenon may be seen in people with OUD with exposure to opioids for a prolonged time who experience more pain with less relief from opioid therapy for treatment of pain. At the time of this publication, researchers continue to explore the physiology and processes involved with opioid-induced hyperalgesia, although the exact mechanism that elicits hyperalgesia remains unknown. This topic is also addressed in Chapter 12.

Pseudoaddiction is a term used to describe behaviors resembling those associated with SUD but occur when pain is ineffectively treated and then resolve when pain is adequately controlled (Greene & Chambers, 2015). The term *pseudoaddiction* was coined in 1989 by Drs. Weissman and Haddox as an "iatrogenic syndrome of abnormal behavior developing as a direct consequence of inadeuqte pain management" (Weissman & Haddox, 1989, p. 363). The originators of the phrase described three phases of the phenomenon as (1) inadequate analgesia, (2) intensification of demands for pain relief with associated changes in behavior, with (3) evolving mutual mistrust between clinicians and patient. Although the concept of pseudoaddiction appears in the medical literature, in a review of 224 articles published through 2014, researchers were unable to identify any empiric studies that examined pseudoaddiction (Greene & Chambers, 2015). There is a need for researchers to examine the concept of pseudoaddiction and differentiate the clinical presentation of pseudoaddiction from that of SUD (Green & Chambers, 2015; Passik, Kirsh, & Webster, 2011).

Ethical Challenges to the Treatment of Pain in Patients With Comorbid Opioid Use Disorder

More than five decades ago when addressing issues of SUD at the 1961 Single Convention on Narcotic Drug convention, members of the United Nations noted that countries must ensure pain medications are available for the medical purpose to relieve pain and suffering for all people (Lohman, Schliefer, & Amon, 2010; United Nations, 1972). OUD and SUD are prevalent among people from all ethnic, socioeconomic, and educational backgrounds. Clinicians have an ethical obligation to withhold judgment and judiciously and appropriately treat people with SUDs/OUDs with compassion and respect. Relative to pain management, the ethical principles of autonomy, beneficence, nonmaleficence, and justice, described in Chapter 2, should be applied when considering decisions about pain management for the patient with OUD or SUD (Oliver et al., 2012) (Table 14.1). The principles of autonomy and beneficence are supported by clinicians' efforts to educate patients and their families about benefits and risks of opioid therapy. Beneficence and nonmaleficence are applied through safe, effective, and individualized multimodal pain management, monitoring for misuse and diversion, and minimizing potential harm while respecting the autonomy and dignity of all patients (justice).

Clinicians are obligated to acknowledge and consider their personal biases about patients with SUDs and OUDs because these biases may potentially result in the lack professionalism and deprivation of *just* care. A balance must be sought in providing compassionate pain care for people with serious illness and pain along with judicious efforts to support them in addressing any misuse of substances (Glod, 2017). Terminology such as *drug seeking* and *frequent flyer* must be avoided when referring to patients. In an effort to reduce stigma, clinicians are encouraged to consider replacing the derogatory term *drug seeking* with the term *comfort seeking* (Quinlan-Colwell & O'Conner-Von, 2014).

Caring for Patients With Pain and Opioid Use Disorder

Clinical Challenges of Treating Pain With Comorbid Opioid Use Disorder

It is important for clinicians to recognize that pain relief may be complicated for individuals with OUD who also have a potentially increased risk for poor outcomes. Patients with OUD are often opioid tolerant. Although the mechanisms of opioid tolerance are complex and not completely understood (Stromer et al., 2013), patients

Table 14.1	Ethical Principles and Application to Clinical Practice	
Ethical Principle	**Application to Clinical Practice**
Autonomy and dignity	Patients must be fully informed of treatment risks, benefits, and alternatives to preserve dignity and autonomy. This includes a complete discussion regarding the use of opioids when the patient has a known substance use disorder.
Beneficence	Requires that care be delivered in the patient's best interest. This includes appropriate screening for addiction risk. If the patient demonstrates an underlying substance use disorder with exposure to controlled substances, a clear plan of care is required.
Nonmaleficence (do no harm)	Requires monitoring for substance use and medication misuse in a stigma-free environment (Gourlay et al., 2005; Heit & Lipman, 2009). Discharging a patient from care without appropriate transfer of care or referral to another provider may lead to patient harm and is deemed to be maleficent.
Justice	Every patient should have equal access to pain management and be treated with the same level of vigilance, dignity, and respect, regardless of a coexisting substance use disorder (Savage, Kirsh, & Passik, 2008).
Fidelity and veracity	Ethical decisions (reasoned and systematic moral decision-making) and behaviors are bound by the moral obligations of veracity (truthfulness) and fidelity (faithfulness) (Beauchamp & Childress, 2009; Brown & Bennett, 2010).

Oliver. J., Coggins, C., Compton, P., Hagen, S., Matteliano, D., Stanton, M., ... Turner, H. N. (2012). American Society for Pain Management Nursing position statement: Pain management in patients with substance use disorders. *Pain Management Nursing, 13,* 169–183.

with OUD may experience increased pain sensitivity; report higher pain intensity, require more postoperative opioid analgesia; and use more anxiolytics than opioid-naïve individuals (Eyler, 2013).

When compared to opioid-free matched controls, adults seeking treatment for heroin dependence (n = 82) had higher pain sensitivity and lower tolerance for pain than those in the opioid-free control group (Compton, Canamar, Hillhouse, & Ling, 2012). In addition to opioid tolerance, individuals with OUD may experience opioid-induced hyperalgesia, anxiety, and withdrawal symptoms (Wachholtz, Foster, & Cheatle, 2015). For patients who have a prolonged abstinence from opioids, pain tolerance may improve, but they may still experience opioid-induced hyperalgesia (Wachholtz & Gonzalez, 2015). Well-designed rigorous research is needed to further explore these relationships.

Multimodal opioid-sparing analgesia, including nonopioid medications and nonpharmacologic interventions, is an important pain management approach for all patients, including those with OUD. It is also important for clinicians to focus the goals of pain treatment plans on functional improvement. Patients need education and support to establish safe and effective goals for pain control that are related to function rather than only to a pain intensity score (Pasero, Quinlan-Colwell, Rae, Broglio, & Drew, 2016). For example, when encouraged to establish a functional goal, one young woman with a long-standing history of intravenous heroin abuse determined that her goal for pain control was to be able to read her electronic tablet pages only once rather than multiple times because of being distracted by pain. On a scale of 0 to 10, she ascribed a pain intensity of 4 as her goal for the intensity with which she was able to comfortably read her electronic tablet and with which she was satisfied.

Risk Factors for Development of Opioid Use Disorder

Knowledge about the risks for developing OUD and addiction has evolved over time. In the past, many clinicians were taught that when opioids were used to treat either acute or chronic pain, the risk for development of OUD was minimal. The broader advocacy for the use of opioids for chronic nonmalignant pain in the late 1990s (Portenoy, 1996; Portenoy & Foley, 1986) was supported by the notion that opioids could be safely used for pain and the risk for addiction was less than 1% in those using opioids for pain relief. That belief emanated from a short letter to the editor summarizing the findings from a review of a database that assessed the risks for addiction among hospitalized patients who received opioids for treatment of acute pain (Porter & Jick, 1980). The conclusion of that letter evolved into a fact used to strongly support the belief that there was very low risk for developing OUD. That fact and belief were promoted and disseminated by advocates for pain management. Since then, the Porter and Jick letter has been cited over 600 times in the literature and at times the conclusions were grossly misrepresented (Leung, MacDonald, Dhalla, & Juurlink, 2017). During recent years, those early claims of negligible risk have been refuted by clinical experiences, studies, statistics, and the national focus on OUD.

Currently, the actual risk for developing OUD as a result of using prescription opioids for the treatment of chronic nonmalignant pain is unknown and estimates vary. Ten fair-quality uncontrolled studies reported prevalence of addiction in patients in pain clinics ranging from 2% to 14%, whereas dependence in primary care settings ranged from 3% to 26% (Chou et al., 2015). Recent studies have not indicated a clear association between the nonmedical use of opioids and the use of heroin but do acknowledge the nonmedical use of opioids is a factor among some people contributing to the progression to use of heroin (Compton, Jones, & Baldwin, 2016). Factors affecting the progression include the low cost of heroin and increased availability of heroin during an era when there is increased scrutiny combined with more restrictions on opioid prescribing (Compton et al., 2016).

In a review of patients receiving opioids for chronic pain in a large U.S. health system, risk factors identified for development of OUD include a history of opioid use, depression, use of psychotropic medications, pain impairment, and age younger than 65 years (Boscarino et al., 2010). At the same time, it is important to remember that others, including older adults may also be at risk for OUD and SUD (Quinlan-Colwell, 2012). The genetic predisposition for addictive disorders is a significant factor and reports from emerging research identified multiple genetic variants that can increase the risk for opioid misuse (Mistry et al., 2014). Risk factors are related to demographic, psychosocial, comorbid psychopathologies, genetics, premorbid SUD, and substance specific characteristics (Kaye et al., 2017a).

Although many opioid risk assessment instruments have been developed to assess for the risk of opioid misuse or abuse before starting opioid therapy and during opioid therapy, no one tool has been shown to be completely reliable (Kaye et al., 2017b). Many opioid risk assessment tools identify factors such as younger age, psychological comorbidities (e.g., depression, anxiety, posttraumatic stress disorder), and history of sexual abuse (Kaye et al., 2017b) (Table 14.2). Clinicians should consider using one of the opioid risk assessment tools along with a comprehensive interview, review of the prescription drug monitoring programs, and urine drug screening before initiating and periodically during prescription of opioid therapy (Kaye et al., 2017b). See Table 14.3 for descriptions of selected risk assessment tools.

Treatment of Opioid Use Disorder

All patients with OUD should receive psychosocial treatment that includes a psychosocial needs assessment, referrals to community services, links to family resources, and supportive counseling (Kampman & Jarvis, 2015). However, a patient's decision to defer or refuse supportive counseling should not be a barrier to the initiation of treatment for OUD (American Society for Addiction Medicine, 2020). Treatment of OUD may include medication-assisted treatment (MAT) with methadone, buprenorphine, or naltrexone. In 2011, approximately 300,000 people received methadone in opioid treatment programs (OTPs) and more than 32,000 individuals were treated with buprenorphine (Alderks, 2013). The number of people receiving MAT with buprenorphine is expected to increase because of the Comprehensive Addiction and Recovery Act (CARA) legislation in 2016. This act expands access to buprenorphine by allowing nurse

Table 14.2	Risk Factors for Opioid Misuse or Abuse[a]	
Demographics	Younger age Men Lower educational level
Pain severity	Disabling chronic pain Higher reported pain severity Increased functional limitations
Psychosocial factors	Past history of substance use disorder Tobacco, alcohol, cannabis, or illicit drug use Psychosocial stressors
Comorbid psychopathology	Depression Anxiety Posttraumatic stress disorder Schizophrenia
Drug-related factors	Self-reported craving High daily dose of opioids Use of short-acting opioids
Genetic factors	Variations in the opioid receptor genes (OPRM1, OPRKQ, OPRD1) Polymorphism preproenkephalin gene (PENK) Variations in multiple stress-related genes

[a] List is not inclusive.
Data from Kaye, A. D., Jones, M. R., Kaye, A. M., Ripoli, J. G., Galen, V., Beaklye, B. D ...Manchikanti, I. (2017a). Prescription opioid abuse in chronic pain: An updated review of opioid abuse predictors and strategies to curb opioid abuse: Part 1. *Pain Physician, 20*, S93–109.

practitioners and physician assistants who complete 24 hours of training to become certified, and register to prescribe buprenorphine for MAT within an office-based setting (American Society of Addiction Medicine, 2016).

Patients receiving MAT may present with painful conditions in different health care settings; therefore clinicians need to understand how to individualize treatment for patients who are receiving such therapy. Table 14.4 summarizes the medications used in MAT. Each of the medications that can be part of MAT are discussed in greater detail in the following paragraphs.

Methadone

Methadone is a biphasic synthetic mu opioid agonist first used in the United States in 1947 as an analgesic medication (Salsitz & Wiegand, 2016) and continues to be used as such for chronic pain management. See Chapter 11 for a description of methadone pharmacology. In 1965, methadone began to be used in *addiction treatment* (Salsitz & Wiegand, 2016). Individuals receiving methadone for the treatment of OUD must participate in a federally licensed OTP. To treat OUD, methadone is scheduled as a daily maintenance dose to reduce craving, block the euphoric effect of short-acting opioids, and prevent withdrawal for at least 24 hours (Kampman & Jarvis, 2015; Salsitz & Wiegand, 2016). The initial dose of methadone is no

Table 14.3 | Opioid Risk Tools

Opioid Risk Assessment Tools	Key Points	
Assess risk for opioid abuse before starting chronic opioid therapy		
Diagnosis, Intractability, Risk, Efficacy (DIRE)	7 items Patient interview	(Belgrade et al., 2006)
Opioid Risk Tool-OUD (ORT-OUD)	9 items Self-administer	(Cheatle et al., 2019)
Screener and Opioid Assessment for Patients with Pain-Revised (SOAPP-R)	24 items Self-administer	(Butler et al., 2008)
CAGE-AID (cutting down, annoyance by criticism, guilty feeling, eye opener adapted to include drugs)	4 items Patient interview Adapted from CAGE tool for alcoholism	(McPherson & Hersch, 2000)
Ongoing assessment tools for patients on opioid therapy		
Addictions Behavior Checklist (ABC)	20 item Self-administer/clinician observed behavior	(Wu et al., 2006)
Current Opioid Misuse Measure (COMM)	17 items Self-administer	(Butler et al., 2007)
Pain Assessment and Documentation Tool (PADT)	41 items (chart note documentation)	(Passik et al., 2004)

Modified and updated from Walsh, A. F., & Broglio, K. (2016). Pain management in the individual with serious illness and comorbid substance use disorder. *Nursing Clinics of North America: Palliative Care, 51,* 433–447.

more than 30 mg with the ability to add an extra 10 mg if withdrawal symptoms persist (Kampman & Jarvis, 2015; Salsitz & Wiegand, 2016). Dosing is then titrated until an appropriate maintenance dose is reached, with usual maintenance doses ranging from 60 to 120 mg/day (Kampman & Jarvis, 2015). Methadone may be the choice when a patient has failed buprenorphine therapy or has concomitant substance use issues such as alcohol or benzodiazepines that may put them at greater risk for adverse effects with self-management of medications at home (Kampman & Jarvis, 2015).

Individuals who choose to participate in methadone MAT generally visit the OTP daily to receive directly observed methadone dosing. However, in certain cases when an individual has demonstrated compliance through clean urine tests and is considered stable with low risk for misuse, methadone doses to be taken at home may be dispensed for a period of 2 to 7 days. For some participants this is a desirable incentive because it reduces the number of required visits to the OTP. When OTPs are not open on the weekend, *take home* methadone doses are provided on Friday to cover the weekend.

Psychological counseling is an integral component of MAT with methadone (Kampman & Jarvis, 2015). Counseling is known to provide an opportunity for participants to review the effect of substances on their lives and consider changing perspective and behaviors while exploring new coping skills (Schukit, 2016). As

with all psychological intervention, variability in benefit depends on the quality of the counseling provided. The benefits of counseling are not well identified in the literature (Kampman & Jarvis, 2015) and is an area in which research is needed.

Methadone can be used safely in people with liver or renal disease, which makes it a good opioid option for those with renal or hepatic comorbidities. However, methadone has more drug-drug interactions than other opioids because of its metabolism through the cytochrome (CYP)P450 enzyme systems (see Chapter 11). (McPherson, Costantino, & McPherson, 2018). To minimize adverse side effects associated with these drug-drug interactions, it may be necessary to adjust the methadone dose, reconsider the dose of the interacting medication, or reconsider use of the interacting medications (Chou et al., 2014; McCance-Katz, Sullivan, & Nallani, 2010; Salsitz & Wiegand, 2016). Clinicians should check drug-drug interactions before starting any new medications concurrently with methadone (McCance-Katz, et al., 2010). Another caution with methadone is the potential to cause electrocardiogram (ECG) QTc interval prolongation (McPherson et al., 2018). Concomitant use with other medications that prolong the QTc interval can place a patient at risk for torsades de pointes, a potentially fatal arrhythmia, thus requiring careful consideration of other medications and closer monitoring for adverse effects. ECGs should be periodically monitored when patients are

Table 14.4 | Medication-Assisted Treatments

Medication	Action	Dose	Where is it Obtained?	Comments
Methadone	Full mu-opioid agonist: can reduce craving for 24 h	Usual: 60–120 mg PO once daily: patient goes to clinic daily for observed dosing	Must be administered through a federal opioid treatment program	Provides analgesia only for 6–12 h; thus if used in MAT, but needing to optimize analgesic effect during hospitalization, more than once-daily dosing necessary for pain management Many drug-drug interactions; can cause QTc prolongation
Buprenorphine/ naloxone Buprenorphine Buprenorphine implants Buprenorphine extended-release product for subcutaneous injectable	Partial mu-agonist: occupies mu receptors, reduces craving; naloxone decreases effect if used intravenously	8–24 mg sublingual/ transmucosal once daily 4 single-rod implants (each containing 74.2 mg of buprenorphine) changed every 6 mo 100 or 300-mg subcutaneous monthly injection	Can be prescribed by physicians, nurse practitioners, and physician assistants who have completed training and have waiver with special DEA number starting with "X" Subdermal implant is office surgical procedure Injection is usually administered in a provider's office	May provide analgesia and if also used for pain benefit, would need to be given in split doses (bid or tid); if mu opioids administered at same time, would need higher doses to have any efficacy Implants can be removed before 6 mo; fewer drug-drug interactions than methadone Additional injectable extended-release products are expected to become available
Naltrexone	Full mu receptor antagonist	50 mg/day PO or 380 mg/mo IM depot injection	Injection can be administered by any clinician licensed to prescribe medications	Also used for alcohol use disorder. Cannot be used if opioids are necessary because will block the effects of opioids

Aboujaoude, E., & Salame, W. O. (2016). Naltrexone: A pan-addiction treatment? *CNS Drugs, 30,* 719–733; Barnwal, P. Das, S., Mondal, S., Ramasamy, A., Maiti, T., & Saha, A. (2017). Probuphine® [buprenorphine implant]: A promising candidate in opioid dependence. *Therapeutic Advances in Psychopharmacology, 7,* 119–134; Kampman, K., & Jarvis, M. (2015). American Society of Addiction Medicine (ASAM) national practice guideline for the use of medications in the treatment of addiction involving opioid use. *Journal of Addiction Medicine, 9,* 358–367; Ling, W., Shoptaw, S., & Goodman-Meza, D. (2019). Depot buprenorphine injection in the management of opioid use disorder: From development to implementation. *Substance Abuse and Rehabilitation, 10,* 69.

taking methadone, with frequency based on baseline QTc intervals, methadone dose, and concomitant use of other medications that can also prolong the QTc interval (Chou et al., 2014).

Buprenorphine

Buprenorphine is a semisynthetic partial mu agonist used for OUD and for pain management (Khanna & Pillarisetti, 2015). Buprenorphine treatment for OUD began in 2002. Treatment formulations include sublingual tablets, transmucosal film combined with naloxone, a 6-month implant (Ling, 2012), or a monthly extended-release subcutaneous injection (Ling, Shoptaw, & Goodman-Meza, 2019). As a partial mu agonist, buprenorphine activates the mu receptor at lower levels by occupying most of the mu opioid receptors and displacing other opioids. Buprenorphine has high affinity for binding to the mu opioid receptor yet only partially activates it. The partial activation is the reason a ceiling effect may occur with buprenorphine, and it

is suggested that when used alone buprenorphine carries less risk for overdose (Phillips & Preston, 2014). It has broad half-life variability and slowly dissociates from the mu opioid receptor (Anderson et al., 2017).

The sublingual and transmucosal formulations of buprenorphine, usually given in doses ranging from 8 to 24 mg/day, are available alone or in combination with naloxone to minimize the risk for tampering and injection (Kampman & Jarvis, 2015; Silverman, 2015). Patients should be taught to allow these formulations to completely dissolve in the mouth and not chew or swallow them. Pregnant women with OUD may be treated with buprenorphine with or without naloxone. The combination product is reported to be safe and effective for use in pregnant women as naloxone is minimally absorbed when taken as directed (American Society for Addiction Medicine, 2020). Buprenorphine implants, which are surgically implanted in an office procedure, are effective for 6 months. The buprenorphine implants deliver about 1.3 mg/day of buprenorphine through 4 or 5 implanted rods and have been comparable in efficacy to patients taking buprenorphine 8 mg daily. Some patients using buprenorphine implants have required additional buprenorphine transmucosally to maintain abstinence. The implants can be surgically removed before 6 months if necessary (Barnwal et al., 2017). Buprenorphine is available in an extended-release product for subcutaneous (peri-umbilical) administration to individuals who have received 8-24mg/day doses of transmucosal buprenorphine for at least 7 days. The 100mg or 300mg peri-umbilical injection is administered monthly under the provider's supervision.

Buprenorphine can be prescribed by physicians, nurse practitioners, and physician assistants who have completed additional training and have obtained a required waiver. The prescribers must complete documentation, easily accessible from the Drug Enforcement Agency (DEA), that outlines the treatment, and they also must ensure that patients are offered or referred to psychological treatment (Phillips & Preston, 2014). These prescribers are issued a (DEA) number beginning with an "X" (Phillips & Preston, 2014). Buprenorphine can be prescribed in general ambulatory care settings and does not require the patient to go to a federally allocated OTP, although some OTPs do prescribe buprenorphine (Kampman & Jarvis, 2015).

Patients are first started on buprenorphine when they have been abstinent from opioids long enough to have observable opioid withdrawal symptoms which may range from 4 hours after the last dose of heroin to 48–72 hours after the last dose of methadone (Hämmig et al., 2016). If a patient is unable to tolerate methadone or chooses to rotate to buprenorphine, methadone should be decreased to 30 to 40mg/day before rotation (Kampman & Jarvis, 2015). If buprenorphine is started when the patient is currently taking opioids, there is a possibility that withdrawal symptoms will be precipitated because of the partial mu agonist effect (Phillips & Preston, 2014). Craving for opioids tend to decrease once the patient is on a stable dose of buprenorphine for a 24-hour period. That dose is continued and self-administered daily, although there has been some research to suggest that every-other-day dosing can be effective (Kampman & Jarvis, 2015). At the onset of therapy, visits are often scheduled weekly to reduce the risks for diversion and may extend to monthly visits once the patient is on a stable dose and not demonstrating evidence of misuse or diversion (Kampman & Jarvis, 2015).

The ability of buprenorphine to block the effect of other opioids makes it a viable treatment option for OUD (Silverman, 2015); however, buprenorphine therapy may not be appropriate for all people with OUD. For some patients who have been on very high doses of opioids, buprenorphine therapy may not reduce the cravings even at maximal dose; thus these patients may require or be considered for methadone maintenance therapy. Patients who are at higher risk for abuse and diversion also may not be appropriate candidates for sublingual or transmucosal buprenorphine therapy (Kampman & Jarvis, 2015). If the patient is not able to safely self-administer buprenorphine on a daily regimen, an extended-release buprenorphine product methadone maintenance therapy may be the better treatment alternative (Kampman & Jarvis, 2015).

Because buprenorphine is only a partial mu agonist, the risk for respiratory depression and oversedation is rarely seen in those on buprenorphine therapy unless there has been concomitant use of other central nervous system depressants (Connery, 2015; Phillips & Preston, 2014), including opioids (Kelty & Hulse, 2017). However, it is important to know that when additional opioids are prescribed or are used in conjunction with buprenorphine, sedation and respiratory depression are possible and assessment is needed. The effects of short-acting transmucosal or sublingual buprenorphine can last 24 to 72 hours, and binding to the mu receptors can result in difficulty in treating pain with pure mu opioid agonists (Bryson, 2014). Buprenorphine is metabolized through the CYP450 3A4 pathway so may have an inhibitory or inducing effect on other medications metabolized through this pathway (McCance-Katz, et al., 2010).

Naltrexone

Naltrexone has been used for many years to treat alcohol dependence and is also approved for use as a mu receptor antagonist to prevent relapse of opioid dependence after completion of opioid detoxification (Sudakin, 2016). Naltrexone blocks the euphoric effects of opioids, can reduce alcohol craving, and has been studied in a variety of addictions (Aboujaoude & Salame, 2016; Barnett, Twycross, Mihalyo, & Wilcock, 2014). Naltrexone has no analgesic properties. It should not be confused with naloxone, which is also a mu receptor antagonist with a shorter half-life, used to reverse opioid-induced respiratory depression (Calas, Wilkins, & Oliphant 2016) (see Chapter 13). Early studies showed that when compared to buprenorphine and methadone, the relapse risk is higher with naltrexone (Kjome & Moeller, 2011). Comparison of relapse rates among available MATs is an area in need of research. As with other MAT selection, individual patient characteristics must be considered.

Naltrexone can be administered in doses of 50 mg/day or three times weekly doses of 100 mg/100 mg/150 mg (Kampman & Jarvis, 2015). Naltrexone can also be administered as a monthly intramuscular depot injection [Vivitrol] of 380 mg (Drugs@FDA: Vivitrol, 2010). Challenges with oral dosing related to medication adherence may be reduced by directly observed daily dosing or use of the monthly injectable formulation, which may be administered by any health care professional (Drugs@FDA: Vivitrol, 2010; Kampman & Jarvis, 2015). Individuals must have completely withdrawn from opioids (usually 7–10 days) before starting naltrexone (Drugs@FDA: Vivitrol, 2010). Monthly dosing of naltrexone may be a feasible option for patients who have transportation or other issues limiting access to a directly observed therapy program or to a prescriber of buprenorphine. However, a barrier for using monthly dosing of naltrexone is the significant expense of the monthly medication. Individuals who receive naltrexone therapy should also receive psychological counseling for OUD (Kampman & Jarvis, 2015).

The most suitable individuals for use of naltrexone are those who are willing to commit to total abstinence from any type of agonist therapy, who in the past have not tolerated agonist therapies, who are highly motivated or work in settings where urine drug testing is routinely conducted, and who may not choose to disclose their previous substance use status (Substance Abuse and Mental Health Services Administration [SAMHSA], 2012). Patients who receive naltrexone therapy must be cautioned that as a result of decreased opioid tolerance, if they relapse and use opioids, when the naltrexone effect is diminished, they will be at increased risk for opioid overdose (Kampman & Jarvis, 2015). If patients rotate from naltrexone to methadone or buprenorphine, the starting doses may be less than for those actively using opioids. For those who have been receiving injectable naltrexone, rotation should not take place until 30 days after the last injection (Kampman & Jarvis, 2015). A small risk for hepatotoxicity has been seen, so judicious monitoring of liver enzymes may be warranted (Kjome & Moeller, 2011).

Pain and Opioid Use Disorder: Acute Care Setting

Screening for Opioid Use Disorder in the Acute Care Setting

Given the increasing reports of misuse and abuse of opioids in the last decade (Center for Behavioral Health Statistics and Quality, 2016), it is incumbent on all clinicians to screen for OUD to prevent unintended withdrawal in the acute care setting and inadequate treatment of pain related to inaccurate estimates of opioid needs during an acute pain event. When possible, an opioid risk assessment should be included with any pain assessment in which opioids are considered as a treatment option. In the acute care setting, conducting a risk assessment is intended to aid the clinician to formulate a safe and effective treatment plan by gaining an understanding of risk for OUD and is not intended to be a means for withholding treatment.

Developing a therapeutically safe rapport with patients is a first step in the screening process and clinical interview. This is important because many patients struggle to report an honest history of substance abuse, especially when previous health care experiences include untreated or undertreated pain (St. Marie, 2014). The clinician may consider starting the assessment with questions related to tobacco or alcohol use and to explain that assessment guides the clinician in providing safe and effective pain management (Walsh & Broglio, 2016). Although opioid risk screening tools (see Table 14.3) have not been validated for use in the acute care setting, they may be beneficial, particularly if opioids will be prescribed on discharge. Other important components of risk assessment are review of the medical records, which may provide beneficial information, and to query the state prescription drug monitoring program (PDMP) (Kaye et al., 2017a). Of note, methadone and buprenorphine obtained through MAT are not included on PDMP reports. Urine drug screening may be appropriate in the inpatient setting to confirm presence or absence of substances (Cooney & Broglio, 2017; Sen et al., 2016). For patients who are receiving MAT, permission to contact the OTP or the prescriber of buprenorphine or naltrexone should be obtained. Communication with MAT clinicians is essential to develop the most appropriate plans for pain management and follow-up care (Savage, 2014).

A physical examination may also provide information that will aid the clinician in developing a safe and effective plan of care. Physical examination includes assessment for excessive drowsiness, pupil constriction, lesions over veins (track marks), or atrophy and erosion of the nares and septum (Bowman, Eiserman, Beletsky, Stancliff, & Bruce, 2013). It is important to recognize signs and symptoms of opioid use and opioid withdrawal.

Acute Pain Management of the Patient With Active Opioid Use Disorder Who Is Not in Active Treatment

The challenge in the treatment of pain in the patient with active OUD is to find the balance between safely and effectively treating pain while minimizing the effects of opioid withdrawal. Clinicians must be able to assess and treat pain, implementing a multimodal approach while simultaneously lessening any withdrawal symptoms. Treatment with opioids may minimize withdrawal effects and, in some situations, the use of methadone or buprenorphine may be helpful (Kampman & Jarvis, 2015; Schuckit, 2016). However, it is necessary to ensure that the use of these medications in the inpatient setting is in accordance with federal and state laws that qualify their use. Both methadone and buprenorphine can be used without a specialty waiver in an acute setting to minimize withdrawal if they are used to maintain or detoxify a person who is hospitalized for medical or surgical conditions not related to addiction. For example, a pregnant patient who has been actively using intravenous heroin and is not receiving MAT, if admitted for urosepsis and develops severe withdrawal symptoms, may receive methadone to reduce severity of withdrawal. Prescribers are advised to refer to specific limitations for methadone and buprenorphine specified by the U.S. Drug Enforcement Administration, Department of Justice (Electronic Code of Federal Regulations, 2018) and by individual state regulations. If methadone is used, there must be an agreeable and established plan in place for care after discharge because methadone for treatment of OUD can be dispensed only at federally licensed OTPs after discharge (Kampman & Jarvis, 2015). Either of these medications, if started in the hospital, will have to be weaned before discharge if the patient will not continue with MAT at an OTP (methadone or buprenorphine) or with a licensed prescriber (buprenorphine).

If opioids are required for treatment of pain during the hospitalization and opioid tolerance is unknown, intravenous patient-controlled analgesia (PCA) may be an option because it will enable the patient to self-administer necessary doses for effective pain relief (Sen et al., 2016). A basal (continuous) infusion of intravenous PCA along with patient-controlled boluses may be necessary to ensure adequate pain control among opioid-tolerant patients (Herndon et al., 2016). Because the degree of opioid tolerance is unknown, it is necessary to ensure close monitoring for effectiveness and signs of adverse effects (see Chapters 12 and 13). In addition, observation precautions are needed to minimize the risk for tampering with the opioid infusion or using illicit drugs in the acute care setting when patients have been actively misusing or abusing substances before admission. Once patients are transitioned to oral medications, the use of scheduled opioids versus as-needed (prn) analgesics can minimize continued reactivation of the reward system in the brain (Vadivelu, Kai, Kodumudi, Zhu, & Hines, 2017). Adequate scheduled analgesia also serves to convey that clinicians think the person has pain and is proactively helping to safely control his or her pain.

Patients who may have been on very high doses of opioids before admission may experience some withdrawal symptoms even with concurrent use of opioids for pain management. Some withdrawal symptoms can be treated to minimize distress with the use of medications such as clonidine and tiZANidine (alpha$_2$-adrenergic agonists), which may help decrease symptoms of autonomic overactivity such as anxiety and piloerection (Gowing, Farrell, Ali, & White, 2014). Other withdrawal symptoms such as diarrhea, nausea and vomiting, and dehydration can be treated with pharmacologic and/or nonpharmacologic supportive care (Schukit, 2016). Nonpharmacologic interventions, including breathing techniques, progressive muscle relaxation, art therapy, music therapy, yoga, tai chi, massage, and therapeutic touch can be effectively used to help manage symptoms of anxiety. See Chapters 22 through 27 for descriptions of nonpharmacologic interventions.

It is important to effectively treat pain before addressing possible interventions for OUD. If the patient is willing to discuss treatment for OUD in the inpatient setting and resources are available, appropriate referrals to clinicians who specialize in SUDs, should be offered. When these services are not available in the hospital setting and the patient is agreeable, attempts should be made to coordinate an immediate referral to an OTP for methadone or a clinician who can prescribe buprenorphine or naltrexone. The involvement of specialists in SUDs, including counselors, social workers, advanced practice nurses, case managers, and physicians can be very valuable in coordinating a solid workable discharge plan for MAT (Quinlan-Colwell, 2017).

If a patient requires treatment with opioids for pain management after discharge from the hospital setting, the safest plan would be for transfer to a specialized facility until the opioids can be weaned off. If this is not feasible, it is important to have a discharge plan in place with an outpatient clinician to treat pain after discharge. If no follow-up plans are in place, the patient may be at increased risk for overdose from illegally obtained opioids, especially if opioid doses in the hospital were much lower than what had been used before admission. Before discharge, it is prudent to counsel patients about the increased risk for overdose and availability of naloxone as a reversal agent if they resume their prehospitalization use of opioids (Kampman & Jarvis, 2015). On discharge it is appropriate to provide a prescription for naloxone for opioid reversal, especially in communities where it is not readily available without prescription (DHHS, 2018). When patients do not agree to immediate referral for OUD treatment, on discharge it is important to provide them with information for resources they can access if they decide to seek treatment at a later date.

Acute Pain Management for Patients on Medication-Assisted Treatment

The recommended approach for effective pain management in patients being treated with MAT incorporates the general principles for treating acute pain with MMA. It is essential for clinicians in the acute care setting to verify that patients are enrolled in MAT; the dose of medication that is prescribed; and the degree of patient compliance with therapy. Such verification is important because the information must be considered in the plan for pain management. The following discussion includes some of the basic considerations when treating acute pain in patients receiving MAT.

Acute Pain Management for Patients on Methadone Maintenance Therapy

When patients who receive methadone maintenance therapy (MMT) are hospitalized, questions may arise about appropriate methadone prescribing and treatment of acute pain. Individuals on MMT should continue their usual daily methadone dose during hospitalization (Bryson, 2014; Wenzel, Schwenk, Baratta, & Viscusi, 2016). In the hospital setting, clinicians are able to prescribe continuation of methadone maintenance doses during hospitalization (Electronic Code of Federal Regulations, 2018).

However, because methadone administered through a treatment program does not appear on PDMP reports, clinicians must contact treatment programs to verify methadone dosage. Although the usual daily methadone dose is generally continued in the hospital setting, conditions such as increased somnolence, prolonged QT/QTc intervals, fever, shock, or hemodynamic instability may necessitate the methadone dose be decreased or held. If the methadone dose or dosing schedule is changed (as with divided daily doses), it is advisable to discuss the changes with the OTP (Taveros & Chuang, 2016).

When it is not possible for the patient to have oral methadone, intravenous methadone (if available) may be administered using an oral to intravenous conversion of 2:1. This conversion with a dose reduction has been recommended, even though methadone has oral bioavailability from 30% to 100% (Sen et al., 2016). Another recommendation is to start the intravenous methadone at 0.8 mg to every 1 mg oral methadone (Mercadante, 2014). When this change is made, clinicians are advised to ensure increased monitoring because there may be side effects (such as myoclonus) with the intravenous route that are not present with oral administration (Mercadante, 2014). If the patient cannot take oral medications and intravenous methadone is not available, the use of intravenous PCA can mitigate the risk for opioid withdrawal. However, when transitioning from methadone to another opioid, equianalgesic dosing is not as predictable as it is with other opioids, and clinicians with expertise should be consulted for guidance. See Chapter 11 for detailed description of methadone dose conversion.

Currently, no consensus guidelines are available to guide treatment of pain in this group of patients. Because of the decreased pain tolerance, increased pain sensitivity, and opioid tolerance with possible hyperalgesia seen in patients receiving methadone MAT, clinicians need to anticipate possible reports of high pain severity scores and the potential need for opioids in higher doses at a greater frequency than in opioid-naïve patients (Bryson, 2014; Macintyre, Russell, Usher, Gaughwin, & Huxtable, 2013). A multimodal approach to pain management needs to be used to minimize opioid needs and manage pain most effectively.

When a patient who is receiving MMT is hospitalized and experiences acute pain, some clinicians may erroneously think the methadone maintenance dose will provide adequate analgesia, and no other pain management interventions are necessary. Although methadone is a pure mu agonist opioid and analgesic, the pain-relieving effects are sustained for only 3 to 12 hours. Therefore the once-daily dose used to treat OUD will not likely provide enough pain relief or adequately manage pain over the 24-hour period (Pasero, Quill, Portenoy, McCaffery, & Rizos, 2011). To optimize its analgesic effects, if possible and agreeable to the patient, the methadone dose can be divided into every 6 to 8 hour dosing during hospitalization (Wenzel et al, 2016). Intravenous PCA with another opioid can be used to provide additional opioids to the patient on MAT and may improve patient satisfaction while reducing the risk for undertreating acute pain (Sen et al., 2016). Assessment of pain, respiratory status, and sedation along with a multimodal approach to pain management targeting the specific source of pain are essential.

Acute Pain Management for Patients on Buprenorphine Therapy

Multiple protocols have been suggested to manage acute pain in patients who are taking buprenorphine as a treatment for OUD, with no consensus as to the best approach (Anderson et al., 2017). Thus clinicians need to work collaboratively with prescribers of buprenorphine therapy to establish approaches to treatment that can address acute pain. Collaboration with the buprenorphine prescriber is particularly important when the buprenorphine is the extended-release injection or the implanted product. In these situations, elective surgery may need to be delayed until the buprenorphine effect is extinguished, or additional consideration must be made to assure adequate analgesia while the buprenorphine effect is present. The following paragraphs apply to management of patient situations involving transmucosal or sublingual buprenorphine.

In preparation for elective surgery, sublingual or transmucosal buprenorphine may be weaned by 2 mg every 3 days and discontinued 72 hours before surgery (Bryson, 2014; Kampman & Jarvis, 2015; Sen et al., 2016). The slow weaning is needed to prevent opioid withdrawal. Considerations for this type of protocol need to be based on patient characteristics, type of surgery, and the duration of time the patient will not be receiving MAT. This approach may not be appropriate if there is a concern about possible relapse during weaning and the time the patient is not on any MAT.

In cases in which a rapid discontinuation is required, buprenorphine can be weaned over 3 days; however, withdrawal symptoms are likely to be experienced with such rapid weaning. Alternatively, if there is intolerable pain or withdrawal symptoms and the risk for relapse is very high, some authors suggest buprenorphine can be converted to methadone at 30 to 40 mg/day and dosing can be increased by 5 to 10 mg/day to prevent withdrawal symptoms (Bryson 2014; Sen et al., 2016).

Another option is to continue buprenorphine through the perioperative period to capitalize on its analgesic effects, with buprenorphine divided into 6- or 8-hour dosing intervals during hospitalization (Bryson, 2014; Kampman & Jarvis, 2015; Sen et al., 2016). It has been postulated that buprenorphine has an analgesic ceiling effect and doses above 32 mg/day sublingually will not provide additional analgesia. To adequately provide pain control, an MMA approach, including nonopioid and nonpharmacologic interventions, is necessary. In some cases, immediate-release opioids also may be used (Bryson 2014; Sen et al, 2016) (Table 14.5).

Table 14.5 | Buprenorphine and Acute Pain Management Strategies[a]

Type of Surgery	Anticipated Pain	Suggested Strategies
Elective surgery	Minimal pain expected	Continue buprenorphine therapy and consider administering in divided doses every 6–8 h to maximize analgesia
Unplanned surgery/ trauma	Minimal pain	Utilize multimodal analgesia
Elective surgery	Moderate to severe pain expected	Wean buprenorphine by 2 mg every 2–3 days and discontinue 72 hours before surgery[b] Use multimodal analgesia and short-acting opioids for acute pain Restart buprenorphine once pain subsides and patient has gone through mild withdrawal
Elective surgery	Moderate to severe pain expected Increased concern about relapse or intolerable pain or withdrawal symptoms	Convert buprenorphine to methadone 30–40 mg/day Increase methadone by 5–10 mg/day to treat withdrawal or craving Use multimodal analgesia and short-acting opioids for acute pain
Elective surgery	Moderate to severe pain expected	Continue buprenorphine therapy and consider divided doses every 6–8 h and can increase dose to maximum of 32 mg/day
Unplanned surgery/ trauma	Desire to continue buprenorphine therapy	Use multimodal analgesia Treat acute pain with mu opioid agonists such as fentaNYL, HYDROmorphone or morphine, or sublingual or intravenous buprenorphine if available
Unplanned surgery/ trauma[c]	Moderate to severe pain expected Clinician plan to discontinue buprenorphine	Use multimodal analgesia Treat acute pain with mu opioid agonists such as fentaNYL, HYDROmorphone, or morphine Anticipate higher doses needed for 72 h until buprenorphine cleared from system Consider monitored setting because may have increased risk for respiratory depression once buprenorphine cleared from system

[a] Collaboration with patient's buprenorphine prescriber should be part of the treatment plan in all cases.
[b] If patient has 6-month implantable buprenorphine, will need to make decision whether to remove before planned surgery.
[c] In cases of unplanned surgery will need to treat with immediate-release opioids potentially at higher doses if patient has implantable buprenorphine.
Anderson, T. A., Quaye, A. N. A., Ward, E. N., Wilens, T. E., Hilliard, P. E., & Brummett, C. M. (2017). To stop or not, that is the question: Acute pain management for the patient on chronic buprenorphine. *Anesthesiology, 126,* 1180–1186; Bryson, E. O. (2014). The perioperative management of patients maintained on medications used to manage opioid addiction. *Current Opinion in Anaesthesiology, 27,* 359–364; Sen, S., Arulkumar, S., Cornett, E. M., Gayle, J. A., Flower, R. R., Fox, C. J., & Kaye, A. D. (2016). New pain management options for the surgical patient on methadone and buprenorphine. *Current Pain Headache Report, 20,* 16.

For patients with severe acute pain, discontinuation of buprenorphine and the administration of opioids such as fentaNYL may be the most appropriate option (Kampman & Jarvis, 2015). However, as clinical experience with buprenorphine increases, different approaches have been recommended. In a small retrospective study (n = 24) of patients continued on buprenorphine who also received intravenous PCA opioids, the additional use of buprenorphine was not seen as a deterrent to pain control, although higher doses of intravenous PCA opioids were necessary (Macintyre et al., 2013). A number of professional organizations, including those with specialties in pain management and anesthesia, recommend that if opioids are required to control severe pain, the oral route is preferred over the intravenous route; the use of PCA is preferred over clinician-administered intravenous injections; and continuous opioid infusions should be avoided (Anderson et al., 2017).

There is no definitive answer or single approach to the management of acute pain in hospitalized patients who are receiving buprenorphine for OUD. If buprenorphine is abruptly discontinued, recognize that the affinity of buprenorphine for mu receptors will persist and can be sustained for 24 to 72 hours after the last dose. This effect may block other opioid binding effects, and the individual may require dramatic upward titration of opioids to overcome the effect of the buprenorphine (Bryson, 2014). If buprenorphine has been discontinued, once the mu binding effect has cleared, the individual may have decreased tolerance to opioids and may be at increased risk for respiratory depression (Bryson, 2014). A monitored setting may be appropriate for these patients, and they may also benefit from using multiple coanalgesic medications to control pain (Anderson et al., 2017).

If buprenorphine was discontinued and pain significantly subsided during the hospitalization, buprenorphine can be restarted on discharge after allowing for a period of mild withdrawal (Bryson, 2014). A critical component of any treatment plan is coordination of care with the patient's buprenorphine prescriber (Anderson et al., 2017). If it is expected that the individual may require opioids for pain control after discharge, collaboration with the buprenorphine prescriber and patient may be beneficial in ensuring the development of a plan for safe and appropriate treatment (Anderson et al., 2017). As has been stressed throughout this book, regardless of whether buprenorphine has been used for the treatment of acute pain, the use of MMA is highly recommended, and the use of nonopioid therapy is particularly important for those individuals with OUD (Anderson et al., 2017).

Acute Pain Management for Patients on Naltrexone

When an individual is admitted for elective surgery, oral naltrexone should be discontinued 72 hours preoperatively and injectable naltrexone should be discontinued 1 month before the elective surgery date (Kampman & Jarvis, 2015). In the case of an unplanned admission such as trauma or acute illness, 10 to 20 times the usual opioid dose may be required to overcome the antagonistic action of naltrexone (Bryson, 2014). Even when high doses of opioids are used, there may be less analgesia, but the risk for side effects may be greater. For safety reasons, individuals need to be placed in a monitored setting during this time (Wenzel et al., 2016). Multimodal pain management is essential, including nonopioid analgesics and regional analgesia when it is appropriate and available (Chou et al., 2016; Wenzel et al., 2016). If patients have been receiving naltrexone, it is important to monitor liver function tests because naltrexone has a small but documented risk for hepatoxicity (Kjome & Moeller, 2011).

Acute Pain Management for Patients With Opioid Use Disorder in Recovery Without Medication-Assisted Treatment

Patients who are in recovery without the use of MAT also need individualized pain management when hospitalized in an acute care setting, particularly when opioid therapy may be necessary. Although the goal of MMA is to target receptors at multiple sites through the use of different classes of analgesics, opioids remain one of the most effective classes of medications for acute, severe pain. Assessment of patients who are in OUD recovery and are not on MAT should include the patient's perceptions or concerns about the use of opioids in the acute pain management situation. Some patients have significant concerns or fears about relapse if using opioids even for a short time. Clinicians should be sensitive to these concerns because many patients may have experienced periods of relapse in the past, and thus their concerns are very realistic. All efforts should be made to respect the patient's wishes, provide reassurance, and use effective nonopioid multimodal pain management. When opioids are necessary to provide effective pain relief, clinicians should use the lowest effective dose; if feasible, an opioid the patient has not previously used should be prescribed;

and a plan for tapering/weaning from the opioid developed with the patient.

Patients should be reassured that if opioids are used, a plan is in place for opioid weaning and additional support can be provided if the wean is difficult. The use of immediate-release opioids, which may stimulate the reward system, should be minimized (Savage, 2014) and if used, should be scheduled rather than used on an as-needed basis. Use of nonopioid and nonpharmacologic pain management approaches and consultation with clinicians who specialize in working with patients with OUD, including psychologists, counselors, behavioral health experts, social workers, and case managers, are important to support the patient and family during this time. A plan for care in the outpatient setting should be negotiated and developed before discharge. Given that patients who are not receiving MAT are at risk for relapse, education and counseling ought to include the increased risk for opioid overdose should the patient relapse into opioid use after discharge (Connery, 2015).

Acute Pain Management: Special Considerations

As discussed, the use of opioids may be necessary as part of an MMA plan of care established between the patient and clinicians with thoughtful consideration in the selection and dosing of medications in patients with OUD. For those unable to take oral medications, intravenous PCA may enable the patient to obtain better pain control through self-administered dosing (Anderson et al., 2017). Multimodal strategies, including acetaminophen, nonsteroidal antiinflammatory drugs, interventional approaches, and nonpharmacologic therapies, may be beneficial.

Coanalgesic medications, further described in Chapter 15, may contribute to effective pain management. Lidocaine may be particularly beneficial and has been shown to decrease opioid requirements (Chou et al., 2016; Stromer et al., 2013). The use of gabapentinoids has become controversial. Although these medications may offer a role in reducing symptoms of opioid withdrawal (Freynhagen et al., 2016; Salehi, Kheirabadi, Maracy, & Ranjkesh, 2011); recent studies indicate they may present risks for misuse and abuse (Evoy, Morrison, & Saklad, 2017; Stein, Kenney, Anderson, Conti, & Bailey, 2020). Alpha-$_2$ agonists, such as dexmedetomidine, may be useful for pain that is refractory to opioid treatment (Schnabel, Meyer-Friessem, Reichl, Zahn, & Pogatzki-Zahn, 2013). CloNIDine, in addition to being used to reduce symptoms related to opioid withdrawal, may be an effective adjunct in pain management (Kowalczyk et al., 2015).

Ketamine may be considered for patients who are opioid tolerant or actively abusing opioids or for those who are refractory to effective pain management with opioid therapy (Vadivelu et al., 2017). Evidence shows that ketamine may be useful for opioid-tolerant surgical patients and may have a role in the prevention of persistent postsurgical pain (Gorlin, Rosenfeld, & Ramakrishna, 2016). However, ketamine is also a substance with known abuse potential (Liu, Lin, Wu, & Zhou, 2016).

An acute event requiring pain management during hospitalization with disruption in the recovery process can cause significant concern for individuals who have been successful with MAT or those in recovery not receiving MAT. Individuals in either group may have increased anxiety, fears, and concerns about relapse if opioids are used for control of pain. In addition, as a result of previous encounters in the health care system, they may have realistic concerns about the potential for undertreatment of pain (St. Marie, 2014). Clinicians need to provide support during this phase, and, if Narcotics Anonymous meetings are available in the hospital setting, patients should be encouraged to attend if possible. Patient access to the support of 12-Step sponsors or sobriety coaches in the acute care setting is important. Coordination of care with practitioners who specialize in working with patients with SUD is optimal. It cannot be emphasized enough that a collaborative interdisciplinary multimodal plan of care is fundamental for effectively managing pain with patients with OUD.

Discharge Planning for Patients With Opioid Use Disorder

No specific guidelines currently exist for using opioids as treatment of acute pain in patients with OUD after hospital discharge. Involvement of the multidisciplinary team, including the community MAT prescriber or OTP, and continuation of an MMA plan that includes the use of nonopioid analgesics, adjuvant agents, and nonpharmacologic therapies are critical to a successful transition to another level of care. When it is anticipated that opioids will be considered after hospital discharge, a well-designed plan coordinated with outpatient support, including significant others, is recommended to ensure safety and recognition of untoward responses. Depending on the individual patient situation and availability of resources, it may be necessary to facilitate an alternative level of care for continued opioid administration. An alternative option might include the engagement of an outpatient clinician to assist in confirming appropriate use and supervision of prescribed opioids. According to recent guidelines, the dose and quantity of opioids prescribed on discharge should be limited to no more than 3 to 5 days (Dowell, Haegerich, & Chou, 2016) and a specific tapering plan should be incorporated in the prescription provided at discharge. If additional medications are needed, follow-up office visits should be arranged for reassessment and management.

If opioids are prescribed on discharge, the use of tamper-resistant or abuse-deterrent extended-release opioids, if available, is preferred (Savage, 2014). However, these medications may not be available on formularies or covered by insurers. In addition, there have not been sufficient research studies to ascertain the efficacy of these opioids in reducing misuse and abuse, even though in some states advocacy efforts are under way to require insurers to provide these medications to patients at risk (Institute for Clinical and Economic Review, 2017). It is imperative to include the community prescriber of MAT or OTP staff in discharge plans that involve opioid prescriptions.

Chronic Pain Management in Patients With Opioid Use Disorder

Chronic pain may be more prevalent among people with OUD and may predate the onset of OUD (Hser et al., 2017). Although clinicians have an ethical imperative to treat pain, evidence for the efficacy of long-term use of opioids is lacking. Because of the paucity of literature regarding the value of opioids for long-term treatment of chronic nonmalignant pain and rising opioid misuse, the Centers for Disease Control and Prevention (Dowell, Haegerich, & Chou, 2016) guidelines recommend nonopioid treatment as the first choice and an acceptable intervention for treatment of chronic pain. The use of opioids according to the guidelines should be reserved for those who cannot achieve effective pain relief with nonopioid therapy, and consideration for treatment should be coupled with a careful assessment for opioid-associated risks for misuse (Dowell et al., 2016). The tenets of MMA outlined in other sections of this book provide the basis for chronic pain management in patients with OUD.

Although nonopioid analgesics, adjuvant medications, and nonpharmacologic therapies for pain management are essential elements of an effective pain management plan, individuals with OUD may also require opioid therapy for chronic pain. It may be appropriate to consider opioid therapy in cases such as severe pain secondary to a trauma that has not resolved, in pain secondary to cancer, or in someone approaching the end of life (Walsh & Broglio, 2016). For those with OUD, consideration of the benefits for use of opioids for chronic pain must be carefully weighed with the potential for harm. If opioids are necessary, it is critical to have safeguards in place to guard against opioid misuse (Dowell et al., 2016; Oliver et al., 2012; Price, Hawkins, & Passik, 2015).

Although a risk assessment may not yield any new information among patients with known OUD, for patients with OUD who are in recovery the use of reassessment tools for safe opioid use may help the clinicians identify if the patient is relapsing into risky opioid use or misuse. Such tools include the Current Opioid Misuse Measure (COMM) and Pain Assessment Documentation Tool (PADT). The additional safeguards of urine drug screening, pill counts, and use of PDMPs may provide additional objective data in addition to a comprehensive reassessment by the clinician.

Chronic Pain Management for Patients With Opioid Use Disorder on Medication-Assisted Treatment: Special Considerations

Methadone Maintenance Therapy

For patients with chronic pain who are enrolled in MMT programs, close collaboration with the patient and OTP team is essential. When considering nonopioids to treat pain, the clinician is obligated to evaluate for drug-drug interactions with methadone that could affect the metabolism and efficacy of the medication. As mentioned previously, methadone can prolong the QTc interval, and clinicians must be aware of the potential of other medications to increase the risk (Leal & January, 2014). If pain is severe and opioids are warranted, the maintenance dose of methadone may not be sufficient to manage the pain of a comorbid disease process such as cancer. In these cases, the OTP may advise continuation of the methadone maintenance dose with the addition of more methadone in divided doses or another opioid appropriate for chronic pain (Kampman & Jarvis, 2015). In addition to coordination with the OTP, it is appropriate for the clinician to follow all precautions, including checking the PDMP, pill counts, and urine drug screening.

Buprenorphine Therapy

The clinician may find it beneficial to discuss plans for pain management with the buprenorphine prescriber. As with methadone, the clinician will need to evaluate for all drug-drug interactions between the chosen analgesic and buprenorphine that could affect either medication metabolism or efficacy. Analgesia for patients on buprenorphine therapy may be improved by increasing the daily dose (to no more than 32 mg/day) and administering it in divided daily doses (Kampman & Jarvis, 2015; Anderson et al., 2017). These changes need to be coordinated with the clinician treating the patient for OUD. If the use of nonopioids and increased buprenorphine doses are not effective for pain and there is a disease process such as cancer, patients on buprenorphine therapy may need to rotate to methadone therapy and, as mentioned earlier, receive additional daily doses of an opioid to adequately control pain (Kampman & Jarvis, 2015).

Naltrexone Therapy

For patients who have been on naltrexone therapy, the use of nonopioids in a multimodal pain management plan will be necessary to treat chronic pain. However, as described earlier, the increased hepatotoxicity risk associated with high-dose naltrexone necessitates awareness of the need for reduced doses or avoidance of other medications such as acetaminophen that can affect liver function. If it is necessary to use opioids, naltrexone must be discontinued and the clinician in collaboration with the naloxone prescriber will need to determine the safest course of OUD treatment. If the patient received a naltrexone injection, it may be necessary to wait for up to 4 weeks after the naltrexone injection for opioids to provide analgesia (see previous discussion of naltrexone).

Chronic Pain Management for Patients in Recovery Without the Use of Medication-Assisted Treatment

Patients with OUD who are in recovery without the use of MAT benefit from a multidisciplinary approach, including input from clinicians with expertise in SUD to provide support and prevent relapse. Chronic pain is most effectively treated by optimizing a multimodal approach, with the goal of avoiding the use of opioids unless absolutely necessary. Multidisciplinary treatment may include referral for physical therapy to restore function if indicated and behavioral health clinicians to address mental health comorbidities or sleep disorders (SAMHSA, 2011). Some patients with significant fear of relapse may refuse opioids, even when pain is severe. When patients endorse that position, clinician support is important in conjunction with nonopioid, coanalgesic therapies, nonpharmacologic therapies, self-care strategies, identifying support systems, and assessing for signs of relapse (SAMHSA, 2011).

Ultimately, if the clinician and patient agree a trial of opioids is appropriate, it is important to develop a plan for close assessment and intervention to minimize risks. When opioids are prescribed, a prescription for naloxone is appropriate because it can serve as an increased safety precaution if relapses occur. With relapse, the risk for overdose is increased because the period of abstinence may result in reduced tolerance to opioids and doses that were previously used.

Chronic Pain Management for Patients With Active Opioid Use Disorder Who Are Not in Recovery

Management of chronic pain among patients who live with active OUD and who are not in a recovery program requires clinicians to have a dual focus. Assessment and consistent management of pain are needed while working with the patients to encourage and hopefully engage them in treatment for the OUD. The tenets of MMA are essential while considering all comorbidities and contraindications to commonly used nonopioid analgesics. Nonopioid analgesics, adjuvant medications, and nonpharmacologic therapies for pain management are essential for effective pain management.

Prescribing opioids for chronic pain in the person with active drug use disorder is usually avoided because the risk generally outweighs any benefit. However, there may be extenuating circumstances, when multimodal pain management may include appropriate opioid therapy despite the fact that the person is not in recovery. Such situations include a serious illness or an end-of-life situation, when special arrangements are made (such as an inpatient hospice, daily visits by home health nurses, or supervised home setting) to ensure safe opioid administration. In these cases, the treatment plan must be carefully crafted to minimize patient harm. Consideration can be given to daily visits by home health nurses and using fentaNYL patches in the home or clinical setting, without dispensing a supply of oral pain medications for those patients (Savage, 2014). However, a careful assessment and education of all involved parties is necessary because it has been shown that the majority of opioids obtained outside of a legitimate prescribing relationship were obtained from family or friends (Center for Behavioral Health Statistics and Quality, 2016). Pain management among patients in this category is best accomplished by clinicians who specialize in pain management and SUD. Unfortunately, such specialists are not accessible in many areas.

Strategies to Reduce Risk

Universal Precautions

A universal precautions approach has been recommended when treating individuals with chronic opioid therapy (Gourlay & Heit, 2009). This approach encourages clinicians to treat all patients as if they may be at risk for misuse, abuse, or OUD. A universal precautions approach reduces the stigma associated with labeling an individual as at risk and ensures appropriate care of patients who may not be perceived as being at risk or having SUD (Savage, 2014). Universal precautions include the following (Gourlay & Heit, 2009):

- Use of informed consent and goals for opioid treatment
- Clear documentation of the treatment plan
- Ongoing reassessment of analgesia effects
- Use of urine drug screening

The use of opioid treatment agreements for patients receiving chronic opioid therapy may be even more salient for patients who have histories of OUD or SUD. Such agreements need to be considered as an opportunity to promote a collaborative trusting approach between the clinician and the patient (Buchman & Ho, 2014; Ho, 2017). It is important for clinicians to remember that the ethical responsibility to treat pain (beneficence) must always be balanced with the ethical responsibility to avoid or minimize harm, including relapse, risk for overdose, and societal risks resulting from diversion (nonmaleficence).

Opioid Selection

The use of opioids in patients with OUD needs careful evaluation and consideration. Mu agonist opioids can trigger the reward system through binding to GABAergic interneurons, which inhibit dopamine production (Savage,

2014). Individuals with current or previous SUD or OUD can experience activation of this reward system, which may trigger craving and thus possibly the misuse of opioids (Savage, 2014). Immediate-release oral opioids or intravenous opioids have a fast onset that can readily trigger the reward system (Savage, 2014). There has not been any robust evidence regarding the superior efficacy of extended-release opioids versus short-acting opioids to manage pain and decrease misuse. However, there is some literature to suggest that extended-release opioids may produce longer periods of stable analgesia, improved sleep, and improved physical function (Nicholson, 2013). When extended-release opioids (i.e., morphine extended release or fentaNYL transdermal) or long-acting opioids (i.e., methadone) are used as directed, and not tampered with for the purposes of injection to insufflation, they may be less likely to trigger the reward system than immediate-release opioids (Savage, 2014). Some extended-release medications have been reformulated to reduce misuse and tampering risks, but obstacles such as cost, high copays, requirements for authorization by insurance companies, and lack of availability in local pharmacies may limit use.

With the escalation of prescription opioid abuse, the U.S Food and Drug Administration has provided guidance to the pharmaceutical industry for future opioid development to ensure that opioids are more tamper-resistant and have reduced drug-liking potential (DHHS, 2015). New formulations of extended-release opioids should incorporate a physical barrier to prevent crushing or contain either antagonists or irritants if the tablet is altered and ingested (Nicholson, 2013; Stanos, 2012). The emergence of formulations that are abuse-deterrent or tamper-resistant may help in minimizing the abuse of opioids, but the results of postmarketing studies are still not available and these medications may be cost prohibitive (Institute for Clinical and Economic Review, 2017).

Designing a Safe Treatment Plan

It is strongly recommended, whenever possible, to refer patients with pain who have an active or prior SUD history, to a pain management specialist, preferably one with a multidisciplinary practice and expertise in managing pain in patients with SUD. Because of the high probability of comorbid mental illness in patients with SUD, an interdisciplinary approach is essential. The team members may include physicians, physician assistants, nurse practitioners, psychiatrists, psychologists, those with a specialty in SUD, registered nurses, social workers, and spiritual care counselors (Price et al., 2015; SAMHSA, 2011; Walsh & Broglio, 2016). For those with chronic pain without a life-limiting illness, participation in counseling or programs such as Narcotics Anonymous should be an expectation (Savage, 2014).

Health care providers have a responsibility to make efforts to minimize misuse, abuse, and diversion of opioids. When working with patients who have OUD it is important that clinicians work together to develop a cohesive, unified plan of care. This plan must be accurately documented in a way that can be easily accessed and understood by all team members (Savage, 2014). As noted, breakthrough immediate-release opioids should be used with caution in this population. It may be necessary to preemptively prescribe immediate-release opioids for patients who undergo a painful procedure or activity (e.g., physical therapy) rather than prescribing opioids based only on reported pain severity as needed (Savage, 2014). For patients at high risk for misuse or abuse, particular care should be taken to ensure that if opioids are appropriate, patient education is provided and the dose and quantity of medications are very limited and individualized (Broglio & Cole, 2014; Savage, 2014). To reduce misunderstanding of instructions, it is critical to provide specific directions regarding the times and frequency of medication dosing (e.g., 7:00 a.m., 3:00 p.m., 11:00 p.m.) versus every 8 hours (Savage, 2014).

Patient and family education are important to ensure a safe home environment by keeping medications safely secured in places such as lockboxes to prevent diversion or theft (Savage, 2014; Walsh & Broglio, 2016). It is often advantageous for one family member to be identified as the person who controls the medication and dispenses the opioid to the patient as prescribed. Education should also include instructions on safe disposal of medications or the use of Drug Enforcement Agency (DEA) take back programs (U.S. Department of Justice, Drug Enforcement Agency, Office of Diversion Control, n.d.; U.S. Food and Drug Administration, 2015).

Overdose Prevention

Individuals and families need to be educated on the safe use of opioids and measures to support the patient during an adverse event secondary to opioid use (SAMHSA, 2013). Patients who have OUD and are in MAT should be given prescriptions for naloxone in the event of accidental overdose and family or caregivers should be educated on its use (Kampman & Jarvis, 2015; DHHS, 2018).

Naloxone has become increasingly available to first responders (police, fire departments, and emergency medical responders), patients, and families when opioid overdose is a concern. In some states, efforts to reduce overdose include increased access to naloxone through the expansion of community services, pharmacist ability to provide naloxone (without individual patient prescriptions) through the use of state-approved standing orders, blanket prescriptions, and protocols (Reynolds, Causey, McKee, Reinstein, & Muzyk, 2017; Thornton, Lyvers, Scott & Dwibedi, 2017).

As of May 2017, all 50 states and the District of Columbia had some type of legislation in place to improve naloxone access (The Network for Public Health Law, 2017). Forty states and the District of Columbia also passed varied forms of Good Samaritan Laws that minimized risks to those who report overdoses (The Network for Public Health Law, 2017). In May 2018, the Surgeon General issued an advisory recommending that naloxone for opioid reversal should be prescribed or available to any patients at risk and their family and friends (DHHS, 2018). See additional discussion of naloxone and community availability in Chapter 28.

Additional Considerations

Although evidence is equivocal or lacking for the use of many complementary therapies for the treatment of chronic pain among those with comorbid SUD (SAMHSA, 2011) and additional research is needed in these areas, such interventions can be important components of MMA. Cognitive-behavioral therapy (see Chapter 22) was found to have some benefit among people with alcohol or illicit drug use disorders, but most of the benefit was seen in those who used marijuana (Magill & Ray, 2009). Exercise (see Chapter 20) has been found to be beneficial in many psychiatric conditions, and literature review showed some benefit for those with alcohol use disorder (Giesen, Deimel, & Bloch, 2015). Although there have been few and inconclusive studies using such nonpharmacologic interventions with people living with SUD, it is possible to extrapolate findings to that population because the potential benefits could far outweigh the risks. To reiterate, successful effective pain management requires a multimodal approach, including both pharmacologic and nonpharmacologic interventions. Effective pain management is individualized for patients and collaboratively developed by the clinician and patient.

As health prescribers continue to explore options for providing safe and optimal pain management while opening doors to opportunities for the treatment of OUD, it is clear that there is no one single solution to these challenges, and the involvement of the multidisciplinary team is critical in the quest for best possible outcomes. As organizations struggle to address these challenges, novel approaches will continue to be developed and these approaches may prove beneficial to patients and providers in other organizations. An example of a novel approach to working with patients with OUD who require prolonged hospitalization is presented in Box 14.2.

Key Points

- Opioid use disorder (OUD), previously known as opioid addiction, is a chronic, complex disorder characterized by periods of exacerbation and remission.
- Health care providers have an ethical imperative to treat all patients with dignity and respect and to provide safe and effective pain management for all patients, including those with substance use disorder (SUD).

| Box 14.2 | Novel Approach to a Clinical Challenge |

A consequence of intravenous substance use is the increased incidence of serious infectious diseases, including bacterial endocarditis, which require surgery and long-term intravenous antibiotics (Fleischauer, Ruhl, Rhea, & Barnes, 2017). Patients who present with these conditions pose ethical and care dilemmas for clinicians who are faced with allocating strained resources and providing extended courses of intravenous antibiotic therapy. Although clinicians want to do good (beneficience) and appropriately treat these patients, they often are concerned about the use of limited resources (justice) for a patient who may continue to use intravenous substances and who may use intravenous access needed for antibiotic therapy to use illegal substances (nonmaleficence). A team of clinicians at New Hanover Regional Medical Center in Wilmington, NC has approached these concerns from an interdisciplinary approach when the patient with a life-threatening infection needs more than 6 weeks of intravenous antibiotic therapy (Quinlan-Colwell, 2017). Operating from an underlying premise that the seriousness of the diagnosis will increase the likelihood that these patients will be motivated to actively work toward sobriety, the interdisciplinary team (physicians, pain management, social workers, substance abuse counselor, nursing case management, and ad hoc members) provides coordinated care, communicating through documentation in the electronic medical record. Preoperatively, patients are educated that their postoperative pain will be believed and treated with a multimodal approach and a plan for opioid weaning will be implemented as healing occurs. A licensed clinical social worker and substance abuse counselors work with the patients to develop plans for sobriety, including coordinating with community medication-assissted treatment and housing before discharge. Substance counselor work groups, Alcoholics Anonymous/Narcotics Anonymous meetings, and yoga and tai chi classes are offered on site during hospitalization. Problem solving, reframing, breathing, and relaxation techniques are taught to expand patient coping abilities. Al-Anon meetings are also available on the hospital campus for family members who are encouraged to attend. Clinical staff are supported in providing care with consistent messages to support recovery efforts. Discharge plans for pain management and opioid use disorder treatment are initiated during hospitalization. During this time, representatives from the local treatment centers assess, engage with, and enroll patients who are agreeable. As this work evolved, a number of hospitalists underwent buprenorphine education and pursued appropriate DEA licensure. They work with patients who are interested in using buprenorphine for MAT and initiate treatment during hospitalization. Follow-up care is coordinated with a prescriber in the community for when the patient is discharged. If necessary the hospitalists insures that the patient has a bridge prescription of buprenorphine until they are able to engage with the community prescriber. Early results have been positive and promising.

- Stereotyping, misconceptions, and stigma are barriers to compassionate, patient-centered care.
- Screening for substance use disorders is an element of the pain assessment. A number of tools may be used for screening purposes.
- Physical signs such as constricted pupils, drowsiness, slurred speech, track marks or lesions over veins, or withdrawal signs and symptoms such as excessive yawning, dilated pupils, sweating, rhinorrhea, piloerection, and gastrointestinal complaints should be addressed because they may suggest an OUD.
- The pathophysiology of OUD is highly complex and multifactorial and is thought to involve neurobiologic, genetic, psychological, social, and environmental processes.
- Opioid-tolerant individuals, including those with OUD and those on medication-assisted treatment (MAT), may have higher pain intensity levels and higher opioid requirements than those who are opioid naïve.

- Treatment of OUD may include MAT with methadone, buprenorphine, or naltrexone.
- Multimodal analgesia, including pharmacologic and nonpharmacologic approaches, and multidisciplinary team involvement are key elements in the effective treatment of pain in those with OUD.
- Psychosocial assessment and treatment is critical to the management of pain in those with OUD.
- Patients on MAT who are taking buprenorphine or naltrexone may have partial or full blockade of their opioid receptors, thus presenting particular challenges to effective pain control.
- Communication with providers during transitions of care is necessary for responsible, safe, and effective pain management.
- Health care providers have an obligation to educate patients, family members, significant others, and the community about OUD and take appropriate precautions to minimize the risks for opioid abuse and diversion.

Case Scenario

Because of fevers, weight loss, and lymphadenopathy, a 34-year-old man, John, was admitted to the hospital for a workup for possible endocarditis. He reports a 16-year history of chronic back pain for which he self-injects carfentanil (illicitly manufactured fentaNYL much more potent than licit fentaNYL) three times daily. He has been evaluated at pain centers in the past and imaging of his spine was negative for any abnormal pathologic condition. He reports inadequate analgesia with the use of buprenorphine/naloxone therapy to treat the pain and OUD. He was discharged from the pain clinic because of comorbid use of alcohol. He has a history of leaving hospitals against medical advice when providers refused to treat his pain. Workup is positive for an epidural abscess, and he will require 6 weeks of intravenous antibiotic therapy. He lives alone in a mobile trailer in a rural county where there is only a small critical access hospital. He is estranged from family and has a very limited social network.

1. What are the challenges for the health care team?
2. When assessing John's pain, how would you address his opioid use disorder?
3. What signs and symptoms may indicate that John is experiencing withdrawal?
4. What pharmacologic and nonpharmacologic interventions could be offered to address John's pain?
5. How could John's opioid use disorder be addressed during his hospitalization?
6. What safe discharge options could be offered to John?

References

Aboujaoude, E., & Salame, W. O. (2016). Naltrexone: A Pan-Addiction Treatment? *CNS Drugs, 30*, 719–733.

Alderks, C. E. (2013). Trends in the use of methadone and buprenorphine at substance abuse treatment facilities: 2003 to 2011. In *The Center for Behavioral Health Statistics and Quality Report*. Rockville (MD): Substance Abuse and Mental Health Services Administration.

American Psychiatric Association. (2013). *Diagnostic and statistical manual of mental disorders: DSM-5*. Washington, D.C: American Psychiatric Association.

American Society of Addiction Medicine. (2016). *Summary of the Comprehensive Addiction and Recovery Act. 2016*. Retrieved from http://www.asam.org/advocacy/issues/opioids/summary-of-the-comprehensive-addiction-and-recovery-act.

American Society of Addiction Medicine. (2020). *The ASAM National Practice Guideline for the Treatment of Opioid Use Disorder: 2020 Focused Update*. Retrieved July 30, 2020 from https://www.asam.org/docs/default-source/quality-science/npg-jam-supplement.pdf?sfvrsn=a00a52c2_2.

Anderson, T. A., Quaye, A. N. A., Ward, E. N., Wilens, T. E., Hilliard, P. E., & Brummett, C. M. (2017). To stop or not, that is the question: Acute pain management for the patient on chronic buprenorphine. *Anesthesiology, 126*, 1180–1186.

Barnwal, P., Das, S., Mondal, S., Ramasamy, A., Maiti, T., & Saha, A. (2017). Probuphine® [buprenorphine implant]: a promising candidate in opioid dependence. *Therapeutic Advances in Psychopharmacology, 7*, 119–134.

Barnett, V., Twycross, R., Mihalyo, M., & Wilcock, A. (2014). Opioid antagonists. *Journal of Pain and Symptom Management, 47*(2), 341–352.

Beauchamp, T. L., & Childress, J. F. (2009). *Principles of Biomedical Ethics* (6th ed., pp. 288–331). New York: Oxford University Press.

Belgrade, M. J., Schamber, C. D., & Lindgren, B. R. (2006). The DIRE score: predicting outcomes of opioid prescribing for chronic pain. *The Journal of Pain, 7*(9), 671–681.

Boscarino, J. A., Rukstalis, M., Hoffman, S. N., Han, J. J., Erlich, P. M., Gerhad, G. S., & Stewart, W. F. (2010). Risk factors for drug dependence among outpatients on opioid therapy in a large US health-care system. *Addiction, 105*, 1776–1782.

Bowman, S., Eiserman, J., Beletsky, L., Stancliff, S., & Bruce, R. D. (2013). Reducing the health consequences of opioid addiction in primary care. *The American Journal of Medicine, 126*(7), 565–571.

Broglio, K., & Cole, B. E. (2014). Prescribing opioids in primary care: Avoiding perils and pitfalls. *The Nurse Practitioner, 39*, 30–37.

Brown, M., & Bennett, P. (2010). Social, political, and ethical forces influencing nursing practice. In Marie BJSt (Ed.), *Core Curriculum for Pain Management Nursing*. 2nd. Dubuque, IA: Kendall Hunt (pp. 181–213). Publishers.

Bryson, E. O. (2014). The perioperative management of patients maintained on medications used to manage opioid addiction. *Current Opinion in Anaesthesiology, 27*, 359–364.

Buchman, D. Z., & Ho, A. (2014). What's trust got to do with it? Revisiting opioid contracts. *Journal of Medical Ethics, 40*, 673–677.

Butler, S. F., Budman, S. H., Fernandez, K. C., Houle, B., Benoit, C., Katz, N., & Jamison, R. N. (2007). Development and validation of the current opioid misuse measure. *Pain, 130*(1-2), 144–156.

Butler, S. F., Fernandez, K., Benoit, C., Budman, S. H., & Jamison, R. N. (2008). Validation of the revised Screener and Opioid Assessment for Patients with Pain (SOAPP-R). *The Journal of Pain, 9*(4), 360–372.

Calas, T., Wilkins, M., & Oliphant, C. M. (2016). Naloxone: An opportunity for another chance. *The Journal of Nurse Practitioners, 12*, 154–160.

Center for Behavioral Health Statistics and Quality. (2016). *Key substance use and mental health indicators in the United States: Results from the 2015 National Survey on Drug Use and Health*. Retrieved from https://www.samhsa.gov/data/sites/default/files/NSDUH-FFR1-2015/NSDUH-FFR1-2015/NSDUH-FFR1-2015.htm.

Centers for Disease Control and Prevention. (2016). *Synthetic opioid data. 2016*. Retrieved from https://www.cdc.gov/drugoverdose/data/fentanyl.html.

Centers for Disease Control and Prevention. (2017). *Heroin overdose data. 2017*. Retrieved from https://www.cdc.gov/drugoverdose/data/heroin.html.

Cheatle, M. D., Compton, P. A., Dhingra, L., Wasser, T. E., & O'Brien, C. P. (2019). Development of the revised opioid risk tool to predict opioid use disorder in patients with chronic nonmalignant pain. *The Journal of Pain, 20*(7), 842–851.

Chou, R., Cruciani, R. A., Fiellin, D. A., Compton, P., Farrar, J. T., Halgney, M. T., & Zeltzer, L. (2014). Methadone safety: a clinical practice guideline from the American Pain Society and College on Problems of Drug Dependence, in collaboration with the Heart Rhythm Society. *The Journal of Pain, 15*, 321–337.

Chou, R., Turner, J. A., Devine, E. B., Hansen, R. N., Sullivan, S. D., Blazina, I., ... Deyo, R. A. (2015). The Effectiveness and Risks of Long-Term Opioid Therapy for Chronic Pain: A Systematic Review for a National Institutes of Health Pathways to Prevention Workshop Effectiveness and Risks of Long-Term Opioid Therapy for Chronic Pain. *Annals of Internal Medicine, 162*(4), 276–286.

Chou, R., Gordon, D. B., de Leon-Casasola, O. A., Rosenberg, J. M., Bickler, S., Brennan, T., ... Griffith, S. (2016). Management of Postoperative Pain: a clinical practice guideline from the American pain society, the American Society of Regional Anesthesia and Pain Medicine, and the American Society of Anesthesiologists' committee on regional anesthesia, executive committee, and administrative council. *The Journal of Pain, 17*(2), 131–157.

Compton, P., Canamar, C. P., Hillhouse, M., & Ling, W. (2012). Hyperalgesia in heroin dependent patients and the effects of opioid substitution therapy. *The Journal of Pain, 13*, 401–409.

Compton, W. M., Jones, C. M., & Baldwin, G. T. (2016). Relationship between nonmedical prescription-opioid use and heroin use. *New England Journal of Medicine, 374*, 154–163.

Connery, H. S. (2015). Medication-assisted treatment of opioid use disorder: Review of the evidence and future directions. *Harvard Review of Psychiatry, 20*, 63–75.

Cooney, M. F., & Broglio, K. (2017). Acute pain management in opioid-tolerant individuals. *The Journal for Nurse Practitioners, 13*, 394–399.

Dowell, D., Haegerich, T. M., & Chou, R. (2016). CDC guideline for prescribing opioids for chronic pain–United States, 2016. *Journal of the American Medical Association, 315*, 1624–1645.

Drugs @ FDA. Vivitrol®. (2010). (naltrexone for extended-release injectable suspension) [Package Insert]. Retrieved June, 26, 2020. https://www.accessdata.fda.gov/drugsatfda_docs/label/2010/021897s015lbl.pdf.

Eisenberg, E., Suzan, E., & Pud, D. (2015). Opioid-induced hyperalgesia (OIH): a real clinical problem or just an experimental phenomenon? *Journal of Pain and Symptom Management, 4*(3), 632–635.

Electronic Code of Federal Regulations. (2018). *Title 21 Food and Drugs, Part 1306 Prescriptions, §1306.07 Administering or dispensing of narcotic drugs.* Retrieved from https://www.ecfr.gov/cgibin/retrieveECFR?gp=&SID=44ac95adaf21d78f1dd1e28e7f-ba5e83&mc=true&r=SECTION&n=se21.9.1306_107.

Evoy, K. E., Morrison, M. D., & Saklad, S. R. (2017). Abuse and misuse of pregabalin and gabapentin. *Drugs, 77*(4), 403–426.

Eyler, E. C. (2013). Chronic and acute pain and pain management for patients in methadone maintenance treatment. *The American Journal on Addictions, 22*, 75–83.

Fleischauer, A. T., Ruhl, L., Rhea, S., & Barnes, E. (2017). Hospitalizations for endocarditis and associated health care costs among persons with diagnosed drug dependence – North Carolina, 2010-2015. *Morbidity and Mortality Weekly, Report, 66*(22), 569–573.

Freynhagen, R., Backonja, M., Schug, S., Lyndon, G., Parsons, B., Watt, S., & Behar, R. (2016). Pregabalin for the treatment of drug and alcohol withdrawal symptoms: a comprehensive review. *CNS Drugs, 30*(12), 1191–1200.

Giesen, E. S., Deimel, H., & Bloch, W. (2015). Clinical exercise interventions in alcohol use disorders: a systematic review. *Journal of Substance Abuse Treatment, 52*, 1–9.

Glod, S. (2017). Perspective: The other victims of the opioid epidemic. *New England Journal of Medicine, 376*, 2101–2102.

Gorlin, A. W., Rosenfeld, D. M., & Ramakrishna, H. (2016). Intravenous sub-anesthetic ketamine for perioperative analgesia. *Journal of Anaesthesiology, Clinical Pharmacology, 32*, 160–167.

Gourlay, D. L., & Heit, H. A. (2009). Universal precautions revisited: Managing the inherited pain patient. *Pain Medicine, 10*, S115-23.

Gowing, L., Farrell, M. F., Ali, R., & White, J. M. (2014). Alpha2-adrenergic agonists for the management of opioid withdrawal. *Cochrane Database Systematic Review, 3*, CD002024.

Greene, M. S., & Chambers, R. A. (2015). Pseudoaddiction: Fact or fiction? An investigation of the medical literature. *Current Addiction Reports, 2*, 310–317.

Hämmig, R., Kemter, A., Strasser, J., von Bardeleben, U., Gugger, B., Walter, M., ... Vogel, M. (2016). Use of microdoses for induction of buprenorphine treatment with overlapping full opioid agonist use: the Bernese method. *Substance Abuse and Rehabilitation, 7*, 99.

Heit, H. A., & Lipman, A. G. (2009). Pain: Substance abuse issues in the treatment of pain. In *Biobehavioral Approaches to pain* (pp. 363–380). New York, NY: Springer.

Herndon, C. M., Arnstein, P., Darnall, B., Hartrick, K., Lyons, M., & Sehgal, N. (2016). *Principles of Analgesic Use.* Chicago, IL: American Pain Society.

Ho, A. (2017). Reconciling patient safety and epistemic humility: An ethical use of opioid treatment plans. *The Hastings Center Report, May-June*, 34–35.

Hser, Y. I., Mooney, L. J., Saxon, A. J., Miotto, K., Bell, D. S., & Huang, D. (2017). Chronic pain among patients with opioid use disorder. Results from electronic health records data. *Journal of Substance Abuse and Treatment, 77*, 26–30.

Institute for Clinical and Economic Review. (2017). *Abuse deterrent formulations of opioids: Effectiveness and value. Draft Evidence Report.* Retrieved from https://icer-review.org/wp-content/uploads/2016/08/NECEPAC_ADF_Draft_Report_05.05.17.pdf.

Kampman, K., & Jarvis, M. (2015). American Society of Addiction Medicine (ASAM) National practice guideline for the use of medications in the treatment of addiction involving opioid use. *Journal of Addiction Medicine, 9*, 358–367.

Kaye, A. D., Jones, M. R., Kaye, A. M., Ripoli, J. G., Galen, V., Beaklye, B. D., ... Manchikanti, L. (2017a). Prescription opioid abuse in chronic pain: An updated review of opioid abuse predictors and strategies to curb opioid abuse: Part 1. *Pain Physician, 20*, S93–109.

Kaye, A. D., Jones, M. R., Kaye, A. M., Ripoli, J. G., Jones, D. E., Galen, V., ... Manchikanti, L. (2017b). Prescription opioid abuse in chronic pain: An updated review of opioid abuse predictors and strategies to curb opioid abuse (Part 2). *Pain Physician, 20*, S11–133.

Kelty, E., & Hulse, G. (2017). Fatal and non-fatal opioid overdose in opioid dependent patients treated with methadone, buprenorphine or implant naltrexone. *International Journal of Drug Policy, 46,* 54–60.

Khanna, I. K., & Pillarisetti, S. (2015). Buprenorphine–an attractive opioid with underutilized potential in treatment of chronic pain. *Journal of Pain Research, 8,* 859.

Koob, G. F., & Volkow, N. D. (2016). Neurobiology of addiction: a neurocircuitry analysis. *The Lancet Psychiatry, 3*(8), 760–773.

Kowalczyk, W. J., Phillips, K. A., Jobes, M. L., Kennedy, A. P., Ghitza, U. E., Agage, D. A., ... Preston, K. L. (2015). Clonidine maintenance prolongs opioid abstinence and decouples stress from craving in daily life: a randomized controlled trial with ecological momentary assessment. *American Journal of Psychiatry, 172,* 760–767.

Kim, S. H., Stoicea, N., Soghomonyan, S., & Bergese, S. D. (2014). Remifentanil-acute opioid tolerance and opioid-induced hyperalgesia: a systematic review. *American Journal of Therapeutics, 22,* 62–74.

Kjome, K. L., & Moeller, F. G. (2011). Long-acting injectable naltrexone for the management of patients with opioid dependence. *Substance Abuse: Research and Treatment, 5,* 1–9.

Kreek, M. J., Levran, O., Reed, B., Schlussman, S. D., Zhou, Y., & Butelman, E. R. (2012). Opiate addiction and cocaine addiction: underlying molecular neurobiology and genetics. *Journal of Clinical Investigation, 122,* 3387–3393.

Leal, M. A., & January, C. T. (2014). Cardiovascular effects of methadone. In R. A. Cruciani, & H. Knotkova (Eds.), *Handbook of Methadone Prescribing and Buprenorphine Therapy (pp. 51–58).* New York, NY: Springer.

Leung, P. T. M., MacDonald, E. M., Dhalla, I. A., & Juurlink, D. N. (2017). Correspondence: A 1980's letter on the risk of opioid addiction. *New England Journal of Medicine, 376,* 2194–2195.

Ling, W. (2012). Buprenorphine implant for opioid addiction. *Pain Management, 2,* 345–350.

Ling, W., Shoptaw, S., & Goodman-Meza, D. (2019). Depot buprenorphine injection in the management of opioid use disorder: From development to implementation. *Substance Abuse and Rehabilitation, 10,* 69.

Liu, Y., Lin, D., Wu, B., & Zhou, W. (2016). Ketamine abuse potential and use disorder. *Brain Research Bulletin, 126,* 68–73.

Lohman, D., Schliefer, R., & Amon, J. J. (2010). Access to pain treatment as a human right. *BMC Medicine.* Retrieved from https://bmcmedicine.biomedcentral.com/articles/10.1186/1741-7015-8-8.

Magill, M., & Ray, L. A. (2009). Cognitive-behavioral treatment with adult alcohol and illicit drug users: a meta-analysis of randomized controlled trials. *Journal of Studies on Alcohol and Drugs, 70,* 516–527.

McCance-Katz, E. F., Sullivan, L. E., & Nallani, S. (2010). Drug interactions of clinical importance among the opioids, methadone and buprenorphine, and other frequently prescribed medications: a review. *American Journal of Addictions, 19,* 4–16.

Macintyre, P. E., Russell, R. A., Usher, K. A. N., Gaughwins, M., & Huxtable, C. A. (2013). Pain relief and opioid requirements in the first 24 hours after surgery in patients taking buprenorphine and methadone opioid substitution therapy. *Anaesthesia and Intensive Care, 41,* 222–230.

McPherson, T. L., & Hersch, R. K. (2000). Brief substance use screening instruments for primary care settings: A review. *Journal of Substance Abuse Treatment, 18*(2), 193–202.

McPherson, M. L., Costantino, R. C., & McPherson, A. L. (2018). Methadone: Maximizing Safety and Efficacy for Pain Control in Patients with Cancer. *Hematology/Oncology Clinics of North America, 32*(3), 405–415.

Mercadante, S. (2014). Intravenous use of methadone: safety and efficacy. In R. A. Cruciani, & H. Knotkova (Eds.), *Handbook of Methadone Prescribing and Buprenorphine Therapy (pp 81–89).* New York, NY: Springer.

Mistry, C. J., Bawor, M., Desai, D., Marsh, D. C., & Samaan, Z. (2014). Genetics of opioid dependence: A review of the genetic contribution of opioid dependence. *Current Psychiatry Reviews, 10,* 156–167.

Nestler, E. J. (2015). Role of the brain's reward circuitry in depression: transcriptional mechanisms. *International Review of Neurobiology. 124* (pp. 151–170). Academic Press.

Nicholson, B. (2013). Primary care considerations of the pharmacokinetics and clinical use of extended-release opioids in treating patients with chronic noncancer pain. *Postgraduate Medicine, 125,* 115–127.

Oliver, J., Coggins, C., Compton, P., Hagen, S., Matteliano, D., Stanton, M., ... Turner, H. N. (2012). American Society for Pain Management Nursing position statement: Pain management in patients with substance use disorders. *Pain Management Nursing, 13,* 169–183.

Pasero, C., Quill, T., Portenoy, R. K., McCaffery, M., & Rizos, A. (2011). Guidelines for opioid drug selection. In C. Pasero & M. McCaffery (Eds.), *Pain Assessment and Pharmacologic Management* (pp. 323–367). St Louis, MO: Mosby.

Pasero, C., Quinlan-Colwell, A., Rae, D., Broglio, K., & Drew, D. (2016). American Society for Pain Management Nursing position statement: Prescribing and administering opioid doses based solely on pain intensity. *Pain Management Nursing, 17*(3), 170–180.

Passik, S. D., Kirsh, K. L., & Webster, L. (2011). Pseudoaddiction revisited: A commentary on clinical and historical considerations. *Pain Management, 1,* 239–248.

Passik, S. D., Kirsh, K. L., Whitcomb, L., Portenoy, R. K., Katz, N. P., Kleinman, L., ... Schein, J. R. (2004). A new tool to assess and document pain outcomes in chronic pain patients receiving opioid therapy. *Clinical Therapeutics, 26*(4), 552–561.

Phillips, K. A., & Preston, K. L. (2014). Buprenorphine in maintenance therapy. In R. A. Cruciani, & H. Knotkova (Eds.), *Handbook of Methadone Prescribing and Buprenorphine Therapy (pp. 139–162).* New York, NY: Springer.

Portenoy, R. K. (1996). Opioid therapy for chronic nonmalignant pain: a review of the critical issues. *Journal of Pain and Symptom Management, 11,* 203–217.

Portenoy, R. K., & Foley, K. M. (1986). Chronic use of opioid analgesics in non-malignant pain: report of 38 cases. *Pain, 25,* 171–186.

Porter, J., & Jick, H. (1980). Addiction rare in patients treated with narcotics. *New England Journal of Medicine, 302,* 123.

Price, J. R., Hawkins, A. D., & Passik, S. D. (2015). Opioid therapy: Managing risks of abuse, addiction, and diversion. In N. I. Cherny, M. Fallon, S. Kaasa, R. K. Portenoy, & D. C. Currow (Eds.), *Oxford Textbook of Palliative Medicine. Fifth Edition ed. (pp. 560–566).* Oxford, UK: Oxford University Press.

Quinlan-Colwell, A. (2012). *Pain Management for Older Adults: A Clinical Guide for Nurses.* NY: Springer Publishing Company.

Quinlan-Colwell, A. (2017). An innovative approach to address serious consequences of opioid substance use disorder. *Southern Pain Society Newsletter, Winter 2017*, (3-4).

Quinlan-Colwell, A., & O'Conner-Von, S. (2014). Shifting the paradigm. Southern Pain Society Newsletter. *Summer 2014*, (2-3).

Reynolds, V., Causey, H., McKee, J., Reinstein, V., & Muzyk, A. (2017). The role of pharmacists in the opioid epidemic: an examination of pharmacist-focused initiatives across the United States and North Carolina. *North Carolina Medical Journal, 78*(3), 202–205.

Salehi, M., Kheirabadi, G. R., Maracy, M. R., & Ranjkesh, M. (2011). Importance of gabapentin dose in treatment of opioid withdrawal. *Journal of Clinical Psychopharmacology, 31*(5), 593–596.

Salsitz, E., & Wiegand, T. (2016). Pharmacotherapy of opioid addiction: "Putting a real face on a false demon". *Journal of Medical Toxicology, 12*, 58–63.

Savage, S. R. (2014). Opioid therapy for pain. In R. K. Ries, D. A. Fiellin, S. C. Miller, & R. Saitz (Eds.), *The ASAM principles of addiction medicine* (5th ed., pp. 1500–1529). Philadelphia, PA: Wolters Kluwer.

Savage, S. R., Kirsh, K. L., & Passik, S. D. (2008). Challenges in using opioids to treat pain in persons with substance use disorders. *Addiction Science & Clinical Practice, 4*, 4–25.

Schnabel, A., Meyer-Friessem, C. H., Reichl, S. U., Zahn, P. K., & Pogatzki-Zahn, E. M. (2013). Is intraoperative dexmedetomidine a new option for postoperative pain treatment? A meta-analysis of randomized controlled trials. *Pain, 154*, 1140–1149.

Schuckit, M. A. (2016). Treatment of opioid-use disorders. *New England Journal of Medicine, 375*, 357–368.

Sen, S., Arulkumar, S., Cornett, E. M., Gayle, J. A., Flower, R. R., Fox, C. J., & Kaye, A. D. (2016). New pain management options for the surgical patient on methadone and buprenorphine. *Current Pain Headache Report, 20*, 16.

Sharma, B., Bruner, A., Barnett, G., & Fishman, M. (2016). Opioid use disorders. *Child and Adolescent Psychiatric Clinics of North America, 25*, 473–487.

Silverman, S. (2015). Buprenorphine for pain and opioid dependence. In A. Kaye, N. Vadivelu, & R. D. Urman (Eds.), *Substance Abuse: Inpatient and Outpatient Management for Every Clinician* (pp. 311–318). New York, NY: Springer.

St. Marie, B. (2014). Health care experiences when pain and substance use disorder coexist: "Just because I'm an addict doesn't mean I don't have pain". *Pain Medicine, 15*, 2075–2086.

Stanos, S. (2012). Continuing evolution of opioid use in primary care practice: Implications of emerging technologies. *Current Medical Research and Opinion, 28*, 1505–1516.

Stein, M. D., Kenney, S. R., Anderson, B. J., Conti, M. T., & Bailey, G. L. (2020). Prescribed and non-prescribed gabapentin use among persons seeking inpatient opioid detoxification. *Journal of Substance Abuse Treatment, 110*, 37–41.

Stromer, W., Michaeli, K., & Sandner-Kiesling, A. (2013). Perioperative pain therapy in opioid abuse. *European Journal of Anaesthesiology, 30*, 55–64.

Substance Abuse and Mental Health Services Administration. (2011). Managing chronic pain in adults with or in recovery from substance use disorders. In *Treatment improvement protocol (TIP) Series 54. HHS Publication No. (SMA)* 12-4671. Rockville, MD: Substance Abuse and Mental Health Services Administration. Retrieved from http://store.samhsa.gov/shin/content/SMA12-4671/TIP54.pdf.

Substance Abuse and Mental Health Services Administration. (2012). *SAMHSA Advisory: an introduction to extended-release injectable naltrexone for the treatment of people with opioid dependence*. Retrieved from http://store.samhsa.gov/shin/content//SMA12-4682/SMA12-4682.pdf.

Substance Abuse and Mental Health Services Administration. (2013). *SAMHSA opioid overdose prevention toolkit. Vol HHS Publication No. (SMA) 13-4742*. Rockville, MD: Substance Abuse and Mental Health Services Administration.

Sudakin, D. (2016, March). Naltrexone: not just for opioids anymore. In *Journal of Medical Toxicology* (Vol. 12, No. 1, pp. 71-75). Springer US.

Taveros, M. C., & Chaung, E. J. (2017). Pain management strategies for patients on methadone maintenance therapy: a systematic review of the literature. *BMJ Supportive and Palliative Care, 7*, 383–389.

Tetrault, J. M., & O'Connor, P. G. (2014). Management of opioid intoxication and withdrawal. In R. K. Ries, D. A. Fiellin, S. C. Miller, & R. Saitz (Eds.), *The ASAM Principles of Addiction Medicine, Fifth Edition (pp. 668-684)*. Philadelphia, PA: Wolters Kluwer.

The Network for Public Health Law. (2017). *Legal interventions to reduce overdose mortality: Naloxone access and overdose Good Samaritan Laws*. Retrieved from https://www.networkforphl.org/_asset/qz5pvn/naloxone-_FINAL.pdf.

Thornton, J. D., Lyvers, E., Scott, V. G. G., & Dwibedi, N. (2017). Pharmacists' readiness to provide naloxone in community pharmacies in West Virginia. *Journal of the American Pharmacists Association, 57*(2), S12–S18.

Turton, S., & Lingford-Hughes, A. (2016). Neurobiology and principles of addiction and tolerance. *Medicine, 44*(12), 693–696.

United Nations. (1972). *Single Convention on Narcotic Drugs, 1961 As amended by the 1972 protocol amending the Single Convention on Narcotic Drugs, 1961*. New York, NY: United Nations.

U.S. Food and Drug Administration. (2015a). *FDA blueprint for prescriber education for extended-release and long-acting opioid analgesics*. Retrieved from http://www.fda.gov/downloads/drugs/drugsafety/postmarketdrugsafetyinformationforpati//entsandproviders/ucm311290.pdf.

U.S. Food and Drug Administration. (2015b). *Medication disposal: Questions and answers*. Retrieved from http://www.fda.gov/Drugs/ResourcesForYou/Consumers/BuyingUsingMedicineSafely/EnsuringSafeUseofMedicine/SafeDisposalofMedicines/ucm186188.htm.

U. S. Department of Health and Human Services, Food and Drug Administration, Center for Drug Evaluation and Research. (2015). *Abuse-deterrent opioids—evaluation and labeling guidance for industry*. Retrieved from http://www.fda.gov/Drugs/GuidanceComplianceRegulatoryInformation/Guidances/default.htm.

U.S. Department of Health and Human Services, Substance Abuse and Mental Health Services Administration. (2013). *Report to Congress on the nation's substance abuse and mental health workforce issues*. Retrieved from https://store.samhsa.gov/shin/content/PEP13-RTC-BHWORK/PEP13-RTC-BHWORK.pdf.

U.S. Department of Health and Human Services, Surgeon General. (2018). *Surgeon General's advisory on naloxone and overdose.* Retrieved from https://www.surgeongeneral.gov/priorities/opioid-overdose-prevention/naloxone-advisory.html.

U.S. Department of Justice, Drug Enforcement Administration. (n.d.a). DEA requirements for DATA waived physicians (DWPs). Retrieved from https://www.deadiversion.usdoj.gov/pubs/docs/dwp_buprenorphine.htm.

U.S. Department of Justice, Drug Enforcement Administration, Office of Diversion Control. (n.d.b). National take-back initiative. Retrieved from http://www.deadiversion.usdoj.gov/drug_disposal/takeback/index.html.

Vadivelu, N., Kai, A. M., Kodumudi, V., Zhu, R., & Hines, R. (2017). Pain management of patients with substance abuse in the ambulatory setting. *Current Pain and Headache Reports*, 21. doi:https://doi.org/10.1007/sl1916-017-0610-3.

Volkow, N. D., & Collins, F. S. (2017). The role of science in addressing the opioid crisis. *New England Journal of Medicine*, 377(4), 391–394.

Volkow, N. D., & McLellan, A. T. (2016). Opioid abuse in chronic pain—misconceptions and mitigation strategies. *New England Journal of Medicine*, 374(13), 1253–1263.

Volkow, N. D., & Warren, K. R. (2014). Drug addiction: the neurobiology of behavior gone awry. In R. K. Ries, D. A. Fiellin, S. C. Miller, & R. Saitz (Eds.), *The ASAM Principles of Addiction Medicine* (5th Ed.). Philadelphia, PA.: Wolters Kluwer.

Wachholtz, A., & Gonzalez, G. (2015). Pain sensitivity and tolerance among individuals on opioid maintenance: Long-term effects. *Drug and Alcohol Dependence*, 146, e14.

Wachholtz, A., Foster, S., & Cheatle, M. (2015). Psychophysiology of pain and opioid use: implications for managing pain in patients with an opioid use disorder. *Drug and Alcohol Dependence*, 146, 1–6.

Walsh, A. F., & Broglio, K. (2016). Pain management in the individual with serious illness and comorbid substance use disorder. In J. Pace, & D. Wholihan, (Eds.), *Nursing Clinics of North America: Palliative Care. 51* (pp. 433–447).

Weissman, D. E., & Haddox, J. D. (1989). Opioid pseudoaddiction–an iatrogenic syndrome. *Pain*, 36, 363–366.

Wenzel, J. T., Schwenk, E. S., Baratta, J. L., & Viscusi, E. R. (2016). Managing Opioid-Tolerant Patients in the Perioperative Surgical Home. *Anesthesiology Clinics*, 34, 287–301.

Wesson, D. R., & Ling, W. (2003). The Clinical Opiate Withdrawal Scale (COWS). *Journal of Psychoactive Drugs*, 35, 253–259.

Wilford, B. B. (2014). Appendix 1: ASAM Addiction Terminology. In R. K. Ries, D. A. Fiellin, S. C. Miller, & R. Saitz (Eds.), *The ASAM Principles of Addiction Medicine* (5th ed.). Philadelphia, PA: Wolters Kluwer.

Wu, S. M., Compton, P., Bolus, R., Schieffer, B., Pham, Q., Baria, A., ... Naliboff, B. D. (2006). The addiction behaviors checklist: validation of a new clinician-based measure of inappropriate opioid use in chronic pain. *Journal of Pain and Symptom Management*, 32(4), 342–351.

Chapter 15 Coanalgesic Medications

Courtney Kominek, Maureen F. Cooney

CHAPTER OUTLINE

Medication Selection, pg. 386

Gabapentinoids, pg. 389

    Mechanism of Action, pg. 389

    Indications and Uses, pg. 389

    Pharmacokinetics, pg. 392

    Dosing and Routes, pg. 393

    Adverse Effects, pg. 393

    Monitoring of Patients, pg. 394

Antidepressants, pg. 394

    Tricyclic Antidepressants, pg. 394

    Serotonin Norepinephrine Reuptake Inhibitors, pg. 396

Alpha-Adrenergic Receptor Agonists, pg. 398

    Mechanism of Action, pg. 398

    Indications and Uses, pg. 398

    Pharmacokinetics, pg. 399

    Dosing and Routes, pg. 399

    Adverse Effects, pg. 400

    Monitoring of Patients, pg. 401

Corticosteroids, pg. 401

    Mechanism of Action, pg. 401

    Indications and Uses, pg. 401

    Dosing and Routes, pg. 402

    Adverse Effects, pg. 402

    Monitoring of Patients, pg. 403

N-Methyl-D-Aspartate Receptor Antagonists, pg. 403

    Dextromethorphan, pg. 403

    Ketamine, pg. 404

    Magnesium, pg. 408

Sodium Channel Blockers: Lidocaine and Mexiletine, pg. 409

    Lidocaine, pg. 409

    Mexiletine, pg. 411

Muscle Relaxants, pg. 412

    Baclofen for Spasticity From Upper Motor Neuron Syndromes, pg. 412

    Skeletal Muscle Relaxants for Muscular Pain and Spasms From Musculoskeletal Conditions, pg. 415

Dronabinol, Nabilone, and Cannabidiol, pg. 416

    Mechanism of Action, pg. 417

    Indications and Uses, pg. 417

    Dosing and Routes, pg. 417

    Adverse Effects, pg. 418

    Monitoring of Patients, pg. 418

Other Coanalgesic Medications, pg. 418

Key Points, pg. 418

Case Scenario, pg. 419

References, pg. 419

COANALGESIC medications, also known as adjuvant analgesics, are defined by the American Pain Society (APS) as a diverse group of medications that may increase analgesia provided by other medications, may independently provide analgesia in certain pain states, or may be used to treat analgesic-related adverse effects (Herndon et al., 2016). For patients with chronic, noncancer pain, nonopioid analgesics (nonsteroidal antiinflammatory drugs [NSAIDs] and acetaminophen) and coanalgesic medications are often considered first-line therapies. In moderate to severe acute and active cancer pain, coanalgesics are often recommended in addition to an opioid regimen.

The APS, the American Society of Regional Anesthesia and Pain Medicine (ASRA), and the American Society of Anesthesiologists (ASA) collaborated to develop guidelines for the management of acute postoperative pain (Chou et al., 2016). The guidelines include recommendations for the use of a number of coanalgesic medications, which are addressed in this chapter. Expanding use of guidelines published by the Enhanced Recovery After Surgery (ERAS) Society with an emphasis on opioid reduction or elimination has led to use of a number of coanalgesics throughout the perioperative period (Beverly, Kaye, Ljungqvist, & Urman, 2017). Similarly, in a guideline addressing the use of opioids for chronic pain, the Centers for Disease Control and Prevention supported the use of multimodal approaches, including nonopioid analgesics and coanalgesics in the treatment of chronic pain (Dowell, Haegerich, & Chou, 2016). The role of coanalgesics in pain management plans of care is summarized in Box 15.1.

Multimodal pain management plans to treat acute and chronic pain that include the use of appropriately selected coanalgesics offer the potential to provide effective and safe pain treatment while reducing opioid reliance. However, despite increasing recognition of the need for use of coanalgesics, some misconceptions about coanalgesic use exist (Table 15.1) and education of clinicians and patients is necessary to address these misconceptions. This chapter will describe factors involved in coanalgesic selection and review various coanalgesic medications, including their indications, mechanisms of action, dosing, adverse effects, and monitoring.

Box 15.1 | Role of Coanalgesic Medications

Coanalgesic medications may be used in addition to other analgesics or alone as distinct primary therapy for certain painful conditions. Most experience with coanalgesic medications has been in the treatment of persistent (chronic) pain, but use of coanalgesic medications is now expanding to include treatment of acute pain.

TWO CLASSES

1. Multipurpose coanalgesic medications useful for persistent pain and symptom management, and in some cases acute pain. Examples of drug classes are as follows:
   a. Antidepressants
   b. Corticosteroids
   c. Alpha-$_2$ adrenergic agonists
   d. Cannabinoids
   e. Topical analgesics
2. Coanalgesic medications may be used for specific types of pain. Examples of pain conditions and recommended classes/medications are as follows:
   a. Persistent neuropathic pain (e.g., anticonvulsants, antidepressants, sodium channel blockers, cannabinoids, topical analgesics)
   b. Persistent bone pain such as bony metastasis or osteoporosis (e.g., bisphosphonates, calcitonin, radiopharmaceuticals)
   c. Malignant bowel obstruction (e.g., anticholinergics, corticosteroids, octreotide)
   d. Musculoskeletal pain (e.g., muscle relaxants, benzodiazepines)
   e. Procedural pain (e.g., propofol, dexmedetomidine, ketamine, local anesthetic)
   f. Goal-directed sedation in the critically ill (propofol, fospropofol, local anesthetic)
   g. Postoperative pain, other types of acute inflammatory pain, prevention of persistent neuropathic postsurgical pain (e.g., anticonvulsants, cloNIDine, ketamine, sodium channel blockers)

From Pasero, C., & McCaffery, M. (2011). *Pain assessment and pharmacologic management* (p. 627). St. Louis, Mosby. © 2011, Pasero, C., & McCaffery, M. May be duplicated for use in clinical practice.

Table 15.1 | Misconceptions About Coanalgesic Medications

Misconception	Correction
Coanalgesics are effective only for neuropathic pain.	Some coanalgesics, such as antidepressants, corticosteroids, alpha-$_2$ adrenergic agonists (e.g., cloNIDine), and cannabinoids are multipurpose analgesics that may be useful for both neuropathic and nociceptive (somatic and visceral) pain.
Coanalgesics are appropriate only for persistent (chronic), not acute, pain.	There is growing evidence to support the role of coanalgesics (e.g., anticonvulsants, sodium channel blockers, ketamine) in the treatment of both acute and persistent pain.
Pain relief from antidepressants depends on their ability to relieve depression in the patient with pain.	The analgesic effects of antidepressants are independent of their antidepressant activity. Patients who are depressed and those who are not depressed with pain report analgesia. Furthermore, the analgesic dose is often lower than that required to treat depression, and the onset of analgesia typically occurs much sooner, usually within 1 week.

Continued

Table 15.1 | Misconceptions About Coanalgesic Medications—cont'd

Misconception	Correction
Antidepressants are more appropriate analgesics for burning neuropathic pain than for stabbing and lancinating (knifelike) neuropathic pain.	Research shows that antidepressants may be effective for both lancinating (knifelike) and continuous neuropathic pain.
Anticonvulsants are only used for persistent neuropathic pain.	Anticonvulsants now have a role in the treatment of acute pain, such as postoperative pain and prevention of persistent neuropathic postsurgical pain, as well as persistent mixed pain syndromes, such as fibromyalgia.
Topical analgesics relieve only superficial pain.	Topical analgesics, such as lidocaine patch 5% and capsaicin, have been shown to be effective in relieving a variety of types of pain including some types of neuropathic pain.
Drugs marketed as muscle relaxants, such as methocarbamol, relieve muscle pain by relaxing the muscle.	Well-controlled research is lacking to demonstrate that muscle relaxants relax skeletal muscle in humans. Muscle relaxants are a heterogenous group of medications with varying mechanisms of action, many of which are unknown or due to sedation.

Modified from Pasero, C., & McCaffery, M. (2011). *Pain assessment and pharmacologic management* (p. 627–628). St. Louis, Mosby. © 2011, Pasero, C., & McCaffery, M. May be duplicated for use in clinical practice.

Medication Selection

Coanalgesic medications are the largest group of analgesic medications and include medications with a variety of mechanisms of action and indications. Strength of evidence to support the use of coanalgesics varies depending on the clinical situation, medication class, individual medications within a class, dosing of the medication, and coadministered medications. Table 15.2 summarizes some of the coanalgesic medications used in the management of pain.

The decision to use coanalgesic medication requires careful patient selection based on a systematic patient assessment with consideration of the source and characteristics of pain and patient comorbidities, organ function, and medication use. Particularly when used to manage chronic pain, it is important to assess the patient's medication use history and response to various medications. There is variability among individuals in response to coanalgesics, including medications in the same class. Characteristics such as age, organ function, and genetic variability in drug metabolism, among other factors, may affect medication efficacy and adverse effects.

Medication selection requires awareness of evidence for use of specific coanalgesics, efficacy, dosing and scheduling, potential drug-drug interactions, pill burden, availability, and cost. It is necessary to consider patient preferences and ability to comply with a medication regimen and any necessary follow-up when selecting coanalgesic medications. Follow-up is needed to assess for improvements or other changes in pain, medication adherence, adverse effects, and impact on function and quality of life. Modifications in coanalgesic use may be needed based on subsequent assessments.

In a systematic review of medication adherence in chronic pain, compliance with the use of pain medications was found to be less with chronic pain regimens than with medication regimens for other chronic conditions (Timmerman, Stronks, Groeneweg, & Huygen, 2016). Many individual patient-related factors were found to contribute to noncompliance, but medication-related factors were also significant. The review showed patient knowledge of the prescribed medication and medication dosing regimen was associated with increased compliance. Factors such as lack of efficacy, the need for multiple daily doses, and the use of multiple medications were related to nonadherence. Interventions recommended to improve compliance were simplification of the analgesic plan, patient education, reminders, and regular follow-up visits (Timmerman et al., 2016).

Some coanalgesics must be started at low doses and slowly increased to a therapeutic effect, whereas others may not exert an immediate beneficial effect but must be taken for a period of time until a therapeutic effect is achieved. Patients need to be educated about these characteristics to optimize compliance with these medication administration recommendations. The coanalgesic medications often considered useful in clinical practice include the gabapentinoids, ketamine, antidepressants, corticosteroids, and alpha-$_2$ agonists. Other medications, such as sodium channel blocker antiarrhythmics, and cannabinoids have evidence to suggest broad application as

Table 15.2 | Coanalgesic Medications: Summary of Clinical Benefits

Drug	Summary of clinical benefits
Ketamine	• Useful adjuvant in painful procedures: Upper abdominal, thoracic, and major orthopedic surgeries (Level I) • Useful adjuvant to PCA (Level I) • Patients with chronic pain issues and on high-dose opioids: Decreases pain intensity and opioid consumption lasting much beyond the perioperative period (Level II) • Opioid-resistant pain: Rescue analgesia (mixed evidence; Level II) • Has preventive but not preemptive analgesic effect (Level I). Studies looking at the role of ketamine in preventing CPSP have shown only mixed effects (Level II)
Pregabalin	• Risk versus benefits probably more acceptable for painful procedures resulting in acute neuropathic pain, requiring large doses of opioids (e.g., cardiothoracic surgery, arthroplasty, or spine surgery) for the reduction in opioid-related side effects to outweigh the side effects. The evidence for this is limited and needs further research. Risks for minor, laparoscopic, or daycare procedures probably outweigh the benefits • Useful preventive analgesic effect
Gabapentin	• Benefits similar to those of pregabalin, but being an older drug has more literature evidence • Improved analgesia at rest and movement (Level I) • Improved functional recovery with better range of movements and pulmonary function (Level II) • Analgesic effect comparable and synergetic with NSAIDS and superior to traMADol • Useful adjuvant to epidural analgesia: Decreased pain scores, epidural analgesic consumption, and patient satisfaction despite an increase in dizziness • In established acute postoperative pain, single-dose gabapentin is superior to placebo but worse than other commonly used analgesic. The NNT was 11 (Cochrane review) • Useful preventive analgesic effect • A small RCT (60 patients undergoing abdominal hysterectomy) showed gabapentin was superior to ketamine in preventing CPSP
Intravenous lidocaine	• Useful in visceral pain and improves postoperative bowel function after abdominal surgery: Reduces pain and opioid requirements, nausea, vomiting, duration of ileus, resulting in decreased time to pass flatus, feces, and earlier intake of enteral food, rehabilitation, and discharge (Level I) • Benefit seen even in patients undergoing laparoscopic colectomy as part of acute rehabilitation program • No proven use in nonabdominal surgeries • Probably has a preventive effect after major abdominal and breast surgery (Level II)
Systemic α_2 agonist	• Moderate analgesic benefit: Probably better than paracetamol but less than that of ketamine and NSAIDS as inferred from nonsystematic indirect comparison • All of these beneficial effects may come at a price of significant hypotension and bradycardia • Useful adjuvant in perioperative care in adults and children because of several useful extra-analgesic benefits, such as sedation, anxiolysis, analgesia, postoperative shivering, PONV, agitation, mitigation of stress response to surgery and tracheal intubation, anesthetic-sparing effect, and as supplement to neuraxial and peripheral nerve blocks • Decreased perioperative mortality and myocardial infarction, especially in high-risk vascular surgeries • No evidence for preventive analgesia

National Health and Medical Research Council: Levels of Evidence

Level I Obtained from a systematic review of all relevant randomized controlled trials

Level II Obtained from at least one properly designed randomized controlled trial

Level III-I Obtained from well-designed pseudo-randomized controlled trials (alternate allocation or some other method)

Lebel III-2 Obtained from comparative studies with concurrent controls and allocation not randomized (cohort studies), case-control studies, or interrupted time series with a control group

Level III-3 Obtained from comparative studies with historical control, two or more single-arm studies, or interrupted time series without a parallel control group

Level IV Obtained from case series, either post-test or pre-test and post-test

CPSP, Chronic postsurgical pain; *NNT,* number needed to treat; *NSAIDs,* nonsteroidal antiinflammatory drugs; *PCA,* patient-controlled analgesia; *PONV,* postoperative nausea and vomiting; *RCT,* randomized controlled trial.

From Ramaswamy, S., Wilson, J. A., & Colvin, L. (2013). Non-opioid-based adjuvant analgesia in perioperative care. *Continuing Education in Anaesthesia, Critical Care & Pain, 13*(5), 152–157.

analgesic agents. Although local anesthetics are important coanalgesic medications, they are more extensively described in Chapters 16 and 18.

Techniques for introduction of coanalgesics vary. For example, in many ERAS protocols, a coanalgesic is selected from one or more classes and initiated, along with nonopioid analgesics (acetaminophen and NSAID), in the preoperative period and continued into the postoperative period. Although there are a number of classes of medications used as coanalgesics, it is important for clinicians to use medications for which there is evidence to support their use. Initial coanalgesics should be selected based on evidence that demonstrates the greatest effectiveness for a particular condition, balanced by an assessment of the benefits and risks of the medication. When additional medications from different classes are added to the initial plan, it is necessary to consider risks for additive or new adverse effects and drug-drug interactions.

Coanalgesic medications for chronic pain, if not initiated when pain was acute, are often introduced over a period when pain is refractory to initial interventions. Several evidence-based guidelines for the treatment of chronic pain, especially neuropathic pain, have been published. Medications from the antidepressant and anticonvulsant classes are recommended as first-line therapy for chronic neuropathic pain (Cruccu & Truini, 2017; Finnerup et al., 2015). As with use of coanalgesics in the treatment of acute pain, it is important to select medications that have been shown to be effective, while balancing the benefits and risks of the medications. For example, among the antidepressants, tricyclic antidepressants (TCAs) have the strongest evidence for effectiveness, but because serotonin norepinephrine reuptake inhibitors (SNRIs) have superior side effect profiles, an SNRI may be selected as the preferred medication (Cruccu & Truini, 2017). Table 15.3 provides a sample of a multimodal approach to the management of a chronic neuropathic pain condition.

Table 15.3 | Guideline for Treatment of Chronic Neuropathic Pain

Central Pain Treatment Algorithm

Step 1. Identify Problems
- Determine existing problems and potential adverse sequelae.
- Identify biologic and psychological contributors to pain and their influence on the individual's pain experience.
- Determine the impact of pain on the patient's function.
- Determine how well the patient has adjusted to the disorder causing their central pain (SCI, stroke, MS).
- Determine the risk for and/or presence of additional consequences of pain and the disorder underlying the central pain (i.e., pressure sores, contractures, adverse drug effects).

Step 2. Determine Reasonable Objectives/Goals for Patient and Treating Physician
- Pain relief/reduction.
- Treatment of spasm: Decrease frequency and/or severity.
- Increase exercise tolerance and improve function.
- Achieve independent living.
- Return to work.

Step 3. Create Multidisciplinary Approach

Pharmacologic	Interventional	Physical and Occupational Therapy	Psychosocial
First line	Specific to condition	Structured therapy and home exercises	Psychiatric therapy
AEDs (gabapentin and pregabalin)	Limited evidence	Postural reeducation	Pharmacologic
	Mainly for refractory cases	Spasticity treatment	Counseling
Second line	Neuromodulation	Bowel and bladder management	CBT
TCAs	SCS	Braces and devices to assist in home and work function	Pain coping skills
SNRIs	DBS	Home or work remodeling	Relaxation
Combinations with AED	MCS	Speech therapy	Family support and education
Third line	Intrathecal therapy		
Opioids	Baclofen		
SSRI	Morphine		
Fourth line	CloNIDine		
Ketamine infusion	Ziconotide		
Lidocaine infusion	Acupuncture		
	Ablative therapies (DREZ, cordotomy)		

NOTE: The treatment of central pain requires a careful assessment of the pain and problems associated with the patient's underlying disorder. Understanding goals and setting expectations are essential to creating an appropriate multidisciplinary treatment plan.

AEDs, Antiepileptic drugs; *CBT,* cognitive-behavioral therapy; *DBS,* deep brain stimulation; *DREZ,* dorsal reentry zone lesioning; *MCS,* motor cortex stimulation; *MS,* multiple sclerosis; *SCI,* spinal cord injury; *SCS,* spinal cord stimulation; *SNRIs,* serotonin-norepinephrine reuptake inhibitors; *SSRIs,* selective serotonin reuptake inhibitors; *TCAs,* tricyclic antidepressants.

From Cohen, S. P., & Raja, S. N. (2016). Pain. In L. Goldman, & A. Schaefer. *Goldman-Cecil medicine* (25th ed.). Philadelphia: Saunders.

Gabapentinoids

Medications in the gabapentinoid class include gabapentin and pregabalin. These medications have been used for their analgesic effect in the treatment of neuropathic pain and are increasingly used in perioperative management of acute postoperative pain (Chincholkar, 2018). A side-by-side comparison of gabapentin and pregabalin is provided in Table 15.4.

Mechanism of Action

Despite their names, gabapentin and pregabalin do not alter γ-aminobutyric acid (GABA) binding, uptake, or degradation but produce GABA-mimetic (GABA-like) effects (Pfizer, 2017a). Gabapentin and pregabalin exert their effects primarily by binding to the α2δ subunit of the voltage-gated calcium channel. Much of this effect occurs in the dorsal route ganglia and results in inhibition of calcium currents (Chincholkar, 2018). This leads to a reduction in the release of excitatory neurotransmitters including glutamate, norepinephrine, and substance P (Dworkin et al., 2007). These excitatory neurotransmitters are discussed in detail in Chapter 3. The gabapentinoids also have supraspinal effects, may activate descending noradrenergic systems, and facilitate release of norepinephrine in the spinal cord and interact with serotonin pathways (Chincholkar, 2018).

Indications and Uses

Several different formulations of gabapentin and pregabalin are available. All include the pain indication for the treatment of postherpetic neuralgia (PHN) (Arbor Pharmaceuticals, 2020; Almatica Pharma, 2020; Pfizer, 2016, 2017a). Gabapentin enacarbil, a prodrug, is approved for the treatment of restless legs syndrome (Arbor Pharmaceuticals, 2020). Other U.S. Food and Drug Administration (FDA)-labeled indications for pregabalin include diabetic peripheral neuropathy (DPN), fibromyalgia, and neuropathic pain associated with spinal cord injury (SCI) (Pfizer, 2016). Pregabalin controlled release (CR) is indicated for PHN and DPN (Pfizer, 2017b). Table 15.5 provides a summary of the indications and dosing for use of the gabapentinoids. There are concerns about potential gabapentinoid abuse that necessitate that clinicians appraise available evidence for a given indication and exercise caution when using the gabapentinoids for conditions for which evidence is lacking (Peckham, Evoy, Ochs, & Covvey, 2018).

Many randomized controlled trials (RCTs) of gabapentin and pregabalin have examined the use of these medications for the treatment of pain in different patient populations and clinical situations. Systematic reviews and meta-analysis of studies involving gabapentin and pregabalin have examined the results of these RCTs, and several are summarized in the following section. Despite the large number of published studies, questions remain about the efficacy of these agents in certain clinical situations, and

Table 15.4 | Comparison of Gabapentin and Pregabalin

	Gabapentin	Pregabalin
Mechanism of action	Binds to α_2-δ subunit of N-type calcium channels in the CNS	Binds to α_2-δ subunit of N-type calcium channels in the CNS
Oral bioavailability	Saturable and dose-dependent ∼60% with a 300-mg dose ∼40% with a 600-mg dose	>90%; independent of dose
Metabolism	None	None
Elimination	Renal	Renal
Dosing range for chronic neuropathic pain	900–3600 mg/day (titration usually required) Target dose is 1800 mg/day Lower initial doses with gradual upward rotation Requires renal dose adjustments	150–600 mg/day (titration may be required) Requires renal dose adjustments
Duration of adequate trial	3–8 weeks	8 weeks
Adverse effects	Somnolence, dizziness, ataxia, dry mouth, blurred vision, peripheral edema, weight gain	Somnolence, dizziness, ataxia, dry mouth, blurred vision, peripheral edema, weight gain

CNS, Central nervous system.
Modified from Golembiewski, J. A. (2007). Postoperative pain management: Is there a role for gabapentin or pregabalin? *Journal of PeriAnesthesia Nursing, 22*(2), 136–138 ; Dworkin, R. H., O'connor, A. B., Backonja, M., Farrar, J. T., Finnerup, N. B., Jensen, T. S., ... & Portenoy, R. K. (2007). Pharmacologic management of neuropathic pain: evidence-based recommendations. Pain, 132(3), 237–251.

Table 15.5 | Gabapentinoid: U.S. Food and Drug Administration–Approved Indications and Dosing

Gabapentinoid Medication	Approved Indications	Dosing	Renal Dose Adjustments Based on Creatinine Clearance
Gabapentin	• PHN • Adjunctive treatment of partial-onset seizures	• Initiate at 100–300 mg PO at bedtime or tid • Doses can be increased by 100–300 mg/day every 1–7 days • Maximum dose 3600 mg/day, but exceeding 1800 mg/day may not provide further benefit owing to saturable nonlinear kinetics	• 60 mL/min or more: No change • 30–59 mL/min: 400–1400 mg/day in two divided doses • >15–29 mL/min: 200–700 mg in one daily dose • 15 mL/min: 100–300 mg in one daily dose • Hemodialysis: Provide supplemental dose based on estimated CrCl
Gabapentin[a] (Gralise) (Almatica Pharma, 2020)	• PHN	• Take once daily with evening meal • Day 1: 300 mg • Day 2: 600 mg • Days 3–6: 900 mg • Days 7–10: 1200 mg • Days 11–14: 1500 mg • Day 15: 1800 mg • Maximum dose: 1800 mg/day	• More than 60 mL/min: None • 30–60 mL/min: 600–1800 mg • <30 mL/min: Do not use • Hemodialysis: Do not use
Gabapentin enacarbil[a,b] (Arbor Pharmaceuticals, 2020)	• Moderate to severe RLS • PHN	Postherpetic Neuralgia (PHN) • 600 mg q a.m. for 3 days, then increase to 600 mg PO bid • Maximum dose 1200 mg/day	Postherpetic Neuralgia (PHN) • More than 60 mL/min: No change • 30–59 mL/min: Initiate at 300 mg q a.m. for 3 days; may increase up to 600 mg bid • 15–29 mL/min: 300 mg in AM on Day 1 and Day 3, may increase to 300 mg bid, if needed • <15 mL/min: 300 mg every other day; may increase to 300 mg q a.m., if needed • Hemodialysis: 300 mg after dialysis; may increase to 600 mg after dialysis
Pregabalin (Pfizer, 2016)	• DPN • PHN • Adjunctive therapy for partial-onset seizures • Fibromyalgia • Neuropathic pain associated with SCI	• Initiate at 150 mg/day in two or three divided doses. Increase dose to 300 mg/day within 1 wk. • Maximum doses vary depending on indications	• More than 60 mL/min: No change needed • 30–60 mL/min: 75–300 mg divided bid or tid • 15–30 mL/min: 25–150 mg divided daily or bid • <15 mL/min: 25–75 mg/day • Hemodialysis: Provide supplemental doses after dialysis based on daily dose
Pregabalin CR (Pfizer, 2017b)	• PHN • DPN	*DPN:* • Initial dose: 165 mg/day • Maximum dose: 330 mg/day *PHN:* • Initial dose: 165 mg/day • Maximum dose: 330–660 mg/day	• Renal dosage adjustments needed • 30–60 mL/min: Reduce usual extended-release dose by 50% • <30 mL/min: Use not recommended, Consider use of immediate-release formulation

[a] Not interchangeable with other gabapentin products.
[b] Dosing for PHN.
CR, Controlled release; *CrCl*, creatine clearance; *DPN*, diabetic peripheral neuropathy; *PHN*, postherpetic neuralgia; *RLS*, restless legs syndrome; *SCI*, spinal cord injury.

the role of these medications in the prevention of post-operative and chronic postsurgical pain (CPSP). In many cases, RCTs include only small numbers of participants, and effect size and potential bias may have a negative impact on findings. In some studies, gabapentin or pregabalin may not have been the only coanalgesic medication included in the treatment plan, making it difficult to determine the effect of the gabapentinoid on study outcomes.

Gabapentinoids and Neuropathic Pain

Gabapentin and pregabalin were included by the Neuropathic Pain Special Interest Group (NeuPSIG) of the International Association for the Study of Pain in a systematic review of RCTs of medications used for the treatment of neuropathic pain (Finnerup et al., 2015). The review included 25 placebo-controlled RCTs of pregabalin (150–600 mg/day), 14 RCTs of gabapentin (900–3600 mg/day), and 6 RCTs of gabapentin extended release or gabapentin enacarbil (1200–3600 mg/day). NeuPSIG recommended these medications as first-line agents for the treatment of neuropathic pain based on a strong rating by the Grading of Recommendations Assessment, Development, and Evaluation (GRADE) system. The GRADE system is an approach used in guideline development to rate the quality of evidence and strength of recommendations (Alhazzani & Guyatt, 2018). In a meta-analysis that included eight controlled and uncontrolled studies, neuropathic pain in those with SCIs was significantly reduced with the use of gabapentin and pregabalin (Mehta, McIntyre, Dijkers, Loh, & Teasell, 2014). Doses of gabapentin ranged up to 3600 mg/day, and pregabalin up to 300 mg/day.

A 2017 update of previous Cochrane reviews of gabapentin use in the treatment of chronic neuropathic pain in adults included 37 studies involving 5914 participants (Wiffen et al., 2017). When compared to placebo in those with PHN, more participants (32%) had substantial improvement (identified as at least 50% pain relief or report of pain as very much improved) with gabapentin doses of 1200 mg or more daily than with placebo (17%). In studies involving painful diabetic neuropathy, 38% had substantial improvement with gabapentin at 1200 mg or more daily than with placebo (21%). Side effects experienced by participants in these studies included dizziness (19%), somnolence (14%), peripheral edema (7%), and gait disturbance (14%). A meta-analysis of 6 RCTs of gabapentin 1800 mg/day used for 4 to 16 weeks in the treatment of PHN demonstrated an improvement in pain relief and safety (Fan et al., 2014). There was no difference in efficacy between once-daily and divided-daily doses, but higher rates of dizziness and somnolence were reported in the divided dose studies.

In a meta-analysis of 12 studies that compared pregabalin to placebo in 6117 patients with neuropathic pain conditions, including DPN, PHN, human immunodeficiency virus-associated distal sensory polyneuropathy (HIV-DSP), SCI, and complex regional pain syndrome (CRPS), pregabalin was associated with a statistically significant decrease in pain intensity rating, but was not found to sta-

tistically affect sleep quality (Wang, Bao, Zhang, Ju, & Yu, 2017). When examining the use of pregabalin in the treatment of patients with herpetic neuralgia, Wang et al. (2017), in a meta-analysis involving 7 clinical studies with 2192 patients, reported pregabalin was associated with lowered pain scores at 8 weeks. Compared to controls, more participants, after 6 weeks of pregabalin treatment, reported a decrease of pain ratings on the visual analogue scale ($P < .05$), reduced sleep interference score, and improvement in patient global impression of change ($P < .05$) (Wang et al., 2017). A meta-analysis of 9 trials involving 2056 participants with painful DPN demonstrated pregabalin was significantly more effective than placebo in reducing mean pain scores ($P < .001$) and improvement in sleep quality (Zhang et al., 2015). In an analysis comparing the effectiveness of pregabalin in patients with neuropathic pain who previously received gabapentin, but had been undertreated, were refractory to, or unable to tolerate gabapentin, to those who had not previously been treated with gabapentin, the groups had similar pain relief and relief of pain-related sleep interference (Markman et al., 2017). The studies included the use of pregabalin in daily doses ranging from 150 to 600 mg over 4- to 6-week intervals.

Not all studies of gabapentinoid use in neuropathic pain have yielded positive results. A recent study did not show benefit for the use of pregabalin for acute or chronic sciatica (Mathieson et al., 2017). Similarly, a meta-analysis reviewing gabapentin and pregabalin in nonspecific low back pain showed that gabapentin and pregabalin are ineffective and may lead to adverse effects; therefore, they are not recommended for this purpose (Shanthanna et al., 2017). The most commonly reported adverse effects in this meta-analysis included dizziness, fatigue, mentation difficulties, and visual disturbances (Shanthanna et al., 2017).

Gabapentinoids and Perioperative Pain

Both gabapentin and pregabalin have been studied in perioperative and acute postoperative pain settings. When used for these indications, the gabapentinoids are often combined with other medications in multimodal plans of care. Overall, the optimal dose and timing of gabapentin and pregabalin for use in acute pain remains unclear (Li et al., 2017; Yu, Ran, Li, & Shi, 2013)

Numerous meta-analyses have addressed the use of gabapentinoids in perioperative multimodal analgesic (MMA) plans of care and have examined benefits on pain scores, opioid doses, and/or reductions in opioid-related side effects. In guidelines for the management of postoperative pain, a panel of experts from the APS, ASRA, and ASA recommend consideration for the inclusion of gabapentin or pregabalin in a multimodal approach (Chou et al., 2016). Gabapentin and pregabalin are often included in ERAS protocols proposed by professional organizations or developed by individual health care organizations. However, the 2017 ERAS Society guidelines state that although these medications have been shown to reduce postoperative opioid requirements when used in MMA plans, evidence is still not convincing enough to require inclusion of either of these medications in routine ERAS Society guidelines (Beverly et al., 2017).

The challenges of inconclusive evidence related to perioperative gabapentin use are illustrated in a retrospective analysis of 228 consecutive postoperative patients in the postanesthesia care unit (PACU) who had been included in ERAS protocols. The researchers found there were no differences among those who had preoperatively received 300 mg of gabapentin, 600 mg of gabapentin, or no gabapentin on hemodynamic stability, opioid consumption, nausea, vomiting, or respiratory depression (Siddiqui et al., 2018). Those in the gabapentin groups had significantly less pain but also had significantly more sedation that resulted in a longer than 2-hour PACU stay (Siddiqui et al., 2018).

A meta-analysis of 17 RCTs involving 1793 patients identified a statistically significant reduction in postoperative opioid use (fentaNYL, morphine, and traMADol) compared to placebo when preoperative gabapentin was administered to patients who underwent mastectomy or spinal, abdominal, or thyroid surgeries. Smaller reductions were seen after thoracotomy, cesarean section, and prostatectomy cases (Arumugam, Lau, & Chamberlain, 2016). The dose, timing, and duration of preoperative gabapentin administration varied among the studies. The most commonly observed postoperative side effect was somnolence, and, despite opioid reductions, common opioid side effects of postoperative nausea and vomiting were not reduced (Arumugam et al., 2016).

In a meta-analysis involving 10 RCTs with 535 patients who underwent spine surgeries, the use of preoperative gabapentin compared to placebo was found to reduce pain scores in the first 48 hours and postoperative opioid consumption in the first 24 hours after surgery (Jiang, Huang, Song, Wang, & Cao, 2017). Pain scores with mobilization were not reduced. There was a significant reduction in nausea, but no difference in somnolence or dizziness (Jiang et al., 2017).

A systematic review and meta-regression analysis of 133 RCTs involving the use of gabapentin (any dose) at any time before the end of surgery on postoperative pain scores and morphine consumption demonstrated statistically significant reductions in pain scores at time intervals after surgery of 1, 2, 6, 12, and 24 hours (Doleman et al., 2015). Morphine equivalent consumption in the first postoperative 24 hours was significantly reduced. There was also a significant reduction in preoperative anxiety and an increase in postoperative patient satisfaction (Doleman et al., 2015).

A meta-analysis of 74 studies by Lam, Choi, Wong, Irwin, and Cheung (2015) examined the effect of preoperative pregabalin compared to placebo on pain scores, morphine consumption, and adverse effects in patients undergoing a variety of surgical procedures. Statistically significant improvements in pain scores were found in all surgical cases: orthopedic; cardiothoracic; spine; gynecologic; ear, nose, and throat (ENT); laparoscopic cholecystectomy; and several miscellaneous procedures. The use of pregabalin was associated with a statistically significant reduction in morphine consumption in the first 24 hours after surgery in gynecologic, orthopedic, spine, laparoscopic cholecystectomy,

and miscellaneous procedures. Sedation after pregabalin administration was a statistically significant side effect in all procedures except ENT, gynecologic, and laparoscopic cholecystectomy, and nausea and vomiting were only significant in the miscellaneous cases (Lam et al., 2015).

A meta-analysis of six RCTs examined perioperative pregabalin use compared to controls for gynecologic surgeries and included 452 patients who received at least one preoperative dose (Yao, Shen, & Zhong, 2015). Pregabalin-treated patients, compared to controls, had significantly less pain and consumed significantly less opioids in the first 24 hours after surgery than controls and did not increase the frequency of adverse events (Yao et al., 2015). Limitations include small study size, variable pregabalin dose, frequency, and variable use of other coanalgesic medications.

Six RCTs including 769 patients who underwent total knee arthroplasties were included in a meta-analysis that compared outcomes of patients who received pregabalin to controls (Dong, Li, & Wang, 2016). The preoperative use of pregabalin, compared to placebo, was associated with statistically significant reductions in postoperative pain scores at rest and during activity at 24 and 48 hours after surgery. Postoperative cumulative morphine use was also significantly reduced at the same time intervals. Pregabalin use was associated with improvements in nausea and vomiting, but sedation and dizziness were increased compared to controls (Dong et al., 2016).

In a meta-analysis of six RCTs with 464 patients, the effect of preoperative administration of pregabalin compared to controls in patients undergoing laparoscopic cholecystectomy was shown to significantly improve postoperative pain scores and reduce fentaNYL use (Zhang, Wang, & Zhang, 2017). There was less sedation in the pregabalin group, but no difference in nausea, vomiting, or headache (Zhang et al., 2017).

Gabapentinoids and Prevention of Chronic Postsurgical Neuropathic Pain

Most CPSP is neuropathic (chronic postsurgical neuropathic pain [CPSNP]), and the gabapentinoids, because of their efficacy in treating neuropathic pain, have been studied to examine their role in the prevention of CPSP and CPSNP. In a systematic review with meta-analysis of RCTs that included 18 studies and 2485 patients, pregabalin was not found to affect the incidence of CPSP development at 3, 6, or 12 months after surgery (Martinez, Pichard, & Fletcher, 2017). Data was insufficient to determine the effect on CPSNP. The authors of this review recommend against systematic perioperative use of gabapentinoids, because benefits have not been shown to outweigh risks, there is a small risk for adverse effects, and moderate-quality evidence does not show an effect on CPSP (Martinez et al., 2017).

Pharmacokinetics

Compared to gabapentin, pregabalin has more favorable pharmacokinetics, including greater bioavailability, greater ability to bind to receptors, and faster onset of action (Schifano, 2014). Bioavailability of gabapentin ranges from 33% to 60% and decreases with increasing doses because of nonlinear pharmacokinetics, whereas pregabalin maintains bioavailability of at least 90% throughout all doses (Pruskowski & Arnold, 2015). The onset for pregabalin is around 25 minutes compared to a range of 1 to 3 hours for gabapentin (Pruskowski & Arnold, 2015). Pregabalin reaches peak serum concentration in 1 hour compared to 3 hours for gabapentin (Chincholkar, 2018).

Dosing and Routes

The gabapentinoids have a wide dosing range. The wide range depends on the indication for use, patient age, and comorbidities. Tables 15.4 and 15.5 include dosing ranges for these medications. The rate of upward dose titration depends on the response to the medication. Some patients experience significant sedation and dizziness when starting gabapentin and thus require more conservative initial dosing. When discontinuing gabapentinoids, a slow taper, over at least 1 week, rather than abrupt discontinuation, is recommended to minimize withdrawal (McQuoid, 2019; Schifano, 2014).

The administration route for gabapentenoids is primarily orally, and some preparations may be administered through a feeding tube. There is some research interest in the use of intranasal gabapentenoids, and compounded preparations may be obtained for topical use, although there is limited evidence of efficacy (Portenoy, 2020). The use of unapproved administration routes has been reported, especially in cases involving substance use disorders (rectal, intravenous) (Elsayed et al., 2019).

Adverse Effects

Typical adverse effects described in the aforementioned studies include dizziness and sedation, both of which can be lessened with slow dosage titration. Peripheral edema may also occur, necessitating the use of caution in patients with congestive heart failure (Stewart & McPherson, 2017). Anticonvulsants, including gabapentin and pregabalin, have been associated with an increased risk for suicidal thoughts and behavior (Pfizer, 2016, 2017a)

Awareness of the potential for misuse and abuse of gabapentin and pregabalin has risen in recent years (Evoy, Covvey, Peckham, Ochs, & Hultgren, 2018). Gabapentin is not listed as a controlled substance by the U.S. Drug Enforcement Agency (DEA) at the time of writing; however, pregabalin is listed as a Schedule V controlled substance because of euphoric effects observed in clinical studies. Gabapentinoids have GABAmimetic properties similar to those of benzodiazepines that may contribute to their abuse (Evoy et al., 2018). Doses of gabapentin and pregabalin are abused at doses 3 to 20 times greater than therapeutic doses and are often taken as one large dose rather than divided throughout the day (Schifano, 2014). Patients with a history of substance use disorder, particularly opioid use disorder, are at higher risk for

gabapentinoid abuse (Evoy, Morrison, & Saklad, 2017; Smith, Havens, & Walsh, 2016). Pregabalin and gabapentin may be abused via the oral route, but are also self-administered through intravenous and rectal methods (Schifano, 2014). Gabapentin, in a systematic review of its misuse, abuse, and diversion, is abused to achieve euphoria, enhance or potentiate opioid effects, and/or mitigate withdrawal from other substances (Smith, Havens, & Walsh, 2016).

Bonnet and Scherbaum (2017) conducted a systematic review including 106 studies to evaluate the addiction potential of the gabapentinoids. They determined the addiction risk of pregabalin is higher than that with gabapentin, and in those without a history of substance use disorder the addiction risk to gabapentinoids is very low. However, the risk is higher in those with a current or past substance use disorder history, especially an opioid use disorder. It is recommended to avoid the use of the gabapentinoids, if possible, in the higher risk population, and if gabapentinoids are needed, use should be carefully monitored (Bonnet & Scherbaum, 2017).

A case-control study was done examining opioid overdoses and concomitant gabapentin use. Cases included patients who were prescribed opioids and died of an opioid-related cause; controls were matched according to several variables and were prescribed opioids but did not die of an opioid-related cause. There were 1256 cases that were matched to 4619 controls. In total, there were 155 cases and 313 controls that were prescribed gabapentin. The odds of an opioid-related death were elevated 49% if the patient was prescribed concomitant gabapentin and an opioid. Moderate gabapentin doses of 800 to 1799 mg/day or high doses of 1800 mg/day or more were associated with even higher odds of opioid-related death. The odds of an opioid-related death increased two-fold with very high doses of 2500 mg or more. There were differences in the number of patients prescribed benzodiazepines between the two groups, however this was deemed not significant (Gomes et al., 2017). In a large, population-based study, similar evidence of a potentially life-threatening drug-drug interaction was noted with concommitant use of pregabalin and opioids (Gomes et al., 2018).

With the increased use of prescribed gabapentenoids, as well as misused and abused gabapentenoids, there is growing awarenesss of potential harms associated with these medications. In 2019, the FDA issued a warning that serious breathing difficulties may occur in those taking gabapentin or pregabalin who have respiratory risk factors. These risk factors include older age, chronic obstructive pulmonary disease or other conditions that reduce lung function, and concomitant use of opioids or other CNS depressants (FDA, 2019).

With concerns related to risks for opioid-related respiratory depression and overdose, it is necessary to consider all of the medications a patient is taking and comorbidities in weighing the potential for serious opioid-related adverse events (Gomes et al., 2017).

Monitoring of Patients

Gabapentin and pregabalin require renal dosage adjustment; therefore, monitoring of renal function is needed. Because of the association of anticonvulsants with suicidal ideation, it is necessary to assess for depressed mood and suicidal thoughts. If practicing in a state that reports gabapentin and/or pregabalin on the prescription drug monitoring program (PDMP), it is necessary for prescribers to check the PDMP before prescribing.

Antidepressants

Antidepressant adjuvant analgesics are usually divided into two major groups: the TCAs and the newer biogenic amine reuptake inhibitors (Table 15.6). Of the latter group, the serotonin-norepinephrine reuptake inhibitors (SNRIs) are the medications with the stronger evidence for use as analgesics, whereas research is lacking or inconsistent regarding the analgesic potential of the selective serotonin reuptake inhibitors (SSRIs).

Tricyclic Antidepressants

TCAs can be subdivided into tertiary and secondary amines. Tertiary amines include amitriptyline and imipramine, which are metabolized to the secondary amines nortriptyline and desipramine. These two subgroups have equal efficacy for pain, but secondary amines have improved tolerability (Watson & Dyck, 2015).

Table 15.6 | Antidepressant Coanalgesic Medications: Classes With Examples of Drugs

Classes	Examples
Tricyclic Antidepressants	
Tertiary amines	Amitriptyline
	ClomiPRAMINE
	Doxepin
	Imipramine
Secondary amines	Desipramine
	Nortriptyline
"Newer" Second-Generation Antidepressants	
Serotonin-norepinephrine reuptake inhibitors (SNRIs)	DULoxetine
	Milnacipran
	Venlafaxine
Selective serotonin reuptake inhibitors (SSRIs)	FLUoxetine
	PARoxetine
SSRIs have very limited evidence for use as coanalgesics	Sertraline

From Pasero, C., & McCaffery, M. (2011). *Pain assessment and pharmacologic management* (p. 637). St. Louis, Mosby. © 2011, Pasero, C., & McCaffery, M. May be duplicated for use in clinical practice.

Mechanism of Action

The analgesic effects of TCAs are independent of their antidepressant effects (Obata, 2017; Dharmshaktu, Tayal, & Kalra, 2012; Mylan Pharmaceuticals, 2016). TCAs interact with numerous other receptors, which are shown in Table 15.7. TCAs block sodium channels, which inhibit abnormal discharges from damaged nerves and neuropathic pain (Obata, 2017). The mechanism of action of TCAs is also related to their ability to bind to norepinephrine and serotonin transporters and thereby inhibit their reuptake in the synaptic cleft. Norepinephrine reuptake inhibition has the more significant role because it acts on α_2-adrenergic receptors in the dorsal horn of the spinal cord to inhibit neuropathic pain (Obata, 2017; Dharmshaktu, Tayal, & Kalra, 2012; Mylan Pharmaceuticals, 2016). The pain pathway is more fully described in Chapter 3.

Indications and Uses

TCAs are FDA-labeled for major depressive disorder (MDD), with the exceptions of clomiPRAMINE (obsessive-compulsive disorder) and imipramine (MDD and childhood enuresis) (Lupin Pharmaceuticals, 2016; Mallincrodt, 2015; Mylan Pharmaceuticals, 2016; Sandoz, 2014; Teva Pharmaceuticals, 2015).

According to several guidelines, TCAs are first-line treatment options for neuropathic pain (Finnerup et al., 2015; Moulin et al., 2014). The American Diabetic Association ranks TCAs as a second-line therapy for diabetic neuropathy because it is an off-label use and associated with significant side effects (Pop-Busui et al., 2017). Evidence also suggests benefit for TCAs in low back pain and fibromyalgia and for migraine prophylaxis (Dharmshaktu et al., 2012).

Although the TCAs are often recommended as first-line agents in the treatment of neuropathic pain, and individual studies in the early 2000s demonstrated efficacy in the

Table 15.7 | Tricyclic Antidepressant Receptor Activity

Medication	Ach M	α_1	H_1	5-HT$_3$	NE
Secondary Amines					
Desipramine	+	+	+	+	++++
Nortriptyline	+	+	+	++	+++
Tertiary Amines					
Amitriptyline	+++	+++	++	++++	++
Doxepin	++	+++	+++	++	++
Imipramine	++	+	+	+++	+++

Ach M, Acetylcholine muscarinic receptor; α_1, alpha-$_1$ adrenergic receptor; H_1, histamine-1 receptor.
Modified from DeBattista, C. (2018). Antidepressant agents. In B. Katzung, S. B. Masters, & A. J. Trevor (Eds.), *Basic and clinical pharmacology* (14th ed.). New York, NY: McGraw-Hill.

use of TCAs for the treatment of neuropathic and other types of chronic pain, more recent systematic reviews have not supported the earlier individual studies. In a 2015 Cochrane review of amitriptyline for the treatment of neuropathic pain, 15 studies from a previous review and two more recent studies were included, involving a total of 1342 participants with seven different types of neuropathic pain conditions (Moore, Derry, Aldington, Cole, & Wiffen, 2015). The authors concluded there was no strong evidence to support a beneficial effect, nor was there strong evidence to show a lack of effect. Although there is a lack of unbiased evidence of efficacy, the authors acknowledge small studies over decades reported successful treatment of neuropathic pain with amitriptyline and therefore conclude amitriptyline may be beneficial for a small number of patients. They also note alternative TCAs may provide different clinical responses (Moore et al., 2015).

Another Cochrane review addressed the use of nortriptyline in the treatment of neuropathic pain conditions. The limited number of studies the researchers identified were of poor methodology and small size. As a result, the authors could not recommend the use of nortriptyline as a first-line agent in the treatment of neuropathic pain (Derry, Wiffen, Aldington, & Moore, 2015b). A Cochrane review on the use of amitriptyline in fibromyalgia consisted of nine studies and 649 participants (Moore et al., 2015). The recommendations from this review were similar to those in the amitriptyline and neuropathic pain review. There is a lack of strong evidence to show effectiveness for the use of amitriptyline in the treatment of fibromyalgia, and there is inadequate evidence to show lack of benefit. Therefore amitriptyline may be one option for the treatment of fibromyalgia with the awareness that it may be beneficial for only a small group of patients (Moore et al., 2015).

A network meta-analysis of four RCTs demonstrated TCAs to have greater efficacy than placebo in reducing pain associated with DPN, but the strength of the evidence was low (Waldfogel et al., 2017). Two studies involved the use of imipramine, but evidence was insufficient to examine the use of alternative TCAs.

Pharmacokinetics

The TCAs have long half-lives and are well absorbed, which account for their ability to be dosed once daily (DeBattista, 2018). They are metabolized in the liver and are cytochrome P450 CYD 2D6 substrates; therefore serum levels may be altered by concurrent administration of enzymes CYP 2D6 inhibitors or inducers. CYP 2D6 genetic polymorphisms may affect the metabolism of the TCAs (DeBattista, 2018).

Dosing Selection

Typical starting doses of TCAs are 25 mg orally (PO) at bedtime. Lower doses of 10 mg at bedtime may be more appropriate for the elderly who are predisposed to adverse reactions (Watson & Dyck, 2015). The dose can be titrated by 25 mg/day every 3 to 7 days up to a max-

imum dose of 150 mg/day; however, doses in excess of 75 mg/day are not advised for adults 65 years or older because of sedative effects, major anticholinergic effects, and fall risks (Gilron, Baron, & Jensen, 2015; Watson & Dyck, 2015). With an even stronger recommendation, the Beers Criteria of inappropriate medication use in older individuals lists TCAs as medications that should be avoided because of the same risks (2019 American Geriatrics Society Beers Criteria® Update Expert Panel, 2019). Side effects often limit the use of higher doses. An analgesic response to TCAs is achieved at lower doses than are used to treat depression (Kremer, Salvat, Muller, Yalcin, & Barrot, 2016). TCAs may provide an analgesic response within a few days to 1 week after TCA initiation, whereas the antidepressant effect may take up to 4 weeks to be noted (Hayashida & Obata, 2019). TCAs are primarily administered through the enteral route, but compounding pharmacies may prepare amitriptyline for topical use (see Chapter 16). An adequate trial of TCAs is considered 6-8 weeks with 2 weeks at maximally tolerated dose (Dharmshaktu et al., 2012; Dworkin et al., 2007).

Adverse Effects

Cardiovascular side effects are particularly concerning with TCAs because they act similarly to class I antiarrhythmics. Additionally, TCAs inhibit alpha-adrenergic receptors and muscarinic-adrenergic receptors. Slowed cardiac conduction, QTc prolongation, arrhythmias, tachycardia, and orthostatic hypotension may occur. Orthostatic hypotension may also contribute to increased risk for falls (Gilron et al., 2015). Doses of greater than 100 mg/day have been associated with sudden cardiac death (Watson & Dyck, 2015).

Anticholinergic side effects are also common and can be problematic, particularly in the elderly. These include dry mouth, urinary retention, constipation, tachycardia, confusion, and blurred vision; therefore TCAs should be avoided in patients with glaucoma, cognitive impairment, or benign prostatic hypertrophy (BPH) (Riediger et al., 2017). Secondary amine TCAs have less interaction with antimuscarinic receptors, which explains their improved tolerability (Watson & Dyck, 2015).

TCAs also inhibit histamine receptors, and this contributes to weight gain and sedation. Weight gain may be dose related and differs from one TCA to another. The antihistaminergic effects may result in sedation, which may be problematic for some patients, particularly as sedation may increase fall risks, but the sedating effect may be desirable for those with insomnia (Riediger et al., 2017). For this reason, TCAs are often administered before bedtime.

Monitoring of Patients

Electrocardiogram (ECG) monitoring may be appropriate before initiating TCAs in older adults and younger patients with cardiac risk factors. In those with risk factors, periodic ECG monitoring may be prudent throughout TCA therapy (Glick & Marcus, 2015). Other monitoring parameters include changes in mood, pain, cognition, sleep, and potential adverse effects such as urinary retention and constipation. Drug levels of TCAs are not typically monitored. Monitor for drug-drug interactions and the potential for serotonin syndrome when combined with other serotonergic medications (e.g., traMADol, triptans, meperidine, linezolid) (Bleakley, 2016). Also monitor for development or exacerbation of anticholinergic side effects when other anticholinergics, such as antihistamines, are used in patients receiving TCA therapy (Kouladjian O'Donnell, Gnjidic, Nahas, Bell, & Hilmer, 2017).

Serotonin Norepinephrine Reuptake Inhibitors

DULoxetine, venlafaxine, milnacipran, and desvenlafaxine are SNRIs that have been considered for the treatment of pain in a variety of conditions. They are among the first-line medications recommended for the treatment of neuropathic pain in adults (Finnerup et al., 2015), are sometimes used as a single analgesic and at other times are incorporated into MMA plans of care.

Mechanism of Action

SNRIs are involved in the modulation of pain because they work by inhibiting the reuptake of serotonin and norepinephrine (see Chapter 3). At lower doses, venlafaxine activity more closely resembles that of an SSRI, but with higher doses venlafaxine is an SNRI (Aiyer, Barkin, & Bhatia, 2017). The analgesic benefits occur regardless of the presence of anxiety or depression, but may be particularly helpful in those with comorbid mental health diagnoses (Trouvin, Perrot, & Lloret-Linares, 2017). These medications exert their effects through inhibition of descending pain pathways (Aiyer et al., 2017).

Indications and Uses

DULoxetine DULoxetine has multiple indications related to pain, including fibromyalgia, chronic musculoskeletal pain (low back pain and osteoarthritis), and DPN pain. Nonpain indications for DULoxetine include MDD and generalized anxiety disorder (Lilly USA, 2016).

Venlafaxine Venlafaxine does not have an FDA-approved indication for pain (Wyeth, 2016a, 2016b); however, in clinical trials, venlafaxine has been shown to relieve neuropathic pain and is recommended by the European Federation of Neurological Societies as a first-line medication for painful diabetic neuropathy (Kremer et al., 2016). Evidence supports the use of venlafaxine for the treatment of fibromyalgia and low back pain (Kus et al., 2016; Trouvin et al., 2017; Waldfogel et al., 2017). There is also weak evidence to support the use of venlafaxine for migraine prophylaxis (Ambrosini & Schoenen, 2016).

Milnacipran The only FDA-approved pain indication for milnacipran is for fibromyalgia (Drugs@FDA: Savella[R], 2016).

SNRIs and Pain-Related Research SNRIs were included in the NeuPSIG systematic review and meta-analysis of pharmacotherapy for neuropathic pain (Finnerup et al., 2015). A total of 14 studies of SNRIs were identified. The majority of studies were with DULoxetine (9 studies) compared to venlafaxine (4 studies). Overall, there were 7 positive DULoxetine studies and 2 positive venlafaxine studies. In the 2 negative venlafaxine studies, low doses were used, which would affect the findings. It was determined that the number needed to treat (NNT) was 7.7 (6.5–9.4) and the number needed to harm (NNH) was 11.8 (9.5–15.2). SNRIs, DULoxetine, and venlafaxine were given strong GRADE recommendations and included as first-line recommended medications for neuropathic pain (Finnerup et al., 2015).

A Cochrane systematic review of double-blind randomized trials was published in 2014 examining the effectiveness of DULoxetine for painful neuropathy, chronic pain, and fibromyalgia. A total of 18 studies involving 6407 participants were included (8 diabetic neuropathy studies, 6 fibromyalgia studies, 3 depression with painful symptoms studies, 1 central neuropathic pain study). It was determined that there was moderate-quality evidence supporting the use of DULoxetine 60 mg and 120 mg for DPN (Lunn, Hughes, & Wiffen, 2014). In regard to fibromyalgia, the authors concluded there was low-quality evidence of benefit for DULoxetine 60 mg and DULoxetine 120 mg for greater than 50% reduction in pain at 12 weeks and painful physical symptoms in depression (Lunn et al., 2014).

A 2015 Cochrane systematic review looked at milnacipran for treating fibromyalgia through six studies with 4238 patients. Milnacipran 100 and 200 mg/day each compared to placebo favored milnacipran for a 30% reduction in pain. The overall NNT was around 7 to 8 (Cording, Derry, Phillips, Moore, & Wiffen, 2015). A systematic review was attempted for milnacipran in neuropathic pain. There was only one study, including 40 participants with chronic low back pain, with a neuropathic component. No differences were found between milnacipran 100 or 200 mg/day versus placebo (Derry, Phillips, Moore, & Wiffen, 2015a).

A later Cochrane systematic review in 2018 examined the efficacy of SNRIs (milnacipran and DULoxetine) in fibromyalgia and involved 18 studies with 7903 patients' findings. There was no benefit for DULoxetine and milnacipran compared to placebo for more than 50% reduction in pain, improvement in health-related quality of life, or fatigue, but the study did show benefit in patient global impression and 30% or more reduction in pain (Welsch, Uceyler, Klose, Walitt, & Hauser, 2018).

Pharmacokinetics

The SNRIs have fairly rapid oral absorption and achieve peak plasma levels within 3 hours. They undergo hepatic metabolism and are renally excreted (DeBattista, 2018). The half-lives of these medications vary (DULoxetine 12–15 hours; venlafaxine 8–11 hours; milnacipran 6–8 hours) and as a result, dosing varies (DeBattista, 2018).

SNRIs are metabolized through CYP450 enzymes CYP2D6 (DULoxetine and venlafaxine) and CYP1A2 (DULoxetine). DULoxetine is a moderate inhibitor of CYP2D6 (Lilly USA, 2016; Wyeth, 2016a). Milnacipran does not have any clinically significant pharmacokinetic drug interactions (Drugs@FDA: Savella[R], 2016).

Dosing and Routes

Usual analgesic doses of SNRIs are summarized in Table 15.8. These medications are administered orally. SNRIs are initiated at low doses, and doses are gradually increased if the medication is well tolerated. Dose reductions are necessary with renal and hepatic impairments. To reduce risks for withdrawal when discontinuing SNRIs, gradual dose reductions are advised.

Adverse Effects

Common side effects of SNRIs include nausea, somnolence, dry mouth, hyperhidrosis, anorexia, erectile dysfunction, and constipation (Drugs@FDA: Savella[R], 2016; Lilly USA, 2016; Wyeth, 2016a). Other SNRI-associated adverse effects include serotonin syndrome, hyponatremia, angle-closure glaucoma, and seizures (Drugs@FDA: Savella[R], 2016; Lilly USA, 2016; Wyeth, 2016a).

Because of the changes in norepinephrine with SNRIs, elevation in blood pressure may occur. Hypertension should be controlled before initiation of an SNRI. Reduced doses or discontinuation of the SNRI may be needed should a patient experience significant elevations in blood pressure (Drugs@FDA: Savella[R], 2016; Lilly USA, 2016; Wyeth, 2016a).

Venlafaxine has been associated with QTc prolongation at both therapeutic and supratherapeutic doses. This is an important consideration because other medications used in MMA plans, such as methadone, may also lead to QTc prolongation. Caution should be used in patients with cardiovascular disease or risk factors for QTc prolongation (Herndon, Lider, & Daniels, 2015; Wenzel-Seifert, Wittmann, & Haen, 2011; Wyeth, 2016a). QTc monitoring before initiation and during therapy in patients at risk for QTc prolongation is prudent but not universally recommended (Herndon et al., 2015).

DULoxetine and milnacipran should be avoided in patients with chronic liver disease or who consume substantial amounts of alcohol because these medications have been associated with worsening of liver function test (LFT) results and liver dysfunction (Drugs@FDA: Savella[R], 2016; Lilly USA, 2016). Also, hepatic dose adjustments are recommended with venlafaxine (Wyeth, 2016a).

Table 15.8	Serotonin Norepinephrine Reuptake Inhibitors (SNRIs) Dosing Information			
Medication	**Dose (Oral)**	**Titration**	**Dose Adjustments**	**Comments**
DULoxetine	30 mg/day to start	Increase after 7 days to 60 mg/day.	Avoid if GFR is < 30 mL/min or with chronic liver disease or cirrhosis.	For elderly, continue 30 mg/day for 2 wk before increasing to 60 mg/day. If discontinuing, gradual dose reductions needed to avoid withdrawal symptoms.
Venlafaxine SA (sustained acting)	37.5 mg/day to start	Increase by 75 mg/day every wk to a max 225 mg/day.	Reduce dose by 25%–50% if mild to moderate renal impairment. Reduce dose by 50% if severe renal impairment or dialysis. Reduce dose by 50% if mild to moderate hepatic impairment; additional reductions for severe hepatic impairment or cirrhosis.	Higher doses are needed for SNRI activity because lower doses of venlafaxine result in SSRI, not SNRI activity. If discontinuing, gradual dose reductions needed to avoid withdrawal symptoms.
Milnacipran	12.5 mg/day on first day	Increase to 12.5 mg bid on days 2 and 3. Increase to 25 mg bid for days 4–7; increase to 50 mg bid after day 7.	Severe renal impairment (CrCl 5–29 mL/min), reduce maintenance dose by 50% to 25 mg bid (max 50 mg). Not recommended for end-stage renal disease Use with caution if severe hepatic impairment.	Maximum dose 200 mg/day. If discontinuing, gradual dose reductions needed to avoid withdrawal symptoms.

CrCl, Creatinine clearance; *GFR,* glomerular filtration rate; *SNRI,* serotonin-norepinephrine reuptake inhibitor; *SSRI,* selective serotonin reuptake inhibitor.
DULoxetine (Lilly USA, L. (2016). Cymbalta: Highlights of prescribing information. Retrieved from http://pi.lilly.com/us/cymbalta-pi.pdf; Venlafaxine (Wyeth, 2016a); Effexor XR: Highlights of prescribing information. Retrieved from http://labeling.pfizer.com/showlabeling.aspx?ID=100); and Milnacipran (Drugs@FDA: Savella[R], 2016). Savella: Highlights of prescribing information. Retrieved from https://media.allergan.com/actavis/actavis/media/allergan-pdf-documents/product-prescribing/Savella_PI_clean_December_2017.pdf .

Data are mixed on the effects of SNRIs and the risk for bleeding. Serotonin is involved in platelet aggregation, and because SNRIs (and SSRIs) reduce the amount of serotonin taken up by the platelet, there is the potential for increased bleeding (Smith et al., 2018). Combining SSRIs or SNRIs with other medications that alter platelets, including NSAIDs, which are often included in MMA plans, or anticoagulants, may further increase risk. Data focusing specifically on DULoxetine found increased risk for bleeding when NSAIDs were used with DULoxetine or placebo, but no significant difference in bleeding between DULoxetine or placebo was found when NSAIDs were not used (Perahia et al., 2013). In contrast, an observational study found no increased risk for upper gastrointestinal (GI) bleeds when DULoxetine was combined with an NSAID or aspirin (Li, Cheng, Ahl, & Skljarevski, 2014).

Monitoring of Patients

Key monitoring for SNRIs include blood pressure, renal function, hepatic function, mood/suicidal ideation, and bleeding. There is the potential for drug-drug interactions with SNRIs. DULoxetine and venlafaxine, because of their CYP450 metabolism, have potential for drug-drug interactions (Lilly USA, 2016; Wyeth, 2016a). Milnacipran does not have any clinically significant pharmacokinetic drug interactions (Drugs@FDA: Savella^R, 2016).

SNRIs should be avoided with monoamine oxidase inhibitors (MAOIs) because of the risk for serotonin syndrome. The risk for serotonin syndrome is also present when SNRIs are combined with other medications with serotonergic mechanisms of action (Drugs@FDA: Savella^R, 2016; Lilly USA, 2016; Wyeth, 2016a). Commonly used medications in multimodal pain management with serotonergic activity include traMADol and triptans.

Alpha-Adrenergic Receptor Agonists

CloNIDine, dexmedetomidine, tiZANidine are alpha-adrenergic receptor agonists that may provide analgesic benefits when used in an MMA plan of care.

Mechanism of Action

There are two subtypes of alpha agonists. Alpha-$_1$ agonists lead to smooth muscle contraction and are not known to have an analgesic effect. Alpha-$_2$ agonists provide analgesia through a combination of central and peripheral mechanisms. Centrally, alpha-$_2$ agonists interact with presynaptic and postsynaptic neurons located within the dorsal horn of the spinal cord. The principle site of action for alpha-$_2$ agonists is the spinal cord, not the brain (Tonner, 2017). Analgesic effects are the result of decreased excitability of primary afferent nerve fibers, decreased release of substance P, and hyperpolarization of dorsal horn neurons. Supraspinal mechanisms thought to be related to increasing norepinephrine in the locus coeruleus also contribute to the analgesic effect (Nguyen, Tiemann, Park, & Salehi, 2017; Zhang & Bai, 2014).

Overall, alpha-$_2$ agonists produce sedative, anxiolytic, and analgesic properties with limited, if any, respiratory depression (Hwang, Lee, Park, & Joo, 2015). The alpha-$_2$ adrenergic agonists vary in their interaction with alpha receptors. In comparison to cloNIDine, dexmedetomidine has approximately 8 times more selectivity for the alpha-$_2$ receptor over the alpha-$_1$ receptor (Tonner, 2017).

The peripheral analgesic effect of alpha-$_2$ agonists is suggested by the ability of these medications to produce analgesia without crossing the blood-brain barrier. The mechanism of peripheral action of alpha-$_2$ agonists is not well understood, and no recent studies are available to further explain the pharmacodynamics. However, increasing interest in the topical and intraarticular use of these medication may yield additional research. When administered to a peripheral nerve, alpha-$_2$ agonists have been shown to relieve hypersensitivity from nerve injury; it is theorized that the nociceptive effects of these medications are due to their ability to reduce proinflammatory cytokines and the number of local leukocytes, which contribute to the inflammatory process (Romero-Sandoval, Bynum, & Eisenach, 2007). Another theory is that the peripheral alpha-$_2$ agonists inhibit C-fibers or may have an effect on mu opioid receptors or α_1-adenosine receptors (Chan, Cheung, & Chong, 2010).

Indications and Uses

CloNIDine

CloNIDine in the oral and patch formulations is indicated for the treatment of hypertension; whereas cloNIDine for injection is labeled for use in combination with opioids for the treatment of severe pain in patients with cancer not adequately treated with opioids alone. When the injection preparation is used, it is administered as a continuous epidural infusion (Boehringer Ingelheim Pharmaceuticals, 2009; PharmaForce, 2009). Additionally, epidural cloNIDine may be best for use in neuropathic pain types compared to other pain types (PharmaForce, 2009). CloNIDine, often in combination with other agents, is also used in intrathecal infusions to optimize pain relief (see Chapter 18) (Rauck, North, & Eisenach, 2015). Topical cloNIDine, more fully described in Chapter 16, has been studied in DPN (Wrzosek, Woron, Dobrogowski, Jakowicka-Wordliczek, & Wordliczek, 2015). Epidural cloNIDine has been studied in neuropathic pain, including CRPS (Duong, Bravo, Todd, Finlayson, & Tran, 2018). CloNIDine, often in combination with morphine or other medications, has been used in the treatment of pain associated with SCIs (Mehta et al., 2016).

CloNIDine also has evidence for analgesia in the postoperative setting with opioid-sparing effects (Nguyen et al., 2017; Tonner, 2017). A variety of routes of administration and range of doses have been studied for cloNIDine in the postoperative setting. However, the packaging information for cloNIDine for injection recommends against the use of cloNIDine in this setting because of risk for hemodynamic instability (PharmaForce, 2009).

Another area in which cloNIDine can be used is for the treatment of opioid withdrawal symptoms. During opioid withdrawal, there is noradrenergic hyperactivity, and cloNIDine inhibits the release of norepinephrine, thereby blunting sympathetic hyperactivity (e.g., tachycardia, hypertension, anxiety, and agitation). A Cochrane review comprising 25 RCTs with 1668 participants showed that cloNIDine was more effective than placebo in the management of opioid withdrawal (Gowing, Farrell, & White, 2014).

TiZANidine

TiZANidine is another alpha-$_2$ adrenergic agonist that may provide analgesic benefits in addition to its effectiveness in relieving spasticity. It is FDA approved for the treatment of spasticity (Acorda Therapeutics, 2013) and has been used in the treatment of some acute and chronic pain conditions. In a prospective, randomized, double-blind study of 60 patients who underwent inguinal hernia repair, when compared to placebo, patients who received tiZANidine 4 mg 1 hour before surgery and continued twice daily for a week had significantly lower pain scores and analgesic requirements (Yazicioglu, Caparlar, Akkaya, Mercan, & Kulaçoglu, 2016). In another prospective, randomized, double-blind study with 70 participants, when compared to placebo, those who received tiZANidine 4 mg 90 minutes preoperatively were noted to have lower pain scores and lower opioid requirements in the PACU (Talakoub, Abbasi, Maghami, & Zavareh, 2016). TiZANidine also has been found to be useful in the treatment of chronic neck and lower back pain, particularly when there is a myofascial component to the pain. TiZANidine was shown in one small double-blind placebo controlled trial to have a role in chronic daily headache (Starling & Dodick, 2015) and may also have a role in the treatment of myofascial pain (Saxena, Chansoria, Tomar, & Kumar, 2015).

Dexmedetomidine

Dexmedetomidine is FDA-approved for sedation of nonintubated patients before or during surgery and other procedures (Akorn, 2014). Its lack of respiratory depression is one of its advantages (Zhang & Bai, 2014). Positive results (patient satisfaction, analgesia, reduced opioid requirements, and/or reduction in opioid side effects) for dexmedetomidine have been shown in various settings, including postcraniotomy pain (Peng, Jin, Liu, & Ji, 2015), post–spinal surgery pain (Hwang, Lee, Park, & Joo, 2015), post–colorectal surgery pain (Cheung et al., 2014), and refractory cancer pain (Liu et al., 2014). Studies have also demonstrated pain reduction in the following conditions: after arthroscopic subacromial decompression (Bengisun, Ekmekci, Akan, Koroglu, & Tuzuner, 2014), after cesarean section (Nie, Liu, Luo, & Huang, 2014), after hysterectomy (Ren et al., 2015), in cardiovascular disease (Zhang & Bai, 2014), and in lung and liver transplantation (Perahia et al., 2013).

Blaudszun et al. (2012) conducted a systematic review and meta-analysis including 30 studies of 1792 surgical patients with 933 patients receiving cloNIDine or dexmedetomidine. No study examined cloNIDine compared to dexmedetomidine. CloNIDine and dexmedetomidine showed reduction in morphine needs at 24 hours, pain intensity at 24 hours, and early nausea. Intraoperative and postoperative hypotension was increased with cloNIDine; dexmedetomidine increased the likelihood of postoperative bradycardia (NNH = 3) (Blaudszun et al., 2012).

In a meta-analysis of 11 RCTs involving 674 neurosurgical patients who had received intraoperative dexmedetomidine (335 patients, 339 controls), pain scores and postoperative opioid requirements in the PACU were significantly less in the treatment group (pain = 0.0001; opioid requirements $p = .05$). Intraoperative opioid use was also significantly reduced in the treatment group ($p = .002$) (Liu et al., 2018)

Pharmacokinetics

CloNIDine is highly lipophilic and well absorbed by the oral route, with a bioavailability near 100%. It reaches a peak effect in 1 to 3 hours after oral dosing, and the oral formulation has a half-life of 6 to 24 hours (Westfall, Macarthur, & Westfall, 2018). TiZANidine has an oral bioavailability of 21% because of extensive first-pass metabolism and has a mean half-life of 3 hours (Granfors, Backman, Laitila, & Neuvonen, 2004). Both cloNIDine and tiZANidine are hepatically metabolized through the CYP450 system. The CYP450 isoforms involved in cloNIDine are not well studied (Claessens et al., 2010); tiZANidine is primarily metabolized by CYP1A2, and both medications are renally excreted (Granfors et al., 2004).

Dexmedetomidine, a highly lipophilic medication, is rapidly redistributed and has a short elimination half-life. It is hepatically metabolized through the CYP450 system and glucuronidation, and its metabolites are renally excreted (Eilers & Yost, 2018).

Dosing and Routes

FDA-approved routes for administration of cloNIDine include oral, transdermal, and epidural routes. Dexmedetomidine has been approved for intravenous and intranasal administration. Other routes of administration have been used in research and recommendations for route and dose information in Tables 15.9 and 15.10 include both approved and nonapproved routes.

Table 15.9 | Routes and Doses of CloNIDine in Acute Pain Management

Route	Dose	Titration	Comments
Oral	2–5 mcg/kg or start at 0.1 mg bid	Increase by 0.1 mg/day every 7 days to max of 2.4 mg/day	
Transdermal patch system	Start at 0.1 mg/day transdermal patch and replace every 7 days	Titrate up based on response; 0.2 mg/day and 0.3 mg/day patches are available	
Epidural	Infusion: 30 mcg/h	Titrate up slowly for pain relief; limited experience with doses above 40 mcg/h	May start at lower doses if increased concerns about hypotension
Peripheral nerve/plexus block	0.5–1 mcg/kg		
Intrathecal	15–150 mcg		

Chan, A. K., Cheung, C. W., & Chong, Y. K. (2010). Alpha-2 agonists in acute pain management. *Expert Opinion in Pharmacotherapy, 11*(17), 2849–2868. https://doi.org/10.1517/14656566.2010.511613; Clonidine. (2019) Drug monographs. Wolters Kluwer Clinical Drug Information, Inc. Nahman-Averbuch, H., Dayan, L., Sprecher, E., Hochberg, U., Brill, S., Yarnitsky, D., & Jacob, G. (2016). Pain modulation and autonomic function: the effect of clonidine. *Pain Medicine, 17*(7), 1292-1301; and Kaye, A. D., Cornett, E. M., Helander, E., Menard, B., Hsu, E., Hart, B., & Brunk, A. (2017). An update on nonopioids: Intravenous or oral analgesics for perioperative pain management. *Anesthesiology Clinics, 35*(2), e55–e71.

CloNIDine

Initially, cloNIDine can be dosed at 0.1 mg PO bid and titrated by 0.1 mg/day every 7 days until at a maximum dose of 2.4 mg/day (Boehringer Ingelheim Pharmaceuticals, 2009). Transdermal patches can be used in place of the oral formulation (Guay, 2001) and are worn for 7 days at a time (Boehringer Ingelheim Pharmaceuticals, 2009). Recommended dosing for continuous epidural infusion is 30 mcg/h (PharmaForce, 2009). Initial dose reductions are needed when starting cloNIDine in a patient with renal dysfunction (Boehringer Ingelheim Pharmaceuticals, 2009; PharmaForce, 2009). Intrathecal dosing of cloNIDine ranges from 15 to 150 mcg.

TiZANidine

TiZANidine is administered orally and typically is started at 2 mg and repeated at 6- to 8-hour intervals up to a maximum of 3 doses in the first 24 hours. Dose titration occurs with increases in 2 to 4 mg/dose every 1 to 4 days. The maximum dose of tiZANidine is 36 mg/day. To prevent withdrawal symptoms, high doses of tiZANidine

Table 15.10 | Routes and Doses of Dexmedetomidine for Acute Pain Management

Route	Dose
Intravenous	Initiate infusion at 0.2 mcg/kg/h and titrate up, if hemodynamically stable, by 0.1 mcg/kg/h every 30 min until pain is controlled to maximum of 1.5 mcg/kg/h
Intranasal	1–1.5 mcg/kg
Adjunct to spinal anesthesia	0.5 mg/kg over 10 min
Intravenous regional anesthesia	1 mcg/kg
Buccal	2.5 mcg/kg
Intramuscular	2.5 mcg/kg
Intraarticular	1 mcg/kg
Epidural	1 mcg/kg
Caudal block (pediatric)	1–2 mcg/kg

Chan, A. K., Cheung, C. W., & Chong, Y. K. (2010). Alpha-2 agonists in acute pain management. *Expert Opinion in Pharmacotherapy, 11*(17), 2849–2868. https://doi.org/10.1517/14656566.2010.511613; Gandhi, K. A., Panda, N. B., Vellaichamy, A., Mathew, P. J., Sahni, N., & Batra, Y. K. (2017). Intraoperative and postoperative administration of dexmedetomidine reduces anesthetic and postoperative analgesic requirements in patients undergoing cervical spine surgeries. *Journal of Neurosurgical Anesthesiology, 29*(3), 258–263.; Lexicomp, 2019 https://www.wolterskluwercdi.com/lexicomp-online/.

(20–28 mg/day) for long durations (≥9 weeks) should be slowly decreased by 2 to 4 mg/day (Acorda Therapeutics, 2013).

Dexmedetomidine

Dexmedetomidine is administered intravenously and is dosed based on body weight. An initial intravenous loading dose is usually administered, followed by a continuous intravenous infusion. Table 15.10 describes the loading dose, bolus dose, and continuous intravenous infusion dosing recommendations. Dosage reduction is recommended for dexmedetomidine in geriatric patients and hepatic impairment. When used in combination with other anesthetics, sedatives, hypnotics, or opioids dosage adjustment for dexmedetomidine or the other concomitant medication may be warranted (Akorn, 2014).

Adverse Effects

CloNIDine

Sedation may occur with cloNIDine because of the presence of alpha-$_2$ receptors in the brainstem; however, this usually occurs with higher doses than those used to treat pain. Generally, when cloNIDine is used as an analgesic, the risks for sedation and respiratory depression are low. The use of other sedative substances, including alcohol or benzodiazepines, can increase the effects. Other common side effects include dry mouth, nausea, confusion, and dizziness (Boehringer Ingelheim Pharmaceuticals, 2009; PharmaForce, 2009).

CloNIDine is an alpha-$_2$ agonist, and thus bradycardia and hypotension are a concern with its use, particularly in patients with baseline cardiac disease or hemodynamic instability. Bradycardia can be treated with atropine, and severe hypotension can be treated with intravenous fluids or EPINEPHrine (Boehringer Ingelheim Pharmaceuticals, 2009; PharmaForce, 2009).

Withdrawal from abrupt cessation of cloNIDine is another concerning adverse effect. Symptoms of cloNIDine withdrawal include nervousness, agitation, headache, tremor, and significant rebound hypertension. People on higher doses of cloNIDine and on concomitant beta-blocker therapy are at increased risk. The profound rebound hypertension can be treated with reintroduction of cloNIDine or phentolamine. If epidural cloNIDine is to be discontinued, it should be tapered over 2 to 4 days to minimize the potential for withdrawal, and, if a beta-blocker is also used, this should be stopped days before the epidural cloNIDine is tapered (Boehringer Ingelheim Pharmaceuticals, 2009; PharmaForce, 2009).

TiZANidine

The most common adverse effects of tiZANidine include dry mouth, somnolence, asthenia, dizziness, urinary tract infections, constipation, vomiting, nervousness, pharyngitis, and rhinitis. Hypotension occurs with tiZANidine and may limit the ability to titrate the dose. It is not recommended to use tiZANidine with other α-$_2$ receptor agonists, and the risk for hypotension is increased when used with other antihypertensives. With a creatinine clearance (CrCl) of less than 25 mL/min, tiZANidine should be used with caution because concentrations can increase 50%. If tiZANidine is stopped abruptly, rebound hypertension tachycardia and hypertonia may occur. The concomitant use of strong CYP1A2 inhibitors is contraindicated and include fluvoxaMINE and ciprofloxacin (Acorda Therapeutics, 2013).

Dexmedetomidine

Common adverse effects of dexmedetomidine include dry mouth, hypotension, and bradycardia. Those with diabetes, hypovolemia, or hypertension and the elderly may be more prone to hypotension and bradycardia. Time-limited hypertension may occur with the loading dose and may necessitate dose reduction. When dexmedetomidine is used beyond 24 hours, tolerance develops, requiring titration of dose that is associated with increased adverse effects (Akorn, 2014).

Monitoring of Patients

It is important to monitor vital signs in patients receiving alpha-$_2$ agonists because of the possibility for hemodynamic changes, especially hypotension and bradycardia.

Routine inspection of pump function and catheter tubing for obstruction or dislodgement is essential to avoid unintended cessation of epidural cloNIDine. It is necessary to seek immediate assistance if there is a sudden disruption in epidural cloNIDine administration because this is a medical emergency (PharmaForce, 2009).

Other medications used commonly in the treatment of pain can increase the potential or severity of α-adrenergic agonist side effects. Hypotension may be worsened when combined with opioids. Sedation is exacerbated when combined with central nervous system (CNS) depressants, including alcohol, barbiturates, benzodiazepines, and opioids (Akorn, 2014; Boehringer Ingelheim Pharmaceuticals, 2009).

There are several important monitoring parameters with tiZANidine. Because of possible liver toxicity, LFTs should be monitored. Renal function also needs to be periodically monitored. With severe renal impairment, tiZANidine levels increase and may increase potential for adverse effects. Because of the risk for hypotension, blood pressure should be monitored (Acorda Therapeutics, 2013).

Corticosteroids

This section will focus on the use of systemic corticosteroids. The use of corticosteroids in regional and intraspinal approaches is discussed in Chapters 18 and 19.

Mechanism of Action

Corticosteroids bind to glucocorticoid and mineralocorticoid receptors that are located throughout the peripheral and central nervous system. They exert their antiinflammatory effects by inhibiting the synthesis of proinflammatory cytokines while also increasing antiinflammatory factors (Balague, Piguet, & Dudler, 2012; Vyvey, 2010). In addition, glucocorticoids alter vascular permeability, leading to reduced tissue edema. Glucocorticoid receptors also play a role in building and maintaining nerves. When glucocorticoids are administered, there is less firing of an unhealthy, damaged nerve (Vyvey, 2010).

Indications and Uses

Corticosteroids are often used in cancer-related pain. The National Comprehensive Cancer Network (NCCN) Guidelines for Adult Cancer Pain suggest a role for corticosteroids in the management of specific cancer pain syndromes (Swarm et al., 2018). NSAIDs and corticosteroids are recommended for pain associated with inflammation. Corticosteroids are recommended for diffuse bone pain not associated with an oncologic emergency. They are also recommended for nerve pain associated with nerve compression or inflammation (Swarm et al., 2018). Other uses of corticosteroids in the palliative care setting include bowel obstruction, raised intracranial pressure (ICP), and superior vena cava obstruction (Leppert & Buss, 2012; Vyvey, 2010). A Cochrane review of 15 randomized or prospective studies including 1926 patients found weak evidence supporting the use of corticosteroids in cancer-related pain, although some studies showed short-term benefit (Haywood et al., 2015).

Corticosteroids are also indicated for the treatment of pain associated with sickle cell disease. A systematic review of treatment options for sickle cell disease identified the use of high-dose corticosteroids added to morphine to treat severe pain associated with sickle cell crisis. It was noted that although corticosteroids may improve analgesia, they may increase adverse outcomes, including infection, hypertension, and metabolic abnormalities (Meremikwu & Okomo, 2010). Additionally, although corticosteroids have been shown to reduce the duration of acute chest syndrome associated with sickle cell crisis, patients who have received corticosteroids have been found to have higher rates of hospital readmission because of rebound sickling (Howard et al., 2015).

Corticosteroids have sometimes been considered for the prevention of PHN. A Cochrane review investigated the role of corticosteroids for this indication. A total of 787 participants from five RCTs were included. The conclusion was that there was moderate-quality evidence that corticosteroids were ineffective in preventing PHN (Han et al., 2013). Therefore corticosteroids are not recommended for PHN.

Corticosteroids are often given for acute radicular low back pain; however, data to support this practice are limited. A randomized, placebo-controlled study was conducted of 82 patients aged 21 to 50 years who presented to the emergency department with low back pain and a positive straight leg raise. There was no significant difference in mean pain improvement between those administered methylPREDNISolone 160 mg IV versus placebo (Friedman et al., 2008). Because of the lack of efficacy data, one group of researchers went as far as to say that the use of systemic corticosteroids for low back pain should be "banned" (Balague et al., 2012).

The American College of Physicians recently completed a systematic review to develop their Noninvasive Treatments for Acute, Subacute, and Chronic Low Back Pain Clinical Practice Guideline. Systemic corticosteroids were not effective for pain or function in acute low back pain according to low-quality evidence. In radicular low back pain, there was moderate-quality evidence to suggest that systemic corticosteroids led to no difference in function compared to placebo (Chou et al., 2018; Qaseem, Wilt, McLean, Forciea, & Clinical Guidelines Committee of the American College of Physicians, 2017). In summary, there is a lack of evidence to support the use of corticosteroids for the treatment of low back pain.

Dosing and Routes

Typically, dexamethasone is the preferred corticosteroid in the treatment of cancer-related pain because of its lower mineralocorticoid effects and long half-life, which allows once-daily dosing. Betamethasone, predniSONE, and predniSOLONE are alternative medications that can be used (Leppert & Buss, 2012; Vyvey, 2010). Equianalgesic dosing of corticosteroids is summarized in Table 15.11. Morning corticosteroid administration is recommended because of the CNS stimulating effects (Swarm et al., 2018).

Doses of dexamethasone for cancer pain vary depending on the indication (Leppert & Buss, 2012). Typical doses of dexamethasone for bone pain and neuropathic pain range from 4 to 8 mg PO once to three times daily (Leppert & Buss, 2012; Vyvey, 2010). For elevated ICP or bowel obstruction, dexamethasone is dosed 8 to 16 mg/day. Dosing for spinal cord compression is dexamethasone 16 to 32 mg/day or 8 to 16 mg bid; doses of 16 to 24 mg or 8 mg bid to tid have been used for superior vena cava obstruction (Leppert & Buss, 2012). Because of the significant side effects that can occur with corticosteroids, the lowest effective dose for the shortest duration should be used (Vyvey, 2010).

The oral route is often used for dexamethasone administration. Dexamethadone and select other corticosteroids are also available in solutions for intravenous, intraarticular, intramuscular, epidural, and soft tissue infiltration (Drugs@FDA. Dexamethasone Sodium Phosphate Injection, USP. 2014)

Adverse Effects

As noted earlier, corticosteroids are associated with multiple short- and long-term side effects. Immediate effects of corticosteroids include immunosuppression, hyperglycemia, and psychiatric changes (Leppert & Buss, 2012).

Table 15.11 | Equivalent Doses of Corticosteroids

Corticosteroid	Equivalent Dose (mg)
Cortisone	25
Hydrocortisone	20
PrednisoLONE	5
PredniSONE	5
MethylPREDNISolone	4
Triamcinolone	4
Dexamethasone	0.75–1
Betamethasone	0.6

From Pasero, C., & McCaffery, M. (2011). *Pain assessment and pharmacologic management* (p. 647). St. Louis: Mosby. Data from Clinical Pharmacology Online. Gold Standard, Inc. Retrieved August 1, 2009 from http://clinicalpharmacology.com. © 2011, Pasero, C., & McCaffery, M. May be duplicated for use in clinical practice.

Psychiatric side effects include anxiety, depression, delirium, and psychosis (Vyvey, 2010). Common side effects include weight gain, increased appetite, muscle weakness, insomnia, and GI upset (Vyvey, 2010). Long-term effects include myopathy, peptic ulcer, osteoporosis, and Cushing's syndrome (Leppert & Buss, 2012). Myopathy and muscle weakness are particularly problematic when using these medications to treat pain; fortunately, myopathy is usually reversible on discontinuation. GI bleeding is more likely if the patient is also on NSAIDs or elderly; however, this can be mitigated with gastroprotection. The use of bisphosphonates may be considered with long-term use of corticosteroids (Leppert & Buss, 2012; Vyvey, 2010).

Long-term use of corticosteroids suppresses the hypothalamic-pituitary-axis. When patients are on high doses or on corticosteroids for more than 2 weeks, the corticosteroid should be tapered to prevent adverse sequelae of adrenal insufficiency. If corticosteroids are stopped abruptly, patients may experience pain, nausea/vomiting, weight loss, depression, fatigue, fever, dizziness, and rebound symptoms (Vyvey, 2010; Zoorob & Cender, 1998).

Monitoring of Patients

When using corticosteroids in the pain management plan, it is important to monitor blood pressure and blood glucose, especially if the patient has diabetes or is receiving high doses of corticosteroids. With long-term use, monitoring for osteoporosis is important.

N-Methyl-D-Aspartate Receptor Antagonists

Dextromethorphan (DXM), ketamine, and magnesium are N-methyl-D-aspartate (NMDA) antagonists that are sometimes used in pain management plans of care.

Dextromethorphan

Mechanism of Action

The ability of DXM to antagonize the NMDA receptors is thought to account for its analgesic effects. DXM binds noncompetitively with low affinity at NMDA receptors as an antagonist (Nguyen et al., 2016). By blocking NMDA receptors, the release of excitatory neurotransmitters and central sensitization is inhibited (Siu & Drachtman, 2007; Weinbroum, Rudick, Paret, & Ben-Abraham, 2000). DXM also has been shown to interact with other receptors; DXM may be an agonist at sigma-1 receptors (receptors that may have antidepressant activity), an antagonist of nicotinic receptors, or a potential antagonist of serotonin transporters and norepinephrine transporters. However, its effects on NMDA receptors and sigma-1 receptors are associated with most of its pharmacologic benefits (Nguyen et al., 2016).

Despite being structurally related to levorphanol, a phenanthrene group opioid, DXM does not have significant activity at opioid receptors (Nguyen et al., 2016). Its antitussive effects are related to increasing the cough threshold within the medulla and not related to activity on opioid receptors (Siu & Drachtman, 2007; Weinbroum et al., 2000).

Indications and Uses

Traditionally, DXM has been used as a cough suppressant. More recently, DXM when combined with quiNIDine has been approved for the treatment of pseudobulbar affect (Avanir Pharmaceuticals, 2010; Nguyen et al., 2016). DXM has been studied extensively in numerous off-label uses. In the setting of pain, DXM has been most studied in postoperative pain and neuropathic pain. Positive effects on analgesia and/or opioid dose requirements have been shown in bowel resection, tonsillectomy, oral surgery, cholecystectomy, mastectomy, and hysterectomy (Weinbroum et al., 2000). However, not all studies in the postoperative setting have had beneficial outcomes (Nguyen et al., 2016; Weinbroum et al., 2000).

King, Ladha, Gelineau, and Anderson (2016) conducted a systematic review of RCTs examining perioperative DXM for postoperative pain. Twenty-one studies of 848 patients were included. DXM was associated with reduction in opioid doses, pain at 1 hour, and pain at 4 to 6 hours, and a few studies showed reduced pain at 24 hours. Overall, DXM was fairly well tolerated. Several studies showed an increase in side effects, including nausea; another group of studies showed no difference in adverse effects (King et al., 2016).

DXM has been studied in several neuropathic pain conditions. DXM 45 mg or 30 mg combined with quiNIDine 30 mg showed statistically significant improvements in pain, interference with sleep, and interference with activities compared to placebo. The DXM 45 mg with quiNIDine 30 mg group showed greater reductions in pain compared to separate DXM 30 mg and quiNIDine 30 mg groups (Shaibani, Pope, Thisted, & Hepner, 2012). In a systematic review of several NMDA antagonists used for the treatment of neuropathic pain, DXM was evaluated in six studies (Aiyer, Mehta, Gungor, & Gulati, 2018). Clinical benefit was demonstrated in four of the six studies, although results were mixed in two of the four studies. In the studies with mixed results, DXM was effective in pain associated with diabetic neuropathy but not with pain associated with PHN (Aiyer et al., 2018).

Pharmacokinetics

Rapid first-pass metabolism occurs with DXM primarily by O-demethylation by CYP2D6, which forms the active metabolite dextrorphan. A minor route of metabolism involves CYP3A4 to form inactive metabolites. Secondary metabolites are then formed by CYP3A4 and CYP2D6 metabolism. Because of the vast amount of first-pass metabolism, minimal amounts of free DXM or dextrorphan remain. The use of a potent CYP2D6 inhibitor such as quiNIDine can be used to increase active components. To further complicate this, CYP2D6 is subject to pharmacogenetic variants, which can be divided into poor metabolizers, intermediate metabolizers, extensive metabolizers, and ultra-rapid metabolizers (Nguyen et al., 2016).

Dosing and Routes

A wide range of DXM doses have been studied. Previous reviews have suggested using doses of DXM between 30 and 90 mg PO. Higher doses of DXM have been used but were associated with adverse effects (Weinbroum et al., 2000). In studies of DXM for analgesia, it has been administered through the oral route.

Adverse Effects

Because of its lower affinity for the NMDA receptors, DXM has fewer side effects compared to other medications with the same mechanism of action (Weinbroum et al., 2000). Generally, DXM is considered to be safe with minimal side effects at therapeutic doses (Siu & Drachtman, 2007). More common side effects include nausea, vomiting, dizziness, hot flushing, drowsiness, heartburn, and headache (Siu & Drachtman, 2007; Weinbroum et al., 2000). Higher doses of DXM (10 mg/kg/day) have been associated with nystagmus, slurred speech, light-headedness, and fatigue (Siu & Drachtman, 2007).

Capitalizing on the activity on NMDA receptors, DXM is sometimes abused at high doses to achieve dissociative effects similar to those of phencyclidine or ketamine (Antoniou & Juurlink, 2014). The types of effects or "plateaus" are determined by dose (Antoniou & Juurlink, 2014; Burns & Boyer, 2013). Lower doses are associated with mild stimulant effects while higher doses are associated with full dissociation (Antoniou & Juurlink, 2014; Burns & Boyer, 2013). Tolerance develops quickly, contributing to dose escalation (Antoniou & Juurlink, 2014). Onset of effects is within 30 and 60 minutes, with the duration of effect lasting around 6 hours (Burns & Boyer, 2013). DXM is not typically identified in urine drug testing (Antoniou & Juurlink, 2014). Treatment of overdose is supportive measures (Antoniou & Juurlink, 2014).

Monitoring of Patients

Monitoring for DXM focuses on assessment of analgesic benefits and monitoring for any adverse effects, including the possibility of DXM abuse.

Ketamine

Ketamine has traditionally been used as an anesthetic medication, but its analgesic properties have resulted in much research and clinical interest for its potential benefit in pain management plans of care.

Mechanism of Action

Ketamine is a dissociative anesthetic originally developed as an alternative to phencyclidine. Ketamine is available in some countries as both racemic ketamine and the S-enantiomer, but only the racemic mixture is available in the United States. Ketamine has been shown to exert a wide range of molecular effects and mechanism of actions. Growing recognition of ketamine's effects has led to the expansion of this medication beyond its original use as an anesthetic agent. Ketamine at subanesthetic doses is used as an analgesic agent for acute and chronic pain conditions (Schwenk et al., 2018). It interacts with numerous receptor types; however, ketamine's primary mechanism of analgesia is through its reversible, noncompetitive inhibition of NMDA receptors in the CNS, where it inhibits the binding of glutamate to this receptor and prevents the release of excitatory neurotransmitters (Cohen et al., 2018; Kurdi, Theerth, & Deva, 2014; Schwenk et al., 2018). Inhibition of NMDA receptors also contributes to ketamine's ability to halt central sensitization (Niesters, Martini, & Dahan, 2014; Schwenk et al., 2018).

At high doses, ketamine has been shown to bind to mu, kappa, and delta opioid receptors, but the effects on the receptors remains unclear and may be dose related (Cohen et al., 2018). The effect of ketamine on opioid receptors may be more significant in chronic pain than acute pain because ketamine has demonstrated ability to reduce opioid tolerance (Sleigh et al., 2014). The effect of ketamine is not reversed by naloxone, thus indicating that its primary analgesic effect is not related to its opioid effect (Cohen et al., 2018). Ketamine also acts by other, non-NMDA pathways and exerts analgesic effects that may account for its effectiveness when used peripherally as a topical analgesic (Cohen et al., 2018).

Ketamine also plays a role in enhancing the inhibition of pain through the descending pain pathway. It inhibits the reuptake of dopamine and serotonin while also increasing the amounts of EPINEPHrine and norepinephrine (Cohen et al., 2018; Gao, Rejaei, & Liu, 2016). The effect on descending pathways may contribute to ketamine's analgesic benefits in nonneuropathic pain conditions (Cohen et al., 2018).

Indications and Uses

Ketamine has been studied in a number of conditions, including the management of pain. Outside of the pain realm, ketamine has been examined in depression, posttraumatic stress disorder, anxiety, and bipolar depression among others (Niesters, Martini, & Dahan, 2014). A nasal spray ketamine product is available and FDA-labeled for treatment-resistant depression when used in combination with an antidepressant (Drugs@FDA: Spravato, 2020). Even within the context of use for analgesia, there are numerous proposed uses, including burn pain, trauma pain, abdominal pain, migraine, and fibromyalgia (Niesters et al., 2014). Ketamine in subanesthetic doses may be of particular interest in the treatment of neuropathic pain (including CRPS), cancer pain, acute postoperative pain, and opioid-induced hyperalgesia (Bell, Eccleston, & Kalso, 2017; Bredlau, Thakur, Korones, & Dworkin, 2013; Hagen & Rekand, 2015; Hardy et al., 2012;

Hirota & Lambert, 1996, 2011; Marchetti et al., 2015; National Health Service of Scotland, 2014; Niesters et al., 2014; Salas et al., 2012; Schwartzman et al., 2009b; Schwenk et al., 2018; Sigtermans et al., 2009).

Acute Pain

Evidence-based guidelines for the use of intravenous ketamine infusions for the treatment of acute pain were developed by a committee of the ASRA, American Academy of Pain (AAP), and ASA (Schwenk et al., 2018). The same group of professional associations published consensus guidelines on the use of intravenous ketamine infusions for chronic pain (Cohen et al., 2018).

In the guidelines for the use of ketamine in the treatment of acute pain, the use of subanesthetic doses of ketamine are supported for the following indications (Schwenk et al., 2018):

- Patients who are expected to have severe postoperative pain, such as those who have undergone abdominal, thoracic, or orthopedic (limb and spine) surgeries
- Opioid-tolerant patients who require surgery
- Opioid-tolerant patients with an acute exacerbation of a chronic pain condition, such as those with sickle cell disease acute pain episodes
- As an adjunct to reduce opioid use for those who are at increased risk for opioid-related adverse outcomes, such as those with obstructive sleep apnea

Yang et al. (2014) conducted a meta-analysis of randomized controlled trials (RCTs) of 266 patients who preoperatively received ketamine or saline in the control group. In those who received ketamine, the time to first analgesic was prolonged compared to placebo. No difference in nausea and vomiting was identified.

Another meta-analysis in the postoperative pain setting looked at RCTs of patients undergoing laparoscopic cholecystectomy. Five studies with 212 patients were included. Analysis demonstrated significant differences between ketamine and placebo for pain scores at 24 and 48 hours. Additionally, opioid use was significantly lower with ketamine at 12, 24, and 48 hours (Ye, Wu, & Zhou, 2017).

The use of ketamine in the treatment of postoperative pain is also of interest, because interventions are sought to reduce the potential for development of persistent postsurgical pain. A systematic review and meta-analysis were conducted to examine the efficacy and safety of ketamine when used for this purpose (McNicol, Schumann, & Haroutounian, 2014). The review included 17 RCTs of ketamine administered perioperatively via any route. Although the overall risk for developing persistent postsurgical pain was not significantly reduced in the ketamine versus placebo group, when RCTs that included the epidural administration route were removed, there was a statistically significant reduction in risk at 3 months ($P = .01$) and 6 months ($P = .04$) postoperatively, and there was no difference in adverse effects between the ketamine and placebo groups (McNicol et al., 2014).

Ketamine has been shown to have an opioid-sparing effect. In a review of the literature that examined continuous ketamine infusion and administration of a single low dose of intravenous ketamine, low-dose ketamine reduced opioid requirements by 40% in patients with postoperative pain; postoperative pain scores were also reduced (Jouguelet-Lacoste, La Colla, Schilling, & Chelly, 2015).

A systematic review and meta-analysis compared the effectiveness and adverse effects of subanesthetic ketamine to intravenous opioids in adults in the emergency department setting with acute pain (Karlow et al., 2018). Three studies were identified, which included 261 patients, that compared the pain scores of patients who received similar doses of ketamine (less than 0.5 mg/kg) to 0.1 mg/kg morphine equivalent doses as the primary outcome and adverse events as the secondary outcome. Ketamine was found to be noninferior to morphine, and although there were more nonsevere adverse effects with ketamine, there were no reported severe adverse effects.

Although no RCTS involving the use of ketamine in the treatment of acute pain associated with vaso-occlusive crisis in sickle cell disease are identified, a number of case reports support the efficacy of ketamine as an analgesic or coanalgesic (Hassell, Ngongo, Montgomery, & Hornick, 2017; Jobanputra, Dixit, & Hussain, 2016; Olivo et al., 2016; Palm, Floroff, Hassig, Boylan, & Kanter, 2018; Uprety, Baber, & Foy, 2014). A survey was conducted to query advanced practice registered nurses about the use of ketamine in the treatment of pain associated with vaso-occlusive crisis in sickle cell disease (Applequist, Daly, Koniaris, & Musil, 2017). Of the 128 returned surveys, only 13 respondents reported use of ketamine for this indication. The most frequently reported reason for the lack of use of ketamine was the lack of awareness of its potential as a treatment option. Given the lack of published studies, RCTs are necessary to examine the use of ketamine in the treatment of vaso-occlusive crisis-associated pain.

Chronic Pain

Evidence-based consensus guidelines for the use of intravenous ketamine infusions for chronic pain were developed by a committee of the ASRA, the AAP, and the ASA (Cohen et al., 2018). Cohen et al. (2018) note the level of evidence for use of intravenous ketamine infusions varies depending on the pain condition and the dose of ketamine used in the studies. Most studies were small, uncontrolled, and unblinded or ineffectively blinded (Cohen et al., 2018). The guidelines include the following recommendations for ketamine infusions in the treatment of chronic pain (Cohen et al., 2018, p. 538):

- "Spinal cord injury pain (weak evidence to support short-term improvement)
- Chronic regional pain syndrome (CRPS) (moderate evidence to support improvement for up to 12 weeks)
- Mixed neuropathic pain, fibromyalgia, cancer pain, ischemic pain, headache, spinal pain (weak or no evidence for immediate improvement)"

Pharmacokinetics

Ketamine, when administered intravenously, achieves rapid maximum plasma concentrations; it has low bioavailability (16%–29%) because of extensive first-pass hepatic metabolism, and peak effect is reached in 20 to 120 minutes (Zanos et al., 2018). Ketamine undergoes extensive hepatic metabolism, catalyzed by CYP450 2B6 and CYP3A4, to an active metabolite, norketamine. Norketamine has antianalgesic and excitatory effects; norketamine is further metabolized to inactive glucuronide (Dershwitz & Rosow, 2018). The half-life of ketamine is 2 to 4 hours, which may be prolonged with repeated administration (Zanos et al., 2018). Ketamine and its metabolite are renally eliminated (Zanos et al., 2018).

Dosing and Routes

Ketamine use is associated with a wide range of doses and routes. Intravenous, oral, subcutaneous, intranasal, topical, and intramuscular routes have all been studied (Bredlau et al., 2013; Connolly, Prager, & Harden, 2015). Intravenous ketamine bolus doses and continuous intravenous infusions are often used in the treatment of acute and chronic pain conditions. Dosing protocols vary, and the following doses are provided for illustration:

Acute Pain:

- IV bolus dose for acute pain up to 0.35 mg/kg.
- IV infusion rate of 1 mg/kg/h or less in non–intensive care settings.
- Infusion rates of 0.5 mg/kg/h (8 mcg/kg/min) or less are used in most acute pain studies.
- Individual pharmacokinetics and pharmacodynamics may necessitate higher doses (Schwenk et al., 2018).

Chronic Pain:

- IV bolus dose for chronic pain is up to 0.35 mg/kg.
- IV infusion rate of 0.5 to 2 mg/kg/h.
- IV infusion rates up to 7 mg/kg/h have been used when pain is refractory and patients are in intensive care settings.
- In some chronic pain conditions, total doses of at least 80 mg over 2 hours or more may be needed (Cohen et al., 2018).

Examples of various ketamine dosing protocols are described in Table 15.12. There is a paucity of RCTs that have examined the use of intravenous patient-controlled analgesia (PCA) ketamine, but studies of ketamine in combination with an opioid in intravenous PCA have shown positive outcomes (Schwenk et al., 2018).

Other routes for ketamine administration are associated with specific challenges. A number of small studies have shown intranasal ketamine administration for acute pain and sedation to be rapid acting, effective, and safe; however, at this time the intranasal formula requires preparation by a compounding pharmacy (Schwenk et al., 2018). Intranasal ketamine formulations are in development but not yet available for commercial use.

Table 15.12	Sample Ketamine Administration Protocols	
Route(s)	**Dose**
Intermittent intravenous infusion	• 0.25–0.5 mg/kg tid
Oral dosing	• 0.25–0.5 mg/kg tid • 0.8 mg/kg/day in divided doses • 4–6 mg/kg (procedural pain) • 10–25 mg/day or 0.5 mg/kg at bedtime (chronic pain)
Subcutaneous dosing	• 0.8 mg/kg/day in divided doses • 0.5 mg/kg subq bolus (chronic pain) • 0.1–1.5 mg/kg/h subq infusion (chronic pain)
Continuous intravenous infusion	• 0.1–0.2 mg/kg/h • 100 mg/day • 10 mg/h with dose titration and continue for median infusion of 4 days • 4 mg/h × 24h, 12 mg/h × 24h, 20 mg/h on day 3–5h • 0.14–0.4 mg/kg/h continuous IV infusion (chronic pain)
Intravenous loading dose and continuous infusion	• 0.3 mg/kg loading dose over 30 min followed by 0.1–0.2 mg/kg/h and titrated to effect
Intravenous bolus or subq bolus for dose finding, then continuous intravenous infusion	• 0.1 mg/kg IV and double IV dose q15 min until pain improves, then continuous intravenous infusion at effective dose • 0.5 mg/kg subq and double subq dose q30–45 min until pain improves, then continuous intravenous infusion at effective dose
Intravenous bolus (procedural pain)	• 0.2–0.8 mg/kg

subq, Subcutaneously.
Pasero, C., & McCaffery, M. (2005). Ketamine: Low doses may provide relief for some painful conditions. *American Journal of Nursing, 105*(4), 60–64; Okon, T. (2007). Ketamine: An introduction for the pain and palliative medicine physician. *Pain Physician, 10*(3), 493–500; and Schwenk, E. S., Viscusi, E. R., Buvanendran, A., Hurley, R. W., Wasan, A. D., Narouze, S., . . . & Cohen, S. P. (2018). Consensus guidelines on the use of intravenous ketamine infusions for acute pain management from the American Society of Regional Anesthesia and Pain Medicine, the American Academy of Pain Medicine, and the American Society of Anesthesiologists. *Regional Anesthesia and Pain Medicine, 43*(5), 456–466.

There is no oral ketamine formulation commercially available, and there have been few studies of oral ketamine use. It has been used off-label by dilution of the intravenous racemic formulation, but bioavailability is limited (Quibell, Fallon, Mihalyo, Twycross, & Wilcock, 2015; Schwenk et al., 2018). Because of its bitter taste, it may be diluted with purified water, simple sugar, or juice to improve the taste tolerability (Bredlau et al., 2013; Quibelle et al., 2015).

The intramuscular route is generally avoided in pain management because of the discomfort associated with intramuscular administration of medications (Bredlau et al., 2013). The use of subcutaneous ketamine is also limited by injection site irritation and need for frequent injection site rotation (Bredlau et al., 2013). Intrathecal administration of ketamine is avoided because the preservative contained in its formulation is associated with neurotoxicity and a preservative-free formulation is unavailable (Bredlau et al., 2013; Connolly et al., 2015).

Adverse Effects

The major contraindications identified for the use of ketamine are related to the high doses when ketamine is used as an anesthetic agent. Contraindications for use of subanesthetic ketamine are not well known because studies are small and are mostly conducted on healthy individuals. The evidence-based guidelines for the use of intravenous ketamine infusions for the treatment of acute pain published by Schwenk et al. (2018) and for the use of intravenous ketamine infusions for the treatment of chronic pain published by Cohen et al. (2018) recommend avoidance of ketamine in pregnancy, poorly controlled cardiovascular disease, active psychosis, and severe liver disease and use with caution in moderate hepatic dysfunction. Both guidelines recommend avoidance of ketamine in patients with elevated ICP and intraocular pressure. However, several reviews have not supported the need for avoidance of ketamine in conditions associated with increased ICP or altered cerebral hemodynamics. A systematic review that analyzed the results of 16 studies, 15 manuscripts, and 1 meeting proceeding concluded there was evidence that ketamine does not increase ICP in patients with non-traumatic neurologic conditions who are sedated and ventilated and that it may contribute to a decrease in ICP (Zeiler, Teitelbaum, West, & Gilman, 2014). In a systemic review of 10 studies that examined effects of ketamine on ICP, neurologic outcomes, intensive care unit length of stay, and mortality, ketamine did not adversely affect any of the outcomes (Cohen et al., 2015), and a meta-analysis of five studies that examined the effects of ketamine on ICP and other cerebral hemodynamics concluded the use of ketamine should not be avoided for ICP-related concerns (Wang et al., 2014).

The acute pain guidelines note there is no evidence to demonstrate the use of a short course of intravenous ketamine in the hospital setting for treatment of acute pain in patients with opioid use disorder and high tolerance increases risks for ketamine addiction; it is recommended to assess risk on an individual basis (Schwenk et al., 2018). The chronic pain guidelines recommend avoidance of ketamine in patients with active substance use disorders because the higher doses used in treatment of chronic pain compared to acute pain may pose greater risks than benefits (Cohen et al., 2018). It is recommended to exercise caution if intravenous ketamine is used to treat chronic pain in patients with substance abuse and use universal precautions in monitoring for use disorder (Cohen et al., 2018).

A systematic review that included 17 studies of ketamine in the treatment of acute postoperative pain showed the adverse effects in the ketamine group to be similar to those in the placebo group (McNicol et al., 2014). Regardless of administration route, ketamine was not associated with an increase in adverse effects in four of five meta-analyses, and in the fifth meta-analysis, adverse effects were mild, reversible, and short-term psychomimetic effects (Jouguelet-Lacoste et al., 2015). In a systematic review of the use of subanesthetic doses of ketamine with opioids in pain treatment plans, ketamine reduced opioid requirements and opioid adverse effects, and no additional adverse effects were attributed to ketamine (Wang et al., 2016).

The most commonly reported adverse effects of subanesthetic doses of ketamine used in the treatment of acute pain are nausea, vomiting, vivid dreams, or hallucinations; in rare cases, dissociative effects have been reported (Schwenk et al., 2018). These side effects can be mitigated with administration of a benzodiazepine or cloNIDine but not antipsychotics (Cohen et al., 2018; Schwenk et al., 2018). Other approaches include reducing the dose or slowing the titration of ketamine (Niesters et al., 2014).

Ketamine use may be associated with cardiac stimulatory effects such as tachycardia, hypertension, and arrhythmias. If cardiovascular side effects occur, dose reduction is recommended (Cohen et al., 2018; Niesters et al., 2014). Ketamine may be associated with hepatotoxicity, which is most commonly manifested as elevations in alanine transaminase, alkaline phosphatase, aspartate transaminase, and γ-glutamyl transferase. The mechanism involved is not fully elucidated. Repeated doses in short periods of time tend to increase risk for hepatic injury. Usually, liver enzymes return back to normal within 3 months (Niesters et al., 2014). Ketamine-associated lower urinary tract dysfunction (bladder pain syndrome and interstitial cystitis) has been associated with chronic repetitive use of ketamine, with most cases reported in those who abuse illicit ketamine (Bredlau et al., 2013; Myers, Bluth, & Cheung, 2016). It is a complex and not well-understood complication that has the potential to cause severe urinary tract destruction (Myers et al., 2016). In some cases, symptoms improve with cessation of ketamine use (Radvansky et al., 2015).

As ketamine has been shown to reduce opioid requirements, it is recommended to reduce opioid doses to reduce opioid-related adverse effects, such as excessive sedation and respiratory depression. Opioid doses are reduced by some practitioners by 25% to 50% when parenteral ketamine is initiated (Quibell et al., 2015). Opioids are titrated based on responses. Further reductions are necessary if excessive sedation or other opioid-related adverse effects develop. It is also important to identify and manage opioid withdrawal if signs and symptoms are noted.

Monitoring of Patients

The monitoring of patients on ketamine includes assessment of pain, sedation, and other CNS side effects. Patients are also assessed for hemodynamic changes by monitoring of vital signs in vulnerable patients or for those on prolonged ketamine therapy, and liver function is assessed through periodic measurement of LFTs. Monitoring parameters differ based on the patient's condition and indication for ketamine use. Examples of ketamine monitoring protocols are shown in Table 15.13.

Magnesium

Magnesium has received research and clinical interest for use in multimodal pain treatment plans because it has been found to provide analgesia in acute postoperative pain and neuropathic pain (Castro & Cooney, 2017; Srebro et al., 2017).

Mechanism of Action

Magnesium binds to NMDA receptors and blocks the release of glutamate and aspartate, thereby altering the perception and duration of pain (De Oliveira, Castro-Alves, Khan, & McCarthy, 2013; Guo et al., 2015; Yousef & Al-deeb, 2013). In addition, magnesium binds to and inhibits calcium channels and modulates potassium channels (Srebro et al., 2017). The mechanism of action in the treatment of migraines is unclear (Chiu, Yeh, Huang, & Chen, 2016). Magnesium may increase opioid effectiveness in neuropathic and inflammatory chronic pain models associated with sensitization and NMDA receptor activity (Bujalska-Zadrożny, Tatarkiewicz, Kulik, Filip, & Naruszewicz, 2017).

Indications and Uses

Intravenous magnesium has been used in a variety of pain conditions as efforts are made to optimize multimodal and opioid-sparing analgesic approaches to various pain conditions. Intravenous magnesium administration intraoperatively, postoperatively, and in nonsurgical pain conditions has gained interest as an analgesic option. It is difficult and premature to draw conclusions about the effectiveness of this modality because many studies are in progress with unpublished data, and published studies have used heterogeneous doses, timing (intraoperative or postoperative), administration techniques, and routes. The literature related to the use of magnesium as analgesic intervention is currently sparse but increasing.

Several systematic reviews or meta-analyses examined the efficacy of intravenous magnesium as an analgesic intervention and described reduction in pain scores and opioid doses. In a meta-analysis of 25 studies that included patients who underwent abdominal surgery (48%), hysterectomy (24%), or orthopedic surgery (24%), intravenous magnesium, administered perioperatively by bolus injection and/or continuous infusion, was compared to placebo (Albrecht, Kirkham, Liu, & Brull, 2013). Perioperative magnesium reduced intravenous morphine consumption by 24% at 24 hours after surgery ($p < .00001$) and significantly reduced numerical pain scores at rest ($p < .0001$) and movement ($p = .009$); there was no significant difference in time to first request for an analgesic or incidence of postoperative nausea or vomiting or pruritus (Albrecht et al., 2013). In another meta-analysis of 20 RCTS with 1257 participants in which intravenous magnesium was administered intraoperatively or postoperatively to patients during a variety of surgical procedures, opioid use was significantly reduced in the magnesium group compared to placebo, and pain scores at rest and movement were reduced during the first 24 postoperative hours (De Oliveira et al., 2013). In a systematic review of

Table 15.13 | Ketamine Patient Monitoring Parameters Examples

	Heart Rate	Blood Pressure	Respiratory Rate
Fitzgibbon, 2005	• Monitor 30 min after initial dose and each dose increase • Subsequent monitoring every 4 h or as clinically required	• Monitor 30 min after initial dose and each dose increase • Subsequent monitoring as clinically required	• Monitor 30 min after initial dose and each dose increase
National Health Service of Scotland, 2013	• Check baseline pulse • Check 1 h after first dose • Check 24 h after first dose • Check daily • If pulse increases to ≥20 beats/min above baseline or >100 beats/min, inform provider	• Check baseline BP • Check 1 h after first dose • Check 24 h after first dose • Check daily • If BP increases ≥20 mm Hg above baseline, notify provider	• If RR decreases to 10 breaths/min, inform provider

BP, Blood pressure; *RR*, respiratory rate.
Fitzgibbon, E. J., & Viola, R. (2005). Parenteral ketamine as an analgesic adjuvant for severe pain: Development and retrospective audit of a protocol for a palliative care unit. *Journal of Palliative Medicine, 8*(1), 49–57. https://doi.org/10.1089/jpm.2005.8.49; and National Health Service of Scotland. (2014). Scotland palliative care guidelines: Ketamine. Retrieved from http://www.palliativecareguidelines.scot.nhs.uk/guidelines/medicine-information-sheets/ketamine.aspx. Accessed 7/7/2020.

27 RCTs that involved 1504 patients, the use of intravenous magnesium compared to placebo during general anesthesia significantly reduced postoperative pain in patients who had undergone urogenital, orthopedic, and cardiovascular surgeries without an increase in adverse effects; similar response was not seen in GI surgery (Guo et al., 2015). Guo et al. identified the need for caution in interpretation of results because magnesium doses and duration of administration varied among the studies, and an additional 18 RCTs were identified that did not yet have published data (Guo et al., 2015).

The effect of intraoperative magnesium, administered by an intravenous bolus dose followed by an infusion, was examined in an RCT of 32 participants who underwent major GI surgery. Postoperative morphine consumption, severe pain ratings, and duration of postoperative ileus were lower in the magnesium group than the placebo group (Moharari et al., 2014). In an RCT that compared the effect of intraoperative magnesium infusions (n = 22) and saline infusions (n = 22) on postoperative pain in patients who underwent staged bilateral total knee replacements, postoperative pain scores, use of PCA, and rescue analgesia were examined during the initial 48 postoperative hours and compared between the two groups and within each group between the two arthroplasties (Shin et al., 2016). In the saline group, postoperative pain scores were significantly higher after the second knee arthroplasty than the first, while in the magnesium group, there was no difference in postoperative pain scores between the first arthroplasty and the second. The magnesium group had significantly reduced use of rescue analgesics and fentanyl in the 48 hours after surgery (Shin et al., 2016).

Magnesium has been examined in other pain states. One pilot study of 10 patients with CRPS type 1 (CRPS-1) described significant improvements in pain, impairment, and quality of life when given intravenous magnesium (Collins, Zuurmond, de Lange, van Hilten, & Perez, 2009). However, Fischer et al. (2013), in a subsequent RCT of 56 patients with CRPS-1 who received intravenous magnesium using doses similar to those in the study by Collins et al. (2009), found no additional benefit of magnesium infusion compared to placebo. The investigators noted results of their study indicated intravenous magnesium may be beneficial if used in patients with shorter duration of CRPS or those with severe sensitization (Fischer et al., 2013). Magnesium has been shown to be effective in the treatment of acute migraine attacks at 15 to 45 minutes, 120 minutes, and 24 hours after the start of the migraine and by the oral route for migraine prophylaxis (Chiu et al., 2016).

Five randomized, placebo-controlled studies involving 386 participants admitted for acute pain crisis from sickle cell disease comparing intravenous magnesium to placebo were included in a Cochrane review. There were no significant differences in groups in pain scores, hospital length of stay, or pediatric quality of life scores (Than, Soe, Palaniappan, Abas, & De Franceschi, 2017).

Dosing and Routes

In the setting of postoperative pain, there is a wide array of doses and duration of treatment. Most often an intravenous bolus of magnesium of 30 to 50 mg/kg is given, followed by 6 to 25 mg/kg continuous infusion for the duration of the surgery or up to 24 hours with total doses ranging from 1.03 to 18.2 g (Albrecht et al., 2013; De Oliveira et al., 2013).

To treat acute migraine, there were a range of doses used, from magnesium sulfate 1 to 2 g IV given over 10 to 20 minutes or 32 mg of magnesium chloride–adenosine disodium triphosphate given over 1 to 1.5 hours. Doses of magnesium for migraine prophylaxis range from 102 to 800 mg/day PO (Chiu et al., 2016).

Doses of magnesium used in a pilot study to treat CRPS were 70 mg/kg magnesium sulfate continuous infusion for 4 hours for 4 days (Collins et al., 2009) or 5 days (Fischer et al., 2013). Patients receiving magnesium for refractory low back pain with a neuropathic component were given magnesium sulfate 1 g IV over 4 hours daily for 2 weeks followed by 400 mg of magnesium oxide PO and 1000 mg of magnesium gluconate PO bid for 4 weeks (De Oliveira et al., 2013).

Adverse Effects

Magnesium is generally well tolerated. Some studies have shown bradycardia, hypotension, or sedation with its use (Albrecht et al., 2013). Flushing and dizziness have been reported during and for up to 4 hours after the intravenous infusion (Fischer et al., 2013). Oral magnesium has led to diarrhea (De Oliveira et al., 2013).

Monitoring of Patients

Monitoring for patients after the administration of magnesium includes measurement of magnesium levels, vital signs, pain assessment, and assessment of other side effects.

Sodium Channel Blockers: Lidocaine and Mexiletine

Lidocaine and mexiletine are sodium channel blocker antiarrhythmic medications that are receiving interest as coanalgesics for use in acute and chronic pain conditions.

Lidocaine

Mechanism of Action

Lidocaine is classified as an anesthetic and is a prototypical class 1b antiarrhythmic (Beaussier, Delbos, Maurice-Szamburski, Ecoffey, & Mercadal, 2018). The primary mechanism of action is through nonselective inhibition of voltage-gated sodium channels leading to a reduction in neuronal pain transmission (Beaussier et al., 2018; Gibbons et al., 2016). It is theorized that sodium channels are upregulated in neuropathic pain states, which may explain its particular benefit in treating neuropathic pain

(Hutson et al., 2015). There are several other proposed mechanisms of action for lidocaine, including blocking NMDA receptors, blocking capsaicin-sensitive afferents, blocking substance P and bradykinin, interacting with glycine receptors in the spinal cord, and altering levels of proinflammatory neurotransmitters (Estebe, 2017; Gibbons et al., 2016).

The mechanism of action of mexiletine is the same as the mechanism described for lidocaine. Mexiletine blocks sodium channels, which leads to a reduction in neuronal signaling, contributing to reduced pain transmission (Dibj-Hajj, Black, & Waxman, 2009).

Indications and Uses

Lidocaine is administered by various routes as an analgesic medication. In this section, the use of intravenous lidocaine in pain management is described; Chapter 16 describes the use of lidocaine as a topical analgesic, and the use of lidocaine in interventional pain management is described in Chapter 18. Intravenous lidocaine has been studied in a variety of pain conditions, including neuropathic pain and perioperative pain (Van der Wal et al., 2016).

Lidocaine has been studied in neuropathic pain conditions such as diabetic neuropathy and PHN (Hutson et al., 2015; Kosharskyy, Almonte, & Shaparin, 2013). Additionally, it has been shown to be beneficial in central pain, SCI, fibromyalgia, painful symptoms associated with multiple sclerosis, and CRPS (Hutson et al., 2015). It has also been used in the treatment of chronic migraine, chronic daily headaches, and medication overuse headaches (Marmura & Goldberg, 2015). Lidocaine has also shown positive outcomes in reducing pain and opioid-analgesic requirements in the treatment of opioid-refractory cancer pain in adult and pediatric patients (Gibbons et al., 2016; Kintzel, Knol, & Roe, 2018; Peixoto & Hawley, 2015).

In the postoperative setting, systematic reviews and/or meta-analyses have shown that lidocaine has been associated with reducing postoperative pain, opioid requirement, opioid-related side effects, and hospital stay and improving patient rehabilitation (Kranke et al., 2015; Marrett, Rolin, Beaussier, & Bonnet, 2008; McCleane, 2007; Vigneault et al., 2011; Zhao et al., 2018). In a meta-analysis of six RCTs in which intravenous lidocaine (n = 178) was compared to placebo (n = 176) in postoperative patients who had undergone laparoscopic cholecystectomies, patients in the lidocaine group had significant reductions in postoperative pain at 12 hours ($p = .014$) and 24 hours ($p = .015$) after surgery (Zhao et al., 2018). Opioid consumption was also significantly lowered at 12 hours ($p = .005$) and 24 hours ($p = .009$) after surgery.

In a Cochrane review that included 68 trials with 4525 randomized participants, the authors were unable to conclude that intravenous lidocaine was beneficial in reducing pain or opioid consumption, because the quality of evidence was limited by poor quality of the studies, imprecise study data, and inconsistencies (Weibel et al., 2018).

Intravenous lidocaine has been a treatment option that has gained interest in the setting of emergency medicine. Intravenous lidocaine was compared to intravenous morphine in patients presenting to the emergency department with renal colic. Lidocaine was shown to significantly reduce pain 5 minutes, 10 minutes, 15 minutes, and 30 minutes after injection (Soleimanpour et al., 2012). A systematic review of the safety and efficacy of intravenous lidocaine examined its use in the treatment of adult patients with acute and chronic pain (e Silva et al., 2018). In six RCTs and two active control studies involving 536 patients, intravenous lidocaine provided pain score reductions similar to that provide by morphine in renal colic and acute, critical limb ischemia; it was not found to be effective in migraine headache relief (e Silva et al., 2018).

Dosing and Routes

Lidocaine undergoes significant first-pass metabolism. Thus it has limited oral bioavailability, preventing the use of oral administration (Sim, 2015). Lidocaine is used topically but will be discussed in Chapter 16. There are a variety of dosing protocols and durations of treatment in the literature. See Table 15.14 for examples of lidocaine dosing practices.

Adverse Effects

The side effects of lidocaine are dose related (Estebe, 2017) and when used at recommended doses are rare (Dunn & Durieux, 2017). Side effects that may occur when lidocaine levels are elevated include perioral numbness, metallic taste, drowsiness, sedation, light-headedness, relaxation, and euphoria (Eipe, Gupta, & Penning, 2016). Toxicity is associated with plasma concentrations greater than 5 mcg/mL. When plasma levels reach the toxicity level, CNS symptoms may develop (Eipe et al., 2016). These symptoms include visual changes, dizziness, lightheadedness, headache, paresthesias, changes in level of consciousness, respiratory depression, and seizures (Aronson, 2016a). Cardiac symptoms of lidocaine toxicity are rarer and are associated with serum levels exceeding 10 mcg/mL (Eipe et al., 2016). Allergic reactions to lidocaine are rare and when they occur, are usually mild (Aronson, 2016a).

Monitoring of Patients

Some studies use therapeutic levels to assist with dosing while others use lidocaine levels to monitor for side effects. Therapeutic plasma levels of lidocaine range from 2.5 to 3.5 mcg/mL with toxicity occurring when levels exceed 5 mcg/mL (Eipe et al., 2016).

Because of the concerns with cardiovascular side effects, baseline and periodic monitoring of vital signs and ECG are common (Gibbons et al., 2016). However, clinical studies have shown intravenous lidocaine can be safely administered with close observation and vital sign monitoring and ECG monitoring may be unnecessary (Eipe et al., 2016; Peixoto & Hawley, 2015). CNS signs

Table 15.14 | Intravenous Lidocaine Dosing

Study	Pain Type	Initial dose	Titrations	Max Dose	Duration of Infusion	Frequency of Infusions
Gibbons, et al., 2016	Opioid-refractory cancer pain	Median: 30 mcg/kg/min	Not reported	36 mcg/kg/min	2.15 days (median)	Not reported
Schwartzman, 2009	Refractory complex regional pain syndrome (CRPS)	60.4 mg/h	Daily titrations if lidocaine blood level <5 mg/L	168 mg/h	5 days	One-time infusion
Peixoto & Hawley, 2015	Cancer pain	5 mg/kg over 1 h	2 mg/kg	10 mg/kg	Not reported	Not reported
Hutson, et al., 2015	Neuropathic pain	16.7 mg/min over 30 min	Individualized	500 mg	Not reported	19.4 days
Marmura, et al., 2008b	Refractory headache	1 mg/min for 4 h	Individualized	4 mg/min	8.5 days (average)	Not reported

Gibbons, K., DeMonbrun, A., Beckman, E. J., Keefer, P., Wagner, D., Stewart, M., . . . Niedner, M. (2016). Continuous lidocaine infusions to manage opioid-refractory pain in a series of pediatric cancer patients. *Pediatric Blood Cancer, 63*, 1168–1174. https://doi.org/10.1002/pbc.25870; Hutson, P., Backonja, M., & Knurr, H. (2015). Intravenous lidocaine for neuropathic pain: A retrospective analysis of tolerability and efficacy. *Pain Medicine, 16*, 531–536; Marmura, M. J., Rosen, N., Abbas, M., & Silberstein, S. (2008b). Intravenous lidocaine in the treatment of refractory headache. *Headache, 49*, 286–291. https://doi.org/10.1111/j.1526-4610.2008.01281.x; Peixoto, R. D., & Hawley, P. (2015). Intravenous lidocaine for cancer pain without electrocardiographic monitoring: a retrospective review. *Journal of Palliative Medicine, 18*(4), 373–377. https://doi.org/10.1089/jpm.2014.0279; and Schwartzman, R. J., Patel, M., Grothusen, J. R., & Alexander, G. M. (2009a). Efficacy of 5 day continuous lidocaine infusion for the treatment of refractory complex regional pain syndrome. *Pain Medicine, 10*(2), 401–412. https://doi.org/10.1111/j.1526-4637.2009.00573.x.

of toxicity usually occur before cardiac toxicity; therefore adverse signs are recognized before ECG changes would develop. In some palliative care settings, ECG monitoring has been forgone (Peixoto & Hawley, 2015).

Dose adjustments may be needed with renal or hepatic impairment because 90% of lidocaine undergoes significant CYP3A4 hepatic metabolism and is partially excreted via the kidneys (Estebe, 2017). Thus monitoring of LFTs and creatinine clearance may be helpful.

During lidocaine infusions, it is important to observe for possible drug-drug interactions. Coadministration of lidocaine with intravenous ketamine has the potential to impair cognitive function, although coadministration of these medications may prevent lidocaine-induced seizures (Estebe, 2017). Administration of intravenous lidocaine during general anesthesia may result in increased lidocaine levels (Estebe, 2017).

Mexiletine

Indications and Uses

Mexiletine is classified as a local anesthetic and a class 1B antiarrhythmic agent. It is similar in structure to lidocaine but has the benefit that it can be used by the oral route. FDA-approved indications for mexiletine include the treatment of documented ventricular arrhythmias. Mexiletine is contraindicated in patients with cardiogenic shock or with second- or third-degree atrioventricular block without a pacemaker (Watson Laboratories, 2006).

In a 2009 overview of guidelines related to treatment of neuropathic pain, it was listed as a fourth-line treatment option (O'Connor & Dworkin, 2009).

Mexiletine has been studied in numerous neuropathic pain states; however, data related to its effectiveness are mixed. It has been used as a coanalgesic medication in multimodal treatment of neuropathic pain, fibromyalgia, and headache, but is not often prescribed for these indications (Romman, Salama-Hanna, & Dwivedi, 2018). In a retrospective cohort study of 74 patients in chronic pain clinics who had received at least one mexiletine prescription in the preceding year, neuropathic pain (64%), which included diabetic neuropathy and radiculopathy, and fibromyalgia (28%) were the most common indications; efficacy and outcomes were not examined (Romman et al., 2018). The researchers noted mexiletine was rarely used as a first-line treatment option but was used when multiple other modalities were ineffective. A review of sodium channel blockers used in the treatment of neuropathic pain listed five clinical studies that yielded positive effects of mexiletine in RCTs that involved DPN, nerve injury, and neuropathy, but four RCTS that did not demonstrate significant benefit in DPN and SCI (Bhattacharya, Wickenden, & Chaplan, 2009). Many of these studies involved small numbers of participants, thus limiting the power of the studies (Bhattacharya et al., 2009). One double-blind, placebo-controlled study in 29 patients with DPN did not show any statistically significant changes in pain scores between mexiletine 600 mg/day and placebo; no statistically significant difference in adverse effects was noted between the groups (Wright, Oki, & Graves, 1997).

Another double-blind, placebo-controlled study of 11 subjects with peripheral nerve injury or dysfunction showed statistically significant reductions in pain with mexiletine 750 mg/day compared to placebo, with mild adverse effects (Chabal, Jacobson, Mariano, Chaney, & Britell, 1992). There is a lack of strong evidence supporting the efficacy and safety of mexiletine as an analgesic, but the limited number of studies have focused its use on the treatment of neuropathic pain. In clinical practice, when used, it is reserved for treatment of refractory neuropathic pain.

Dosing and Routes

Compared to lidocaine, mexiletine has limited first-pass metabolism and systemic absorption of around 90%, allowing oral administration of the medication (Marmura, 2010). Typical dosing for mexiletine is 200 mg PO tid (Watson Laboratories, 2006). The dose can be titrated up to a maximum of 1200 mg/day (Marmura, 2010; Marmura et al., 2008a).

Adverse Effects

The most common side effects of mexiletine include nausea, vomiting, and heartburn, which may occur in nearly 40% of patients and is ameliorated with taking the medication with food. Dizziness, lightheadedness, paresthesias, tremor or nervousness, coordination issues, palpitations, chest pain, changes in sleep, headache, and blurred vision are fairly common. Mexiletine can worsen arrhythmias (Marmura, 2010; Haroutounian & Finnerup, 2018; Watson Laboratories, 2006).

There are several rare but concerning possible side effects. A rare consequence of mexiletine treatment is hepatotoxicity. Liver enzyme elevation occurs in 1% to 2% of patients treated with mexiletine (Haroutounian & Finnerup, 2018). If significant elevations in LFTs occur, discontinuing mexiletine may be necessary. Blood dyscrasias such as leukopenia and agranulocytosis have occurred (Haroutounian & Finnerup, 2018). However, patients had comorbid conditions or were taking other medications associated with blood dyscrasias. If there are significant changes in blood counts, mexiletine should be discontinued (Watson Laboratories, 2006).

Monitoring of Patients

To monitor for adverse reactions, check LFTs and complete blood count periodically. An ECG before and during treatment is also recommended (Watson Laboratories, 2006). Therapeutic levels of mexiletine are 0.5 to 2 mcg/mL, with levels exceeding 2 mcg/mL leading to toxicity (Marmura, 2010).

Muscle Relaxants

The group of medications known as muscle relaxants are a heterogeneous group of medications that have different chemical structures and mechanisms of action. There is a lack of research comparing the efficacy of muscle relaxants as coanalgesic medications, and available evidence is derived from studies of variable quality. Although these medications are classified as muscle relaxants, evidence of their ability to actually relax muscle is lacking, and their analgesic effects may be nonspecific. There are two major groups of muscle relaxants; one group is used to treat spasticity from upper motor neuron syndromes such as SCI and cerebral palsy (baclofen and dantrolene); the other group of muscle relaxants is used to treat skeletal muscle spasms, which are often associated with pain (cyclobenzaprine, metaxalone, methocarbamol, orphenadrine, carisoprodol); and other medications (diazePAM and tiZANidine) are used for both antispasticity and antispasmodic effects (Cohen & Warfield, 2015; Witenko et al., 2014). Table 15.15 summarizes several muscle relaxants.

Baclofen for Spasticity From Upper Motor Neuron Syndromes

Mechanism of Action

Baclofen is a GABA-receptor agonist that works mainly through inhibition of nociceptive transmission at the level of the dorsal horn through activation of $GABA_B$ receptors. $GABA_B$ receptor activation results in inhibition of calcium channel activity and inhibition of the release of excitatory neurotransmitters such as substance P and glutamate (Malcangio, 2018). Baclofen provides analgesia through a pathway independent from the opioid system.

Indications and Uses

A primary indication for the use of baclofen is in the treatment of spasticity of spinal origin such as in SCI and cerebral palsy. When used for spinal spasticity, it is most effective when administered intrathecally, and implanted intrathecal infusion pumps are used for long-term baclofen therapy. Intrathecal baclofen is also used as an analgesic for chronic pain associated with SCI-related spasticity and in oral or intrathecal formulations for the treatment of neuropathic pain that is refractory to other treatment options (Malcangio, 2018). Two small studies have supported the efficacy of oral baclofen in the treatment of pain associated with trigeminal neuralgia (Di Stefano, Truini, & Cruccu, 2018). In a Cochrane review of the treatment of trigeminal neuralgia, there is consensus that baclofen may have efficacy in the treatment of patients with multiple sclerosis who develop trigeminal neuralgia, but no RCTs were identified to support its use in the general treatment of trigeminal neuralgia (Zakrzewska & Linskey, 2014). Baclofen also has been used as a treatment option in the management of pain associated with dystonia in CRPS (Williams, Guarino, & Raja, 2018). In animal studies, it has shown antihyperalgesic benefits in cancer-related bone pain (Zhou et al., 2017).

Table 15.15 | Skeletal Muscle Relaxants

Medication	Indication	Common Oral Dosage	Metabolism	Adverse Effects	Comments
Antispasticity					
Baclofen (Lioresal)	Spasticity	5 mg bid to tid, max 80 mg/day (use lowest effective dose)	Hepatic (15%)	CNS depression	**Black box warning:** Avoid abrupt discontinuation due to risk of withdrawal Avoid CrCl <30 mL/min
Dantrolene (Dantrium)	Spasticity (also used intravenously for malignant hyperthermia)	Initial: 25 mg/day Maintenance: 25–100 mg up to 4 times/day	Hepatic (extensive) CYP3A4	Major hepatic impairment, hepatitis, CNS depression, difficulty swallowing	**Black Box warning:** Oral dantrolene carries potential for hepatotoxicity, including overt hepatitis Not recommended for routine use; has a direct inhibitory effect on skeletal muscle and no CNS effect Discontinue if no benefit within 45 days
Antispasmodic Agents					
Carisoprodol (Soma)	Acute musculoskeletal pain No longer recommended because of potential for abuse/addiction	250–350 mg tid and at bedtime, max 1400 mg/day *Liver disease:* Use lower initial dose and increase gradually as needed/tolerated	Hepatic (2C19) Active metabolite: Meprobamate	Drowsiness, dizziness, headaches, somnolence, seizure Respiratory depression, especially when used with other CNS depressants Idiosyncratic allergic reactions	**Schedule IV** Beers Criteria Abuse, addiction, withdrawal potential; controlled medication Avoid use
Chlorzoxazone (Parafon Forte DSC)	Acute musculoskeletal pain	375–750 mg tid-qid, max	Hepatic (glucuronidation)	CNS depression; rare but serious idiosyncratic and unpredictable hepatotoxicity	Beers Criteria Periodic LFTs during chronic use
Cyclobenzaprine (Amrix)	Acute musculoskeletal pain	IR: 5 mg tid, max 10 mg tid ER: 15 mg/day, max 30 mg/day	Hepatic (CYP3A4, CYP1A2, CYP2D6)	Anticholinergic effects, CNS depression, rare arrhythmias	Beers Criteria Use with caution with elderly and with liver disease Similar structure to that of TCAs Limit use to 2–3 weeks and do not use within 14 days of MAOIs
Metaxalone (Skelaxin)	Acute musculoskeletal pain	800 mg tid to qid	Hepatic (CYP1A2. 2D6, 2E1, 3A4)	CNS depression, nausea, vomiting Rare: Jaundice, hemolytic anemia, elevated LFTs	Beers Criteria Sedating Take with food Contraindicated in severe hepatic and renal dysfunction Monitor liver function in mild to moderate liver dysfunction

Continued

Table 15.15 | Skeletal Muscle Relaxants—cont'd

Medication	Indication	Common Oral Dosage	Metabolism	Adverse Effects	Comments
Methocarbamol (Robaxin)	Acute musculoskeletal pain	*Initial: (oral)* 1500 mg qid for 2–3 days *Maintenance:* 750 mg qid, 1500 mg tid, or 1000 mg qid, max 4 g/day Lower initial doses and gradual increases as tolerated in older adults and liver and renal impairment	Conjugation, dealkylation, and hydroxylation	Dizziness, headache, lightheadedness	Beers Criteria May be associated with CNS depression May turn urine brown, black, or green Available for intravenous (and intramuscular administration, which should be avoided because of injection pain) Parenteral dose maximum 1g every 8 hours, not to exceed 3 days; may be repeated after a drug-free interval of 48 h
Orphenadrine (Norflex)	Acute musculoskeletal pain	100 mg bid	Hepatic (extensive)	Anticholinergic effects	Beers criteria Use cautiously with heart failure Do not crush Parenteral dose 60 mg IV (or IM) every 12 h Euphoric and analgesic properties Taper with chronic use Avoid with GI obstruction or ulcers

Antispasticity and Antispasmodic Agents

Medication	Indication	Common Oral Dosage	Metabolism	Adverse Effects	Comments
DiazePAM (Valium)	Relief of skeletal muscle spasm	2–10 mg tid to qid, maximum dose 40 mg/day Hepatic disease: Decrease by 50% Older adults: 2–2.5 mg/day to bid, slow titration	Hepatic (2C19, 3A4)	Drowsiness, fatigue, ataxia Abuse potential Withdrawal with abrupt cessation	Schedule IV Beers Criteria Long elimination half-life 20–50 h, active metabolites up to 100 h Available for intravenous and intramuscular administration, which should be avoided because of injection pain Taper after extended therapy
TiZANidine (Zanaflex)	Spasticity	Initial: 2–4 mg up to 3 times/day; may titrate to optimal effect in 2- to 4-mg increments as needed to a max of three doses (24 mg) in 24 h	Hepatic (1A2)	Somnolence, xerostomia, and weakness	Older adults: Use with caution because of reduced clearance Monitor effect on blood pressure May cause additive sedation if used with other psychotropic medications Contraindicated with ciprofloxacin and fluvoxamine Renal: Use with caution if CrCl <25mL/min; hepatic, avoid use in severe impairment; monitor liver function; avoid rapid discontinuation

CNS, Central nervous system; *CrCl,* creatinine clearance rate; *ER,* extended release; *IR,* immediate release; *LFT,* liver function test; *MAOIs,* monoamine oxidase inhibitors; *Max,* maximum; *TCAs,* tricyclic antidepressants.
Modified from Witenko et al., 2014.

Dosing and Routes

Oral baclofen is usually initiated at 5 mg bid to tid and titrated up to doses as high as 80 mg/day in divided doses (Aronson, 2016b; Drugs@FDA: Ozobax™, 2019). Side effects often limit upward dose titration. Baclofen is very hydrophilic and has limited penetration across the blood-brain barrier. Intrathecal administration is often used because oral doses may not be effective or may be limited by side effects (Dinakar, 2016). A single intrathecal bolus dose of baclofen 50 to 100 mcg may be administered as a test dose to assess benefits (Drugs@FDA: LioresalR Intrathecal, 2011). The dose of intrathecal baclofen administered through implanted pumps is titrated to achieve optimal effects with minimal side effects. The use of baclofen in an implanted intrathecal pump is further discussed in Chapter 19. There is interest in the use of baclofen as a topical medication for the treatment of localized neuropathic pain. It is more commonly used in topical preparations compounded as a cream and combined with other medications, as described in Chapter 16, but two case reports of baclofen as a single compounded topical medication for the treatment of neuropathic pain have been published (Casale, Symeonidou, & Bartolo, 2017).

Adverse Effects

The most commonly reported side effects associated with baclofen use are drowsiness, dizziness, fatigue, nausea, confusion, and hypotension (Aronson, 2016b). Alteration in mental status is a major adverse effect, and other CNS effects such as seizures and abnormal movements are possible. The intrathecal route is often preferred to reduce the risks for systemic adverse effects. However, adverse effects may be associated with intrathecal implantation surgery, misprogramming, or pump malfunction (Jamison, Cohen, & Rosenow, 2018). One of the most serious and potentially life-threatening effects associated with the use of baclofen is withdrawal that results from a decline in CNS levels of baclofen over a short period. Abrupt discontinuation of intrathecal baclofen can result in hallucinations, altered mental state, psychosis, tonic-clonic seizures, neuroleptic malignant-like syndrome, increased spasticity, and hyperthermia (Alvis & Sobey, 2017; Aronson, 2016b). Case reports of withdrawal associated with sudden cessation of oral baclofen also have been reported (Alvis & Sobey, 2017; Nasti & Brakoulias, 2011). Withdrawal is treated with replacement of baclofen; if intrathecal delivery is interrupted, oral baclofen is initiated, but doses may not be adequate and there is no consistent oral-to-intrathecal conversion rate (Jamison et al., 2018). Benzodiazepines, dantrolene, skeletal muscle relaxants, and tiZANidine have been used to treat baclofen withdrawal (Saulino, 2018). Baclofen overdose can lead to altered mental status, including somnolence and confusion, severe hypotonia, respiratory depression, apnea, arrhythmias, hypothermia, hypotension, and coma (Aronson, 2016b). Treatment of overdose requires cessation of baclofen administration and emergency respiratory and cardiac support; physostigmine and flumazenil have been used to reduce CNS effects (Saulino, 2018).

Monitoring of Patients

Patients receiving baclofen are monitored for efficacy in addressing the indication for which baclofen is prescribed. Patients are also monitored for side effects. Dose adjustments are made based on efficacy and development of adverse effects. It is particularly important to assess for signs and symptoms of baclofen withdrawal if a patient is unable to take oral medication because of interruption in enteral medications or if there is an interference or disruption in intrathecal baclofen delivery. Intrathecal baclofen is briefly addressed in Chapter 19.

Skeletal Muscle Relaxants for Muscular Pain and Spasms From Musculoskeletal Conditions

Skeletal muscle relaxants are often used for the treatment of muscular pain and spasms arising from peripheral musculoskeletal conditions such as mechanical low back pain, neck pain, and myofascial pain, although high-quality evidence is lacking. This group of medications includes antihistamines (orphenadrine), tricyclic compounds that are structurally similar to TCAs (cyclobenzaprine), benzodiazepines (diazePAM), and other types of medications such as carisoprodol, methocarbamol, and metaxalone. Often, after 1 to 2 weeks of use, the effects of skeletal muscle relaxants become more central rather than peripheral; therefore it is preferred that they be used for short periods to minimize the potential for abuse of these medications (Herndon et al., 2016).

There are few head-to-head studies comparing the skeletal muscle relaxants. Limited research has compared the efficacy of muscle relaxants to that of NSAIDS or acetaminophen. In a prospective observational study of 300 patients with low back pain, researchers reported that those who received a combination of skeletal muscle relaxants with NSAIDs had better analgesia than those who received NSAIDs alone or NSAIDs or muscle relaxants with other coanalgesics (Patel et al., 2015). When skeletal muscle relaxants are indicated, factors such as duration and severity of symptoms, previous response to medications, side effect profiles of individual medications, comorbidities, cost, and treatment goals, and other factors are considered in medication selection (Witenko et al., 2014).

In the early 2000s, cyclobenzaprine, carisoprodol, and metaxalone were the most frequently prescribed muscle relaxants in the United States. Carisoprodol is a muscle relaxant that has a metabolite known as meprobamate. Meprobamate is a barbiturate prescribed several decades ago as an anxiolytic that fell out of favor because of its abuse potential, adverse effect profile, and availability of benzodiazepines (James, Nicholson, Hill, & Bearn, 2016; Kumar & Dillon, 2015). Carisoprodol accounted for 21% of all prescribed muscle relaxants in 2000. More recently, carisoprodol has been shown to have addictive properties and abuse potential; it has been associated with unintended psychological effects and may result in a severe withdrawal syndrome (Kumar & Dillon, 2015). As a result of recognition of its abuse potential, carisoprodol was designated as a controlled substance (schedule IV) at the federal level (Cohen & Warfield, 2015).

Mechanism of Action

The skeletal muscle relaxants are a heterogenous group with different mechanisms of action, and the exact mechanism of action for the various medications is not completely understood (Jackson, Argoff, & Dubin, 2014). Most of these medications decrease muscle spasms through changes in conduction within the dorsal horn through a variety of mechanisms and therefore have an indirect effect on relaxation of muscle tissue (Jackson et al., 2014). Benzodiazepines inhibit transmission on the GABA neurons while the nonbenzodiazepine medications inhibit impulse transmission in the brainstem and spinal cord (Witenko et al., 2014).

Indications and Uses for Skeletal Muscle Relaxants for Peripheral Conditions

Skeletal muscle relaxants are used to treat acute and chronic pain associated with a variety of skeletal muscle conditions. They are frequently used in the treatment of low back pain, although there is limited evidence of efficacy and concerns for adverse effects and diversion (Abdel Shaheed, Maher, Williams, & McLachlan, 2017). A systematic review and meta-analysis of the efficacy and tolerability of muscle relaxant use for low back pain was published by Abdel Shaheed et al. in 2017. This review of 15 trials with 3362 participants included 5 trials (n = 496) with high-quality evidence that muscle relaxants offer clinically significant analgesia when used over the short term for acute low back pain. Evidence for outcomes of long-term use was lacking, and efficacy for use in chronic pain is not known (Abdel Shaheed et al., 2017). Of note, there was no evidence to support the use of benzodiazepines in the treatment of low back pain.

In a review that included treatment of neck pain, Cohen (2015) identified two large RCTs (n = 1405) that demonstrated cyclobenzaprine at 15 or 30 mg/day is more effective than placebo in alleviating acute neck pain. It was also recommended to avoid use of benzodiazepines because they fail to demonstrate greater efficacy than other muscle relaxants and are associated with potential for abuse. The review included a recommendation for limitation of benzodiazepine use to situations in which other muscle relaxants are ineffective and for use only with clearly defined goals, time frames, and adequate monitoring (Cohen, 2015).

Skeletal muscle relaxants such as methocarbamol have received research interest because they are sometimes included in the MMA plan for patients who have pain associated with traumatic rib fractures. In a retrospective cohort study of 592 patients with closed traumatic rib fractures, those who received methocarbamol (n = 329) had an average of a 3-day shorter time to hospital discharge and a greater likelihood of discharge than the nonmethocarbamol cohort (Patanwala, Aljuhani, Kopp, & Erstad, 2017). Methocarbamol also has been shown to reduce pain and opioid consumption compared to placebo in a clinical trial of 72 patients who underwent inguinal hernia surgery (Mogharabian, Asadpour, Sohrabi, & Karimi, 2018).

Dosing and Routes

Most skeletal muscle relaxants are administered by the oral route, although diazepPAM, methocarbamol, and orphenadrine have parenteral formulations. Refer to Table 15.15 for additional information.

Adverse Effects

Skeletal muscle relaxants have been associated with CNS-related adverse effects, and in an older systematic review they were associated with a 50% increased risk for adverse effects (Van Tulder, Touray, Furlan, Solway, & Bouter, 2003). These adverse effects include headaches, blurred vision, and potential dependency (Witenko et al., 2014). A number of skeletal muscle relaxants are among the medications listed on the Beers List because of increased safety concerns if administered to older adults. Table 15.15 includes specific adverse effects for some skeletal muscle relaxants.

Monitoring of Patients

All patients receiving skeletal muscle relaxants should have ongoing assessments of the efficacy of the medication, effects on function, and development of side effects. Data to support use of muscle relaxants for treatment of chronic pain are limited, and therefore monitoring of effectiveness and readiness for discontinuation of the medication should be considered. Table 15.15 provides specific monitoring recommendations for the different skeletal muscle relaxants.

Dronabinol, Nabilone, and Cannabidiol

Much controversy surrounds the use of medical marijuana for the treatment of chronic pain despite documentation of its medicinal use for centuries (Kim & Fishman, 2017). Although many states across the United States have legalized the use of medical marijuana, its use remains illegal on a federal level. Botanical marijuana produces more than 100 cannabinoid compounds, and medical marijuana products, which have not met the rigorous FDA approval requirements, vary in the range of cannabinoids that make up the products. This section will focus on the FDA-approved products; when they are used for pain, it is considered an off-label use. Additional information related to the use of cannabinoids, including cannabinoid compounds, is presented in Chapter 26.

Mechanism of Action

Cannabinoids bind to the cannabinoid 1 (CB1) and cannabinoid 2 (CB2) receptors located in the peripheral and central nervous system. δ-9-Tetrahydrocannabinol (THC) is a partial agonist of CB1 and CB2 receptors. The psychological and analgesic effects are primary the result of activation of CB1 receptors found in neuron terminals, reducing the release of neurotransmitters, including glutamate and GABA. CB2 receptors are mostly located in the periphery, but also at low levels in the brain microglia. They are responsible for immunomodulation in the periphery and may contribute to modulation of inflammatory and neuropathic pain (Kim & Fishman, 2017; Tsang & Giudice, 2016).

Indications and Uses

Dronabinol is synthetic THC that is the primary psychoactive component in marijuana and is a Schedule III controlled substance. It is labeled for use in the treatment of anorexia associated with weight loss with acquired immunodeficiency syndrome (AIDS) and nausea and vomiting associated with cancer chemotherapy in patients who have failed traditional treatment options. Caution is advised in patients with a history of psychiatric conditions, including substance use disorder, cardiac disorders, and seizure disorders and in the elderly (AbbVie, 2017).

The other FDA-approved synthetic cannabinoid similar in chemical structure and activity to THC is nabilone, a Schedule II controlled substance (Meda, 2013). Nabilone is 10 times more potent than dronabinol (Kim & Fishman, 2017). Nabilone is labeled for the treatment of nausea and vomiting associated with chemotherapy that is inadequately treated with conventional antiemetics. It is important to evaluate risks and benefits in patients with hypertension or heart disease; current or history of psychiatric disorders, including substance use disorders; and use of other medications that depress the CNS, because these conditions precluded patients from participating in studies for pain (Meda, 2013; Tsang & Giudice, 2016).

Overall, there are mixed results for dronabinol and nabilone in the treatment of pain. Issues identified with studies examining nabilone included small sample size, short duration, limited studies using an active control, varying dosing, use as an adjunctive treatment, and failure to disclose concomitant analgesics (Tsang & Giudice, 2016). Nabilone has been studied in acute postoperative pain, cancer pain, chronic noncancer pain, DPN, fibromyalgia, multiple sclerosis–induced neuropathic pain, nonspecific neuropathic pain, spasticity related to SCI, and medication overuse headache (Beaulieu, 2006; Berlach, Shir, & Ware, 2006; Pini et al., 2012; Tsang & Giudice, 2016; Wissel et al., 2006). A Cochrane review of cannabinoids for fibromyalgia was attempted. Nabilone was the only cannabinoid with RCTs that met inclusion criteria, with two studies that showed no significant difference from placebo for pain, mood, or health-related quality of life. Six patients receiving nabilone experienced dizziness, nausea, dry mouth, and/or dizziness (Walitt, Klose, Fitzcharles, Phillips, & Hauser, 2016). Another systematic review studied nabilone and its role in the management of pain across multiple origins. Several studies showed significant differences in pain scores, whereas others showed no difference. There were also data suggestive of benefits of nabilone for sleep and anxiety (Tsang & Giudice, 2016).

Dronabinol has been studied in chronic pain, neuropathic pain associated with SCI, and central pain associated with multiple sclerosis (Lynch & Campbell, 2011; Rintala, Fiess, Tan, Holmes, & Bruel, 2010; Svendsen, Jensen, & Bach, 2004). Dronabinol, nabilone, and nabiximols (not available in the United States) were studied in neuropathic pain in a systematic review. The majority of studies involved nabiximols (seven trials), with three trials using nabilone, and one trial with dronabinol. Overall, there was a small but statistically significant reduction in pain scores with cannabinoids compared to placebo. When examining the three trials that used nabilone, there was no significant reduction in pain scores compared to placebo or dihydrocodeine (Meng, Johnston, Englesakis, Moulin, & Bhatia, 2017).

Nabilone was studied as an add-on medication to gabapentin in multiple sclerosis–induced neuropathic pain in an RCT. Patients who failed gabapentin 1800 mg/day were randomized to nabilone or placebo. There was a significant reduction in pain scores with nabilone compared to placebo. The most common side effects were dizziness and drowsiness (Turcotte et al., 2015).

A cannabis-derived product from the C. Sativa plant, cannabidiol (CBD), is available in an oral solution recently approved by the FDA as a Schedule V for the treatment of seizures in Dravet syndrome and Lennox-Gastaut syndrome (Drugs@FDA: Epidiolex[R], 2018). This product is a pharmaceutical derivative of cannabis in which the CBD has been isolated from the cannabis plant to provide targeted therapeutic benefit without the psychoeffective impact (Urits et al., 2019). Analgesic and anti-inflammatory effects have been shown in pre-clinical studies of this medication (Boehnke & Clauw, 2019; Boyaji et al., 2020; Bruni et al., 2018).

Several guidelines weigh in on the role of synthetic cannabinoids in the management of pain. A trial of dronabinol or nabilone may be considered for patients with fibromyalgia and may be especially helpful for those with sleep disturbance according to the Canadian Guidelines for Diagnosis and Management of Fibromyalgia Syndrome in Adults (Fitzcharles et al., 2012). The Pharmacological Management of Chronic Neuropathic Pain: Revised Consensus Statement from the Canadian Pain Society lists cannabinoids, including dronabinol and nabilone, as third-line agents (Moulin et al., 2014).

Dosing and Routes

A variety of doses and dosing schedules were used for nabilone in the treatment of pain, making it challenging to provide a specific dose recommendation. A reasonable approach is to start at a low dose of dronabinol (2.5–5 mg/day PO) or nabilone (1 mg/day PO). Titrate the dose by 2.5 mg of dronabinol or 0.5 mg of nabilone every 1 to 2 days until analgesic benefit or until intolerable side effects occur. Should intolerable side effects occur, reduce the dose by increments of dronabinol 2.5 mg or nabilone 0.5 mg. Typical dosing of dronabinol is 5 to 30 mg/day and of nabilone is 1 to 4 mg/day (Grotenhermen & Muller-Vahl, 2012). Both dronabinol and nabilone should be tapered to discontinuation because of the potential for a withdrawal syndrome (AbbVie, 2017; Tsang & Giudice, 2016). The effective therapeutic dose of the CBD-derived product for pain is unclear due to the paucity of research (Boyaji et al., 2020).

Adverse Effects

Typical adverse effects of dronabinol include abdominal pain, dizziness, euphoria, nausea, paranoid reaction, somnolence, abnormal thinking, and vomiting (AbbVie, 2017). Dose reduction can be attempted if a patient has nausea, vomiting, or abdominal pain; otherwise the medication will have to be discontinued. Those with cardiovascular diseases may encounter hypotension, hypertension, syncope, or tachycardia. There have been reports of seizures and seizure-like activity with dronabinol; therefore risks versus benefits should be considered before initiation of dronabinol in a patient with a baseline seizure disorder. There is also the potential for misuse and abuse (AbbVie, 2017).

Drowsiness, vertigo, dry mouth, euphoria, ataxia, headache, and concentration difficulties were common adverse effects reported with nabilone. Nabilone also has a potential for abuse. Tachycardia and postural hypotension may occur, and the elderly and those with hypertension are particularly at-risk. There is the potential for worsening of psychiatric disorders, including depression, manic depression, and schizophrenia (Meda, 2013). Overall, tolerance develops with time to most of the adverse effects that occur with dronabinol and nabilone (Tsang & Giudice, 2016).

The approved CBD-based product has been associated with elevations in liver transaminases, therefore requiring baseline and regular monitoring of liver function. In addition to hepatocellular injury during use, other adverse effects include somnolence, sedation, suicidal behavior, and ideation (Drugs@FDA: Epidiolex[R], 2018). Patients who take this medication for anticonvulsant use are advised to gradually taper the medication for planned discontinuation to reduce the risk for increased seizure frequency and status epilepticus (Drugs@FDA: Epidiolex[R], 2018).

Monitoring of Patients

To monitor the effects of prescribed cannabinoids, vital signs and mood changes are periodically assessed. Urine drug monitoring may be considered in patients prescribed cannabinoids. Nabilone will not lead to a positive result on the THC immunoassay because it has unique metabolites (Moeller, Kissack, Atayee, & Lee, 2017). A positive THC result would be indicative of other THC substances (Tsang & Giudice, 2016). Dronabinol, on the other hand,

does lead to a positive result on the THC immunoassay because toxicology tests are unable to distinguish between synthetic and plant THC (Moeller et al., 2017). The CBD-derived product will produce positive results on cannabis drug screens (Drugs@FDA: Epidiolex[R], 2018).

Other Coanalgesic Medications

In addition to the coanalgesic medications addressed in this chapter, other medications are used as coanalgesic medications for specific pain conditions in MMA plans. For example, the NCCN, in the 2018 guidelines for the management of cancer pain, support the use of many of the medications mentioned in this chapter as coanalgesic medications to treat cancer pain and also suggest the use of bisphosphonates (zoledronic acid, ibandronate) and denosumab as coanalgesics in the management of bone pain (Swarm et al., 2018).

Bone pain associated with the use of granulocyte-colony stimulating factor (G-CSF) can be severe and difficult to treat with opioids and other frequently used coanalgesics, and medications such as NSAIDs are often contraindicated in patients who require G-CSF. Because bone pain associated with G-CSF is proposed to be due to histamine release from an inflammatory response, the use of antihistamines to treat bone pain associated with G-CSF has received attention. Few studies have examined the efficacy of this approach, and results have been conflicting. Several published case reports have supported the use of loratadine in treating G-CSF bone pain that is poorly responsive to opioids and other analgesics (Lambertini, Del Mastro, Bellodi, & Pronzato, 2014; Moore & Haroz, 2017; Romeo, Li, & Copeland, 2015). In a small (n = 17) retrospective cohort study of patients who received a combination of two antihistamines (loratadine and famotidine), the use of double antihistamines before G-CSF administration resulted in lower pain scores (Gavioli & Abrams, 2017). Large, well-designed studies are needed to further examine the effectiveness of this treatment approach.

In addition to cancer pain, there are other pain conditions that may be treated with coanalgesic medications not included in this chapter. Clinicians may review clinical practice guidelines and studies specific to these conditions for identification of other coanalgesic medications that may be useful in the management of pain associated with these conditions.

Key Points

- Coanalgesic medications are essential components in the management of pain.
- Many coanalgesics are considered first-line options for the management of specific pain types.
- Gabapentinoids, tricyclic antidepressants, and serotonin-norepinephrine reuptake inhibitors are widely used in the management of neuropathic pain.

- Coanalgesics are beneficial components of multimodal perioperative pain management plans because they may provide improvements in pain, lower opioid requirements, and reduce opioid-related adverse effects.
- Coanalgesic use requires consideration of patient-specific factors, including comorbidities, concomitant medications, and renal and hepatic function to determine appropriateness of use.
- Monitor patients who receive coanalgesic medications for analgesic benefits, drug-drug interactions, and other adverse effects.

Case Scenario

Mr. L., a 64-year-old with a history of diabetes, osteoarthritis, and chronic low back pain is scheduled for an elective total knee replacement. His knee pain has increased over the past year and is limiting his mobility. When reconciling his medications, he reports daily use of pregabalin and DULoxetine. He is very concerned about postoperative pain and asks many questions about options for his perioperative pain management plan. He is very interested in minimizing his opioid use.

- What questions should be asked about Mr. L.'s home medications?
- What are the possible reasons Mr. L. may be prescribed pregabalin and DULoxetine?
- What factors should be considered in the patient assessment based on his home medication use?
- Describe coanalgesic medications that may be appropriate for use in a multimodal pain management plan for Mr. L.
- If Mr. L. is unable to take oral medications in the immediate postoperative period, what coanalgesic medications are available to optimize his pain control?

References

AbbVie. (2017). *Highlights of prescribing information: Marinol.* Retrieved July 18, 2020 from http://www.rxabbvie.com/pdf/marinol_PI.pdf.Abdel Shaheed, C., Maher, C. G., Williams, K. A., & McLachlan, A. J. (2017). Efficacy and tolerability of muscle relaxants for low back pain: Systematic review and meta-analysis. *European Journal of Pain*, 21(2), 228–237.

American Geriatrics Society Beers Criteria® Update Expert Panel, Fick, D. M., Semla, T. P., Steinman, M., Beizer, J., Brandt, N., & Flanagan, N. (2019). American Geriatrics Society 2019 updated AGS Beers Criteria® for potentially inappropriate medication use in older adults. *Journal of the American Geriatrics Society*, 67(4), 674–694.

Acorda Therapeutics. (2013). *Zanaflex: highlights of prescribing information.* Retrieved July 18, 2020 from https://www.accessdata.fda.gov/drugsatfda_docs/label/2006/020397s021,021447s002lbl.pdf.

Aiyer, R., Barkin, R. L., & Bhatia, A. (2017). Treatment of neuropathic pain with venlafaxine: a systematic review. *Pain Medicine*, 18(10), 1999–2012.

Aiyer, R., Mehta, N., Gungor, S., & Gulati, A. (2018). A systematic review of NMDA receptor antagonists for treatment of neuropathic pain in clinical practice. *The Clinical Journal of Pain*, 34(5), 450–467.

Akorn, I. (2014). *Dexmedetomidine: highlights of prescribing information.* Retrieved July 18, 2020 from https://dailymed.nlm.nih.gov/dailymed/drugInfo.cfm?setid=8fb7886c-7762-4b72-989b-0fe8e963b4b8.

Albrecht, E., Kirkham, K. R., Liu, S. S., & Brull, R. (2013). Perioperative intravenous administration of magnesium sulphate and postoperative pain: a meta-analysis. *Anaesthesia*, 68(1), 79–90.

Alhazzani, W., & Guyatt, G. (2018). An overview of the GRADE approach and a peek at the future. *The Medical Journal of Australia*, 209(7), 291–292.

Almatica Pharma. (2020). Gralise Full Prescribing Information. *Retrieved from August*, 15, 2020. https://www.gralise.com/pdfs/gralise-prescribing-information.pdf.

Alvis, B. D., & Sobey, C. M. (2017). Oral baclofen withdrawal resulting in progressive weakness and sedation requiring intensive care admission. *The Neurohospitalist*, 7(1), 39–40. https://doi.org/10.1177/1941874416637404.

Ambrosini, A., & Schoenen, J. (2016). Preventive Episodic Migraine Treatment. In *Pharmacological Management of Headaches* (pp. 63–79). Cham, Switzerland: Springer.

Antoniou, T., & Juurlink, D. N. (2014). Dextromethorphan abuse. *Canadian Medical Association Journal*, 186(16), E631. https://doi.org/10.1503/cmaj.131676/-/DC1.

Applequist, H., Daly, B. J., Koniaris, C., & Musil, C. M. (2017). An Assessment of the Use, Perceived Benefits, and Outcomes of Ketamine in Sickle Cell Vaso-Occlusive Crisis in the United States. *Journal of Hospice & Palliative Nursing*, 19(1), 75–81.

Arbor Pharmaceuticals, (2020). Horizant: Highlights of prescribing information. Retrieved from https://www.horizant.com/pdf/Horizant-Prescribing-Information.pdf.

Aronson, J. K. (2016b). Baclofen. In J. K. Aronson (Ed.), *Meyle's Side Effects of Drugs* (pp. 809–816). Waltham, MA: Elsevier.

Aronson, J. K. (2016a). Lidocaine. In J. K. Aronson (Ed.), *Meyler's Side Effects of Drugs* (pp. 565–576). Waltham, MA: Elsevier.

Arumugam, S., Lau, C. S., & Chamberlain, R. S. (2016). Use of preoperative gabapentin significantly reduces postoperative opioid consumption: a meta-analysis. *Journal of Pain Research*, 9, 631.

Avanir Pharmaceuticals, I. (2010). *Nuedexta: highlights of prescribing information.* Retrieved July 18, 2020 from https://www.nuedexta.com/sites/default/files/pdfs/Prescribing_Information.pdf.

Balague, F., Piguet, V., & Dudler, J. (2012). Steroids for LBP – from rationale to inconvenient truth. *Swiss Medical Weekly*, 142(w13566), 1–7. https://doi.org/10.4414/smw.2012.13566.

Beaulieu, P. (2006). Effects of nabilone, a synthetic cannabinoid, on postoperative pain. *Canadian Journal of Anesthesiology*, 53(8), 769–775.

Beaussier, M., Delbos, A., Maurice-Szamburski, A., Ecoffey, C., & Mercadal, L. (2018). Perioperative Use of Intravenous Lidocaine. *Drugs*, 1–18.

Bell, R. F., Eccleston, C., & Kalso, E. A. (2017). Ketamine as an adjuvant to opioids for cancer pain. *Cochrane Database Syst Rev*, (6). https://doi.org/10.1002/14651858.CD003351.pub3.

Bengisun, Z. K., Ekmekci, P., Akan, B., Koroglu, A., & Tuzuner, F. (2014). The effect of adding dexmedetomidine to levobupivacaine for interscalene block for postoperative pain management after arthroscopic shoulder surgery. *Clin J Pain*, 30(12), 1057–1061. https://doi.org/10.1097/ajp.0000000000000065.

Berlach, D. M., Shir, Y., & Ware, M. A. (2006). Experience with synthetic cannabinoids in chronic noncancer pain. *Pain Medicine*, 7(1), 25–29.

Beverly, A., Kaye, A. D., Ljungqvist, O., & Urman, R. D. (2017). Essential elements of multimodal analgesia in Enhanced Recovery After Surgery (ERAS) guidelines. *Anesthesiology Clinics*, 35(2), e115–e143.

Bhattacharya, A., Wickenden, A. D., & Chaplan, S. R. (2009). Sodium channel blockers for the treatment of neuropathic pain. *Neurotherapeutics*, 6(4), 663–678. https://doi.org/10.1016/j.nurt.2009.08.001.

Blaudszun, G., C.H., L, Elia, N., & Tramer, M. R. (2012). Effect of perioperative systemic alpha-2 agonists on postoperative morphine consumption and pain intensity: systematic review and meta-analysis of randomized controlled trials. *Anesthesiology*, 116(6), 1312–1322.

Bleakley, S. (2016). Antidepressant drug interactions: evidence and clinical significance. *Progress in Neurology and Psychiatry*, 20(3), 21–27.

Boehringer Ingelheim Pharmaceuticals, I. (2009). Catapress: prescribing information. Retrieved July 18, 2020 from https://www.accessdata.fda.gov/drugsatfda_docs/label/2009/017407s034lbl.pdf.

Boehnke, K. F., & Clauw, D. J. (2019). Brief commentary: cannabinoid dosing for chronic pain management. *Annals of Internal Medicine*, 170(2), 118.

Boyaji, S., Merkow, J., Elman, R. N. M., Kaye, A. D., Yong, R. J., & Urman, R. D. (2020). The role of cannabidiol (CBD) in chronic pain management: an assessment of current evidence. *Current Pain and Headache Reports*, 24(2), 4.

Bruni, N., Della Pepa, C., Oliaro-Bosso, S., Pessione, E., Gastaldi, D., & Dosio, F. (2018). Cannabinoid delivery systems for pain and inflammation treatment. *Molecules*, 23(10), 2478.

Bonnet, U., & Scherbaum, N. (2017). How addictive are gabapentin and pregabalin? A systematic review. *European Neuropsychopharmacology*, 27(12), 1185–1215.

Bredlau, A. L., Thakur, R., Korones, D. N., & Dworkin, R. H. (2013). Ketamine for pain in adults and children with cancer: a systematic review and synthesis of the literature. *Pain Med*, 14(10), 1505–1517. https://doi.org/10.1111/pme.12182.

Bujalska-Zadrożny, M., Tatarkiewicz, J., Kulik, K., Filip, M., & Naruszewicz, M. (2017). Magnesium enhances opioid-induced analgesia–What we have learnt in the past decades? *European Journal of Pharmaceutical Sciences*, 99, 113–127.

Burns, J. M., & Boyer, E. W. (2013). Antitussives and substance abuse. *Subst Abuse Rehabil*, 4, 75–82. https://doi.org/10.2147/SAR.S36761.

Casale, R., Symeonidou, Z., & Bartolo, M. (2017). Topical treatments for localized neuropathic pain. *Current Pain and Headache Reports*, 21(3), 15.

Castro, J., & Cooney, M. F. (2017). Intravenous Magnesium in the Management of Postoperative Pain. *Journal of PeriAnesthesia Nursing*, 32(1), 72–76.

Chabal, C., Jacobson, L., Mariano, A., Chaney, E., & Britell, C. W. (1992). The use of oral mexiletine for the treatment of pain after peripheral nerve injury. *Anesthesiology*, 76(4), 513–517.

Chan, A. K., Cheung, C. W., & Chong, Y. K. (2010). Alpha-2 agonists in acute pain management. *Expert Opin Pharmacother*, 11(17), 2849–2868. https://doi.org/10.1517/14656566.2010.511613.

Cheung, C. W., Qiu, Q., Ying, A. C., Choi, S. W., Law, W. L., & Irwin, M. G. (2014). The effects of intra-operative dexmedetomidine on postoperative pain, side-effects and recovery in colorectal surgery. *Anaesthesia*, 69(11), 1214–1221. https://doi.org/10.1111/anae.12759.

Chincholkar, M. (2018). Analgesic mechanisms of gabapentinoids and effects in experimental pain models: a narrative review. *British Journal of Anaesthesia.*, 120(6), 1315–1334.

Chiu, H. Y., Yeh, T. H., Huang, Y. C., & Chen, P. Y. (2016). Effects of Intravenous and Oral Magnesium on Reducing Migraine: A Meta-analysis of Randomized Controlled Trials. *Pain Physician*, 19(1). E97-112.

Chou, R., Deyo, R., Friedly, J., Skelly, A., Weimer, M., Fu, R., … Grusing, S. (2018). Systemic pharmacologic therapies for low back pain: a systematic review for an American College of Physicians Clinical Practice Guideline. *Annals Internal Medicine*, 166, 480–492.

Chou, R., Gordon, D. B., de Leon-Casasola, O. A., Rosenberg, J. M., Bickler, S., Brennan, T., … Griffith, S. (2016). Management of Postoperative Pain: a clinical practice guideline from the American Pain Society, the American Society of Regional Anesthesia and Pain Medicine, and the American Society of Anesthesiologists' committee on regional anesthesia, executive committee, and administrative council. *The Journal of Pain*, 17(2), 131–157.

Claessens, A. J., Risler, L. J., Eyal, S., Shen, D. D., Easterling, T. R., & Hebert, M. F. (2010). CYP2D6 mediates 4-hydroxylation of clonidine in vitro: implication for pregnancy-induced changes in clonidine clearance. *Drug Metabolism and Disposition*, 38(9), 1393–1396.

Cohen, L., Athaide, V., Wickham, M. E., Doyle-Waters, M. M., Rose, N. G., & Hohl, C. M. (2015). The effect of ketamine on intracranial and cerebral perfusion pressure and health outcomes: a systematic review. *Annals of Emergency Medicine*, 65(1), 43–51.

Cohen, S. P. (2015, February). Epidemiology, diagnosis, and treatment of neck pain. *Mayo Clinic Proceedings*, 90(2), 284–299.

Cohen, R. I., & Warfield, C. A. (2015). Role of Muscle Relaxants in the Treatment of Pain. In *Treatment of Chronic Pain by Medical Approaches (pp. 67-75)*. New York, NY: Springer.

Cohen, S. P., Bhatia, A., Buvanendran, A., Schwenk, E. S., Wasan, A. D., Hurley, R. W., … Lubenow, T. R. (2018). Consensus guidelines on the use of intravenous ketamine infusions for chronic pain from the American Society of Regional Anesthesia and Pain Medicine, the American Academy of Pain Medicine, and the American Society of Anesthesiologists. *Regional Anesthesia and Pain Medicine*, 43(5), 521–546.

Collins, S., Zuurmond, W. W., de Lange, J. J., van Hilten, B. J., & Perez, R. S. (2009). Intravenous magnesium for complex regional pain syndrome type 1 (CRPS 1) patients: a pilot study. *Pain Med*, 10(5), 930–940. https://doi.org/10.1111/j.1526-4637.2009.00639.x.

Connolly, S. B., Prager, J. P., & Harden, R. N. (2015). A systematic review of ketamine for complex regional pain syndrome. *Pain Med, 16*(5), 943–969. https://doi.org/10.1111/pme.12675.

Cording, M., Derry, S., Phillips, T., Moore, R. A., & Wiffen, P. J. (2015). Milnacipran for pain in fibromyalgia in adults. *Cochrane Database Syst Rev*(10), CD008244. doi:https://doi.org/10.1002/14651858.CD008244.pub3.

Cruccu, G., & Truini, A. (2017). A review of neuropathic pain: from guidelines to clinical practice. *Pain and Therapy, 6*(1), 35–42.

De Oliveira, G. S., Castro-Alves, L. J., Khan, J. H., & McCarthy, R. J. (2013). Perioperative systemic magnesium to minimize postoperative pain a meta-analysis of randomized controlled trials. *Anesthesiology, 119*(1), 178–190.

DeBattista, C. (2018). Antidepressant Agents. In B. Katzung, S. B. Masters, & A. J. Trevor (Eds.), *Basic and Clinical Pharmacology (14th ed.). New York.* New York: McGraw-Hill.

Depomed. (2012). *Gralise Full Prescribing Information.* Retrieved from https://www.gralise.com/sites/default/files/GRALISE_PI_DEC2012.pdf.

Derry, S., Phillips, T., Moore, R. A., & Wiffen, P. J. (2015a). Milnacipran for neuropathic pain in adults. *Cochrane Database Syst Rev, 7.* https://doi.org/10.1002/14651858.CD011789.

Derry, S., Wiffen, P. J., Aldington, D., & Moore, R. A. (2015b). Nortriptyline for neuropathic pain in adults. *The Cochrane Library., 1*(1), CD011209.

Dershwitz, M., & Rosow, C. E. (2018). Intravenous anesthetics. In D. E. Longnecker, S. C. Mackey, M. F. Newman, W. S. Sandberg, & W. M. Zapol (Eds.), *Anesthesiology, 3e.* New York, NY: McGraw-Hill.

Dharmshaktu, P., Tayal, V., & Kalra, B. S. (2012). Efficacy of antidepressants as analgesics: a review. *J Clin Pharmacol, 52*(1), 6–17. https://doi.org/10.1177/0091270010394852.

Dibj-Hajj, S. D., Black, J. A., & Waxman, S. G. (2009). Voltage gated sodium channels therapeutic targets for pain. *Pain Medicine, 10*(7), 1260–1269. https://doi.org/10.1111/j.1526-4637.2009.00719.x.

Dinakar, P. (2016). Principles of pain management. In R. B. Daroff, J. Jankovic, J. C. Mazziotta, & S. L. Pomeroy (Eds.), *Bradley's Neurology in Clinical Practice* (pp. 720–741). London: Elsevier.

Di Stefano, G., Truini, A., & Cruccu, G. (2018). Current and Innovative Pharmacological Options to Treat Typical and Atypical Trigeminal Neuralgia. *Drugs,* 1–10.

Doleman, B., Heinink, T. P., Read, D. J., Faleiro, R. J., Lund, J. N., & Williams, J. P. (2015). A systematic review and meta-regression analysis of prophylactic gabapentin for postoperative pain. *Anaesthesia, 70*(10), 1186–1204.

Dong, J., Li, W., & Wang, Y. (2016). The effect of pregabalin on acute postoperative pain in patients undergoing total knee arthroplasty: a meta-analysis. *International Journal of Surgery, 34,* 148–160.

Dowell, D., Haegerich, T. M., & Chou, R. (2016). CDC guideline for prescribing opioids for chronic pain—United States, 2016. *JAMA, 315*(15), 1624–1645.

Drugs@FDA. Dexamethasone Sodium Phosphate Injection, USP [Package Insert]. (2014). Retrieved July 15, 2020 from https://www.accessdata.fda.gov/drugsatfda_docs/label/2014/040572s002lbl.pdf.

Drugs@FDA. Epidiolex® (cannabidiol) oral solution. [Package Insert]. (2018). Retrieved Sept. 24, 2020 from https://www.accessdata.fda.gov/drugsatfda_docs/label/2018/210365lbl.pdf.

Drugs@FDA. Lioresal^R Intrathecal (baclofen injection) [Package Insert]. (2011). Retrieved July 12, 2020, from https://www.accessdata.fda.gov/drugsatfda_docs/label/2011/020075s021lbl.pdf.

Drugs@FDA. Ozobax™ (Baclofen) oral solution [Package Insert]. (2019). Retrieved July 12, 2020. In *from.* https://www.accessdata.fda.gov/drugsatfda_docs/label/2019/208193s000lbl.pdf.

Drugs@FDA. Savella^R (milnacipran HCL) Tablets [Package Insert]. (2016). Retrieved July 12, 2020 from https://www.accessdata.fda.gov/drugsatfda_docs/label/2016/022256s022lbl.pdf.

Drugs@FDA. Spravato™ (esketamine) [Package Insert]. (2020). Retrieved July 15, 2020 from https://www.accessdata.fda.gov/drugsatfda_docs/label/2020/211243s003lbl.pdf.

Dunn, L. K., & Durieux, M. E. (2017). Perioperative use of intravenous lidocaine. *Anesthesiology: The Journal of the American Society of Anesthesiologists, 126*(4), 729–737.

Duong, S., Bravo, D., Todd, K. J., Finlayson, R. J., & Tran, D. Q. (2018). Treatment of complex regional pain syndrome: an updated systematic review and narrative synthesis. *Canadian Journal of Anesthesia/Journal canadien d'anesthésie, 65*(6), 658–684.

Dworkin, R. H., O'Connor, A. B., Backonja, M., Farrar, J. T., Finnerup, N. B., Jensen, T. S., ... Wallace, M. S. (2007). Pharmacologic management of neuropathic pain: evidence-based recommendations. *Pain, 132*(3), 237–251. https://doi.org/10.1016/j.pain.2007.08.033.

Eilers, H., & Yost, S. (2018). General anesthetics. In B. Katzung, S. B. Masters, & A. J. Trevor (Eds.), *Basic and Clinical Pharmacology (14th ed.). New York.* New York: McGraw-Hill.

Eipe, N., Gupta, S., & Penning, J. (2016). Intravenous lidocaine for acute pain: an evidence-based clinical update. *BJA Education, 16*(9), 292–298.

e Silva, L. O. J., Scherber, K., Cabrera, D., Motov, S., Erwin, P. J., West, C. P., ... Bellolio, M. F. (2018). Safety and Efficacy of Intravenous Lidocaine for Pain Management in the Emergency Department: A Systematic Review. *Annals of Emergency Medicine, 72*(2), 135–144.

Estebe, J. P. (2017). Intravenous lidocaine. *Best practice & research Clinical anaesthesiology, 31*(4), 513–521.

Elsayed, M., Zeiss, R., Gahr, M., Connemann, B. J., & Schönfeldt-Lecuona, C. (2019). Intranasal Pregabalin Administration: A Review of the Literature and the Worldwide Spontaneous Reporting System of Adverse Drug Reactions. *Brain Sciences, 9*(11), 322.

Evoy, K. E., Morrison, M. D., & Saklad, S. R. (2017). Abuse and misuse of pregabalin and gabapentin. *Drugs, 77*(4), 403–426.

Evoy, K. E., Covvey, J. R., Peckham, A. M., Ochs, L., & Hultgren, K. E. (2018). Reports of gabapentin and pregabalin abuse, misuse, dependence, or overdose: an analysis of the Food and Drug Administration Adverse Events Reporting System (FAERS). *Research in Social and Administrative Pharmacy., 15*(8), 953–958.

Fan, H., Yu, W., Zhang, Q., Cao, H., Li, J., Wang, J., ... Hu, X. (2014). Efficacy and safety of gabapentin 1800 mg treatment for post-herpetic neuralgia: a meta-analysis of randomized controlled trials. *Journal of Clinical Pharmacy and Therapeutics, 39*(4), 334–342.

Finnerup, N. B., Attal, N., Haroutounian, S., McNicol, E., Baron, R., Dworkin, R. H., ... Wallace, M. (2015). Pharmacotherapy for neuropathic pain in adults: a systematic review and meta-analysis. *The Lancet Neurology, 14*(2), 162–173. https://doi.org/10.1016/s1474-4422(14)70251-0.

Fischer, S. G., Collins, S., Boogaard, S., Loer, S. A., Zuurmond, W. W., & Perez, R. S. (2013). Intravenous magnesium for chronic complex regional pain syndrome type 1 (CRPS-1). *Pain Medicine, 14*(9), 1388–1399.

Fitzcharles, M., Ste-Marie, P. A., Govldenberg, D. L., Pereira, J. X., Abbey, S., Choiniere, M., ... Shir, Y. (2012). *2012 Canadian Guidelines for Diagnosis and Management of Fibromyalgia Syndrome.* Retrieved July 18, 2020 from http://fmguidelines.ca/.

Fitzgibbon, E. J., & Viola, R. (2005). Parenteral ketamine as an analgesic adjuvant for severe pain: development and retrospective audit of a protocol for a palliative care unit. *J Palliat Med, 8*(1), 49–57. https://doi.org/10.1089/jpm.2005.8.49.

Food and Drug Administration. (2019). FDA warns about serious breathing problems with seizure and nerve pain medicines gabapentin (Neurontin, Gralise, Horizant) and pregabalin (Lyrica, Lyrica CR). *12-29-2019 FDA Drug Safety. Communication.* Retrieved July 15, 2020 from https://www.fda.gov/drugs/drug-safety-and-availability/fda-warns-about-serious-breathing-problems-seizure-and-nerve-pain-medicines-gabapentin-neurontin.

Friedman, B. W., Esses, D., Solorzano, C., Choi, H. K., Cole, M., Davitt, M., ... Gallagher, E. J. (2008). A randomized placebo-controlled trial of single-dose IM corticosteroid for radicular low back pain. *Spine (Phila Pa 1976), 33*(18), E624–E629. https://doi.org/10.1097/BRS.0b013e3181822711.

Gao, M., Rejaei, D., & Liu, H. (2016). Ketamine use in current clinical practice. *Acta Pharmacologica Sinica, 37*(7), 865.

Gavioli, E., & Abrams, M. (2017). Prevention of granulocyte-colony stimulating factor (G-CSF) induced bone pain using double histamine blockade. *Supportive Care in Cancer, 25*(3), 817–822.

Gibbons, K., DeMonbrun, A., Beckman, E. J., Keefer, P., Wagner, D., M., S, ... Niedner, M. (2016). Continuous lidocaine infusions to manage opioid-refractory pain in a series of pediatric cancer patients. *Pediatric Blood Cancer, 63*, 1168–1174. https://doi.org/10.1002/pbc.25870.

Gilron, I., Baron, R., & Jensen, T. (2015, April). Neuropathic pain: principles of diagnosis and treatment. *Mayo Clinic Proceedings, 90*(4), 532–545.

Glick, R. M., & Marcus, D. A. (2015). Chronic Pain Management. In J. E. South-Paul, S. C. Matheny, & E. L. Lewis (Eds.), *CURRENT Diagnosis & Treatment: Family Medicine, 4e.* New York, NY: McGraw-Hill.

Gomes, T., Greaves, S., van den Brink, W., Antoniou, T., Mamdani, M. M., Paterson, J. M., ... Juurlink, D. N. (2018). Pregabalin and the risk for opioid-related death: a nested case–control study. *Annals of Internal Medicine, 169*(10), 732–734.

Gomes, T., Juurlink, D. N., Antoniou, T., Mamdani, M. M., Paterson, J. M., & van den Brink, W. (2017). Gabapentin, opioids, and the risk of opioid-related death: A population-based nested case-control study. *PLoS Med, 14*(10). https://doi.org/10.1371/journal.pmed.1002396.

Gowing, L., Farrell, M. F., & White, J. M. (2014). Alpha2-adrenergic agonists for the management of opioid withdrawal. *Cochrane Database Syst Rev, 31*(3), CD002024.

Granfors, M. T., Backman, J. T., Laitila, J., & Neuvonen, P. J. (2004). Tizanidine is mainly metabolized by cytochrome p450 1A2 in vitro. *British Journal of Clinical Pharmacology, 57*(3), 349–353.

Grotenhermen, F., & Muller-Vahl, K. (2012). The therapeutic potential of cannabis and cannabinoids. *Dtsch Arztebl Int, 109*(29-30), 495–501. https://doi.org/10.3238/arztebl.2012.0495.

Guay, D. R. P. (2001). Adjunctive agents in the management of chronic pain. *Pharmacotherapy, 21*(9), 1070–1081.

Guo, B. L., Lin, Y., Hu, W., Zhen, C. X., Bao-Cheng, Z., Wu, H. H., ... Qu, Y. (2015). Effects of Systemic Magnesium on Postoperative Analgesia: Is the Current Evidence Strong Enough? *Pain Physician, 18*(5), 405–418.

Hagen, E. M., & Rekand, T. (2015). Management of Neuropathic Pain Associated with Spinal Cord Injury. *Pain Ther, 4*(1), 51–65. https://doi.org/10.1007/s40122-015-0033-y.

Han, Y., Zhang, J., Chen, N., He, L., Zhou, M., & Zhu, C. (2013). Corticosteroids for preventing postherpetic neuralgia. *Cochrane Database Syst Rev*(3), CD005582. https://doi.org/10.1002/14651858.CD005582.pub4.

Hardy, J., Quinn, S., Fazekas, B., Plummer, J., Eckermann, S., Agar, M., ... Currow, D. C. (2012). Randomized, double-blind, placebo-controlled study to assess the efficacy and toxicity of subcutaneous ketamine in the management of cancer pain. *J Clin Oncol, 30*(29), 3611–3617. https://doi.org/10.1200/jco.2012.42.1081.

Haroutounian, S., & Finnerup, N. B. (2018). Recommendations for pharmacologic therapy of neuropathic pain. In H. Benzon, S. Raja, N. Srinivasa, S. Liu, S. Fishman, & S (Eds.), *Cohen Essentials of Pain Medicine* (4th Ed., pp. 445–456). Philadelphia, PA: Elsevier. Chapter 50.

Hassell, K., Ngongo, W., Montgomery, R., & Hornick, L. (2017). Ketamine infusion as an analgesic adjunct in the management of severe pain in patients with sickle cell disease. *The Journal of Pain, 18*(4), S68.

Hayashida, K. I., & Obata, H. (2019). Strategies to treat chronic pain and strengthen impaired descending noradrenergic inhibitory system. *International Journal of Molecular Sciences, 20*(4), 822.

Haywood, A., Good, P., Khan, S., Leupp, A., Jenkins-Marsh, S., Rickett, K., & Hardy, J. R. (2015). Corticosteroids for the management of cancer-related pain in adults. *Cochrane Database Syst Rev, 4*. https://doi.org/10.1002/14651858.CD010756.pub2.

Herndon, C., Lider, J. M., & Daniels, A. M. (2015). QT Intervals and Antidepressants. *Practical Pain Management,* (10), 15.

Herndon, C. M., Arnstein, P., Darnall, B., Hartrick, C., Hecht, K., Lyons, M., & Seghal, N. (2016). *Principles of Analgesic Use.* Chicago, Ill: American Pain Society.

Hirota, K., & Lambert, D. G. (1996). Ketamine its mechanism(s) of action and unusual clinical uses. *British Journal of Anaesthesiology., 77*(4), 441–444.

Hirota, K., & Lambert, D. G. (2011). Ketamine: new uses for an old drug? *Br J Anaesth, 107*(2), 123–126. https://doi.org/10.1093/bja/aer221.

Howard, J., Hart, N., Roberts-Harewood, M., Cummins, M., Awogbade, M., Davis, B., & BCSH Committee. (2015). Guideline on the management of acute chest syndrome in sickle cell disease. *British Journal of Haematology, 169*(4), 492–505.

Hutson, P., Backonja, M., & Knurr, H. (2015). Intravenous lidocaine for neuropathic pain: a retrospective analysis of tolerability and efficacy. *Pain Medicine, 16*, 531–536.

Hwang, W., Lee, J., Park, J., & Joo, J. (2015). Dexmedetomidine versus remifentanil in postoperative pain control after spinal surgery: a randomized controlled study. *BMC Anesthesiol, 15*. https://doi.org/10.1186/s12871-015-0004-1.

Jackson, K. C., Argoff, C. E., & Dubin, A. (2014). Skeletal muscle relaxants. In *Practical Management of Pain (Fifth Edition)* (pp. 569-574). Philadelphia: Mosby.

James, A. O., Nicholson, T. R., Hill, R., & Bearn, J. (2016). Something old, something new: a successful case of meprobamate withdrawal. *BMJ case reports, 2016*, bcr2015213606.

Jamison, D. E., Cohen, S. P., & Rosenow, J. (2018). Implanted Drug Delivery Systems for Control of Chronic Pain. In H. Benzon, S. Raja, N. Srinivasa, S. Liu, S. Fishman, & S (Eds.), *Cohen Essentials of Pain Medicine (Fourth Edition)* (pp. 693–702). Philadelphia, PA: Elsevier.

Jiang, H. L., Huang, S., Song, J., Wang, X., & Cao, Z. S. (2017). Preoperative use of pregabalin for acute pain in spine surgery: a meta-analysis of randomized controlled trials. *Medicine, 96*(11).

Jobanputra, A., Dixit, D., & Hussain, S. (2016). 1858: Intravenous ketamine for refractory sickle cell pain crisis management in the medical icu. *Critical Care Medicine, 44*(12), 540.

Jouguelet-Lacoste, J., La Colla, L., Schilling, D., & Chelly, J. E. (2015). The use of intravenous infusion or single dose of low-dose ketamine for postoperative analgesia: a review of the current literature. *Pain Medicine, 16*(2), 383–403.

Karlow, N., Schlaepfer, C. H., Stoll, C. R., Doering, M., Carpenter, C. R., Colditz, G. A., … Schwarz, E. S. (2018). A Systematic Review and Meta-analysis of Ketamine as an Alternative to Opioids for Acute Pain in the Emergency Department. *Academic Emergency Medicine, 25*(10), 1086–1097.

Kaye, A. D., Cornett, E. M., Helander, E., Menard, B., Hsu, E., Hart, B., & Brunk, A. (2017). An update on nonopioids: intravenous or oral analgesics for perioperative pain management. *Anesthesiology Clinics, 35*(2), e55–e71.

Kim, P. S., & Fishman, M. A. (2017). Cannabis for Pain and Headaches: Primer. *Curr Pain Headache Rep, 21*(4). https://doi.org/10.1007/s11916-017-0619-7.

King, M. R., Ladha, K. S., Gelineau, A. M., & Anderson, T. A. (2016). Perioperative Dextromethorphan as an Adjunct for Postoperative Pain: A Meta-analysis of Randomized Controlled Trials. *Anesthesiology, 124*(3), 696–705. https://doi.org/10.1097/ALN.0000000000000950.

Kintzel, P. E., Knol, J. D., & Roe, G. (2018). Intravenous Lidocaine Administered as Twice Daily Bolus and Continuous Infusion for Intractable Cancer Pain and Wound Care Pain. *Journal of Palliative Medicine., 22*(3), 343–347.

Kosharskyy, B., Almonte, W., & Shaparin, N. (2013). Intravenous infusions in chronic pain management. *Pain Physician, 16*, 231–249.

Kouladjian O'Donnell, L., Gnjidic, D., Nahas, R., Bell, J. S., & Hilmer, S. N. (2017). Anticholinergic burden: considerations for older adults. *Journal of Pharmacy Practice and Research, 47*(1), 67–77.

Kranke, P., Jokinen, J., Pace, N. L., Schnabel, A., Hollmann, M. W., Hahnenkamp, K., … Weibel, S. (2015). Continuous intravenous perioperative lidocaine infusion for postoperative pain and recovery. *Cochrane Database Syst Rev, 7*. https://doi.org/10.1002/14651858.CD009642.pub2.

Kremer, M., Salvat, E., Muller, A., Yalcin, I., & Barrot, M. (2016). Antidepressants and gabapentinoids in neuropathic pain: mechanistic insights. *Neuroscience, 338*, 183–206.

Kumar, M., & Dillon, G. H. (2015). Carisoprodol: update on abuse potential and mechanism of action. *Molecular and Cellular Pharmacology, 7*(1), 1–10.

Kurdi, M. S., Theerth, K. A., & Deva, R. S. (2014). Ketamine: current applications in anesthesia, pain, and critical care. *Anesthesia, essays and researches, 8*(3), 283.

Kus, T., Aktas, G., Alpak, G., Kalender, M. E., Sevinc, A., Kul, S., … Camci, C. (2016). Efficacy of venlafaxine for the relief of taxane and oxaliplatin-induced acute neurotoxicity: a single-center retrospective case-control study. *Support Care Cancer, 24*(5), 2085–2091. https://doi.org/10.1007/s00520-015-3009-x.

Lam, D. M., Choi, S. W., Wong, S. S., Irwin, M. G., & Cheung, C. W. (2015). Efficacy of pregabalin in acute postoperative pain under different surgical categories: a meta-analysis. *Medicine, 94*(46).

Lambertini, M., Del Mastro, L., Bellodi, A., & Pronzato, P. (2014). The five "Ws" for bone pain due to the administration of granulocyte-colony stimulating factors (G-CSFs). *Critical Reviews in Oncology/Hematology, 89*, 112–128. https://doi.org/10.1016/j.critrevonc.2013.08.006.

Leppert, W., & Buss, T. (2012). The role of corticosteroids in the treatment of pain in cancer patients. *Curr Pain Headache Rep, 16*(4), 307–313. https://doi.org/10.1007/s11916-012-0273-z.

Li, H., Cheng, Y., Ahl, J., & Skljarevski, V. (2014). Observational study of upper gastrointestinal tract bleeding events in patients taking duloxetine and nonsteroidal anti-inflammatory drugs: a case-control analysis. *Drug Healthc Patient Saf, 6*, 167–174. https://doi.org/10.2147/DHPS.S66835.

Li, S., Guo, J., Li, F., Yang, Z., Wang, S., & Qin, C. (2017). Pregabalin can decrease acute pain and morphine consumption in laparoscopic cholecystectomy patients: A meta-analysis of randomized controlled trials. *Medicine (Baltimore), 96*(21). https://doi.org/10.1097/MD.0000000000006982.

Lilly USA, L. (2016). *Cymbalta: highlights of prescribing information*. Retrieved from http://pi.lilly.com/us/cymbalta-pi.pdf.

Liu, H. J., Gao, X. Z., Liu, X. M., Xia, M., Li, W. Y., & Jin, Y. (2014). Effect of intrathecal dexmedetomidine on spinal morphine analgesia in patients with refractory cancer pain. *J Palliat Med, 17*(7), 837–840. https://doi.org/10.1089/jpm.2013.0544.

Liu, Y., Liang, F., Liu, X., Shao, X., Jiang, N., & Gan, X. (2018). Dexmedetomidine reduces perioperative opioid consumption and postoperative pain intensity in neurosurgery: a meta-analysis. *Journal of Neurosurgical Anesthesiology, 30*(2), 146–155.

Lunn, M. P., Hughes, R. A., & Wiffen, P. J. (2014). Duloxetine for treating painful neuropathy, chronic pain or fibromyalgia. *Cochrane Database Syst Rev, (1)*. https://doi.org/10.1002/14651858.CD007115.pub3.

Lupin Pharmaceuticals, I. (2016). *Imipramine: prescribing information*. Retrieved July 18, 2020 from https://dailymed.nlm.nih.gov/dailymed/drugInfo.cfm?setid=55311747-710c-43c4-821d-76323ff2520e.

Lynch, M. E., & Campbell, F. (2011). Cannabinoids for treatment of chronic non-cancer pain; a systematic review of randomized trials. *British Journal of Pharmacology, 72*(5), 735–744. https://doi.org/10.1111/bph.2011.163.issue-1.

Malcangio, M. (2018). GABAB receptors and pain. *Neuropharmacology, 136*, 102–105.

Mallincrodt. (2015). *Clomipramine: prescribing information*. Retrieved July 18, 2020 from https://dailymed.nlm.nih.gov/dailymed/drugInfo.cfm?setid=d7cee3fa-d05c-4702-8f75-f446627bdb49.

Marchetti, F., Coutaux, A., Bellanger, A., Magneux, C., Bourgeois, P., & Mion, G. (2015). Efficacy and safety of oral ketamine for the relief of intractable chronic pain: A retrospective 5-year study of 51 patients. *Eur J Pain, 19*(7), 984–993. https://doi.org/10.1002/ejp.624.

Markman, J. D., Jensen, T. S., Semel, D., Li, C., Parsons, B., Behar, R., & Sadosky, A. B. (2017). Effects of Pregabalin in Patients with Neuropathic Pain Previously Treated with Gabapentin: A Pooled Analysis of Parallel-group, Randomized, Placebo-controlled Clinical Trials. *Pain Practice*, 17(6), 718–728.

Marmura, M. J. (2010). Intravenous lidocaine and mexiletine in the management of trigeminal autonomic cephalalgias. *Current Pain and Headache Reports*, 14, 145–150. https://doi.org/10.1007/s11916-010-0098-6.

Marmura, M. J., & Goldberg, S. W. (2015). Inpatient management of migraine. *Current Neurology and Neuroscience Reports*, 15(4), 13.

Marmura, M. J., Passero, F. C., Jr., & Young, W. B. (2008a). Mexiletine for refractory chronic daily headache: a report of nine cases. *Headache*, 48(10), 1506–1510. https://doi.org/10.1111/j.1526-4610.2008.01234.x.

Marmura, M. J., Rosen, N., Abbas, M., & Silberstein, S. (2008b). Intravenous Lidocaine in the Treatment of Refractory Headache. *Headache*, 49, 286–291. https://doi.org/10.1111/j.1526-4610.2008.01281.x.

Marrett, E., Rolin, M., Beaussier, M., & Bonnet, F. (2008). Meta-analysis of intravenous lidocaine and postoperative recovery after abdominal surgery. *British Journal of Surgery*, 95, 1331–1338. https://doi.org/10.1002/bjs.6375.

Martinez, V., Pichard, X., & Fletcher, D. (2017). Perioperative pregabalin administration does not prevent chronic postoperative pain: systematic review with a meta-analysis of randomized trials. *Pain*, 158(5), 775–783.

Mathieson, S., Maher, C. G., McLachlan, A. J., Latimer, J., Koes, B. W., Hancock, M. J., … Lin, C. C. (2017). Trial of Pregabalin for Acute and Chronic Sciatica. *N Engl J Med*, 376(12), 1111–1120. https://doi.org/10.1056/NEJMoa1614292.

McCleane, G. (2007). Intravenous lidocaine: an outdated or underutilized treatment for pain. *J Palliat Med*, 10(3), 798–805. https://doi.org/10.1089/jpm.2006.0209.

McNicol, E. D., Schumann, R., & Haroutounian, S. (2014). A systematic review and meta-analysis of ketamine for the prevention of persistent post-surgical pain. *Acta Anaesthesiologica Scandinavica*, 58(10), 1199–1213.

McQuoid, P. (2019). Switching from gabapentin to pregabalin. *The New Zealand Medical Journal (Online)*, 132(1491), 101–103.

Meda, P. (2013). *Cesamet (nabilone) capsules for oral administration*. Retrieved July 18, 2020 from http://www.cesamet.com/pdf/Cesamet_PI_50_count.pdf.

Mehta, S., McIntyre, A., Dijkers, M., Loh, E., & Teasell, R. W. (2014). Gabapentinoids are effective in decreasing neuropathic pain and other secondary outcomes after spinal cord injury: a meta-analysis. *Archives of Physical Medicine and Rehabilitation*, 95(11), 2180–2186.

Mehta, S., McIntyre, A., Janzen, S., Loh, E., Teasell, R., & Team, S. C. I. R. E. (2016). Systematic review of pharmacologic treatments of pain after spinal cord injury: an update. *Archives of Physical Medicine and Rehabilitation*, 97(8), 1381–1391.

Meng, H., Johnston, B., Englesakis, M., Moulin, D. E., & Bhatia, A. (2017). Selective Cannabinoids for Chronic Neuropathic Pain: A Systematic Review and Meta-analysis. *Anesth Analg*, 125(5), 1638–1652. https://doi.org/10.1213/ane.0000000000002110.

Meremikwu, M. M., & Okomo, U. (2010). Sickle cell disease. *Clinical Evidence.*, 2, 1–19.

Moeller, K. E., Kissack, J. C., Atayee, R. S., & Lee, K. C. (2017, May). Clinical interpretation of urine drug tests: What clinicians need to know about urine drug screens. *Mayo Clinic Proceedings*, 92(5), 774–796.

Mogharabian, N., Asadpour, A., Sohrabi, M. B., & Karimi, M. (2018). Effect of methocarbamol on postoperative pain following inguinal hernia surgery. *European Urology Supplements*, 17(2), e1567.

Moharari, R. S., Motalebi, M., Najafi, A., Zamani, M. M., Imani, F., Etezadi, F., … Khajavi, M. R. (2014). Magnesium can decrease postoperative physiological ileus and postoperative pain in major non laparoscopic gastrointestinal surgeries: a randomized controlled trial. *Anesthesiology and Pain Medicine*, 4(1). https://doi.org/10.5812/aapm.12750.

Moore, K., & Haroz, R. (2017). When hydromorphone is not working, try loratadine: an emergency department case of loratadine as abortive therapy for severe pegfilgrastim-induced bone pain. *The Journal of Emergency Medicine*, 52(2), e29–e31.

Moore, R. A., Derry, S., Aldington, D., Cole, P., & Wiffen, P. J. (2015). Amitriptyline for fibromyalgia in adults. *The Cochrane Library.*, 7, CD008242.

Moulin, D., Boulanger, A., Clark, A. J., Clarke, H., Dao, T., Finley, G. A., … Williamson, O. D. (2014). Pharmacological management of chronic neuropathic pain: revised consensus statement from the Canadian Pain Society. *Pain Research and Management*, 19(6), 328–335.

Myers, F. A., Bluth, M. H., & Cheung, W. W. (2016). Ketamine: A cause of urinary tract dysfunction. *Clinics in Laboratory Medicine*, 36(4), 721–744.

Mylan Pharmaceuticals, I. (2016). *Amitriptyline: prescribing information*. Retrieved July 18, 2020 from https://dailymed.nlm.nih.gov/dailymed/drugInfo.cfm?setid=61d2da8d-b435-4ada-a013-401786f7cace.

Nasti, J. J., & Brakoulias, V. (2011). Chronic baclofen abuse and withdrawal delirium. *Australian and New Zealand Journal of Psychiatry*, 45(1), 86–87.

National Health Service of Scotland, N. H. S. (2014). *Scotland Palliative Care Guidelines: ketamine*. Retrieved from Ketamine website http://www.palliativecareguidelines.scot.nhs.uk/guidelines/medicine-information-sheets/ketamine.aspx.

National Health Service of Scotland, N. H. S. (2014). *Scotland Palliative Care Guidelines: ketamine*. Retrieved July 18, 2020 from Ketamine website http://www.palliativecareguidelines.scot.nhs.uk/guidelines/medicine-information-sheets/ketamine.aspx.

Nguyen, L., Thomas, K. L., Lucke-Wold, B. P., Cavendish, J. Z., Crowe, M. S., & Matsumoto, R. R. (2016). Dextromethorphan: An update on its utility for neurological and neuropsychiatric disorders. *Pharmacol Ther*, 159, 1–22. https://doi.org/10.1016/j.pharmthera.2016.01.016.

Nguyen, V., Tiemann, D., Park, E., & Salehi, A. (2017). Alpha-2 agonists. *Anesthesiology Clinics*, 35(2), 233–245.

Nie, Y., Liu, Y., Luo, Q., & Huang, S. (2014). Effect of dexmedetomidine combined with sufentanil for post-caesarean section intravenous analgesia: a randomised, placebo-controlled study. *Eur J Anaesthesiol*, 31(4), 197–203. https://doi.org/10.1097/EJA.0000000000000011.

Niesters, M., Martini, C., & Dahan, A. (2014). Ketamine for chronic pain: risks and benefits. *Br J Clin Pharmacol*, 77(2), 357–367. https://doi.org/10.1111/bcp.12094.

Obata, H. (2017). Analgesic mechanisms of antidepressants for neuropathic pain. *International Journal of Molecular Sciences, 18*(11), 2483.

O'Connor, A. B., & Dworkin, R. H. (2009). Treatment of neuropathic pain: an overview of recent guidelines. *Am J Med, 122*(10), S22–S32. https://doi.org/10.1016/j.amjmed.2009.04.007. Suppl.

Okon, T. (2007). Ketamine: an introduction for the pain and palliative medicine physician. *Pain Physician, 10*(3), 493–500.

Olivo, M. G., Sin, B., Liu, M., Inamasu, K., Cheng, D., & DeSouza, S. (2016). 232 The Use of Sub-dissociative Ketamine For Sickle Cell Pain in the Emergency Department. *Annals of Emergency Medicine, 68*(4), S91.

Palm, N., Floroff, C., Hassig, T. B., Boylan, A., & Kanter, J. (2018). Low-Dose Ketamine Infusion for Adjunct Management during Vaso-occlusive Episodes in Adults with Sickle Cell Disease: A Case Series. *Journal of Pain & Palliative Care Pharmacotherapy, 32*(1), 20–26.

Pasero, C., & McCaffery, M. (2005). Ketamine: low doses may provide relief for some painful conditions. *American Journal of Nursing, 105*(4), 60–64.

Patanwala, A. E., Aljuhani, O., Kopp, B. J., & Erstad, B. L. (2017). Methocarbamol use is associated with decreased hospital length of stay in trauma patients with closed rib fractures. *The American Journal of Surgery, 214*(4), 738–742.

Patel, I. B., Bairy, K. L., Bhat, S. N., Shetty, D. J., Shalini, A., & Esha, R. (2015). Efficacy of Non-Steroidal Anti-Inflammatory Drugs (NSAIDs), Muscle Relaxants and Neurotropic Drugs in Patients with Low Back Pain. *American Journal of PharmTech Research, 5*(1), 633–641.

Peckham, A. M., Evoy, K. E., Ochs, L., & Covvey, J. R. (2018). Gabapentin for off-label use: evidence-based or cause for concern?. *Substance Abuse: Research and Treatment, 12*, 1178221818801311.

Peixoto, R. D. A., & Hawley, P. (2015). Intravenous lidocaine for cancer pain without electrocardiographic monitoring: a retrospective review. *Journal of Palliative Medicine, 18*(4), 373–377.

Peng, K., Jin, X. H., Liu, S. L., & Ji, F. H. (2015). Effect of Intraoperative Dexmedetomidine on Post-Craniotomy Pain. *Clin Ther, 37*(5). https://doi.org/10.1016/j.clinthera.2015.02.011. 1114-1121.e1111.

Perahia, D. G., Bangs, M. E., Zhang, Q., Cheng, Y., Ahl, J., Frakes, E. P., ... Martinez, J. M. (2013). The risk of bleeding with duloxetine treatment in patients who use nonsteroidal anti-inflammatory drugs (NSAIDs): analysis of placebo-controlled trials and post-marketing adverse event reports. *Drug Healthc Patient Saf, 5*, 211–219. https://doi.org/10.2147/DHPS.S45445.

Pfizer. *Lyrica: once-daily treatment option*. Retrieved July 18, 2020 from https://www.lyrica.com/pain-after-shingles/lyrica-cr.

Pfizer. (2016). *Lyrica: Highlights of prescribing information*. Retrieved July 18, 2020 from http://labeling.pfizer.com/showlabeling.aspx?id=561.

Pfizer. (2017a). *Neurontin: highlights of prescribing information*. Retrieved July 18, 2020 from http://labeling.pfizer.com/ShowLabeling.aspx?id=630.

Pfizer. (2017b). U.S. FDA approves Lyrica® CR (pregabalin) extended-release tablets CV [press release]. Retrieved July 18, 2020 from http://www.pfizer.com/news/press-release/press-release-detail/u_s_fda_approves_lyrica_cr_pregabalin_extended_release_tablets_cv.

PharmaForce, I. (2009). *Clonidine hydrochloride injection, solution: prescribing information*. Retrieved July 18, 2020 from https://dailymed.nlm.nih.gov/dailymed/drugInfo.cfm?setid=6E562C90-2E37-47AC-9C3F-12460F96DC33.

Pini, L. A., Guerzoni, S., Cainazzo, M. M., Ferrari, A., Sarchielli, P., Tiraferri, I., ... Zappaterra, M. (2012). Nabilone for the treatment of medication overuse headache: results of a preliminary double-blind, active-controlled, randomized trial. *J Headache Pain, 13*(8), 677–684. https://doi.org/10.1007/s10194-012-0490-1.

Pop-Busui, R., Boulton, A. J., Feldman, E. L., Bril, V., Freeman, R., Malik, R. A., ... Ziegler, D. (2017). Diabetic Neuropathy: A Position Statement by the American Diabetes Association. *Diabetes Care, 40*(1), 136–154. https://doi.org/10.2337/dc16-2042.

Portenoy, R. K. (2020). A Practical Approach to Using Adjuvant Analgesics in Older Adults. *Journal of the American Geriatrics Society, 68*(4), 691–698.

Pruskowski, J., & Arnold, R. M. (2015). A comparison of pregabalin and gabapentin in palliative care #289. *J Palliat Med, 18*(4), 386–387. https://doi.org/10.1089/jpm.2015.1022.

Qaseem, A., Wilt, T. J., McLean, R. M., Forciea, M. A., & Physicians, C. G. C.o.t. A. C.o. (2017). Noninvasive treatments for acute, subacute, and chronic low back pain: a clinical practice guideline from the American College of Physicians. *Annals Internal Medicine, 166*, 514–530.

Quibell, R., Fallon, M., Mihalyo, M., Twycross, R., & Wilcock, A. (2015). Ketamine. *Journal of pain and symptom management, 50*(2), 268–278.

Radvansky, B. M., Shah, K., Parikh, A., Sifonios, A. N., Le, V., & Eloy, J. D. (2015). Role of ketamine in acute postoperative pain management: a narrative review. *BioMed research international, 2015*. https://doi.org/10.1155/2015/749837.

Rauck, R. L., North, J., & Eisenach, J. C. (2015). Intrathecal clonidine and adenosine: effects on pain and sensory processing in patients with chronic regional pain syndrome. *Pain, 156*(1), 88–95.

Ren, C., Chi, M., Zhang, Y., Zhang, Z., Qi, F., & Liu, Z. (2015). Dexmedetomidine in Postoperative Analgesia in Patients Undergoing Hysterectomy: A CONSORT-Prospective, Randomized, Controlled Trial. *Medicine (Baltimore), 94*(32). https://doi.org/10.1097/MD.0000000000001348.

Riediger, C., Schuster, T., Barlinn, K., Maier, S., Weitz, J., & Siepmann, T. (2017). Adverse effects of antidepressants for chronic pain: a systematic review and meta-analysis. *Frontiers in neurology, 8*, 307.

Rintala, D. H., Fiess, R. N., Tan, G., Holmes, S. A., & Bruel, B. M. (2010). Effect of dronabinol on central neuropathic pain after spinal cord injury: a pilot study. *Am J Phys Med Rehabil, 89*(10), 840–848. https://doi.org/10.1097/PHM.0b013e3181f1c4ec.

Romeo, C., Li, Q., & Copeland, L. (2015). Severe pegfilgrastim-induced bone pain completely alleviated with loratadine: A case report. *Journal of Oncology Pharmacy Practice, 21*, 301–304. https://doi.org/10.1177/1078155214527858.

Romero-Sandoval, A., Bynum, T., & Eisenach, J. C. (2007). Analgesia induced by perineural clonidine is enhanced in persistent neuritis. *Neuroreport, 18*, 67–71.

Romman, A., Salama-Hanna, J., & Dwivedi, S. (2018). Mexiletine Usage in a Chronic Pain Clinic: Indications, Tolerability, and Side Effects. *Pain Physician, 21*(5), E573–E579.

Salas, S., Frasca, M., Planchet-Barraud, B., Burucoa, B., Pascal, M., Lapiana, J. M., ... Baumstarck, K. (2012). Ketamine analgesic effect by continuous intravenous infusion in refractory cancer pain: considerations about the clinical research in palliative care. *J Palliat Med*, 15(3), 287–293. https://doi.org/10.1089/jpm.2011.0353.

Sandoz. (2014). *Desipramine: prescribing information*. Retrieved July 18, 2020 from https://dailymed.nlm.nih.gov/dailymed/drugInfo.cfm?setid=7ec5f73f-32b6-48c3-b16e-891d06edf6eb.

Saulino, M. (2018). Intrathecal baclofen therapy for the control of spasticity. In E. S. Krames, P. Hunter Peckham, & A. R. Rezai (Eds.), *Neuromodulation* (2nd edn, pp. 889–900). Philadelphia, PA: Elsevier-Saunders.

Saxena, A., Chansoria, M., Tomar, G., & Kumar, A. (2015). Myofascial pain syndrome: an overview. *Journal of Pain & Palliative Care Pharmacotherapy*, 29(1), 16–21.

Schifano, F. (2014). Misuse and abuse of pregabalin and gabapentin: cause for concern? *CNS Drugs*, 28(6), 491–496. https://doi.org/10.1007/s40263-014-0164-4.

Schwartzman, R. J., Patel, M., Grothusen, J. R., & Alexander, G. M. (2009a). Efficacy of 5 day continuous lidocaine infusion for the treatment of refractory complex regional pain syndrome. *Pain Medicine*, 10(2), 401–412. https://doi.org/10.1111/j.1526-4637.2009.00573.x.

Schwartzman, R. J., Alexander, G. M., Grothusen, J. R., Paylor, T., Reichenberger, E., & Perreault, M. (2009b). Outpatient intravenous ketamine for the treatment of complex regional pain syndrome: a double-blind placebo controlled study. *Pain*, 147(1-3), 107–115. https://doi.org/10.1016/j.pain.2009.08.015.

Schwenk, E. S., Viscusi, E. R., Buvanendran, A., Hurley, R. W., Wasan, A. D., Narouze, S., ... Cohen, S. P. (2018). Consensus guidelines on the use of intravenous ketamine infusions for acute pain management from the American Society of Regional Anesthesia and Pain Medicine. *the American Academy of Pain Medicine, and the American Society of Anesthesiologists.*, 43(5), 456–466.

Shaibani, A. I., Pope, L. E., Thisted, R., & Hepner, A. (2012). Efficacy and safety of dextromethorphan-quinidine at two dosage levels for diabetic neuropathic pain. *Pain Medicine*, 13, 243–254.

Shanthanna, H., Gilron, I., Rajarathinam, M., AlAmri, R., Kamath, S., Thabane, L., ... Bhandari, M. (2017). Benefits and safety of gabapentinoids in chronic low back pain: A systematic review and meta-analysis of randomized controlled trials. *PLoS Med*, 14(8). https://doi.org/10.1371/journal.pmed.1002369.

Shin, H. J., Kim, E. Y., Na, H. S., Kim, T. K., Kim, M. H., & Do, S. H. (2016). Magnesium sulphate attenuates acute postoperative pain and increased pain intensity after surgical injury in staged bilateral total knee arthroplasty: a randomized, double-blinded, placebo-controlled trial. *BJA: British Journal of Anaesthesia*, 117(4), 497–503.

Siddiqui, N. T., Yousefzadeh, A., Yousuf, M., Kumar, D., Choudhry, F. K., & Friedman, Z. (2018). The effect of gabapentin on delayed discharge from the postanesthesia care unit: a retrospective analysis. *Pain Practice*, 18(1), 18–22.

Sigtermans, M. J., van Hilten, J. J., Bauer, M. C., Arbous, M. S., Marinus, J., Sarton, E. Y., & Dahan, A. (2009). Ketamine produces effective and long-term pain relief in patients with Complex Regional Pain Syndrome Type 1. *Pain*, 145(3), 304–311. https://doi.org/10.1016/j.pain.2009.06.023.

Sim, D. S. M. (2015). Drug Absorption and Bioavailability. In Y. K. Chan, K. P. Ng, & D. S. M. Sim (Eds.), *Pharmacological Basis of Acute Care (pp. 17-26)*. Cham, Switzerland: Springer.

Siu, A., & Drachtman, R. (2007). Dextromethorphan: a review of N-methyl-D-aspartate receptor antagonism in the management of pain. *CNS Drug Reviews*, 13(1), 96–106.

Sleigh, J., Harvey, M., Voss, L., & Denny, B. (2014). Ketamine—More mechanisms of action than just NMDA blockade. *Trends in Anaesthesia and Critical Care*, 4(2), 76–81.

Smith, R. V., Havens, J. R., & Walsh, S. L. (2016). Gabapentin misuse, abuse and diversion: a systematic review. *Addiction*, 111(7), 1160–1174.

Smith, M. M., Smith, B. B., Lahr, B. D., Nuttall, G. A., Mauermann, W. J., Weister, T. J., ... Barbara, D. W. (2018). Selective Serotonin Reuptake Inhibitors and Serotonin–Norepinephrine Reuptake Inhibitors Are Not Associated With Bleeding or Transfusion in Cardiac Surgical Patients. *Anesthesia & Analgesia*, 126(6), 1859–1866.

Soleimanpour, H., Hassanzadeh, K., Vaezi, H., Golzari, S. E., Esfanjani, R. M., & Soleimanpour, M. (2012). Effectiveness of intravenous lidocaine versus intravenous morphine for patients with renal colic in the emergency department. *BMC Urol*, 12. https://doi.org/10.1186/1471-2490-12-13.

Srebro, D., Vuckovic, S., Milovanovic, A., Kosutic, J., Savic Vujovic, K., & Prostran, M. (2017). Magnesium in pain research: state of the art. *Current Medicinal Chemistry*, 24(4), 424–434.

Starling, A. J., & Dodick, D. W. (2015, March). Best practices for patients with chronic migraine: burden, diagnosis, and management in primary care. *Mayo Clinic Proceedings*, 90(3), 408–414.

Stewart, D., & McPherson, M. L. (2017). Symptom management challenges in heart failure: pharmacotherapy considerations. *Heart Failure Reviews*, 22(5), 525–534.

Svendsen, K. B., Jensen, T. S., & Bach, F. W. (2004). Does the cannabinoid dronabinol reduce central pain in multiple sclerosis? Randomised double blind placebo controlled crossover trial. *BMJ*, 329(7460), 253. https://doi.org/10.1136/bmj.38149.566979.AE.

Swarm, R. A., Anghelescu, D. L., Are, M., Bruce, J. Y., Buga, S., Chwistek, M., ... Youngwerth, J. M. (2018). *NCCN Clinical Practice Guidelines in Oncology: Adult Cancer Pain*. Retrieved July 18, 2020 from https://www.nccn.org/professionals/physician_gls/pdf/pain.pdf.

Talakoub, R., Abbasi, S., Maghami, E., & Zavareh, S.M.H.T. (2016). The effect of oral tizanidine on postoperative pain relief after elective laparoscopic cholecystectomy. *Advanced Biomedical Research*, 5, 19. https://doi.org/10.4103/2277-9175.175905.

Teva Pharmaceuticals USA, I. (2015). *Nortriptyline: prescribing information*. Retrieved July 18, 2020 from https://dailymed.nlm.nih.gov/dailymed/drugInfo.cfm?setid=b58d473a-b19f-4d2a-b1ae-dd398d7a29e1.

Than, N. N., Soe, H. H. K., Palaniappan, S. K., Abas, A. B., & De Franceschi, L. (2017). Magnesium for treating sickle cell disease. *Cochrane Database Syst Rev*, 4. https://doi.org/10.1002/14651858.CD011358.pub2.

Timmerman, L., Stronks, D. L., Groeneweg, J. G., & Huygen, F. J. (2016). Prevalence and determinants of medication non-adherence in chronic pain patients: a systematic review. *Acta Anaesthesiologica Scandinavica*, 60(4), 416–431.

Tonner, P. H. (2017). Additives used to reduce perioperative opioid consumption 1: Alpha2-agonists. *Best Practice & Research Clinical Anaesthesiology*, 31(4), 505–512.

Trouvin, A. P., Perrot, S., & Lloret-Linares, C. (2017). Efficacy of venlafaxine in neuropathic pain: a narrative review of optimized treatment. *Clinical Therapeutics, 39*(6), 1104–1122.

Tsang, C. C., & Giudice, M. G. (2016). Nabilone for the Management of Pain. *Pharmacotherapy, 36*(3), 273–286. https://doi.org/10.1002/phar.1709.

Turcotte, D., Doupe, M., Torabi, M., Gomori, A., Ethans, K., Esfahani, F., … Namaka, M. (2015). Nabilone as an adjunctive to gabapentin for multiple sclerosis-induced neuropathic pain: a randomized controlled trial. *Pain Med, 16*(1), 149–159. https://doi.org/10.1111/pme.12569.

Uprety, D., Baber, A., & Foy, M. (2014). Ketamine infusion for sickle cell pain crisis refractory to opioids: a case report and review of literature. *Annals of Hematology, 93*(5), 769–771.

Urits, I., Borchart, M., Hasegawa, M., Kochanski, J., Orhurhu, V., & Viswanath, O. (2019). An update of current cannabis-based pharmaceuticals in pain medicine. *Pain and Therapy, 8*(1), 41–51.

van der Wal, S. E., van den Heuvel, S. A., Radema, S. A., van Berkum, B. F., Vaneker, M., Steegers, M. A., … Vissers, K. C. (2016). The in vitro mechanisms and in vivo efficacy of intravenous lidocaine on the neuroinflammatory response in acute and chronic pain. *European Journal of Pain, 20*(5), 655–674.

Van Tulder, M. W., Touray, T., Furlan, A. D., Solway, S., & Bouter, L. M. (2003). Muscle relaxants for nonspecific low back pain: a systematic review within the framework of the cochrane collaboration. *Spine, 28*(17), 1978–1992.

Vigneault, L., Turgeon, A. F., Cote, D., Lauzier, F., Zarychanski, R., Moore, L., … Fergusson, D. A. (2011). Perioperative intravenous lidocaine infusion for postoperative pain control: a meta-analysis of randomized controlled trials. *Canadian Journal of Anesthesiology, 58*, 22–37. https://doi.org/10.1007/s12630-010-9407-0.

Vyvey, M. (2010). Steroids as pain relief adjuvants. *Canadian Family Physician, 56*, 1295–1297.

Waldfogel, J. M., Nesbit, S. A., Dy, S. M., Sharma, R., Zhang, A., Wilson, L. M., … Robinson, K. A. (2017). Pharmacotherapy for diabetic peripheral neuropathy pain and quality of life: A systematic review. *Neurology, 88*(29), 1958–1967.

Walitt, B., Klose, P., Fitzcharles, M. A., Phillips, T., & Hauser, W. (2016). Cannabinoids for fibromyalgia. *Cochrane Database Syst Rev,* (7). https://doi.org/10.1002/14651858.CD011694.pub2.

Wang, D., Bao, J. B., Zhang, K., Ju, L. F., & Yu, L. Z. (2017). Pregabalin for the treatment of neuropathic pain in adults: a systematic review of randomized controlled trials. *International Journal of Clinical and Experimental Medicine, 10*(1), 16–29.

Wang, L., Johnston, B., Kaushal, A., Cheng, D., Zhu, F., & Martin, J. (2016). Ketamine added to morphine or hydromorphone patient-controlled analgesia for acute postoperative pain in adults: a systematic review and meta-analysis of randomized trials. *Canadian Journal of Anesthesia/Journal canadien d'anesthésie, 63*(3), 311–325.

Wang, S. L., Wang, H., Nie, H. Y., Bu, G., Shen, X. D., & Wang, H. (2017). The efficacy of pregabalin for acute pain control in herpetic neuralgia patients: A meta-analysis. *Medicine, 96*(51), e9167.

Wang, X., Ding, X., Tong, Y., Zong, J., Zhao, X., Ren, H., & Li, Q. (2014). Ketamine does not increase intracranial pressure compared with opioids: meta-analysis of randomized controlled trials. *Journal of anesthesia, 28*(6), 821–827.

Watson, J. C., & Dyck, P. J. B. (2015, July). Peripheral neuropathy: a practical approach to diagnosis and symptom management. *Mayo Clinic Proceedings, 90*(7), 940–951. Watson Laboratories, I. (2006). Mexiletine: prescribing information. Retrieved July 18, 2020 from https://dailymed.nlm.nih.gov/dailymed/drugInfo.cfm?setid=ab73778b-6794-441c-b127-610a6d0733ea.

Weibel, S., Jelting, Y., Pace, N. L., Helf, A., Eberhart, L. H., Hahnenkamp, K., … Kranke, P. (2018). Continuous intravenous perioperative lidocaine infusion for postoperative pain and recovery in adults. *Cochrane Database of Systematic Reviews, 6*(6), CD009642.

Weinbroum, A. A., Rudick, V. V., Paret, G., & Ben-Abraham, R. (2000). The role of dextromethorphan in pain control. *Canadian Journal of Anesthesiology, 47*(6), 585–596.

Welsch, P., Uceyler, N., Klose, P., Walitt, B., & Hauser, W. (2018). Serotonin and noradrenaline reuptake inhibitors (SNRIs) for fibromyalgia. *Cochrane Database Syst Rev,* (2). https://doi.org/10.1002/14651858.CD010292.pub2.

Wenzel-Seifert, K., Wittmann, M., & Haen, E. (2011). QTc prolongation by psychotropic drugs and the risk of torsades de pointes. *Dtsch Arztebl Int, 108*(41), 687–693. https://doi.org/10.3238/arztebl.2011.0687.

Westfall, T. C., Macarthur, H., & Westfall, D. P. (2018). Adrenergic agonists and antagonists. In L. L. Brunton, R. Hilal-Danda, & B. C. Knollman (Eds.), *Goodman and Gilman's The Pharmacological Basis of Therapeutics* (13th ed.). New York, N.Y.: McGraw-Hill Education.

Wiffen, P. J., Derry, S., Bell, R. F., Rice, A. S., Tölle, T. R., Phillips, T., & Moore, R. A. (2017). Gabapentin for chronic neuropathic pain in adults. *The Cochrane Library, 6*(6), CD007938.

Williams, K., Guarino, A., & Raja, S. N. (2018). Complex regional pain syndrome. In H. Benzon, S. Raja, N. Srinivasa, S. Liu, S. Fishman, & S. Cohen (Eds.), *Essentials of Pain Medicine* (4th edition, pp. 223–232). Philadelphia, PA: Elsevier.

Wissel, J., Haydn, T., Muller, J., Brenneis, C., Berger, T., Poewe, W., & Schelosky, L. D. (2006). Low dose treatment with the synthetic cannabinoid nabilone significantly reduces spasticity-related pain : a double-blind placebo-controlled cross-over trial. *J Neurol, 253*(10), 1337–1341. https://doi.org/10.1007/s00415-006-0218-8.

Witenko, C., Moorman-Li, R., Motycka, C., Duane, K., Hincapie-Castillo, J., Leonard, P., & Valaer, C. (2014). Considerations for the appropriate use of skeletal muscle relaxants for the management of acute low back pain. *Pharmacy and Therapeutics, 39*(6), 427.

Wright, J. M., Oki, J. C., & Graves, L., 3rd. (1997). Mexiletine in the symptomatic treatment of diabetic peripheral neuropathy. *Ann Pharmacother, 31*(1), 29–34. https://doi.org/10.1177/106002809703100103.

Wrzosek, A., Woron, J., Dobrogowski, J., Jakowicka-Wordliczek, J., & Wordliczek, J. (2015). Topical clonidine for neuropathic pain. *Cochrane Database of Systematic Reviews, 8*, CD010967.

Wyeth. (2016a). *Effexor XR: highlights of prescribing information.* Retrieved July 18, 2020 from http://labeling.pfizer.com/showlabeling.aspx?ID=100.

Wyeth. (2016b). *Pristiq: highlights of prescribing information.* Retrieved July 18, 2020 from http://labeling.pfizer.com/showlabeling.aspx?id=497.

Yang, L., Zhang, J., Zhang, Z., Zhang, C., Zhao, D., & Li, J. (2014). Preemptive analgesia effects of ketamine in patients undergoing surgery. A meta-analysis. *Acta Cir Bras*, 29(12), 819–825. https://doi.org/10.1590/s0102-86502014001900009.

Yao, Z., Shen, C., & Zhong, Y. (2015). Perioperative pregabalin for acute pain after gynecological surgery: a meta-analysis. *Clinical therapeutics*, 37(5), 1128–1135.

Yazicioglu, D., Caparlar, C., Akkaya, T., Mercan, U., & Kulaçoglu, H. (2016). Tizanidine for the management of acute postoperative pain after inguinal hernia repair: a placebo-controlled double-blind trial. *European Journal of Anaesthesiology*, 33(3), 215–222.

Ye, F., Wu, Y., & Zhou, C. (2017). Effect of intravenous ketamine for postoperative analgesia in patients undergoing laparoscopic cholecystectomy: A meta-analysis. *Medicine*, 96(51). https://doi.org/10.1097/MD.0000000000009147.

Yousef, A. A., & Al-deeb, A. E. (2013). A double-blinded randomised controlled study of the value of sequential intravenous and oral magnesium therapy in patients with chronic low back pain with a neuropathic component. *Anaesthesia*, 68(3), 260–266. https://doi.org/10.1111/anae.12107.

Yu, L., Ran, B., Li, M., & Shi, Z. (2013). Gabapentin and pregabalin in the management of postoperative pain after lumbar spinal surgery: a systematic review and meta-analysis. *Spine (Phila Pa 1976)*, 38(22), 1947–1952. https://doi.org/10.1097/BRS.0b013e3182a69b90.

Zakrzewska, J. M., & Linskey, M. E. (2014). Trigeminal neuralgia. *BMJ*, 348, g474.

Zanaflex Highlights of Prescribing Information. *Acorda Therapeutics*. Retrieved July 18, 2020 from https://dailymed.nlm.nih.gov/dailymed/drugInfo.cfm?setid=413ee468-c7e8-4283-8e2b-b573dcc1f607.

Zanos, P., Moaddel, R., Morris, P. J., Riggs, L. M., Highland, J. N., Georgiou, P., ... Gould, T. D. (2018). Ketamine and ketamine metabolite pharmacology: insights into therapeutic mechanisms. *Pharmacological Reviews*, 70(3), 621–660.

Zeiler, F. A., Teitelbaum, J., West, M., & Gillman, L. M. (2014). The ketamine effect on intracranial pressure in nontraumatic neurological illness. *Journal of Critical Care*, 29(6), 1096–1106.

Zhang, S. S., Wu, Z., Zhang, L. C., Zhang, Z., Chen, R. P., Huang, Y. H., & Chen, H. (2015). Efficacy and safety of pregabalin for treating painful diabetic peripheral neuropathy: a meta-analysis. *Acta Anaesthesiologica Scandinavica*, 59(2), 147–159.

Zhang, X., & Bai, X. (2014). New therapeutic uses for an alpha2 adrenergic receptor agonist- -dexmedetomidine in pain management. *Neurosci Lett*, 561, 7–12. https://doi.org/10.1016/j.neulet.2013.12.039.

Zhang, Y., Wang, Y., & Zhang, X. (2017). Effect of pre-emptive pregabalin on pain management in patients undergoing laparoscopic cholecystectomy: A systematic review and meta-analysis. *International Journal of Surgery*, 44, 122–127.

Zhao, J. B., Li, Y. L., Wang, Y. M., Teng, J. L., Xia, D. Y., Zhao, J. S., & Li, F. L. (2018). Intravenous lidocaine infusion for pain control after laparoscopic cholecystectomy: A meta-analysis of randomized controlled trials. *Medicine (Baltimore)*, 97(5), e9771.

Zhou, Y. Q., Chen, S. P., Liu, D. Q., Manyande, A., Zhang, W., Yang, S. B., ... Ye, D. W. (2017). The role of spinal GABAB receptors in cancer-induced bone pain in rats. *The Journal of Pain*, 18(8), 933–946.

Zoorob, R. J., & Cender, D. (1998). A different look at corticosteroids. *American Family Physician*, 58(2), 443–450.

Chapter 16 Topical Analgesics for the Management of Acute and Chronic Pain

Elsa Wuhrman, Maureen F. Cooney, Thien C. Pham

CHAPTER OUTLINE

Benefits of Topical Analgesics, pg. 429

Types of Topical Analgesics, pg. 431

    Counter-irritants, pg. 431

    Local Anesthetics, pg. 436

    Nonsteroidal Antiinflammatory Drugs, pg. 438

Compound Analgesics, pg. 441

    Ketamine, pg. 441

    Amitriptyline, pg. 442

    Ketamine and Amitriptyline Combination, pg. 442

    CloNIDine, pg. 442

    Gabapentin, pg. 442

    Baclofen, pg. 443

    Opioids, pg. 443

Key Points, pg. 443

Case Scenario, pg. 443

References, pg. 444

chapter is to identify indications and benefits for topical analgesics and describe various types of topical analgesics, including counter-irritants, local anesthetics, nonsteroidal antiinflammatory drugs (NSAIDs), and compound analgesics.

The formulation terms *topical* and *transdermal* are sometimes erroneously used interchangeably. Topical medications are applied externally and absorbed into the skin to exert their pharmacologic effects at or near the application site with little systemic absorption (Fig. 16.2). Transdermal formulations of analgesics (e.g., fentaNYL transdermal patch, buprenorphine transdermal patch) are designed to use the deeper, subcutaneous layer of the skin as a depot or vehicle for medication to be gradually absorbed into the systemic circulation (Fig. 16.3). This type of delivery system results in serum concentration of medication similar to oral or parenteral administration, thereby resulting in systemic activity (Leppert, Malec-Milewska, Zajaczkowska & Wordliczek, 2018). The focus of this chapter is topical, local medication delivery; transdermal medications are addressed in Chapter 11.

Different medications display varying degrees of dermal penetration through the dense layer of the stratum corneum of the epidermis and may require vehicles or solvents to enhance permeability to allow adequate absorption into the tissues (Derry, Wiffen et al., 2017). Molecular weight, degree of lipophilicity, aqueous solubility, and drug formulation are important pharmacokinetic factors that can affect drug permeability across membrane tissues and allow for adequate absorption (Derry, Wiffen et al., 2017; Nastiti et al., 2017). Table 16.1 summarizes pharmacokinetic properties of various topical analgesics.

Benefits of Topical Analgesics

Benefits of topical analgesics include (1) avoidance of first-pass metabolism and other variable factors associated with the gastrointestinal (GI) tract (e.g., pH, gastric emptying time), (2) localized targeted drug delivery, (3) controlled and sustained drug delivery over a period of time, (4) improved patient acceptance and adherence with

TOPICAL analgesics are a viable treatment strategy in the management of acute and chronic pain. Topical analgesics provide a means for localized targeted drug delivery with controlled and sustained delivery over a period of time. Some of these medications are available over the counter (OTC) (e.g., capsaicin, lidocaine, menthol/methylsalicylate), and others are prescribed. Topical medications may be used for musculoskeletal aches, sprains and strains, chronic conditions such as osteoarthritis, and neuropathic pain, alone and/or as part of a multimodal analgesia plan. There are various topical formulations available, including creams, foams, gels, lotions, ointments, patches, and solutions. Fig. 16.1 illustrates the anatomy and physiology of the skin and potential action sites of several analgesic medications. The purpose of this

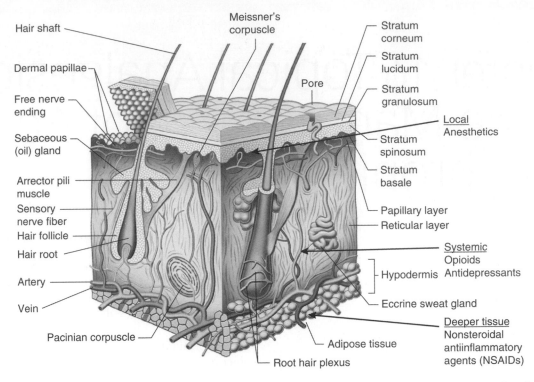

Fig. 16.1 | Anatomy and physiology of the skin: potential sites of analgesic action. (From Pasero, C., & McCaffery, M. [2011]. *Pain Assessment and Pharmacologic Management*, St. Louis, Mosby.)

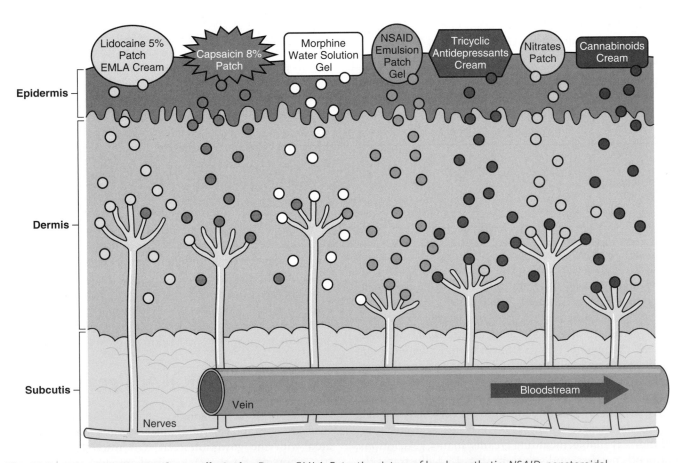

Fig. 16.2 | **Topical Application for Locally Acting Drugs.** *EMLA,* Eutectic mixture of local anesthetic; *NSAID,* nonsteroidal antiinflammatory drug. (Redrawn from Leppert, W., Malec-Milewska, M., Zajaczkowska, R., & Wordliczek, J. [2018]. Transdermal and topical drug administration in the treatment of pain. *Molecules (Basel, Switzerland), 23*[3], 681. https://doi.org/10.3390/molecules23030681.)

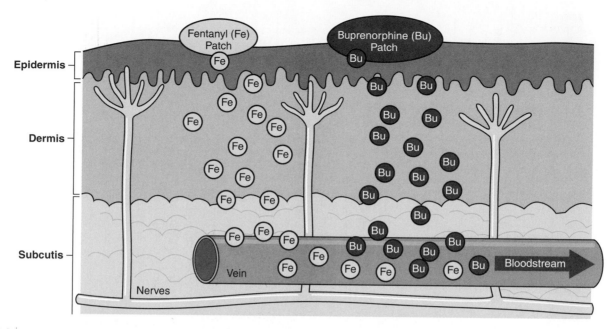

Fig. 16.3 | Transdermal Formulation for Systemically Acting Drugs. (Redrawn from Leppert, W., Malec-Milewska, M., Zajaczkowska, R., & Wordliczek, J. [2018]. Transdermal and topical drug administration in the treatment of pain. *Molecules (Basel, Switzerland), 23*[3], 681. https://doi.org/10.3390/molecules23030681.)

Table 16.1 | Pharmacokinetic Properties of Common Topical Analgesic Agents

Drug	Pharmacologic Category	Half-Life ($T_{1/2}$, Hours)
Amitriptyline	Tricyclic antidepressant	10–50
Baclofen	Muscle relaxant	2.5–4
Bupivacaine	Local anesthetic	2.7
Capsaicin	Counterirritant	1.64
CloNIDine	Alpha-2 adrenergic agent	6–20
Diclofenac	NSAID	2
Gabapentin	Anticonvulsant	5–7
Ketamine	General anesthetic	2.5–3
Lidocaine	Local anesthetic	1.82
Methylsalicylate	Counter-irritant NSAID	2–12

Data from Kim, S., Thiessen, P. A., Bolton, E. E., Chen, J., Fu, G., Gindulyte, A., . . . & Bryant, S. H. (2016) and PubChem substance and databases. *Nucleic Acids Research, 44*(D1), D1202–1213. https://doi.org/10.1093/nar/gkv951; Derry, S., Matthews, P. R., Wiffen, P. J., & Moore, R. A. (2014). Salicylate-containing rubefacients for acute and chronic musculoskeletal pain in adults. *Cochrane Database of Systematic Reviews, 11.* https://doi.org/10.1002/14651858.CD007403.pub3.

ease of use, (5) ease of medication discontinuation in the event of adverse effects, (6) reduction in potential adverse effects and medication interactions because of generally limited systemic absorption, and (7) alternative route of medication administration, especially when the oral route is not feasible (Anitescu, Benzon, & Argoff, 2013; Brown, Martin, & Jones, 2006; Leppert et al., 2018; Sarbacker, 2015).

Although studies do not reveal markedly superior efficacy, topical analgesics are increasingly recommended in clinical practice guidelines because they may provide safer options for medication administration to special populations such as the elderly and those with cardiovascular disease, hepatic disease, and/or renal insufficiency (Leppert et al., 2018).

Types of Topical Analgesics

Several different categories of medications are used as topical analgesics. Table 16.2 presents a comparison of topical analgesics used in acute and chronic pain.

Counter-irritants

Capsaicin

Capsaicin is an active ingredient found in chili peppers. It acts as a neuropeptide (substance P and tachykinin), releasing mediators of C fibers within primary sensory peripheral neurons, and inducing a "hot" sensation when exposed to skin (Derry, Rice, Cole, Tan, & Moore, 2017; Derry, Wiffen et al., 2017) and other epithelial tissues such as the conjunctiva. Capsaicin binds to nociceptors within the skin primarily at the transient receptor potential cation channel subfamily V member 1 (TRPV1) receptor (also known as the capsaicin nociceptor receptor), which facilitates an influx of sodium and calcium ions across the cell membrane causing

Table 16.2 | Comparison of Select Topical Analgesics

Drug	Formulation	Dose Concentrations	Mechanism of Action	Site of Action	Pain Pathology	Frequency of Application
CloNIDine	Compounded	0.1%	Alpha-2 receptor agonist, I2 imidazoline receptor agonist	A-delta and C fibers	Diabetic peripheral neuropathy	Apply up to 3 times/day
Gabapentin	Compounded	2%–6%	GABA analogue, voltage-gated calcium channel inhibitor, glutamate antagonist	C fibers	Vulvodynia	—
Capsaicin	Cream	0.025%–0.1%	TRPV1 receptor agonist with reversible superficial nerve degeneration	A-delta and C fibers	Neuropathic pain, muscle/joint pain, postherpetic neuralgia, HIV distal sensory polyneuropathy, cervical radiculopathy, lumbar radiculopathy, diabetic peripheral neuropathy	Apply up to 3–5 times/day
	Patch	8%	TRPV1 receptor agonist with reversible superficial nerve degeneration	A-delta and C fibers	Postherpetic neuralgia	Apply for 60 min, repeated every 3 mo
Ketamine	Compounded	0.5%–5%, 10%	NMDA receptor antagonist	A-delta and C fibers	Postherpetic neuralgia, diabetic peripheral neuropathy, complex regional pain syndrome, radiculopathy, neuropathic pain	—
Bupivacaine	Compounded	—	Voltage-gated sodium channel inhibitor	A-delta and C fibers	—	—

Drug	Formulation	Concentration	Mechanism	Fiber/tissue target	Indication	Dosing
Lidocaine	Patch	5%	Voltage-gated sodium channel inhibitor	A-delta and C fibers	Postherpetic neuralgia, diabetic peripheral neuropathy, cervical radiculopathy, neuropathic pain	Up to 12 hours on within a 24-hour period[a]
Baclofen	Compounded	0.01%, 5%	$GABA_B$ receptor agonist	C fibers	—	—
Diclofenac	Gel	1%, 3%	COX2 inhibitor Antinociception TRPV1, TRPA1	A-delta and C fibers Superficial tissues	Osteoarthritis of joints	2–4 g 4 times/day
	Patch	1.3%	COX2 inhibitor Antinociception TRPV1, TRPA1	A-delta and C fibers Superficial tissues	Acute muscle/joint pain	1 patch 2 times/day
	Solution	2%	COX2 inhibitor Antinociception TRPV1, TRPA1	A-delta and C fibers Superficial tissues	Osteoarthritis of the knees	2 pump actuations 2 times/day
Methylsalicylate	Cream, patch	10%–30%	Counterirritant COX inhibitor	Superficial tissues	Muscle/joint pain	Apply up to 3–5 times/day
Amitriptyline	Compounded	1%–10%	SNRI, SSRI, alpha-2 adrenergic, adenosine, cholinergic, histaminergic, muscarinic, nicotinic, and NMDA receptors	Aδ and C fibers	Neuropathic pain, postherpetic neuralgia, diabetic peripheral neuropathy	—

[a] Postmarketing research has established the safety of using up to four patches at a time, 24 hours per day for 3 days in healthy adults (Gammaitoni, Alvarez & Galer, 2003).

Data from Casale, R., Symeonidou, Z., & Bartolo, M. (2017). Topical treatments for localized neuropathic pain. Current Pain and Headache Reports, 21(3), 15. https://doi.org/10.1007/s11916-017-0615-y; Cline, A. E., & Turrentine, J. E. (2016). Compounded topical analgesics for chronic pain. Dermatitis, 27(5), 263–271. https://doi.org/10.1097/der.0000000000000216; Derry, S., Matthews, P. R., Wiffen, P. J., & Moore, R. A. (2014). Salicylate-containing rubefacients for acute and chronic musculoskeletal pain in adults. Cochrane Database of Systematic Reviews, 11. https://doi.org/10.1002/14651858.CD007403.pub3; and Gammaitoni, A., Alvarez, N., & Galer, B. (2003). Safety and tolerability of the lidocaine patch 5%, a targeted peripheral analgesic: A review of the literature. The Journal of Clinical Pharmacology, 43, 111–117. https://doi.org/10.1177/0091270002239817.

depolarization and an action potential that results in burning sensations of the skin and other tissues (Derry, Rice et al., 2017; Derry, Wiffen et al., 2017; National Center for Biotechnology Information [NCBI], n.d.f.). TRPV1 is predominantly expressed in A-delta and C fibers, where depolarization and action potentials send impulses to the central nervous system (CNS) resulting in capsaicin-mediated effects, such as warming, tingling, itching, stinging, and burning sensations followed by a period of "desensitization" of these capsaicin nociceptors (Chung & Campbell, 2016; NCBI, n.d.f). Capsaicin is also associated with many cellular changes that impair nociceptor function for prolonged periods (Anand & Bley, 2011; Evangelista, 2015; NCBI, n.d.f.). This process has been termed *defunctionalization* (Evangelista, 2015).

Topical capsaicin creams at low concentrations ranging from 0.025% to 0.1% intended for repeated (3–5 times per day) applications are commonly used to treat a variety of chronic pain conditions such as postherpetic neuralgia (PHN), diabetic peripheral neuropathy (DPN), osteoarthritis, and rheumatoid arthritis (Derry, Rice et al., 2017; Derry, Wiffen et al., 2017). Topical capsaicin is sometimes used as a coanalgesic or as the only analgesic when there are limitations to the use of other medications. Derry and Moore (2012), in a Cochrane Review of low-concentration topical capsaicin in the treatment of chronic pain, indicated all studies available for review were conducted before 1996. The available studies failed to provide sufficient data to determine efficacy for the treatment of various types of neuropathic pain; local skin irritation was a common effect of these medications (Derry & Moore, 2012).

Higher concentration of capsaicin, such as capsaicin delivered in the 8% patch, provides an enhanced rate of drug delivery to the skin that allows for rapid defunctionalization, as described earlier, and in turn improves tolerability and medication adherence as the patch is only reapplied after 3 months if necessary (Derry, Rice et al., 2017; Derry, Wiffen et al., 2017).

High-concentration capsaicin is superior to low-concentration capsaicin in PHN with analgesic benefit for 2 to 12 weeks, according to a meta-analysis of high-dose capsaicin treatment (Derry, Rice et al., 2017). The meta-analysis involved eight randomized controlled trials (RCTs) comparing high-dose capsaicin to either placebo treatment or "low"-dose (0.4%) capsaicin topical therapy (Derry, Rice et al., 2017). Most of the studies had been included in a 2013 review, but two additional studies were added for this updated review; per the analysis, studies ranged from providing very low evidence quality to evidence that was of moderate quality (Derry, Rice et al., 2017). In this same meta-analysis, limited evidence was found to support analgesic benefit from high-concentration capsaicin in DPN and human immunodeficiency virus (HIV) distal sensory polyneuropathy (Derry, Rice et al., 2017).

A systematic review and network meta-analysis was conducted in the Netherlands comparing capsaicin 8% patch and oral neuropathic pain medications for the treatment of painful diabetic peripheral neuropathy (PDPN) (van Nooten, Treur, Pantiri, Stoker, & Charokopou, 2017). The review was pharmacy industry supported but included 25 RCTs published in peer-reviewed journals. Capsaicin 8% patch was compared to oral medications (pregabalin, gabapentin, DULoxetine, and amitriptyline) used for the treatment of PDPN. Outcome measures included the proportion of patients with pain relief of more than 30%, proportion of patients with pain relief of more than 50%, and tolerability (common adverse events). After allowing for a certain amount of heterogeneity in the studies (using indicated statistical methods) and lack of data concerning amitriptyline, the authors concluded pain relief with capsaicin 8% patch is in line with relief obtained by pregabalin, DULoxetine, and gabapentin for treatment of PDPN. However, these oral medications were more often associated with somnolence, dizziness, and discontinuation because of adverse events compared with placebo, which did not occur in the capsaicin group.

Derry, Rice et al., 2017 suggest that because of the high cost of high-concentration capsaicin and need for repeated clinic visit applications, clinicians may elect to reserve this medication for treatment of PHN when conventional measures have failed and analgesic benefit should be determined before continuation of therapy. Similarly, the decision to use capsaicin 8% for the treatment of PDPN is based on the individual patient's situation. Factors that should be considered when weighing the decision to use high-concentration capsaicin include patient comorbidities that might contraindicate the use of traditional oral coanalgesics, insurance coverage and medication costs, and time commitment required for application of capsaicin 8%.

Capsaicin Application, Dosing, and Monitoring

Cream preparations of capsaicin are available in varying concentrations and should be applied only to intact uncompromised skin 3 to 5 times daily. Pain relief depends on routine capsaicin use and required rubbing with each application to achieve an analgesic effect (Derry, Rice et al., 2017).

The capsaicin 8% transdermal patch (179 mg/patch) is approved by the U.S Food and Drug Administration for the treatment of PHN with recommended application to be performed by a trained health care professional under the supervision of a physician (Drugs@FDA: Qutenza, 2020). To anesthetize the skin, local anesthetic cream should be applied to the intended painful intact and unbroken skin area before patch application. Nitrile gloves should be used by the health care professional when applying capsaicin patches (up to a maximum of four) for 60 minutes because latex gloves do not provide enough protection for health care providers. After

Box 16.1 | Use of Topical Capsaicin 8% Patch

DESCRIPTION

- Capsaicin 8% patch is a single-use patch stored in a sealed pouch.
- Each patch contains a total of 179 mg of capsaicin (640 mcg/cm^2).
- Cleansing gel is provided in a 50-g tube.

INDICATIONS

- Neuropathic pain associated with postherpetic neuralgia.

CONTRAINDICATIONS

- None.

DOSING RECOMMENDATIONS

- Apply a single, 60-minute application of up to four patches.
- Treatment with capsaicin 8% patch may be repeated every 3 months or as warranted by the return of pain (not more frequently than every 3 months).

STORAGE

- Store carton between 20° to 25° C (68° to 77° F). Excursions between 15° and 30° C (59° and 86° F) are allowed.
- Keep the patch in the sealed pouch until immediately before use.

APPLICATION INSTRUCTIONS

Prepare

- Put on nitrile gloves.
- Inspect the pouch.
- Do not use if the pouch has been torn or damaged.

Identify

- The treatment area (painful area, including areas of hypersensitivity and allodynia) must be identified by a prescriber and marked on the skin.
- If necessary, clip hair (do not shave) in and around the identified treatment area to promote patch adherence.
- Capsaicin 8% patch can be cut to match the size and the shape of the treatment area.
- Gently wash the treatment area with mild soap and water and dry thoroughly.

Anesthetize

- Pretreat with a topical anesthetic to reduce discomfort associated with the application of capsaicin 8% patch.
- Apply topical anesthetic to the entire treatment area and surrounding 1 to 2 cm, and keep the local anesthetic in place until the skin is anesthetized before the application of the capsaicin 8% patch.
- Remove the topical anesthetic with a dry wipe.

- Gently wash the treatment area with mild soap and water and dry thoroughly.

Apply

- Tear open the pouch along the three dashed lines, remove the capsaicin 8% patch.
- Inspect the capsaicin 8% patch and identify the outer surface backing layer with the printing on one side and the capsaicin-containing adhesive on the other side.
  - The adhesive side of the patch is covered by a clear, unprinted, diagonally cut release liner.
- Cut capsaicin 8% patch before removing the protective release liner.
- The diagonal cut in the release liner is to aid in its removal.
- Peel a small section of the release liner back, and place the adhesive side of the patch on the treatment area.
- While you slowly peel back the release liner from under the patch with one hand, use your other hand to smooth the patch down on to the skin.
- Once capsaicin 8% patch is applied, leave in place for 60 minutes.
- To ensure capsaicin 8% patch maintains contact with the treatment area, a dressing, such as rolled gauze, may be used.
- Instruct the patient not to touch the patch or treatment area.

Remove

- Remove capsaicin 8% patch by gently and slowly rolling them inward.

Cleanse

- After removal of the capsaicin 8% patch, generously apply cleansing gel to the treatment area and leave on for at least 1 minute.
- Remove cleansing gel with a dry wipe and gently wash the area with mild soap and water and dry thoroughly.
- Dispose of all treatment materials as described.
- Inform the patient that the treated area may be sensitive for a few days to heat (e.g., hot showers/baths, direct sunlight, vigorous exercise).

DISPOSAL INSTRUCTIONS

- Capsaicin 8% patch is capable of producing severe irritation of eyes, skin, respiratory tract, and mucous membranes.
- Do not dispense capsaicin 8% patch to patients for self-administration.
- It is critical that health care professionals who administer capsaicin 8% patch have completely familiarized themselves with proper dosing, handling, and disposal procedures before handling capsaicin 8% patch to avoid accidental or inadvertent capsaicin exposure to themselves or others.

Continued

Box 16.1   Use of Topical Capsaicin 8% Patch—cont'd

- Do not touch capsaicin 8% patch, treatment areas, and all used supplies or other materials placed in contact with the treatment area without wearing nitrile gloves.
  - Wear nitrile gloves at all times while handling capsaicin 8% patch and cleaning treatment areas.
  - Do NOT use latex gloves because latex gloves do not provide enough protection for the health care provider
- Do not hold capsaicin 8% patch near eyes or mucous membranes.

- Immediately after use, dispose of used and unused patches, patch clippings, unused cleansing gel and associated treatment supplies in accordance with local biomedical waste procedures.

Modified from Drugs@FDA. Qutenza® (Capsaicin patch)[Package Insert]. May, 2020. Retrieved July 29, 2020 from https://www.accessdata.fda.gov/drugsatfda_docs/label/2020/022395s018lbl.pdf.

---

the patch is removed, a cleansing gel (included with each patch) is applied for 1 minute and then removed, and the skin is wiped dry (Drugs@FDA: Qutenza, 2020). If the patch is determined to be effective and without significant adverse effects, the medication may be reapplied no more frequently than every 3 months. Box 16.1 presents a summary of the use of capsaicin 8% patch.

Common side effects from topical capsaicin include burning, erythema, and stinging at the application site (Derry, Rice et al., 2017). Transient increases in blood pressure may occur during and shortly after application of the capsaicin 8% patch (Derry, Rice et al., 2017). The manufacturer recommends monitoring blood pressure during and after the treatment procedure (Derry, Rice et al., 2017). Further research and long-term clinical use are needed to further evaluate the safety and effectiveness of this novel formulation.

Salicylates

Salicylates are pharmacologically similar to aspirin and NSAIDs and therefore could be placed in the NSAID section of this chapter. However, unlike NSAIDs, which penetrate the skin and underlying tissues to provide localized antiinflammatory effects, salicylates are thought to provide analgesia by acting as counter-irritants to the skin when used topically (Derry, Matthews, Wiffen, & Moore, 2014). Salicylates, as a type of rubefacient, provide analgesia for musculoskeletal pains by causing skin reddening secondary to local vasodilation. This vasodilation then results in a soothing warm sensation. Additionally, irritation of the sensory nerve endings is postulated to offset pain in the surrounding joints and muscles (Derry et al., 2014).

Derry et al. (2014) conducted an update of their 2009 meta-analysis of the effects of topical salicylate–containing rubefacients on acute and chronic musculoskeletal pain in adults. Studies included in the analysis, which had one additional study not present in the 2009 review, were randomized, double-blind, placebo- or active-controlled clinical trials. The authors concluded the current evidence does not support the use of salicylates for acute and chronic musculoskeletal pain because the studies were of low to very low level of evidence, including a high risk for bias secondary to the low number of study participants (Derry et al., 2014). Local irritation at the application site, greater than with placebo, was noted in several studies, but salicylate-containing rubefacients seemed well tolerated in the short term. For this reason, as with other topical agents, one may consider its use for patients with serious comorbidities or in which other topical or systemic medications may not be suitable.

Menthol

Menthol is an organic compound synthetically developed or extracted from peppermint oils. It has a counter-irritant effect on skin and mucous membranes, thereby providing local analgesic and/or anesthetic effects (NCBI, n.d.a.). Recently, another receptor in the transient receptor potential (TRP) family (see earlier discussion of capsaicin) has been identified and has been nicknamed the "menthol" receptor (Pergolizzi, Taylor, LeQuang, & Raffa, 2018). This receptor, TRPM8, is activated by cold temperatures (less than 26° C [78.8° F]) and by certain chemicals, among them menthol.

Menthol applied topically acts as a counter-irritant by inducing a cooling sensation and by initially stimulating nociceptors and then causing desensitization to those same nociceptors. Pergolizzi et al. (2018) describe several small-scale pilot studies in varied pain conditions. Results indicate positive analgesic effects and little risk for significant adverse effects. Further studies are needed.

Menthol, especially as an OTC topical agent, is used both alone and in combination with other counter-irritants (Terrie, 2013).

Local Anesthetics

Several topical local anesthetic medications (e.g., benzocaine, lidocaine, prilocaine, tetracaine) are available by prescription or OTC formulations, including creams, gels, ointments, solutions, sprays, and patches, alone or in combination. The primary purpose of local anesthetics is to provide temporary complete or near complete numbing of the skin or mucous membranes. It is important to note that benzocaine, often used for gum, dental, and/or throat pain, is associated with a risk for methemoglobinemia (U.S. Food and Drug Administration [FDA], 2018).

This section focuses on the use of lidocaine patch as a local anesthetic medication to provide analgesia in a topical formulation.

Lidocaine

Lidocaine is a synthetic aminoethylamide local anesthetic that stabilizes neuronal membranes by inhibiting voltage-gated sodium channels responsible for ionic fluxes necessary for the induction and transmission of impulses (NCBI, n.d.f) (see Chapter 15). Topical lidocaine is hypothesized to produce analgesia by reducing ectopic discharges in A-delta and C fibers within the peripheral sensory afferent neurons (Cline & Turrentine, 2016; Derry, Rice et al., 2017). Topical lidocaine may demonstrate other peripheral actions through desensitization and activation of irritant receptors TRPV1 and TRPA1, which may contribute to its nonanesthetic analgesic effects (Casale, Symeonidou, & Bartolo, 2017; Derry, Rice et al., 2017).

As a topical analgesic used for neuropathic and musculoskeletal pain, lidocaine is delivered to the skin in patch (known in Europe as a "plaster") formulation (Baron et al., 2016). Although approved by the FDA only for PHN, a comprehensive topical analgesic review cited studies that consistently found lidocaine patch 5% to be superior to placebo and similar or superior to oral gabapentin in the treatment of both PHN and PDPN (Argoff, 2013). In this review, the author also notes the results of a randomized, placebo-controlled crossover trial of 40 patients with focal neuropathic pain, primarily PHN or postsurgical neuralgia. Patches (lidocaine or placebo) were applied for 12 hours per day as an adjuvant to other analgesic medications such as opioids or tricyclic antidepressants. The lidocaine patch was found to produce significant ongoing pain reduction, compared to placebo, for 8 hours after application (Argoff, 2013).

Pasero and McCaffery (2011) noted many studies conducted in the late 1990s or early 2000s supported the use of lidocaine patches for a variety of painful conditions, both chronic and acute. Finnerup et al. (2015) also conducted a meta-analysis of pharmacotherapy for the treatment of neuropathic pain in adults. Although this review covered numerous therapies, their findings concerning lidocaine were similar, indicating that the efficacy trials included were of low quality but safety and tolerability were rated high. Lidocaine patch was identified as a second-line agent in the treatment of neuropathic pain in adults, despite the fact that the strength of recommendation for use was listed as weak.

Baron et al. (2016), in an examination of the inclusion of lidocaine 5% patch in international treatment guidelines, noted that if guideline recommendations were based on quality-of-life end-points such as general activity, mood,

work, and sleep, the patch would be more frequently recommended as first-line treatment for localized neuropathic pain. They concluded that the lidocaine 5% patch has been demonstrated to be effective in treating a variety of localized peripheral neuropathies in short- and long-term treatment and has an excellent safety profile. With the proviso that further study is needed, they strongly recommend the use of the lidocaine patch in the treatment of peripheral neuropathies either alone or as part of a multimodal regimen.

Lidocaine patches for the treatment of acute, postoperative, myofascial, and osteoarthritis pain states has also been studied and found to have varied results. Some older studies and case reports indicated significantly positive effects with the use of topical lidocaine (Affaitati, 2009; Gilhooly, McGarvey, O'Mahony, & O'Connor, 2011; Kwon et al., 2012; Zink, Mayberry, Peck & Schreiber, 2011), whereas others did not find statistical significance for pain relief, though patients may have attributed pain relief to its use (Khanna, Peters, & Singh, 2012).

More recent research does not support the use of lidocaine as a first-line agent. In a randomized, placebo-controlled, double-blinded study comparing lidocaine patch 5% application after robotic cardiac surgery to a placebo patch, with evaluation at 1 week, 1 month, 3 months, and 6 months, acute pain scores, opioid usage, and incidence of persistent pain were low in both the treatment group and the placebo group (Vrooman et al., 2015). A meta-analysis of prospective controlled trials in which lidocaine patch was used for various acute pain states, including postoperative pain, suggests lidocaine patch is not effective either alone or as an adjuvant in acute pain states (Bai, Miller, Tan, Law, & Gan, 2015). The authors noted that despite an initial review of over 80 studies, only 5 were ultimately considered in the meta-analysis.

Despite the inconclusive findings regarding the efficacy of lidocaine patch in varied pain states, all studies indicated it is both safe and well tolerated. Therefore, as with any therapy, it is important to consider its potential use for any individual patient based on his or her comorbidities and response to a lidocaine patch trial. Although not recommended as a first-line agent in general, it may be a good therapy if other medications cannot be used and/or as a supplemental therapy when first-line agents alone do not provide satisfactory analgesia.

The official insert of the lidocaine 5% patch (Lidoderm, 2015) states a maximum duration of application time as 12 hours. However, in patients for whom lidocaine patch is a useful therapy, it often can be applied for longer. Studies conducted soon after the lidocaine patch came to market (Gammaitoni, Alvarez, & Galer, 2003) established the safety of applying up to four patches at a time, up to 24 hours per day for 3 consecutive days with little systemic increase beyond the already low systemic absorption found in healthy adults. No subsequent research has been identified.

Lidocaine Application, Dosing, and Monitoring

Box 16.2 details the administration of lidocaine 5% patch.

BOX 16.2   Use of Topical Lidocaine 5% Patch

DESCRIPTION

- Lidocaine 5% patch comprises an adhesive material containing 5% lidocaine, which is applied to a nonwoven polyester felt backing and covered with a polyethylene terephthalate (PET) film release liner.
- The release liner is removed before application to the skin.
- The size of the patch is 10 × 14 cm.
- Each patch is packaged into individual child-resistant envelopes.

INDICATIONS

- Pain associated with postherpetic neuralgia.

CONTRAINDICATIONS

- Known history of sensitivity to local anesthetics of the amide type or to any other component of the product.

WARNINGS

- Consider the amount of lidocaine that is absorbed when used concomitantly with other local anesthetics.
- Local anesthetics may cause methemoglobinemia, especially when used along with some other medications (see product insert).

DOSING RECOMMENDATIONS

- Apply the prescribed number of patches (maximum of three), only once for up to 12 hours within a 24-hour period.[a]

STORAGE

- Store at 25° C (77° F); excursions permitted to 15° to 30° C (59° to 86° F).

APPLICATION INSTRUCTIONS

- Apply lidocaine 5% patch to intact skin to cover the most painful area.

- Patches may be cut into smaller sizes with scissors before removal of the release liner.
- Clothing may be worn over the area of application.
- Smaller areas of treatment are recommended in a debilitated patient or a patient with impaired elimination.
- If irritation or a burning sensation occurs during application, remove the patch(es) and do not reapply until the irritation subsides.
- When lidocaine 5% patch is used concomitantly with other products containing local anesthetic agents, the amount absorbed from all formulations must be considered.
- Lidocaine 5% patch may not stick if it gets wet. Avoid contact with water, such as bathing, swimming, or showering.

DISPOSAL INSTRUCTIONS

- Hands should be washed after the handling of lidocaine 5% patch, and eye contact with lidocaine 5% patch should be avoided.
- Do not store patch outside the sealed envelope.
- Apply immediately after removal from the protective envelope.
- Fold used patches so that the adhesive side sticks to itself and safely discard used patches or pieces of cut patches where children and pets cannot get to them.
- Lidocaine 5% patch should be kept out of the reach of children.

Modified from Endo Pharmaceuticals. (2018). Lidoderm Prescribing Information. Retrieved July 28, 2020 from https://www.endo.com/File%20Library/Products/Prescribing%20Information/LIDODERM_prescribing_information.html.
[a]Postmarketing research has established the safety of using up to four patches at a time, 24 hours per day for 3 days in healthy adults (Gammaitoni, Alvarez, & Galer, 2003).

Nonsteroidal Antiinflammatory Drugs

Antiinflammatory medications are a common component of analgesic therapy for numerous painful conditions, either alone or as part of a multimodal plan. However, in oral formulations there may be significant adverse effects. Included among these are GI distress, cardiovascular events, renal toxicity, and, though less common, hepatic toxicity (Altman, Bosch, Brun, Patrignani, & Young, 2015; Barkin, 2015; LiverTox, n.d.).

Topical formulations of NSAIDs, however, are associated with fewer systemic effects than their oral counterparts (Altman et al., 2015; Barkin, 2015).

Topical NSAIDs are intended to inhibit cyclooxygenase (COX) enzymes locally and peripherally while minimizing systemic absorption. Less systemic absorption from the use of topical NSAIDs may be better tolerated and improve adherence to therapy while also potentially providing a viable and safer option in patients with cardiovascular, GI, and renal comorbidities (Barkin, 2015). This desired effect of limited absorption also therefore limits the clinical utility of topical NSAID treatment to joint and skeletal muscle areas (Derry, Rice et al., 2017).

In a 2015 update of an earlier meta-analysis of randomized, double-blinded studies, Derry, Moore, Gaskell, McIntyre, and Wiffen (2015) found topical NSAIDs effective for treatment of acute musculoskeletal pain. The review involved 5311 participants who were treated with a topical NSAID (several medications included in the study) and 3470 participants who received a placebo, for the treatment of acute musculoskeletal pain. Patients treated with a topical NSAID had statistically significant higher rates of clinical success (defined as "at least a 50% reduction in pain or equivalent measure, such as a 'very good' or 'excellent' global assessment of treatment or 'none' or 'slight' pain on rest or movement," [Derry et al., 2015, p. 7]) than matching topical placebo without the NSAID. In this same meta-analysis use of a topical NSAID did not increase local adverse skin reactions compared with placebo. Similarly, the rate of withdrawal because of adverse events was not associated with topical NSAID treatment. Systemic adverse events were, per the authors, not common for either the treatment or the placebo groups. There were few data comparing oral to topical NSAIDs in this study, but the available data indicated fewer systemic adverse effects for topical NSAID than oral NSAID therapy.

The literature also supports use of topical NSAID therapy for the treatment of chronic musculoskeletal pain, specifically osteoarthritis. Similar to the meta-analysis update conducted for acute musculoskeletal pain, an update to a 2012 meta-analysis reviewing data on topical NSAID treatment for osteoarthritis was published in 2016 (Derry, Conaghan, Da Silva, Wiffen, & Moore, 2016). This meta-analysis reviewed the results from 39 studies, in which there were 10,631 participants. The authors report that in studies lasting 6 to 12 weeks, topical diclofenac and topical ketoprofen were significantly more effective at reducing pain than carrier alone (placebo). The review did note, however, that many people did respond positively to the carrier without NSAID added (the placebo topical agent).

Loveless and Fry (2016) note topical NSAIDs are generally effective within 2 to 3 days and reach steady state in 2 to 5 days. Consistent with findings described previously, they also indicate systemic adverse effects are uncommon compared to those of oral NSAID medications. They do add, however, that despite this fact, the topical formulations carry the same black box warnings concerning GI and cardiovascular risks as oral NSAID medications. As with oral formulations it is recommended that within 4 to 8 weeks of initiating topical diclofenac liver function studies are done because of the hepatotoxicity risk. Finally, they specify topical NSAID medication should be applied only to intact skin.

The studies in the previous paragraphs examined the use of different topical NSAID medications. Availability of topical NSAIDs varies by country. Ibuprofen and ketoprofen topical formulations are available in Europe (Barkin, 2015), but only topical diclofenac, also available in Europe, is approved for use in the United States.

Diclofenac

Diclofenac is an acetic acid NSAID that reversibly inhibits the enzyme COX (NCBI, n.d.c.). There are two isoforms of COX, COX-1 and COX-2, both of which mediate the production of prostaglandins and thromboxane A2 (Derry, Rice et al., 2017). When an inflammatory response arises as a result of peripheral nerve damage, prostaglandin production (prostaglandin G_2 and H_2) from arachidonic acid is increased, which then heightens the influx of sodium and calcium currents within peripheral nociceptive neurons, central neurotransmitter release is then increased, and depolarization of second-order nociceptive neurons occur (Casale et al., 2017; Herndon et al., 2008). Inhibition of COX-2 plays a vital role within this pathway through its antiinflammatory and analgesic effects to interrupt the progression of this painful stimulus (Casale et al., 2017; Derry, Rice et al., 2017). Chapter 10 provides a more detailed explanation of the mechanism of action of NSAIDs.

Diclofenac Application, Dosing, and Monitoring

Diclofenac is available in several commercial formulations: gel, patch, and solution. Diclofenac sodium 2% topical solution is formulated with dimethyl sulfoxide (DMSO). DMSO is a highly polar organic solvent with membrane-penetrating ability as a vehicle to enhance diffusion of topical drug applications (Drugs@FDA: Diclofenac Sodium Topical Solution 2%; McPherson & Cimino, 2013; NCBI, n.d.c.). Formulations of topical diclofenac have a reported maximum 0.4% to 2.2% serum concentration attainable with oral diclofenac, thus resulting in considerably lower systemic distribution (McPherson & Cimino, 2013). For examples of diclofenac topical formulations, see summaries of diclofenac epolamine 1.3% topical patch and diclofenac sodium diclofenac 2% solution in Boxes 16.3 and 16.4.

Box 16.3 | Use of Topical Diclofenac 1.3% Patch

DESCRIPTION

- Diclofenac epolamine patch (10 × 14 cm) containing 180 mg of diclofenac epolamine in an aqueous base (13 mg of active per gram of adhesive or 1.3%).

INDICATIONS

- Acute pain resulting from minor strains, sprains, and contusions in adults and pediatric patients 6 years of age and older.

CONTRAINDICATIONS

- Known hypersensitivity (e.g., anaphylactic reactions and serious skin reactions) to diclofenac or any components of the drug product.
- History of asthma, urticaria, or other allergic-type reactions after taking aspirin or other nonsteroidal antiinflammatory drugs (NSAIDs).
- Severe, sometimes fatal, anaphylactic reactions to NSAIDs have been reported in such patients.

Continued

Box 16.3 Use of Topical Diclofenac 1.3% Patch—cont'd

- In the setting of coronary artery bypass graft (CABG) surgery.
- Diclofenac epolamine patch is contraindicated for use on nonintact or damaged skin resulting from any cause, including exudative dermatitis, eczema, infection lesions, burns, or wounds.

DOSING RECOMMENDATIONS

- Apply (1) patch to the most painful area twice a day.

STORAGE

- Store at 20° to 25° C (68° to 77° F); excursions permitted between 15° C to 30° C (59° to 86° F).

APPLICATION INSTRUCTIONS

- Inform patients that if the diclofenac epolamine patch begins to peel off, the edges of the patch may be taped down.
  - If problems with adhesion persist, patients may overlay the patch with a mesh netting sleeve, if appropriate (e.g., to secure patches applied to ankles, knees, or elbows).

- The mesh netting sleeve (e.g., Curad Hold Tite, Surgilast Tubular Elastic Dressing) must allow air to pass through and not be occlusive (nonbreathable).
- Do not apply diclofenac epolamine patch to nonintact or damaged skin resulting from any cause.
  - For example, exudative dermatitis, eczema, infected lesion, burns, or wounds.
- Do not wear a diclofenac epolamine patch when bathing or showering.
- Wash your hands after applying, handling, or removing the patch.
- Avoid eye contact.
- Do not use combination therapy with diclofenac epolamine patch and an oral NSAID unless the benefit outweighs the risk, and conduct periodic laboratory evaluations.

DISPOSAL INSTRUCTIONS

- Discard in the same manner as other pharmaceutical waste in health care institutions.

Modified from Pfizer. (2019). Flector patch prescribing information. Retrieved August 2020 from http://labeling.pfizer.com/ShowLabeling.aspx?id=829.

Box 16.4 Use of Topical Diclofenac 2% Solution

DESCRIPTION

- Clear, colorless to faintly pink or orange solution containing 20 mg of diclofenac sodium per gram of solution, in a white polypropylene-dose pump bottle with a clear cap.
- Each pump actuation delivers 20 mg of diclofenac sodium in 1 g of solution.

INDICATIONS

- Treatment of the pain of osteoarthritis of the knee(s).

CONTRAINDICATIONS

- Known hypersensitivity to diclofenac or any components of the drug product.
- History of asthma, urticaria, or allergic-type reactions after taking aspirin or other nonsteroidal antiinflammatory drugs.
- In the setting of coronary artery bypass graft (CABG) surgery.

DOSING RECOMMENDATIONS

- 40 mg of diclofenac sodium (2 pump actuations) on each painful knee, 2 times a day.

STORAGE

- Store at 25° C (77° F); excursions permitted to 15° to 30° C (59° to 86° F).

APPLICATION INSTRUCTIONS

- Use the lowest effective dosage for the shortest duration consistent with individual patient treatment goals.
- Apply diclofenac topical solution to clean, dry skin.
- The pump must be primed before first use.
- While holding the bottle in an upright position, fully depress the pump mechanism (actuation) 4 times.
  - This portion should be discarded to ensure proper priming of the pump.
  - No further priming of the bottle should be required.

Box 16.4	Use of Topical Diclofenac 2% Solution—cont'd

- After the priming procedure, diclofenac topical solution is properly dispensed by completely depressing the pump 2 times to achieve the prescribed dosage for one knee.
- Deliver the product directly into the palm of the hand and then apply evenly around front, back, and sides of the knee.
- Dispense 40 mg (2 pump actuations) directly onto the knee or first into the hand and then onto the knee.
  - Spread evenly around front, back, and sides of the knee.
- Wash hands completely after administering the product.
- Wait until the area is completely dry before covering with clothing or applying sunscreen, insect repellent, cosmetics, topical medications, or other substances.
- Avoid skin-to-skin contact between other people and the treated knee(s) until completely dry.
- Do not get diclofenac topical solution in the eyes, nose, or mouth.

DISPOSAL INSTRUCTIONS

- Discard in the same manner as other pharmaceutical waste in health care institutions.

Data from Drugs@FDA. Qutenza® (Capsaicin patch)[Package Insert]. May, 2020. Retrieved July 29, 2020 from https://www.access-data.fda.gov/drugsatfda_docs/label/2020/022395s018lbl.pdf. Endo Pharmaceuticals. (2015). Lidoderm Prescribing Information. Retrieved July 28, 2020 from http://www.endo.com/File Library/Products/Prescribing Information/LIDODERM_prescribing_information.html. Gammaitoni, A., Alvarez, N., & Galer, B. (2003). Safety and tolerability of the lidocaine patch 5%, a targeted peripheral analgesic: A review of the literature. *The Journal of Clinical Pharmacology, 43,* 111–117. Pfizer. (2016). Flector Patch Prescribing Information. Retrieved August 2020 from http://labeling.pfizer.com/ShowLabeling.aspx?id=829. Drugs@FDA: Diclofenac Sodium Topical Solution 2%. (Highlights of Prescribing information). 2016. Retrieved August, 2020 from https://www.accessdata.fda.gov/drugsatfda_docs/label/2017/207238ORig-1s000lbl.pdf.

In a meta-analysis specifically focused on the effects of topical diclofenac on osteoarthritis pain (Deng et al., 2016), diclofenac was found to be effective for pain relief and improvement of function.

Like the general class of topical NSAIDs, topical diclofenac, compared to oral diclofenac, is associated with better tolerability and decreased risks for diclofenac-related adverse GI and cardiac effects and abnormal laboratory values. The most common adverse effect associated with topical diclofenac is minor, localized skin irritation (Tieppo Francio, Davani, Towery, & Brown, 2017).

Compound Analgesics

Topical analgesia is increasingly accepted among clinicians for personalized, targeted therapy, although there is insufficient evidence to recommend or support its routine use at this time.

There are limited numbers of commercially available single-medication and combination topical products; thus compounding pharmacists are in a position to formulate single-medication products not commercially available or medication combinations in vehicles that can be applied topically to provide pain relief (Peppin et al., 2015). Combinations of medications that work on different pain pathways in a topical product is an example of a multi-modal analgesic therapy. Compounded analgesics can be targeted to treat various sites of pain with tailored doses

and formulations for a specific individual for the management of chronic pain (Cline & Turrentine, 2016).

Ketamine

Ketamine has unique yet complex pharmacologic analgesic and anesthetic properties. It is a glutamate N-methyl-D-aspartate (NMDA) receptor antagonist that, systemically, inhibits the release of L-glutamate and excites glutamate transmission at α-amino-3-hydroxy-5-methyl-4-isoxazolepropionic acid (AMPA) receptors (Kopsky et al., 2015). Topical ketamine acts on the NMDA receptor (Cline & Turrentine, 2016; Knezevic, Tverdohleb, Nikibin, & Candido, 2017; Kopsky et al., 2015). This and other related ionotropic glutamate receptors can be found on the hairy skin of humans. Inflammation increases the number of NMDA receptors on peripheral nerve fibers (Cline & Turrentine, 2016) and other pain-related peripheral receptors (Kopsky et al., 2015)

Ketamine's interaction with mu and kappa opioid receptors helps delay desensitization while also increasing resensitization of mu receptors to prevent the development of opioid tolerance as well as opioid-induced hyperalgesia (Kopsky et al., 2015). (See Chapter 15 for a more complete discussion of ketamine.).

Topical ketamine has been used in various compounded formulations as a single agent in concentrations ranging from 0.5% to 20% or in combination with other coanalgesics for pain (Cline & Turrentine, 2016; Knezevic et al., 2017; Kopsky et al., 2015). Various types of studies, including short-term RCTs, case reports, and retrospective studies, have not regularly found statistically significant improvement in neuropathic or acute pain when ketamine is used as a single agent (Cline & Turrentine, 2016; Knezevic et al., 2017; Kopsky et al., 2015; Mercadante, 2015). Studies of blood ketamine levels after topical application have indicated minimal absorption and minimal adverse side effects (Cline & Turrentine, 2016; Knezevic et al., 2017; Kopsky et al., 2015), making topical ketamine a relatively safe agent. Similar to other topical agents, trial for a patient with refractory pain and/or health risks associated with usual oral medications may therefore be of benefit.

Amitriptyline

Amitriptyline is a first-generation tricyclic dibenzocycloheptadiene antidepressant with antinociceptive activities through inhibition of norepinephrine and serotonin reuptake within the CNS, or in the periphery by blocking sodium, potassium, calcium voltage-gated ion channels, and alpha-$_2$ adrenergic, adenosine, cholinergic, histaminergic, muscarinic, nicotinic, and NMDA receptors (Casale et al., 2017; Cline & Turrentine, 2016) (see Chapter 15). Studies of single-agent topical applications of 1% to 5% amitriptyline in various neuropathic pain conditions such as postherpetic neuralgia (PHN), DPN, posttraumatic neuropathic pain, and painful peripheral neuropathy, did not show statistical significance in the reduction of pain with a medium level of evidence (Casale et al., 2017, p. 14). Although some case reports and uncontrolled trials showed some analgesic benefit, controlled clinical trials of topical amitriptyline failed to display significant reduction in pain compared with that of placebo (Knezevic et al., 2017; Thompson & Brooks, 2015). Therefore there is insufficient evidence to support the use of topical amitriptyline for the treatment of peripheral neuropathic pain (Thompson & Brooks, 2015).

Ketamine and Amitriptyline Combination

Although topical ketamine and topical amitriptyline have not been found particularly effective as single agents, results of studies investigating compounded combination topical ketamine and amitriptyline have been mixed. Kopsky et al. (2015) identified several mostly short-term (6 weeks or less) studies of various design. A double-blinded RCT was conducted for 360 patients with PHN. The study compared a combination cream of ketamine 2% and amitriptyline 4%, 4 g twice daily, with oral gabapentin 1800 mg/day, placebo cream, and placebo capsules during a 4-week period. This study showed statistically significant pain reduction in the combination cream and the oral gabapentin groups versus placebo.

Sawynok and Zinger (2016) also reviewed trials comparing ketamine-amitriptyline (which they termed AmiKet) combinations. Findings in RCTs and open-label and other types of studies supported the potential use of AmiKet for PHN, similar to the 2015 finding of Kopsky et al. (2015). Safety and side effect profile were favorable in all studies for use of AmiKet.

CloNIDine

CloNIDine is a presynaptic alpha-$_2$ adrenergic and imidazoline receptor agonist with potent antinociceptive properties similar to or greater than those of morphine (Wrzosek, Woron, Dobrogowski, Jakowicka-Wordliczek, & Wordliczek, 2015). Epidural, intravenous, and intrathecal use of cloNIDine have been shown to be effective in the treatment of acute and chronic pain (Wrzosek et al., 2015) (see Chapter 15). Unfortunately, systemic use of cloNIDine may be limited by its intolerable side effects of dry mouth, hypotension, rebound hypertension, and sedation (Wrzosek et al., 2015).

CloNIDine is lipophilic and displays good topical penetration that may be beneficial with its local antinociceptive properties while potentially limiting systemic side effects (Wrzosek, et al., 2015). It is important to note topical cloNIDine is a compounded product and should be distinguished from the commercially available transdermal cloNIDine product, which has systemic effects (see Chapter 15). There is limited evidence from low- to medium-quality studies suggesting benefit with topical cloNIDine in DPN, but no evidence has been found to support its effectiveness in other neuropathic pain syndromes (Wrzosek et al., 2015). With this limited evidence, clinicians should reserve the use of topical cloNIDine for treatment of DPN when all other treatment options have been exhausted or are unavailable (Wrzosek et al., 2015).

Gabapentin

Gabapentin is a synthetic analogue of the neurotransmitter γ-aminobutyric acid (GABA) with anticonvulsant activity. Although its exact mechanism of action in treating pain is unclear, gabapentin appears to inhibit voltage-gated calcium channels and exert glutamate antagonism, resulting in inhibition of excitatory neuron activity with analgesia (Cline & Turrentine, 2016; NCBI, n.d.d.). (See Chapter 15 for additional information related to the mechanism of action and use of oral gabapentin.) Topical gabapentin has been used as a single agent or in combination with other coanalgesics for neuropathic pain, exhibiting potential benefit for vulvodynia (Cline & Turrentine, 2016). In animal studies, gabapentin gel has been found to be effective in several induced pain states, and researchers advocate for additional studies to determine the benefits of topical gabapentin on different neuropathic pain syndromes (Shahid et al., 2017; Shahid et al., 2019). To date, one of the limitations of topical gabapentin use has been the lack of evidence to identify the optimal vehicle, or formulation, of topical gabapentin to facilitate penetration of the medication across human skin (Martin, Alcock, Hiom, & Birchall, 2017).

Baclofen

Baclofen is a synthetic chlorophenyl-butanoic acid derivative muscle relaxant that functions as a GABA agonist at $GABA_B$ receptors causing a decrease in calcium membrane conductivity and an increase in potassium. This causes hyperpolarization of primary afferent fibers resulting in inhibition of both monosynaptic and polysynaptic transmission at the spinal cord level, which is beneficial in the treatment of spasticity and pain (Cline & Turrentine, 2016; NCBI, n.d.b.) (see Chapter 15). Topical baclofen has shown some benefit for vulvodynia and chemotherapy-induced neuropathy with symptomatic improvements in the hands for cramping, tingling, and burning/shooting pain sensations (Cline & Turrentine, 2016). Similar to other compounded topical analgesics, baclofen is commonly formulated in combination with other coanalgesics (Casale et al., 2017).

Opioids

Since peripheral mu opioid receptors were first described over two decades ago there has been hope that topical opioids might provide analgesia without systemic side effects and addiction potential. Many early, small sample size, pilot studies and/or case reports using different opioids for various types of skin wounds support this premise when used in inflamed tissues (Sehgal, Smith, & Manchikanti, 2011). These have been noted in several reviews (Farley, 2011; Graham, et al., 2013; LeBon, Zeppetella, & Higginson, 2009) and individually reported case reports (Miyazaki, Satou, Ohno, Yoshida & Nishimura, 2014; Tennant, 2012). All of the authors note that more robust studies with larger sample sizes and greater consistency are needed before conclusions can be drawn. However, few subsequent studies have been identified.

In an RCT of 44 patients undergoing surgery for skin grafting (Zaslansky et al., 2014), patients with topical morphine did not report statistically significant lower pain scores than those receiving placebo nor did the study group use less supplemental opioids than the control group.

Although efficacy of topical opioid treatment has not been established, in all the studies found in the literature, few adverse effects and systemic absorption have been reported (Farley, 2011; Graham et al., 2013; Ribeiro, Joel, & Zeppetella, 2004). Ribeiro et al. (2004) cautioned that systemic absorption is likely to increase and could potentially cause systemic side effects when topical morphine is applied to large surface area wounds, but, overall, systemic absorption as measured by blood levels was low. In the case report series discussed by Graham et al. (2013), methadone systemic absorption was variable. Similar to Ribeiro's cautions concerning morphine, it was postulated that absorption of methadone likely depended on surface area and also the presence of eschar tissue.

As with other topical agents, robust research is lacking; definitive support for topical opioids has not been established. However, systemic absorption and adverse skin reactions are generally mild. Therefore, in individual cases in which other therapies do not provide sufficient analgesia and/or patient comorbidities limit the use of traditional medications or routes, an "N of 1 trial should be encouraged" (LeBon et al., 2009, p. 913).

Key Points

- Topical analgesics provide a means for localized targeted drug delivery with controlled and sustained delivery over a period of time.
- Topical medications have been found to have, at best, fair efficacy but generally excellent safety profiles.
- Topical medications may be considered when patients are not able to take oral medications, are not responding to oral or other traditional analgesics, as a supplemental agent, and/or when patient comorbidities make use of more typical analgesic medications potentially unsafe.
- Benefits of topical analgesics include avoidance of first-pass metabolism, improved patient acceptance and adherence, fewer systemic adverse effects, and fewer potential drug interactions.
- Although compounded topical medications are increasingly available, there is insufficient evidence to recommend or support their routine use at this time.

Case Scenario

Mrs. R is an 84-year-old woman with a history of severe osteoarthritis of the knees and recent recovery from herpes zoster, which involved painful lesions on her chest wall. She has a history of breast cancer at age 72, was treated with chemotherapy and a lumpectomy, and is disease-free. She lives alone in a single-family ranch home and is trying to continue to independently perform most of her activities of daily living. Since her herpes zoster outbreak, she has had pain along the site of the lesions and has been less active. She previously enjoyed walking outdoors in her neighborhood, but since her zoster outbreak, she has been less active and has had more stiffness and pain in her knees and hips.

1. What are some reasons Mrs. R may benefit from the use of topical medications?
2. What types of topical medications may be appropriate to treat Mrs. R's pain conditions?
3. Mrs. R's daughter is concerned that her mother will have significant side effects with the use of topical medications because she usually never tolerates oral medications well. Explain the possible side effects of the medications that have been selected for Mrs. R.

4. Mrs. R tells you she heard the staff in the hospital talking about a new compounding pharmacy opening in the community, and she wants to know what a compounding pharmacy is, and what she can buy there. What would you tell her?
5. Several years ago, Mrs. R was prescribed a fentaNYL patch during treatment for breast cancer. She experienced severe nausea and vomiting with the fentaNYL patch and is afraid that she will have similar symptoms with the topical medications. Discuss how you would address these concerns.

References

Affaitati, G., Fabrizio, A., Savini, A., Lerza, R., Tafuri, E., Costantini, R., & Giamberardino, M. A. (2009). A randomized, controlled study comparing a lidocaine patch, a placebo patch, and anesthetic injection for treatment of trigger points in patients with myofascial pain syndrome: Evaluation of pain and somatic pain thresholds. *Clinical Therapeutics, 31*(4), 705–720.

Altman, R., Bosch, B., Brun, K., Patrignani, P., & Young, C. (2015). Advanced in NSAID development: Evolution of diclofenac products using pharmaceutical technology. *Drugs, 75*, 859–877. https://doi.org/10.1007/s40265-015-0392-z.

Anand, P., & Bley, K. (2011). Topical capsaicin for pain management: therapeutic potential and mechanisms of action of the new high-concentration capsaicin 8% patch. *British Journal of Anaesthesia, 107*(4), 490–502.

Anitescu, A., Benzon, H. T., & Argoff, C. E. (2013). Advances in Topical Analgesics. *Current Opinion in Anesthesiology, 26*, 555–561. https://doi.org/10.1097/01.aco.0000432514.00446.22.

Argoff, C. (2013). Topical analgesics in the management of acute and chronic pain. *Mayo Clinic Proceedings, 88*(2), 195–205. https://dx.doi.org/10.1016/j.mayocp.2012.11.015.

Bai, Y., Miller, T., Tan, M., Law, L. S., & Gan, T. J. (2015). Lidocaine patch for acute pain management: a meta-analysis of prospective controlled trials. *Current Medical Research and Opinion, 31*(3), 575–581. https://doi.org/10.1185/03007995.2014.973484.

Barkin, R. (2015). Topical nonsteroidal anti-inflammatory drugs: The importance of drug, delivery, and therapeutic outcome. *American Journal of Therapeutics, 22*(5), 388–407.

Baron, R., Allegri, M., Correa-Illanes, G., Hans, G., Serpell, M., Mick, G., & Mayoral, V. (2016). The 5% lidocaine-medicated plaster: Its inclusion in international treatment guidelines for treating localized neuropathic pain, and clinical evidence supporting its use. *Pain and Therapy, 5*, 149–169. https://doi.org/10.1007/s40122-016-0060-3.

Brown, M. B., Martin, G. P., & Jones, S. A. (2006). Dermal and transdermal drug delivery systems: Current and future prospects. *Drug Delivery, 13*(3), 175–187.

Casale, R., Symeonidou, Z., & Bartolo, M. (2017). Topical treatments for localized neuropathic pain. *Current Pain and Headache Reports, 21*(3). https://doi.org/10.1007/s11916-017-0615-y.

Chung, M. K., & Campbell, J. N. (2016). Use of Capsaicin to Treat Pain: Mechanistic and Therapeutic Considerations. *Pharmaceuticals (Basel, Switzerland), 9*(4), 66. https://doi.org/10.3390/ph9040066.

Cline, A. E., & Turrentine, J. E. (2016). Compounded topical analgesics for chronic pain. *Dermatitis, 27*(5), 263–271. https://doi.org/10.1097/der.0000000000000216.

Deng, C. H., Zeng, C., Yang, Y., Li, Y. S., Wei, J., Yang, T., & Lei, G. H. (2016). Topical diclofenac therapy for osteoarthritis: a meta-analysis of randomized controlled trials. *Clinical Rheumatology, 35*, 1253–1261. https://doi.org/10.1007/s10067-015-3021-z.

Derry, S., Matthews, P. R., Wiffen, P. J., & Moore, R. A. (2014). Salicylate-containing rubefacients for acute and chronic musculoskeletal pain in adults. *Cochrane Database of Systematic Reviews, 11*. https://doi.org/10.1002/14651858.CD007403.pub3. CD007403.

Derry, S., Conaghan, P., Da Silva, J., Wiffen, P., & Moore, R. (2016). Topical NSAIDS for chronic musculoskeletal pain in adults (Review). *Cochrane Database of Systematic Reviews, 4*(4). https://doi.org/10.1002/14651858.CD007400.pub3.

Derry, S., & Moore, R. A. (2012). Topical capsaicin (low concentration) for chronic neuropathic pain in adults. *The Cochrane database of systematic reviews, 2012*(9), CD010111. https://doi.org/10.1002/14651858.CD010111.

Derry, S., Moore, R. A., Gaskell, H., McIntyre, M., & Wiffen, P. J. (2015). Topical NSAIDs for acute musculoskeletal pain in adults (Review). *Cochrane Database of Systematic Reviews, 6*. https://doi.org/10.1002/14651858.CD007402.pub3.

Derry, S., Rice, A. S., Cole, P., Tan, T., & Moore, R. A. (2017). Topical capsaicin (high concentration) for chronic neuropathic pain in adults. *Cochrane Database of Systematic Reviews, 1*(1). https://doi.org/10.1002/14651858.CD007393.pub4.

Derry, S., Wiffen, P. J., Kalso, E. A., Bell, R. F., Aldington, D., Phillips, T., ... & Moore, R. A. (2017). Topical analgesics for acute and chronic pain in adults - an overview of Cochrane Reviews. *Cochrane Database of Systematic Reviews, 5*(5). https://doi.org/10.1002/14651858.CD008609.pub2.

Drugs@FDA: Diclofenac Sodium Topical Solution 2%. (Highlights of Prescribing information). 2016. Retrieved August, 2020 from https://www.accessdata.fda.gov/drugsatfda_docs/label/2017/207238ORig1s000lbl.pdf.

Drugs@FDA. Qutenza® (Capsaicin patch)[Package Insert]. May, 2020. Retrieved July 29, 2020 from https://www.accessdata.fda.gov/drugsatfda_docs/label/2020/022395s018lbl.pdf.

Evangelista, S. (2015). Novel therapeutics in the field of capsaicin and pain. *Expert Review of Clinical Pharmacology, 8*(4), 373–375. https://doi.org/10.1586/17512433.2015.1044438.

Farley, P. (2011). Should topical opioid analgesics be regarded as effective and safe when applied to chronic cutaneous lesions? *Journal of Pharmacy and Pharmacology, 63*(6), 747–756. https://doi.org/10.1111/j.2042-7158.2011.01252.x.

Finnerup, N., Attal, N., Haroutounian, S., McNicol, E., Baron, R., Dworkin, R., & Wallace, M. (2015). Pharmacotherapy for neuropathic pain in adults: a systematic review and meta-analysis. *The Lancet. Neurology, 14*(2), 162–173. https://doi.org/10.1016/S1474-4422(14)70251-0.

Gammaitoni, A., Alvarez, N., & Galer, B. (2003). Safety and tolerability of the lidocaine patch 5%, a targeted peripheral analgesic: A review of the literature. *The Journal of Clinical Pharmacology, 43*, 111–117. https://doi.org/10.1177/0091270002239817.

Gilhooly, D., McGarvey, B., O'Mahony, H., & O'Connor, T. C. (2011). Topical lidocaine patch 5% for acute postoperative pain control. *BMJ Case Reports*. https://doi.org/10.1136/bcr.06.2010.3074.

Graham, T., Grocott, P., Probst, S., Wanklyn, S., Dawson, J., & Gethin, G. (2013). How are topical opioids used to manage painful cutaneous lesions in palliative care? A critical review. *Pain, 154*(10), 1920–1928.

Herndon, C. M., Hutchison, R. W., Berdine, H. J., Stacy, Z. A., Chen, J. T., Farnsworth, D. D., & Fermo, J. D. (2008). Management of chronic nonmalignant pain with nonsteroidal anti- inflammatory drugs. Joint opinion statement of the Ambulatory Care, Cardiology, and Pain and Palliative Care Practice and Research Networks of the American College of Clinical Pharmacy. *Pharmacotherapy, 28*(6), 788–805. https://doi.org/10.1592/phco.28.6.788.

Khanna, M., Peters, C., & Singh, J. R. (2012). Treating pain with the lidocaine patch 5% after total knee arthroplasty. *Physical Medicine and Rehabilitation, 4*, 642–646. https://dx.doi.org/10.1016/j.pmrj.2012.06.003.

Knezevic, N. N., Tverdohleb, T., Nikibin, F., Knezevic, I., & Candido, K. (2017). Management of chronic neuropathic pain with single and compounded topical analgesics. *Pain Management, 7*(6), 537–558.

Kopsky, D. J., Keppel Hesselink, J. M., Bhaskar, A., Hariton, G., Romanenko, V., & Casale, R. (2015). Analgesic effects of topical ketamine. *Minerva Anestesiologica, 81*(4), 440–449.

Kwon, Y. S., Kim, J. B., Jung, H. J., Koo, Y. J., Lee, I. H., Im, K. T., ... & Im, K. S. (2012). Treatment for postoperative wound pain in gynecologic laparoscopic surgery: Topical lidocaine patches. *Journal of Laparoendoscopic and Advanced Surgical Techniques, 22*(7), 668–673.

LeBon, B., Zeppetella, G., & Higginson, I. (2009). Effectiveness of topical administration of opioids in palliative care: A systematic review. *Journal of Pain and Symptom Management, 37*(5), 913–917.

Leppert, W., Malec-Milewska, M., Zajaczkowska, R., & Wordliczek, J. (2018). Transdermal and topical administration in the treatment of pain. *Molecules, 23*(3). https://doi.org/10.3390/molecules23030681.

Lidoderm® package insert. (January, 2015). Retrieved from: https://www.accessdata.fda.gov/drugsatfda_docs/label/2015/020612s012lbl.pdf.

LiverTox. (n.d.). Retrieved on November 19, 2018 from: https://livertox.nih.gov/NonsteroidalAntiinflammatoryDrugs.htm.

Loveless, M., & Fry, A. (2016). Pharmacologic therapies in musculoskeletal conditions. *Medical Clinics of North America, 100*, 869–890.

Martin, C. J., Alcock, N., Hiom, S., & Birchall, J. C. (2017). Development and Evaluation of Topical Gabapentin Formulations. *Pharmaceutics, 9*(3), 31. https://doi.org/10.3390/pharmaceutics9030031.

McPherson, M. L., & Cimino, N. M. (2013). Topical NSAID formulations. *Pain Medicine, 14*, S35–S39. https://doi.org/10.1111/pme.12288. *Supplement 1.*

Mercadante, S. (2015). Topical amitriptyline and ketamine for the treatment of neuropathic pain. *Expert Review of Neurotherapeutics, 15*(11), 1249–1253. https://doi.org/10.1586/14737175.2015.1101347.

Miyazaki, T., Satou, S., Ohno, T., Yoshida, A., & Nishimura, K. (2014). Topical morphine gel for pain management in head and neck cancer patients. *Auris Nasus Larynx, 41*(5), 496–498.

Nastiti, C., Ponto, T., Abd, E., Grice, J. E., Benson, H. A. E., & Roberts, M. S. (2017). Topical nano and microemulsions for skin delivery. *Pharmaceutics, 9*(4), 37. https://doi.org/10.3390/pharmaceutics9040037.

National Center for Biotechnology Information. PubChem Compound Database; CID = 1254. (n.d.a.). Retrieved January 22, 2019, from: https://pubchem.ncbi.nlm.nih.gov/compound/1254.

National Center for Biotechnology Information. PubChem Compound Database; CID = 2284. (n.d.b.). Retrieved January 22, 2019, from https://pubchem.ncbi.nlm.nih.gov/compound/2284.

National Center for Biotechnology Information. PubChem Compound Database; CID = 3033. (n.d.c.). Retrieved November 11, 2018, from https://pubchem.ncbi.nlm.nih.gov/compound/3033.

National Center for Biotechnology Information. PubChem Compound Database; CID = 3446. (n.d.d.). Retrieved October 29, 2018, from https://pubchem.ncbi.nlm.nih.gov/compound/3446.

National Center for Biotechnology Information. PubChem Compound Database; CID = 1548943. (n.d.f.). Retrieved October 29, 2018, from https://pubchem.ncbi.nlm.nih.gov/compound/1548943.

Pasero, C., & McCaffery, M. (2011). Chapter 24. Topical analgesics for persistent (chronic) pain. *Pain assessment and pharmacologic management* (pp. 684–695). St. Louis, MO: Mosby, Inc.

Peppin, J. F., Albrecht, P. J., Argoff, C., Gustorff, B., Pappagallo, M., Rice, F. L., & Wallace, M. S. (2015). Skin matters: a review of topical treatments for chronic pain. Part two: treatments and applications. *Pain and Therapy, 4*(1), 33–50.

Pergolizzi, J. V., Taylor, R., LeQuang, J. A., & Raffa, R. B. (2018). The role and mechanism of action of menthol in topical analgesic products. *Journal of Clinical Pharmacy and Therapeutics, 43*(3), 313–319.

Ribeiro, M., Joel, S. P., & Zeppetella, G. (2004). The bioavailability of morphine applied topically to cutaneous ulcers. *Journal of Pain and Symptom Management, 27*(5), 434–439.

Sarbacker, G. B. (2015). Topical therapies for chronic pain management: A review of diclofenac and lidocaine. *US Pharm, 40*(3), 35–38.

Sawynok, J., & Zinger, C. (2016). Topical amitriptyline and ketamine for post-herpetic neuralgia and other forms of neuropathic pain. *Expert Opinion on Pharmacotherapy, 17*(4), 601–609. https://doi.org/10.1517/14656566.2016.1146691.

Sehgal, N., Smith, H., & Manchikanti, L. (2011). Peripherally acting opioids and clinical implications for pain control. *Pain Physician, 14*(3), 249–258.

Shahid, M., Subhan, F., Ahmad, N., Ali, G., Akbar, S., Fawad, K., & Sewell, R. D. (2017). Topical gabapentin gel alleviates allodynia and hyperalgesia in the chronic sciatic nerve constriction injury neuropathic pain model. *European journal of pain (London, England), 21*(4), 668–680. https://doi.org/10.1002/ejp.971.

Shahid, M., Subhan, F., Ahmad, N., & Sewell, R. (2019). Efficacy of a topical gabapentin gel in a cisplatin paradigm of chemotherapy-induced peripheral neuropathy. *BMC pharmacology & toxicology, 20*(1), 51. https://doi.org/10.1186/s40360-019-0329-3.

Tennant, F. (2012). Topical morphine. Practical Pain Management, 8 (8). Retrieved on January 23, 2019 from: https://www.practicalpainmanagement.com/treatments/pharmacological/non-opioids/topical-use-morphine?page=0,1.

Terrie, Y. (2013). *Pain control using nonprescription analgesics. Pharmacy Times.* Retrieved on January 23, 2019 from https://www.pharmacytimes.com/publications/otc/2013/otcguide-2013/pain-control-using-nonprescription-analgesics.

Thompson, D. F., & Brooks, K. G. (2015). Systematic review of topical amitriptyline for the treatment of neuropathic pain. *Journal of Clinical Pharmacy and Therapeutics, 40*(5), 496–503. https://doi.org/10.1111/jcpt.12297.

Tieppo Francio, V., Davani, S., Towery, C., & Brown, T. L. (2017). Oral versus topical diclofenac sodium in the treatment of osteoarthritis. *Journal of Pain & Palliative Care Pharmacotherapy, 31*(2), 113–120.

U.S. Food and Drug Administration (FDA) (May 31, 2018). Risk of serious and potentially fatal blood disorder prompts FDA action on oral over-the-counter benzocaine products used for teething and mouth pain and prescription local anesthetics. Retrieved on June 8, 2019 from: https://www.fda.gov/drugs/drug-safety-and-availability/risk-serious-and-potentially-fatal-blood-disorder-prompts-fda-action-oral-over-counter-benzocaine.

van Nooten, F., Treur, M., Pantiri, K., Stoker, M., & Charokopou, M. (2017). Capsaicin 8% patch versus oral neuropathic pain medications for the treatment of painful diabetic peripheral neuropathy: A systematic literature review and network meta-analysis. *Clinical Therapeutics, 39*(4), 787–803. 803.e1-803.e18.

Vrooman, B., Kapural, L., Sarwar, S., Mascha, E., Mihaljevic, T., Gillinov, M., & Sessler, D. (2015). Lidocaine 5% patch for treatment of acute pain after robotic cardiac surgery and prevention of persistent incisional pain: A randomized, placebo-controlled, double-blind trial. *Pain Medicine, 16,* 1610–1621.

Wrzosek, A., Woron, J., Dobrogowski, J., Jakowicka-Wordliczek, J., & Wordliczek, J. (September 2, 2015). Topical clonidine for neuropathic pain. *Cochrane Database of Systematic Reviews,* 9. https://doi.org/10.1002/14651858.CD010967.pub2.

Zaslansky, R., Ben-Nun, O., Ben-Shitrit, S., Ullmann, Y., Kopf, A., & Stein, C. (2014). A randomized, controlled, clinical pilot study assessing the analgesic effect of morphine applied topically onto split-thickness skin wounds. *Journal of Pharmacy and Pharmacology, 66,* 1559–1566. https://doi.org/10.1111/jphp.12284.

Zink, K., Mayberry, J., Peck, E., & Schreiber, M. (2011). Lidocaine patches reduce pain in trauma patients with rib fractures. *The American Surgeon, 77*(4). 483-442.

Chapter 17 Patient-Controlled Analgesia

Ann Quinlan-Colwell

CHAPTER OUTLINE

General Concepts, pg. 447

    Advantages of Use, pg. 448

    Indications for Use, pg. 448

Optimize Safety Within the Patient-Controlled Analgesia Process, pg. 449

    Clinician Education, pg. 449

    Patient and Family Education, pg. 450

    Appropriate Prescription, pg. 451

    Patient Selection, pg. 451

Prescription Components, pg. 455

    Modes of Administration, pg. 455

    Medications Administered, pg. 455

    Technical Components of Prescription, pg. 456

Routes of Administration, pg. 458

    Intravenous Route, pg. 459

    Epidural Route, pg. 459

    Regional Route, pg. 459

    Subcutaneous Route, pg. 459

    Transdermal Route, pg. 460

    Oral or Enteral Route, pg. 460

    Intranasal Route, pg. 461

    Sublingual Route, pg. 461

    Inhalation Route, pg. 461

Patient Assessment and Monitoring to Optimize Safety, pg. 462

    Respiratory Assessment, pg. 462

    Sedation Assessment, pg. 462

    Monitoring With Equipment, pg. 463

Evaluating Equipment to Optimize Patient Safety, pg. 464

    Infusion Tubing, pg. 464

Authorized Agent–Controlled Analgesia, pg. 465

    Family-Controlled or Caregiver-Controlled Analgesia, pg. 465

    Nurse-Controlled Analgesia, pg. 466

Key Points, pg. 468

Case Scenario, pg. 468

References, pg. 468

General Concepts

IN the purest of senses, any medication a patient self-administers for pain is patient-controlled analgesia (PCA). However, this chapter will address PCA as an interactive method of pain management that enables patients to treat their pain by self-administering individual doses of analgesic medications using a specialized delivery system, as prescribed by a clinician (Cox & Cooney, 2018; Smith & Goldberg, 2012; Surprise & Simpson, 2014). Since 1976, these devices, in accordance with clinician orders, are programmed to administer small amounts of prescribed medication within certain time parameters, which are delivered through the identified route when activated by the patient (Lien & Youngwerth, 2012) (Fig. 17.1). PCA has been used to effectively deliver opioids and other medications through a variety of routes of administration, including oral (PO), intravenous (IV), subcutaneous (subcut), and epidural (Pasero & McCaffery, 2011). It is important to remember there is no need to choose between multimodal analgesia (MMA) and PCA. Rather, PCA can be used as an effective component of an MMA plan of care, particularly among patients who are not able to take medication orally and those who are in an enhanced recovery program after surgery (Nelson et al., 2016).

The PCA approach recognizes that only the patient can feel the pain being experienced and only the patient knows how much analgesia will relieve the pain (Pasero & McCaffery, 1993; Pasero, Portenoy, & McCaffery, 1999). Consistent with that concept, it is essential to accurately assess the patient, the reported pain intensity, and the characteristics of the pain as described by the patient (Fernandes et al., 2017). By enabling patients to determine the frequency of dosing, PCA addresses the variations of analgesia needed by each person at different times during the day and the significant variations in analgesic requirements among individuals (Pasero & McCaffery, 2011; Pasero, Quinlan-Colwell, Rae, Broglio, & Drew, 2016). Moderate-quality data support PCA as being more effective than non-PCA in reducing pain intensity, with patients using PCA also reporting being more satisfied (P = .002) (McNicol, Ferguson, & Hudcova, 2015).

PCA requires patients to recognize pain is being experienced and analgesia is needed; thus PCA is similar to the clinician responding with as-needed (prn) dosing of medication to a patient recognizing pain and requesting to receive analgesia (Pasero & McCaffery, 2011). See Chapter 9 for discussion of nurse-administered prn dosing of analgesia. However, compared to the patient calling a nurse to administer a dose of medication, with PCA the patient activates the device (i.e., pressing a button) to deliver a bolus dose of medication. Because the patient, rather than a caregiver, administers the analgesic, any delay in waiting for a caregiver's response to the request for analgesia is eliminated. Thus the analgesic effect can be attained in a more timely manner. Just as with effective prn dosing, patients are reminded to use the PCA device to maintain a relatively steady analgesic level and administer doses at a reasonable level at which they can function (e.g., deep breath, cough, turn, ambulate) and prevent pain from progressing to a severe level.

Advantages of Use

Using PCA has several important advantages. First, as reported in various research studies, pain can be well controlled with the use of PCA (Lien & Youngwerth, 2012). Second, patient satisfaction is frequently improved because patients not only have control over when they receive their medication but they also do not have to wait for it be prepared and administered (Elliott, 2016; Fernandes et al., 2017). Third, the PCA delivery device can be programmed to address the analgesic needs, physiology, and other pertinent characteristics of the individual patient more specifically (Elliott, 2016; Lien & Youngwerth, 2012). Fourth, PCA often provides less fluctuation in plasma concentration of analgesia, with less potential for inadequate analgesia and untoward effects (Elliott, 2016). Fifth, included in the design of the equipment are important safety measures that require patients to be alert to process information about their pain and be able to activate the machine to control it, thus preventing excessive administration (Lien & Youngwerth, 2012). Finally, PCA use is associated with less opioid use, fewer opioid side effects, faster postoperative activity, fewer postoperative complications, and shorter hospital stays (Elliott, 2016).

Indications for Use

PCA is used to manage all types of pain in a variety of settings. It is commonly used to control acute pain in the acute inpatient setting (Pasero & McCaffery, 2011),

particularly after surgery or trauma. It is also used effectively in acute care for patients with cancer who are admitted to the hospital with uncontrolled or poorly controlled pain (Martin et al., 2017). PCA is used in the same way with patients who experience acute exacerbation of sickle cell disease (Peterson, Selvaggi, Scullion, & Blinderman, 2018). At times, PCA is started in the emergency department (ED), such as with patients experiencing a sickle cell crisis (Lovett, Sule, & Lopez, 2014; Tanabe, Freiermuth, Cline, & Silva, 2017) (Box 17.1).

Use of PCA for pain management in the ED is receiving increasing attention. One large multisite study (N = 636) compared PCA with intravenous administration in patients who were opioid naïve experiencing acute pain with no history of chronic pain (Bijur et al., 2017). Among those patients, the ones using PCA reported statistically greater satisfaction and analgesia improved more quickly (P < 0.001). Despite that, the authors concluded "the findings did not favor patient-controlled analgesia over usual ED care for acute pain management" (Bijur et al., 2017, p. 809). They based their conclusion on the speed of analgesia not achieving the threshold they expected for clinical significance and on the occurrence of more adverse events with PCA use (seven adverse events [2.3%]) compared with usual care (one adverse event [0.04%]). In addition to four patients with hypotensive episodes, the seven adverse events included three patients with reductions in pulse oximetry between 93% and 88% among those with PCA, compared with one pulse oximetry reduction of 88% in the usual care group.

Procedural sedation also has been delivered by PCA (Pasero & McCaffery, 2011). When sedation with propofol administered by PCA was compared with intravenous infusion during orthopedic surgery performed under regional analgesia (N = 60), those who received PCA (n = 30) used less medication (Ekin, Donmez, Taspinar, & Dikmen, 2013). In that study, the participants who used PCA also reported greater satisfaction even though 76% of that group reported injection site pain.

Even though it is most frequently associated with hospital use, PCA is also effective in the home setting with patients with painful chronic conditions and has been used in that location since 1988 (Kerr et al., 1988). Although use of PCA, by at least some patients who are living with chronic pain, may facilitate better analgesia and avoid hospitalization for acute exacerbations, use at home has not been well addressed or studied (Pergolizzi, Taylor, & Muniz, 2011). Research is needed to identify which patients living with chronic pain may benefit, evaluate the risks versus benefits among different patients, identify safety issues and precautions, and develop educational resources for patients, families, and nurses. PCA is generally used less often in the home setting with nonhospice cancer pain because most cancer pain can be managed with oral opioid analgesics (Martin et al., 2017). However, in a small retrospective study with children living with cancer (N = 33), pain was managed well using

PCA devices with no adverse events even when there were changes in dosage and medication (Mherekumombe & Collins, 2015). PCA is increasingly used to safely manage pain experienced by both adult and pediatric hospice patients living at home (Anghelescu, Zhang, Faughnan, & Pei, 2015; Mherekumombe & Collins, 2015; Shah, Homel, & Breznay, 2016). In fact, analysis of data from the National Home and Hospice Care Survey, showed that PCA is significantly used among patients receiving hospice care (Shah et al., 2016). Often, the subcutaneous route is used for PCA among patients living at home while receiving hospice care.

Optimize Safety Within the Patient-Controlled Analgesia Process

PCA is an effective method for delivering opioids and/or local analgesia through several routes of administration. However, adverse events that occurred among patients using PCA have led to concern for safe use (Cohen, Weber, & Moss, 2006; ECRI, 2017). When concerns arose, many efforts were made to correct problems and improve safety when using intravenous PCA (Institute for Safe Medication Practices [ISMP], 2008, 2013, 2016). Safe PCA use is facilitated when factors known to contribute to adverse events are identified, considered, modified, or eliminated (see Box 17.1). The following discussion addresses the factors and measures advised to improve safety when PCA is used in an MMA plan of care.

Clinician Education

General Concepts

All clinicians who prescribe and/or administer medication using PCA need to be aware of the general principles involved, appropriate prescription requirements, equipment currently used, safety concerns, monitoring requirements, and patient education needs (ECRI, 2017; Paul et al., 2010; Pasero & McCaffery, 2011). To best educate patients, it is important for clinicians to understand the various concepts, considerations and safety needs involved with administration of PCA. It is recommended for clinicians to receive standardized education regarding the electronic ordering system where applicable, monitoring guidelines, and safe operation of the equipment used in the organization in which they work. It is also recommended that clinicians demonstrate competency in providing safe patient care using PCA.

The six rights of medication administration—right patient, right medication, right dose, right time, right route, and right documentation—is an important foundational concept of all medication prescription and administration (Pasero & McCaffery, 2011). With PCA it is prudent to adhere to eight rights by adding *right concentration* and *right lockout interval*.

Equipment-Related Education

Human error is a significant source of adverse events involving PCA, with administering an incorrect medication, misprogramming the pump (equipment), and inappropriate prescription of PCA as significant sources of

---

| **BOX 17.1** | Current Therapy: Potential Sources of Patient-Controlled Analgesia–Related Mishaps |

OPERATOR ERRORS

- Inappropriate patient selection
- Selection of inappropriate medication
- Inappropriate prescribed dosing parameters
- Insertion of wrong syringe into PCA device
- PCA pump misprogramming
- Improper loading of syringe into PCA device
- Failure to clamp or unclamp PCA tubing
- Failure to turn on PCA machine after syringe change
- PCA key displacement
- Inadequate training of staff regarding PCA and setup
- Failure to respond to device or monitor alarms

PATIENT ERRORS

- Failure to understand PCA therapy or use of device
- Confusion between PCA button and nurse call button

- Physical inability to activate demand button
- PCA by proxy
- Intentional device tampering

MECHANICAL PROBLEMS

- Electrical failure/battery failure
- Short circuiting of PCA device
- Siphoning of medication
- Alarm malfunctions
- Tubing defects/lack of antireflux valves
- Accumulation of drug in tubing dead space
- Hardware or software failure in PCA machine

From Elliott, J. A. (2009). Patient-controlled analgesia. In H. S. Smith (Ed.), *Current therapy in pain*, (pp. 73–78). Philadelphia, PA: Saunders.

errors (Tran, Ciarkowski, Wagner, & Stevenson, 2012). It is important for clinicians who are prescribing PCA to understand how to appropriately prescribe the various components involved with PCA prescription, including medication, concentration, dose, lockout interval, and 1-hour or 4-hour limit (ECRI, 2017). Further, it is critical to provide front-line clinician education in the proper use and troubleshooting of the equipment and how to optimize patient safety, including how to intervene when equipment malfunctions. It is advised that all clinical staff demonstrate competency in administering analgesia by PCA and using the devices approved in the organization in which they are working.

PCA by Proxy

The Institute for Safe Medication Practices (ISMP) cautions that an important patient safety need is to repeatedly educate and remind all staff of the danger of *PCA by proxy*, which occurs when people other than the patient activate PCA delivery systems when they do not have official authorization (ISMP, 2016; Pasero & McCaffery, 2011). (See the later discussion of nurse-controlled analgesia [NCA] and family-controlled analgesia [FCA].) Unauthorized activation of the PCA device by someone other than the patient is a continuing danger in which one of the prime safety features of PCA is overridden. Intrinsic in PCA use and safety is for the alert patient to recognize the need for analgesia, understand he or she is self-administering analgesia by a PCA system, and then activate that system to deliver the medication. When another person activates the system and the patient is not awake and not in pain, the risk for oversedation with subsequent respiratory depression is significantly increased. An alternative method of analgesia needs to be provided whenever a family member or visitor continues to compromise the safety of the patient by activating the PCA device despite being cautioned not do to do so (ISMP, 2016).

Patient and Family Education

Patient and family education is an important component of ensuring safe use of PCA, and it is thought education is most effective when done when the patient is alert before surgery (ISMP, 2016). This education begins with explaining PCA, including what it is, how it functions, why it is being used, and the role and responsibility of the patient in the PCA process. Device safety features need to be explained, including dose limits, lockout intervals, hourly maximum dosing, and the reasons for using them (Box 17.2). It is imperative to reinforce to patients with diagnosed sleep apnea the importance of using their continuous positive airway pressure (CPAP) equipment at all times as prescribed during PCA therapy (Eksterowicz & DiMaggio, 2018).

The patient and family need to be educated about reasonable expectations for controlling pain (i.e., pain control versus eliminating pain). Often, reasonable expectations for pain control are best explained when incorporated with the concept of being able to function as optimally as possible (ECRI, 2017). From that perspective function goals for PCA can be identified. For example, the patient can be taught to activate the PCA device a few minutes before what is anticipated to be a painful activity (e.g., coughing, deep breathing, participating in physical therapy). Another important concept is for patients to know clinicians strive to help them be as comfortable as possible while keeping them as safe as possible. Patients and family members need to know nurses and other staff will assess and monitor the patient as well as the related equipment (e.g., PCA device, pulse oximetry, capnography) to ensure safety of the patient during therapy (ECRI, 2017).

Patients also need to know when to call the nurse, including when they experience inadequate analgesia or side effects and when any alerts sound or malfunctions of the delivery device occur. An extremely important aspect of patient and family/visitor education before initiation

---

Box 17.2 | Education Points for Teaching Patients About Patient-Controlled Analgesia

- Define PCA and the concepts supporting it.
- Explain the reasonable expectations for pain and functioning while using PCA.
- Teach how to use the PCA device to best control pain (e.g., when to use it).
- Explain PCA safety depends on only the patient using the device to control pain.
- Teach that no one other than the patient should ever use the device (e.g., press the button).
- Explain it may be advisable to activate the device a few minutes before an activity or procedure that is known or expected to be painful.

- Teach that clinicians and equipment will monitor the patient to ensure safety. This may mean the patient will be awakened to be assessed.
- Educate the patient when to call the nurse (e.g., pain not being controlled, untoward side effects, equipment malfunction).
- If the patient uses continuous positive airway pressure (CPAP) equipment at home, explain why it is important to use CPAP equipment while using PCA.

of PCA and throughout therapy is that PCA by proxy is a clear danger and *under no circumstances is anyone other than the patient to activate the PCA delivery device unless authorized to do so* (Brown et al., 2015; Cohen et al., 2006; ECRI, 2017; Elliott, 2016; ISMP, 2013, 2016; Pasero & McCaffery, 2011; San Diego Patient Safety Council [SDPSC], 2014; Se et al., 2016). (See discussion of FCA later in this chapter.)

Appropriate Prescription

In a review of PCA-related medication errors that occurred between 2005 and 2015 (N = 1948), more than half (58%) involved improper dose or quantity of medication delivered, with another 15% specifically related to errors in prescribing (Mohanty, Lawal, & Katz, 2017). Safe pain management using PCA begins with an appropriate PCA prescription. Historically, errors related to prescriber handwriting were a source of error, but, with the onset of electronic medical records (EMR) this is much less of an issue.

Although not foolproof, standardized order sets within the EMR have incorporated many safety factors with regard to PCA. Optimally, order sets provide a standardization of analgesic choices while also providing options to address the particular needs of each patient (ECRI, 2017). For example, an order set may default to a 10-minute lockout but provide options for a 15- or 20-minute lockout. Clinicians continue to be responsible for appropriate prescribing, including ensuring the right medication is prescribed at the right dose with the right parameters for the right patient. Fundamental in safe prescribing is to prescribe only for patients for whom use of PCA devices are appropriate.

Patient Selection

Great care must be taken to ensure PCA is an appropriate analgesic option for the patient and to ensure that only patients who are deemed able to use PCA safely and effectively are selected for PCA therapy. Several factors need to be considered in determining whether a patient is an appropriate candidate for PCA (Box 17.3). These factors can be considered from cognitive, psychological, and physical perspectives.

Cognitive Factors to Consider

Patients must have adequate cognitive ability to understand the concepts of PCA administration, including how to operate the PCA equipment (Elliott, 2016; Lien & Youngwerth, 2012). A basic requirement is that the patient must understand the relationships among pain, activating the PCA equipment (pushing the PCA button), and achieving pain relief (Pasero, Portenoy, & McCaffery, 1999). Clinicians may hesitate to prescribe PCA for children, thinking they are too young to understand the concepts of PCA and how to use the delivery device appropriately.

However, PCA has been used effectively and safely in developmentally normal children as young as 4 years of age (Wellington & Chia, 2009). The researchers of a very large retrospective study with surgical (n = 45,445) and nonsurgical (63,511) patients, taking place over 4 years, compared use of intravenously nurse-administered morphine with morphine administered by PCA in hospitalized children ranging in age from 5 to 21 years (Faerber et al., 2017). In that study, no increased risk for events requiring cardiopulmonary resuscitation or mechanical ventilation were reported when PCA was used and there was slightly improved safety reported with PCA use.

It is important for clinicians to regularly assess an individual's ability to self-administer analgesia after PCA is initiated. Patients who are originally deemed appropriate candidates for the therapy may, over time, prove to be unable or unwilling to maintain adequate analgesia with this method. Research has shown older patients tend to self-administer less opioid by PCA than younger patients (Gagliese et al., 2008). When that occurs, the patient can be encouraged to appropriately use the PCA device and educated with regard to PCA safety features. However, if patients are unable or unwilling to use PCA, it should be discontinued and alternative methods for managing pain, such as nurse-administered scheduled around-the-clock (ATC) or prn doses, should be promptly initiated (Pasero & McCaffery, 2011).

Psychological Factors to Consider

Although patient independence in controlling pain has been described as a benefit of PCA, for many years, research and clinical experience has shown not all patients want this responsibility (Salmon & Hall, 2001). Further, it has been noted that several factors influence the variation seen in a patient's ability to use PCA successfully (Katz, Buis, & Cohen, 2008). Patients who are anxious about self-administering medication or using the equipment are not likely to be successful with PCA (Elliott, 2016). For example, some patients may fear adverse effects or mistrust the technology. People who have an external locus of control (e.g., prefer nurse-administered medication) are not likely to be good candidates for PCA (Elliott, 2016).

Physiologic Factors to Consider

It is essential the patient has adequate finger dexterity to be able to activate dosing by pressing the button or other standard delivery device (Elliott, 2016; Lien & Youngwerth, 2012; Surprise & Simpson, 2014). For patients who do not have finger dexterity, such as patients who have a spinal cord injury, there are some PCA devices with a delivery mechanism that can be activated by a pressure device.

In addition, physical comorbidities are important safety considerations of patient selection. From a patient safety perspective, patients who are obese, have obstructive sleep apnea (see Chapters 8 and 13), or have other respiratory

Box 17.3 | Use of Intravenous Patient-Controlled Analgesia

PATIENT SELECTION

- For patients with cancer and noncancer pain, oral and other noninvasive routes produce unmanageable and intolerable adverse effects.
- For patients with acute pain (e.g., surgery, trauma), the oral and other noninvasive routes have been considered and are not an option because they would produce unmanageable and intolerable adverse effects at the anticipated doses required for adequate analgesia, or the oral route is not an option because the patient is fasting (NPO).
- In the patient with persistent cancer or noncancer pain or who is terminally ill, the patient's need for parenteral administration of an opioid analgesic is expected to be longer than 1 or 2 days.
- Patient is able to understand the relationships among pain, pushing the PCA button, and pain relief; is motivated to manage his or her pain; and is cognitively and physically able to self-administer a PCA dose using the available equipment.

OTHER CONSIDERATIONS

- Pumps are available.
- Cost is not prohibitive.
- Staff (or family) is trained to explain, assess, manage, and document intravenous PCA analgesia, adverse effects, and complications.

SURGICAL PROCEDURES FOR WHICH IV PCA IS PRESCRIBED

- Cesarean section when epidural anaesthesia/analgesia is not used
- Abdominal, vaginal hysterectomy
- Anterior and posterior repair
- Bladder surgery
- Ureteral reimplantation
- Penile implant
- Radical prostatectomy
- Mastectomy
- Gastroplasty
- Abdominoplasty
- Inpatient rectal surgeries
- Major plastic surgeries and skin grafts
- Major hand, ankle, or foot repair
- Joint replacement
- Long bone surgery
- Laminectomy
- Shoulder repair
- Radical neck surgery

MEDICAL CONDITIONS FOR WHICH IV PCA IS PRESCRIBED

- Cancer pain
- Sickle cell pain
- Burn pain
- HIV pain
- Fractures
- Pancreatitis
- Nephrolithiasis

From Pasero, C., & McCaffery, M. (2011). *Pain assessment and pharmacologic management* (p. 315). St. Louis, MO: Mosby. Data from Cashman, J. N. (2006). Patient-controlled analgesia. In G. Shorten, D. B. Carr, D. Harmon, M. Puig, & J. Browne (Eds.), *Postoperative pain management: An evidence-based guide to practice*, Philadelphia, PA: Saunders; Grass, J. A. (2005). Patient-controlled analgesia. *Anesthesia and Analgesia, 101*(Suppl. 1), S44–S61; Lehmann, K. A. (2005). Recent developments in patient-controlled analgesia. *Journal of Pain and Symptom Management, 29*(Suppl. 5), S72–S89; Macintyre, P. E., & Coldrey, J. (2008). Patient-controlled analgesia. In R. S. Sinatra, O. A. de Leon-Casasola, B. Ginsberg, E. R. Viscusi (Eds.), *Acute pain management*, Cambridge, New York, Cambridge University Press; Macintyre, P. E., & Coldrey, J. (2008). Patient-controlled analgesia. In P. E. Macintyre, S. M. Walker, & D. J. Rowbotham. (Eds.), *Clinical pain management: Acute pain* (2nd ed.). London: Hodder Arnold; Sherman, B., Enu, I., & Sinatra, R. S. (2009). Patient-controlled analgesia devices and analgesic infusion pumps. *Acute Pain Management*, 302–322. © 2011, Pasero C, & McCaffery M. May be duplicated for use in clinical practice.
HIV, Human immunodeficiency virus; *IV*, intravenous; *PCA*, patient-controlled analgesia.

---

diseases are not ideal candidates for pain management using PCA (Craft, 2010). Patients who have renal failure and those who are receiving sedative medications (e.g., muscle relaxants, antiemetics, benzodiazepines) also are not considered ideal candidates for using PCA therapy (Cohen et al., 2006; Marks & Rodgers, 2014). If PCA is prescribed for patients with these comorbidities, it is advised that additional caution be exerted with appropriate and more frequent monitoring, including pulse oximetry (Marks & Rodgers, 2014) or capnography. (See Chapter 13 for detailed discussion of opioid-induced respiratory depression.)

An important aspect of patient history is the use of opioids before administration. There is very little evidence to determine what PCA bolus dose is appropriate for patients who are opioid naïve (Pasero & McCaffery, 2011). (See Chapters 11 and 14 for other discussion of pain management among patients who are opioid tolerant and opioid naïve.) To ensure patient safety with opioid-naïve patients it is best to use the rule to *start low and go slow* (Box 17.4). This is particularly important with opioid-naïve older adults (e.g., those age 65 years and older) who may require a reduction of 25% of what

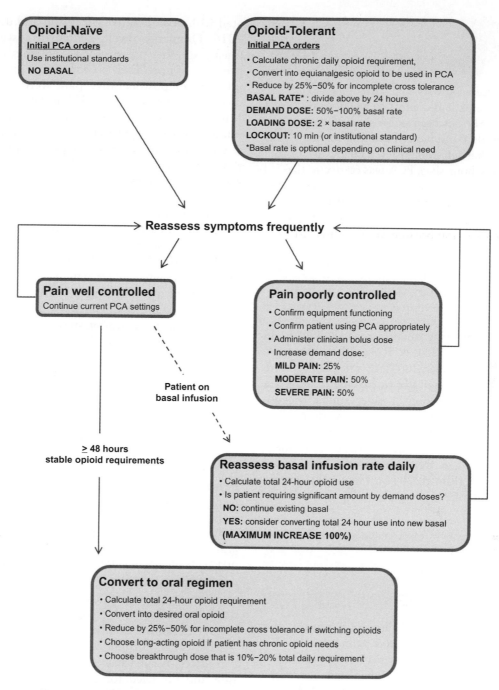

Opioid-Naïve
<u>Initial PCA orders</u>
Use institutional standards
NO BASAL

Opioid-Tolerant
<u>Initial PCA orders</u>
• Calculate chronic daily opioid requirement,
• Convert into equianalgesic opioid to be used in PCA
• Reduce by 25%–50% for incomplete cross tolerance
BASAL RATE* : divide above by 24 hours
DEMAND DOSE: 50%–100% basal rate
LOADING DOSE: 2 × basal rate
LOCKOUT: 10 min (or institutional standard)
*Basal rate is optional depending on clinical need

→ **Reassess symptoms frequently** ←

Pain well controlled
Continue current PCA settings

Pain poorly controlled
• Confirm equipment functioning
• Confirm patient using PCA appropriately
• Administer clinician bolus dose
• Increase demand dose:
  MILD PAIN: 25%
  MODERATE PAIN: 50%
  SEVERE PAIN: 50%

Patient on
basal infusion

≥ 48 hours
stable opioid requirements

Reassess basal infusion rate daily
• Calculate total 24-hour opioid use
• Is patient requiring significant amount by demand doses?
  NO: continue existing basal
  YES: consider converting total 24 hour use into new basal
(MAXIMUM INCREASE 100%)

Convert to oral regimen
• Calculate total 24-hour opioid requirement
• Convert into desired oral opioid
• Reduce by 25%–50% for incomplete cross tolerance if switching opioids
• Choose long-acting opioid if patient has chronic opioid needs
• Choose breakthrough dose that is 10%–20% total daily requirement

Fig. 17.1 | **Patient-Controlled Analgesia Overview.** (From Lien, C., & Youngwerth, J. [2012]. Patient-controlled analgesia. *Hospital Medicine Clinics, 1*[3], e386–e403.)

would be considered a safe starting bolus dose for an opioid-naïve younger adult (Pasero & McCaffery, 2011).

Determining the appropriate PCA doses for patients who are opioid tolerant can be challenging. There are many definitions of what characteristics determine when a person is opioid tolerant. One definition from the ISMP is the person consumes 60 mg or more of morphine or an equivalent for at least 7 days prior (ECRI, 2017; FDA, 2015). For such patients, it may be necessary for the majority of analgesia to be delivered by an appropriately determined equianalgesic continuous infusion with larger

bolus doses and longer lockout intervals than would be prescribed for opioid-naïve patients (Pasero & McCaffery, 2011) (Box 17.5).

Although one report cautioned PCA is not appropriate for older patients in the ED setting (Motov & Nelson, 2016), that has not been substantiated by other findings. Rather, for many years, intravenous PCA has been shown to be safe in older patients (Pasero & McCaffery, 2011). Even so, clinicians often do not prescribe it for fear of producing confusion in older patients. However, many factors can contribute to confusion in hospitalized older adults,

Box 17.4	Patient Example: Opioid Naïve

After total hip replacement, Mrs. G. is managing her pain with intravenous patient-controlled analgesia (PCA) HYDROmorphone. She has been stable since surgery 7 hours earlier. She is alert and has a respiratory rate of 16 breaths/min. She has self-administered an average of four PCA doses every hour since PCA was started in the postanesthesia care unit. She rates her pain as 4 on a scale of 0 to 10, has a comfort-function goal of 2 on a scale of 0 to 10 to turn and deep breathe. Her respiratory status has been stable, and she has experienced no more than mild sedation.

From Pasero, C., & McCaffery, M. (2011). *Pain assessment and pharmacologic management.* St. Louis, MO: Mosby.

with only one of them being opioids, regardless of route of administration (Bagri, Rico, & Ruiz, 2008; Pasero & McCaffery, 2011; Redelmeier, 2007). It is not appropriate and can delay accurate diagnosis to assume opioids are the primary cause of confusion in older adults, because confusion may not be related to either the medication or the delivery approach (Pasero & McCaffery, 2011).

There is some evidence that alterations in mental status may occur less frequently when opioids are administered by PCA (Elliott, 2016). This is reasonable, because poorly controlled or unrelieved pain is associ-

Box 17.5	Patient Example: Opioid Tolerant

Mrs. S. has been receiving a subcutaneous infusion of morphine 30 mg/h to control her cancer pain. While in the hospital, the nurses offer her subcutaneous breakthrough bolus doses every 2 hours. Often, Mrs. S. has been tolerating pain rather than asking the nurses for breakthrough doses. Her family is concerned that this pattern will continue at home. Her nurse discusses the concept of patient-controlled analgesia (PCA) with Mrs. S. and her family. They are receptive to the idea of using subcutaneous PCA to control Mrs. S.'s breakthrough pain. Her PCA bolus dose is calculated at 8 mg (~25% of the hourly morphine dose) with a lockout interval of 15 minutes. Mrs. S. self-administers doses readily, reports better pain control, and is significantly more satisfied with her pain treatment plan once she has PCA. She remains alert and her activity level improves.

From Pasero, C., & McCaffery, M. (2011). *Pain assessment and pharmacologic management.* St. Louis, MO: Mosby.

ated with postoperative confusion and delirium (Elliott, 2016; Quinlan-Colwell, 2012). In a study with older (mean age 74) postoperative patients (N = 333) the presence of unrelieved postoperative pain and increased intensity of postoperative pain were independent predictors of postoperative delirium (Vaurio, Sands, Wang, Mullen, & Leung, 2006). There was also an ordered relationship between the severity of preoperative persistent pain and the risk for postoperative delirium in that study. The patients with severe preoperative pain were at greater risk than those with moderate preoperative pain. It is interesting to note naloxone administration does not improve postoperative delirium, further suggesting opioids often are not a primary underlying cause (Redelmeier, 2007).

Considering the available research, in cases in which PCA is warranted, older patients should not be denied access to this modality simply because of their age. In fact, the smaller, more frequent doses delivered by PCA with lower serum concentration may be more appropriate for older adults (McKeown, 2015). Rather, older adults need to be carefully screened to ascertain if they have the cognitive and physical ability to manage their pain by using PCA therapy. Careful monitoring with close attention to dosing patterns is important to help ensure adequate pain relief with PCA (Pasero & McCaffery, 2011). It is important to note intravenous PCA also has been used effectively with some older patients with cognitive impairment who were cautiously selected (Licht, Siegler, & Reid, 2009). Further research in that subpopulation of older adults using PCA is warranted before any recommendations can be made.

As with many medications used with older adults a good rule is to start low and go slow (Quinlan-Colwell, 2012). With older adults, it is also prudent practice to start with a dose that is half what would be started in a younger patient with the same (or longer) interval for dose availability and avoid continuous infusions (basal rates) (McKeown, 2015).

Physical comorbidities are another consideration that can affect the pharmacokinetics of the selected medication and the need for dosing adjustments, particularly among older adults (Elliott, 2016). Related to comorbidities is the need to consider other medications the patient is taking to control those conditions. Patients who are taking medications with sedating side effects may not be appropriate candidates for using PCA (Ritter, 2011). Such patients may be at increased risk for sedation and respiratory depression and may not be able to adequately manage pain using the PCA because of sedation. If used, close monitoring of sedation level and respiratory status during PCA therapy needs to be implemented.

The *body habitus* of a patient is most likely the least important criterion to use when deciding on the appropriate dose for PCA analgesia. Although at times intravenous opioid PCA is prescribed based on weight (e.g., milligram of opioid per kilogram of body weight), there is no evidence this is beneficial (Wellington & Chia, 2009). Dosing opioids based on total body weight can lead to excessive medication with resultant adverse effects (Budiansky, Margarson, & Eipe, 2017). Excessive sedation has occurred in patients who are obese using PCA (Ritter, 2011). It is not clear if weight-based dosing or another reason is the cause of these adverse events. For these reasons weight-based dosing is not advised. Rather, among individuals who are obese, with increased adipose tissue compared to lean body weight, it may be safest to decrease the quantity of the dose that would be considered appropriate for someone with a lean body weight (Leykin, Miotto, & Pellis, 2011).

Prescription Components

A valuable aspect of using PCA as part of an MMA plan of care is the extensive variability of mode of administration, medication options, dosing parameters, and route. Selection of the most appropriate option for each of these components facilitates the availability of analgesia specific to the needs of the individual patient (Surprise & Simpson, 2014).

Modes of Administration

PCA can be delivered by two modes: PCA bolus doses with a continuous infusion (basal rate) or PCA bolus doses alone with no continuous infusion (Fernandes et al., 2017). The components of the modes of PCA are presented in Table 17.1. Typically, a specialized infusion pump is used to deliver PCA by the particular route of administration. In this context, PCA refers to the bolus dose the patient controls when pressing a button on the device or attached to the device.

Medications Administered

The medication needs to be selected based on the requirements of the individual patient considering current pain, history with effectiveness of opioids, allergic responses, and tolerability of side effects. Patient comorbidities are another important consideration that may affect medication choice (Ritter, 2011) (see Chapters 9 and 11). The frequently prescribed medications for PCA administration are opioids and local anesthetics. Other medications, including ketamine, are less frequently or rarely prescribed by PCA. From a comprehensive perspective, all of the medications used are discussed here.

Medications Frequently Administered by PCA

Mu Agonist Opioids Mu agonist opioid analgesics, specifically morphine, HYDROmorphone, and fentaNYL, are the most common analgesics administered by intravenous and subcutaneous PCA (Smith & Goldberg, 2012). They are also frequently used either alone or in combination with local anesthetics by patient-controlled epidural analgesia (PCEA) (Gupta et al., 2016). (See Chapter 11 for detailed discussion of mu opioids.)

Very rarely, methadone is used in PCA, primarily with people with chronic pain, those living with cancer, and those receiving palliative care (Flory, Wiesenthal, Thaler, Koranteng, & Moryl, 2016). However, a recent study assessed it being used in acute postoperative pain

Table 17.1	Components of Patient-Controlled Analgesia
Medication and concentration	The name and concentration of the prescribed medication to be administered (e.g., 0.5 mg/mL versus 1 mg/mL HYDROmorphone).
Loading dose	Amount of medication prescribed to be administered by clinician when PCA is initiated to rapidly achieve an adequate serum level of analgesia and patient comfort.
Demand dose	The prescribed and preprogrammed amount of medication that is delivered to the patient each time the patient activates the delivery device. Also called patient bolus dose.
Continuous infusion	Dose of medication prescribed and programmed to be delivered during 1 hour by the microprocessor-control in the PCA infusion device. This is not under the control of the patient and is accessed without any action by the patient. It is delivered in addition to the demand doses.
Lockout interval	Period (often 6–15 min) between available doses when medication cannot be accessed or delivered. This prevents stacking of medication and allows for the patient to appreciate the effect of the analgesia delivered.
Hourly maximum dose	Maximum amount of medication that can be delivered within 1 hour. In some instances a 4 hour maximum is used that limits the amount of medication that can be delivered in 4 hours.
Clinician rescue or bolus dose	An additional dose of medication that can be administered by the clinician when the patient is experiencing breakthrough or unrelieved pain to help increase the level of analgesia. These doses generally are twice the medication amount as the demand dose.

management (Neto et al., 2014). In that study, when compared to patients receiving morphine PCA, those who received methadone PCA reported significantly less pain at rest and after movement and consuming less opioid. Although drowsiness, nausea, and vomiting occurred more frequently among those with the methadone PCA, the instances were not statistically different. Methadone has a long elimination half-life (e.g., 5–59 hours), so there is concern for accumulation over time with increased risk for serious side effects such as respiratory depression (Modesto-Lowe, Brooks, & Petry, 2010). This concern is particularly significant for people such as older adults who may have slower metabolism of methadone. The long elimination half-life of methadone is an important reason why it is not recommended to be used in the treatment of acute pain. Clinicians need to be aware there is some evidence of increased risk for hypoglycemia with PCA use (Flory et al., 2016). In addition, because of the unique pharmacokinetic properties of methadone, it should be used only by clinicians who are experienced with using it (Polomano et al., 2017).

Local Anesthetics Local anesthetics, which are an important component of MMA, are the principle medication used for patient-controlled regional analgesia (PCRA) (Pasero & McCaffery, 2011). Frequently, local anesthetics (ropivacaine, bupivacaine, and levobupivacaine) also are used alone or in combination with an opioid for epidural analgesia by PCEA (Chou et al., 2016; Ong, Kirthinanda, Loh, & Sng, 2016). Use of local anesthetics in regional and epidural infusions is considered safe, with only rare incidences of local anesthetic toxicity, which recent data indicate are further declining (Neal et al., 2018). Local anesthetics are also used in combination with opioids for intrathecal PCA (ITPCA). (See Chapters 18 and 19 for detailed information on local anesthetics.)

Medications Not Frequently Administered by PCA

CloNIDine At times the alpha$_2$-adrenergic drug cloNIDine is added to a local anesthetic and opioid for analgesia by PCEA (Chou et al., 2016). When cloNIDine (e.g., 2 mcg/mL) was used with SUFentanil and levobupivacaine in PCEA with women in labor, analgesia was improved and there was less need for rescue analgesia (Wallet et al., 2010). However, use of cloNIDine is not widespread for two reasons (Ong et al., 2016). First, the safety challenge when using cloNIDine is to balance analgesia while maintaining adequate blood pressure and avoiding sedation. Second, it is important to remember the use of cloNIDine for this purpose is an off-label use and safety is not established (Paech & Pan, 2009). (See Chapter 15 for more information on cloNIDine.)

Neostigmine Neostigmine has been used at times in PCEA with reports of local anesthetic–sparing effect (Ross et al., 2009). However, with neostigmine there were

also reports of increased nausea, vomiting, and anxiety with slowed heart rate. There is no evidence the slight improvement in reducing local anesthetic need is worth the negative factors, and it is also an off-label use with no established safety (Ong et al., 2016; Paech & Pan, 2009).

Ketamine Ketamine was studied in PCA in conjunction with opioids (e.g., morphine and HYDROmorphone). The authors of a systematic review and meta-analysis (N = 36 studies; n = 2502 subjects) reported that when ketamine was added to opioid intravenous PCA, there was a small improvement in pain relief with some sparing of opioid dose but no difference in length of stay (Wang et al., 2016). In a pilot study (N = 20) ketamine PCA was compared with HYDROmorphone PCA among trauma patients in an intensive care unit (ICU) setting (Takieddine et al., 2018). In that study, those who received ketamine required less total opioids and supplemental oxygen but they experienced more hallucinations. Additional research is needed to assess the benefits versus risks of using ketamine by PCA. (See Chapter 15 for more information regarding ketamine.)

Dexmedetomidine Dexmedetomidine has been studied as an adjunct with opioids in intravenous PCA. The authors of a meta-analysis (N = 7 studies) concluded combining dexmedetomidine is effective to achieve lower pain intensity scores (P = .002), less opioid analgesic use (P = .0001), less nausea (P = .0001), and fewer side effects, with greater patient satisfaction with pain control (P = .02) (Peng, Liu, Wu, Cheng, & Ji, 2015). In a subsequent randomized double-blind controlled study, the effect of dexmedetomidine plus SUFentanil intravenous PCA was compared with that of SUFentanil intravenous PCA to evaluate the quality of recovery after laparotomy surgery (n = 93) (Xin et al., 2017). In that study, the participants who received SUFentanil plus dexmedetomidine reported significantly lower pain intensity scores (P < .05) and that nausea occurred less frequently. Yet, there was no difference in activation of the intravenous PCA device or rescue doses of opioid. In addition, there were no adverse events of respiratory depression, hypotension, or bradycardia. The data to date suggests the addition of dexmedetomidine to an opioid delivered by PCA may provide better analgesia in a safe manner; however, additional research with more diverse populations is needed to provide more evidence to evaluate safety and effectiveness (Peng et al., 2015; Xin et al., 2017). (See Chapter 15 for more information on dexmedetomidine.)

Technical Components of Prescription

Regardless of the route of administration the prescription for PCA by a mechanical delivery system requires a number of components to be specifically prescribed by the clinician. Despite PCA therapy being used extensively since first marketed in 1973 (Evans, MacCarthy, Rosen,

& Hogg, 1976), it is surprising that there is very little evidence to support how best to prescribe the various components of a PCA prescription (Pasero & McCaffery, 2011). Although guidelines for prescribing PCA are available, it is essential that the prescription be based on the individual patient factors, needs, and comorbidities (SDSPC, 2014) (Table 17.2). Optimal PCA therapy depends on adjustment of the various components based on the needs of the patient as determined by assessment and reassessment. It is also recommended to include a prescription for naloxone in case it is needed (see Chapters 11, 13, and 28).

Medication Concentration

Medications used in PCA devices are prepared in a variety of concentrations. The concentration of medication is prescribed either in milligrams per milliliter or micrograms per milliliter of solution. One source of serious error is when the concentration of medication is administered or programmed incorrectly (ISMP, 2008). To help ensure patient safety, it is recommended only one standard concentration of each medication is routinely accessible for administration, with different concentrations available only through specific pharmacy request (ISMP, 2009; Lien & Youngwerth, 2012) or restricted to particular units (e.g., palliative care). In addition, many hospitals require an independent double-check of the programming of the PCA by another clinical professional to ensure patient safety. An independent double-check requires two clinicians, with each clinician independently verifying the concentration of the medication in the PCA device is the same as what was prescribed.

Clinician Rescue Dose and Loading Dose

A clinician-administered dose is prescribed to enable the clinician to administer a prescribed amount of medication in addition to what the patient can self-administer. This may be prescribed specifically as a single or as multiple loading dose(s) to be administered by the clinician at the initiation of the PCA to provide for more rapid relief of pain when there may not yet be any serum opioid level (Elliott, 2009). This is important because a key point when using PCA is initiating it when the patient has reasonably good pain relief, with the intention of continuing good pain control (Elliott, 2009; Pasero & McCaffery, 2011). The *clinician rescue dose(s)* also may be prescribed as rescue doses to be administered when the patient has an escalation of pain, has breakthrough pain, or needs additional analgesia for a painful procedure (Lien & Youngwerth, 2012).

Bolus Dose or Demand Dose

The PCA bolus dose, also called demand dose, is the amount of medication prescribed for the patient to self-administer by the infusion device (Elliott, 2009). To a significant degree the success of PCA depends on appropriate prescription of the PCA bolus dose in conjunction with the lockout interval (see later). Patient pain, perception, analgesia requirements, general health, body habitus, previous experiences, and tolerance are highly individualized; thus it is not possible to create a formula for PCA dosing. Guidance is provided in Table 17.2. The intent is for the patient to self-administer relatively small doses of medication as needed to manage pain (Pasero & McCaffery, 2011). This is consistent with the concept of *minimal effective analgesic concentration* (MEAC), which is the minimal concentration of serum analgesia required to effectively relieve pain (Lien & Youngwerth, 2012). With the patient in control of managing the subjective sensations of pain, it is possible to maintain this level of analgesia, avoiding troughs and breakthrough pain; however, clinicians must remember that adjustments to the bolus dose may still be needed. Although *bolus dose* is the term used most often as a synonym for demand dose, in some locations it is used to describe an extra dose of medication that can be administered by a clinician as a

---

Table 17.2 | Starting Intravenous Patient-Controlled Analgesia Prescription Parameters for Opioid-Naïve Adult Patients

Medication	Concentration Strength	Loading Dose/ Clinician Dose*	PCA Dose	Lockout Interval (Min)	Hourly Maximum
Morphine	1 mg/mL	2.5 mg	0.5–2 mg	8–10	**
HYDROmorphone	0.2 mg/mL	0.4 mg	0.1–0.4 mg	8–10	**
FentaNYL	10–20 mcg/mL	25 mcg	5–25 mcg	6–10	**
OxyMORphone	0.25 mg/mL	0.4 mg	0.25–0.5 mg	8–10	**

*The number of loading doses and whether the clinician dose is a one time dose or may be repeated PRN depends upon what is prescribed in the orders.
**Hourly maximum needs to be the total amount of the loading plus clinician doses plus the number of PCA doses available within an hour (e.g., if a PCA is set with one 2-mg loading dose plus one 2-mg clinician dose of morphine plus 1 mg PCA every 10 min, in 1 h the patient may receive 2 mg + 2 mg + 6 mg or a total of 10 mg, which is the hourly maximum). If the device requires a 4-h maximum, the hourly maximum is multiplied × 4 or in the case above 40 mg per 4 h.
From Pasero, C., & McCaffery, M., (2011). *Pain assessment and pharmacologic management* (p. 463). St. Louis, MO: Mosby. Lien, C., & Youngwerth, J. (2012). Patient-controlled analgesia. *Hospital Medicine Clinics, 1*(3), e386–e403, 390; and San Diego Patient Safety Council (2014). *Tool kit patient controlled analgesia (PCA) guidelines of care for the opioid naïve patient* (p. 5). San Diego, CA: San Diego Patient Safety Council.

rescue dose, similar to a loading dose (Elliott, 2009). This underscores the importance of all clinicians fully understanding the exact meaning of the terminology used in the facility where they are currently working.

Lockout Interval

The lockout interval is the prescribed period to be programmed into the device to ensure adequate time elapses between doses (Elliott, 2009). There is a balance involved with establishing the lockout interval. The timing needs to be long enough for the patient to appreciate the effect of the analgesia and avoid stacking of doses, which can occur if a second dose is activated before the first taking full effect. It also needs to be short enough for the person to be able to self-administer the analgesia when needed, particularly before and during activities (Pasero & McCaffery, 2011) (see Table 17.2). During the lockout interval, no medication can be delivered despite the patient attempting to activate the demand device. Thus this is one inherent safety component within the system (Elliott, 2009). However, it is critical to remember that neither this nor any other component of the PCA prescription guarantee that the therapy is failsafe. As mentioned, the safety of PCA therapy depends on systematic assessment, reassessment, and prescription adjustment based on patient needs.

Hourly Maximum

The hourly maximum is the total amount of medication that can be administered to the patient within the 1-hour or 4-hour period depending on the PCA device (Pasero & McCaffery, 2011). This amount includes the clinician-administered doses and the PCA bolus doses the patient can self-administer. If a morphine IV PCA is set with one 2 mg loading dose, plus one PRN 2 mg clinician bolus dose, plus 1 mg PCA dose every 10 minutes, the patient can receive as much as one 2 mg loading dose + one PRN 2 mg clinician bolus dose + 6 mg self-administered bolus doses (1 mg on each of six occasions) equaling a total of 10 mg (i.e., 2 mg + 2 mg + 1 mg x 6 = 10), which is the 1 hour maximum during the first hour. However, after the first hour the hourly maximum is just 8 mg to allow for the patient administered boluses available every 10 minutes, totaling 6 mg plus the possible PRN administration of the one clinician bolus of 2 mg. If the device requires a 4-hour maximum, the hourly maximum is multiplied by 4 or in the case mentioned previously, after the one time loading dose there is a 4 hour maximum that includes 26 mg to allow for 6 patient administered bolus doses (1 mg each) per hour x 4, plus one possible PRN clinician bolus dose of 2 mg (i.e., 1 mg x 6 [doses per hour] = 6 mg x 4 [hours] = 24 mg +2 mg [clinician bolus dose] = 26 mg). Of note, the clinician may prescribe an hourly maximum that is less than the summed maximum amount that can be delivered by the device. For instance, in the previous example, if the clinician does not think it is safe for the patient to receive morphine 10 mg/h, the hourly maximum could be established at a lower rate (e.g., 8 mg). In that case, once the hourly maximum (e.g., 8 mg) is reached the patient is "locked out" and cannot access additional medication until that hour has elapsed.

Basal or Continuous Infusion Rate

A basal or continuous infusion rate is the amount of medication prescribed to be programmed to infuse continuously by the device, regardless of any action by the patient or clinician (Lien & Youngwerth, 2012). No clear research evidence demonstrates benefit, there is a fivefold increased risk for respiratory depression when an infusion is continuously infused, and basal or continuous infusions must be used with caution (George et al., 2010; ISMP, 2009). It is recommended to avoid continuous infusions with opioid-naïve patients (Chou et al., 2016; ECRI, 2017; ISMP, 2009; Lien & Youngwerth, 2012; Ritter, 2011). However, when patients who are opioid naïve are in a setting with close and continuous monitoring such as an ICU, this caution may not be applicable. Although there is no strong evidence regarding effectiveness of basal or continuous infusions in patients who are opioid tolerant, this method may be beneficial for avoiding inadequate analgesia and preventing opioid withdrawal (Chou et al., 2016). When a basal or continuous infusion is in place, close monitoring by the nurse is essential. Some institutions require continuous pulse oximetry or capnography monitoring on all patients when they are prescribed a continous infusion (ISMP, 2013, 2016).

Routes of Administration

Traditionally, the term patient-controlled analgesia refers to the patient self-administering doses of opioids by intravenous, subcutaneous (Smith & Goldberg, 2012), perineural (PCRA) (Eksterowicz & DiMaggio, 2018), epidural (PCEA) (Stroud, Tulanont, Coates, Goodney, & Croitoriu, 2014), intrathecal (Brogan, Winter, & Okifuji, 2015), and intranasal (Pasero & McCaffery, 2011) routes of administration. Although patients have always controlled oral medication administration at home, less commonly there is also oral or enteral PCA in the inpatient setting (Eksterowicz & DiMaggio, 2018). Iontophoretic transdermal systems (ITSs) provide another route of PCA (Sinatra et al., 2015). Each of these routes will be discussed individually.

Regardless of the route of administration, it is important to understand each patient is unique with varying patterns of resolution of pain as he or she recovers from acute pain situations (Pasero & McCaffery, 2011). Often, as patients recover, they use less medication by a PCA, and it may be necessary to assist the patient with tapering the amount of analgesia (ECRI, 2017). Because it is advisable postoperatively to discontinue the intravenous PCA once normal gastrointestinal function reactivates, an important consideration is transitioning the patient from an intravenous PCA to oral opioid medication (Pasero & McCaffery, 2011). (See Chapter 11 for equianalgesic dosing.)

Intravenous Route

Intravenous PCA uses the intravenous route of administration with a specified PCA delivery system connected to intravenous tubing. In many settings, intravenous PCA has been considered the standard of care for postoperative pain management (Winer, Sfakianos, Puttanniah, & Bochner, 2015). Unless otherwise noted, content discussed previously in this chapter applies to intravenous PCA. Interestingly, the majority of the recent literature reporting research involving intravenous PCA is written with the intravenous PCA being the gold standard against which the effectiveness of other routes of PCA are compared (Katz, Takyar, Palmer, & Liedgens, 2017). Even the concept of MMA is compared to intravenous PCA as an effective method of pain management (Park et al., 2015). That comparison is curious because intravenous PCA is often an important component within a multimodal approach of pain management.

Intravenous PCA is appropriate for patients who can safely use a patient-controlled system of analgesia and who are expected to require parenteral opioid analgesia for 1 day or longer. This may be due to the person not being able to take anything by mouth (NPO) or to experiencing intolerable side effects with oral administration of opioids. Suitable patients may have postoperative pain (e.g., abdominal, thoracic, neurologic, orthopedic, gynecologic, urologic), pain related to trauma (e.g., fractures, burns, etc.) or pain related to medical conditions (e.g., cancer, burns, sickle cell crisis, pancreatitis, nephrolithiasis) (Pasero & McCaffery, 2011).

Two criticisms of intravenous PCA is that it is viewed as awkward and limiting for patients who are able to be active and participate in physical therapy and it is labor intensive for nurses (Schechter & Finkelstein, 2015). Clinical staff can be taught to assist with managing equipment in patients using intravenous PCA who need to participate in physical therapy or who are otherwise active. Some older studies have assessed nursing time involved with PCA use (Koh & Thomas, 1994). Recent studies indicate greater nursing time is involved with intravenous PCA compared to patient-controlled iontophoretic transdermal PCA (see later) (Evans et al., 2007; Pestano, Lindley, Ding, Danesi, & Jones, 2017; Viscusi, 2008). Research is needed to collect and analyze data to compare staff time involved with administration of intravenous PCA with other current analgesic options and considering clinician responsibilities for overall patient care. If intravenous PCA proves to be more labor intensive, yet it is the best method of analgesia for a specific patient with pain, staffing modifications are needed.

Epidural Route

Along with intravenous PCA, PCEA is one of the most frequently used PCA routes (Argoff, 2014). In a retrospective review, when PCEA was compared with intravenous PCA (n = 308), those patients who had analgesia by PCEA reported statistically significant lower pain intensity on postoperative days 1 ($P = .0001$) and 2 ($P = .004$) and less total opioid use during postoperative days 1 through 3 ($P = .0001$) (Winer et al., 2015). A benefit of PCEA is that less opioid is required by the epidural route than is required by the intravenous route; thus there is less risk for dose-related adverse events (Elliott, 2009).

PCEA may either be used in the acute care setting (e.g., postoperatively) or for long-term management of chronic pain. When used in an acute care situation, the catheter extends from the epidural space through the skin, where it is secured and connected to the delivery device. When used over an extended period, the catheter can be tunneled through the subcutaneous tissue (usually along the flank area), where it exits and is secured on the abdomen then connected to the delivery device (Paz & Quinlan, 2014). (For detailed information on epidural analgesia see Chapter 18.)

Regional Route

PCRA is delivered by a catheter that is inserted into a particular anatomic area traditionally near a peripheral nerve (Paz & Quinlan, 2014). More recently, PCRA has been successfully used with catheters inserted either within the surgical wound or intraarticularly (into a joint) (Kaye, Ali, & Urman, 2014). PCRA can be beneficial when using MMA with patients who have undergone thoracotomy (paravertebral block), abdominal procedures (transversus abdominis plane block), and total joint replacement surgeries (Chou et al., 2016). In one study comparing the local anesthetic ropivacaine with placebo via PCRA, the patients who self-administered ropivacaine via PCRA after open carpal tunnel surgery, reported less pain and required significantly less rescue analgesia ($P = .001$) (Argoff, 2014). Patient satisfaction is reported to be high for PCRA, and it can be used in the home setting with disposable delivery systems continued after discharge (Elliott, 2009). (For detailed information on regional analgesia see Chapter 18.)

Subcutaneous Route

With the onset of more sophisticated technology that expands options for delivery of analgesia, the subcutaneous route is not used as frequently today as it was in the past (Sharma & de Leon-Cassola, 2014). Today, subcutaneous PCA is most frequently used in palliative care and as part of comfort measures at the end of life, often with a continuous basal infusion (Müller-Schwefe et al., 2014). This route also continues to be useful when managing pain in both children and adults in the home setting, where it is not generally reasonable to continue long-term peripheral intravenous therapy (Coyle & Glajchen, 2014; Suresh & Shah, 2014). Small-caliber needles are generally used for access (e.g., 27-gauge butterfly), but larger needles also can be used for infusion (Suresh & Shah, 2014). The subcutaneous route also has been used successfully with hospitalized patients with sickle cell disease who may have limited intravenous access (Dampier, 2014; Myers & Eckes, 2012). Although some may disagree, one perceived benefit of the subcutaneous route is that the site is rotated frequently, thus avoiding distress in any one administration site (Martin et al., 2016). Often the site is changed every 3 days to prevent possible irritation and ensure optimal absorption.

When using the subcutaneous route, it is important to remember that although they are effective, when boluses are administered they have a slower onset of action and the peak effect is lower compared to boluses delivered by the intravenous route (Fine & Bekanich, 2014). One study reported HYDROmorphone administered by subcutaneous PCA had approximately 80% bioavailability and within 24 hours steady-state concentrations were achieved (Martin et al., 2016). Those findings support the belief that subcutaneous infusions are equivalent to those by the intravenous route (Suresh & Shah, 2014). Most patients can tolerate subcutaneous infusions of 2 or 4 mL/h with little difficulty or pain at the site of infusion (Martin et al., 2016). However, infusions as high as 10 mL/h are often generally absorbed and tolerated as well (Fine & Bekanich, 2014). Because the amount of volume by subcutaneous infusion is limited, the opioid concentration used is often much higher than in the standard concentration available to enable adequate analgesia with a lower volume infusion. It is important to remember the risk for respiratory depression does not appreciably differ when the subcutaneous route is used (Hanna, Ouanes, & Tomas, 2014).

Transdermal Route

Patient-controlled transdermal analgesia (PCTA) currently uses a fentaNYL ITS, which was approved by the U.S. Food and Drug Administration (FDA) in 2006 (Argoff, 2014). The delivery system consists of a needleless system that is attached with adhesive backing typically to either the outer upper arm or chest, and by iontophoresis the medication is delivered and absorbed across the intact skin (Paz & Quinlan, 2014). The current device is preset with a 40-mcg dose of fentaNYL that can be self-administered by the patient as frequently as every 10 minutes, which is the standard preset lockout interval for the device. Thus a maximum of 80 doses may be delivered during a 24-hour period. This system is not intended to be used for more than 72 hours (Polomano et al., 2017).

In a multicenter randomized, active-controlled study (n = 506), PCTA with a 40-mcg fentaNYL ITS dose was compared with morphine intravenous PCA with 1-mg PCA dose (Minkowitz et al., 2007). In that study, analgesic benefit, pain intensity, patient satisfaction, and adverse events were comparable with the two delivery systems.

The one difference reported by both nurses and patients was that the fentaNYL ITS was easier to use. The author of a review of fentaNYL ITS used among acute postoperative patients concluded fentaNYL ITS is equivalent in analgesia to morphine IV PCA with the benefit that it enabled patients to be more mobile during use (Scott, 2016). In three trials, nurses reported superior ease of care using fentaNYL ITS compared with IV PCA (Pestano et al., 2017). PCTA has potential to be effective for use by people living with chronic pain (Indermun et al., 2014). However, that use is not currently FDA approved and needs further research.

After most surgical procedures, the fentaNYL ITS is described as a safe alternative to intravenous PCA regardless of the sex of the patient or type of anesthesia (Mattia, Coluzzi, Sonnino, & Anker-Møller, 2010). The fentaNYL ITS is described as having less risk for errors because of equipment or operation malfunction and no risk for intravenous line infection (Argoff, 2014). One of the safety concerns is the preset 40-mcg dose and 10-minute lockout (Scott, 2016). Although it is true that when these components are predetermined the chance for error in programming is reduced, a major disadvantage of that system is that because the dose is predetermined the ability of the prescriber to individualize the dose and lockout interval for each patient is not possible. It also prohibits safe use in patients for whom 40 mcg of fentaNYL is too large a PCA dose. For this reason, patients must be monitored closely to help ensure safety and adequacy of analgesia.

Oral or Enteral Route

A vast number of individuals in society self-administer their own medications at home, sometimes multiple times daily. This could be defined as oral PCA and described as the most common method by which medications are administered. However, this section describes the use of oral or enteral PCA as an analgesic therapy for patients with pain that can be managed by self-administration of analgesics generally in a hospital setting. The oral or enteral device is a newer version of PCA. In the United States, oral PCA currently is available as a portable delivery unit that is attached to a radiofrequency identification (RFID) bracelet or wristband that uniquely identifies the patient who wears it (Palmer & Miller, 2010; Palmer, Royal, & Miller, 2014). The RFID bracelet is preprogrammed to allow the medication to be accessed only at certain time intervals (Fernandes et al., 2017). An additional feature with this device is that the patient records the perceived pain intensity score in the device when accessing the medication (Fernandes et al., 2017). After the patient records pain intensity and swipes the bracelet, it is possible for the patient to rotate the tray to access a dose of medication (Palmer et al., 2014).

The investigators of an industry-sponsored and industry-led pilot study evaluating the use of the oral

PCA device among oncology patients (N = 20) reported that 95% of patients described better pain control and they preferred the oral PCA to nurse-administered prn medication (Rosati et al., 2007). In addition, in that pilot study, 80% of nurses reported satisfaction with the device and 90% reported good patient pain control among the patients using it. Recently, a European version of the oral PCA was developed and tested (n = 27) under industry sponsorship, with 90% of those using the oral PCA reporting satisfaction and significantly lower pain intensity ($P < .05$) compared to those in the control group who received nurse-administered prn oral analgesia. Interestingly, in that study the patients using oral PCA used 67% more doses of medication than those in the control group (Wirz, Conrad, Shtrichman, Schimo, & Hoffmann, 2017). No adverse events were reported in either industry-supported study, and both sets of investigators reported oral PCA as safe and effective (Rosati et al., 2007; Wirz et al., 2017). An independent study (N = 60) used the oral PCA device with patients who had undergone total knee arthroplasty (Lambert & Cata, 2014). In that study, compared to patients who received nurse-administered prn oral analgesia (n = 30), the patients with the oral PCA (n = 30) reported improved pain control with greater activity, including participation in physical therapy. When nurses and patients were questioned regarding satisfaction with use in a 4-week trial, the patients reported more favorable experience with oral PCA than did the nurses (Riemondy, Gonzalez, Gosik, Ricords, & Schirm, 2016). In that study, more than half of the nurses did not think the device was easy to set up or that it was easy to find data within the device and did not think it functioned reliably. More than half of the nurses also did not think it saved nursing time and did not want to use the oral PCA with other patients.

Intranasal Route

Although opioids, particularly fentaNYL and morphine, can be effectively delivered by the intranasal route, this is not a common delivery route in the United States. The first use of opioids delivered by a patient-controlled intranasal analgesia (PCINA) administration system was in Germany in a pilot study reported in 1996 (Striebel, Olmann, Spies, & Brummer, 1996). When using the intranasal route, opioids are administered by syringe, spray, dropper, or nebulized inhaler with a pump-type apparatus modified for PCINA administration (Paz & Quinlan, 2014). When fentaNYL delivered by PCINA was compared to intravenous PCA the effectiveness and patient satisfaction among both groups were comparable (Toussaint, Maidl, Schwagmeier, & Striebel, 2000). Satisfactory analgesia with fentaNYL PCINA was reported with women during childbirth (N = 32) (Kerr, Taylor, & Evans, 2015); however, respiratory depression was a particular concern for the neonates born to the women who received fentaNYL by PCINA during childbirth. The nonsteroidal antiinflammatory medication ketorolac was studied in a PCINA formulation among postoperative patients (Argoff, 2014). The patients who received ketorolac 30 mg by PCINA reported less pain and used less opioid.

Disadvantages of PCINA are the upper respiratory tract side effects (e.g., irritation, congestion, rhinitis, epistaxis, infection) (Argoff, 2014; Fernandes et al., 2017). The technical limitation of using PCINA is that to date equipment designed specifically for administration of intranasal therapy has not been developed, and IV PCA administration devices have been modified for PCINA use (Toussaint et al., 2000). This route seems to be effective, is noninvasive, and warrants further research. Such research needs to include development of equipment designed specifically for administration of intranasal opioids with programmed doses and lock out intervals to ensure safe patient-controlled administration (Fernandes et al., 2017).

Sublingual Route

Although sublingual PCA is currently available in Europe through a SUFentanil sublingual tablet system (SSTS), it has not been approved by the FDA for use in the United States (AcelRx Pharmaceuticals, 2017). In comparison with morphine intravenous PCA the sublingual system had quicker onset of action with greater patient satisfaction and was considered easier to use by clinicians and patients (Frampton, 2016). The authors of a systematic review comparing SSTS with morphine intravenous PCA and the fentaNYL PCTS, reported the onset of analgesic effect was quicker, pain intensity was less but not significant, and side effects were fewer among those who received fentaNYL PCTS (Katz et al., 2017). Additional research is needed to explore cost effectiveness and comparison of clinical effectiveness with other needle-free PCA systems (Frampton, 2016).

Inhalation Route

Patient-controlled inhalation analgesia (PCIA) is rarely used. Inhalation as a delivery route of medications is not new and has been reported in the literature at least since 1847, when Simpson used it to ease the pain of labor during childbirth (Rosen, 2003). Since then morphine and fentaNYL have been evaluated for inhalation during childbirth (Cipolla, 2016). PCIA was used with sevoflurane at subanesthetic concentration to provide adequate analgesia (Yeo, Holdcroft, Yentis, Stewart, & Bassett, 2006). When inhaled morphine was compared with intravenous morphine in patients who had undergone bunionectomies (N = 89), the effectiveness was comparable for the two therapies (Thipphawong et al., 2003). However, to date the inhalation route has not been well researched and has not garnered much interest.

Patient Assessment and Monitoring to Optimize Safety

Successful PCA therapy depends on the systematic assessment by clinicians of the patient's pain, adverse effects, and use of the technology. With time, this needs to be followed by adjustments in the prescription if necessary to optimize pain control and ensure patient safety (Marks & Rodgers, 2014; Pasero & McCaffery, 2011). In one study with older adults, the authors reported pain was not optimally controlled because patients were not aware of how often they could activate the device (Brown et al., 2015). This study underscores the importance of proper patient education and thorough education before initiation of therapy. It also supports the need to assess patients during therapy, including assessment to determine if the patient continues to understand the PCA concepts and is willing and able to use the equipment.

PCA is not a substitute for the critical role of the nurse as the primary pain manager of the patient (Pasero & McCaffery, 2011). Patients using PCA need to be assessed at least every 2 to 4 hours, during nighttime hours, and more frequently throughout the first 24 hours (ISMP, 2009). Pulse oximetry and capnography are useful tools for assessing respiratory status (Cohen et al., 2006), yet they are not intended to replace the respiratory assessment by the clinician. The American Patient Safety Foundation (APSF) recommends limiting supplemental oxygen during PCA administration, particularly if the only technology used to monitor for hypoventilation is pulse oximetry (Weinger, 2009). Pulse oximetry can yield false high oxygen saturation levels in patients receiving supplemental oxygen. In addition, clinicians need to be aware pulse oximetry readings may remain within a normal range for several minutes after cessation of breathing (ISMP, 2013) and is usually the last sign of systemic distress.

Respiratory Assessment

An accurate respiratory assessment is done by observing respirations before disturbing or stimulating the patient (Cohen et al., 2006). Assessing respiratory function in this way prevents assessing an artificially deep breath or increased respiratory rate as a result of stimulation. Respiratory assessment includes evaluating the rate, quality, depth, pattern, and sound of respirations (Table 17.3). It is important to also note the presence of snoring. Any abnormality in the respiratory assessment warrants arousing a sleeping patient for further evaluation. In addition, respiratory function and oxygen saturation may be monitored using pulse oximetry equipment or end-tidal carbon dioxide equipment. It is important to know that oxygen desaturation recorded on pulse oximetry may be a late indicator of respiratory compromise and that end-tidal carbon dioxide monitoring detects this sooner (Elliott, 2009; ISMP, 2013). Thus, despite the perceived benefits of pulse oximetry, there are limitations. (Also see Chapters 12 and 13 for discussion of opioid-induced respiratory depression.)

Sedation Assessment

Currently, the level of sedation can be accurately determined only by clinical assessment. The ISMP recommended each institution adapt or develop a standard assessment scale to monitor and document the level of sedation (Cohen et al., 2006). One such tool is the Pasero Opioid Sedation Scale (POSS) (Pasero & McCaffery, 2011) (Box 17.6). An excellent way to ensure sedation is assessed on a regular basis is to incorporate the selected sedation tool into the EMR in a location that is adjacent to pain assessment. As with assessing respiratory status, to assess sedation as accurately as possible it is advised to use a minimal amount of stimulation (verbal or tactile) when assessing sedation (ISMP, 2009). (Also see Chapters 12 and 13.)

Table 17.3	Respiratory Assessment
Rate of respirations	The number of complete breaths in 60 seconds. A rate of ≤ 10 per minute warrants notifying clinician and indicates possible discontinuation of PCA.
Depth of respirations	Assess if the breaths are normal, shallow, or deep. Assess if there is increased (deep) movement with use of accessory muscles needed for breathing.
Pattern of respirations	Assess if the breaths are regular or irregular.
Quality of respirations	Assess if breathing is comfortable, effortless, or labored (necessary for patient to work to move air on inhalation and exhalation).
Sound of respirations	Assess the sound of breathing: clear, blocked (stuffed sound) noisy, snoring (partially blocked sounds), gurgling (fluids in airway), or stridor (harsh, noisy sounds). Remember snoring indicates breathing difficulty, not sound sleeping.

From Institute for Safe Medication Practices (ISMP). (2013). Fatal PCA adverse events continue to happen. . . . Better patient monitoring is essential to prevent harm. *Acute Care—ISMP Medication Safety Alert.* Horsham, PA: Institute for Safe Medication Practices; San Diego Patient Safety Council (2014). *Tool kit patient controlled analgesia (PCA) guidelines of care for the opioid naïve patient.* San Diego, CA: The Council.

Box 17.6 | Pasero Opioid Sedation Scale

S = Sleep, easy to arouse
   Acceptable; no action necessary; may increase opioid dose if needed

1 = Awake and alert
   Acceptable; no action necessary; may increase opioid dose if needed

2 = Slightly drowsy, easily aroused
   Acceptable; no action necessary; may increase opioid dose if needed

3 = Frequently drowsy, arousable, drifts off to sleep during conversation
   Unacceptable; monitor respiratory status and sedation level closely until sedation level is stable at less than 3 and respiratory status is satisfactory; decrease opioid dose 25% to 50% or notify primary or anesthesia provider for orders; consider administering a nonsedating, opioid-sparing nonopioid, such as acetaminophen or a nonsteroidal antiinflammatory drug, if not contraindicated; ask patient to take deep breaths every 15 to 30 minutes.

4 = Somnolent, minimal or no response to verbal and physical stimulation
   Unacceptable; stop opioid; consider administering naloxone; call rapid response team (code blue), if indicated by patient status; stay with patient, stimulate, and support respiration as indicated by patient status; or anesthesia provider; monitor respiratory status and sedation level closely until sedation level is stable at less than 3 and respiratory status is satisfactory.

From Pasero, C., & McCaffery, M. (2011). *Pain assessment and pharmacologic management* (p. 510). St. Louis, MO: Mosby. Data from American Pain Society. (2003). *Principles of analgesic use in the treatment of acute pain and chronic cancer pain* (5th ed.). Glenview, IL, The Society; Pasero, C. (2009). Assessment of sedation during opioid administration for pain management. *Journal of PeriAnesthesia Nursing*, 24(3), 186–190; Pasero, C., & McCaffery, M. (2002). Monitoring sedation. *American Journal of Nursing*, 102(2), 67–69. Reliability and validity information for the Pasero Opioid Sedation Scale (POSS) can be found in Dempsey, S. J., Davidson, J., Cahill, D., et al. (2008). Selection of a sedation assessment scale for clinical practice: Inter-rater reliability, ease of use, and applicability testing of the Richmond-Agitation-Sedation and Pasero Opioid-Induced Sedation Scale. Poster presentation, National Association of Orthopedic Nurses Congress, Tampa, FL, May 6–10; Nisbet, A. T., & Mooney-Cotter, F. (2009). Selected scales for reporting opioid-induced sedation. *Pain Management Nursing*, 10(3), 154–164. ©1994, Pasero C. May be duplicated for use in clinical practice.

Monitoring With Equipment

It is generally not feasible or possible for clinicians to continually assess and monitor each patient. In an effort to improve safety with enhanced monitoring, equipment is often used to augment clinician assessment. (Also see Chapter 13.)

Pulse Oximetry

Pulse oximetry can be used either intermittently or continuously. It is abundantly available, simple to use, nonintrusive, and comparatively inexpensive (Ritter, 2011). With a sophisticated system using pulse oximetry as part of a patient surveillance system, when there is an abnormal reading, the nurse is alerted through a pager system (Taenzer, Pyke, McGrath, & Blike, 2010). In one study using that system, there was a significant ($P = .01$) reduction in rescue events when pulse oximetry with patient surveillance system was used.

Despite the perceived benefits of pulse oximetry, there are limitations. It is important for clinicians to be aware that reductions in pulse oximetry readings can be a late finding (Pasero & McCaffery, 2011). Patients have experienced fatal hypercarbia while still recording oxygen saturation within normal levels; this is particularly true when patients are receiving supplemental oxygen (Maddox & Williams, 2012). Another concern is that pulse oximetry can provide a false sense of security.

Capnography

Capnography measures the amount of carbon dioxide through one of two systems (Lam et al., 2017). *End-tidal carbon dioxide (ETCO2) capnography* measures the partial pressure of carbon dioxide gases that are exhaled. *Transcutaneous capnography* measures the partial pressure of carbon dioxide through an electrochemical sensor that is heated and applied topically to skin. Recent technologic advancement has resulted in PCA devices that include capnography monitoring equipment (ECRI, 2017).

The APSF, The Joint Commission, the American Society of Anesthesiologists, and the American Society of Regional Anesthesia and Pain Medicine have all endorsed the use of capnography (ECRI, 2017). The APSF specifically recommends whenever supplemental oxygen is being administered, to use capnography to monitor the postoperative patient (Geralemou, Probst, & Gan, 2016). In one health system, capnography was found to alert clinicians of respiratory depression as long as 2 hours earlier than more traditional measures (e.g., nursing assessment and pulse oximetry) (Maddox & Williams, 2012). The authors of a recent systematic review and meta-analysis (N = 9 studies) concluded capnography identifies postoperative respiratory depression earlier than oxygen desaturation. This is particularly true in the presence of supplemental oxygen (Lam et al., 2017).

Although capnography is beneficial with the early identification of respiratory distress, there are some challenges associated with using it. It restricts the mobility of the patient, it can be dislodged, the alarms are sensitive and trigger false alerts, and patients may not be compliant with using the devices (Maddox & Williams, 2012). Even though transcutaneous capnography allows for enhanced mobility, the site may need to be changed frequently, it may cause skin irritation, and the equipment needs recalibration (Lam et al., 2017). Clearly there is a critical need for improvement in capnography technology. With either capnography system, clinicians need to be educated and be able to demonstrate competency with using the equipment. Research is still needed to determine if capnography affects the need for rescue team responses, transfers to an ICU, and patient mortality (Lam et al., 2017) (see also Chapter 13).

Evaluating Equipment to Optimize Patient Safety

Although manufacturers of PCA devices have worked to improve their safety over the years, it is still important with each use to evaluate the equipment to ensure proper functioning to prevent inadequate or excessive delivery of medication. See Box 17.1 for common mechanical hazards.

It is advisable for organizations to establish policy and guidelines during which all PCA devices being used are independently double-checked by the primary nurse and another professional at specified times (e.g., initiation of PCA, on adjustment of the prescription, with refill of medication, with nursing handoffs) (Pasero & McCaffery, 2011). This independent double-check involves two clinicians autonomously, without prompting or interference, verifying the medication and device settings with what is in the prescription to ascertain accuracy (Paul et al., 2010). The review of device settings and of prescriber orders needs to be done without distraction and with adequate lighting to ensure accuracy. During verification, the eight rights of PCA administration are evaluated: right patient, right medication, right dose, right time, right route, right concentration, right lockout interval, and right documentation.

Verifying the PCA device is operating appropriately and accurately is also important. There have been reported instances when the device was not plugged into the wall and when batteries were not functioning (SDPSC, 2014). A case report from Korea described a situation in which the button used to activate a PCA device malfunctioned and was continuously activating resulting in the administration of 221 mcg of fentaNYL within 30 minutes of initiation of the PCA (Yi, Kang, & Hwang, 2013). Although a unique occurrence, this underscores the importance of assessing both patients and equipment with an awareness that unexpected malfunctions can occur with equipment.

Because programming the incorrect concentration is a significant source of error when PCA is used, it is advisable for only one standard concentration for each medication be available for use for PCA (ISMP, 2008; Paul et al., 2010). It is best to minimize the use of nonstandard concentrations and limit their use to specialized areas such as a palliative care unit (ISMP, 2008).

Whenever possible it is advisable to use PCA equipment with *dose error reduction system* (DERS) technology (ECRI, 2017). The DERS, or smart pumps, which are so called because they store predetermined limits for PCA prescribing components such as dose and concentration, compare what is being programmed with the stored limits and alert the clinician if the limits are exceeded (Ritter, 2011). As beneficial as this technology is, it is important to know that although using smart pumps is associated with a reduction in errors, they do not eliminate errors in programming (Ohashi, Dalleur, Dykes, & Bates, 2014).

Infusion Tubing

It is important to assess for defects or obstructions that may occur in the tubing connecting the PCA device to the patient (Elliott, 2009). Such obstructions can result in inadequate medication and then excessive medication when the line is cleared if the patient has been activating the device while the tubing was obstructed. In that case it is advisable to disconnect the tubing before clearing the obstruction and flush or clear the tubing to avoid the infusion of excessive medication.

Solution tubing has been incorrectly connected or reconnected (SDPSC, 2014). Among other misconnections, there have been instances of epidural tubing being inadvertently connected to an intravenous connection with intravenous tubing being connected to the epidural connection, which results in the wrong medication being delivered by the wrong route (The Joint Commission [TJC], 2014). These misconnections have caused serious injuries and even death (Block, Horn, & Schlesinger, 2012). It is prudent to assess all solution tubing by tracing lines from the patient back to the point of origin before connecting or reconnecting the infusion or device, whenever transitioning the setting or transitioning to a different device and whenever transferring care of the patient (TJC, 2014) (Box 17.7).

Using color to identify tubing for one purpose rather than another is often considered to be a safety technique. However, clinicians are cautioned that color coding of tubing can be a source of false security and an actual source of error. This is likely when the meaning of a color is not standardized, when color use is not consistent, when multiple colors are used, and when not all clinicians are aware of which colors are considered standard for which purpose. Color coding is best used to differentiate one item rather than using it to identify many different items (Grissinger, 2013). An example of this is to use a yellow stripe to identify tubing used for epidural infusions, but not use different colored stripes for other tubing. Using a number of different colored stripes for different types of tubing can actually increase the risk for error.

Box 17.7 | Steps to Improve Patient-Controlled Analgesia Infusion Tubing Safety

1. Trace all solution tubing lines from the patient to their point of origin with all patient changes of medication and transfer of care.
2. Standardize the process for "line reconciliation."
3. Employ a high reliability practice such as STAR: Stop, Think, Act, Review.
4. Standardize directions for tubing and catheters.
5. When there is more than one type of tubing and/or medication, label all lines both close to the patient and near the source of solution.
6. Solution tubing used to administer medication by the epidural, regional, intrathecal, or arterial routes should not have any ports for access.
7. Implement processes of independent double-check of solution tubing for all high-risk medications, routes, and delivery systems.
8. Use different delivery devices with different types of tubing for medications being delivered by the intravenous and epidural or intrathecal routes.
9. Use different delivery devices with different types of tubing for medications being delivered by the intravenous, epidural, and intrathecal routes.
10. Immediately after connecting the tubing, assess patient vital signs.
11. Educate all clinicians of potential solution tubing hazards.

From The Joint Commission. (2014). Managing risk during transition to new ISO tubing connector standards. Sentinel Event Alert,#53, 1-6, pp. 3, 4.

Authorized Agent–Controlled Analgesia

Although PCA delivery systems are designed for use by the patient to self-administer medication as needed, the devices have advantages for use by others who are authorized to administer medications to the patient. The devices also enable the administration of preprogrammed doses of medication and the delivery of a continuous infusion within a secure (locked) system. It is important to remember that when the devices are authorized or prescribed to be used by others to help the person manage pain, the method of delivery is no longer PCA. Rather a PCA delivery system is being used by an authorized agent. The two situations in which this occurs is with *family-controlled analgesia* or *caregiver-controlled analgesia* and *nurse-controlled analgesia*. It is important to clarify that authorized agent–controlled anesthesia (AACA) is totally different from *PCA by proxy*, which occurs when someone other than the patient is administering boluses of medication when they are *not* authorized to do so (Cox & Cooney, 2018; Pasero, 2015). The American Society for Pain Management Nursing (ASPMN), which supports AACA, provides guidelines in a position paper for implementing AACA therapy (Cooney et al., 2013).

There are two main types of AACA. These are family-controlled analgesia (FCA) or caregiver-controlled analgesia (CCA) and nurse-controlled analgesia (NCA), or nurse-activated dosing (NAD) (Pasero & McCaffery, 2011) (Table 17.4). Either type of AACA should be used only for the patient who is not able to self-administer analgesia and when the authorized agent has been properly educated (Eksterowicz & DiMaggio, 2018). This may occur because the patient is unable to comprehend the concepts involved with PCA (e.g., a young child or an adult with cognitive impairment), because the patient is physically unable to activate the device (e.g., paralysis or finger immobility), or when the patient is at the end of life.

Family-Controlled or Caregiver-Controlled Analgesia

FCA or CCA may be appropriate when the patient needs small doses of analgesia to be administered as needed but is unable to self-administer the medication (Pasero & McCaffery, 2011). It is optimal for the organization overseeing care of the patient to have a policy and education to guide FCA or CCA. With FCA or CCA only *one* person in the family or caregiving circle is identified as the primary pain manager for the patient and assumes responsibility for activating the device. It is advisable for a second person to be identified as the secondary pain manager to enable respite for the primary pain manager. A critical safety component is that only one person manages the pain during any given period (Pasero & McCaffery, 2011).

Both the care nurse and the authorized agent have responsibilities to ensure as much safety as possible with AACA therapy. The ASPMN position paper identifies four responsibilities of the adult caregiver who agrees to be the authorized agent (Cooney et al., 2013). First the person agrees to actively participate in education regarding safe application of AACA, understands the education,

Table 17.4 | Nurses Responsibilities With Authorized Agent–Controlled Analgesia

Education	Inform the patient, if possible, family, and others involved with patient what AACA is and how it is different from PCA by proxy which is dangerous.
	Instruct the authorized agent: • How to recognize behaviors that indicate pain. • How to recognize behaviors that indicate sedation, respiratory depression, or a medical emergency. • How to activate the analgesic delivery device. • To activate analgesic dosing device when the patient is awake and expressing pain either verbally or by behavior, when pain is anticipated (e.g., before turning or wound care), or based on patient specific criteria. • To not activate the device at other times (e.g., during sleep, to promote sleep or reduce anxiety, or for abnormal breathing). • What to do when pain is not being relieved, side effects are excessive, or other patient-specific needs. • How to stimulate the patient in an emergency situation and notify the nurse or emergency responders.
Assess the authorized agent	The ability of the person chosen to be the AACA to carry out the responsibilities and understand the education provided.
Assess the patient	Assess the patient for continuing effective pain control; opioid-related sedation and respiratory distress.
Communicate	Verbally and in writing or electronically convey to all other clinicians that patient is receiving AACA and who is the authorized agent. Report to the nurse to whom care is transferred: • Patient responses to AACA. • The adequacy of safe and effective care provided by the authorized agent.
Document	What has been taught to the patient, authorized agent, and family members. Appropriately record and document the quantity of opioid administered by the authorized agent.

Data from Cooney, M. F., Czarnecki, M., Dunwoody, C., Eksterowicz, N., Merkel, S., Oakes, L., & Wuhrman, E. (2013). American Society for Pain Management Nursing position statement with clinical practice guidelines: Authorized agent-controlled analgesia. *Pain Management Nursing, 14*(3), 176–181.

and will adhere to the education provided. Second, the person agrees to alert staff of any concerns about the AACA process and if the person is not able to continue as an authorized agent. Third, the authorized agent agrees to inform and reinforce to other family members that the other members cannot activate the PCA system and safety depends on only one person (the authorized agent) doing so at a time. Fourth, there must be agreement to not try to reprogram the infusion device or in any way violate the integrity of the system. Box 17.8 presents the nursing responsibilities with AACA.

FCA is known to be safe and effective when used by parents or surrogates to help manage pain among children with cancer even with very painful situations such as bone marrow and stem cell transplantation (Vasquenza et al., 2015). The effectiveness and safety of FCA with children and young adults with cancer in the home setting was tested (N = 45), reporting a complication rate of 4 in 1100 PCA days with good analgesia (Anghelescu et al., 2015). It is important to note that the willingness of family members to participate in FCA varies. Although many family members appreciate being involved in helping to control pain of a loved one, some family members prefer for the nurse to administer the medications (Czarnecki, Hainsworth, Jacobson, Simpson, & Weisman, 2015).

Increasingly, FCA is being used with adults in palliative care settings. In addition to facilitating adequate analgesia for the person in pain, when AACA is used, the caregiver(s) are more directly able to participate in care and provide comfort for the person with pain. When follow-up was done with family caregivers who had used AACA with a loved one who was dying (N = 118), all of them reported satisfaction with pain control (Webb & Shelton, 2015).

Nurse-Controlled Analgesia

NCA or NAD occurs when the primary nurse caring for the patient assumes the responsibility of activating the PCA delivery system for the patient (Pasero & McCaffery, 2011). It is advisable for the institution to have a policy in place with criteria for identifying which patients are appropriate for NCA, monitoring guidelines, and education of nursing staff (Pasero, 2015). The authors of a large prospective study in the United Kingdom, which assessed NCA used with children with pain (N = 10,079), reported good or very good analgesia in the clear majority (98%), with low incidence of any side effects and only 0.4% of serious side effects (Howard et al., 2010). When used in a critical care unit, the patients who received analgesia by AACA experienced less pain (Messing et al., 2015).

BOX 17.8	Authorized Agent-Controlled Analgesia: Unconventional Use of the Patient-Controlled Analgesia Pump[a,b,c]

PATIENT SELECTION (ANY ONE OF THE FOLLOWING)

- Patient is unable to understand the relationships among pain, pushing the PCA button, and pain relief.
- Patient is not cognitively or physically able to self-administer a PCA dose using the available equipment.
- Patient is not motivated to manage his or her own pain.

NURSE-ACTIVATED DOSING (NAD)

- The patient's primary nurse is designated to be the patient's primary pain manager (the primary nurse is the only person who presses the PCA button during that nurse's shift).
- The nurse is competent in the use of the equipment used to deliver NAD.
- This method may be used:
  - In addition to a basal rate. Patients are assessed every 30 to 60 minutes for the need for a bolus dose for breakthrough pain.
  - Without a basal rate as a means of maintaining analgesia with ATC bolus doses.
  - To administer prn bolus doses before painful procedures.

FAMILY-CONTROLLED ANALGESIA (FCA) OR CAREGIVER-CONTROLLED ANALGESIA (CCA)

- *One* family member or significant other is designated to be the patient's primary pain manager and has the responsibility of pressing the PCA button.
- Guidelines for selecting a primary pain manager for FCA:
  - Spends a significant amount of time with the patient.
  - Is willing to assume responsibility of being primary pain manager.
  - Is willing to accept and respect patient's reports of pain (if able to provide) as the best indicator of how much pain the patient is experiencing.
  - Demonstrates understanding of the educational content below.

EDUCATION OF THE PAIN MANAGER (FCA, CCA)

- Select and teach the pain manager the appropriate method for assessment of the patient's pain (see Chapters 6 and 7 for appropriate tools).
  - If the patient is able to report, teach the pain manager to use a numerical scale of 0 to 10, the Wong-Baker Faces Pain Rating Scale, or another self-report tool appropriate to the patient's ability.
  - If the patient is unable to report, a behavioral assessment tool may be used.
- Discuss the purpose and goals of the patient's pain management plan.
- Explain the concept of maintaining a steady analgesic blood level.

- Teach the pain manager to look for adverse effects, such as nausea, sedation, and respiratory depression, before administering a bolus dose. Explain when it is safe and unsafe to administer a PCA bolus dose and to promptly notify the staff if any adverse effects are detected.
- Explain that sedation precedes opioid-induced respiratory depression and that the patient's sedation level should be assessed using a sedation scale that includes appropriate interventions at each level of sedation such as the one shown below.[c] Provide the pain manager with a copy of the sedation scale with interventions as a reference during therapy.

PASERO OPIOID-INDUCED SEDATION SCALE (POSS) (MODIFIED FOR AACA)

S = Sleep, easy to arouse
  Action: Awaken patient to determine arousability (1 to 4 below) before administering a PCA bolus dose
1 = Awake and alert
  Action: Acceptable; may administer PCA bolus dose
2 = Slightly drowsy, easily aroused
  Action: Acceptable; may administer a PCA bolus dose
3 = Frequently drowsy, arousable, drifts off during conversation
  Action: Unacceptable; notify nurse immediately.
4 = Somnolent, minimal or no response to physical stimulation
  Action: Unacceptable; notify nurse immediately.

TREATMENT OF EXCESSIVELY SEDATED PATIENT[c,d]

- Treat life-threatening significant respiratory depression if present.
- Decrease opioid dose; stop basal infusion if in use.
- Increase monitoring until sedation level is 2 or lower; consider capnography.
- Evaluate pain manager's (FCA, CCA) ability to manage pain safely and effectively.
- Promptly switch to an alternative pain management approach if increased sedation is thought to be related to the family member's or caregiver's inability to manage pain safely.

---

[a]Before the use of AACA, institutional policies and procedures should be approved and staff (and patients and families when indicated) trained to assess and manage the therapies. Note that AACA is not PCA; policies and procedures, orders, and teaching materials should be entitled with the correct name of the therapy (e.g., family-controlled analgesia; caregiver-controlled analgesia, nurse-activated dosing).
[b]In all cases of AACA, the control of analgesia is returned to patients (i.e., PCA) if and as soon as they are able to assume it.
[c]This guideline should be adjusted as appropriate for patient condition. For example, the suggested level of monitoring and actions for treatment of sedation may need to be adjusted for terminally ill patients.
[d]See Chapter 13 for discussion of opioid-induced sedation and respiratory depression.

Continued

ATC, Around the clock.
From Pasero, C., & McCaffery, M. *Pain assessment and pharmacologic management* (pp. 318–319). St. Louis, MO: Mosby. Data from Nisbet, A. T., & Mooney-Cotter, F. (2009). Selected scales for reporting opioid-induced sedation. *Pain Management Nursing, 10*(3), 154–164; Pasero, C., & McCaffery, M. (1993). Unconventional PCA: Making it work for your patient. *American Journal of Nursing, 93*(9), 38–41; Pasero, C., & McCaffery, M. (2005). Authorized and unauthorized use of PCA pumps.

Am J Nurs, 105(7), 30–33; Pasero, C., Portenoy, R. K., & McCaffery, M. (1999). Opioid analgesics. In M. McCaffery, & C. Pasero. *Pain: Clinical manual* (2nd ed.). St. Louis, MO: Mosby; and Wuhrman, E., Cooney, M. F., Dunwoody, C. J., et al. (2007). Authorized and unauthorized ("PCA by proxy") dosing of analgesic infusion pumps: Position statement with clinical practice recommendations. *Pain Management Nursing, 8*(1), 4–11. © 2011, Pasero, C., & McCaffery, M. May be duplicated for use in clinical practice.

Key Points

- PCA does not negate clinician responsibilities to monitor for analgesia and safety while helping the patient control pain.
- Only the patient can activate the PCA device (press the button)!
- PCA should be initiated when the patient has reasonably good pain relief with the intention of achieving and maintaining good pain control.
- Smart pump technology supports clinicians in keeping patients safe, but it is not fool proof.
- Supplemental oxygen does not provide a safety net for preventing respiratory depression.
- Patients receiving supplemental oxygen may be at greater risk for respiratory depression.
- Pulse oximetry can yield false high oxygen saturation in patients who are receiving supplemental oxygen.
- There are eight rights for PCA administration (the right patient, medication, dose, time, route, concentration, lockout interval, and documentation).
- When AACA is being used, only one family member or caregiver can be an authorized agent at any given time.

Case Scenario

Mindy is scheduled for spinal fusion surgery in 2 weeks. She arrives for her preadmission testing and education and tells you that she is worried about having a lot of pain and is very confused about all the different types of pain control she was told about in the surgeon's office. She said they talked about some types of analgesia that she would control herself. She thinks it sounds interesting, and she likes the idea of not having to wait for pain medicine, but she is confused and wants to know if it is safe.

1. What do you tell Mindy about PCA?
2. How do you explain to her the different components of PCA?
3. What routes of PCA might be appropriate for Mindy?
4. What do you tell her about PCA safety?
5. What is important for her surgeon to know about transitioning Mindy to oral medication after using her PCA?

References

AcelRx Pharmaceuticals. (2017). *AcelRx pharmaceuticals receives complete response letter from the FDA for DSUVIATM NDA.* PRN Newswire. October 12 https://www.prnewswire.com/news-releases/acelrx-pharmaceuticals-receives-complete-response-letter-from-the-fda-for-dsuvia-nda-300535506.html. (Accessed 2 March 2018).

Anghelescu, D. L., Zhang, K., Faughnan, L. G., & Pei, D. (2015). The safety and effectiveness of patient-controlled analgesia in outpatient children and young adults with cancer: a retrospective study. *Journal of Pediatric Hematology/Oncology, 37*(5), 378–382.

Argoff, C. E. (2014). Recent management advances in acute postoperative pain. *Pain Practice, 14*(5), 477–487.

Bagri, A. S., Rico, A., & Ruiz, J. G. (2008). Evaluation and management of the elderly patient at risk for postoperative delirium. *Clinics in Geriatric Medicine, 24*(4), 667–686.

Bijur, P. E., Mills, A. M., Chang, A. K., White, D., Restivo, A., Persaud, S., ... Birnbaum, A. J. (2017). Comparative effectiveness of patient-controlled analgesia for treating acute pain in the emergency department. *Annals of Emergency Medicine, 70*(6), 809–818.

Block, M., Horn, R. J., & Schlesinger, M. D. (2012). Reducing risk of epidural-intravenous misconnections. *APSF Newsletter, 26,* 63–65.

Brogan, S. E., Winter, N. B., & Okifuji, A. (2015). Prospective observational study of patient-controlled intrathecal analgesia: Impact on cancer-associated symptoms, breakthrough pain control, and patient satisfaction. *Regional Anesthesia and Pain Medicine, 40*(4), 369–375.

Brown, A., Boshers, B., Chapman, L. F., Huckaba, K., Pangle, M., Pogue, L. C., ... MacArthur, S. (2015). Do elderly patients use patient-controlled analgesia medication delivery systems correctly? *Orthopaedic Nursing, 34*(4), 203–208.

Budiansky, A. S., Margarson, M. P., & Eipe, N. (2017). Acute pain management in morbid obesity–an evidence based clinical update. *Surgery for Obesity and Related Diseases*, 13(3), 523–532.

Chou, R., Gordon, D. B., de Leon-Casasola, O. A., Rosenberg, J. M., Bickler, S., Brennan, T., & Wu, C. L. (2016). Management of Postoperative Pain: A Clinical Practice Guideline From the American Pain Society, the American Society of Regional Anesthesia and Pain Medicine, and the American Society of Anesthesiologists' Committee on Regional Anesthesia, Executive Committee, and Administrative Council. *Journal of Pain*, 17(2), 131–157. https://doi.org/10.1016/j.jpain.2015.12.008.

Cipolla, D. (2016). Will pulmonary drug delivery for systemic application ever fulfill its rich promise? *Expert Opinion on Drug Delivery*, 13(10), 1337–1340.

Cohen, M., Weber, R. J., & Moss, J. (2006). *Patient-controlled analgesia: Making it safer for patients* (pp. 1–12). Philadelphia, PA: Institute for Safe Medication Practices.

Cooney, M. F., Czarnecki, M., Dunwoody, C., Eksterowicz, N., Merkel, S., Oakes, L., & Wuhrman, E. (2013). American Society for Pain Management Nursing position statement with clinical practice guidelines: authorized agent controlled analgesia. *Pain Management Nursing*, 14(3), 176–181.

Cox, D., & Cooney, M. F. (2018). Key terms and definitions for pain management nursing. In H. Turner, & M. Czarnecki (Eds.), *Core Curriculum for Pain Management Nursing* (3rd ed., pp. 83–93). Elsevier.

Coyle, N., & Glajchen, M. (2014). Pain management in the home: Using cancer patients as a model. In H. Benzon, J. P. Rathmell, C. L. Wu, D. Turk, C. E. Argoff, & R. W. Hurley (Eds.), *Practical Pain Management* (5th ed., pp. 1040–1048.e2). St. Louis, MO: Elsevier.

Craft, J. (2010). Patient-controlled analgesia: Is it worth the painful prescribing process? *Baylor University Medical Center Proceedings*, 23(4), 434–438. https://doi.org/10.1080/08998280.2010.11928666.

Czarnecki, M. L., Hainsworth, K. R., Jacobson, A. A., Simpson, P. M., & Weisman, S. J. (2015). Opioid Administration for Postoperative Pain in Children with Developmental Delay: Parent and Nurse Satisfaction. *Journal of Pediatric Surgical Nursing*, 4(1), 15–27.

Dampier, C. (2014). The management of pain from Sickle Cell Disease. In H. Benzon, J. P. Rathmell, C. L. Wu, D. Turk, C. E. Argoff, & R. W. Hurley (Eds.), *Practical Pain Management* (5th ed., pp. 997–1002.e2). St. Louis, MO: Elsevier.

ECRI Institute. (2017). *ECRI Institute PSO Deep Dive Opioid Use in Acute Care*. Plymouth Meeting, PA: ECRI Institute.

Ekin, A., Donmez, F., Taspinar, V., & Dikmen, B. (2013). Patient-controlled sedation in orthopedic surgery under regional anesthesia: a new approach in procedural sedation. *Brazilian Journal of Anesthesiology (English Edition)*, 63(5), 410–414.

Eksterowicz, N., & DiMaggio, T. J. (2018). Acute pain management. In H. Turner, & M. Czarnecki (Eds.), *Core Curriculum for Pain Management Nursing* (3rd ed., pp. 238–278). Elsevier.

Elliott, J. A. (2009). Patient-controlled analgesia. In H. S. Smith (Ed.), *Current Therapy in Pain* (pp. 73–78). Philadelphia, PA: Saunders.

Elliott, J. A. (2016). Patient-controlled analgesia in the management of acute pain. In J. A. Elliott, & H. S. Smith (Eds.), *Handbook of Acute Pain Management* (pp. 110–125). Boca Raton, FL: CRC Press Taylor & Francis Group.

Evans, C., Schein, J., Nelson, W., Crespi, S., Gargiulo, K., Horowicz-Mehler, N., & Panchal, S. (2007). Improving patient and nurse outcomes: a comparison of nurse tasks and time associated with two patient-controlled analgesia modalities using delphi panels. *Pain Management Nursing*, 8(2), 86–95.

Evans, J. M., MacCarthy, J., Rosen, M., & Hogg, M. I. J. (1976). Apparatus for patient-controlled administration of intravenous narcotics during labour. *The Lancet*, 307(7949), 17–18.

Faerber, J., Zhong, W., Dai, D., Baehr, A., Maxwell, L. G., Kraemer, F. W., & Feudtner, C. (2017). Comparative Safety of Morphine Delivered via Intravenous Route vs. Patient-Controlled Analgesia Device for Pediatric Inpatients. *Journal of Pain and Symptom Management*, 53(5), 842–850.

Federal Drug Administration (FDA). Extended-release (ER) and long-acting (LA) opioid analgesics Risk Evaluation and Mitigation Strategy (REMS). Reference ID: 3784602. p. 1–11. www.fda.gov/downloads/drugs/drugsafety/postmarketdrugsafetyinformationforpatientsandproviders/ucm311290.pdf. Accessed July 10, 2020.

Fernandes, M. T. P., Hernandes, F. B., de Almeida, T. N., Sobottka, V. P., Poli-Frederico, R. C., & Fernandes, K. B. P. (2017). Patient-Controlled Analgesia (PCA) in Acute Pain: Pharmacological and Clinical Aspects. In *In Pain Relief-From Analgesics to Alternative Therapies* InTechOpen. https://www.intechopen.com/books/pain-relief-from-analgesics-to-alternative-therapies/patient-controlled-analgesia-pca-in-acute-pain-pharmacological-and-clinical-aspects. Accessed July 10, 2020.

Fine, P. G., & Bekanich, S. J. (2014). Pain management at the end of life. In H. Benzon, J. P. Rathmell, C. L. Wu, D. Turk, C. E. Argoff, & R. W. Hurley (Eds.), *Practical Pain Management* (5th ed., pp. 1023–1039.e4). St. Louis, MO: Elsevier.

Flory, J. H., Wiesenthal, A. C., Thaler, H. T., Koranteng, L., & Moryl, N. (2016). Methadone use and the risk of hypoglycemia for inpatients with cancer pain. *Journal of Pain and Symptom Management*, 51(1), 79–87.

Frampton, J. E. (2016). Sublingual sufentanil: a review in acute postoperative pain. *Drugs*, 76(6), 719–729.

Gagliese, L., Gauthier, L. R., Macpherson, A. K., Jovellanos, M., & Chan, V. W. (2008). Correlates of postoperative pain and intravenous patient-controlled analgesia use in younger and older surgical patients. *Pain Medicine*, 9(3), 299–314.

George, J. A., Lin, E. E., Hanna, M. N., Murphy, J. D., Kumar, K., Ko, P. S., & Wu, C. L. (2010). The effect of intravenous opioid patient-controlled analgesia with and without background infusion on respiratory depression: a meta-analysis. *Journal of Opioid Management*, 6(1), 47–54.

Geralemou, S., Probst, S., & Gan, T. J. (2016). The role of capnography to prevent postoperative respiratory adverse events. *Anesthesia Patient Safety Foundation Newsletter*, 10 (5), 1–2.

Grissinger, M. (2013). Preventing Mixups With Color-Tinted Intravenous Tubing. *Pharmacy and Therapeutics*, 38(4), 187–189.

Gupta, K., Mitra, S., Kazal, S., Saroa, R., Ahuja, V., & Goel, P. (2016). IV paracetamol as an adjunct to patient-controlled epidural analgesia with levobupivacaine and fentanyl in labour: a randomized controlled study. *BJA: British Journal of Anaesthesia*, 117(5), 617–622.

Hanna, M. N., Ouanes, J.-P. P., & Tomas, V. G. (2014). Postoperative pain and other acute pain syndromes. In H. Benzon, J. P. Rathmell, C. L. Wu, D. Turk, C. E. Argoff, & R. W. Hurley (Eds.), *Practical Pain Management* (5th ed., pp. 271–297.e11). St. Louis, MO: Elsevier.

Howard, R. F., Lloyd-Thomas, A., Thomas, M., Glyn Williams, D., Saul, R., Bruce, E., & Peters, J. (2010). Nurse-controlled analgesia (NCA) following major surgery in 10 000 patients in a children's hospital. *Pediatric Anesthesia, 20*(2), 126–134.

Indermun, S., Choonara, Y. E., Kumar, P., Du Toit, L. C., Modi, G., Luttge, R., & Pillay, V. (2014). Patient-controlled analgesia: therapeutic interventions using transdermal electro-activated and electro-modulated drug delivery. *Journal of Pharmaceutical Sciences, 103*(2), 353–366.

Institute for Safe Medication Practices (ISMP). (2008). Misprogramming PCA concentration leads to dosing errors. In *Acute Care – ISMP Medication Safety Alert.* Horsham, PA: Institute for Safe Medication Practices.

Institute for Safe Medication Practices (ISMP). (2009). Beware of basal opioid infusions with PCA therapy. In *Acute Care – ISMP Medication Safety Alert.* Horsham, PA: Institute for Safe Medication Practices.

Institute for Safe Medication Practices (ISMP). (2013). Fatal PCA adverse events continue to happen …. Better patient monitoring is essential to prevent harm. In *Acute Care – ISMP Medication Safety Alert.* Horsham, PA: Institute for Safe Medication Practices.

Institute for Safe Medication Practices (ISMP). (2016). Worth repeating …. Recent PCA by proxy event suggests reassessment of practices that may have fallen by the wayside. In *Acute Care – ISMP Medication Safety Alert.* Horsham, PA: Institute for Safe Medication Practices.

Katz, J., Buis, T., & Cohen, L. (2008). Locked out and still knocking: predictors of excessive demands for postoperative intravenous patient-controlled analgesia. *Canadian Journal of Anesthesia, 55*(2), 88–99.

Katz, P., Takyar, S., Palmer, P., & Liedgens, H. (2017). Sublingual, transdermal and intravenous patient-controlled analgesia for acute post-operative pain: systematic literature review and mixed treatment comparison. *Current Medical Research and Opinion, 33*(5), 899–910.

Kaye, A. D., Ali, S. I. Q., & Urman, R. D. (2014). Perioperative analgesia: Ever-changing technology and pharmacology. *Best Practice & Research Clinical Anaesthesiology, 28*(1), 3–14.

Kerr, D., Taylor, D., & Evans, B. (2015). Patient-controlled intranasal fentanyl analgesia: a pilot study to assess practicality and tolerability during childbirth. *International Journal of Obstetric Anesthesia, 24*(2), 117–123.

Kerr, I. G., Sone, M., DeAngelis, C., Iscoe, N., MacKenzie, R., & Schueller, T. (1988). Continuous narcotic infusion with patient-controlled analgesia for chronic cancer pain in outpatients. *Annals of Internal Medicine, 108*(4), 554–557.

Koh, P., & Thomas, V. J. (1994). Patient-controlled analgesia (PCA): does time saved by PCA improve patient satisfaction with nursing care? *Journal of Advanced Nursing, 20*(1), 61–70.

Lam, T., Nagappa, M., Wong, J., Singh, M., Wong, D., & Chung, F. (2017). Continuous Pulse Oximetry and Capnography Monitoring for Postoperative Respiratory Depression and Adverse Events: A Systematic Review and Meta-analysis. *Anesthesia & Analgesia, 125*(6), 2019–2029.

Lambert, T. L., & Cata, D. M. (2014). The traditional method of oral as-needed pain medication delivery compared to an oral patient-controlled analgesia device following total knee arthroplasty. *Orthopaedic Nursing, 33*(4), 217–223.

Leykin, Y., Miotto, L., & Pellis, T. (2011). Pharmacokinetic considerations in the obese. *Best Practice & Research Clinical Anaesthesiology, 25*(1), 27–36.

Licht, E., Siegler, E. L., & Reid, M. C. (2009). Can the Cognitively Impaired Safely Use Patient Controlled Analgesia? *Journal of Opioid Management, 5*(5), 307–312.

Lien, C., & Youngwerth, J. (2012). Patient-controlled analgesia. *Hospital Medicine Clinics, 1*(3), e386–e403.

Lovett, P. B., Sule, H. P., & Lopez, B. L. (2014). Sickle cell disease in the emergency department. *Emergency Medicine Clinics, 32*(3), 629–647.

Maddox, R. R., & Williams, C. K. (2012). Clinical experience with capnography monitoring for PCA patients. *Anesthesia Patient Safety Foundation Newsletter, 26*(4), 47–50.

Marks, A. D., & Rodgers, P. E. (2014). Diagnosis and management of acute pain in the hospitalized patient. *Hospital Medicine Clinics, 3*(3), e396–e408.

Martin, C., De Baerdemaeker, A., Poelaert, J., Madder, A., Hoogenboom, R., & Ballet, S. (2016). Controlled-release of opioids for improved pain management. *Materials Today, 19*(9), 491–502.

Martin, E. J., Roeland, E. J., Sharp, M. B., Revta, C., Murphy, J. D., Fero, K. E., & Yeung, H. N. (2017). Patient-Controlled Analgesia for Cancer-Related Pain: Clinical Predictors of Patient Outcomes. *Journal of the National Comprehensive Cancer Network, 15*(5), 595–600.

Mattia, C., Coluzzi, F., Sonnino, D., & Anker-Møller, E. (2010). Efficacy and safety of fentanyl HCl iontophoretic transdermal system compared with morphine intravenous patient-controlled analgesia for postoperative pain management for patient subgroups. *European Journal of Anaesthesiology (EJA), 27*(5), 433–440.

McKeown, J. L. (2015). Pain management issues for the geriatric surgical patient. *Anesthesiology Clinics, 33*(3), 563–576.

McNicol, E. D., Ferguson, M. C., & Hudcova, J. (2015). Patient controlled opioid analgesia versus non-patient controlled opioid analgesia for postoperative pain (Review). *The Cochrane Library,* (6), CD003348.

Messing, J., Aburahma, J., Amdur, R., Hernandez, M., Sirajuddin, S., Davison, D., & Sarani, B. (2015). 613: Authorized Agent Controlled Analgesia improves pain control in critically ill adult patients. *Critical Care Medicine, 43*(12), 155.

Mherekumombe, M. F., & Collins, J. J. (2015). Patient-controlled analgesia for children at home. *Journal of Pain and Symptom Management, 49*(5), 923–927.

Minkowitz, H. S., Rathmell, J. P., Vallow, S., Gargiulo, K., Damaraju, C. V., & Hewitt, D. J. (2007). Efficacy and safety of the fentanyl iontophoretic transdermal system (ITS) and intravenous patient-controlled analgesia (IV PCA) with morphine for pain management following abdominal or pelvic surgery. *Pain Medicine, 8*(8), 657–668.

Modesto-Lowe, V., Brooks, D., & Petry, N. (2010). Methadone deaths: risk factors in pain and addicted populations. *Journal of General Internal Medicine, 25*(4), 305–309.

Mohanty, M., Lawal, D., & Katz, N. (2017). (358) Medication errors associated with intravenous patient controlled analgesia: a descriptive analysis of 2005-2015 MEDMARX database. *The Journal of Pain, 18*(4), S64.

Motov, S. M., & Nelson, L. S. (2016). Advanced concepts and controversies in emergency department pain management. *Anesthesiology Clinics, 34*(2), 271–285.

Müller-Schwefe, G., Ahlbeck, K., Aldington, D., Alon, E., Coaccioli, S., Coluzzi, F., ... Kress, H. G. (2014). Pain in the cancer patient: different pain characteristics CHANGE pharmacological treatment requirements. *Current Medical Research and Opinion*, 30(9), 1895–1908.

Myers, M., & Eckes, E. J. (2012). A novel approach to pain management in persons with sickle cell disease. *Medsurg Nursing*, 21(5), 293.

Neal, J. M., Barrington, M. J., Fettiplace, M. R., Gitman, M., Memtsoudis, S. G., Mörwald, E. E., ... Weinberg, G. (2018). The third American Society of Regional Anesthesia and Pain Medicine practice advisory on local anesthetic systemic toxicity: executive summary 2017. *Regional Anesthesia and Pain Medicine*, 43(2), 113–123.

Nelson, G., Altman, A. D., Nick, A., Meyer, L. A., Ramirez, P. T., Achtari, C., ... Acheson, N. (2016). Guidelines for postoperative care in gynecologic/oncology surgery: Enhanced Recovery After Surgery (ERAS®) Society recommendations—Part II. *Gynecologic Oncology*, 140(2), 323–332.

Neto, J. O. B., Machado, M. D. T., de Almeida Correa, M., Scomparim, H. A., Posso, I. P., & Ashmawi, H. A. (2014). Methadone patient-controlled analgesia for postoperative pain: a randomized, controlled, double-blind study. *Journal of Anesthesia*, 28(4), 505–510.

Ohashi, K., Dalleur, O., Dykes, P. C., & Bates, D. W. (2014). Benefits and risks of using smart pumps to reduce medication error rates: a systematic review. *Drug Safety*, 37(12), 1011–1020.

Ong, J., Kirthinanda, D., Loh, S. K. N., & Sng, B. L. (2016). Strategies to reduce neuraxial analgesia failure during labour. *Trends in Anaesthesia and Critical Care*, 7, 41–46.

Paech, M., & Pan, P. (2009). New recipes for neuraxial labor analgesia: simple fare or gourmet combos? *International Journal of Obstetric Anesthesia*, 18(3), 201–203.

Palmer, P. P., & Miller, R. D. (2010). Current and developing methods of patient-controlled analgesia. *Anesthesiology Clinics*, 28(4), 587–599.

Palmer, P. P., Royal, M. A., & Miller, R. D. (2014). Novel delivery systems for postoperative analgesia. *Best Practice & Research Clinical Anaesthesiology*, 28(1), 81–90.

Park, A. J., Ahn, J., Buvanendran, A., Leblang, S., Kurd, M. F., Massel, D. H., ... Phillips, F. M. (2015). Multimodal versus Intravenous Patient Controlled Analgesia for Minimally Invasive Transforaminal Lumbar Interbody Fusion: A Prospective Randomized Study. *The Spine Journal*, 15(10), S262.

Pasero, C. (2015). Unconventional Use of a PCA Pump: Nurse-Activated Dosing. *Journal of PeriAnesthesia Nursing*, 30(1), 68–70.

Pasero, C., & McCaffery, M. (1993). Unconventional PCA: Making it work for your patient. *American Journal of Nursing*, 93(9), 38–41.

Pasero, C., & McCaffery, M. (2011). *Pain assessment and pharmacologic management*. St Louis: Mosby.

Pasero, C., Portenoy, R. K., & McCaffery, M. (1999). Opioid analgesics. In M. McCaffery, & C. Pasero (Eds.), *Pain: Clinical Manual* (Ed 2). St. Louis: Mosby.

Pasero, C., Quinlan-Colwell, A., Rae, D., Broglio, K., & Drew, D. (2016). American Society for Pain Management Nursing position statement: Prescribing and administering opioid doses based solely on pain intensity. *Pain Management Nursing*, 17(3), 170–180.

Paul, J. E., Bertram, B., Antoni, K., Kampf, M., Kitowski, T., Morgan, A., & Thabane, L. (2010). Impact of a comprehensive safety initiative on patient-controlled analgesia errors. *Anesthesiology: The Journal of the American Society of Anesthesiologists*, 113(6), 1427–1432.

Paz, J. C., & Quinlan, D. (2014). Acute pain management. In J. C. Paz, & M. P. West (Eds.), *Acute Care Handbook for Physical Therapists* (4th ed., pp. 457–465). St. Louis, MO: Saunders.

Peng, K., Liu, H. Y., Wu, S. R., Cheng, H., & Ji, F. H. (2015). Effects of combining dexmedetomidine and opioids for postoperative intravenous patient-controlled analgesia: a systematic review and meta-analysis. *The Clinical Journal of Pain*, 31(12), 1097–1104.

Pergolizzi, J. V., Jr., Taylor, R., Jr., & Muniz, E. (2011). The role of patient-controlled analgesia in the management of chronic pain. *European Journal of Pain Supplements*, 5(2), 457–463.

Pestano, C. R., Lindley, P., Ding, L., Danesi, H., & Jones, J. B. (2017). Meta-Analysis of the Ease of Care from the Nurses' Perspective Comparing Fentanyl Iontophoretic Transdermal System (ITS) Vs Morphine Intravenous Patient-Controlled Analgesia (IV PCA) in Postoperative Pain Management. *Journal of PeriAnesthesia Nursing*, 32(4), 329–340.

Peterson, S. E., Selvaggi, K. J., Scullion, B. F., & Blinderman, C. D. (2018). Pain management and antiemetic therapy in hematologic disorders. In R. Hoffman, E. J. Benz, L. E. Silberstein, J. I. Weitz, J. Anastasi, & S. A. Abutalib (Eds.), *Hematology Basic Principles and Practice* (7th ed., pp. 1473–1487). Philadelphia, PA: Elsevier.

Polomano, R. C., Fillman, M., Giordano, N. A., Vallerand, A. H., Nicely, K. L. W., & Jungquist, C. R. (2017). Multimodal analgesia for acute postoperative and trauma-related pain. *AJN The American Journal of Nursing*, 117(3), S12–S26.

Quinlan-Colwell, A. (2012). *Pain Management for Older Adults: A Clinical Guide for Nurses*. NY: Springer Publishing Company.

Redelmeier, D. (2007). New thinking about postoperative delirium. *Canadian Medical Association Journal*, 177(4), 424–424.

Riemondy, S., Gonzalez, L., Gosik, K., Ricords, A., & Schirm, V. (2016). Nurses' Perceptions and Attitudes Toward Use of Oral Patient-Controlled Analgesia. *Pain Management Nursing*, 17(2), 132–139.

Ritter, H. T. M. (2011). Making patient-controlled analgesia safer for patients. *Pennsylvania Patient Safety Advisory*, 8(3), 94–99.

Rosati, J., Gallagher, M., Shook, B., Luwisch, E., Favis, G., Deveras, R., & Conley, S. (2007). Evaluation of an oral patient-controlled analgesia device for pain management in oncology inpatients. *Journal Supportive Oncology*, 5(9), 443–448.

Rosen, M. (2003). Another choice for Queen Victoria? *International Journal of Obstetric Anesthesia*, 12(2), 71–73.

Ross, V. H., Pan, P. H., Owen, M. D., Seid, M. H., Harris, L., Clyne, B., & Eisenach, J. C. (2009). Neostigmine decreases bupivacaine use by patient-controlled epidural analgesia during labor: a randomized controlled study. *Anesthesia and Analgesia*, 109(2), 524–531.

Salmon, P., & Hall, G. M. (2001). PCA: patient-controlled analgesia or politically correct analgesia? The Board of Management and Trustees of the British Journal of Anesthesia. *Editorial III*, 87(6), 815–818.

San Diego Patient Safety Council (SDPSC). (2014). *Tool Kit Patient Controlled Analgesia (PCA) Guidelines of Care for the Opioid Naïve Patient.* San Diego, CA: San Diego Patient Safety Council.

Schechter, L. N., & Finkelstein, L. (2015). Nurse, physical therapist and patient ease-of-care: a meta-analysis comparing fentanyl iontophoretic transdermal system (ITS) versus intravenous patient-controlled analgesia (IV PCA) in postoperative pain management. *Journal of PeriAnesthesia Nursing, 30*(4), e44–e45.

Scott, L. J. (2016). Fentanyl iontophoretic transdermal system: a review in acute postoperative pain. *Clinical Drug Investigation, 36*(4), 321–330.

Se, H., Ho, C. C., Zainah, M., Jaafar, M. Z., Choy, Y. C., & Ismail, M. S. (2016). Structured Education Programme on Patient Controlled Analgesia (PCA) for Orthopaedic Patients. *Medicine and Health,* 62–71.

Shah, N., Homel, P., & Breznay, J. (2016). Use of Medical Devices in Hospice for Symptom Management. *American Journal of Hospice and Palliative Medicine®, 33*(10), 929–934.

Sharma, V., & de Leon-Cassola, O. (2014). Cancer pain. In H. Benson, J. P. Rathmell, C. L., Wu, D. Turk, C. E. Argoff, & R. W. Hurley (Eds.), *Practical Pain Management* (5th ed., pp. 335–345.e3). St. Louis, MO: Elsevier.

Sinatra, R. J., Viscusi, E. R., Ding, L., Danesi, H., Jones, J. B., & Grond, S. (2015). Meta-analysis of the efficacy of the fentanyl iontophoretic transdermal system versus intravenous patient controlled analgesia in postoperative pain management. *Expert Opinion Pharmacotherapy, 16*(11), 1607–1613.

Smith, C. B., & Goldberg, G. R. (2012). How should patient controlled analgesia be used in patients with serious illness and those experiencing postoperative pain? In N. E. Goldstein, & R. S. Morrison (Eds.), *Evidence-Based Practice of Palliative Medicine E-Book. Elsevier Health Sciences* (pp. 14–17).

Striebel, H. W., Olmann, T., Spies, C., & Brummer, G. (1996). Patient-controlled intranasal analgesia (PCINA) for the management of postoperative pain: a pilot study. *Journal of Clinical Anesthesia, 8*(1), 4–8.

Stroud, A. M., Tulanont, D. D., Coates, T. E., Goodney, P. P., & Croitoru, D. P. (2014). Epidural analgesia versus intravenous patient-controlled analgesia following minimally invasive pectus excavatum repair: a systematic review and meta-analysis. *Journal of Pediatric Surgery, 49*(5), 798–806.

Suresh, S., & Shah, R. (2014). Pediatric chronic pain management. In H. Benzon, J. P. Rathmell, C. L. Wu, D. Turk, C. E. Argoff, & R. W. Hurley (Eds.), *Practical Pain Management* (5th ed., pp. 449–466). St. Louis, MO: Elsevier. e6.

Surprise, J. K., & Simpson, M. H. (2014). PCA: Is that Patient-or Provider-Controlled Analgesia? *Journal of Radiology Nursing, 33*(1), 18–22.

Taenzer, A. H., Pyke, J. B., McGrath, S. P., & Blike, G. T. (2010). Impact of pulse oximetry surveillance on rescue events and intensive care unit transfers: A before-and-after concurrence study. *Anesthesiology: The Journal of the American Society of Anesthesiologists, 112*(2), 282–287.

Takieddine, S. C., Droege, C. A., Ernst, N., Droege, M. E., Webb, M., Branson, R. D., ... Mueller, E. W. (2018). Ketamine versus hydromorphone patient-controlled analgesia for acute pain in trauma patients. *Journal of Surgical Research, 225,* 6–14.

Tanabe, P., Freiermuth, C. E., Cline, D. M., & Silva, S. (2017). A prospective emergency department quality improvement project to improve the treatment of vaso-occlusive crisis in sickle cell disease: lessons learned. *The Joint Commission Journal on Quality and Patient Safety, 43*(3), 116–126.

The Joint Commission. (2014). Managing risk during transition to new ISO tubing connector standards. *Sentinel Event Alert,#53,* 1–6.

Thipphawong, J. B., Babul, N., Morishige, R. J., Findlay, H. K., Reber, K. R., Millward, G. J., & Otulana, B. A. (2003). Analgesic efficacy of inhaled morphine in patients after bunionectomy surgery. *Anesthesiology: The Journal of the American Society of Anesthesiologists, 99*(3), 693–700.

Toussaint, S., Maidl, J., Schwagmeier, R., & Striebel, H. W. (2000). Patient-controlled intranasal analgesia: effective alternative to intravenous PCA for postoperative pain relief. *Canadian Journal of Anesthesia, 47*(4), 299–302.

Tran, M., Ciarkowski, S., Wagner, D., & Stevenson, J. G. (2012). A case study on the safety impact of implementing smart patient-controlled analgesic pumps at a tertiary care academic medical center. *Joint Commission Journal on Quality and Patient Safety, 38*(3), 112–119.

Vasquenza, K., Ruble, K., Chen, A., Billett, C., Kozlowski, L., Atwater, S., & Kost-Byerly, S. (2015). Pain management for children during bone marrow and stem cell transplantation. *Pain Management Nursing, 16*(3), 156–162.

Vaurio, L. E., Sands, L. P., Wang, Y., Mullen, E. A., & Leung, J. M. (2006). Postoperative delirium: the importance of pain and pain management. *Anesthesia & Analgesia, 102*(4), 1267–1273.

Viscusi, E. R. (2008). Patient-controlled drug delivery for acute postoperative pain management: a review of current and emerging technologies. *Regional Anesthesia and Pain Medicine, 33*(2), 146–158.

Wallet, F., Clement, H. J., Bouret, C., Lopez, F., Broisin, F., Pignal, C., ... Aubrun, F. (2010). Effects of a continuous low-dose clonidine epidural regimen on pain, satisfaction and adverse events during labour: a randomized, double-blind, placebo-controlled trial. *European Journal of Anaesthesiology (EJA), 27*(5), 441–447.

Wang, L., Johnston, B., Kaushal, A., Cheng, D., Zhu, F., & Martin, J. (2016). Ketamine added to morphine or hydromorphone patient-controlled analgesia for acute postoperative pain in adults: a systematic review and meta-analysis of randomized trials. *Canadian Journal of Anesthesia/Journal Canadien d'Anesthésie, 63*(3), 311–325.

Webb, R. J., & Shelton, C. P. (2015). The benefits of authorized agent controlled analgesia (AACA) to control pain and other symptoms at the end of life. *Journal of Pain and Symptom Management, 50*(3), 371–374.

Weinger, M. B. (2009). Dangers of postoperative opioids-is there a cure? *Anesthesia Patient Safety Foundation (APSF) Newsletter, 24,* 25–26.

Wellington, J., & Chia, Y. Y. (2009). Patient variables influencing acute pain management. In R. S. Sinatra, O. A. De Leon-Cassasola, E. Viscusi, & B. Ginsberg (Eds.), *Acute Pain Management* (pp. 33–40). New York: University of Rochester Medical Center. Cambridge, UK: Cambridge University Press.

Winer, A. G., Sfakianos, J. P., Puttanniah, V. G., & Bochner, B. H. (2015). Comparison of perioperative outcomes for epidural versus intravenous patient-controlled analgesia after radical cystectomy. *Regional Anesthesia and Pain Medicine, 40*(3), 239–244.

Wirz, S., Conrad, S., Shtrichman, R., Schimo, K., & Hoffmann, E. (2017). Clinical Evaluation of a Novel Technology for Oral Patient-Controlled Analgesia, the PCoA® Acute Device, for Hospitalized Patients with Postoperative Pain, in Pilot Feasibility Study. *Pain Research and Management*. https://doi.org/10.1155/2017/7962135.

Xin, J., Zhang, Y., Zhou, L., Liu, F., Zhou, X., Liu, B., & Li, Q. (2017). Effect of dexmedetomidine infusion for intravenous patient-controlled analgesia on the quality of recovery after laparotomy surgery. *Oncotarget*, *8*(59), 100371–100383.

Yeo, S. T., Holdcroft, A., Yentis, S. M., Stewart, A., & Bassett, P. (2006). Analgesia with sevoflurane during labour: ii. Sevoflurane compared with Entonox for labour analgesia. *BJA: British Journal of Anaesthesia*, *98*(1), 110–115.

Yi, Y., Kang, S., & Hwang, B. (2013). Drug overdose due to malfunction of a patient-controlled analgesia machine-A case report. *Korean Journal of Anesthesiology*, *64*(3), 272–275.

Chapter 18 Regional Analgesia, Local Infiltration, and Pain Management

Maureen F. Cooney, Christine Peltier, Ann Quinlan-Colwell

CHAPTER OUTLINE

Neuraxial Analgesia, pg. 475

Principles of Neuraxial Analgesia, pg. 475

Neuraxial Anatomy, pg. 475

Neuraxial Analgesic Interventions, pg. 477

Beneficial Effects of Neuraxial Analgesia, pg. 478

Contraindications to Neuraxial Analgesia, pg. 482

Neuraxial Analgesia Techniques, pg. 482

Medications Used In Neuraxial Analgesia, pg. 486

Multimodal Analgesia Using Neuraxial Opioids and Local Anesthetics, pg. 493

Coanalgesic Medications Used in Neuraxial Analgesia, pg. 494

Administration of Neuraxial Medications, pg. 495

Unintended Effects of Neuraxial Analgesics, pg. 496

Unintended Effects of Neuraxial Local Anesthetics, pg. 498

Other Potential Complications Related to Neuraxial Analgesia, pg. 502

Neurologic Complications Associated With Neuraxial Analgesia, pg. 504

Regional Analgesia, pg. 510

Overview of Truncal and Peripheral Regional Analgesia, pg. 510

Peripheral Nerve Block Interventions, pg. 510

Beneficial Effects of Peripheral Nerve Blocks, pg. 511

Contraindications and Risks Associated With Peripheral Nerve Blocks, pg. 511

Medications for Peripheral Nerve Blocks, pg. 512

Administration of Peripheral Nerve Block Medications, pg. 513

Management of Peripheral Nerve Block Catheters and Infusions, pg. 513

Peripheral Nerve Blocks: Truncal Approaches, pg. 513

Peripheral Nerve Blocks: Extremity Approaches, pg. 515

Adductor Canal, pg. 517

Regional Analgesia Infusion Systems, pg. 518

Tapering and Discontinuing Regional Analgesia Catheters, pg. 518

Catheter Removal, pg. 518

Preventing and Managing Regional Analgesia Infusion System Complications, pg. 520

Minimizing Errors in Administration of Regional Anesthesia, pg. 520

Local Infiltration Analgesia, pg. 520

Additional Analgesic Procedures Involving Use of Local Anesthetics, pg. 524

Key Points, pg. 525

Case Scenario, pg. 526

References, pg. 526

REGIONAL anesthesia, often used to provide intraoperative anesthesia, can also be used to provide analgesia for postoperative and acute pain management. Regional analgesia involves the use of local anesthetics (LAs), opioids, and coanalgesics in doses less than those used for regional anesthesia to provide effective pain relief (Brull, Macfarlane, & Chan, 2015a). When LAs are administered in regional analgesia, the procedure is often described as a *block* because the LA acts to block propagation and conduction of nerve impulses. Regional techniques include neuraxial (spinal and epidural) and truncal/peripheral nerve blocks, which are performed in a variety of acute settings. An interdisciplinary expert panel commissioned by the American Pain Society developed clinical practice guidelines for the management of postoperative pain. The guidelines recommend clinicians offer neuraxial analgesia for major thoracic and abdominal surgery, particularly in patients with pulmonary or cardiac complications or at risk for prolonged ileus, and, depending on the type of surgery, consider surgical site–specific regional techniques (Chou et al., 2016). The use of local infiltration of analgesics (LIAs) into a surgical wound, joint, or site of tissue injury is another technique used in a multimodal approach to pain management. In recent years, different combinations of medications have been used for infiltration into surgical wounds to optimize analgesia (Baldini & Miller, 2018).

This chapter addresses the use of a variety of regional analgesic approaches, including neuraxial and peripheral nerve blocks, for the management of acute pain, including acute postoperative pain. Regional analgesia offers significant benefits in the multimodal approach to acute pain management. Medications used in regional analgesia, potential adverse effects, and management of catheters and infusion systems used in the delivery of regional analgesia are addressed. LIAs into a surgical wound or other site of tissue injury is also briefly described, because this technique offers another route for delivery of multimodal analgesia (MMA), which, with continued research and product development, is an area for potential expansion. Management of chronic pain with interventional therapies is addressed in Chapter 19.

Neuraxial Analgesia

Principles of Neuraxial Analgesia

Neuraxial analgesia pertains to epidural or spinal techniques used to deliver analgesic medications by injection or infusion into the neuraxial space. The medications are administered either into an area of fatty tissue that surrounds nerve roots as they exit the spine, known as the epidural space, or into the cerebrospinal fluid (CSF), which surrounds the spinal cord, referred to as the subarachnoid or intrathecal (IT) space (Benzon et al., 2014). Neuraxial techniques are used for pain control in many settings, including the preoperative, intraoperative, postoperative, and peripartum periods, as well as for the management of pain related to cancer or injury. The aim of neuraxial analgesia is to relieve pain by taking advantage of the endogenous pharmacology, reducing the afferent transmission of nociceptive signaling, and aiding in prevention of the development of central sensitization (See Chapter 3) (Argoff, 2013). In the literature, the word *spinal* may also be used when referring generally to all of the routes of administration near or within the spinal meninges. *Intrathecal* is often used synonymously with *subarachnoid,* but anatomically the intrathecal space includes the subdural space (see the following paragraphs on functional spinal anatomy). Similarly, the term *intraspinal* is used to describe administration of medication by the epidural or intrathecal route. The word *spinal,* which is used in this chapter, is interchangeable with the word *intrathecal* when referring to route of administration.

Neuraxial Anatomy

Neuraxial anatomy pertaining to epidural and intrathecal anesthesia-analgesia consists of the vertebral column, ligaments, spinal cord, spinal canal, and spinal nerves.

Vertebral Column

The vertebral column in humans consists of 33 individual vertebrae referred to by their location: (1) 7 cervical, (2) 12 thoracic, and (3) 5 lumbar; at the caudal end are (4) 5 sacral (fused into one bone, the sacrum) and (5) 4 coccygeal (fused into one bone, the coccyx) (Fig. 18.1). Vertebrae consist of an anterior body, the laminae that protect the lateral spinal cord, and spinous processes that project outwardly and posteriorly from the laminae. The vertebrae become larger as they descend in the vertebral column. The bones of the laminae are bound together by a number of discs and ligaments (e.g., the dense and elastic ligamentum flavum) (Fig. 18.2).

The spinal cord is a continuous structure extending from the foramen magnum and terminating at approximately the lower border of L1-L2 level in adults. In infants, the spinal cord extends to the lower border of L3 intervertebral disc level and moves up with age. The spinal cord tapers and ends as the *conus medullaris*. Distal to the conus medullaris is a tangle of nerve roots known as the *cauda equina* ("horse's tail") that exit the spine and extend to the lower part of the sacrum. Because the spinal cord ends at L1-L2 intervertebral disc level, performing spinal anesthesia is not recommended at or above this level.

The spinal cord is located within and protected by the bony vertebral canal and covered by three membranes of connective tissue, the spinal meninges. Moving from the outside toward the spinal cord is the dura mater, arachnoid mater, and the pia mater. These membranes divide the vertebral canal into three compartments referred to as spaces: the epidural space, subdural space, and subarachnoid space.

The epidural space extends from the base of the skull to the sacral hiatus, an opening formed by incomplete posterior fusion of the fifth sacral vertebrae. The epidural space lies between the spinal meninges and the sides of the vertebral canal. It lies outside and surrounds the dura mater anteriorly, laterally, and posteriorly and is bound posteriorly by the ligamentum flavum. The ligamentum flavum is not one continuous ligament, but rather is composed of right and left ligament flava, which meet in the middle (see Fig. 18.2). Next is the dura mater that together with the arachnoid mater forms the dural sac, and between these membranes is the subdural space. The subdural space contains serous fluid and is "potential" space that can be expanded by injecting air or liquid to separate the layers (Orebaugh & Cruz Eng, 2020).

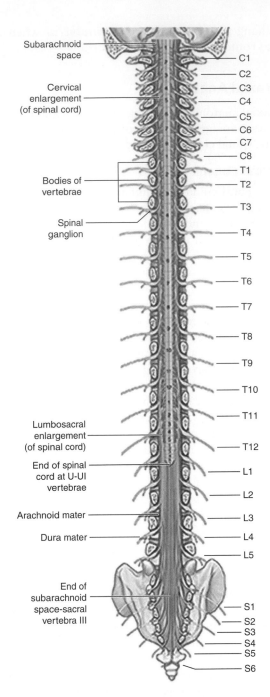

Fig. 18.1 | Vertebral Column. The human spinal column consists of 33 individual vertebrae referred to by their location: (1) 7 cervical, (2) 12 thoracic, (3) 5 lumbar; at the caudal end are (4) 5 caudal or sacral (fused into one bone, the sacrum) and (5) 4 coccygeal (fused into one bone, the coccyx). At each vertebral body level, nerve roots exit from the spinal cord bilaterally. Specific skin areas are innervated by a single spinal nerve or group of spinal nerves. (From Drake, R. L., Vogl, W., & Mitchell, A. M. W. [2019]. *Gray's anatomy for students* [4th ed.]. London: Elsevier.)

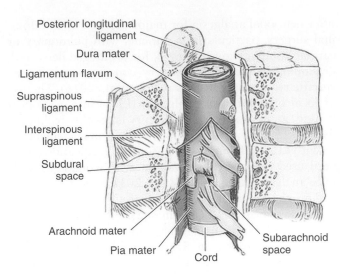

Fig. 18.2 | Spinal Anatomy. The spinal cord is a continuous structure extending from the foramen magnum to approximately the first or second lumbar (L1-L2) vertebral interspace in adults and the lower border of L3 in infants and moves up with age. The subarachnoid space (also called the *intrathecal space* in the caudal part of the spine) surrounds the spinal cord, separated by the pia mater. The subarachnoid space is filled with CSF that continuously circulates and bathes the spinal cord. The dura is composed of the arachnoid and dura mater membranes and separates the epidural space from the subarachnoid space. The epidural space is a potential space filled with vasculature, fat, and a network of nerve extensions. (From Pellegrini, J. [2018]. *Nurse anesthesia* [6th ed.]. Philadelphia: Elsevier.)

The epidural space is composed of layers of fat, connective tissue, an extensive venous plexus and is traversed by spinal nerve roots. The layers of fat and texture of the epidural space allows inconsistent paths where the epidural solution will flow, ultimately creating less uniform flow and variable paths. This concept provides a possible rationale for less than optimal results of epidural analgesia (Gill, Nagda, Aner, & Simopoulos, 2016).

The space closest to the spinal cord is the subarachnoid space, also called the *intrathecal space,* distally in the caudal part of the spine. It lies between the arachnoid and pia mater. The subarachnoid space contains clear, colorless CSF that continually circulates and bathes the spinal cord and dorsal and ventral nerve roots; it also transmits blood to and from the spinal cord through blood vessels. The dural sac, subarachnoid, and subdural spaces usually extend to S2 in adults and often S3 in children; because of this, performing caudal epidural administration in children with smaller body size carries a greater risk for subarachnoid injection than it does in adults. The pia mater forms the inner layer that lies on the surface of the spinal cord (Orebaugh & Cruz Eng, 2020).

Spinal Nerves

Thirty-one pairs of spinal nerves exit from the spinal cord below the skull and between each vertebral body level bilaterally. The regional number of each nerve is used to identify its association with the adjacent vertebrae. Ventral nerve roots are responsible for motor and varying degrees of sympathetic input and blockade. A specific area on the surface of the skin that is innervated by a single dorsal (sensory) root of the spinal nerve is known as a dermatome (see (Fig. 18.3). There is overlap of dermatome territories between adjacent segmental nerves.

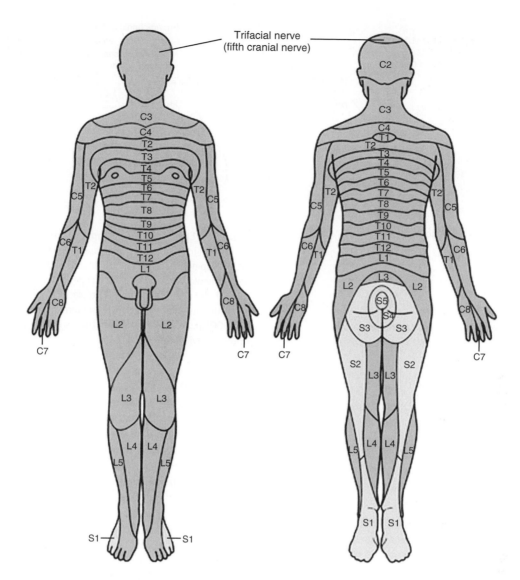

Fig. 18.3 | Dermatomes. Segmental dermatome distribution of spinal nerves to the front, back, and side of the body. *C,* Cervical segments; *L,* lumbar segments; *S,* sacral segments; *T,* thoracic segments. Dermatomes are specific skin areas innervated by a single spinal nerve or group of spinal nerves. Dermatome assessment is done to determine the level of spinal anesthesia for surgical procedures and postoperative analgesia when epidural local anesthetics are used. (From Pellegrini, J. [2018]. *Nurse anesthesia* [6th ed.]. Philadelphia: Elsevier.)

The pattern of innervation is variable from patient to patient; thus dermatome diagrams serve more as a guide than a fixed map. Although dermatome assessment of nerve innervation to the trunk is more straightforward, assessment of innervation to the neck, extremities, and pelvis is more complex because the ventral rami of the segmental nerve branches out and forms a nerve plexus in these areas. There are four major nerve plexuses: cervical, brachial, lumbar, and sacral plexus (Carrera et al., 2020).

Neuraxial Analgesic Interventions

Delivery of analgesics by the neuraxial route can be accomplished by inserting a needle into the subarachnoid space (for intrathecal analgesia, also known as spinal anesthesia or spinal block), or into the epidural space.

The medications are administered as a single injection or by threading a small flexible catheter through the needle, removing the needle, then taping the catheter in place temporarily for intermittent bolus dosing or continuous administration of analgesic medications (Figs. 18.4 to 18.6). Patient selection guidelines and considerations for neuraxial analgesia are presented in Box 18.1.

Neuraxial approaches, both spinal and epidural needle and catheter insertion, for analgesia usually are performed by an anesthesiologist or certified registered nurse anesthetist (CRNA). Nurses who are appropriately educated often assist with the procedure by preparing supplies and monitoring and supporting the patient during the procedure. The risks and benefits must be explained and informed consent obtained by the provider before the procedure whenever neuraxial analgesia is planned.

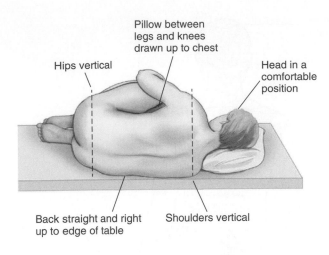

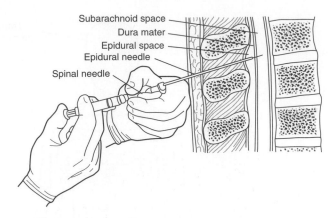

Fig. 18.5 | **Epidural Needle and Catheter Placement.** Performing an epidural involves the needle passing through the skin, subcutaneous fat, intraspinous ligament, and ligamentum flavum into the epidural space *(shown)* and injecting the analgesic or threading a catheter through the needle and taping it in place temporarily for bolus dosing or continuous administration. (From Birnbach, D. J., Gatt, S. P., & Datta, S. [2000]. [Eds.], *Textbook of obstetric anesthesia* [p. 166]. Philadelphia: Churchill Livingstone.

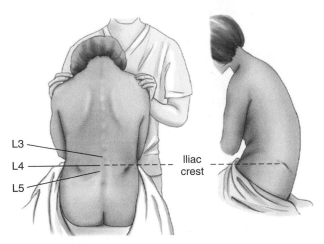

Fig. 18.4 | **Patient Positioned for Catheter Placement.** This figure shows two positions patients can assume for the epidural catheter placement procedure. (From Pasero, C., & McCaffery, M. [2011]. *Pain assessment and pharmacologic management* [p. 409]. St. Louis: Mosby. May be duplicated for use in clinical practice.)

Neuraxial Analgesia

Spinal, epidural, combined spinal-epidural, and caudal techniques are used to provide central neuraxial analgesia. LAs are often administered by one of these techniques to provide analgesia through disruption of nerve transmission in the spinal cord, spinal nerve roots, and the dorsal route ganglia (Macfarlane, Brull, & Chan, 2018). LAs block sodium channels in sympathetic and somatic (sensory and motor) nerve membranes and prevent propagation and conduction of neural impulses, referred to as a *block* (Nathan & Wong, 2014). Opioids are also frequently administered using these techniques and facilitate neuraxial blockade and analgesia. Details related to medications used in neuraxial analgesia are provided in a subsequent section of this chapter.

Spinal analgesia for acute pain involves the administration of medications as a single injection directly into the CSF in the subarachnoid space, thus avoiding absorption by the epidural fat and blood vessels. Epidural analgesia for acute pain involves delivery of analgesic medications

directly into the epidural space. To obtain continuous epidural analgesia, a temporary indwelling epidural catheter is attached to an external infusion pump that controls the delivery of epidural medication. "Continuous epidural infusion of local anesthetic with or without opioids is a cornerstone of multimodal anesthesia" (Lukof et al., 2017). Epidural catheters for acute pain management are usually placed at the lumbar or thoracic vertebral level depending on the surgical site. To reduce the risk for catheter-related infections, continuous infusions of LA, opioid, and other medications into the epidural space usually infuse for 2 to 3 days and rarely longer than 5 days. Tunneled neuraxial catheters are sometimes used to minimize risks for neuraxial infection or allow the catheter to be used for a longer period. Table 18.1 shows some of the persistent misconceptions related to epidural analgesia.

Clinicians are responsible to ensure appropriate patient education related to spinal and epidural analgesia. See Box 18.2 for an example of patient preparation and education related to epidural placement that may also be applied to spinal needle insertion. This information may be helpful in reinforcing the anesthesia provider's explanation of the procedure to patients.

Beneficial Effects of Neuraxial Analgesia

The benefits of neuraxial anesthesia are well documented in the literature. For example, Guay et al. (2014) analyzed 9 Cochrane systematic reviews that included neuraxial blockade consisting of epidural, caudal, spinal, or combined spinal-epidural as a bolus or by continuous infusion. In that analysis, outcomes, including death, chest infection, myocardial infarction, and/or serious adverse events, were examined. The reviewers compared neuraxial blockade versus general anesthesia alone and neuraxial

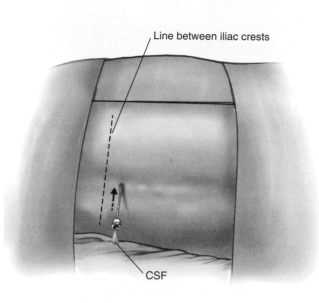

Location of spinal needle placement with confirmation by CSF

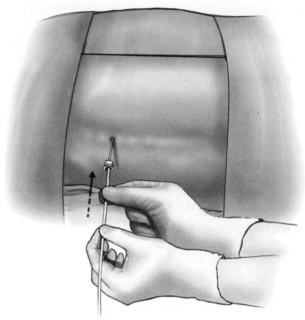

Insertion of spinal catheter for medication administration

Fig. 18.6 | Spinal (Subarachnoid or Intrathecal) Needle and Catheter Placement. Performing spinal blockade by midline approach involves the needle passing through the skin, subcutaneous fat, interspinous ligament, ligamentum flavum, dura mater, subdural space, arachnoid mater, and into the subarachnoid space. When placement is via paramedian approach passage through the interspinous ligament is eliminated. *CSF*, cerebrospinal fluid.

| **Box 18.1** | Patient Selection for Use of Epidural Anesthesia and Analgesia |

INDICATIONS

The decision to use this epidural technique should be determined based on the needs of the patient. *Examples:*
- The patient has a painful condition or surgical procedure for which the benefits of epidural analgesia are likely to outweigh the risks.
- The patient has acute pain (e.g., surgery, trauma). The systemic routes have been considered and pose the risks for unmanageable and intolerable adverse effects at the anticipated doses required for adequate analgesia.
- Epidural preemptive analgesia could prevent or reduce the severity of a persistent postsurgical pain syndrome (e.g., phantom limb pain, postthoracotomy pain).
- Epidural anesthesia for surgery and a single bolus dose before removal of needle or catheter will may produce acceptable postoperative analgesia (e.g., preservative-free epidural morphine or extended-release epidural morphine for cesarean section or hip replacement).
- The patient has a pain syndrome that may be responsive to a specific therapy such as local anesthetics, cloNIDine, or corticosteroids, that is delivered by the epidural route

(e.g., neuropathic pain unresponsive to systemic and topical adjuvant analgesics).
- The patient has persistent cancer or noncancer pain. Pain is uncontrolled and/or adverse effects are unmanageable and intolerable with systemic analgesics.

CONTRAINDICATIONS

- **Absolute contraindications** to needle or catheter placement include patient refusal, uncorrected hypovolemia, increased intracranial pressure, indeterminate neurologic disease, infection at the site of injection, and true allergy to local anesthetics and/or opioids.
- **Relative contraindications** include iatrogenic or idiopathic coagulopathy; anticoagulants should be withheld based on mechanism of action and duration of the medication, unstable neurologic disease, anatomic abnormalities of the spine, immunocompromise, sepsis, and signs of infection distinct from the anatomic puncture site; if the patient is treated with antibiotics and vital signs are stable, then epidural may be considered.

Continued

Box 18.1 Patient Selection for Use of Epidural Anesthesia and Analgesia—cont'd

OTHER CONSIDERATIONS

- Appropriate equipment and supplies are available for therapy.
- Staff is trained to assess and manage epidural analgesia.
- Clinical support systems are available ATC if needed.

COMMON SURGICAL APPLICATIONS

- Obstetrics (cesarean section, labor analgesia)
- Open thoracic surgeries
- Vascular surgery of the lower extremities
- Major hip/knee joint replacement
- Lower limb amputation
- Large open upper abdominal surgery (e.g., open cholecystectomy, pancreatectomy, nephrectomy, hepatic resection, gastrectomy, esophagectomy, abdominal aortic aneurysm repair)
- Large open lower abdominal surgery (e.g., small bowel, mesentery, colon)
- Urogenital and gynecologic (cystectomy, radical prostatectomy, open hysterectomy)

COMMON MEDICAL CONDITIONS

- Chest trauma
- Intractable cancer pain
- Intractable neuropathic pain
- Myocardial ischemia unresponsive to conventional treatment

ATC, Around the clock.

From Pasero, C., & McCaffery, M. (2011). *Pain assessment and pharmacologic management* (p. 406). St. Louis: Mosby. Data from American Society of Anesthesiologists Committee on Standards and Practice Parameters. (2017). Practice advisory for the prevention, diagnosis and management of infectious complications associated with neuraxial techniques: An updated report by the American Society of Anesthesiologists Task Force on infectious complications associated with neuraxial techniques and the American Society of Regional Anesthesia and Pain Medicine. *Anesthesiology, 126*(4), 585–601; Cashman, J. (2008). Routes of administration. In P. E. Macintyre, S. M. Walker, & D. J. Rowbotham (Eds.), *Clinical pain management: Acute pain* (2nd ed.). London: Hodder Arnold; Deschner, B., Allen, M., & de Leon O. (2007). Epidural blockade. In A. Hadzic (Ed.), *Textbook of regional anesthesia and acute pain management* (pp. 229–267). New York: McGraw Hill; and Hsu, E., & Cohen, S. P. (2013). Postamputation pain: Epidemiology, mechanisms, and treatment. *Journal of Pain Research 6*, 121–136. © 2011, Pasero, C., & McCaffery, M. May be duplicated for use in clinical practice.

Table 18.1 | Misconceptions: Epidural Analgesia

Misconception	Correction
• Compared with parenteral opioid administration, the incidence of opioid-induced respiratory depression is higher when opioids are administered by the epidural route.	• The incidence of respiratory depression associated with the various methods of pain management is not firmly established because of a lack of consensus on definitions and well-controlled research. According to updated practice guidelines by American Society of Anesthesiologists (2016) a meta-analysis of RCTs indicates there is no significant difference in the frequency of respiratory depression and less somnolence or sedation with single-injection epidural opioid than that of intramuscular opioid injections and inconsistent findings when compared with intravenous opioid administration. The incidence of respiratory depression and hypoxemia is equivocal in RCTs when comparing opioid patient-controlled epidural analgesia (PCEA) with intravenous PCA opioid. Meta-analysis of RCTs for continuous infusion of epidural opioid indicate less respiratory depression, when compared with intravenous infusion of opioids, and findings are equivocal when evaluating differences in hypercarbia, somnolence, and sedation. Clinically significant opioid-induced respiratory depression can be avoided by slow titration, careful monitoring of sedation levels, adequacy of ventilation, oxygenation, and opioid dose reduction versus cessation when increased sedation is detected (see Chapter 13).
• Patients receiving epidural analgesia must be cared for in intensive care settings where their respiratory status can be mechanically monitored.	• Patients receiving epidural analgesia have been cared for safely outside of the high dependency and intensive care setting for many years. Though increased monitoring is warranted in patients at high risk for respiratory depression (e.g., those with obstructive sleep apnea, chronic pulmonary disease), assessment of pain, sedation level, adequacy of ventilation, and oxygenation is reliable and the most common method for monitoring most patients receiving epidural analgesia (see Chapter 13).

Table 18.1 | Misconceptions: Epidural Analgesia—cont'd

Misconception	Correction
• Epidural local anesthetics cause excessive and disabling sensory and motor blockade.	• Local anesthetics are administered in low (subanesthetic) doses (e.g., 0.05%–0.125% bupivacaine, 0.1%–0.2% ropivacaine) for epidural analgesia. Higher doses are required to produce significant motor and sensory blockade (0.5%–0.75% bupivacaine, 0.75%–1.0% ropivacaine). Patients receiving epidural analgesia are able to ambulate and perform all the routine recovery activities expected of them to the extent their medical or surgical condition allows. The occasional occurrence of minor temporary numbness of lower extremities is resolved easily by decreasing the dose or removing the local anesthetic from the epidural analgesic solution.
• Thoracic epidural catheter is usually avoided because it is technically more difficult and is usually associated with adverse outcomes.	• Thoracic epidural administration is frequently used for postoperative pain control involving the thorax and abdomen. Anesthesia providers are trained in the techniques for thoracic epidural catheter placement and with adequate training and repeated procedures, become proficient in thoracic epidural catheter placement.

PCA, Patient-controlled analgesia; *RCT,* randomized controlled trial.
Note: In spite of widespread use, misconceptions related to epidural analgesia persist. This table corrects some of these misconceptions.
From Pasero, C., & McCaffery, M. (2011). Pain assessment and pharmacologic management (p. 405). St. Louis, MO: Mosby. Data from American Society of Anesthesiology Committee on Practice Standards. (2016). Practice Guidelines for the prevention, detection and management of respiratory depression associated with neuraxial opioid administration: An updated report by the American Society of Anesthesiologists task force on neuraxial opioids and the American Society of Regional Anesthesia and Pain Medicine. *Anesthesiology, 124*(3), 535–552; Schreiber, M. L. (2015). Nursing care considerations: The epidural catheter. *MedSurg Nursing, 24*(4), 273; Toledano, R. D., & Van De Velde, M. (2017). Epidural anesthesia and analgesia. In A. Hadzic. *Hadzic's textbook of regional and acute pain management* (pp. 380–445). New York: McGraw-Hill Education; and Warren, D. T., Nelson, K., Neal, J. M. (2018). Neuraxial anesthesia. In D. E. Longnecker, S. C. Mackey, M. F. Newman, W. S. Sandberg, & W. M. Zapol. *Anesthesiology,* New York: McGraw-Hill. © 2011, Pasero, C., & McCaffery, M. May be duplicated for use in clinical practice.

Box 18.2 | Preparation and Education of the Patient for Epidural Analgesia: Patient Example

Mr. Z. and his wife want to know everything about the epidural catheter placement procedure he is going to receive later today. His nurse reinforces the anesthesia provider's explanation by offering the following information: "You'll either be in a sitting position or lying on your side for the procedure. The provider will be behind you, facing your back. First, he'll wash a small area on your back with a sponge. This may feel cool. Next, he'll put drapes on your back to keep the area as clean as possible. You'll need to roll your shoulders inward and push your back out slightly. The provider will use a local anesthetic to numb the place where the catheter will go. Sometimes injecting the local anesthetic produces a burning, stinging sensation that lasts less than a minute. It usually takes the provider about 2 or 3 minutes to insert the needle into the epidural space. This will feel like dull pressure against your back. Then, the provider inserts the catheter through the needle into the epidural space, which usually takes less than a minute. As he inserts the catheter, you may feel some spark-like sensations in your legs and feet. These will go away very quickly. The provider will remove the epidural needle, then secure the catheter in place with a clear occlusive adhesive dressing and tape up your back to your shoulder. After the catheter is taped in place, you'll be able to move and turn and lie on your back like you did before the procedure. The whole procedure usually takes less than 30 minutes. You may feel a very slight irritation for an hour or two after the procedure just at the site where the catheter goes into your back. If you feel any more discomfort in your back than that at any time while the catheter is in place, you'll need to let us know. Can I answer any questions?"

blockade plus general anesthesia versus general anesthesia for surgical anesthesia involving any type of open or endoscopic surgical procedure. Based on 5 of the studies with 400 participants using neuraxial blockade alone, there was a 55% reduced risk for developing pneumonia (chest infection), and in 9 studies involving 2433 participants, there was 30% reduced risk for developing pneumonia when neuraxial blockade was added to general anesthesia. Based on 20 studies with 3006 participants, the 0 to 30-day risk for dying was reduced by approximately 29% when epidural or spinal block was used to replace general anesthesia. When neuraxial blockade was added to general anesthesia to reduce quantity of other medications required during general anesthesia, the mortality risk was not affected.

Neuraxial techniques are also beneficial for optimizing pain relief outside the operative setting. MMA plans including subanesthetic doses of LAs, opioids, and other additives administered using spinal and/or epidural techniques can provide effective pain relief. Examples of situations in which neuraxial techniques are used for pain relief include labor and delivery, orthopaedic surgery, open abdominal surgeries, thoracotomies, and rib fractures. More detail is provided in the following section.

Contraindications to Neuraxial Analgesia

Absolute contraindications to neuraxial analgesia include patient refusal, localized sepsis, allergy to medications planned for neuraxial administration, inability to remain still and follow directions during neuraxial needle insertion, and increased intracranial pressure (Brull et al., 2015a). Relative contraindications are weighed against the potential benefits and may be related to anatomic risks and/or risks associated with medications used in neuraxial analgesia. Relative contraindications include preexisting neurologic deficits or conditions such as spinal stenosis, spine surgery, multiple sclerosis, spina bifida, aortic stenosis, or hypovolemia; use of antithrombotic, thrombolytic, or antiplatelet therapy; inherited coagulopathies; or infections (Brull et al., 2015a).

Another relative contraindication for use of neuraxial analgesia is risk for compartment syndrome. Worsening pain is a symptom of compartment syndrome, and although evidence is sparse, some clinicians avoid the use of neuraxial analgesia in orthopaedic patients at risk for compartment syndrome because of concerns for delays in recognition and treatment of ischemic pain (Driscoll et al., 2016; Hunter, Kim, Mariano, & Harrison, 2019).

Neuraxial Analgesia Techniques

Spinal (Subarachnoid or Intrathecal) Analgesia

Spinal analgesia is commonly used for acute pain related to obstetric, gynecologic, hernia repair, genitourinary, and lower extremity orthopedic surgeries. This technique is often used for rapid, dense, and predictable anesthesia; a single injection (bolus dose) of medication may be injected to treat acute pain. Administration of a continuous infusion of spinal medications may be used in chronic pain treatment plans (see Chapter 19). Spinal analgesia is effective because it involves injection of medications into the subarachnoid space between the arachnoid and pia mater where the spinal nerves and CSF are located. The spinal analgesia administration technique is described in Box 18.3.

Epidural Analgesia

In contrast to spinal analgesia, epidural analgesia provides segmental analgesia effective for thoracic, abdominal, obstetric, gynecologic, urologic, and lower extremity orthopedic surgeries. Analgesia is most effective when epidural analgesic medication is administered in an epidural

---

| **BOX 18.3** | Technique for Administration of Spinal Anesthesia |

- Spinal anesthesia may be performed with the patient in the sitting, side-lying, or prone position through a midline or paramedian approach.
- First, the superior aspects of the iliac crest are identified and a line is drawn between them to mark the location of the L5 spinous process or the L4-5 interspace between lumbar vertebrae.
- Then the soft area between the spinous processes is located to help locate the interspace.
- Depending on the type of surgery and the ability to feel the interspace, the spinal needle is introduced through L3-4 or L4-5 interspace.
- When performing a spinal block using the midline approach, the skin of the insertion site is first infiltrated with local anesthetic (LA).
- An introducer needle is placed midline and advanced with slightly cephalad angulation traversing through the subcutaneous fat.
- As the needle passes through the ligamentum flavum an increase in resistance followed by a loss of resistance and a characteristic "pop" indicating the penetration of the dura mater, subdural space, arachnoid mater, and entry into the subarachnoid space.
- The stylet is removed from the spinal needle, and free cerebrospinal fluid (CSF) flow is noted.
- On obtaining free flow of CSF, the syringe containing LA with additive is attached to the spinal needle hub and injected.
- With the paramedian approach, the spinal introducer insertion site is approximately one fingerbreadth lateral to the midline approach.
- The length of the spinal cord must always be considered because inadvertent injection into the spinal cord can result in severe neurologic complications or paralysis.
- Because the spinal cord ends at the L1-2 level in adults and L3 in children, spinal anesthesia is usually not advised at or above this level to avoid potential needle trauma to the spinal cord.

From Brull, R., MacFarlane, A. J. R., & Chan, V. W. S. (2015a). Spinal, epidural, and caudal anesthesia. In: R. D. Miller (Ed.). *Miller's anesthesia*, (8th ed., pp 1684–1720).; and Nathan, N., & Wong, C. A. (2014). Spinal, epidural, and caudal anesthesia: Anatomy, physiology, and technique. In: D. Chestnut, C. Wong, L. Tsen, W. D. Ngan Kee, Y. Beilin, & J. Mhyre (Eds.). *Chestnut's obstetric anesthesia: Principles and practice* (5th Ed., pp. 229–261). Philadelphia: Saunders.

---

location that corresponds to the dermatomes affected by the surgical incision (Hurley, Murphy, & Wu, 2015). Table 18.2 presents recommended epidural catheter insertion levels based on the location of injury or incision that is causing pain.

Table 18.2 | Recommended Epidural Catheter Insertion Levels

Location of Incision or Injury	Examples of Surgical Procedures	Congruent Epidural Catheter Placement
Thoracic	Lung reduction, radical mastectomy, thoracotomy	T4-8
Upper abdominal	Cholecystectomy, esophagectomy, gastrectomy, Whipple procedure	T6-8
Middle abdominal	Cystoprostatectomy, nephrectomy	T7-10
Lower abdominal	Abdominal aortic aneurysm repair, colectomy, radical prostatectomy, total abdominal hysterectomy	T8-11
Lower extremity	Femoral-popliteal bypass, total hip or total knee replacement	L1-4

L, Lumbar level; *T,* thoracic level.
Modified from Hurley, R. W., Murphy, J. D., & Wu, C. L. (2015). Acute postoperative pain. In R. D. Miller (Ed.), *Miller's anesthesia* (pp. 2974–2998). Philadelphia: Saunders.

Use of epidural analgesia is associated with attenuation of certain pathophysiologic responses to surgery and may be correlated with reduction in morbidity and mortality when compared to systemic opioid use. Perioperative epidural anesthesia and analgesia may be associated with superior pain relief, opioid-sparing effects, and possible improved surgical outcomes (Ray, Schmidt, & Ottestad, 2018). The physiologic effects of epidural delivery and blockade on different organ systems depends on the spinal level and number of segments blocked. For example, thoracic epidural analgesia (TEA) has been shown to improve bowel motility by causing a sympathectomy, which enhances parasympathetic innervation of the intestines and may reduce the duration of postoperative ileus (Liu & Wu, 2007; Miller & Moon, 2018).

Continuous epidural infusions used for acute postoperative pain allow flexibility in the density and duration of analgesia (Macfarlane et al., 2018). The technique for placing a temporary epidural catheter varies among practitioners; techniques for epidural catheter placement are described in Box 18.4. Once the catheter is placed, the practitioner verifies placement using several techniques described in Box 18.5.

Box 18.4 | Technique for Administration of Epidural Analgesia

Three approaches that may be used for epidural technique are *midline, paramedian* (or lateral), and *Taylor* (or lumbosacral) (Macfarlane, Brull, & Chan, 2018).

- If the *midline* approach is used, the needle passes through the intraspinous ligament in a slightly cephalad (upward) direction and exits through the ligamentum flavum into the epidural space.
- For the *paramedian* approach, after identifying the spinous process, the needle is positioned 1 cm lateral and 1 cm inferior from the spinous process, then directed toward the middle of the interspace, with the ligamentum flavum usually being the first resistance identified.
- On occasion, when the other approaches are not successful or cannot be performed, the Taylor approach, which is a paramedian approach directed toward the L5-S1 interspace, is performed.

Once the approach is selected:

- The epidural needle is inserted with the bevel of the needle directed upward to facilitate threading the epidural catheter in a cephalad (toward the head) direction.
- During placement into the epidural space, the needle is advanced slowly through the interspinous ligament stopping at the point of resistance.
- Most anesthesia providers are able to recognize this point of resistance, which represents the ligamentum flavum.

Once the needle penetrates the dense ligamentum flavum (see Fig. 18.2) there is a loss of resistance.

- Three alternative techniques make it possible to identify the tip of the needle has entered the epidural space: loss of resistance (LOR), "hanging drop," and ultrasonography. The LOR is the most preferred method.
  - LOR technique
    - A subcutaneous LA wheal is performed, and the epidural needle with a stylet or introducer in place is passed slowly through the subcutaneous tissue until increased tissue resistance is felt (this is the ligamentum flavum).
    - The stylet or introducer is removed, and a glass syringe filled with 2 to 3 mL of saline or air is attached to the hub of the needle.
    - The epidural space exerts a negative pressure, which is registered by a loss of resistance in the syringe attached to the needle.
    - The needle is slowly advanced with continuous pressure exerted on the plunger.
    - As the needle tip enters the epidural space, there is a sudden loss of resistance, and injection is easy.
    - When the plunger cannot be compressed, the needle probably is not past the ligamentum flavum (Butterworth, Mackey, & Wasnick, 2018).

Continued

Box 18.4 | Technique for Administration of Epidural Analgesia—cont'd

- Once the LOR to air or saline has occurred, the ligamentum flavum is penetrated, the needle is not advanced further if the epidural space is the desired location.
- If advanced further, the needle will inadvertently penetrate the dura and enter the subarachnoid space. If the subarachnoid space is inadvertently accessed, free-flowing CSF can be aspirated. If a blood vessel is entered during placement, blood often can be aspirated (McClymont & Celnick, 2018).
- Hanging drop technique
  - The "hanging drop" technique is done once the interspinous ligament has been entered, and the stylet is removed.

- The spinal needle and hub are filled with saline so that a drop hangs from the outside opening of the hub.
- The epidural needle is pushed forward, and as soon as it passes through the ligamentum flavum and the epidural space has been entered, the drop of fluid at the needle hub is absorbed into ("sucked into") the needle; this is due to the lower pressure in the epidural space (Larson & Jaffe, 2017).
- Ultrasonography
  - Ultrasonography may be used to guide access to the epidural space. Ultrasound may allow more accurate identification of vertebral level, optimal interspace selection, and guide needle insertion (McClymont & Celnick, 2018).

Box 18.5 | Verification of Epidural Placement

- Once placement of the epidural needle is reasonably certain, the person who has placed the needle confirms that neither CSF nor blood is flowing or aspirated from the needle, which would indicate inadvertent subarachnoid or intravascular placement.
- Needle placement is then often confirmed by injecting a test dose of lidocaine with EPINEPHrine (if there is no contraindication to EPINEPHrine). A test dose is designed to detect both intravascular and subarachnoid injection.
  - If the needle is intravascular, the EPINEPHrine will cause noticeable sudden increase in the patient's heart rate ($\geq$20%) with or without change in blood pressure (BP). (There is the potential for false positives and false negatives. For example, in a pregnant patient, a uterine contraction might cause pain or an increase in heart rate during a test dose, making it difficult to interpret whether variability in heart rate is in response to EPINEPHrine or to uterine blood flow and contractions. Bradycardia or exaggerated elevation in blood

pressure can occur in response to EPINEPHrine in patients taking beta-blockers.)
  - If the needle accidentally penetrates the dura mater and arachnoid membrane, it will be in the subarachnoid space. If the lidocaine is injected in this space (intrathecally) it will produce marked spinal anesthesia that should be rapidly apparent.
- If the patient does not exhibit either of these changes, the needle is thought to be in the epidural space and the catheter is threaded through the needle approximately 5 cm beyond the needle tip.
  - A meta-analysis of results of 31 studies involving use of neuraxial ultrasound for placement of lumbar epidural identified that performance of landmark identification with use of ultrasound as an extension of physical examination enhances accuracy of landmark identification and accurately measures depth of epidural space when compared to palpation of surface landmarks alone (Perlas, Chaparro, & Chin, 2016).

Thoracic Epidural Analgesia

TEA can significantly benefit treatment of acute pain after thoracic or upper abdominal surgery and rib fractures (Toledano & Van de Velde, 2017). Key components of TEA in acute pain management include superior perioperative analgesia compared with systemic opioid analgesia, decrease in pulmonary complications, and duration of mechanical ventilation (Guay & Kopp, 2016) and decreased duration of postoperative ileus (Guay, Nishimori, & Kopp, 2016). TEA is not usually recommended for min-

imally invasive laparoscopic or thoracoscopic procedures because the benefits of TEA are unclear in these procedures (Toledano & Van de Velde, 2017).

High thoracic epidural LA administration (blocks above T5) and extensive epidural blockade result in major physiologic effects on the cardiovascular system as a result of more profound sympathetic block. Segmental neural blockade of thoracic dermatomes that occurs with the use of LA in TEA inhibits nociceptive afferent and sympathetic efferent activity while not affecting vagal parasympathetic innervation.

Sympathetic and nociceptive afferent inhibition may result in arterial and venous vasodilation, reduced systemic vascular resistance, and changes in heart rate and contractility, which alter cardiac output and blood pressure. The level of the block, number of dermatomes involved, and concentration and dose of LA are factors that influence the type and degree of cardiovascular effect (Toledano & Van de Velde, 2017).

In a meta-analysis of studies that compared outcomes of cardiac surgery with and without thoracic epidural anesthesia, the use of thoracic epidural anesthesia showed significant reduction in supraventricular tachyarrhythmias and respiratory complications (Svircevic et al., 2013). Another meta-analysis comparing the efficacy of TEA with or without general anesthesia to general anesthesia alone in those who underwent cardiac surgery showed those who received TEA had significantly fewer ($P < .05$) complications, including supraventricular arrhythmias, respiratory complications, and pain; TEA was also associated with shorter lengths of stay in the intensive care unit and hospital and time to tracheal extubation (Zhang, Wu, Guo, & Ma, 2015).

Lumbar Epidural Analgesia

Lumbar epidural analgesia using LA medications is a technique frequently used during labor; after lumbar anesthetic injection, LAs spread caudally more than toward the head, thereby providing an anesthetic effect over the spinal areas associated with pain in labor (T11-L1 and S3-S5) (McClymont & Celnick, 2018). Lumbar epidural analgesia also may be used for pain associated with injury and major orthopedic surgeries of the lower extremities and painful conditions and surgeries involving the lower abdomen, pelvis, and perineum.

Combined Spinal-Epidural

Combined spinal-epidural anesthesia involves needle placement into the subarachnoid space for injection of medication and, as part of the same procedure, placement of a catheter into the epidural space. This technique is especially useful for patients in labor. The combined spinal-epidural administration technique is described in Box 18.6.

The rationale for combining the epidural and spinal routes is to provide rapid relief of pain or induction of spinal analgesia with the rapid onset of the spinal medication and continued analgesia by administration of medication through the epidural catheter to prolong the duration of pain relief (Ranasinghe, Davidson, & Birnbach, 2017). Another advantage of this technique is that the use of combined spinal-epidural analgesia allows administration of a lower than usual dose of intrathecal (spinal) LA with the ability to extend the LA effect by use of the epidural catheter; an infusion of saline or LA into the epidural catheter may cause compression of the dural sac and increase the height of the spinal block (Brull et al., 2015a). This makes combined spinal-epidural anesthesia a particularly useful option for obstetrics and an option for other surgical procedures, including pelvic and hip surgeries (Tummala, Rao, Vallury, & Sanapala, 2015).

Box 18.6	Combined Spinal-Epidural Technique

- During the needle-through-needle technique, an epidural needle is placed in the epidural space, then a longer, much smaller gauge spinal needle is passed through the epidural needle into the subarachnoid space.
- A distinct pop is felt as the dura is penetrated.
- Spinal needle placement is confirmed by aspiration of cerebrospinal fluid, and the spinal block is performed using intrathecal opioid and/or local anesthetic.
- The spinal needle is then removed, and an epidural catheter is inserted.
- The catheter is threaded into position, and the epidural needle is withdrawn.
- The epidural catheter is left in place and should be aspirated carefully.
- As needed supplemental doses of medications to prolong block and provide ongoing analgesia are administered into the epidural catheter and titrated slowly and incrementally to avoid inadvertent intrathecal injection.

From Warren, D. T., Nelson, K. E., Neal, J. M. (2018). Neuraxial anesthesia. In D. E. Longnecker, S. C. Mackey, M. F. Newman, W. S. Sandberg, & W. M. Zapol (Eds.), *Anesthesiology*. New York: McGraw-Hill.

A meta-analysis of combined spinal-epidural anesthesia versus traditional epidural involving 27 trials with 3274 parturient women indicated that combined spinal-epidural anesthesia had faster onset of effective analgesia from time of injection and less need for rescue analgesia; other clinically significant data reflected no difference in mother's satisfaction, pruritus, ability to mobilize during labor, maternal hypotension, rate of cesarean section birth, or adverse events for the newborn when compared with low-dose epidural anesthesia (Simmons, Taghizadeh, Dennis, Hughes, & Cyna, 2012).

Caudal Anesthesia

Caudal anesthesia is most commonly administered to younger children (up until puberty), because the use of lumbar epidural administration in adults provides similar areas of anesthetic coverage, with more reliable spread (Candido, Tharian, & Winnie, 2017). Caudal anesthesia may be preferred over lumbar epidural administration in adults when sacral nerve spread of LAs, rather than lumbar nerve spread is preferred (Candido et al., 2017). A caudal anesthetic approach is also used to manage pain associated with perineal, anal, or rectal region procedures or when a lumbar scar or mass prevents lumbar epidural access (Macfarlane et al., 2018).

Medications Used In Neuraxial Analgesia

Safe and effective use of neuraxial analgesia for pain management requires knowledge and understanding of pharmacology, as well as analgesic techniques, new analgesic agents, drug delivery systems, and multimodal approaches. The two most widely used analgesics administered neuraxially to treat acute pain are opioids and LAs. Opioids produce analgesia through inhibition of target cell activity by binding to opioid receptors (see Chapter 11). LA agents produce analgesia through reversible conduction blockade of impulses in peripheral and central nerves (see Chapter 15). Either analgesic may be used alone in neuraxial analgesia, but they are often used in combination as multimodal therapies.

Basic Pharmacology of Neuraxial Opioid Analgesics

Bioavailability

Bioavailability refers to the distribution of a medication from the site of administration to its site of action. In contrast to medications administered systemically, medications administered neuraxially are more potent (i.e., relatively small doses and volume are effective) because distribution of the medication brings it close to the action site (opioid receptors in the dorsal horn of the spinal cord). This is particularly true when opioids are delivered by the intrathecal route, by which they are carried by the CSF to the dorsal horn. Opioids administered into the epidural space are distributed by three main pathways: (1) neural diffusion through the dura and arachnoid membranes into the CSF, then into the spinal cord and directly to receptors in the dorsal horn of the spinal cord; (2) vascular uptake by the vessels in the epidural space into systemic circulation; and (3) uptake by the fat in the epidural space, where a medication depot is created from which the medication enters the systemic circulation (Macfarlane et al., 2018).

Compared to systemic opioid administration, the more direct delivery of neuraxial opioids to the site of analgesic action explains why the dose of an opioid by the neuraxial route is lower than that required by the parenteral route to produce equianalgesia; the closer the opioid is delivered to the opioid receptors, the lower is the required analgesic dose.

Solubility

Medication solubility and ability to traverse diffusion barriers (e.g., the dura mater) influence absorption and bioavailability by the neuraxial routes. The more lipid-soluble (readily dissolved in fatty tissue) the medication, the more readily it moves through membranes, resulting in faster absorption. For example, when administered by single epidural injection, lipid-soluble (lipophilic) opioids, such as fentaNYL, rapidly traverse the dura into the CSF, and then exit the aqueous CSF and easily penetrate the lipid-rich spinal tissue and surrounding vasculature (Conlin, Grant, & Wu, 2018; Hernandez, Grant, & Wu,

2018). This contributes to the rapid onset of fentaNYL (5 minutes) and also accounts for its short duration of effect (2 hours) because it is easily removed by the vasculature or remains trapped within the fat of the epidural space (Bujedo, 2015). In contrast, water-soluble (hydrophilic) opioids such as morphine and HYDROmorphone readily dissolve in aqueous solution; therefore they have more difficulty traversing the dura and take longer to reach the aqueous CSF. By either the epidural or intrathecal route, once in the aqueous CSF, hydrophilic medications prefer to remain there. Eventually, high enough concentration of the medication is reached in the CSF and it then moves into the spinal cord to the opioid receptors. This helps explain the slow onset of action of neuraxial morphine (30–60 minutes) and longer duration of action (Conlin et al., 2018; Hernandez et al., 2018).

Because morphine is hydrophilic, it tends to remain within the aqueous CSF. This ensures continued opioid receptor binding by replenishing molecules that dissociate and are cleared from the spinal action sites and helps explain morphine's large volume of distribution, greater bioavailability than lipid-soluble opioids (fentaNYL and SUFentanil), and exceptionally long duration of analgesia from a single neuraxial injection (e.g., 12–24 hours).

When extended pain relief is necessary, the highly lipophilic opioids may be administered by continuous infusion to prolong limited duration of action. Once a steady state is reached by continuous infusion, the various opioids have similar duration. The differences in hydrophilic and lipophilic opioids need to be considered to optimize analgesia, and minimize side effects, taking into account the surgical procedure, comorbidities, and health care setting (inpatient versus outpatient or ambulatory surgery).

Equianalgesic Dose Conversions

Differences in lipid solubility of an opioid result in variation in the opioid analgesic conversion ratio as different opioid administration routes are considered. When administering the less lipid-soluble opioids (e.g., morphine) by the epidural route, the medication is more likely to move more slowly from the epidural area to the CSF in the intrathecal space. There is a paucity of evidence to guide the conversion of an opioid dose when moving from the parenteral route to neuraxial doses or from the neuraxial routes to the intravenous route.

Despite the lack of evidence, it is necessary for clinicians to consider the differences in opioid solubility and doses, as situations arise when a patient will need a change in opioid administration route. For example, a patient who requires high doses of intravenous opioids for cancer pain may have an implanted intrathecal infusion pump placed to facilitate discharge to home. The reverse situation may occur when the patient with an intrathecal morphine pump runs out of medication in the pump while in the hospital and requires intravenous opioids to replace the intrathecal medication. Although there are no strong studies to support the conversion ratios, expert opinion related to conversions involving morphine is fairly consistent. In a survey of pain specialists' practices related to the conversion of high-dose intravenous morphine to neuraxial doses, Gorlin et al. (2016) found the most commonly used ratio for morphine conversions is 100 mg IV:10 mg epidural:1 mg IT. Morphine is the least lipid-soluble medication, so it has the greatest difference in dose required to produce similar analgesic effect.

Consensus regarding conversions from intravenous to epidural and intrathecal routes of fentaNYL and HYDROmorphone is lacking. FentaNYL is highly lipid-soluble. Therefore, intravenous and epidural fentaNYL administered at similar doses may result in similar plasma levels (Gorlin et al., 2016). One of the popular opioid calculators cites an intravenous-to-epidural ratio for fentaNYL as 10:7 but does not address an intrathecal dose. Instead, some calculators and experts simply suggest intrathecal fentaNYL starting doses and suggested titration for effect. The initial intrathecal is 5 to 25 mcg and the typical epidural dose is 25 to 100 mcg (Herndon et al., 2016; Yaksh & Wallace, 2017). Because of variability in dose conversion calculators, conservative dose conversions and close assessment of the patient's response to the opioid switch is important to minimize risks for adverse effects.

HYDROmorphone is slightly more lipid soluble than morphine, but less soluble than fentaNYL, and some suggest it is appropriate to calculate a conversion ratio somewhere between the ratios of the other two medications. Herndon et al. (2016) suggest a range of 0.8 to 1.5 mg of hydromorphone for a single epidural dose. Although there are few available studies, a conversion ratio from epidural HYDROmorphone to intravenous HYDROmorphone of 1:2 is found in older literature (Murray & Hagen, 2005). A table of morphine equivalents used at Memorial Sloan Kettering Cancer Center, published by Foley (1985), identified HYDROmorphone equivalents as 8 mg oral (PO) = 2 mg IV = 0.4 mg epidural = 0.08 mg IT.

Given the lack of strong evidence, when converting between an oral or parenteral route for opioid administration and the neuraxial route, it is important to consider medication solubility and use conservative dosing, starting at the lower dose range and with titration based on the patient's response. During the dose finding period, patients should be carefully monitored for signs of advancing sedation and respiratory depression.

Distribution

An opioid medication deposited into the CSF or diffusing into the CSF from the epidural space distributes throughout the neuroaxis with the movement of the CSF (Bujedo, 2015, 2017). The extent to which the medication moves rostrally toward the brain or caudally toward the lower end of the thecal sac depends on the medication's clearance rate from the CSF (Bujedo, 2017). Hydrophilic medications such as morphine and HYDROmorphone tend to remain in the CSF and produce a broad spread of analgesia (Conlin et al., 2018). Longer acting opioids can be given by intermittent bolus or continuous infusion (Macintyre & Schug, 2015). The opposite is true of lipophilic opioids such as fentaNYL and SUFentanil, which are rapidly cleared from the CSF into plasma or the epidural space tends to be transported for shorter distances and produce what is called *segmental* analgesia. By rapidly leaving the CSF and redistributing into spinal cord tissue, epidural fat, and vasculature, these lipophilic opioids have little rostral spread (Bujedo, 2017). Lipophilic opioids require a continuous infusion because of their short duration of action (Macintyre & Schug, 2015). When using the lipophilic opioids, their analgesic effect is more segmental in a dermatomal band of distribution consistent with the level of the injection; therefore, it is particularly important to position the epidural catheter tip at the spinal level where there is a high level of nociceptive input (Macintyre & Schug, 2015).

Appropriate placement of the catheter is especially important if lipophilic medications (e.g., fentaNYL, SUFentanil, LAs) are used. It is well understood that hydrophilic opioids ascend in the CSF and are likely to cover the spinal segments receiving input from the injured or incisional dermatomes irrespective of catheter placement, whereas lipophilic opioids such as fentaNYL and SUFentanil may not ascend to the necessary spinal level, leading to a situation in which the analgesia is produced largely by systemic redistribution (movement of the dose from the CSF into the bloodstream and then back to sites of action in the brain and spinal cord) rather than by local action of the medication at the spinal cord level. With lipophilic opioids, analgesia associated with epidural administration is primarily the result of the systemic uptake, and epidural administration does not offer any benefits over parenteral administration when a lipophilic opioid is the only medication placed in the epidural space (Bujedo, 2015).

Selected Opioid Analgesics

The mu agonist opioids (morphine, fentaNYL, HYDROmorphone, and SUFentanil) are the most common opioids administered by the neuraxial route. Table 18.3 describes the properties of commonly administered opioids. Tables 18.4 and 18.5 provide examples of common neuraxial opioid administration regimens. The most common side effects of neuraxial opioids include sedation, respiratory depression, pruritus, nausea, vomiting, and urinary retention (see Chapters 12 and 13 for treatment of opioid-induced adverse effects). Older adults are more sensitive to CNS effects of neuraxial opioids; therefore, the initial dose must be reduced based on patient age and condition, and then subsequent dosing should be titrated to effect (Macintyre & Schug, 2015). Given the unique pharmacokinetic characteristics of various opioids when administered neuraxially, the American Society of Anesthesiologists (ASA, 2016) recommends matching

Table 18.3 | Properties of Neuraxial Opioids

Property	Lipophilic Opioids	Hydrophilic Opioids
Common drugs	FentaNYL, SUFentanil	Morphine, HYDROmorphone
Onset of analgesia	Rapid onset (5–10 min)	Delayed onset (30–60 min)
Duration of analgesia[a]	Shorter duration (2–4 h)	Longer duration (6–24 h)
CSF spread	Minimal CSF spread	Extensive CSF spread
Site of action	Spinal ± systemic	Primarily spinal ± supraspinal
Side Effects		
Nausea and vomiting	Lower incidence with lipophilic than with hydrophilic opioids	
Pruritus	Lower incidence with lipophilic than with hydrophilic opioids	
Respiratory depression	Primarily early; minimal delay	Both early (< 6 h) and delayed (> 6 h) possible

CSF, Cerebrospinal fluid.
[a]Duration of analgesia is variable.
From Hurley, R. W., Murphy, J. D., & Wu, C. L. (2015). Acute postoperative pain. In R. D. Miller (Ed.), *Miller's Anesthesia (pp. 2974–2998)*. Philadelphia, PA: Saunders.

the appropriate duration of monitoring with the medications used.

Morphine Morphine is a widely used hydrophilic opioid that produces excellent selective spinal-mediated analgesia by the epidural and intrathecal routes and can be administered as a bolus, as a continuous infusion, or in patient-controlled epidural analgesia (PCEA) systems. Morphine is an effective opioid for acute postoperative pain; however, its slow onset (> 30 minutes), particularly long duration of action (up to 24 hours in the opioid-naïve patient or as long as 48 hours with extended-release epidural morphine), and risk for delayed respiratory depression from rostral spread require careful patient selection and dosing and vigilant monitoring protocols. It is not recommended for use in outpatient or ambulatory surgery patients (Hernandez et al., 2018).

Because of slow rostral spread in the CSF, large-volume bolus doses (> 5 mg) of epidural morphine have been known to produce delayed respiratory depression (approximately 6–12 hours after lumbar injection, corresponding with the rate of CSF flow from the spinal level to the brainstem) (Hurley et al., 2015). Earlier respiratory depression at 5 to 10 minutes and before 2 hours also can occur as a result of vascular uptake of morphine. Fear of late respiratory depression has caused some clinicians to avoid using epidural morphine in opioid-naïve patients; however, rostral spread and late respiratory depression are uncommon when epidural morphine is administered in smaller doses and appropriate monitoring is provided.

Table 18.4 | Examples of Epidural Opioid Regimens

Opioid	Single-Injection Dose Range[a]	Onset[b] (min)	Peak[b] (min)	Analgesic[b-d] (h)	Half-Life (h)	Solubility	Continuous Infusion
Morphine	1–5 mg	30–60	90–120	Up to 24 48 (EREM)	2–3	Hydrophilic	0.1–1 mg/h
HYDROmorphone	0.5–1 mg	15–30	45–60	6–7; up to 18	2–3	Hydrophilic (10 times less water soluble than morphine)	0.1–0.2 mg/h
FentaNYL	50–100 mcg	5–15	10–20	2–4	3–4	Lipophilic	25–100 mcg/h
SUFentanil	10–35 mcg	5–10	10	2–4	2–4	Very lipophilic (2 times more lipid soluble than fentaNYL)	10–20 mcg/h

EREM, Extended-release epidural morphine.
[a]The lowest effective dose should be administered to minimize risk for respiratory depression.
[b]Onset, peak, and duration are based on single-injection administration.
[c]Duration of analgesia is dose dependent; the higher the dose, usually the longer is the duration.
[d]When steady state is reached by continuous infusion, the various opioids differ little in terms of duration.
From Pasero, C., & McCaffery, M. (2011). *Pain assessment and pharmacologic management* (pp. 418–419). St. Louis: Mosby. Data from American Society of Anesthesiologists Committee on Practice Standards. (2016). Practice Guidelines for the prevention, detection and management of respiratory depression associated with neuraxial opioid administration: An updated report by the American Society of Anesthesiologists task force on neuraxial opioids and the American Society of Regional Anesthesia and Pain Medicine. *Anesthesiology, 124*(3), 535–552; Bujedo, B. M. (2015). Clinical use of spinal opioids for postoperative pain. *Journal of The Analgesics 3*(2), 17–23; Bujedo, B. M., Santos, S. G., & Azpiazu, A. U. (2012). A review of epidural and intrathecal opioids used in the management of postoperative pain. *Journal of Opioid Management 8*(3), 177–192; Data Epidural neural blockade. In M. J. Cousins, & P. O. Bridenbaugh (Eds.), *Neural blockade in clinical anesthesia and management of pain*. Philadelphia: Lippincott-Raven; Dabu-Bondoc, S., Franco, S. A., & Sinatra, R. S. (2009). Neuraxial analgesia with hydromorphone, morphine, and fentanyl: Dosing and safety guidelines. In R. S. Sinatra, O. A. de Leon-Casasola, B. Ginsberg, et al. (Eds.), *Acute pain management*, Cambridge, NY, Cambridge University Press; Grape, S., & Schug, S. A. (2008). Epidural and spinal analgesia. In P. E. Macintyre, S. M. Walker, & D. J. Rowbotham (Eds.), *Clinical pain management: Acute pain* (2nd ed.). London: Hodder Arnold; and Maalouf, D. B., & Liu, S. S. (2009). Clinical application of epidural analgesia. In R. S. Sinatra, O. A. de Leon-Casasola, B. Ginsberg, et al. (Eds.), *Acute pain management*. (pp. 221–229). Cambridge, NY, Cambridge University Press. © 2011, Pasero, C., & McCaffery, M. May be duplicated for use in clinical practice.

Table 18.5 | Examples of Intrathecal Opioid Analgesic Regimens

Opioid	Single-injection Dose Range[a]	Onset (min)	Peak (min)	Duration (h)
Morphine	0.1–0.3 mg	30–60	60	Up to 24
HYDROmorphone	—			
FentaNYL	5–25 mcg	5	10	2–4
SUFentanil	2–10 mcg	5	15–20	2–4

[a] The lowest effective dose should be administered to minimize risk of respiratory depression
© 2011, Pasero, C., & McCaffery, M. May be duplicated for use in clinical practice.

In a systematic review, including 78 articles and 18,455 patients, of neuraxial morphine and diamorphine (available in the United Kingdom) associated with respiratory depression after cesarean delivery, the prevalence of clinically significant respiratory depression was low and ranged from 1.63 in 10,000 to 1.08 per 10,000 (Sharawi et al., 2018).

Extended-Release Epidural Morphine

Extended-release epidural morphine (EREM) is distinguished from conventional epidural morphine by its unique delivery system, which consists of multiple microscopic, liposomal (fat-based) particles; the liposomes contain aqueous chambers that encapsulate preservative-free morphine (Bulbake, Doppalapudi, Kommineni, & Khan, 2017). After epidural injection, the liposomes slowly release morphine over a period of 48 hours by erosion or reorganization of the lipid membranes (Toledano & Van de Velde, 2017). EREM should be administered in the lumbar epidural space only. Primary advantages of this formulation are that it allows up to 48 hours of pain relief without the use of an indwelling catheter, which can pose a risk for infection, impede mobility, and raise concerns about postoperative anticoagulant therapy (Rodriguez-Aldrete, Candiotti, Janakiraman, & Rodriguez-Blanco, 2016). Furthermore, concerns regarding infusion device programming errors are eliminated with this approach.

Most studies related to use of EREM were conducted in the early 2000s and demonstrated efficacy and safety of this morphine delivery system. A more recent study in which the EREM medication was compared to an injection of the same dose of preservative-free epidural morphine in 60 patients who underwent lumbar spine surgery demonstrated similar analgesic benefits and adverse effects, but the group receiving the EREM product were less likely to require naloxone or supplemental oxygen, and experienced less nausea or fever but were more likely to have hypotension (Vineyard, Toohey, Neidre, Figel, & Joyner, 2014). Box 18.7 presents guidelines in the care of patients receiving EREM. (See Chapters 12 and 13 for treatment of opioid-related unintended effects.)

Box 18.7 | Care of the Patient Receiving Extended-Release Epidural Morphine

- Ensure that staff is adequately trained regarding EREM before introducing therapy in the organization.
- Develop a standardized order set and policy that includes:
  - EREM dose and time of administration
  - Monitoring parameters
  - Activity, ambulation
  - IV access (e.g., heparin lock) maintained while patient hospitalized and receiving opioid analgesics
  - Management of breakthrough pain
  - Treatment of adverse effects
  - When to notify anesthesia provider (e.g., unrelieved pain, excessive adverse effects)
  - Implement measures that alert staff that EREM has been administered (e.g., colorful patient wristband or brightly colored label or sign on the bed).
- Assess pain with every new report of pain; assess well-controlled pain at least q4h.
- Monitor sedation and respiratory status q1h × 12h, q2h × q12h, then q4h if stable after EREM injection, then q4h for the next 24 hours, then per routine in stable patients.
- Monitor other vital signs q4h for 48 hours then per routine in stable patients (evaluate need to monitor blood pressure more often in some patients).
- Be aware that many of the medications commonly used to treat opioid-induced adverse effects, such as antihistamines for pruritus and antiemetics for nausea, can produce an additive sedating effect.

EREM, Extended-release epidural morphine; *h*, hour; *q*, every. From Pasero, C., & McCaffery, M. (2011). *Pain assessment and pharmacologic management* [p. 422]. St. Louis: Mosby. Data from Pasero, C., & McCaffery, M. (2005). Extended-release epidural morphine (Depodur™). *Journal of PeriAnesthesiology Nursing, 20*(5), 345–350; and Pasero, C., Eksterowicz, N., Primeau, M., Cowley, C. (2007). ASPMN position statement: Registered nurse management and monitoring of analgesia by catheter techniques. *Pain Management Nursing, 8*(2), 48–54. © 2011, Pasero, C., & McCaffery, M. May be duplicated for use in clinical practice.

HYDROmorphone

HYDROmorphone has gained acceptance as a first-line opioid for epidural administration. Many references related to use of neuraxial HYDROmorphone are dated because it has been studied and used over the past two decades or more. Its lipid solubility is intermediate between those of morphine and fentaNYL. Because it is more lipophilic than morphine, its onset of analgesia (5–10 minutes) is faster and its duration of action (4–6 hours) is shorter than those of morphine (Bujedo, 2013) (see Table 18.4). HYDROmorphone is associated with intermediate rostral spread, compared to morphine with high spread. Epidural HYDROmorphone is associated with a lower risk for respiratory depression than epidural morphine, but the risk for delayed respiratory depression after large epidural bolus administration must be considered (Bujedo, 2013).

Epidural HYDROmorphone is more potent than epidural morphine; however, use caution when converting patients from morphine to HYDROmorphone because the exact potency ratio by neuraxial administration is unknown. The switch to any new opioid should be done slowly with appropriate monitoring as described in Chapter 13.

The efficacy and safety of a single injection of intrathecal HYDROmorphone with or without LA in enhanced recovery pathways in colon and rectal surgeries were examined in a retrospective review (Merchea et al., 2018). Of the 601 patients included in the review, 91% received intrathecal HYDROmorphone without LA, and there was no significant difference in length of stay between the groups. Most patients (71%) received 76 to 100 mcg IT HYDROmorphone; other dose ranges were less than 50 mcg, 76 to 100 mcg, and greater than 100 mcg. Pain scores did not differ in any dose range, and the oral morphine equivalents of additional postoperative opioids did not differ in the intrathecal HYDROmorphone dose ranges. The authors concluded intrathecal HYDROmorphone doses of 50 to 75 mcg was comparable to analgesia provided at higher doses, and all the reviewed intrathecal regimens and doses were similarly effective in achieving short lengths of stay, low pain scores, and a low incidence of adverse effects (Merchea et al., 2018). Similarly, in a prospective comparison of intrathecal morphine and intrathecal HYDROmorphone for post–cesarean section analgesia, the 90% effective dose of intrathecal HYDROmorphone was found to be 75 mcg (Sviggum et al., 2016).

Epidural HYDROmorphone is used by continuous infusion and PCEA to provide analgesia in obstetric patients and after major surgery. A 2016 retrospective study of women who underwent cesarean delivery was done in which effectiveness of intrathecal and epidural morphine and HYDROmorphone were compared. The study included 450 patients who received 200 mcg IT morphine, 387 patients who received 60 mcg IT HYDROmorphone, 81 patients who received 3 mg epidural morphine, and 102 patients who received 0.6 mg epidural HYDROmorphone. The time to first request for rescue opioid was 17 hours in the intrathecal morphine group compared to 14.6 hours in the intrathecal HYDROmorphone group ($P < .0001$), and the intrathecal HYDROmorphone group used significantly more rescue opioids ($P < .001$) than the intrathecal morphine group; side effects were similar in the intrathecal groups. Similarly, the epidural morphine group had a significantly ($P = .0007$) longer time to first request for rescue opioids (20.1 hours) compared to the epidural HYDROmorphone group (13 hours). The epidural groups had similar side effects, and there was no significant difference in rescue opioid doses (Marroquin et al., 2017).

FentaNYL

FentaNYL is a highly potent lipophilic opioid used extensively for anesthesia and to provide postoperative analgesia. Single-injection neuraxial doses of fentaNYL provide rapid-onset analgesia (intrathecal: 5–10 minutes; epidural: 10–15 minutes) and relatively short duration (2–5 hours) making this method of administration appropriate only for very short-term pain control, such as after ambulatory surgery and when rapid analgesia is desired (Hurley et al., 2015). Diluting the epidural dose (typically 50–100 mcg) in 10 mL of preservative-free normal saline helps prolong analgesia and increase the initial spread and diffusion of the medication (Hurley et al., 2015). Because lipid-soluble opioids such as fentaNYL have a short duration of analgesia, administration by continuous infusion or PCEA rather than intermittent bolus dosing is preferred for extended pain control (Hurley et al., 2015). Epidural fentaNYL does not provide effective analgesia at sites distant from the site of epidural administration; therefore, epidural injection or catheter tip placement needs to be near the spinal level associated with pain.

FentaNYL is 800 times more lipid-soluble than morphine. The concentration of fentaNYL that can be measured in the blood after epidural delivery is very close to that attained from the same parenteral dose, suggesting that much of the effect of fentaNYL results from systemic uptake from the vasculature in the epidural space. FentaNYL also exhibits close structural similarity to LA, with clearly apparent effect on primary afferent C-fibers that may promote analgesia (Bujedo, 2015). FentaNYL is often used in PCEA because it allows for rapid titration of analgesia and is administered in small doses with LAs for spinal anesthesia and included in epidural analgesia for acute postoperative pain with LA (e.g., ropivacaine or bupivacaine) as continuous infusion (Hernandez et al., 2018). However, although hydrophilic opioids and LA combinations have shown a synergistic effect, it is unclear whether the fentaNYL and LA combination provides similar synergy and the benefit of this combination has been questioned (Hurley et al., 2015).

SUFentanil

SUFentanil is two times more lipid-soluble than fentaNYL, with quality of analgesia similar to that of fentaNYL. When given epidurally, SUFentanil's analgesic effect, like that of fentaNYL, is mainly systemic because of its lipophilicity; therefore administration epidurally as a sole agent is not better than parenteral use (Bujedo, 2014). Combined use of SUFentanil with LAs, similarly to fentaNYL, aids in lowering total dose of each medication, as well as severity of adverse effects, and enhances epidural analgesic effect (Bujedo, 2014). Many studies have shown that single-injection neuraxial (i.e., intrathecal or epidural) fentaNYL and SUFentanil when combined with LA for continuous epidural infusion and at appropriate dosing can be used in place of other opioids for epidural analgesia without increasing the risk for respiratory depression (Bujedo, 2013).

Local Anesthetics

LAs are used in regional, neuraxial, and truncal/peripheral analgesia techniques, to inhibit neural transmission of acute pain. Safe use requires understanding the chemical structure of LAs and basic pharmacodynamic and pharmacokinetic concepts, including potency, duration, and onset of action. When considering the feasibility of use of LAs, essential factors include information about the individual patient's medical condition and clinical situation, taking into account the anatomic location of actual or potential pain, desired duration of analgesia, and appropriate dosing. Specific content related to truncal/peripheral LA use is presented in a later section.

Mechanism of Action

LAs work by reversibly binding and inhibiting the voltage-gated sodium channel, preventing activation and sodium influx that is associated with membrane depolarization, propagation of an action potential, and subsequent nerve transmission (Butterworth, 2020; Lirk, Picardi, & Hollman, 2014). Much of the clinical application of LAs involves their ability to produce analgesia through temporary blockade of sodium channels in afferent and efferent neuronal membranes, thereby inhibiting the neural transmission of pain (see Chapter 15; Berde & Strichartz, 2015; Lirk et al., 2014).

When used for neuraxial blockade, LAs block voltage-gated sodium and potassium channels in the dorsal horn neurons. Blockade of voltage-gated calcium channel in the spinal cord along nerve axons produce reversible conduction blockade of neural transmission in the peripheral and central nerves producing intense analgesic action. LA administered in the epidural space is distributed into the CSF and carried to the dorsal root ganglion of the spinal nerve fibers immediately adjacent to their site of administration (see Figs. 18.3 and 18.5). This results in *segmental analgesia,* which is influenced by the location of catheter placement and dose and volume of the LA.

Effects of Local Anesthetics

Effects on Sensation and Motor Activity

LAs are associated with *differential inhibition of sensory and motor activity,* which is the ability to block sensation before motor activity occurs because LAs block nerve conduction in small nerve fibers faster and at lower concentrations than in large fibers (Brull et al., 2015a). It is possible to give very low doses of neuraxial LAs to block the impulses on the A-delta and C fibers without blocking the larger fibers that affect sensory and motor function (Patel & Sadoughi, 2015). The speed and the degree of nerve blockade are related to the size, surface area, and myelination of the nerve fibers that come in contact with the LA. Smaller nerve fibers are more sensitive to LAs because they have larger ratios of membrane surface area to axon unit. Sensory nerve fibers are smaller than motor fibers; therefore sensation is blocked before motor function; C fibers, which conduct cold and pain, are smaller than A-delta fibers, which conduct pinprick sensation, and A-delta fibers are smaller than A-beta fibers which conduct touch. Therefore, among the sensory fibers, cold sensation will be diminished before sharp pinprick sensation, and sharp pinprick will be diminished before touch. Motor fibers, A-alpha fibers, are larger than the sensory fibers, and therefore motor block does not occur until after sensory block. Reversal or resolution of block occurs in the reverse order because motor block resolves first, followed by touch, pinprick, and cold sensation (Brull et al., 2015a).

Vasodilatation

With the exception of cocaine, which is an LA with vasoconstrictor effects, most LAs have biphasic effects on the vasculature (Patel & Sadoughi, 2015). At lower doses they cause vasoconstriction, but with higher doses, they cause vasodilation. The more vasodilation that occurs, the faster the absorption and the shorter the duration of LA effect (Patel & Sadoughi, 2015). EPINEPHrine is sometimes added to LA solutions to reduce this vasodilatory effect.

Basic Chemical Structure

LAs are classified as amino-ester or amino-amide compounds and are similar in chemical structure (Butterworth, 2020). The chemical structure of a typical LA molecule consists of a hydrophilic amine at one end and a lipophilic (membrane-liking) aromatic (benzene) ring system at the other end. These two parts are linked by an intermediate chain that is either an amide or ester bond. The bond between the benzene ring and the linkage determines the classification of an LA and whether it is an amino-*ester* or amino-*amide* compound (Columb, Cegielski, & Haley, 2017). The type of linkage is clinically relevant because it has implications in pharmacologic effects, including metabolism, duration of action, and hypersensitivity reaction potential. An easy way to distinguish the chemical class that an LA belongs to is to remember that the amino-esters have one letter *i* in their generic name and the amino-amides

Table 18.6 | Classifications of Local Anesthetics

Local Anesthetic	Classification	Onset	Duration of Action
Chloroprocaine	Amino-ester	Very quick	Short
Procaine[a]	Amino-ester	Slow	Short
Tetracaine[a]	Amino-ester	Slow	Long
Lidocaine	Amino-amide	Quick	Intermediate
Mepivacaine	Amino-amide	Quick	Intermediate
Prilocaine	Amino-amide	Quick	Intermediate
Ropivacaine	Amino-amide	Slow	Long
Bupivacaine	Amino-amide	Slow	Long
Etidocaine	Amino-amide	Quick	Long

[a]Not generally used for epidural block because produce poor-quality blockade.
Culp, Jr., W. C., & Culp, W. C. (2011). Practical application of local anesthetics. *Journal of Vascular Interventional Radiology, 22,* 111–118; and Butterworth, J. IV (2020). Local Anesthetics: Clinical pharmacology of local anesthetics. *New York School of Regional Anesthesia (NYSORA).* Retrieved from https://www.nysora.com/foundations-of-regional-anesthesia/pharmacology/ clinical-pharmacology-local-anesthetics/. Retrieved August 19, 2020.

have two. Table 18.6 lists the classification of commonly used LAs.

Amino-esters typically have a shorter half-life and duration of action than amino-amides because they are more quickly degraded in the body. Amino-esters are metabolized primarily by plasma esterase. Amino-amides are metabolized by hepatic cytochrome P450–linked enzymes (CYP1A2 and CYP3A4) in the liver.

Physiologic and Chemical Activity

Factors that determine the ability of LAs to cross the membrane into the cell include the lipid solubility, intrinsic affinity for protein binding, diffusion properties, and percentage of ionized and nonionized forms.

- Lipid solubility is an important characteristic with a strong relationship to potency.
- Potency is increased as lipid solubility is increased. The greater the lipid solubility, the greater is the ability of the drug to penetrate, bind, and block the sodium channels. For example, bupivacaine is more lipid soluble and therefore has more potency than lidocaine.
- Lipid solubility is associated with plasma protein binding. Duration of action is determined by the degree of binding of the LA with the sodium channel. The more firmly bound an LA is to the sodium channel, the longer is the duration. For example, bupivacaine and ropivacaine are highly protein bound and have longer durations of action than less protein-bound medications such as lidocaine and prilocaine, which have moderate durations of action, and procaine, which has a very short duration of action.

- Speed of onset of the block is related to the diffusion properties. LAs are weak bases (pKa ~ 8–9) that exist in both ionized and nonionized forms, and the proportions vary based on the pH of the environment. The nonionized form of an LA is the form that is best able to diffuse across cell membranes. When the pH of the LA is similar to the pH of the tissues (7.35–7.45), there is a more nonionized form of LA and the onset of action will be rapid. If the pH of the tissues decreases (becomes more acidic), more of the LA becomes ionized, resulting in a delayed onset of action. Sodium bicarbonate ($NaHCO_3$) is often added to LAs to enhance the onset and blockade (Patel & Sadoughi, 2015).

Absorption and Distribution

Absorption of LA is directly related to drug mass and concentration, contact surface area, lipid content, and local tissue vascular supply (Brull et al., 2015a). The greater the vascularity of the area of LA administration, the greater the absorption. For example, LA concentration in the blood is highest after intercostal nerve blockade, lower in the epidural space, and even lower in the brachial plexus and subcutaneous tissue. To reduce potential LA toxicity, EPINEPHrine is sometimes administered along with LA to cause vasoconstriction and reduce vascular absorption (Berde & Strichartz, 2015).

Distribution, like absorption of LAs, is also affected by vascularity in the region of LA administration. LAs are distributed throughout all body tissues from injection sites, and well-perfused organs have higher concentrations than poorly perfused organs. LA distribution is of particular concern when used in neuraxial analgesia.

Absorption and distribution of LA affect the speed of onset of the LA effect. Onset of blockade by intrathecal (spinal) route is within a very few minutes after drug injection. When the epidural route is used, the onset of blockade usually can be detected within 5 minutes in dermatomes surrounding the injection site because LAs are delivered in the immediate vicinity of the spinal cord and spinal nerve roots (action sites).

When LA is used in spinal analgesia, it is distributed in the CSF through diffusion from areas of high concentration to areas of lower concentration. There is rostral spread of LA (from the injection site up toward the head) at the speed of CSF circulation flow, which is usually within 10 to 20 minutes.

Epidural LA may be distributed through one or more mechanisms. LA may cross the dura mater into the subarachnoid space, spread longitudinally (rostrally and caudally) up and down from the epidural space, spread within the epidural space circumferentially, leave the epidural space through the intervertebral foramina, bind to epidural fat, and/or be absorbed into epidural blood vessels (Brull et al., 2015a). Longitudinal spread is more likely when larger volumes of LA are used; leakage of LA through the intervertebral foramina is more common in the elderly, those with spinal stenosis, and those with increased epidural pressure as in pregnancy (Brull et al., 2015a). The direction of distribution is influenced by the level of epidural administration. Lumbar and low thoracic injection usually leads to distribution toward the head, and high thoracic injection leads to caudal distribution (Brull et al., 2015a). Awareness of the potential variability in LA distribution is important because it aids in explaining reasons for inadequate analgesia and anticipating and identifying possible LA-associated adverse effects.

Dose and baricity of the selected LA are the most significant factors that affect the distribution and height of neuraxial block, although other factors such as volume, concentration, and temperature also have a role. LA dose is a main determinant in the quality of neuraxial analgesia; as the dose is increased, time to onset, effectiveness, and duration are also increased. Dose can be increased by administering a larger volume of the medication or by using a more concentrated solution. The volume of medication used with epidural administration can influence the spread of the LA. For example, administration of 30 mL of 1% lidocaine will spread at least four dermatomes higher than 10 mL of 3% lidocaine, providing a broader area of analgesia (Berde & Strichartz, 2015).

Baricity refers to the ratio of the density (heaviness) of the LA to the density of the CSF (Brull et al., 2015a). Isobaric medications have the same density as CSF, and the spread of isobaric medications in the spinal canal is not influenced by gravitational forces; hypobaric LAs have lower density than CSF and will spread to nondependent areas of the spinal canal, whereas hyperbaric LAs with higher density than that of the CSF will spread to dependent areas of the spinal canal because of gravitational forces (Brull et al., 2015a). For example, if a hyperbaric LA was used in spinal analgesia, and the patient is placed in a right side-lying position, the LA will spread to the dependent area of the spinal canal and the patient will have a greater block on the right side.

Metabolism and Excretion of Local Anesthetics LA metabolism varies according to the medication's chemical structure. Amino esterases are metabolized primarily by plasma pseudocholinesterases; amino-amide type LAs are mostly metabolized in the liver and excreted by the kidneys (Lehman, 2017).

Local Anesthetic Choices

Many different LAs are available for neuraxial analgesia. The choice of LA is largely determined by the administration route, desired intensity of block, desired time to onset, and duration of LA effect. LAs can be categorized into short-, intermediate-, and long-acting (see Table 18.6). Long-acting LAs provide analgesia for 3 to 4 hours after administration versus 1 to 2 hours after intermediate-acting medications. Duration of the effect of short- and intermediate-acting LAs can be prolonged by the addition of 1:200,000 EPINEPHrine. In some cases,

Table 18.7 | Local Anesthetics for Epidural Analgesia

Drug	Concentration (%)	Onset Time (min)	Duration (min)
2-Chloroprocaine	3	5–15	30–90
Lidocaine	2	10–20	60–120
Bupivacaine	0.0625–0.5	15–20	160–220
Ropivacaine	0.1–0.75	15–20	140–220
Levobupivacaine	0.0625–0.5	15–20	150–225

Duration of blockade can be prolonged by addition of epinephrine, typically 1:200:000 to 1:400:000.
From Hadzic, A. (2017). *Textbook of regional anesthesia and acute pain management.* New York: McGraw-Hill Medical.

Table 18.8 | Recommended Epidural Infusion Rate of Local Anesthetics

Thoracic epidural	3–6 mL/h
Lumbar epidural	6–10 mL/h

From Hadzic, A. (2017). *Textbook of regional anesthesia and acute pain management.* New York: McGraw-Hill Medical.

when a more prolonged duration of LA effect is desired, a catheter for continuous LA infusion, rather than a single-shot injection of LA may be appropriate.

Although any of the LAs can be used for neuraxial analgesia, low concentrations of the lipid-soluble, amide-type LAs bupivacaine (e.g., 0.05%–0.125%) and ropivacaine (e.g., 0.05%–0.2%) are often used for epidural anesthesia/analgesia. Ropivacaine is less lipophilic and its potency is 0.6 that of bupivacaine. Ropivacaine is less likely to produce motor blockade than an equivalent dose of bupivacaine and is also associated with less cardiac toxicity than bupivacaine (Bindra, Singh, & Gupta, 2017; Brull et al., 2015a). Table 18.7 provides a summary of the pharmacokinetics of commonly used neuraxial LAs for single-shot epidural injection. Table 18.8 summarizes recommended epidural infusion rates of LA based on spinal placement levels.

Multimodal Analgesia Using Neuraxial Opioids and Local Anesthetics

The use of a combination of neuraxial opioid and LA may offer greater benefits than either medication alone; combination of these medications, a form of MMA, provides better analgesia, may prolong the local analgesic effect of sensory blockade, and may reduce the dose of LA (Hurley et al., 2015). Studies are needed to determine the most beneficial combination and doses of these medications in various acute pain conditions.

Table 18.9 | Examples of Patient-Controlled Epidural Analgesia Regimens

Analgesic Solution	Continuous Rate (mL/h)	Demand Dose (mL)	Lockout Interval (min)
General Regimens			
0.05% bupivacaine + 4 μg/mL fentaNYL	4	2	10–20
0.0625% bupivacaine + 5 μg/mL fentaNYL	4–8	3–5	10–20
0.1% bupivacaine + 5 μg/mL fentaNYL	6	2	10–20
0.2% ropivacaine + 5 μg/mL fentaNYL	5	2	20
Thoracic Surgery			
0.0625%–0.125% bupivacaine + 5 μg/mL fentaNYL	3–4	2–3	10–20
Abdominal Surgery			
0.0625% bupivacaine + 5 μg/mL fentaNYL	4–8	3–5	10–20
0.125% bupivacaine + 0.5 μg/mL SUFentanil	3–5	2–3	10–20
0.1%–0.2% ropivacaine + 2 μg/mL fentaNYL	3–5	2–5	10–20
Lower Extremity Surgery			
0.0625%–0.125% bupivacaine + 5 μg/mL fentaNYL	4–8	3–5	10–20

From Hurley, R. W., Murphy, J. D., & Wu, C. L. (2015). Acute postoperative pain. In R. D. Miller (Ed.), *Miller's anesthesia* (pp. 2974–2998). Philadelphia: Saunders.

Table 18.9 provides examples of patient-controlled epidural analgesia regimens and concentrations of analgesic solutions containing neuraxial opioids and LAs.

Coanalgesic Medications Used in Neuraxial Analgesia

Several types of medications may be added to neuraxial infusions for acute pain management, but there is not widespread use. Alpha$_2$-adrenergic agonists (cloNIDine and dexmedetomidine) are used neuraxially, and EPINEPHrine is used epidurally to improve postoperative pain. All of these medications can be given alone or in combination with other medications. The rationale for combining medications is that, as components of a multimodal analgesic plan of care, they work synergistically to provide better analgesia and fewer adverse effects at lower doses. Although there has been interest in the use of ketamine as a neuraxial medication, this route is avoided because of possible negative effects on CNS development in children, and neurotoxicity and psychomimetic effects in adults (Gallagher & Grant, 2018).

Epinephrine

Epidural EPINEPHrine has been shown to improve postoperative analgesia and can improve sensory blockade at doses of 2 to 5 mcg/mL (Brull et al., 2015a). EPINEPHrine may be used in combination with LA to intensify and prolong the effect of LA, especially when administered with lidocaine and 2-chloroprocaine, but has less of an effect when used with bupivacaine, and even less effect when used with ropivacaine (Warren, Nelson, & Neal, 2018). EPINEPHrine is also used to test for inadvertent intravascular injection when an epidural injection or catheter placement is attempted. The addition of 15 mcg of EPINEPHrine to LA would result in a rapid increase in heart rate and systolic blood pressure if the test dose is injected into the intravascular compartment (Warren, Nelson, & Neal, 2018).

Alpha$_2$-Adrenergic Agonists (CloNIDine and Dexmedetomidine)

CloNIDine, an alpha$_2$-adrenergic agonist, is used in neuraxial analgesia to attenuate nociceptive input from A-delta and C-fibers (see Chapter 15). When added neuraxially in small doses, it improves pain control, produces dose-sparing effects, and prolongs duration of analgesia without major side effects (Allen, Mishriky, Klinger, & Habib, 2018). In a 2018 systematic review and meta-analysis that examined the efficacy of perioperative neuraxial cloNIDine alone or in combination with LAs and/or opioids during elective cesarean sections, neuraxial cloNIDine reduced morphine use in the first 24 hours postoperatively and prolonged time to the first analgesic request compared to the placebo group (Allen et al., 2018). Use of neuraxial cloNIDine in the treatment of acute pain is limited by its side effects, which include hypotension, bradycardia, and sedation (Hurley et al., 2015). Additionally, when used in combination with opioids, an exacerbation of side effects can occur, making it important to require close monitoring throughout the infusion and the first few hours after discontinuation of the infusion.

Another alpha$_2$-adrenergic agonist, dexmedetomidine, exerts its sedative and analgesic-sparing effects through central actions in the higher centers in the brain and the dorsal horn of the spinal cord. Dexmedetomidine has analgesic and sedative effects when given postoperatively as an adjuvant to ropivacaine in low-dose epidural infusions (Kiran, Jinjil, Tandon, & Kar, 2018). Further research and clinical experience with dexmedetomidine in this setting is needed to define a role in epidural analgesia.

In a prospective double-blind randomized trial that included 80 patients who underwent abdominal hysterectomies, epidural cloNIDine was compared to epidural dexmedetomidine as an LA adjunct. The dexmedetomidine group had significantly ($P < .05$) earlier onset and more prolonged analgesia and was associated with more stable cardiopulmonary parameters than the cloNIDine group (Chiruvella, Donthu, Nallam, & Salla, 2018).

Administration of Neuraxial Medications

In addition to single bolus injection of neuraxial medication, the other methods for administration of neuraxial medications are (1) continuous infusion or basal rate administered through an infusion pump, (2) clinician-administered intermittent bolus, (3) PCEA, and (4) programmed intermittent epidural bolus (PIEB). In caring for patients with neuraxial catheters, including management and monitoring, the registered nurse (RN) should practice as defined by the hospital's policies and procedures and in accordance with the board of nursing in the state in which the RN practices.

Continuous Infusion

Providing continuous pain control with neuraxial analgesia can be accomplished by using an external infusion pump to deliver a continuous infusion (also called *basal rate*) of an analgesic solution. During continuous infusions of neuraxial analgesics, assessment of the patient's response to the infusion, including pain assessment and assessment for development of unintended effects, is necessary. Continuous epidural infusions are usually delivered through an externalized catheter that is connected to an infusion pump dedicated for use with regional analgesia. When a patient is approaching end of life or in other situations in which longer use is needed, a special type of tunneled epidural catheter may be used to allow longer use of the infusion (Patel, 2015).

Clinician-Administered Intermittent Bolus

Intermittent bolus may be administered by a clinician when an epidural catheter is in place. It may be given as a single injection or along with a continuous infusion for breakthrough pain. The incidence of breakthrough pain usually determines how frequently the bolus is ordered.

Clinician-administered intermittent epidural analgesic bolus as a single injection is used less today with advances in infusion delivery devices that allow for continuous infusion, PCEA, and PIEB of analgesic therapy required for pain control. Refer to Box 18.8 for guidelines for administering intermittent bolus doses through a temporary epidural catheter.

When a spinal is performed for acute pain, a single injection of analgesic medication is administered intrathecally by an anesthesiologist, specially trained physician, or credentialed advanced practice provider. Additional patient monitoring is needed during and after a bolus of neuraxial medications to identify and address unintended effects associated with the type of medication administered.

Patient-Controlled Epidural Analgesia

PCEA allows individualization of analgesic requirements through preset programmed doses of the infusion that the patient may self-administer to meet individual analgesic requirements. PCEA may offer several advantages over continuous epidural infusions, including lower medication use, reduction in undesirable side effects, and greater patient satisfaction (Soffin & Liu, 2018). In contrast to intravenous patient-controlled analgesia (PCA), PCEA usually involves the use of a basal infusion, usually an LA with or without an opioid, to maintain continuous segmental sensory block, and the patient-controlled bolus doses are used to manage breakthrough pain (Soffin & Liu, 2018). (See Chapter 17 for more information related to the use of PCA and Table 18.9 for examples of PCEA infusion regimens.)

Programmed Intermittent Epidural Bolus

PIEB that supports automated administration of epidural solution boluses by a programmed pump is increasingly used in labor and delivery. The pump is preprogrammed to deliver a specific volume at specific time intervals. In the setting of labor and delivery, where this technique is often used, the automated bolus technique is proposed to provide better distribution of LA solution in the epidural space, thereby providing an effective mode of pain control during labor. In a prospective, randomized, blinded–end-point study of 130 pregnant women, Nunes, Nunes, Viega, Cortez, and Seifert (2015) found PIEB was associated with a significantly reduced incidence of cesarean delivery (more vaginal deliveries), high maternal satisfaction, and no adverse outcomes. No differences in motor block, instrumental delivery rate, and neonatal outcomes were observed.

Although PIEB has been predominantly studied in patients during labor, there is research related to its use in other patient populations. In a study of women who had open gynecologic surgeries under combined general-epidural anesthesia, when ropivacaine with fentaNYL solutions were administered by PIEB (n = 28) compared to continuous epidural infusions (CEIs) (n = 29), and ropivacaine epidural bolus rescue doses were available, the PIEB group required significantly less LA ($P = .016$)

Box 18.8 | Intermittent Boluses by a Short-Term Epidural Catheter by the Registered Nurse

- Requires institutional policy and procedure and state board of nursing that supports intermittent bolus via epidural catheters by the registered nurse (RN).
- Administer only preservative-free solutions that are labeled safe for spinal use.
- Before injecting, verify with another RN and the electronic medical record that the preservative-free medication, dose, and volume are in accordance with anesthesia provider's order.
- Before injecting, verify that the catheter to be injected is the epidural catheter. (Most catheters are color-coded to prevent errors, but this should always be checked before injection.)
- To prevent exerting too much pressure on injection, administer analgesic in at least a 10-mL syringe.
- The use of indwelling epidural filters depends on institutional policy (see text). A filter straw or needle should be used to draw solutions from glass ampules; if solutions are drawn unfiltered from glass ampules, they always should be injected through a 0.22-micron filter.
- Maintain sterility of the epidural system when removing catheter port cap, attaching syringes, and replacing port cap. (Some institutions require disinfecting connection before removing port cap. Use only nonneurotoxic agents to disinfect the epidural catheter connections or ports (alcohol should not be used to disinfect catheter connections or ports).
- Before injecting analgesic, gently aspirate catheter; allow time for fluid/air to travel up catheter[a] and into the syringe.
- Minimal fluid return (e.g., < 0.5 mL) or an air bubble in the syringe indicates catheter is in the epidural space.
  - Steadily (speed of injection depends on resistance met during injection) inject analgesic through catheter filter (if filter is used).
- Free-flowing clear fluid (cerebrospinal fluid) return indicates catheter may be in the intrathecal space.
  - Do not administer analgesic; notify anesthesia provider.

- Bloody aspirate indicates catheter may be in a blood vessel.
  - Do not administer analgesic; notify anesthesia provider.
- Do not inject solution if patient reports pain on steady injection; notify anesthesia provider.
- Some resistance during injection is normal, but if strong resistance is met during injection, reposition the patient so that the spine is flexed. If resistance continues, stop and notify anesthesia provider.
- Do not flush epidural catheter after injecting solution unless specifically ordered to do so.

When moderate to severe pain is expected to be constant for more than 24 hours, the epidural catheter is sometimes left in place to provide intermittent analgesic bolus doses. A majority of patients require epidural opioid bolus doses every 8 hours. Patients should be assessed systematically because frequency varies depending on analgesic requirement and opioid characteristics; some patients may require dosing more often (e.g., every 6 hours), whereas others may require boluses every 12 to 24 hours.

[a] Some anesthesia providers require the administration of a small test dose of local anesthetic (e.g., bupivacaine or ropivacaine) containing EPINEPHrine to rule out intravascular or intrathecal migration before bolus administration; check with the state board of nursing before performing this function.

From Pasero, C., & McCaffery, M. (2011). *Pain assessment and pharmacologic management* (p. 414). St. Louis: Mosby. Data from email communication and review on August 13, 2009, by Carol Mulvenon, MS, RN-BC, AOCN, ACHPN, Clinical Nurse Specialist, Pain Management-Palliative Care-Oncology, St. Joseph Medical Center, Kansas City, MO. Additional information from DuPen, S. L., & DuPen, A. R. (1998). Spinal analgesia. In M. A. Ashburn, & L. J. Rice (Eds.), *The management of pain*, New York: Churchill Livingstone; Grape, S., & Schug, S. A. (2008). Epidural and spinal analgesia. In P. E. Macintyre, S. M. Walker, & D. J. Rowbotham (Eds.), *Clinical pain management: Acute pain* (2nd ed.). London: Hodder Arnold; Maalouf, D. B., & Liu, S. S. (2009). Clinical application of epidural analgesia. In R. S. Sinatra, O. A. de Leon-Casasola, & B. Ginsberg, et al. (Eds.), *Acute pain management.* (pp. 221–229). Cambridge, NY; Cambridge University Press; Pasero, C., Eksterowicz, N., Primeau, M., & Cowley, C. (2007). ASPMN position statement: Registered nurse management and monitoring of analgesia by catheter techniques. *Pain Management Nursing, 8*(2), 48–54. © 2011, Pasero, C., & McCaffery, M. May be duplicated for use in clinical practice.

at the end of the 40-hour postsurgery study period; pain scores measured throughout the study period were significantly lower for the PIEB group at all study measurement points (Satomi et al., 2018). In a similar type of study in which 110 patients who had undergone colon, pancreatic, or gynecologic surgeries were randomized to either a PIEB or CEI group, the PIEB group required significantly lower amounts of LA rescue epidural bolus doses, but there were no clinically significant differences in pain scores or morphine use between the two groups (Wiesmann et al., 2018).

Unintended Effects of Neuraxial Analgesics

Medications administered by the neuraxial route may be associated with adverse effects ranging from minor in severity to very severe and life threatening. It is important to assess patients for development of these unintended effects and address them promptly. The adverse effects associated with commonly administered neuraxial analgesics, opioids and LAs, are addressed in the following paragraphs.

Neuraxial Opioid Adverse Effects

In an updated 2016 report on practice guidelines for the prevention, detection, and management of respiratory depression associated with neuraxial opioid administration, the American Society of Anesthesiologists Task Force on Neuraxial Opioids and the American Society of Regional Anesthesia and Pain Medicine (ASRA) reported that in a meta-analysis of RCTs, less respiratory depression is associated with the continuous infusion of epidural opioids than continuous infusion of intravenous opioids, and continuous epidural opioids are preferred over parenteral opioids to reduce the risk for respiratory depression (ASA Committee on Practice Standards, 2016). Although it is estimated that the risk for respiratory depression may be as low as 0.07%, there is still a need for assessment of patients for advancing sedation and respiratory depression (Solanki & Akhouri, 2017). Risk factors for opioid-related respiratory depression associated with neuraxial opioids are similar to risk factors associated with opioid administration addressed in Chapter 13. To prevent respiratory depression associated with neuraxial opioids, interventions such as those addressed in Chapter 13 may be appropriate. Consideration should be given to the use of noninvasive positive pressure ventilation and choice of opioid (lipophilic versus hydrophilic) (ASA Committee on Practice Standards, 2016).

Lipophilic epidural opioids such as fentaNYL are associated with earlier onset of respiratory depression (within 2–4 hours after administration) than hydrophilic opioids such as morphine (6–12 hours after administration) (Hernandez et al., 2018). The earlier onset of respiratory depression with lipophilic epidural opioids is explained by rapid systemic absorption of the medication from the epidural venous plexus with circulation to the brain; hydrophilic medication is not systemically absorbed, and therefore respiratory depression occurs later as the medication spreads slowly and rostrally in the CSF to the brain (Hernandez et al., 2018). Because of the delayed risk for respiratory depression and longer duration of action of hydrophilic opioids, it is recommended to avoid use of neuraxial morphine or HYDROmorphone in surgical patients undergoing outpatient procedures (ASA Committee on Practice Standards, 2016).

Respiratory depression associated with administration of epidural opioids may necessitate treatment with intravenous naloxone. Although a dose in the range of 0.1 to 0.4 mg is often effective, when reversing the effects of hydrophilic opioids, a continuous naloxone infusion (0.5–5 mcg/kg/h) may be necessary because of the long duration of action of the hydrophilic opioid (Hernandez et al., 2018).

To promptly identify and intervene to prevent neuraxial opioid-related respiratory depression, frequent and close monitoring of sedation level and respiratory status, including oxygenation and ventilation, is necessary. The frequency and duration of monitoring are based on the patient's clinical condition, opioid-related risk factors, type of opioid, duration of action of the opioid, delivery technique, and administration of other medications (Jungquist et al., 2020). For example, the use of EREM requires an extended monitoring period, 48 hours or longer, because of its hydrophilicity and extended duration of action. A single injection of a lipophilic opioid such as fentaNYL will have a short duration of action, so in many cases, closer monitoring may be discontinued after 2 hours (ASA Committee on Practice Standards, 2016). When continuous epidural infusions of opioids are administered, close monitoring is continued during the infusion and until the effect of the opioid has resolved. Table 18.10 summarizes minimum monitoring recommendations. Once the effect of the neuraxial opioid has resolved, monitoring of sedation level and respiratory status returns to baseline as necessitated by the patient's condition and use of concurrent medications.

Similar to parenteral opioid unintended effects, other neuraxial opioid unintended effects include nausea, vomiting, pruritus, and urinary retention. Nausea and vomiting may result from direct exposure of the chemoreceptive trigger zone in the medulla to the opioid. The incidence with a single dose of epidural opioid is 20% to 50% and increases to 45% to 80% with continuous epidural infusion (Ray et al., 2018). Nausea and vomiting may be dose-dependent and are more commonly associated with neuraxial hydrophilic opioids, especially morphine (Ray et al., 2018). Treatment options include naloxone, droperidol, metoclopramide, ondansetron, dexamethasone, and transdermal scopolamine (Hernandez et al., 2018).

Pruritus occurs more often with spinal opioids than epidural opioids (Toledano & Van de Velde, 2017). The incidence of pruritus with epidural opioids is 30% to 100%, compared to 15% to 18% with intravenous opioids, and the incidence is similar in lipophilic and hydrophilic opioids (Tubog, Harenberg, Buszta, & Hestand, 2018). The cause of pruritus with epidural opioids is unclear, but not related to peripheral histamine release; therefore antihistamines do not provide relief. The cause of pruritus with epidural opioids is thought to have a central (CNS) origin and mu antagonists (naloxone) and mixed mu antagonist/kappa agonists (nalbuphine and butorphanol) are the most effective treatment options (Bujedo, 2016; Hernandez et al., 2018). Serotonin 5HT3 receptor antagonists (e.g., ondansetron) may be useful in preventing and treating central pruritus. Urinary retention with epidural opioids, with an incidence as high as 80%, may be due to increased detrusor muscle strength contraction from activation of spinal opioid receptors (Hernandez et al., 2018).

Many of the neuraxial opioid unintended effects described earlier may be lessened or eliminated by dose reductions or rotations to a different medication; the use of low-dose intravenous naloxone may be effective, but the benefits must be weighed against the risk for analgesia reversal (Hernandez et al., 2018). (Chapter 12 provides a more in-depth description of the unintended effects of opioids.)

Table 18.10	Neuraxial Opioids: Recommended Minimum Monitoring	
Type of Neuraxial Opioid and Administration Technique	**Minimum Monitoring Recommendations**
Lipophilic opioid: Single neuraxial injection (e.g., fentaNYL, SUFentanil)	Monitor continuously for first 20 minutes after administration. Monitor every hour for a minimum of 2 hours. Return to usual monitoring after 2 hours or as indicated by patient condition and concurrent medications.
Continuous epidural infusion or patient controlled-epidural analgesia with lipophilic opioids	Continual monitoring for first 20 minutes. Then monitor at least hourly for total 12 hours. Then monitor at least once every 2 hours for next 12 hours. After 24 hours, monitor at least once every 4 hours. After discontinuation, return to usual monitoring or as indicated by patient condition and concurrent medications.
Hydrophilic opioid: Single neuraxial injection (e.g., morphine or HYDROmorphone) Does not include sustained- or extended-release epidural morphine	Monitor at least hourly for the first 12 hours after administration. Then monitor at least once every 2 hours for next 12 hours. After 24 hours, return to usual monitoring or as indicated by patient condition and concurrent medications.
Continuous epidural infusion or patient-controlled epidural analgesia with hydrophilic opioids	Monitor at least hourly for the first 12 hours after initiation of the infusion. Then monitor at least once every 2 hours for next 12 hours. After 24 hours, monitor at least once every 4 hours. After discontinuation of the infusion, return to usual monitoring or as indicated by patient condition and concurrent medications.
Sustained- or extended-release epidural morphine	Monitor at least hourly for the first 12 hours after administration. Then monitor at least once every 2 hours for next 12 hours. After 24 hours, monitor at least once every 4 hours for a minimum of 48 hours. Then return to usual monitoring or as indicated by patient condition and concurrent medications.

From American Society of Anesthesiology Committee on Practice Standards. (2016). Practice Guidelines for the prevention, detection and management of respiratory depression associated with neuraxial opioid administration: An updated report by the American Society of Anesthesiologists task force on neuraxial opioids and the American Society of Regional Anesthesia and Pain Medicine. *Anesthesiology, 124*(3), 535–552.

Unintended Effects of Neuraxial Local Anesthetics

The use of neuraxial LAs is associated with potential adverse effects and complications. In addition to the CNS, neuraxial LAs may be associated with unintended effects on other organ systems (Catterall & Mackie, 2018). The unintended effects may range from predictable and mild to significant and life threatening. Table 18.11 summarizes common unintended effects of epidural LAs, causes, assessment, and recommendations for reporting to anesthesia/pain specialists.

Allergic Reaction

True immunoglobulin E (IgE)-mediated allergy to LAs is uncommon, occurring in fewer than 1% of all LA-related reactions and more commonly associated with amino-ester anesthetics (see Table 18.6); the cause of the hypersensitivity is thought to be metabolization of amino-ester to para-aminobenzoic acid (PABA), which is a known allergen (Patel & Sadoughi, 2015). Although rare, allergic reactions to amino-amide type LAs may result, particularly

from the use of multidose vials of amino-amide LAs that contain PABA as a preservative (Butterworth, 2020).

Local Anesthetic Neurotoxicity

The direct effects of LAs on the nervous system tissue at the site of injection can cause LA-related neurotoxicity. Cauda equina syndrome is an example of a serious condition that may result from LA toxicity. It is characterized by the acute loss of neurologic function below the termination (conus) of the spinal cord as a result of damage to the spinal nerve roots. The cauda equina consists of nerves that are partially unmyelinated and have increased exposed surface area, making them prone to contact with neurotoxic agents such as LAs. Maldistribution and excessive LA dose concentration in the CSF may contribute to cauda equina syndrome (Chin & van Zundert, 2017).

Transient neurologic symptoms are another clinical representation of LA neurotoxicity. They are characterized by radicular pain without motor deficit that occurs after spinal anesthesia and spontaneously resolves typically within 72 hours; the majority of cases result in complete resolution (Verlinde et al., 2016). Pain is mild to

Table 18.11 | Assessment of Unintended Effects of Epidural Local Anesthetics

Unwanted Effect	Cause and Comments	Assessment	What to Report
Sensory and/or motor deficit	Many factors, including vertebral location of the epidural catheter, local anesthetic concentration and dose, and variability in patient response, can result in patients experiencing unwanted sensory and/or motor deficit. The lower the level of epidural catheter placement, the lower the affected dermatome.	*Sensory deficit:* At least every shift, ask patients to point to numb and tingling skin areas (numbness and tingling at the incision site is common and usually normal). An alcohol swab may be brushed lightly on the skin to determine level of sensation as well. *Motor deficit:* At least every shift, ask patients to bend their knee and lift the buttocks off the mattress. Most are able to do this without difficulty. Determine patient ability to bear weight and ambulate. Ask patients to remain in bed if unable to bear weight. Provide assisted ambulation as needed.	Complete loss of sensation in a skin area Muscle weakness, inability to move extremities or bear weight Numbness and tingling in areas distant to the nociceptive site Changes in sensory or motor deficit from last assessment (e.g., a lower location or increased intensity) Unresolved deficits after changes in therapy have been made
Urinary retention	When epidural analgesics are delivered close to the micturation center, located in the lower segments of the spinal cord, there is a risk of urinary retention. The combination of epidural local anesthetics and opioids can cause relaxation of the detrusor muscle. An opioid-induced increase in sphincter tone can make urination difficult. The central effects of opioids and motor and sensory blockade can interfere with perception of bladder fullness and the patient's attention to bladder stimuli.	Regularly assess for bladder distention; in and out or Foley catheterization if needed.	Persistent urinary retention
Local anesthetic toxicity	Toxicity can result from vascular uptake or injection or infusion of local anesthetic directly into the systemic circulation. Older adults and patients with hepatic impairment may be at higher risk for toxicity from accumulation because most have a decreased ability to clear local anesthetics.	Regularly assess for and ask patients about signs of local anesthetic toxicity: Circumoral tingling and numbness, ringing in the ears, metallic taste, slow speech, irritability, twitching, seizures, and cardiac dysrhythmias. Stop local anesthetic administration if signs are present.	Signs of local anesthetic toxicity
Adverse hemodynamic effects	Because local anesthetics block nerve fibers, they affect the sympathetic nervous system and cause vasodilation. Mild hypotension is common. Some patients receiving neuraxial local anesthetics experience significant hypotension and bradycardia, especially when rising from a prone position or after large dose increases or boluses. Thoracic placement of the epidural catheter is associated with fewer hemodynamic disturbances.	Regular assessment of heart rate and blood pressure, including orthostatic blood pressure before ambulation until dose is stabilized and it is clear that bradycardia and hypotension are not problems.	Symptomatic hypotension and/or bradycardia Persistent hypotension and/or bradycardia Symptomatic orthostatic hypotension

Note: Epidural local anesthetics can produce some unwanted effects. This table lists the causes of some of these effects and how to assess and when to report them.
From Pasero, C., & McCaffery, M. (2011). *Pain assessment and pharmacologic management* (pp. 428–429). St. Louis: Mosby. Data from Dabu-Bondoc, S., Franco, S. A., & Sinatra, R. S. (2009). Neuraxial analgesia with hydromorphone, morphine, and fentanyl: Dosing and safety guidelines. In R. S. Sinatra, O. A. de Leon-Casasola, B. Ginsberg, et al. (Eds.), *Acute pain management.* (pp. 230–244). Cambridge, NY: Cambridge University Press; Grape, S., & Schug, S. A. (2008). Epidural and spinal analgesia. In P. E. Macintyre, S. M. Walker, & D. J. Rowbotham (Eds.), *Clinical pain management: Acute pain* (2nd ed.). London: Hodder Arnold; and Maalouf, D. B., & Liu, S. S. (2009). Clinical application of epidural analgesia. In R. S. Sinatra, O. A. de Leon-Casasola, B. Ginsberg, et al. (Eds.), *Acute pain management.* (pp. 221–229). Cambridge, NY: Cambridge University Press. © 2011, Pasero, C., & McCaffery, M. May be duplicated for use in clinical practice.

severe and may be bilateral or unilateral, occurring in the buttocks and radiating to the leg(s). It is more common with intrathecal injections of lidocaine or mepivacaine and less common with bupivacaine or epidural procedures (Brull et al., 2015a).

Local Anesthetic Systemic Toxicity

All LAs are capable of producing local and systemic toxicity when excessively high plasma concentrations of LA exist. LA systemic toxicity (LAST) is related to the rate of entry of LA into systemic circulation, redistribution of LA to tissue sites, and LA clearance, which depends on the type, initial LA dose, and injection site vascularity. Reduced elimination and slow metabolic degradation can also contribute to LAST (Patel & Sadoughi, 2015), The use of EPINEPHrine with LA administration can reduce LA systemic toxicity because the vasoconstriction caused by the EPINEPHrine can delay LA absorption.

Risk Factors for LAST

The most common cause of LAST is inadvertent intravascular injection during placement of regional anesthesia-analgesia procedures. Clinically toxic blood levels can also occur when there is excessive absorption from the injection site (no intravascular injection). Other factors affecting toxicity are body weight, age, physical status of the patient (renal, hepatic, cardiac failure, and pregnancy), and drug-drug interactions. The risk for adverse reactions is directly proportional to the amount of LA in systemic circulation; therefore prevention by careful selection of patient, medication, concentration, and volume is necessary (Neal et al., 2018b). When assessing for risk for toxicity, the potency of the LA must be taken into consideration because LAs may differ in potency by approximately 40% to 50%. In animal models, when taking this equipotency into account, there was no difference between bupivacaine and ropivacaine in reaching the toxic LA threshold and eliciting CNS symptoms.

Signs and Symptoms of LAST

Early CNS signs of systemic toxicity include ringing in the ears, metallic taste, circumoral or tongue numbness or tingling, metallic taste, diplopia, dizziness, abrupt onset of excitation (e.g., anxiety, agitation, confusion, muscle twitching). Late signs include seizures, generally tonic and clonic, and depressed level of consciousness (drowsiness, obtundation, coma, or apnea) (Noble, 2015). Signs of cardiotoxicity initially include transient hypertension, tachycardia and ventricular arrhythmia that progress to hypotension, conduction block, bradycardia or asystole, and cardiovascular collapse. Although the usual LAST initial manifestation involves CNS signs with or within a minute of LA administration, atypical manifestation of cardiovascular signs without CNS changes, CNS signs combined with cardiovascular signs and symptoms, and delayed manifestation (several minutes up to 60 minutes after LA injection) have been reported (Neal et al., 2018b). Although rare, LAST can be a catastrophic complication of regional anesthesia/analgesia; therefore, techniques for reducing risk and treatment protocols are essential.

Strategies to Reduce Risks for LAST

Several interventions can be used to optimize safety and reduce the risks associated with LAST. It is important to have access to appropriate monitors and have resuscitation equipment in place whenever regional anesthesia is performed. Measures to reduce risks for LAST include the following (Neal et al., 2018b):

- Use lowest effective dose of LA.
- Use ultrasound imaging for regional analgesia, including epidural anesthesia-analgesia.
- Use fractional LA dosing with multiple aspirations in divided aliquots, slow LA injection speed, and a LA test dose (usually containing EPINEPHrine) to determine accurate needle placement into epidural space or perineurally at insertion or to reassess if catheter migration is suspected.
- Avoid repeated injections of LAs over a short time interval.

Treatment of LAST

On recognition of signs and symptoms of LAST, it is recommended to ensure prompt and effective management of the airway followed by the administration of lipid emulsion therapy (Neal et al., 2018b). Previously, it was thought that use of lipid emulsion therapy was unnecessary unless the patient experienced a cardiac arrhythmia, prolonged seizures, or rapid clinical deterioration. In more recent guidelines, as a result of recognition that lipid emulsion therapy is most effective if administered early in the onset of LAST, early lipid emulsion therapy is advised (Neal et al., 2018b).

Lipid emulsion therapy involves the administration of 20% intravenous lipids, which act to carry the lipophilic LAs to sites for storage and detoxification. In addition, the lipid emulsion is thought to increase cardiac output through volume enhancement and direct cardiotonic effects (Gitman, Fettiplace, Weinberg, Neal, & Barrington, 2019). Box 18.9 provides recommendations for treatment of LAST, including use of lipid emulsion therapy (Neal, Woodward, & Harrison, 2018a).

Cardiovascular Unintended Effects

Hypotension

LAs used in neuraxial analgesia can block sympathetic nerve fibers and lead to decreased systemic vascular resistance, vasodilation, and hypotension. This is a particular concern in patients with high sensory block height (level of T5 or higher) and in those who are dehydrated or experiencing volume depletion from other causes.

Box 18.9 | Treatment of Local Anesthetic Systemic Toxicity

1. Prompt and effective airway management
2. Lipid emulsion therapy:
   a. 20% lipid emulsion BOLUS (propofol is not a substitute for lipid emulsion)
      1) 100 mL over 2 to 3 min if over 70 kg
      2) 1.5 mL/kg over 2 to 3 min if less than 70 kg
   b. 20% lipid emulsion infusion
      1) 200 to 250 mL over 15 to 20 min if over 70 kg
      2) 0.25 mL/kg/min if less than 70 kg
   c. If circulatory instability not achieved after the previous step, repeat bolus or increase infusion to 0.5 mL/kg/min
   d. Continue infusion for at least 10 minutes after circulatory stability is attained
   e. Upper dosing limit is 12 mL/kg
3. Seizure control
   a. Benzodiazepines (lipid emulsion or *small* doses of propofol if benzodiazepines unavailable; propofol may further depress cardiac function)
   b. If seizures persist, small doses of succinylcholine or another neuromuscular blocker
4. Cardiac arrest
   a. Small initial doses of EPINEPHrine (≤ 1 mcg/kg)
   b. Vasopressin not recommended
   c. Avoid calcium channel and beta-adrenergic receptor blockers
   d. Amiodarone for ventricular arrhythmias; avoid local anesthetics
5. Treatment failure: If inadequate response to lipid emulsion and vasopressors, initiate cardiopulmonary bypass
6. Subsequent monitoring
   a. Monitor for at least 2 hours after symptoms that resolve quickly and are limited to central nervous system
   b. Monitor for at least 4 to 6 hours after recovery from significant cardiovascular event

Modified from Neal, J. M., Barrington, M. J., Fettiplace, M. R., Gitman, M., Memtsoudis, S. G., Mörwald, E. E., . . . & Weinberg, G. (2018b). The third American Society of Regional Anesthesia and Pain Medicine practice advisory on local anesthetic systemic toxicity: Executive summary 2017. *Regional Anesthesia and Pain Medicine, 43*(5), 113–123; and Neal, J. M., Woodward, C. M., & Harrison T. K. (2018a). The American Society of Regional Anesthesia and Pain Medicine checklist for managing local anesthetic systemic toxicity: 2017 version. *Regional Anesthesia and Pain Medicine, 43*(2), 150–153.

Treatment of noncritical hypotension includes correction of factors contributing to hypotension, such as fluid volume replacement, and reduction in the rate or concentration of LA infusion (Hurley et al., 2015). If hypotension is significant and does not correct with more conservative measures, vasopressors, including alpha-adrenergic medications such as phenylephrine, may be necessary (O'Neill & Helwig, 2016). Patients should be assisted with position changes and ambulation until hypotension resolves to reduce risks for falls.

Bradycardia

Bradycardia is another cardiac-related side effect associated with neuraxial LA administration. It is associated with blockade of the sympathetic cardiac accelerator fibers that are located at the T1-T4 spinal levels and result from a compensatory response to reduced cardiac filling pressures from decreased venous return (O'Neill & Helwig, 2016). Bradycardia usually resolves with diminished LA effect and discontinuation of the LA, but if bradycardia is severe (heart rate <40/min), it is treated with atropine to prevent cardiac arrest (O'Neill & Helwig, 2016).

Urinary Retention

LA administration at the lumbar level resulting in neuraxial blockade of the S2-S4 nerve roots can lead to urinary retention. The urinary retention resolves when the effect of the LA is resolved (Gill et al., 2016; Toledano & Van de Velde, 2017).

Motor Block

Neuraxial administration of LAs may lead to development of motor block of the lower extremities in up to 3% of the patients (Hurley et al., 2015). Lower limb weakness is a known complication of epidural LA administration. In a study of 123 adult patients who received epidural analgesia with bupivacaine and fentaNYL for postoperative pain after abdominal surgery, 36.5% of the patients developed lower extremity weakness (Ahmed & Baig, 2016). The majority (92%) received bupivacaine 0.1% with fentaNYL 2 mcg/mL; infusion rates varied from 6 to 14 mL/h (Ahmed & Baig, 2016). Motor block was more common among those who received lumbar epidurals compared to low thoracic epidurals. Motor block of the lower extremities is associated with increased risk for falls. In addition to motor block, sensory block may also place patients at risk for unintended injuries. Injuries may result from sensory blockade when patients are unable to sense pain as a warning of ischemic, thermal, or mechanical injuries. Fall risk and risks associated with sensory blockade are further described later in this chapter because similar risks are present with the use of LAs administered in peripheral nerve blocks.

Box 18.10	Modified Bromage Scale

0: No motor block
1: Inability to raise extended leg; able to move knees and feet
2: Inability to raise extended leg and move knee; able to move feet
3: Complete block of motor limb

From Brull, R., Macfarlane, A. J. R., & Chan, V. W. S. (2015). Spinal, epidural, and caudal anesthesia. In R. D. Miller, N. H. Cohen, L. I. Eriksson, J. Wiener-Kronish, N. Cohen, & W. Young (Eds.), *Miller's anesthesia* (8th ed., Box 56-1). Philadelphia: Saunders.

Patients receiving neuraxial LAs require frequent neurologic assessments to identify development of sensory and/or motor blocks. The modified Bromage scale (Box 18.10) is a tool recommended to measure lower limb weakness during neuraxial analgesia (Brull et al., 2015a). An increasing motor block can indicate an excessive dose of LA and can be addressed by temporarily stopping the LA infusion if the block is intense; by reducing the infusion rate or concentration of LA; or, if one extremity is affected, by positioning the patient so the affected site is nondependent (up). If the block fails to improve in 2 hours, further evaluation is necessary to rule out development of an epidural hematoma (Ahmed & Baig, 2016). Assessment and management of epidural hematoma is discussed in the following section.

Other Potential Complications Related to Neuraxial Analgesia

Although neuraxial techniques are effective in reducing acute pain, therapies are not always successful and may be associated with complications. The benefits of spinal and epidural anesthesia-analgesia must be weighed against risks associated with these techniques. The risks associated with neuraxial technique can be procedure-related or catheter-related and may result in neurologic complications and other adverse effects.

Procedure-Related Complications

Ineffective, Partial, or Incomplete Neuraxial Analgesia

Ineffective, partial, or incomplete neuraxial analgesia is commonly associated with catheter placement problems; placement of the catheter deeper than 5 cm into the epidural space results in suboptimal epidural analgesia (Nathan & Wong, 2014). When an assessment of the patient's sensory level indicates the block is partial, incomplete, or ineffective, the partial withdrawal of the catheter, or infusion of additional medication are troubleshooting interventions that may improve the effectiveness of the epidural.

Dural Puncture and Postdural Puncture Headache

Dural puncture occurs intentionally when the dura is punctured for intrathecal medication administration or for diagnostic procedures such as a spinal tap. Dural puncture is a relatively common complication of epidural analgesia that occurs when the dura is inadvertently punctured during epidural injection or catheter placement (often referred to as *wet tap*). The anesthesia provider usually knows when an inadvertent dural puncture has occurred and will attempt needle placement at a higher vertebral interspace.

Any dura puncture may result in a postdural puncture headache (PDPH), which is associated with loss of CSF (Gaiser, 2017). The exact mechanism underlying the development of PDPH is not clear. Box 18.11 presents factors that increase the risk for PDPH. The incidence of PDPH is influenced by the experience of the anesthesia provider and the technique used to place the needle, the size and orientation of the needle, and patient characteristics (Brull et al., 2015a; Gaiser, 2017). Rarely, more serious complications can occur from a dural puncture, such as infection and pneumocephalus if air is used during epidural injection using the loss-of-resistance technique; the use of saline rather than air is recommended to prevent pneumocephalus (Toledano & Van de Velde, 2017).

Signs and Symptoms of PDPH

After a dural puncture, patients should be monitored for development of headache. Some patients experience no symptoms after a dural puncture, yet for others, the leakage of CSF through the hole created in the dura characteristically results in a headache within 5 days of the dural puncture that resolves spontaneously within 1 to 2 weeks or after an epidural blood patch (Brull et al., 2015a; Gaiser, 2017). Symptoms include a frontal or occipital headache that is absent or mild, dull, aching, or throbbing when the patient is supine; may worsen to moderate

Box 18.11	Risk Factors for Development of Postdural Puncture Headache

- Younger age
- Female
- Pregnancy
- Use of a larger needle
- Placement of needle bevel
- Multiple dural punctures
- Use of air versus saline in loss-of-resistance technique

From Toldeano, R. D. & Van de Velde, M. (2017). Epidural anesthesia and analgesia. In A. Hadzic. *Hadzic's textbook of regional and acute pain management* (pp. 380–445). New York: McGraw-Hill Education.

to severe when sitting up or standing; and may improve with return to supine position. Other symptoms such as neck or back soreness or stiffness, photophobia, visual disturbances, hearing loss, nausea, and vomiting may also be present. The decrease in CSF pressure as a result of the dural puncture and traction on the meninges and meningeal blood vessels is thought to be the reason patients routinely report that the headache worsens when they move into a sitting or standing position and improves when they lie down (Gaiser, 2017).

Treatment of PDPH

Initial treatment of PDPH is usually symptomatic and conservative, consisting of hydration, including caffeinated beverages, supine positioning, cold and/or heat therapy, oral analgesics, and reassurance that the headache will most likely resolve within a week (Warren et al., 2018).

A small systematic review of 13 randomized controlled trials (RCTs) (479 participants) evaluating oral and intravenous caffeine, subcutaneous SUMAtriptan, oral gabapentin, oral pregabalin, oral theophylline, intravenous hydrocortisone, intravenous cosyntropin, and intramuscular adrenocorticotropic hormone (ACTH) concluded that treatment with intravenous caffeine sodium benzoate resulted in a significant decrease in the number of people with PDPH and the requirement for supplementary interventions when compared to placebo; SUMAtriptan and ACTH did not show any relevant effect on pain visual analogue scale (VAS); gabapentin, theophylline, and hydrocortisone were more effective with better pain VAS scores than conservative treatment alone or placebo; and no important side effects of these medications were reported (Ona, Osorio, & Cosp, 2015). Although there is no pharmacologic rationale or strong evidence for treatment of PDPH with caffeine, it is thought to relieve symptoms by producing cerebral vasoconstriction (Gaiser, 2017). Caffeine benzoate 300 mg/day PO or 500 mg/day or bid IV are the usual doses recommended for PDPH (Lexicomp, 2018). If caffeine benzoate is unavailable, drinking caffeinated beverages may be useful, but the caffeine level will vary.

Interventional treatment for PDPH involves the placement of an epidural blood patch. A blood patch consists of aseptic withdrawal of 15 to 20 mL of the patient's venous blood followed immediately by aseptic injection of the blood into the epidural space at or one level below the previous dural puncture. The blood is distributed both caudally and cephalad and forms a clot over the defect in the dura at puncture site as well as cephalad displacement of the CSF (Gaiser, 2017). The blood patch is thought to act as a mass lesion compressing the dural sac and raising intracranial pressure, and because the thecal sac is compressed, the CSF leak is stopped (Gaiser, 2017). Complications from the blood patch procedure are very rare and include infection, transient bradycardia, bleeding, facial palsy, lumbovertebral syndrome, and, very rarely, cauda equina syndrome (Tsui, Dryden, & Finucane, 2018). Patients may

report back pain during the injection of blood into the epidural space (Booth, Pan, Thomas, Harris, & D'Angelo, 2017). Contraindications for the procedure are similar to epidural contraindications (see Box 18.1).

Direct Needle Trauma

Trauma to neural tissue from neuraxial needles and catheters is extremely rare (paraplegia and cauda equina syndrome each occur in 0.1/10,000 cases); case reports suggest that direct spinal cord trauma is most often the result of excessively caudad termination of the spinal cord or inaccurate determination of bony landmarks (Neal et al., 2018b). Nerve root trauma is also rare and usually is indicated by patient reports of pain that is severe, sharp, and radiating along a nerve when the needle is placed; current literature suggests the majority of nerve injuries occurring during the perioperative period are unrelated to regional anesthesia (Verlinde et al., 2016).

Epidural Catheter–Related Complications

Epidural Catheter Migration

Epidural catheter migration can occur at any time during epidural analgesia therapy despite correct catheter placement. Epidural catheters can migrate out of the epidural space through the dura into the subarachnoid space, into the vascular system through an epidural blood vessel, or into the subcutaneous space. The incidence of intrathecal or intravascular migration of an epidural catheter during epidural analgesia is less frequent than the failure rate of epidural analgesia (Hurley et al., 2015), and in an earlier publication, the rate of intrathecal migration was cited to be as low as 0.15% to 0.18% and intravascular migration as low as 0.18% (Maalouf & Liu, 2009). Multiple case reports describe migration of epidural catheters; strategies to optimally verify catheter position and ensure catheter securement continue to be sought (Dirscherl, Leschka, & Filipovic, 2017; Odor, Bampoe, Hayward, Chis Ster, & Evans, 2016; Smith, & Anderson, 2016; Uchino et al., 2016). Box 18.12 describes clinical presentation of patients with migration of epidural catheters.

Signs and Symptoms of Epidural Catheter Migration

Signs and symptoms of epidural catheter migration are more pronounced when analgesia is administered by the bolus method. Intrathecal injection of an epidural dose of LA or opioid can result in a high block and life-threatening respiratory depression requiring aggressive intervention and support (Hurley et al., 2015). At the time of catheter insertion and whenever migration is suspected, the catheter is tested with the administration of a small dose of EPINEPHrine-containing LA in fractionated doses. An approved clinician aspirates the catheter for blood or CSF to identify possible migration before administration of an epidural bolus or continuous infusion to rule out intravascular or intrathecal migration (Hurley et al., 2015). Intravascular or intrathecal epidural catheter migration during continuous epidural infusion or PCEA may be difficult to detect, because signs

Box 18.12 | Neuraxial Catheter Displacement or Migration

Promptly report any of the following to the anesthesia or pain management provider:

INDICATIONS OF DISPLACED INTRATHECAL OR EPIDURAL CATHETER

- Inadequate pain relief (e.g., a previously comfortable patient reports loss of pain control).
- No pain reduction occurs with increase in opioid dose.

INDICATIONS OF EPIDURAL CATHETER MIGRATION INTO SUBARACHNOID SPACE

- Unexplained increase in opioid-induced adverse effects (e.g., a previously alert patient is excessively sedated or has nausea).
- Widespread sensory and/or motor block (possible if solution contains local anesthetics).
- Catheter migration is confirmed by aspiration of cerebrospinal fluid from epidural catheter and/or sensory blockade when local anesthetic test dose is administered.

INDICATIONS OF INTRAVASCULAR MIGRATION

- Inadequate pain relief (e.g., a previously comfortable patient reports loss of pain control).
- Unexplained increase in opioid-induced adverse effects (e.g., a previously alert patient is sedated or has nausea [increase in adverse effects is possible even though the

patient is being underdosed after intravascular migration because the opioid is being delivered systemically]).
- Signs and symptoms of local anesthetic systemic toxicity (e.g., metallic taste, ringing ears, circumoral numbness, slow speech, irritability [possible if solution contains local anesthetics]).
- Intravascular migration is confirmed by aspiration of blood from catheter and/or transient tachycardia when small test dose of local anesthetic (e.g., bupivacaine, ropivacaine) containing EPINEPHrine is injected.

NOTE: *Displacement* of temporary neuraxial catheters during analgesic therapy is a common occurrence and is often caused by patients accidentally pulling them out. Catheter migration can occur at any time during epidural analgesia therapy and despite correct catheter placement. Epidural catheters can migrate out of the epidural space through the dura into the subarachnoid space or into the vascular system through an epidural blood vessel.
From Pasero, C., & McCaffery, M. (2011). *Pain assessment and pharmacologic management* (433). St. Louis: Mosby. Data from Grape, S., & Schug, S. A. (2008). Epidural and spinal analgesia. In P. E. Macintyre, S. M. Walker, & D. J. Rowbotham (Eds.), *Clinical pain management: Acute pain* (2nd ed. pp. 255–270). London: Hodder Arnold; Maalouf, D. B., & Liu, S. S. (2009). Clinical application of epidural analgesia. In R. S. Sinatra, O. A. de Leon-Casasola, B. Ginsberg, et al. (Eds.), *Acute pain management* (pp. 221–229). Cambridge, NY, Cambridge University Press; and Pasero, C., Eksterowicz, N., Primeau, M., & Cowley, C. (2007). ASPMN position statement: Registered nurse management and monitoring of analgesia by catheter techniques. *Pain Management Nursing*, 8(2), 48–54. © 2011, Pasero, C., & McCaffery, M. May be duplicated for use in clinical practice.

and symptoms are more subtle. During continuous infusion or PCEA, migration is suspected when there is a change in the patient's pain control or sensation and motor changes since the previous assessment. Whenever there is concern about catheter position, the patient should be evaluated by an anesthesia provider or the pain management clinicians responsible for managing the epidural catheter. Box 18.13 presents an example of a patient case involving migration of an epidural catheter.

Neurologic Complications Associated With Neuraxial Analgesia

Injection or Infusion of Neurotoxic Agents

Generally, LAs and opioids administered in clinically recommended doses are safe in the majority of patients; however, infrequently, some patients will be susceptible to neuraxial injury from neurotoxicity related to the administration of these medications. High concentrations of LAs can cause neurotoxicity; use of medications containing preservatives, alcohol, phenol, or their additives can be neurotoxic (Brull, Hadzic, Reina, & Barrington, 2015b). Medications commonly used in skin preparation

for neuraxial injection such as chlorhexidine, alcohol, and povidone-iodine may be potentially neurotoxic, and therefore complete drying of the skin after cleansing is recommended to reduce risks for neurotoxicity (Schulz-Stübner, Pottinger, Coffin, & Herwaldt, 2017). Accidental injection of medications not proven to be safe for neuraxial administration may result in neurotoxicity and neuraxial injury. Measures must be taken to minimize risks for medication errors resulting in accidental injection of neurotoxic medications such as antiseptic solution, antibiotics, potassium chloride, and total parenteral nutrition (Kreutzträger, Kopp, & Liebscher, 2017; Liu, Tariq, Liu, Yan, & Kaye, 2017). Use of bar code medication administration technology may be helpful in reducing medication errors (Shah, Lo, Babich, Tsao, & Bansback, 2016).

All medications and solutions injected or infused neuraxially must be sterile, preservative-free, and regarded safe for administration. To prevent errors, all infusions of LAs should be distinctly labeled; have a special infusion pump dedicated for continuous infusion; and have an infusion line that is color-coded, without an injection port. Box 18.14 lists measures to minimize risks for neurotoxicity.

| Box 18.13 | Intrathecal Migration of Epidural Catheter: Patient Example |

Mr. E. had a nephrectomy yesterday morning and is receiving a continuous epidural infusion of morphine and bupivacaine for his postoperative pain. During previous assessments, Mr. E. has been alert and comfortable, with a pain rating no higher than 4 on a scale of 0 to 10 and ambulating without assistance. This time, Mr. E. rates his pain as 0. He is oriented but very drowsy, with a respiratory rate of 18 breaths/min. The nurse knows that the only sedating medication Mr. E. is receiving is the epidural morphine, and Mr. E. confirms that he has taken only the medications the nurse has given him. The nurse checks the epidural infusion pump and finds it is programmed correctly and functioning properly. Mr. E. tells the nurse that he cannot ambulate because his "legs are numb." The nurse suspects the epidural catheter has migrated into the subarachnoid space. (Intrathecal infusion of an epidural dose of opioid would explain the increase in Mr. E.'s sedation level, and intrathecal infusion of an epidural dose of bupivacaine would explain Mr. E.'s report of lower extremity sensory loss.) The nurse stops the epidural infusion and takes Mr. E.'s blood pressure, which is 120/70 mm Hg, only slightly lower than his baseline. The nurse stays with Mr. E. and takes vital signs every 5 minutes (the high dose of opioid could cause respiratory depression and the high dose of bupivacaine could cause adverse hemodynamic effects) and asks a co-worker to notify the pain service. The pain service nurse arrives and easily aspirates 5 mL cerebrospinal fluid from the catheter, confirming that it is in the subarachnoid space. The catheter is removed, and Mr. E. recovers without difficulty.

Infection

Although rare, infectious complications are a potential with any regional analgesic technique. Of greatest concern are infections associated with neuraxial anesthesia and analgesia because of the potentially severe and disabling adverse sequelae. Infectious complications associated with neuraxial techniques include, but are not limited to, epidural, spinal, subdural abscesses, and meningitis (Brull et al., 2015a).

Risk Factors for Neuraxial Infection
Predisposing factors for neuraxial infection are impaired immune response, diabetes, and cancer (Dale & Checketts, 2016). In addition, neuraxial infections may be related to pre-existing infections, pancreatitis, gastrointestinal bleeding, and drug or alcohol abuse (American Society of Anesthesiologists, 2017). Most clinicians recognize that alternatives to neuraxial technique should be determined on an individual basis for patients at risk for infectious complication. Some clinicians

| Box 18.14 | Prevention of Neurotoxicity |

The following measures may be helpful in preventing inadvertent neuraxial injection or infusion of neurotoxic medications:

- Do not use medications from a multidose vial; it is wise to assume that all multidose vials contain preservatives that may be harmful if injected into the neuraxial region.
- Use only nonneurotoxic agents to disinfect intrathecal or epidural infusion lines, catheter connections, and ports (e.g., alcohol often is used to cleanse skin of secretions, but should not be used to disinfect catheter connections or implanted ports).
- Use infusion pump specifically designated for regional analgesia. Use color-coded infusion lines to identify analgesic infusions.
- Do not use infusion lines with injection ports for local anesthetic infusion.
- Boldly label indwelling pain management catheters.
- Label all infusion lines when patients have several.
- Double-check the medication label on the medication reservoir for wording that indicates the solution used for neuraxial analgesia is both preservative-free and prepared for intrathecal or epidural use.
- Return to the pharmacy medication reservoirs and agents that are unclearly labeled, cloudy, or contain particulate matter.

Modified from Pasero, C., & McCaffery, M. (2011). *Pain assessment and pharmacologic management* (p. 434). St. Louis: Mosby. © 2011, Pasero, C., & McCaffery, M. May be duplicated for use in clinical practice.

suggest that regional anesthesia may be acceptable in those at higher risk if appropriate antibiotic therapy is initiated, the patient has shown response to antibiotic therapy, and vital signs are stable before neuraxial technique is considered (American Society of Anesthesiologists, 2017; Schulz-Stübner, Pottinger, Coffin, & Herwaldt, 2020).

Strategies to Reduce Risk for Neuraxial Infection
Use of aseptic techniques during the placement of neuraxial needles and catheters is important in prevention of infectious complications. Bacterial contamination of the skin, respiratory tract, or water are the most common sources of neuraxial infections (Schulz-Stübner et al., 2017), and many preventive strategies address these potential sources. The American Society of Anesthesiologists (2017), in their Practice Advisory, provides recommendations for interventions to prevent, diagnose, and manage infections associated with neuraxial techniques, which are summarized in Box 18.15.

Nicolotti, Iotti, Fanelli, and Compagnone (2016), in a systematic review of the literature related to perineural

Box 18.15	American Society of Anesthesiologists Recommendations to Prevent Neuraxial Infections

PREPLACEMENT

- Obtain history and perform physical examination, including laboratory studies to identify increased infection risks.
- Avoid neuraxial techniques when patients are at high risk for infection.
- Administer preprocedure antibiotic if neuraxial approach is needed in patient with bacteremia.
- Avoid lumbar puncture if known epidural abscess.

ASEPTIC PLACEMENT

- Remove jewelry from the hands.
- Perform thorough hand washing before placement and manipulation of epidural catheter.
- Use sterile gloves.
- Wear a mask covering the mouth and nose (now required by the Centers for Disease Control and Prevention [2011]).
- Wear a cap.
- Apply sterile draping of the patient and consider use of sterile gowns.
- Perform skin preparation with nonneurotoxic bactericidal solution with rapid onset and long duration of action.[a]
- Little consensus about the preferred antiseptic skin preparation solution, but chlorhexidine with alcohol, allowing for adequate drying time, is preferred by the American Society of Anesthesiologists over povidone-iodine and aseptic preparation without alcohol (American Society of Anesthesiologists, 2017).

AFTER PLACEMENT

- Apply sterile occlusive dressings over catheter placement site.
- Use bacterial filters when continuous epidural infusion is planned for an extended time.
- Limit opening, disconnection, and reconnection of neuraxial infusion system.
- Avoid frequent and unnecessary medication and reservoir and tubing changes.
- Use strict aseptic technique when handling equipment and supplies used for catheter placement, when placing intrathecal and epidural catheters, and when connecting medication reservoir to infusion tubing, administering supplemental boluses, and refilling reservoirs.[a]
- Report catheter disconnections immediately to the anesthesia provider:
  - Wrap the free end of the intrathecal or epidural catheter with a sterile 4 × 4.
  - Anesthesia provider will determine whether the catheter is to be removed or repaired and the infusion continued.
  - Obtain an order for interim analgesia.

- Approved clinician should remove catheter when an unwitnessed disconnection occurs.
- Minimize duration of placement of neuraxial catheters; remove catheters as soon as no longer clinically necessary.
- Perform minimum of daily assessment for signs and symptoms of infectious complications.
  - Assess for neurologic deficits (motor, sensory changes).
  - Check temperature (usually every 4 hours).
  - Immediately report to anesthesia provider signs and symptoms of infection (fever, backache, headache), including infection thought to be unrelated to neuraxial catheterization (e.g., wound, urinary, and pulmonary infections).
  - Assess insertion site and identify early signs and symptoms of infection: Inflammation, erythema, edema, drainage, warmth or tenderness at insertion site.
  - Immediately report unexplained changes in sensory or motor deficit since last assessment, particularly increase in symptoms in spite of decreases in the analgesic infusion rate.
  - Obtain samples for blood tests if infection suspected (white blood count, sedimentation rate, C-reactive protein).
- Approved clinician removes catheter promptly if infection is suspected.
- Administer antibiotic therapy at earliest sign or symptom of serious infection.
- Obtain infectious disease expert consultation.
- Obtain surgical consultation for abscess treatment.

AFTER REMOVAL

- If catheter removed and infection suspected, send catheter tip for culture; obtain additional cultures as needed (blood, skin, abscess, cerebrospinal fluid).
- If abscess suspected and neurologic deficit is present, obtain imaging studies.

From Pasero, C., & McCaffery, M. (2011). *Pain assessment and pharmacologic management* (p. 437). St. Louis: Mosby. American Society of Anesthesiologists Committee on Standards and Practice Parameters. (2017). Practice advisory for the prevention, diagnosis and management of infectious complications associated with neuraxial techniques: An updated report by the American Society of Anesthesiologists task force on infectious complications associated with neuraxial techniques and the American Society of Regional Anesthesia and Pain Medicine. *Anesthesiology, 126*(4), 585–601.
[a] Use only nonneurotoxic agents to disinfect catheter connections or ports. Alcohol may be used to cleanse skin of secretions but should not be used to disinfect catheter connections or ports.

catheter infection, reported the type of dressings used to cover perineural catheter insertion sites should minimize dislodgement and prevent microbial access from the skin. Impermeable transparent dressings and antiseptic chlorhexidine-impregnated dressings are techniques used to reduce infection risk. It is suggested to avoid routine dressing changes because they have been associated with increased infection risk (Nicolotti et al., 2016).

Guidelines to direct the frequency with which neuraxial infusion systems (solution and tubing) should be changed (also called *hang time*) are lacking. References often used by pharmacists, such as *Trissel's Stability of Compounded Formulations*, or the individual medication manufacturer's recommendations for the beyond use date may be useful in guiding selection of hang times; when compounded solutions are used, the typical beyond use date for medication is 30 hours (Trissel, Ashworth, & Ashworth, 2018). Nicolotti et al. (2016), based on their systematic review, suggest a 72-hour hang time for solutions prepared according to United States Pharmacopeia guidelines to reduce contamination risks associated with the number of line disconnections, manipulations, and bag changes.

The literature and clinical practice over the years support maintaining the integrity of the infusion system after therapy is initiated (American Society of Anesthesiologists, 2017), and efforts should be made to minimize entry into the system to prevent inadvertent introduction of bacteria. Because there are no guidelines, practice varies widely with regard to neuraxial analgesic infusion hang time, tubing changes, and dressing changes. In some practice settings, neuraxial infusion systems are not entered unless the solution container (bag or bottle) is empty and a new one must be added. Because neuraxial infusions are used for a short period, often 5 days or less, tubing and dressings are not routinely changed unless a problem is noted. Individual organizational policies should be followed to reduce infection-related risks.

Signs and Symptoms of Neuraxial Infection

Early signs and symptoms of a neuraxial infection can be difficult to detect. Systematic assessment is necessary. The absence of erythema at the injection site and localized tenderness do not negate the possibility of neuraxial infection (Sayed & Diwan, 2015). Symptoms may differ somewhat depending on location and extent of the infection. Early signs of infection include spiking fever, increasing backache, headache, and redness and tenderness at the injection site; infection should be considered if there are changes in sensory and motor function (Toledano & Van de Velde, 2017). Serious signs of infection include neck stiffness, photophobia, fatigue, confusion, altered mental status, nausea, vomiting, and Kernig sign, which are often associated with meningitis and may result from epidural or intrathecal techniques (Toledano & Van de Velde, 2017). Other serious signs include increasing radicular pain, advancing motor deficit, and other neurologic changes (Sayed & Diwan, 2015). Bowel or bladder dysfunction may be associated with epidural abscess and cauda equina syndrome (Malik & Nelson, 2018). Intrathecal infection often leads

to meningeal irritation and may be associated with cerebral signs of bacterial encephalitis (Sayed & Diwan, 2015). Any one of these signs should immediately arouse suspicion and prompt further investigation. Increased white blood cell count, increased erythrocyte sedimentation rate (ESR), and increased C-reactive protein in CSF are often present with neuraxial infections (Sayed & Diwan, 2015; Toledano & Van de Velde, 2017). Box 18.16 lists the signs and symptoms of neuraxial infection.

Box 18.16	Signs and Symptoms of Neuraxial Infection

Skin infection at catheter entry site, implanted port, or implanted pump site
- Inflammation, erythema, edema, drainage, warmth at catheter entry site, implanted port, or implanted pump site.
- Patient reports soreness around catheter entry site, implanted port, or implanted pump site.

Epidural or intrathecal space infection[a]
- Constant diffuse back pain or tenderness.
- Pain or paresthesia during bolus injection.
- Decreased pain relief despite no decrease in analgesic.
- Sensory and/or motor deficit (particularly unexplained changes since last assessment).
- Bowel and bladder dysfunction may or may not be present.
- Skin infection around catheter entry site may or may not be present.
- Fever may or may not be present.

Signs of acute bacterial infection[b]
- Fever
- Headache
- Nuchal rigidity
- Brudzinski's and Kernig's signs
- Altered mental status
- Convulsions

From Pasero, C., & McCaffery, M. (2011). *Pain assessment and pharmacologic management* (p. 437). St. Louis: Mosby. Data from American Society of Anesthesiologists Committee on Standards and Practice Parameters. (2017). Practice advisory for the prevention, diagnosis and management of infectious complications associated with neuraxial techniques: An updated report by the American Society of Anesthesiologists Task Force on infectious complications associated with neuraxial techniques and the American Society of Regional Anesthesia and Pain Medicine. *Anesthesiology, 126*(4), 585–601. © 2011, Pasero, C., & McCaffery, M. May be duplicated for use in clinical practice.

[a] Because the signs of neuraxial infection can occur after patients are released from the hospital, it is imperative that discharge teaching include the signs and symptoms of neuraxial infection and what to do if these are detected.

[b] Neuraxial infection is rare, and early signs and symptoms can be difficult to detect. This box lists the signs and symptoms of neuraxial infection and precautions that can be taken to prevent neuraxial infection in patients who receive neuraxial analgesia.

Signs and symptoms of meningitis usually manifest within 6 to 36 hours after a neuraxial procedure, but an epidural infection may manifest later, within 7 days, and may be delayed for 60 days or longer (Toledano & Van de Velde, 2017). Because the signs of an epidural infection can occur after patients are released from the hospital and can occur even if the course of neuraxial analgesia was short and uneventful, it is imperative that discharge teaching include the signs and symptoms and to report them immediately if detected. Patients should know that it may be necessary to remind the primary care provider that they received neuraxial analgesia during hospitalization because this sometimes is overlooked as a possible cause of symptoms.

Treatment of Neuraxial Infection

The mainstay of treatment for neuraxial infection is antibiotics, which should not be delayed. Broad-spectrum intravenous antibiotics are initiated, and antibiotic selection is reconsidered when culture results are received. A delay in treatment, often due to delayed or initial misdiagnosis can result in sepsis and serious neurologic outcomes. If an epidural abscess is suspected, gadolinium-enhanced MRI is the preferred diagnostic tool; neurosurgical consult and possible surgery may be necessary to treat an epidural abscess and reduce the risk for spinal cord compression and potential paralysis (Toledano & Van de Velde, 2017).

Epidural Hematoma

One of the most devastating serious adverse events associated with neuraxial analgesia are bleeding complications, such as an epidural hematoma, with resultant permanent spinal cord damage. The complication of epidural hematoma is rare, and the incidence of epidural hematoma associated with epidural catheter placement or removal is reported to range from 0.01% to 0.03% (Gulur, Tsui, Pathak, Koury, & Lee, 2015). An analysis of serious complications related to the use of epidural analgesia from 1998 to 2010 in the United States identified the incidence of spinal hematoma in obstetric patients as 0.6 per 100,000 epidural catheterizations and epidural abscess was absent; in nonobstetric patients, the incidence of spinal hematoma was 18.5 per 100,000 and epidural abscess was 18.5 per 100,000 epidural catheterizations (Rosero & Joshi, 2016).

Risk Factors for Epidural Hematoma

Risk factors for epidural hematoma include difficult or traumatic neuraxial needle or catheter placement, advanced age, female sex, and coagulopathy (Macfarlane et al., 2018). Antithrombotic and thrombolytic therapy increase risks for epidural hematoma; thrombocytopenia, which may result from a variety of conditions, is also a risk factor (Hurley et al., 2015; Toledano & Van de Velde, 2017). The timing of neuraxial procedures, including insertion and removal of epidural catheters, are high-risk periods for hematoma formation, especially in the setting of anticoagulation, and

despite numerous studies, there are no absolute conclusions about the safety of anticoagulation and neuraxial procedures (Hurley et al., 2015). A multidisciplinary approach in which physicians, nurses, pharmacists, and laboratory clinicians work together to recognize conditions such as abnormal laboratory results or medications that increase risks for harm are essential to avoid potential consequences.

To address risks related to neuraxial hematoma, the ASRA published an updated evidence-based guideline in patients receiving antithrombotic, antiplatelet, and thrombolytic therapy for use by anesthesiologists and other health care providers involved in managing patients receiving neuraxial and peripheral regional anesthetic/analgesic blockade (Horlocker et al., 2018). Horlocker et al. (2018) also cite the need for awareness of bleeding risks associated with the use of herbal medications such as garlic, gingko, and ginseng, and potential ginseng-warfarin interactions, but do not recommend mandatory discontinuation of these medications or avoidance of neuraxial techniques if these medications have been administered. As new antithrombotic, antiplatelet, and thrombolytic medications continue to be introduced, and new evidence is published, it is important for clinicians to refer to the most recent evidence-based guidelines for recommendations related to use of these medications in relation to neuraxial analgesic procedures and timing of neuraxial catheter placement and removal. Incorporation of evidence-based guideline recommendations into electronic medical records (EMRs), and automatic warnings in EMRs related to neuraxial techniques and medications that increase epidural hematoma risk may support risk reduction efforts. Box 18.17 presents a summary of measures to reduce risk and facilitate early recognition of epidural hematoma.

Signs and Symptoms of Epidural Hematoma

Like epidural infection, early detection of epidural hematoma is difficult because symptoms are often subtle. If a patient who underwent a neuraxial analgesic procedure at any time in the preceding 48 hours develops new or progressive neurologic symptoms such as increasing numbness and motor block, the anesthesia or pain team should be called for further clinical evaluation.

Epidural hematoma may manifest with severe, acute axial back pain at the level of the dermatomes corresponding to the site of the hematoma; as the hematoma increases in size, sensory or motor deficits and urinary or fecal incontinence may develop; lower extremity weakness is a common sign (Nelson, Benzon, & Jabri, 2017). Percussion over the spine, coughing, sneezing, and straining may increase the pain (Nelson et al., 2017). Any of these signs and symptoms should immediately arouse suspicion and further investigation.

Diagnosis of Epidural Hematoma

Patient recovery without neurologic injury from epidural hematoma related to neuraxial analgesia depends

Box 18.17	Measures to Reduce Risks and Provide Early Recognition of Epidural Hematoma

- Regularly assess motor and sensory function and promptly report deficits to the anesthesia or pain management team.
- Promptly report abnormal laboratory values, including low platelet counts, abnormal liver function, and prolonged clotting and bleeding times.
- Question and clarify orders for antithrombotics, thrombolytics, and antiplatelet medications before, during, and after neuraxial analgesia.
- Implement automatic warnings in electronic medication systems when neuraxial medications are ordered for patients with abnormal laboratory values or who have orders for medications that increase risks for epidural hematoma.
- Teach patients to recognize the signs and symptoms of epidural hematoma and advise to seek medical attention if they experience them after discharge, because epidural hematoma may occur even if the course of neuraxial analgesia was short and uneventful.
- Advise patents to remind the primary care provider that they received neuraxial analgesia during hospitalization, because this sometimes is overlooked as a possible cause of symptoms.

Box 18.18	Assessment for Possible Epidural Hematoma Patient Example

Mrs. U. has been receiving a continuous epidural infusion of HYDROmorphone and bupivacaine for the last 36 hours for her postoperative hysterectomy pain. Her epidural site is clean and dry, without edema, redness, or drainage. Mrs. U. says that the area around the epidural site in her back is "tender." She also reports numbness and tingling of her thighs. She has been afebrile, and all of her vital signs have been stable since surgery. Her pain rating is 2 on a scale of 0 to 10. Mrs. U.'s nurse knows that early signs of an epidural abscess or hematoma often are subtle. The cardinal sign of both of these complications is diffuse back pain or tenderness. Although lumbar epidural administration of bupivacaine can cause temporary numbness and tingling of the lower extremities, they could be signs of neurocompression caused by an epidural abscess or hematoma. The nurse asks the anesthesia provider to assess Mrs. U. as soon as possible. The anesthesiologist's examination is negative. Mrs. U.'s back tenderness resolves without treatment, and her thigh numbness and tingling resolve with a slight decrease in the epidural infusion rate.

C. Pasero, C., & McCaffery, M. (2011). *Pain Assessment and Pharmacologic Management.* St. Louis, MO: Mosby.

on early recognition and aggressive treatment. Epidural hematoma should be suspected if sensory or motor deficit develop after the patient recovered from the effects of neuraxial block. If a continuous epidural infusion with LA is running and the patient develops progressive numbness or motor block, the infusion should be turned off with the catheter left in place, and the anesthesia or pain team should be called for evaluation and reevaluation for return of sensory and motor function (Nelson et al., 2017). If improvement is not noted, prompt imaging is obtained. Epidural hematoma is confirmed by magnetic resonance imaging (MRI) or computed tomography (CT), and a neurology or neurosurgery consultation is requested for further management. If an epidural catheter is in place, it is usually removed before MRI because the catheter may not be MRI compatible. CT may identify an epidural hematoma, but false negatives are possible (Nelson et al., 2017). Box 18.18 presents a scenario involving assessment for possible epidural hematoma.

Treatment of Epidural Hematoma

Epidural hematomas are usually treated by immediate laminectomy and hematoma evacuation to prevent progression of spinal cord compression and potential paralysis. Nonoperative treatment with positive outcomes has been reported with hematomas at the level of the cauda equina and if the neurologic deficits are mild (Nelson et al., 2017). In a review of the literature, Zhang, Geng, Wang, Zhang, and Du (2018) reported cases of spontaneous resolution of epidural hematoma; most resolutions involved hematomas of the upper thoracic and cervical spine and resolved from several hours to days after onset of symptoms. Conservative treatment is recommended only when symptoms improve significantly over a short period and imaging demonstrates possible hematoma disintegration (Zhang et al., 2018). When spinal cord compromise is present, the prognosis for complete recovery depends on the level of preoperative neurologic deficit and timing of the intervention. In a review of 647 cases, of which 387 patients had spinal hematoma, the neurologic outcome was better when surgical decompression of the hematoma occurred within 12 hours of clinical diagnosis (Bos et al., 2018). Recovery has been shown in cases involving epidural hematoma if surgery occurs within 48 hours of an incomplete motor deficit and within 36 hours of complete motor deficit (Kim et al., 2012; Nelson et al., 2017).

Regional Analgesia

Overview of Truncal and Peripheral Regional Analgesia

Truncal and peripheral regional analgesia refers to the temporary block of nerve impulses by LA injection or infusion to a selected area of the body, thus blocking sensation and reducing pain. These blocks allow LAs to be administered close to specific nerves involved in the surgical (or traumatic) site, inhibit neural conduction from the pain site to the spinal cord, and decrease spinal cord sensitization (Hunter et al., 2019). Truncal regional analgesia involves blockade of nerves located in the trunk outside of the neuraxial space and includes paravertebral, erector spinae plane, transversus abdominis plane (TAP), and quadratus lumborum nerve blocks (Rahangdale, Tureanu, & Benzon, 2018). Both truncal and peripheral regional analgesia are often categorized as peripheral nerve blocks (PNBs) (Ilfeld, 2017), and for the remainder of this section, unless specified, PNB will apply to blocks of the trunk or extremities. This section will provide an overview of PNBs and describe benefits, risks, techniques, descriptions, and indications for some of the more common PNBs.

Peripheral Nerve Block Interventions

Nerve block techniques are usually performed preoperatively to provide anesthesia and analgesia but may also be placed intraoperatively or postoperatively (Hunter et al., 2019). They are also used for nonsurgical pain, including pain resulting from trauma (Gadsden & Warlick, 2015). The block can be performed as a single injection, or a catheter can be placed for continuous infusion. A single injection involves the injection of a specific LA intended to block a specific nerve distribution. When a continuous catheter infusion is used, it involves percutaneous insertion of an indwelling catheter through a needle in the proximity of the target peripheral nerve or nerves, followed by LA infusion by an infusion device that is connected to the indwelling catheter (Ilfeld, 2017; Joshi, Gandhi, Shah, Gadsden, & Corman, 2016b; Pasero & McCaffery, 2011). Continuous infusion is usually indicated for patients having surgical procedures or nonsurgical pain that is not expected to resolve by the time a single injection of LA would be expected to wear off. The area affected by the block will vary based on the LA and where it is injected or infused. Table 18.12 provides examples of LA dosing regimens used in truncal or peripheral regional analgesia.

Table 18.12	Upper and Lower Extremity Regional Analgesia Dosing Regimens[a,b]			
Type of Block	**Type of Surgery**	**Continuous Infusion**	**Patient-Controlled Regional Analgesia (PCRA)**	
Interscalene block	Surgery around the shoulder	Ropivacaine 0.2% 5 mL/h	Ropivacaine 0.2% 5 mL/h Or: continuous basal infusion of 4–8 mL/h with bolus of 2–5 mL/h and lockout of 20–60 min	
Supraclavicular or infraclavicular block	Surgery around elbow, wrist, and hand	Ropivacaine 0.2% 5 mL/h	Ropivacaine 0.2% 5 mL/h Or: continuous basal infusion of 4–8 mL/h with bolus of 2–5 mL/h and lockout of 20–60 min	
Sciatic nerve block	Posterior cruciate ligament repair, foot and ankle surgery	Ropivacaine 0.2% 5 mL/h	Ropivacaine 0.2% 5 mL/h Or: continuous basal infusion of 4–8 mL/h with bolus of 2–5 mL/h and lockout of 20–60 min	
Femoral nerve block	Knee arthroplasty, anterior cruciate ligament repair	Ropivacaine 0.1% 5 mL/h	Ropivacaine 0.1% 5 mL/h Or: continuous basal infusion of 4–8 mL/h with bolus of 2–5 mL/h and lockout of 20–60 min	
Paravertebral block (thoracic)	Breast surgery	Ropivacaine 0.2% 5 mL/h	Ropivacaine 0.2% 5 mL/h Or: continuous basal infusion of 4–8 mL/h with bolus of 2–5 mL/h and lockout of 20–60 min	

Note: Depending on the type of surgery, multiple nerves may need to be blocked to get good postoperative pain relief. It is necessary to consider the total dose of local anesthetic administered to reduce risk of toxicity. When using catheter techniques, disposable pumps with prefilled local anesthetics may be given to the patient with suitable written and verbal instructions.

[a]Doses are approximations, with lower doses recommended when using ultrasound techniques.

[b]All doses on this chart are approximations and adjusted based on patient condition/risks, catheter tip placement, total amount of local anesthetics used, and patient responses. From Gupta, A., & Smith, I. (2011). Local and regional anesthesia. In I. Smith, D. McWhinnie, I. Jackson (Eds.), *Oxford specialist handbook of day surgery* (pp. 93–108). London: Oxford University Press; Ilfelf, B.M., Renehan, E.M., & Enneking, F.K. (2017). Continuous peripheral nerve blocks in outpatients. In A. Hadzic (Ed.), *Hadzic's Textbook of Regional Anesthesia and Acute Pain Management, 2e.* New York, N.Y.: McGraw-Hill Education; Monahan, A.M., & Ilfeld, B.M. (2017) Continuous peripheral nerve blocks: local anesthetic solutions and infusion strategies. In A. Hadzic (Ed.), *Hadzic's Textbook of Regional Anesthesia and Acute Pain Management, 2e.* New York, N.Y.: McGraw-Hill Education.

Historically, peripheral and plexus nerves were localized using electrical nerve stimulation before single injection of LA and for guidance during catheter placement for continuous nerve block infusion (Ilfeld, 2017). More recently, the use of ultrasound-guided technique has become increasingly prevalent and, in some institutions, both techniques (peripheral nerve stimulation and ultrasound are combined to provide dual guidance (Lewis, Price, Walker, McGrattan, & Smith, 2015). Ultrasound guidance has become more popular for a number of reasons, including visualization in real time, allowing nerves to be seen and injectable solution to be deposited around them more quickly and accurately, and the ability to visualize the distribution of the LA on the ultrasound screen during the actual procedure (Orebaugh & Kirkham, 2017). With the use of ultrasonography for nerve blocks, significantly less LA volume is needed to achieve analgesia.

Beneficial Effects of Peripheral Nerve Blocks

Many benefits have been associated with the use of PNBs. Joshi et al. (2016a), in a review of the benefits, risks, and opportunities associated with PNB, report the use of PNB in a multimodal postanesthesia analgesia plan is associated with greater patient satisfaction, improved analgesia, reduced opioid use, reduced lengths of hospital stay, prevention of hospital readmissions, reduced nausea and vomiting, faster movement through the anesthesia recovery process, and earlier participation in physical therapy. In practice guidelines for the management of acute postoperative pain (Chou et al., 2016), the efficacy of surgical site–specific peripheral regional anesthetic techniques is supported by high-quality evidence.

Kessler, Marhofer, Hopkins, and Hollman (2015), in their review of 189 articles that included 143 RCTs (total n = 12,379), report there is good evidence for short-term benefit when evaluating peripheral regional anesthesia. They cite efficacy in terms of pain reduction, reduced demand for systemic analgesics, reduced general anesthesia requirement, and patient satisfaction. The studies indicated overall greater patient satisfaction, and/or earlier hospital discharge for patients who had truncal blocks, including cervical plexus, intercostal, rectus sheath, and ilioinguinal/iliohypogastric blocks. As a result of their review, Kessler et al. (2015) conclude the majority of peripheral nerve blocks have been shown to produce benefit, suggesting efficiency and economic benefit, excluding supraclavicular block and TAP, for where there was insufficient or conflicting evidence on associated benefits. Information on long-term outcomes, such as functional improvement and chronic pain associated with surgery, is inadequate to inform clinical decisions. Additionally, permanent complications are rare, and accurate estimate of incidence is yet to be elucidated.

Contraindications and Risks Associated With Peripheral Nerve Blocks

Contraindications for the use of truncal and peripheral nerve blocks are relative and must be considered in terms of each individual situation. For example, when it is essential to monitor a patient's sensation and strength of an extremity, a peripheral nerve block might prevent adequate assessment. Absolute contraindications for continuous peripheral nerve blockade include infection at the catheter insertion site, LA allergy, and patient refusal; relative contraindications include coagulopathy, use of anticoagulants, systemic infections, preexisting neuropathy, fall risks, and the need for neurovascular examinations (Monahan & Ilfeld, 2017).

The relative contraindication for use of anticoagulants and other medications that increase bleeding risks (antithrombotics, antiplatelet medications) reflects the lack of strong evidence related to the risks of truncal and peripheral nerve blocks in anticoagulated patients. The ASRA guidelines related to anticoagulation in patients with neuraxial anesthetic techniques (described in the neuraxial section) cite increased risk when blocks are performed in deep, noncompressible truncal/peripheral nerve sites and recommend exercising the same precautions as listed in the neuraxial guidelines for perineuraxial, deep plexus, or deep peripheral blocks (Horlocker et al., 2018). For other plexus or peripheral nerve blocks, it is recommended to exercise judgment based on the compressibility, vascularity, and consequences of bleeding associated with the block site (Horlocker et al., 2018). Dietary supplements and herbal therapies that may increase bleeding risks or interact with anticoagulants include garlic, gingko biloba, ginseng, Asian ginseng, Danshen, and Dong quai; fish oil and vitamin E also may have an impact on coagulation. Bleeding risks associated with PNBs and use of these therapies and supplements should also be considered (Narouze et al., 2018). Other relative contraindications are specific to the proposed block site and are addressed in subsequent sections.

As with all invasive procedures, truncal or peripheral nerve blocks and continuous catheter insertions are associated with risks for bleeding, infection, or neurologic injury. Risks include unintentional injection or placement of the catheter into the intravascular or intraneural spaces. In recent years, there have been few complications associated with block insertion, which may be related to the increased use of ultrasound guidance. Specific risks are related to the site of the block. For example, risks associated with an interscalene catheter or block with LA infusion is the development of hoarseness, dyspnea, and respiratory distress.

There is a risk for inadvertent cutting or breakage of the nerve catheter, which poses risks for overheating and tissue damage during an MRI if the retained part is not removed. Other risks include potential for catheter dislodgement and leakage from the catheter insertion site, although the use of 2-octyl cyanoacrylate glue has reduced this risk (Ilfeld, 2017).

The risk for LA toxicity with PNBs is very low; the risk for significant hematoma formation is also low, but risk versus benefit of block/catheter placement is weighed when there are bleeding risks (see contraindication section).

Single injection of LA in a peripheral nerve block has not been associated with infection. However, bacterial colonization risk exists with placement of catheters (Joshi et al., 2016a). Although catheter colonization rates have been reported as high as 58%, the rate of clinically significant infection has been reported as 3% or less (Ilfeld, 2011). In a 7-year analysis of regional anesthesia catheter infection rates, in 36,300 peripheral catheters the incidence of infection was reported as 3%, with severe infection occurring in 0.07% of the cases (Bomberg et al., 2018). Risk factors for infection included diabetes, type of surgery, catheter site, multiple skin punctures, body mass index, and American Society of Anesthesiologists' physical status (Bomberg et al., 2018). In this study, the risk for infection was noted to increase after day 4 of peripheral nerve catheter insertion.

The rate of postoperative neurologic symptoms (PONS) associated with PNBs is unclear, because there are a number of confounding variables which could contribute to PONS and well-designed RCTs are lacking (Ilfeld, 2017). It is not possible to point to nerve blocks as the cause of PONS because the surgical procedure itself, positioning, tourniquet use during surgery, or other variables could contribute to PONS. Available data do not suggest the increased use of ultrasound for placement has affected the rate of PONS. In a study of 1182 interscalene and femoral nerve blocks, 0.3% of patients developed PONS and the incidence for PONS lasting more than 6 months was greater for those with continuous infusions than for those with single-injection peripheral nerve blocks (Sites et al., 2012). Transient neurologic symptoms have been associated with continuous catheters at a rate of 1.4%, and in a study of 3500 catheters, 0.2% had neurologic symptoms lasting more than 6 weeks (Monahan & Ilfeld, 2017).

Potential for falls is a risk associated with PNBs of the lower extremities. Single-injection femoral nerve blocks do not seem to increase risk, but continuous femoral or psoas compartment infusions are associated with increased fall risks (Ilfeld, 2017). Recognition of these risks has resulted in replacement of femoral nerve blocks with adductor canal blocks because the adductor canal blocks are less likely to cause weakness of the quadriceps and subsequent falls (Ilfeld, 2017). It is important to ensure that patients are assessed for fall risk and that preventive measures are undertaken. Physical therapy evaluation and interventions may be helpful in risk assessment and fall prevention. Patients and their care providers need to be educated about peripheral nerve blocks and potential for weakness rend impairment of proprioception and balance (Hunter et al., 2019).

In addition to fall risks related to peripheral nerve blocks, measures are also necessary to prevent and recognize injuries. It is important to ensure position changes are done to prevent excessive pressure and assess for developments of pressure areas on the skin, especially if splints or casts have been used, because pain may not warn the patient of excessive pressure (Hunter et al., 2019). Similarly, peripheral nerve blocks may increase risks for thermal damage if ice or heat is applied to areas affected by the block. Patients and their care providers need to be educated about the importance of protecting body parts affected by nerve blocks from trauma because injury may be undetected until the sensory block resolves.

Medications for Peripheral Nerve Blocks

LAs are the class of medications generally used for truncal and peripheral nerve analgesia. The pharmacology of LA is addressed in the neuraxial analgesia section of this chapter. The choice of LA is largely determined by the desired intensity of block and desired time to onset and duration of LA effect. The onset of blockade in truncal/peripheral nerve blocks varies depending on the type of LA and absorption and distribution of LA. Times of onset of up to 14 minutes for lidocaine and mepivacaine and 23 minutes for bupivacaine for peripheral blocks have been reported (Patel & Sadoughi, 2015). When LA is used for a peripheral nerve block of the lower extremity, and the goal is to have the patient ambulate with physical therapy shortly after recovery from anesthesia, an LA with a shorter duration of action such as lidocaine or mepivacaine may be preferred over an LA with a longer duration of effect such as ropivacaine. As a result of more precise localization of nerves because of the use of ultrasound, there is increased use of bupivacaine (at smaller doses) to maximize duration of block given its slightly longer duration of action than that of ropivacaine (Butterworth, 2020). The maximum duration of a single injection of a truncal/peripheral nerve block ranges from 8 to 24 hours (Monahan & Ilfeld, 2017). When a more prolonged duration of LA effect is desired, a catheter for continuous LA infusion, rather than single-shot injection of LA may be appropriate.

The effectiveness and risks of LA administration in PNBs are influenced by injection site, dose, and properties of the medication, as described in the neuraxial section. Injection site is particularly important with truncal and peripheral nerve blocks because of variability in tissue vascularity. Highly vascular areas such as the intercostal region promote rapid LA absorption, resulting in higher blood levels with greater potential for LA toxicity, with the following in descending order in terms of vascularity and risk for LA toxicity: caudal, epidural, brachial plexus, sciatic, and subcutaneous injection (Suzuki, Gerner, & Lirk, 2019). Tissue inflammation will also increase LA absorption (Berde & Strichartz, 2015; Butterworth, 2020;

Lirk et al., 2014). Unlike with neuraxial analgesia, the addition of EPINEPHrine to LAs in PNBs has not been shown to improve efficacy (Kolettas et al., 2015).

Administration of Peripheral Nerve Block Medications

In addition to single-bolus injection of LA, the other methods for administration of PNB medications are (1) continuous infusion or basal rate administration through an infusion pump, (2) clinician-administered intermittent bolus, (3) patient-controlled PNB administered by the patient using a programmed infusion pump, and (4) programmed intermittent bolus (PIB) technique for administration of PNB analgesia. These techniques are similar to the neuraxial medication administration techniques described in the earlier part of this chapter. Disposable systems for continuous infusion of LA for peripheral regional analgesia are sometimes used for ambulatory or short hospital stay patients. These systems, which contain a reservoir of LA filled in the hospital setting, have a programmable flow rate for basal infusion, and some allow programming for a patient-controlled bolus volume with a lockout interval; technology to allow remote (internet) communication and pump setting control is under development (Ilfeld, 2017). Disposable infusion systems allow patients to be discharged home with continued regional analgesia for a limited number of days until the reservoir is depleted or the patient returns to the outpatient office for follow-up. Before hospital discharge, patients are taught how to remove the catheter when the infusion is completed or are scheduled to visit the outpatient practice for removal.

PIB involves the delivery of a volume of LA on an intermittent basis into a peripheral nerve catheter as a preprogrammed bolus. PIB is theorized to provide better LA spread around the targeted nerves. Cost of PIB infusion devices has limited its use in many practice settings, and few published studies are available to support its use. In a systematic review of RCTs comparing PIB to continuous infusion of LA in continuous peripheral nerve blocks, the evidence from nine RCTs involving 448 patients showed PIB provided modest reductions in pain scores at 6 and 12 hours postoperatively but did not provide a significant difference in pain scores at subsequent time points (Chong, Wang, Dhir, & Lin, 2017).

As with neuraxial regional analgesia, the care of patients with PNB catheters, including management and monitoring, requires the RN to practice as defined by the hospital's policies and procedures and in accordance with the board of nursing in the state in which the RN practices.

Management of Peripheral Nerve Block Catheters and Infusions

Guidelines for the management of PNB catheter infusion systems are lacking. As described in the neuraxial section, aseptic practices are used to minimize risks for infection.

Aseptic practices are used during catheter insertion and with handling of the infusion system (solution and tubing). As with neuraxial infusions, clinical practice supports maintaining the integrity of the infusion system after therapy is initiated (American Society of Anesthesiologists, 2017). This means that every effort should be made to minimize entry into the system to prevent inadvertent introduction of bacteria. Because there are no guidelines, practice varies widely with regard to infusion hang time, tubing changes, or dressing changes. Typically, infusion systems are not entered unless the solution container (bag or bottle) is empty and a new one must be added. Because infusions are used for a short period, often 5 days or less, tubing and dressings are not routinely changed unless a problem is noted.

To prevent errors, all infusions of LAs should be distinctly labeled, have a dedicated infusion pump available for continuous infusion, and have an infusion line that is color-coded, without an injection port.

Peripheral Nerve Blocks: Truncal Approaches

Paravertebral Block

Anatomy

The paravertebral space is an anatomic wedge-shaped compartment between the heads and necks of the ribs and extends from the cervical to sacral spine. The boundaries are formed posteriorly by the plane of the transverse process and the costotransverse ligaments that travel between the processes and the ribs, anterolaterally by the parietal pleura, and medially by the lateral surface of the vertebral body and intervertebral disc (Karmakar, Greengrass, Latmore, & Levin, 2020). Within this space, outside the neuraxial space, the spinal nerve root emerges from the intervertebral foramina and divides into two rami: the dorsal rami, which reflects posteriorly and innervates the skin and muscles of the back and neck; and the ventral rami, which innervates the muscles and skin over the anterolateral body and limbs (Gill, 2017). Segmental analgesia will be ipsilateral; that is, the area of analgesia will depend on the spinal level and the side of the body in which the paravertebral LA is administered (Fig. 18.7).

Indications

Paravertebral block (PVB) provides perioperative analgesia for certain thoracic, chest wall, and abdominal surgeries, such as thoracotomy, video-assisted thoracic surgery (VATS), minimally invasive cardiac surgery to the chest, breast surgery, reconstructive breast surgery, laparoscopic cholecystectomy, nephrectomy, appendectomy, pancreas surgery (e.g., Whipple), and hernia repair. PVB is also a well-established technique for pain management with rib fractures and chest tubes.

Technique

The patient can be positioned in a sitting or lateral decubitus position. Needle placement is performed once the transverse processes, posterior ribs at the appropriate

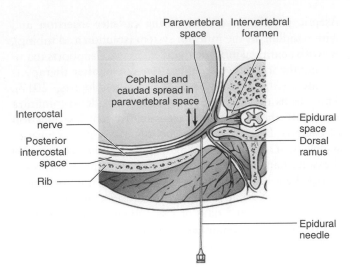

Fig. 18.7 | **Paravertebral Anatomy.** (From Rahangdale, R., Tureanu, L., and Benzon, H. [2018]. *Essentials of pain medicine* [4th ed.]. Philadelphia: Elsevier.)

level of the spine, and paravertebral space are identified. Depending on the type of surgery or chest trauma, there is unilateral or bilateral needle placement into the paravertebral space and sometimes a catheter is threaded through the needle and left in place. The paravertebral space communicates with the epidural space by the intervertebral foramen; consequently, LA injection can spread to the epidural space and result in unilateral or bilateral epidural anesthesia. The paravertebral space also communicates with the intercostal spaces, so LA administration can result in intercostal blockade, making it beneficial for pain related to chest trauma (Vandepitte et al., 2017).

Considerations

Thoracic PVB can be considered when there is concern for sympathetic blockade associated with thoracic epidural; however, bilateral spread can occur because of close proximity and spread of LA along the sympathetic chain ganglion. According to ASRA guidelines for antithrombotic, thrombolytic therapy, the same precautions should be taken with placement of PVB catheters as with neuraxial approaches; however, the complication of significant bleeding in the paravertebral space is less likely to spread to the epidural space and cause a hematoma and associated neurologic deficit (Horlocker et al., 2018). Complications are rare. The major potential adverse event of a thoracic-level approach is pneumothorax, whereas retroperitoneal structures are at risk with a lumbar-level approach. Other potentially serious adverse events with this technique include inadvertent vascular puncture, major bleeding, hematoma, infection, epidural or intrathecal spread, and LAST. Hypotension and urinary retention may occur with lower incidence of side effects than has been associated with the epidural approach (Latmore, Levine, & Gadsden, 2017).

Yeung, Gates, Naidu, Wilson, & Gao Smith (2016) reviewed the evidence regarding paravertebral block versus thoracic epidural in 14 studies with 689 total patients undergoing thoracotomy. Findings were that paravertebral blocks were as effective as thoracic epidural blockade for management of acute pain; moreover, paravertebral blockade reduced the risks for developing complications when compared to thoracic epidural blockade. However, there were no differences in 30-day mortality, major complications, or length of hospital stay, and data were insufficient to make a determination on hospital costs and prevention of persistent pain. The authors concluded that the RCTs included in the review lacked details of randomization, blinding of participants, or outcome assessors, thus increasing potential for bias. Therefore future studies are needed that are adequately powered RCTs and focus not only on acute pain, but also include complications, chronic pain, length of hospital stay, and costs.

Erector Spinae Plane

Indications

The erector spinae plane block is very similar to paravertebral block, but is considered less invasive because anatomically there are no structures at risk for needle injury in the immediate vicinity where the needle is placed; thus there is less potential for serious complications. Potential uses include thoracic neuropathic pain (herpes, malignant rib lesions), pain resulting from rib fractures, breast reconstruction and mastectomy, and thoracic surgery. The erector spinae muscle extends the length of the thoracolumbar spine and thus spread of analgesia with craniocaudal spread covers multiple dermatomes.

Technique

The erector spinae muscle and erector spinae plane lie superior to the laminae and extend from cervical to lumbar to spine. Landmarks for regional anesthesia block placement include the trapezius, rhomboids, and erector spinae paraspinal muscles and T5 transverse process at which LA is injected beneath the muscle plane and spreads to the paravertebral space. The extent of the sensory block after injection of LA involves dermatomes T3-T9. Insertion of an indwelling catheter allows for continuous nerve block infusion (Forero, Adhikary, Lopez, Tsui, & Chin, 2016).

Considerations

Erector spinae plane block is described as safer than PVB because paraspinal injection and catheter placement are far from critical structures involved in paravertebral approach.

Pectoralis

Indications

Available evidence indicates nerves derived from the brachial plexus may be blocked to provide anesthesia and analgesia to the anterolateral chest wall and axilla while avoiding blockade to brachial plexus nerves that innervate the arm (Woodworth, Ivie, Nelson, Walker, & Maniker, 2017). Although mainly used for breast cancer surgery, including mastectomy and breast reconstruction, a few case reports have been written on the use of pectoralis (PEC) blocks for rib fracture and postoperative pain control after thoracotomy (Thiruvenkatarajan, Eng, & Adhikary, 2018; Yalamuri et al., 2017).

Conclusions from a systematic review by Singh, Borle, Kaur, Trikha, & Sinha (2018) were favorable, showing significant opioid-sparing analgesia intraoperatively and analgesic benefit during the first 24 hours after surgery when PEC nerve block was performed as an adjunct to general anesthesia for breast surgery. Limitations identified in the meta-analysis included high heterogeneity (lack of standard technique) and differences in drug doses and volumes leading to high variation in block efficacy.

Technique

The advent of newer blocks such as the PEC I and PEC II blocks has evolved with increasing use of ultrasonography that can identify tissue layers in particular fascial layers. PEC I block targets the fascial plan between the pectoralis major and minor muscles to anesthetize the medial and lateral pectoral nerves, which innervate the pectoralis muscle; PEC II block is an extension of PEC I block and targets the plane between the pectoralis minor and serratus anterior muscles, so injected LA provides blockade to the upper intercostal nerves (Blanco & Barrington, 2017).

Considerations

PEC is a newer ultrasound-guided interfacial thoracic plane block providing analgesia without the potential risks of a neuraxial block.

Transversus Abdominis Plane

Indications

The TAP block is used for many abdominal surgical procedures. The goal of the TAP block is to anesthetize to provide somatic analgesia to part of or the entire abdominal wall (Elsharkawy & Bendtsen, 2017).

Technique

TAP block is a nonspecific term used to describe a group of approaches that mainly differ in location of needle insertion and injection, but all approaches lead to injection of LA into the neurovascular fascial plane, which is between the rectus abdominis sheath and the transversus abdominis muscle. This block to the anterior abdominal wall covers T7-L1 spinal nerves (Chin et al., 2017). The subcostal approach blocks intercostal nerves T6-T9 and the lower lateral classic TAP area blocks intercostal nerves T10-T11 and subcostal nerve T12 (Elsharkawy & Bendtsen, 2017). When the TAP block is not possible, a rectus sheath block may be performed. The rectus sheath is the location of the ventral branches of the T6-L1 thoracolumbar nerves. The rectus sheath block technique involves passing the needle through the anterior rectus

sheath and then through the rectus abdominis muscle to access the posterior wall of the rectus sheath where LA solution is injected to provide postoperative analgesia in upper abdominal surgery (Yarwood & Berrill, 2010).

In a recent meta-analysis by Baeriswyl, Kirkham, Kern, and Albrecht (2015) of 31 controlled trials with total 1611 adult participants, the TAP block was found to provide statistically significant but only modest postoperative analgesic benefit. The mean reduction in intravenously administered morphine at 6 hours was 6 mg and at 24 hours was 11 mg in adult patients who underwent abdominal laparotomy or laparoscopy or cesarean delivery. The authors note these results should be interpreted with caution in view of the heterogeneity of the included studies and the subsequent analysis.

Considerations

Ultrasound-guidance is used to identify TAP space for administering nondermatomal field block (Tsai et al., 2017). TAP blockade is commonly performed for surgery involving the abdominal wall to provide somatic analgesia.

Quadratus Lumborum

Indications

The quadratus lumborum (QL) block is used for postoperative pain involving abdominal and hip surgeries. Indications are for surgical procedures with abdominal wall midline incisions covering dermatomes T6 and as far caudally as L1. QL provides somatic and visceral analgesia to the abdominal wall and lower portion of the thoracic wall, making it a viable option for selected abdominal surgeries.

Technique

The QL block involves the QL muscle along the posterior abdominal wall. It is a variation of the TAP block. The needle passes through the fascial plane between the QL and psoas major muscles. The injected LA travels from the injection site to the thoracic paravertebral space with the goal to provide T4-L1 somatic and visceral analgesia. Bilateral block is required. Extent of the block results in wider sensory blockade than TAP block. There is evidence that this block improves visceral pain (Elsharkawy, 2017; Elsharkawy & Bendtsen, 2017).

Considerations

Patients who receive QL block, depending on block technique, may experience sensory block over the thigh with the QL1 block and the L2 dermatome with the QL block, so precautions for risk for quadriceps weakness and fall injury risk must be considered.

Peripheral Nerve Blocks: Extremity Approaches

Upper extremity peripheral blocks that provide blockade of the brachial plexus include interscalene for surgery involving the shoulder or proximal humerus, supraclavicular, infraclavicular, and axillary nerve block for surgeries that are distal to the mid-humerus (Ottestad & Gowda, 2017). The choice of block is determined based on the type of surgery and individual patient characteristics. For example, a patient with pulmonary disease and respiratory compromise will be less likely to receive an interscalene block because of concerns related to the risk for phrenic nerve block or hemidiaphragmatic paralysis (Tran, Elgueta, Aliste, & Finlayson, 2017).

Lower extremity peripheral blocks are common techniques for surgical anesthesia and analgesia. The lumbosacral plexus provides motor and sensory innervation to the lower abdomen and lower extremity. The lumbar plexus is formed by L1-3 and the superior branch of L4. The major nerve branches of the lumbar plexus are the iliohypogastric (L1), ilioinguinal (L1), genitofemoral (L1, L2), lateral femoral cutaneous (L2, L3), obturator and femoral (L2, L3, L4) nerves (Orebaugh & Cruz Eng, 2020). The inferior branch of L4 and all of L5 plus S1-S3 supply the sacral plexus. The main nerves of the sacral plexus are the sciatic nerve and the pudendal nerve. When blocked at the level of the lumbar plexus, the majority of the anterior leg to the knee, including the anterolateral thigh, medial thigh, and saphenous below the knee, are covered. The sciatic nerve provides innervation to the posterior thigh and the bulk of innervation below the knee except the medial leg, which is supplied by the saphenous nerve (terminal branch of the femoral nerve) (Wasson & Fisher, 2017).

Interscalene Nerve Block

Indications
The interscalene nerve block approach to the brachial plexus is typically indicated for procedures involving shoulder, clavicle or upper arm (i.e., proximal humerus), and elbow. It is not appropriate for procedures at or distal to the elbow (Gautier, Vandepitte, & Gadsden, 2017).

Interscalene Anatomy
The brachial plexus provides innervation to the upper extremity and passes through the interscalene groove bordered by the anterior and middle scalene muscles at about the level C6 vertebrae.

Technique
With the patient's head turned 30 degrees to the contralateral side, a needle is inserted into the interscalene groove at approximately the level of the cricoid and directed in an anteromedial trajectory through the middle scalene muscle and into the interscalene groove near the cervical transverse process.

Considerations
Blockade at this level is around the C5 and C6 nerve roots and can occasionally spread to the cervical plexus and cervical sympathetic chain and results in Horner's syndrome (Wasson & Fisher, 2017). This is not considered a complication and can happen with any brachial plexus block but is most common with interscalene and supraclavicular blocks. Symptoms include miosis (decreased pupil size), ptosis (drooping eyelid), and anhidrosis (decreased sweating) on the affected side of the face (Wasson & Fisher, 2017). These symptoms resolve as the block wears off. Recurrent laryngeal nerve palsy may produce hoarseness. A properly performed interscalene block may also result in ipsilateral (same side of the body) hemidiaphragm paralysis because of the proximity of the phrenic nerve (C3-5) to the interscalene groove (Wasson & Fisher, 2017). Hemidiaphragmatic paralysis in most patients does not significantly compromise lung function, and the patient may need reassurance that the feeling of shortness of breath is transient; however, careful consideration must be given to patients with underlying lung disease (Borgeat, Levine, Latmore, Van Boxstael, & Blumenthal, 2017). Relative contraindications for interscalene block include compromised pulmonary function and preexisting paresis of contralateral phrenic or recurrent laryngeal nerves (Borgeat et al., 2017).

Complications
Early complications soon after the block is performed include risk for LA injection into the vertebral artery leading to LAST; spread of LA into intrathecal, subdural, and epidural space; and risk for pneumothorax because of the close proximity to the pleura. Late complications include neuropathy, plexus nerve injury, and infection (Borgeat et al., 2017).

Supraclavicular

Indications
The supraclavicular block is similar to the interscalene block. This nerve block does not reliably cover the shoulder and is ideal for procedures of the upper extremity from mid-humeral level down to the hand.

Technique
The brachial plexus arrangement is most compact at this location, so there is an increased likelihood of blocking all the branches, resulting in rapid onset and dense, predictable blockade. The brachial plexus is encountered superior to the clavicle at the lateral border of the sternocleidomastoid muscle.

Considerations
Many of the same precautions as with interscalene blocks are taken with patient selection for supraclavicular blocks. Horner's syndrome and recurrent laryngeal nerve palsy may occur. In addition, subclavian artery puncture and pneumothorax remain potential risks (Bendtsen, Lopez, & Vandepitte, 2017)

Infraclavicular

Indications
The infraclavicular block is indicated for pain located in the upper extremity from the mid-humeral level down to the hand. Distribution is similar to the supraclavicular block. It does not cover the shoulder (Albert, Altman, & Doan, 2015).

Technique

This block is typically achieved by advancing the block needle in a caudad direction through the pectoralis muscles and toward the axillary artery, reaching the level of the cords of the brachial plexus. Advantages of this block when compared to supraclavicular block is a reduced risk for pneumothorax and avoidance of cervical vascular structures. It does not affect respiratory function (Albert et al., 2015). Patient selection should include avoiding this approach in any patient with a vascular catheter in the subclavian region, and patients with a pacemaker on the same side as the intended block.

Considerations

This block may be difficult to perform in patients who are obese or cachectic because it may be difficult to visualize the nerve or safely place the needle, thus requiring an alternative block (Wasson & Fisher, 2017). The infraclavicular region is considered a noncompressible area, and therefore this block may not be appropriate for patients who are on anticoagulation drugs or who have coagulopathies. Potential complications include hematoma if a medial approach is used (Wasson & Fisher, 2017).

Axillary

Indications

The axillary block is the most distal brachial plexus block and provides blockade for procedures at the elbow, forearm, wrist, and hand (Gill, 2017). Because of the distal location it has minimal risk for respiratory compromise related to pneumothorax or phrenic nerve blockade.

Technique

The approach involves identification of the axillary artery high in the axilla region; once the landmark is identified the needle is inserted superior to the axillary artery. Injection of LA around the artery will provide effective blockade (Vandepitte, Lopez, & Jalil, 2020).

Considerations

Major neurologic complications with this block are rare; possible complications include neuritis, intravascular injection, and hematoma (Gill, 2017).

Femoral

Indications

The femoral nerve block provides analgesia to the anterior thigh, most of the femur, and the knee; therefore it is often used for femur or knee surgery, hip fractures, and anterior thigh, knee, and quadriceps tendon repair (Vloka, Hadzic, & Gautier, 2017).

Technique

The femoral nerve innervates the main flexor muscles of the hip and the extensor muscles of the knee and also the hip, knee, and ankle joints. Distribution of LA allows for anesthetic coverage to the anterior and medial thigh down to the knee, as well as a variable strip of skin on the medial thigh down to the knee, but no coverage for the posterior knee (Vloka et al., 2017). Placement of the block is done with the patient in the supine position; the femoral/inguinal crease is identified, and then the needle inserted in a plane in a lateral to medial orientation and advanced toward the femoral nerve (Atchabahian, Leunen, Vandepitte, & Lopez, 2017b).

Considerations

Femoral nerve blocks have relatively few risks and contraindications. Contraindications include local infection, previous vascular grafting, and local adenopathy. Femoral nerve blocks result in sensory and motor nerve blockade and can cause weakness of the quadriceps muscles that may contribute to patient falls and impair effective rehabilitation (Vloka et al., 2017).

Fascia Iliaca

Indications

The fascia iliaca block is an alternative to a femoral nerve or lumbar plexus block and is commonly performed for procedures and injuries involving the hip, anterior thigh, and knee. Motor function may be affected, leading to lower extremity weakness (Atchabahian et al., 2017a).

Technique

The fascia iliaca nerve block, sometimes called the fascia iliaca compartment block is similar to the femoral nerve block. This block usually provides blockade to the femoral, lateral femoral cutaneous, and obturator nerves. Distribution of LA in a sufficient volume results in anesthesia of the anterolateral thigh and anteromedial thigh to knee and variable reduced sensation to the skin on the medial leg and foot (Atchabahian et al., 2017a).

Considerations

Anesthesia and amount of analgesia depend on the spread of the LA; this block requires a large volume of LA (30–40 mL) to ensure spread of medication under the fascia iliaca (Atchabahian et al., 2017a). Blockade can result in quadriceps weakness, so fall precautions must be considered.

Adductor Canal

Indications

The adductor canal block provides for analgesia of the knee and medial leg. Compared to the femoral nerve block, this procedure blocks sensation but spares motor function and balance (Madison & Ilfeld, 2018).

Technique

The adductor canal block is actually the saphenous nerve block performed in the adductor canal. Ultrasound guidance facilitates administration of LA to block the saphenous nerve within the adductor canal, distal to the region where most motor nerves of the femoral nerve arise (Madison & Ilfeld, 2018).

Considerations

The adductor canal block preserves quadriceps strength, maintaining lower extremity motor function (Meier et al., 2018).

Sciatic Nerve Block

Indications

The primary indications for sciatic nerve blocks are for ankle and foot surgery, knee surgery involving the posterior compartment, and below knee amputation surgery; the sciatic nerve also may be blocked for surgery involving the hip and thigh (Madison & Ilfeld, 2018).

Technique

The sciatic nerve is composed of spinal nerve roots L4 to S3, supplying motor and sensory innervation to the posterior thigh and the entire lower leg, except the medial leg just below the knee. Because the nerve is so large, it can be blocked from more than one location along the lower extremity. The sciatic nerve can be blocked from several different approaches, including posterior, subgluteal, and anterior or popliteal approaches (Hadzic, Lopez, Vandepitte, & Sala-Blanch, 2017).

Considerations

The sciatic block carries the risk for femoral artery or vein damage and therefore individual patient risks related to vascular grafting, anticoagulation, and coagulopathy are considered (Madison & Ilfeld, 2018).

Ankle Block

Indications

Ankle block is a sensory nerve block performed for all types of foot surgery; because an ankle block does not cause motor blockade, patients are able to ambulate but crutches or other assistive devices may be necessary because of possible proprioceptive deficit or instability (Grant, 2019).

Technique

Ankle block involves five peripheral nerves of the foot, including the tibial, deep peroneal, sural, superficial peroneal, and saphenous nerves. The tibial nerve innervates the heel and sole of the foot; the deep peroneal nerve provides innervation to the ankle extensor muscles, the ankle joint, and the web spaces between the first and second toes; the sural nerve innervates the lateral margin of the foot and ankle; the superficial peroneal nerve innervates the dorsum of the foot; and the saphenous nerve (derived from the femoral nerve) provides innervation to the medial malleolus and a variable portion of the medial aspect of the leg below the knee (Vandepitte, Lopez, Van Boxstael, & Jalil, 2020). The patient is usually positioned supine with support

underneath the calf. The block involves needle placement with the tip of the needle directly adjacent to each of the five nerves so the injected LA can spread around each nerve (Vandepitte, Lopez, Van Boxstael, & Jalil, 2020).

Considerations

The ankle block is a technically challenging block (Grant, 2019). The use of EPINEPHrine in the block solution is avoided because of the potential risk for ischemic complication of the foot (Madison & Ilfeld, 2018).

Regional Analgesia Infusion Systems

Tapering and Discontinuing Regional Analgesia Catheters

For patients with acute pain who are receiving regional analgesia, plans are necessary for smoothly tapering continuous infusions as pain decreases or the patient is able to use a less invasive route of administration. Although most patients experience less pain as the days pass after surgery or injury, it should not be assumed that all patients will follow this pattern. It is best to evaluate patients individually and taper analgesic doses on the basis of patients' reports of pain and ability to perform recovery activities rather than a preconceived notion of when analgesics should be discontinued.

In preparation for discharge, transition to multimodal oral analgesia should be started as soon as the patient is able to tolerate oral/enteral intake and pain is well controlled. As function returns and pain lessens, the rate of the regional catheter infusion can be reduced gradually over the course of the day. When regional analgesia involves the use of continuous infusions for epidural opioids, to make the transition from epidural analgesia to oral analgesia as smooth as possible, the characteristics of the epidural opioid are considered before the epidural is discontinued. When patients are receiving lipophilic epidural LA with or without opioids that have a short duration (e.g., fentaNYL), the oral analgesic can be administered before discontinuing epidural analgesia to optimize patient comfort during the transition. Because analgesia tends to last longer after discontinuing hydrophilic epidural opioids (e.g., morphine, HYDROmorphone), these patients can be informed of the availability of oral analgesia and reminded to ask for it as soon as they feel pain return and before it becomes severe. In all cases, patients should be comfortable before epidural analgesia is discontinued. Frequent pain assessment during the transition provides an opportunity to evaluate and adjust the new analgesic regimen.

Catheter Removal

Removing short-term indwelling neuraxial and PNB block catheters is within the scope of practice for RNs in many U.S. states. Many state boards of nursing have approved this activity by RNs who possess the knowledge and skill to do so and where institutional policy and procedure support it. The procedure for removing epidural catheters varies; Box 18.19 lists important steps and considerations that can be generalized to most situations.

Rarely, catheters break on removal. It is at the discretion of the anesthesia/pain clinician involved in catheter placement to determine whether efforts should be made to remove the retained catheter. If a decision is made to allow the catheter to be retained, the patient is informed of the complication and observed over time. MRI compatibility of the retained portion of the catheter should be determined because catheters may contain coiled wire that poses a risk for heating and tissue damage (Ilfeld, 2017). CT may be helpful in identifying the location of the retained catheter. The incidence of catheter migration or other delayed sequelae appears to be low (Ilfeld, 2017).

Box 18.19 | Removal of Short-Term Epidural Catheters

REQUIREMENTS OF NURSE REMOVAL OF AN EPIDURAL CATHETER

- Institutional policy and procedure and state board of nursing that supports removal of epidural catheters by the registered nurse.
- Knowledge and skills necessary to remove an epidural catheter gained by completing institutional competency requirements.
- Order from anesthesia or pain management provider to remove the epidural catheter.

CONSIDERATIONS *BEFORE* REMOVAL OF AN EPIDURAL CATHETER

- If warranted (e.g., if patient is receiving or received anticoagulants during epidural therapy), platelet count and coagulation studies have been checked and abnormal findings reported to anesthesia or pain management provider. Medication administration record has been reviewed to ensure medications that affect coagulation status have been appropriately held. If questions, confirm with anesthesia or pain management provider. (See Table 18.8.)
- Signs of infection have been reported to anesthesia or pain management provider.
- Pain is under control.
- Appropriate analgesia by alternative route (e.g., oral, intravenous) has been ordered/given to the patient who is receiving epidural analgesia with short-duration opioid (e.g., fentaNYL, SUFentanil) so pain control is maintained when epidural analgesia is discontinued.
- The procedure has been explained to the patient, including the alternative analgesic regimen that will replace the epidural analgesia.

CONSIDERATIONS RELATED TO REMOVING AN EPIDURAL CATHETER

- Universal precautions should be used for the removal of the epidural catheter.
- Removal of the epidural catheter is facilitated when the patient assumes a position similar to the one suggested for catheter placement (i.e., sitting or side-lying with the back arched out toward the person removing the catheter). This position helps to spread the vertebrae apart.
- Although gentle traction is necessary to remove the catheter, it should come out easily and painlessly. If resistance is met or the patient reports pain or unusual sensations (e.g., tingling or a "catch in the back"), the procedure is terminated and the pain management provider is notified.
  - If position change is not successful, the pain management provider may tape the catheter under tension to the patient's back and leave it undisturbed for several hours. The catheter usually works its way out and is then easy to remove.
- After the catheter is removed, the catheter tip is checked for the presence of a black or blue mark. This indicates that the catheter was removed intact. If the tip has no mark, notify pain management provider.
- After cleaning the entry site and surrounding skin with the institution's recommended solution (usually mild soap and water), the insertion site is covered with an adhesive bandage.
- Signs of catheter entry site infection are reported to the pain management provider.

DOCUMENTATION

- Patient tolerance of the procedure, presence of mark on catheter tip, condition of epidural catheter entry site and surrounding area, and specifics of a difficult or unusual removal.

From Pasero, C., & McCaffery, M. (2011). *Pain assessment and pharmacologic management* (p. 441). St. Louis: Mosby. Data from Pasero C, Eksterowicz N, Primeau M, & Cowley C. (2007). ASPMN position statement: Registered nurse management and monitoring of analgesia by catheter techniques. *Pain Management Nursing, 8*(2), 48–54; and Sawhney, M., Chambers, S., & Hysi, F. (2018). Removing epidural catheters: A guide for nurses. *Nursing2019, 48*(12), 47–49. © 2011, Pasero, C., & McCaffery, M. May be duplicated for use in clinical practice.

Preventing and Managing Regional Analgesia Infusion System Complications

Regional analgesia often involves the administration of medications using infusion systems to deliver the medications into a temporary catheter. The system involves a reservoir that contains the medication, tubing, an infusion pump, and a temporary catheter that is placed into a neuraxial, truncal, or peripheral nerve. A number of problems associated with components of the infusion system can place the patient at risk for adverse effects or complications. Measures such as those described in Table 18.13 and Box 18.20 can be taken to minimize risks and prevent patient harm.

Minimizing Errors in Administration of Regional Anesthesia

Operator (human) errors, particularly incorrect loading and programming of infusion pumps, have been identified as a major cause of significant patient injuries and deaths over the years (Institute for Safe Medication Practices, 2011). The use of devices that are not approved for pain management is another potential source of patient injury. The development of smart pump technology with drug libraries has been shown to reduce errors, but mechanical problems, including system malfunctions, software problems, and tubing and connector problems may be encountered despite the technologic advances (Vecchione, 2014). Several patient safety organizations, including the Institute for Safe Medication Practices (ISMP) and the Anesthesia Patient Safety Foundation (APSF) as well as the Joint Commission have published recommendations to optimize safety. Although a number of safety alerts and recommendations were published over 5 years ago, the recommendations remain timely as potential for similar human and technologic risks remain. Many of the recommendations for safe practices related to PCA and epidural medication administration are applicable to medication administration by the neuraxial or truncal/peripheral routes. Table 18.14 presents recommendations to avoid potentially dangerous regional analgesia infusion-related errors.

Local Infiltration Analgesia

In some situations, it is not possible to provide neuraxial or peripheral nerve regional analgesic approaches for patients with acute pain. Lack of availability of skilled procedurists, patient refusal, patient comorbidities and contraindications, and lack of organizational resources to support neuraxial or peripheral nerve regional analgesic techniques are some reasons neuraxial or peripheral nerve analgesic approaches may not be used. Another interventional option for the prevention and treatment of acute pain is the use of local infiltration analgesia.

Local infiltration analgesia (LIA), which primarily involves the use of LAs, administered alone or in a mixture with other analgesics and EPINEPHrine into

the surgical site, has become an alternative to neuraxial or peripheral nerve blocks and catheters, especially in patients undergoing joint replacements and is used as an MMA strategy (Baldini & Miller, 2018). However, research that demonstrates the superiority of this technique over peripheral nerve blockade is lacking (Baldini & Miller, 2018). Orthopedists have supported the use of intraoperative injection of multimodal medications into the surgical joint because some studies have shown LIA lowers postoperative opioid requirements, improves patient satisfaction, and is associated with minimal risks for the first 24 hours after surgery (Hu et al., 2016).

A major benefit of LIA in orthopedic surgery is that, unlike some neuraxial or peripheral nerve blocks, LIA does not cause motor block, and because it is motor sparing, it may permit early mobility and reduce fall risks (Ganapathy, Howard, & Sondekoppam, 2017). There is a lack of standardized LIA techniques. Types of medications and doses vary among studies. In a meta-analysis of 16 RCTs that included 1206 patients who underwent total knee arthroplasties, LIA provided better analgesia than regional blocks at rest and preserved motor function of the quadriceps; the varied techniques used for LIA, and the variety of analgesic medications, dosages, and different administration techniques may have added bias to the study results (Hu et al., 2016).

LIA primarily includes the use of LAs. Nonsteroidal inflammatory drugs (NSAIDs), cyclooxygenase 2 inhibitor, corticosteroids, opioids, and ketamine have been used in LIA, and although not well studied, EPINEPHrine and cloNIDine are also sometimes used (Raeder & Spreng, 2017). EPINEPHrine is included for its vasoconstriction effect, which may prolong the duration of the locally active medications by reducing clearance from the site (Raeder & Spreng, 2017). In addition to use in orthopedic procedures, LIA is used in other surgical procedures, including laparoscopic colectomy, other abdominal surgeries, gynecologic surgeries, and breast surgeries (Hayden et al., 2017; Park et al., 2015; Soliman, 2018; Tam et al., 2015). Increased awareness of the role of the inflammatory process associated with pain in abdominal surgeries has led to use of techniques such as LA infiltration and infusion by catheters into the peritoneum. The musculofascial and subdermal abdominal tissue planes are also often infiltrated with LA to reduce nociceptive pain arising from the abdominal wall (Joshi et al., 2016b).

A major drawback of LIA is the limited duration of effect. The usual duration of effect of LAs such as ropivacaine and bupivacaine is usually 6 to 8 hours (Joshi, Gandhi, Shah, Gadsden, & Corman, et al., 2016a). Because LAs are the main ingredient in most LIA, there is much interest in exploring new formulations of medications and vehicles to deliver analgesics with longer durations of action for use in local infiltration. For example, in open abdominal surgeries, some surgeons have continuously infused solutions of LA into the wound by catheters

Table 18.13 | Minimizing Errors Related to Regional Analgesia Infusions

Risk	Potential Harm	Preventive Measures
Contamination of regional analgesic medication/solution and reservoirs	Infection, neuraxial or truncal peripheral localized or systemic	1. Use commercially available medication preparations, or if not available, outsource preparation, or prepare under appropriate conditions in the pharmacy.
Regional (epidural or truncal/peripheral) line misconnections resulting in wrong route of medication administration.	Local anesthetic could inadvertently be administered intravenously, or intravenous medications could be administered by a regional route.	1. Use distinctly different infusion pumps for different infusion routes. For example, regional medication infusions should be run on infusion pumps that are recognizably different from pumps used for intravenous infusions. 2. Use connectors specifically designed for individual types of infusion devices according to ISO connector standards, which would prevent misconnections of tubing. 3. Always trace tubing or catheter from patient to infusion device before connecting or reconnecting, at any transition in care, in all handoffs. 4. Use yellow-lined tubing to distinguish regional analgesia medication tubing. 5. Route catheter with different purposes in different standardized directions (e.g., epidural tubing and infusion devices are always placed on the patient's left side; intravenous tubing on the left). 6. Label tubing at distal and proximal ends. 7. Label catheter. Do not use tubing with injection ports. 8. Infuse regional analgesics on a dedicated infusion pump; do not run intravenous infusions on same pump unit.
Incorrect patient, medication, dose, settings, or route of regional medication administration.	Patient may be overdosed or underdosed with the prescribed medication or given the wrong medication.	1. Use barcode technology to verify patient and medication. 2. Require independent double check at the bedside of all regional medication infusions, including verification of pump settings at initiation of infusion and any setting changes. 3. Use smart pump technology In approved infusion devices to minimize medication errors. 4. Require independent verification of pump settings, lines, and infusions at all handoffs, including change of shift. 5. Avoid distractions and interruptions during setup, setting changes, and verification of regional analgesic infusion pumps. 6. Ensure clear labeling of regional medication bags and syringes to identify correct administration route and prevent accidental intravenous administration. For example, label infusion bags and syringes that contain epidural medications with labels that state "For Epidural Use Only" in large, readily identified font. 7. Hang infusion bags or load syringes into pump with the label facing outward so it can be easily read. 8. Store regional analgesia medications (bags/syringes) in separate locations to avoid mix-ups.
Pump malfunction	Overdose or underdose of regional analgesic medication with potential adverse effects	1. Avoid use of infusion pumps not approved for use in infusion of regional analgesia; use only devices/infusion pumps approved for the administration of regional analgesia medications. 2. Monitor pump function during patient rounds. 3. Replace pumps that do not appear to be functioning correctly and remove them from service for examination by clinical engineering. 4. In general, regional analgesia infusion devices should not be used in MRI or hyperbaric chambers. Check with manufactures before use in these settings. 5. Sequester pumps for examination and analysis by clinical engineering in the event of an unanticipated poor patient outcome, such as a rapid response or cardiac arrest.

ISO, International Organization for Standardization.

From Anesthesia Patient Safety Foundation. (2012). Reducing risk of epidural-intravenous misconnections. *apsf Newsletter, 26* (3). Retrieved from https://www.apsf.org/article/reducing-risk-of-epidural-intravenous-misconnections; Institute for Safe Medication Practices. Epidural-IV route mix-ups: reducing the risk of deadly errors. (2008). Retrieved from https://www.ismp.org/resources/epidural-iv-route-mix-ups-reducing-risk-deadly-errors; Joint Commission. (2014). Sentinel event alert issue 53: Managing risk during transition to new ISO tubing connector standards. Retrieved from https://www.jointcommission.org/assets/1/6/SEA_53_Connectors_8_19_14_final.pdf; and Ohashi, K., Dalleur, O., Dykes, P. C., & Bates, D. W. (2014). Benefits and risks of using smart pumps to reduce medication error rates: A systematic review. *Drug Safety, 37*(12), 1011–1020.

Box 18.20 | Key Points in Optimizing Epidural Safety

- Check coagulation status before epidural catheter insertion and removal.
- Verify that medications that could affect coagulation status are appropriately held for epidural insertion, during therapy, and for epidural removal.
- Follow guidelines such as those published by the American Society of Regional Anesthesia and Pain Medicine (ASRA) for use and timing of anticoagulants and antiplatelet medication administration and monitoring of laboratory values for bleeding risks.
- Assess sensory and motor block level on a regular basis, especially if patient is experiencing increased pain.

From Horlocker, T. T., Vandermeuelen, E., Kopp, S. L., Gogarten, W., Leffert, L. R., & Benzon, H. T. (2018). Regional anesthesia in the patient receiving antithrombotic or thrombolytic therapy: American Society of Regional Anesthesia and Pain Medicine evidence-based guidelines (fourth edition). *Regional Anesthesia and Pain Medicine, 43*(3), 263–309.

to prolong the LA effect and optimize pain relief (Baldini & Miller, 2018).

In response to the need for opioid-sparing multimodal analgesics, progress has been made in the development of longer acting LAs (Balocco, Van Zundert, Gan, Gan, & Hadzic, 2018). In 2011 the U.S. Food and Drug Administration (FDA) approved the use of liposomal bupivacaine, a novel delivery system of bupivacaine, for infiltration of surgical wounds in bunion and hemorrhoidectomy surgeries; in 2015, approval was expanded to local surgical infiltration, which included transabdominal plane blocks (Malik, Kaye, Kaye, Belani, & Urman, 2017). Subsequently, in 2018 the FDA approved its use in interscalene brachial plexus nerve blocks to provide postoperative analgesia for shoulder surgeries (Balocco et al., 2018).

Liposomal bupivacaine is an extended-release injectable suspension of bupivacaine that is encapsulated in biodegradable liposomes; it is administered as a one-time injection for tissue infiltration during surgery or for an interscalene nerve block (Balocco et al., 2018). Plain bupivacaine hydrochloride may be mixed in the same syringe with liposomal bupivacaine (at 50% or less of the liposomal bupivacaine dose) if it is anticipated that additional plain bupivacaine is needed to provide faster

Table 18.14 | Regional Analgesia Infusion System Catheter-Related Complications

Problem/Symptoms	Usual Causes	Prevention	Nursing Actions	Anesthesia/Approved Clinician Interventions
Regional analgesia is infusing but inadequate analgesia, partial or incomplete block effect	Incorrect catheter placement; may occur if catheter is more than 5 cm into epidural space, or catheter position may have been altered. May be caused by pump problem, tubing disconnection, catheter dislodgement.	Optimize and verify catheter placement if possible. Verify pump settings and function, secured connections, and assess insertion site.	Assess patient. Check insertion site to ensure catheter is not dislodged. Assess sensation for change/loss of block if local anesthetic has been infusing. If epidural catheter, assess sensation at targeted dermatome levels. Notify anesthesia/approved clinician. Assess pump and tubing connections to ensure proper function.	Pull back to partially withdraw catheter if safe based on anticoagulation status. Bolus catheter/infuse additional medication. Replace catheter if catheter placement is incorrect. Verify anticoagulation status. Provide alternative analgesia option while correcting problem.
Regional analgesia catheter dislodgement; decrease or loss of analgesia block effect. For epidural catheter migration through dura into subarachnoid space, or into vascular system, see text.	Accidental dislodgement, especially during activity.	Dress catheter with clear, occlusive dressing. Secure catheter with tape or device. Educate patient and clinicians about presence of catheter and need for caution with positioning and activity.	Assess patient. Note and record catheter depth based on markings at time of placement. Assess catheter depth every shift or per policy. Assess insertion site for signs of dislodgement.	Tunneling of catheter to reduce risk for migration and dislodgement. Ensure secure dressing at time of insertion. Provide alternative analgesia option while correcting problem.

Table 18.14 | Regional Analgesia Infusion System Catheter-Related Complications—cont'd

Problem/Symptoms	Usual Causes	Prevention	Nursing Actions	Anesthesia/Approved Clinician Interventions
Regional analgesia catheter disconnection from tubing; decrease or loss of analgesia block effect	Loosening of tubing-catheter connection.	Check connections during patient assessments and tighten loosened connections. Assess for tightness before mobilization, and recheck after activity.	Assess patient. When disconnection noted, wrap ends in sterile gauze. Notify anesthesia/approved clinician.	If *epidural catheter* disconnection is known to have occurred within 8 hours and fluid column is static, approved clinician may immerse catheter ≥10 inches from disconnected end in povidone-iodine for 3 minutes. Dry thoroughly, using sterile technique, cut in center of cleansed area and reconnect with a sterile connector. If duration of disconnection is unknown or if nonstatic fluid state, catheter removal is advised. If *truncal/peripheral* catheter disconnection, may follow previous recommendations. Provide alternative analgesia option while correcting problem.
Air in tubing/infusion temporarily stopped, resulting in decrease or loss of analgesia block effect.	Solution container may have emptied.	Assess for adequate volume of solution in infusion container.	Assess patient. Ensure adequate volume of solution in infusion container. Small bubbles of air/small amount not problematic; clear tubing to stop alarms and restart infusion.	If infusion has been off for a time, a bolus of solution may be needed to restore analgesia/block. Provide alternative analgesia option while correcting problem.
Infusion pump alarm.	Air in line, tubing kink, low volume in reservoir, low battery.	Ensure adequate reservoir volume, correct pump and alarm settings, proper tubing connections.	Assess patient. Assess for decrease or loss of analgesia block effect. Check entire system from patient and insertion site back through tubing to pump and reservoir.	

From Hebl, J. R., & Niesen, A. D. (2011). Infectious complications of regional anesthesia. *Current Opinion in Anesthesiology, 24*(5), 573–580; Langevin, P. B., Gravenstein, N., Langevin, S. O., & Gulig, P. A. (1996). Epidural catheter reconnection. Safe and unsafe practice. *Anesthesiology 85*(4), 883–888; and Nathan, N., & Wong, C. A. (2014). Spinal, epidural, and caudal anesthesia: anatomy, physiology, and technique. In D. Chestnut, C. Wong, L. Tsen, W. D. Ngan Kee, Y. Beilin, & J. Mhyre. *Chestnut's obstetric anesthesia: Principles and practice* (5th ed., pp. 229–261). Philadelphia: Saunders.

onset to complement the early analgesia provided by the liposomal formulation (Balocco et al., 2018; Gadsden & Long, 2016; Joshi et al., 2016b). Although liposomal bupivacaine results in plasma levels of bupivacaine for 96 hours after local infiltration and 120 hours after interscalene brachial plexus nerve block, plasma levels have not been shown to correlate with local efficacy (Exparel, 2018). Based on Phase III clinical trials, in 2014 the FDA issued a warning to the manufacturers of the product that pain control beyond 24 hours had not been demonstrated (Uskova & O'Connor, 2015).

Published studies have reported on the use of liposomal bupivacaine in a variety of surgical conditions. A systematic review of its use in several different types of plastic surgery cases involving 405 patients demonstrated safety and efficacy and similar or more effective analgesia compared to traditional pain management procedures (Vyas et al., 2016). In a meta-analysis of 16 trials of patients undergoing total knee arthroplasties by Singh et al. (2017), benefits of the use of intraarticular liposomal bupivacaine compared to other conventional analgesic regimens (periarticular conventional LAs, femoral nerve blocks with conventional LAs, and multimodal intravenous analgesia) were examined. The clinical advantage of liposomal bupivacaine was reported to be questionable because lengths of stay were marginally shortened. The liposomal bupivacaine group showed better pain relief in overall comparison to the other analgesic regimens, but the difference in pain scores was found to be relatively small, especially on the second postoperative day. Superiority or inferiority of liposomal bupivacaine could not be determined for opioid use or range of motion because of the small number in the pooled sample (Singh et al., 2017). The authors noted that many variables, including administration techniques, affected the analgesia outcomes, and high heterogeneity had an impact on the analysis of date (Singh et al., 2017).

In a meta-analysis of four RCTs that included 510 patients who underwent total shoulder arthroplasty, when compared to interscalene nerve block, liposomal bupivacaine infiltration provided comparable results in terms of pain scores and opioid consumption during the first 48 hours postoperatively (Wang & Zhang, 2017). In a systematic review and meta-analysis of seven studies involving patients who underwent colorectal resections, liposomal bupivacaine, administered as a TAP block or local infiltration to 538 patients, was associated with shortened lengths of stay and decreased intravenous opioid use compared to the 470 patients in the control group. The authors recognized multiple limitations in their results, including the paucity of RCTs, and recommend caution in interpretation of results (Raman, Lin, & Krishnan, 2018). A systematic review and meta-analysis of nine RCTs involving 770 patients compared postsurgical pain of patients who underwent a variety of surgical procedures and received either surgical site injections of liposomal bupivacaine or LAs (bupivacaine or ropivacaine) (Kendall, Castro Alves, & De Oliveira, 2018. The authors found there was no significant difference in the outcomes of postsurgical pain at rest (measured by pain scores) at 24 or 48 hours after surgery or postoperative opioid consumption at 24, 48, or 72 hours after surgery in the liposomal bupivacaine group compared to the plain LA group; similar results were found in patients who had orthopedic procedures or non-orthopedic procedures (Kendall et al., 2018). The authors note several limitations of the review and recognize the high heterogeneity of the analysis.

In terms of liposomal bupivacaine safety, it is necessary to consider the potential risks for cardiovascular and neurologic toxic effects. Toxicity risks of LAs are additive, and risks increase when LAs are coadministered with liposomal bupivacaine. Caution is taken not to exceed recommended doses of liposomal bupivacaine, and it is recommended to avoid administration of LAs for 96 hours after use of liposomal bupivacaine (Exparel, 2018).

Many other studies and reviews of the use of liposomal bupivacaine have been published in a variety of patient populations examining different techniques and study outcomes. Studies differ in their quality and conflicting outcomes have been reported. It is important to consider the FDA recommendations for the use of liposomal bupivacaine to guide use of this product. As Kendall and colleagues (2018) note, care must be taken to ensure adequate postoperative pain relief and use of more conventional multimodal approaches, including regional approaches, until strong and convincing evidence of the superiority of liposomal bupivacaine or other analgesic options become available. New formulations of LAs with sustained release and prolonged duration of action are in stages of active development (Balocco et al., 2018). The research and clinical interest in liposomal bupivacaine and these other developing products provide future opportunities for use of safe and effective therapies to reduce postoperative pain and reliance on opioid use.

Additional Analgesic Procedures Involving Use of Local Anesthetics

Infiltration anesthesia involves the injection of LA alone or in combination with other medications to optimize the analgesic effect. With infiltration anesthesia, the LA is injected directly into the tissue in a region of pain or potential pain without consideration for the location of the cutaneous nerves. It does not involve use of anatomical landmarks or ultrasound and is minimally invasive. A disadvantage of infiltrative anesthesia is that it may cause temporary distortion of the tissue as it is injected directly into the painful area. Use of LA to infiltrate the site of a wound or laceration sustained in a traumatic event, to ease discomfort during suturing, or to facilitate placement of a chest tube are examples of situations in which infiltration anesthesia is used to optimize comfort and reduce opioid requirements. Infiltration anesthesia can be superficial, involving injection only into the skin, or deep, involving structures such as the intra-abdominal organs (Catterall & Mackie, 2018; Mankowitz, 2017).

Lidocaine 0.5%–0.25% is the most commonly used LA for infiltration anesthesia because of its rapid onset (<2 minutes) and short duration of action (<30 minutes), which is what is usually adequate for most of these procedures. Bupivacaine 0.125%–0.25% is also used in infiltration anesthesia, especially when the pain associated with the procedure is expected to last several hours. It has a longer onset (10 minutes) and duration of action (up to 7 hours) and is slightly more painful than lidocaine with the initial injection (Mankowitz, 2017). The benefits of each of these LAs may be optimized by combining lidocaine with bupivacaine in a single syringe to achieve both rapid onset and longer duration of action. When a patient has an allergy to either of these amide LAs, procaine (an ester) is an alternative LA with a rapid onset (2–5 minutes) and intermediate duration (2 hours). Epinephrine is sometimes added to the LA because the vasoconstrictory effect may allow reduction in the dose of LA and extension of the LA action.

Field block anesthesia involves the subcutaneous infiltration of LA solution (usually the amide LAs) around the border of a well-circumscribed wound, lesion (cyst), or surgical (procedural) field (Latham & Martin, 2014). The LA is injected in a diamond or square shape circumferentially around the targeted field. This technique offers the advantage of injection outside of the targeted field and therefore does not distort the wound or lesion landmarks. It may have a longer duration of action than infiltrative anesthesia.

LAs are also used in peripheral soft tissue, bursa, and intra-articular injections in inpatient and outpatient practice settings to facilitate diagnosis and treatment of peripheral joint-mediated pain. The injections usually include LA in conjunction with corticosteroid. The LA has a rapid onset, which eases the pain of the procedure and aids in promptly determining whether the injected structure is the source of the patient's pain. The corticosteroid provides a potent anti-inflammatory effect, which may take several days to provide maximum effect. Injections are performed using surface anatomy landmarks, and with increased availability of imaging, fluoroscopy or ultrasound are used to optimize effectiveness and safety (Berger & Dangaria, 2014).

Although these LA injection procedures are generally considered safe, as in neuraxial and peripheral nerve blocks, the volume or amount of LA administered must be considered to avoid risks of LA toxicity. Additionally, because LAs are weak acids, they may be painful upon injection. To ease the discomfort, lidocaine may be buffered by mixing 9 mL of lidocaine with 1 mL of 8.4% sodium bicarbonate. Warming lidocaine and using a small needle (30-gauge) can also be used to reduce the discomfort of injection. Other techniques, such as injecting the LA through the wound edges rather than intact skin, may reduce the injection pain (Crystal, McArthur, & Harrison, 2007; Mankowitz, 2017). When time allows, the application of a topical LA over the planned sites for LA injections has also been found to reduce injection site pain.

Key Points

- Regional analgesia is an effective method for managing a variety of types of pain.
- Regional analgesia is a primary analgesic method for some types of postoperative pain and may provide relief for some patients with refractory persistent pain.
- Regional analgesia can be delivered by neuraxial and truncal or peripheral nerve approaches.
- Neuraxial analgesia involves the delivery of analgesic medications by single-bolus injection or continuous infusion into the epidural or spinal (intrathecal) space.

- Preservative-free opioids and local anesthetics (LAs) are the main medications used in neuraxial analgesia. Other preservative-free coanalgesic medications such as cloNIDine also have a role in neuraxial analgesia.
- Complications of neuraxial analgesia can be serious and are procedure and medication related.
- Serious complications of neuraxial analgesia, including epidural hematoma, infection and abscess formation, and neurotoxicity, require frequent patient assessment for early recognition and prompt intervention.
- Regional analgesia requires special consideration of risks and benefits in patients with increased bleeding risks, including those who require anticoagulants, thrombin inhibitors, and other medications that increase bleeding risks.
- Local anesthetic systemic toxicity (LAST) is a potential complication of regional anesthesia, requiring prompt recognition of LAST and administration of lipid rescue.
- Regional analgesia using truncal and peripheral nerve approaches provide safe and effective analgesic options, while reducing some of the risks associated with neuraxial analgesia.
- Improvements in technology and availability of ultrasound have reduced risks and increased accuracy in placement of peripheral and truncal nerve blocks and catheters.
- Truncal and peripheral nerve blocks and catheters require patient assessment for complications, including those associated with bleeding, infection, and nerve damage.
- Skillful assessment of neurologic status, including sensation and motor strength, is important in determining effectiveness of regional analgesia and in promptly recognizing and addressing development of complications.
- Patient education is important to ensure that patients understand risks associated with regional analgesia, including mobility limitations and fall risks.
- Local infiltration analgesia (LIA), which primarily involves the use of LAs, administered alone or in a mixture with other analgesics and EPINEPHrine into the surgical site, has become an alternative to neuraxial or peripheral nerve blocks and catheters and is used as a multimodal analgesic strategy.
- Unique formulations of LAs, such as those used in liposomal delivery systems, may increase the duration of effect of LAs and provide other clinical advantages.
- Local anesthetics, sometimes combined with corticosteroids or other medications, are used for infiltration of superficial soft tissue, deeper tissues, and joints to facilitate analgesia for wounds and injuries and in preparation for invasive procedures. These injections do not target individual or specific nerves and often do not require the use of imaging techniques.

Case Scenario

Mr. G., a 76-year-old with a medical history of atrial fibrillation and coronary artery disease, is admitted after a motor vehicle crash that resulted in fractures of the right 3 to 7 posterior ribs, a right humerus fracture, and an open right femur fracture. He is stabilized in the trauma unit, but there are concerns about his ability to maintain adequate ventilation because he is breathing shallowly as a result of pain from his rib fractures. He reports allergies to penicillin and procaine.

1. What regional analgesia techniques may be appropriate for Mr. G.?
2. What contraindications for regional analgesia can be identified for Mr. G.?
3. Mr. G. asks whether regional analgesia provides any benefits over the use of systemic opioids. What response can be provided?
4. Considering his medication allergies, what are the local anesthetic options for Mr. G.?
5. If Mr. G. undergoes neuraxial analgesia with a continuous epidural infusion of fentaNYL with ropivacaine, what adverse effects are possible?
6. What assessments should be made if Mr. G., who has a paravertebral catheter, reports increasing pain in his right chest near his rib fracture sites?
7. Mr. G. has a lumbar plexus catheter that is infusing ropivacaine 0.2% at 12 mL/h. He is complaining of numbness in his right leg that has increased in the past 2 hours. What are the possible causes and appropriate interventions?

References

Ahmed, A., & Baig, T. (2016). Incidence of lower limb motor weakness in patients receiving postoperative epidural analgesia and factors associated with it: An observational study. *Saudi Journal of Anaesthesia, 10*(2), 149.

Albert, D. B., Altman, R., & Doan, L. (2015). Supraclavicular and Infraclavicular Nerve Blocks. In S. Diwan, & P. S. Staats (Eds.), *Atlas of Pain Medicine Procedures*. New York: McGraw-Hill. Retrieved 8/20/2020 from https://accessanesthesiology.mhmedical.com/content.aspx?sectionid=64179291&bookid=1158.

Allen, T. K., Mishriky, B. M., Klinger, R. Y., & Habib, A. S. (2018). The impact of neuraxial clonidine on postoperative analgesia and perioperative adverse effects in women having elective Caesarean section: a systematic review and meta-analysis. *British Journal of Anaesthesia, 120*(2), 228–240.

American Society of Anesthesiologists Committee on Standards and Practice Parameters. (2017). Practice advisory for the prevention, diagnosis and management of infectious complications associated with neuraxial techniques: An updated report by the American Society of Anesthesiologists task force on infectious complications associated with neuraxial techniques and the American Society of Regional Anesthesia and Pain Medicine. *Anesthesiology, 126*(4), 585–601. Retrieved 8/20/20 from https://www.asra.com/content/documents/practice-advisory-for-the-prevention-diagnosis-and-management-of-infectious-complications.pdf.

American Society of Anesthesiology (ASA) Committee on Practice Standards. (2016). Practice Guidelines for the prevention, detection and management of respiratory depression associated with neuraxial opioid administration: An Updated Report by the American Society of Anesthesiologists Task Force on Neuraxial Opioids and the American Society of Regional Anesthesia and Pain Medicine. *Anesthesiology, 124*(3), 535–552. https://doi.org/10.1097/ALN.0000000000000975.

Argoff, C. E. (2013). Recent management advances in acute postoperative pain. *Pain Practice, 14*(5), 477–487. https://doi.org/10.1111/papr.12108.

Atchabahian, A., Leunen, I., Vandepitte, C., & Lopez, A. M. (2017a). Ultrasound-guided fascia iliaca block. In A. Hadzic (Ed.), *Hadzic's Textbook of Regional Anesthesia and Acute Pain Management, 2e*. New York, N.Y.: McGraw-Hill Education.

Atchabahian, A., Leunen, I., Vandepitte, C., & Lopez, A. M. (2017b). Ultrasound-guided femoral nerve block. In A. Hadzic (Ed.), *Hadzic's Textbook of Regional Anesthesia and Acute Pain Management, 2e*. New York, N.Y.: McGraw-Hill Education.

Baeriswyl, M., Kirkham, K. R., Kern, C., & Albrecht, E. (2015). The analgesic efficacy of ultrasound-guided transversus abdominis plane block in adult patients: A meta-analysis. *Anesthesia & Analgesia, 121*(6), 1640–1654. https://doi.org/10.1213/ANE.0000000000000967.

Baldini, G., & Miller, T. (2018). Enhanced recovery protocols & optimization of perioperative outcomes. In J. F. Butterworth IV, D. C. Mackey, & J. D. Wasnick (Eds.), *Morgan & Mikhail's clinical anesthesiology, 6e*. New York, NY: McGraw-Hill.

Balocco, A. L., Van Zundert, P. G. E., Gan, S. S., Gan, T. J., & Hadzic, A. (2018). Extended release bupivacaine formulations for postoperative analgesia: an update. *Current Opinion in Anaesthesiology, 31*(5), 636–642.

Bendtsen, T. F., Lopez, A. M., & Vandepitte, C. (2017). Ultrasound-guided supraclavicular brachial plexus block. In *New York School of Regional Anesthesia [NYSORA] Based on Hadzic's textbook of RAPM* (2nd ed.). Retrieved 8/20/20 from https://www.nysora.com/ultrasound-guided-supraclavicular-brachial-plexus-block-2.

Benzon, H. T., Rathmell, J. P., Wu, C. L., Turk, D. C., Argoff, C. E., & Hurley, R. W. (Eds.). (2014). *Practical management of pain* (5th ed.). Philadelphia, PA: Mosby.

Berde, C. B., & Strichartz, G. R. (2015). Local anesthetics. In R. D. Miller (Ed.), *Miller's Anesthesia* (8th ed.). Philadelphia, PA: Elsevier.

Berger, J. S., & Dangaria, H. T. (2014). Joint injections & procedures. Chapter 40. In I. B. Maitin, & E. Cruz (Eds.), *CURRENT Diagnosis & Treatment: Physical Medicine & Rehabilitation*. New York, NY: McGraw-Hill.

Bindra, T. K., Singh, R., & Gupta, R. (2017). Comparison of postoperative pain after epidural anesthesia using 0.5%, 0.75% ropivacaine and 0.5% bupivacaine in patients undergoing lower limb surgery: A double-blind study. *Anesthesia, essays and researches, 11*(1), 52.

Blanco, R., & Barrington, M. J. (2017). Pectoralis and serratus plane blocks. In *NYSORA based on Hadzic's Regional Anesthesia and Pain Medicine* (2nd ed.). Retrieved 8/20/20 from https://www.nysora.com/pectoralis-serratus-plane-blocks.

Bomberg, H., Bayer, I., Wagenpfeil, S., Kessler, P., Wulf, H., Standl, T., … Spies, C. (2018). Prolonged catheter use and infection in regional anesthesia: A retrospective registry analysis. *Anesthesiology: The Journal of the American Society of Anesthesiologists*, 128(4), 764–773.

Booth, J. L., Pan, P. H., Thomas, J. A., Harris, L. C., & D'Angelo, R. (2017). A retrospective review of an epidural blood patch database: the incidence of epidural blood patch associated with obstetric neuraxial anesthetic techniques and the effect of blood volume on efficacy. *International Journal of Obstetric Anesthesia*, 29, 10–17.

Borgeat, A., Levine, M., Latmore, M., Van Boxstael, S., & Blumenthal, S. (2017). Interscalene Brachial Plexus Block. In A. Hadzic (Ed.), *Hadzic's Textbook of Regional Anesthesia and Acute Pain Management, 2e*. New York, N.Y.: McGraw-Hill Education.

Bos, E. M. E., Haumann, J., De Quelerij, M., Vandertop, W. P., Kalkman, C. J., Hollmann, M. W., & Lirk, P. (2018). Haematoma and abscess after neuraxial anaesthesia: a review of 647 cases. *British Journal of Anaesthesia*, 120(4), 693–704.

Brull, R., Macfarlane, A. J. R., & Chan, V. W. S. (2015a). Spinal, epidural, and caudal anesthesia. In R. D. Miller (Ed.), 2. *Miller's anesthesia* (8th ed., pp. 1684–1720). Philadelphia, PA: Elsevier.

Brull, R., Hadzic, A., Reina, M. A., & Barrington, M. J. (2015b). Pathophysiology and etiology of nerve injury following peripheral nerve blockade. *Regional Anesthesia & Pain Medicine*, 40(5), 479–490. https://doi.org/10.1097/AAP.0000000000000125.

Bujedo, B. M. (2013). Recommendations for spinal opioids clinical practice in the management of postoperative pain. *Journal of Anesthesiology & Clinical Science*, 2013. https://doi.org/10.7243/2049-9752-2-28. Retrieved 8/20/20 from http://www.hoajonline.com/journals/pdf/2049-9752-2-28.pdf.

Bujedo, B. M. (2014). Spinal opioid bioavailability in postoperative pain. *Pain Practice*, 14(4), 350–364.

Bujedo, B. M. (2015). Clinical use of spinal opioids for postoperative pain. *Journal of The Analgesics*, 3(2), 17–23. https://doi.org/10.20941/2311-0317.2015.03.02.1.

Bujedo, B. M. (2016). An Update on neuraxial opioid-induced pruritus prevention. *Journal of Anesthesia & Critical Care, Open Access*, 6(2), 00226.

Bujedo, B. M. (2017). Physiology of spinal opioids and its relevance for pain management selection. *Open Journal of Pain Medicine*, 1(1), 021–026.

Bujedo, B. M., Santos, S. G., & Azpiazu, A. U. (2012). A review of epidural and intrathecal opioids used in the management of postoperative pain. *Journal of Opioid Management*, 8(3), 177–192. https://doi.org/10.5055/jom.2012.0114.

Bulbake, U., Doppalapudi, S., Kommineni, N., & Khan, W. (2017). Liposomal formulations in clinical use: an updated review. *Pharmaceutics*, 9(2), 12.

Butterworth, J. IV. (2020). Local Anesthetics: Clinical pharmacology of local anesthetics. *New York School of Regional Anesthesia (NYSORA)*. Retrieved from https://www.nysora.com/foundations-of-regional-anesthesia/pharmacology/clinical-pharmacology-local-anesthetics/. Retrieved August 19, 2020.

Butterworth, J. F., IV, Mackey, D. C., & Wasnik, J. D. (2018). Spinal, Epidural, & Caudal Blocks. In J. F. Butterworth IV, D. C. Mackey, & J. D. Wasnik (Eds.), *Morgan & Mikhail's clinical anesthesiology, 6e*. New York, NY: McGraw-Hill.

Candido, K. D., Tharian, A. R., & Winnie, A. P. (2017). Caudal anesthesia. In A. Hadzic (Ed.), *Hadzic's Textbook of Regional Anesthesia and Acute Pain Management, 2e*. New York, N.Y.: McGraw-Hill Education.

Carrera, A., Lopez, A. M., Sala-Blanch, X., Kapur, E., Hasanbegovic, I., & Hadzic, A. (2020). Functional regional anesthesia anatomy. *NYSORA*. Retrieved from https://www.nysora.com/essentials-of-regional-anesthesia-anatomy. Retrieved August 20, 2020.

Catterall, W. A., & Mackie, K. (2018). Local anesthetics. In L. L. Brunton, R. Hilal-Dandan, & B. C. Knollmann (Eds.), *Goodman & Gilman's: The Pharmacological Basis of Therapeutics, 13e*. New York, NY: McGraw-Hill.

Centers for Disease Control and Prevention [CDC]. (2011). CDC clinical reminder: Spinal injection procedures performed without a facemask pose risk for bacterial meningitis. Retrieved 8/20/20 from https://www.cdc.gov/injectionsafety/spinalinjection-meningitis.html.

Chin, A., & van Zundert, A. (2017). Spinal anesthesia. In A. Hadzic. *Hadzic's Textbook of Regional Anesthesia and Acute Pain Management, 2e*, New York, N.Y.: McGraw-Hill Education.

Chin, K. J., McDonnell, J. G., Carvalho, B., Sharkey, A., Pawa, A., & Gadsden, J. (2017). Essentials of our current understanding: Abdominal wall blocks. *Regional Anesthesia and Pain Medicine*, 42(2), 133–183. https://doi.org/10.1092/AAP.0000000000000545.

Chiruvella, S., Donthu, B., Nallam, S. R., & Salla, D. B. (2018). Postoperative analgesia with epidural dexmedetomidine compared with clonidine following total abdominal hysterectomies: A prospective double-blind randomized trial. *Anesthesia, Essays and Researches*, 12(1), 103.

Chong, M. A., Wang, Y., Dhir, S., & Lin, C. (2017). Programmed intermittent peripheral nerve local anesthetic bolus compared with continuous infusions for postoperative analgesia: a systematic review and meta-analysis. *Journal of Clinical Anesthesia*, 42, 69–76.

Chou, R., Gordon, D. B., de Leon-Casasola, O. A., Rosenberg, J. M., Bickler, S., Brennan, T., … Wu, C. L. (2016). Guidelines on the management of postoperative pain. *The Journal of Pain*, 17(2), 131–157. https://doi.org/10.1016/j.jpain.2015.12.008.

Columb, M. O., Cegielski, D., & Haley, D. (2017). Local anaesthetic agents. *Anaesthesia & Intensive Care Medicine*, 18(3), 150–154.

Conlin, N., Grant, M. C., & Wu, C. L. (2018). Intrathecal Opioids for Postoperative Pain. In H. T. Benzon, S. N. Raja, S. S. Liu, S. M. Fishman, & S. P. Cohen (Eds.), *Essentials of Pain Medicine* (4th Ed., pp. 123–128). Philadelphia: Elsevier.

Crystal, C. S., McArthur, T. J., & Harrison, B. (2007). Anesthetic and procedural sedation techniques for wound management. *Emergency Medicine Clinics of North America*, 25(1), 41–71.

Culp, Jr., W. C., & Culp, W. C. (2011). Practical application of local anesthetics. *Journal of Vascular Interventional Radiology*, 22, 111-118. doi: https://doi.org/10.1016/j.vir.2010.10.0005.

Dabu-Bondoc, S., Franco, S. A., & Sinatra, R. S. (2009). Neuraxial analgesia with hydromorphone, morphine, and fentanyl: Dosing and safety guidelines. In R. S. Sinatra, O. A. de Leon-Casasola, B. Ginsberg, & E. R. Viscusi (Eds.), *Acute pain management* (pp. 230–244). Cambridge, New York: Cambridge University Press.

Dale, M. C., & Checketts, M. R. (2016). Complications of regional anaesthesia. *Anaesthesia & Intensive Care Medicine*, 17(4), 175–178.

Deschner, B., Allen, M., & de Leon O. (2007) Epidural blockade. In A. Hadzic (Ed.), *Textbook of regional anesthesia and acute pain management* (pp. 229–267). New York, NY: McGraw Hill.

Dirscherl, K. R., Leschka, S., & Filipovic, M. (2017). Transforaminal migration of an epidural catheter. *Canadian Journal of Anesthesia/Journal canadien d'anesthésie*, 64(4), 428–429.

Driscoll, E. B., Maleki, A. H., Jahromi, L., Hermecz, B. N., Nelson, L. E., Vetter, I. L., … Riesenberg, L. A. (2016). Regional anesthesia or patient-controlled analgesia and compartment syndrome in orthopedic surgical procedures: a systematic review. *Local and Regional Anesthesia*, 9, 65–81.

Elsharkawy, H. (2017). Quadratus lumborum blocks. *Advances in Anesthesia*, 35(1), 145–157. https://doi.org/10.1016/j.aan.2017.07.007.

Elsharkawy, H., & Bendtsen, T. (2017). Ultrasound-guided transversus abdominis plane and quadratus lumborum blocks. In *Hadzic's Textbook of Regional Anesthesia and Acute Pain Medicine* (2nd ed.). NYSORA. Retrieved 8/20/20 from https://www.nysora.com/ultrasound-guided-transversus-abdominis-plane-quadratus-lumborum-blocks.

Exparel (bupivacaine liposome injectable suspension). (2018). *Full prescribing information*. Retrieved 8/20/20 from https://www.accessdata.fda.gov/drugsatfda_docs/label/2018/022496s9lbl.pdf.

Foley, K. M. (1985). The treatment of cancer pain. *New England Journal of Medicine*, 313(3), 84–95.

Forero, M., Adhikary, S. D., Lopez, H., Tsui, C., & Chin, K. J. (2016). The erector spinae plane block: A novel analgesic technique in thoracic neuropathic pain. *Regional Anesthesia and Pain Medicine*, 41(5), 621–627. https://doi.org/10.1097/AAP.0000000000000451.

Gadsden, J., & Long, W. J. (2016). Time to analgesia onset and pharmacokinetics after separate and combined administration of liposome bupivacaine and bupivacaine HCl: considerations for clinicians. *The Open Orthopaedics Journal*, 10, 94–104.

Gadsden, J., & Warlick, A. (2015). Regional anesthesia for the trauma patient: improving patient outcomes. *Local and Regional Anesthesia*, 8, 45–55.

Gaiser, R. R. (2017). Postdural puncture headache: an evidence-based approach. *Anesthesiology Clinics*, 35(1), 157–167.

Gallagher, M., & Grant, C. R. (2018). Adjuvant agents in regional anaesthesia. *Anaesthesia & Intensive Care Medicine*, 19(11), 615–618.

Ganapathy, S., Howard, J. L., & Sondekoppam, R. V. (2017). Local Infiltration Analgesia for Orthopedic Joint Surgery. In *Complications of Regional Anesthesia* (pp. 381–398). Cham, Switzerland: Springer.

Gautier, P. E., Vandepitte, C., & Gadsden, J. (2017). Ultrasound-guided interscalene brachial plexus block. In *New York School of Regional Anesthesia [NYSORA] Based on Hadzic's textbook of RAPM* (2nd ed.). Retrieved 8/20/20 from https://www.nysora.com/ultrasound-guided-interscalene-brachial-plexus-block-2017.

Gill, J. S. (2017). Peripheral nerve blocks. In Z. H. Bajwa, R. Wootton, & C. A. Warfield (Eds.), *Principles and Practice of Pain Medicine*, 3e. New York, NY: McGraw-Hill.

Gill, J., Nagda, J., Aner, M., & Simopoulos, T. (2016). Cervical epidural contrast spread patterns in fluoroscopic antero-posterior, lateral, and contralateral oblique view: a three-dimensional analysis. *Pain Medicine*, 18(6), 1027–1039.

Gitman, M., Fettiplace, M. R., Weinberg, G. L., Neal, J. M., & Barrington, M. J. (2019). Local anesthetic systemic toxicity: A narrative literature review and clinical update on prevention, diagnosis, and management. *Plastic and Reconstructive Surgery*, 144(3), 783–795.

Gorlin, A. W., Rosenfeld, D. M., Maloney, J., Wie, C. S., McGarvey, J., & Trentman, T. L. (2016). Survey of pain specialists regarding conversion of high-dose intravenous to neuraxial opioids. *Journal of Pain Research*, 9, 693–700.

Grant, C. R. (2019). Lower limb nerve blocks. *Anaesthesia & Intensive Care Medicine*, 20(4), 219–223.

Grape, S., & Schug, S. A. (2008). Epidural and spinal anesthesia. In P. Macintyre, S. Walker, & D. Rowbotham (Eds.), *Clinical pain management: Acute pain* (2nd ed., pp. 255–270). Boca Raton, FL: CRC Press.

Guay, J., & Kopp, S. (2016). Epidural pain relief versus systemic opioid–based pain relief for abdominal aortic surgery. *Cochrane Database of Systematic Reviews 2016*, . https://doi.org/10.1002/14651858.CD005059.pub4. Issue 1. Art. No.: CD005059. DOI:.

Guay, J., Nishimori, M., & Kopp, S. (2016). Epidural local anaesthetics for prevention of gastrointestinal paralysis, vomiting and pain. *Cochrane Database of Systematic Reviews*. https://doi.org/10.1002/14651858.CD001893.pub2. Issue 7. Art. No.: CD001893.

Guay, J., Choi, P., Suresh, S., Albert, N., Kopp, S., & Pace, N. L. (2014). Neuraxial blockade for prevention of postoperative mortality and major morbidity: An overview of Cochrane systematic reviews. *Cochrane Database of Systematic Reviews*. https://doi.org/10.1002/14651858.CD010108.pub2. Issue 1. Art. No.: CD010108. doi:.

Gulur, P., Tsui, B., Pathak, R., Koury, K. M., & Lee, H. (2015). Retrospective analysis of the incidence of epidural haematoma in patients with epidural catheters and abnormal coagulation parameters. *British Journal of Anaesthesia*, 114(5), 808–811. https://doi.org/10.1093/bja/aeu461.

Hadzic, A., Lopez, A. M., Vandepitte, C., & Sala-Blanch, X. (2017). Ultrasound-guided popliteal sciatic block. NYSORA. In *Based on Hadzic's Textbook of RAPM* (2nd Ed). Retrieved 8/20/20 from https://www.nysora.com/ultrasound-guided-popliteal-sciatic-block-2.

Hayden, J. M., Oras, J., Karlsson, O. I., Olausson, K. G., Thörn, S. E., & Gupta, A. (2017). Post-operative pain relief using local infiltration analgesia during open abdominal hysterectomy: a randomized, double-blind study. *Acta Anaesthesiologica Scandinavica*, 61(5), 539–548.

Hebl, J. R., & Niesen, A. D. (2011). Infectious complications of regional anesthesia. *Current Opinion in Anesthesiology*, 24(5), 573–580. https://doi.org/10.1097/ACO.0b013e32834a9252.

Hernandez, G. A., Grant, M. C., & Wu, C. L. (2018). Epidural Opioids for Postoperative Pain. In H. T. Benzon, S. N. Raja, S. S. Liu, S. M. Fishman, & S. P. Cohen (Eds.), *Essentials of Pain Medicine* (4th Ed., pp. 129–134). Philadelphia: Elsevier.

Herndon, C. M., Arnstein, P., Darnall, B., Hartrick, C., Hecht, K., Lyons, M., & Seghal, N. (2016). *Principles of Analgesic Use*. Chicago, IL: American Pain Society.

Horlocker, T. T., Vandermeulen, E., Kopp, S. L., Gogarten, W., Leffert, L. R., & Benzon, H. T. (2018). Regional anesthesia in the patient receiving antithrombotic or thrombolytic therapy: American Society of Regional Anesthesia and Pain Medicine evidence-based guidelines (fourth edition). *Regional Anesthesia and Pain Medicine, 43*(3), 263–309. https://doi.org/10.1097/AAP.0000000000000763.

Hu, B., Lin, T., Yan, S. G., Tong, S. L., Yu, J. H., Xu, J. J., & Ying, Y. M. (2016). Local infiltration analgesia versus regional blockade for postoperative analgesia in total knee arthroplasty: a meta-analysis of randomized controlled trials. *Pain Physician, 19*(4), 205–214.

Hunter, O. O., Kim, T. E., Mariano, E. R., & Harrison, T. K. (2019). Care of the Patient With a Peripheral Nerve Block. *Journal of PeriAnesthesia Nursing, 34*(1), 16–26.

Hurley, R. W., Murphy, J. D., & Wu, C. L. (2015). Acute postoperative pain. In R. D. Miller (Ed.), *Miller's Anesthesia* (pp. 2974–2998). Philadelphia, PA: Saunders.

Ilfeld, B. M. (2011). Continuous peripheral nerve blocks: a review of the published evidence. *Anesthesia & Analgesia, 113*(4), 904–925.

Ilfeld, B. M. (2017). Continuous peripheral nerve blocks: an update of the published evidence and comparison with novel, alternative analgesic modalities. *Anesthesia & Analgesia, 124*(1), 308–335.

Ilfelf, B. M., Renehan, E. M., & Enneking, F. K. (2017). Continuous peripheral nerve blocks in outpatients. In A. Hadzic (Ed.), *Hadzic's Textbook of Regional Anesthesia and Acute Pain Management, 2e.* New York, NY.: McGraw-Hill Education.

Institute for Safe Medication Practices (ISMP). (2011). *ISMP Medication Safety Alert! Latent Failures.* Retrieved 8/20/20 from https://medcom.uiowa.edu/annsblog/wp-content/uploads/2011/05/May-6-2011.pdf.

Joshi, G., Gandhi, K., Shah, N., Gadsden, J., & Corman, S. L. (2016a). Peripheral nerve blocks in the management of postoperative pain: challenges and opportunities. *Journal of Clinical Anesthesia, 35*, 524–529.

Joshi, G. P., Janis, J. E., Haas, E. M., Ramshaw, B. J., Nihira, M. A., & Dunkin, B. J. (2016b). Surgical site infiltration for abdominal surgery: a novel neuroanatomical-based approach. *Plastic and Reconstructive Surgery Global Open, 4*(12), e1181.

Jungquist, C. R., Quinlan-Colwell, A., Vallerand, A., Carlisle, H. L., Cooney, M., Dempsey, S. J., ... Sawyer, J. (2020). American Society for Pain Management Nursing Guidelines on Monitoring for Opioid-Induced Advancing Sedation and Respiratory Depression: Revisions. *Pain Management Nursing, 21*(1), 7–25.

Karmakar, M. K., Greengrass, R. A., Latmore, M., & Levin, M. (2020). Thoracic paravertebral block. *NYSORA.* Retrieved 8/20/20 from https://www.nysora.com/regional-anesthesia-for-specific-surgical-procedures/abdomen/thoracic-lumbar-paravertebral-block/.

Kendall, M. C., Castro Alves, L. J., & De Oliveira, G. (2018). Liposome bupivacaine compared to plain local anesthetics to reduce postsurgical pain: an updated meta-analysis of randomized controlled trials. *Pain Research and Treatment.* Article ID 5710169 https://doi.org/10.1155/2018/5710169.

Kessler, J., Marhofer, P., Hopkins, P. M., & Hollmann, M. W. (2015). Peripheral regional anaesthesia and outcome: Lessons learned from the last 10 years. *British Journal of Anaesthesia, 114*(5), 728–745. https://doi.org/10.1093/bja/aeu559.

Kim, T., Lee, C. H., Hyun, S. J., Yoon, S. H., Kim, K. J., & Kim, H. J. (2012). Clinical outcomes of spontaneous spinal epidural hematoma: a comparative study between conservative and surgical treatment. *Journal of Korean Neurosurgical Society, 52*(6), 523–527.

Kiran, S., Jinjil, K., Tandon, U., & Kar, S. (2018). Evaluation of dexmedetomidine and fentanyl as additives to ropivacaine for epidural anesthesia and postoperative analgesia. *Journal of Anaesthesiology, Clinical Pharmacology, 34*(1), 41–45.

Kolettas, A., Lazaridis, G., Backa, S., Mpoukovinas, I., Karavasilis, V., Kioumis, I., ... Zarogoulidis, P. (2015). Postoperative pain management. *Journal of Thoracic Disease, 7*(Suppl 1), s62–s72. https://doi.org/10.3978/j.issn.2072-1439.2015.01.15.

Kreutzträger, M., Kopp, M. A., & Liebscher, T. (2017). Acute transient spinal paralysis and cardiac symptoms following an accidental epidural potassium infusion: a case report. *BMC Anesthesiology, 17*(1), 135.

Latham, J. L., & Martin, S. N. (2014). Infiltrative anesthesia in office practice. *American Family Physician, 89*(12), 956–962.

Larson, C. P., & Jaffe, R. A. (2017). Epidural Anesthesia: The Best Technique. *Practical Anesthetic Management* (pp. 125–128). New York: Springer.

Latmore, M., Levine, M., & Gadsen, J. (2017). Regional Anesthesia and Systemic Disease. In A. Hadzic (Ed.), *Hadzic's Textbook of Regional Anesthesia and Acute Pain Management, 2e.* New York, N.Y.: McGraw-Hill Education.

Lehman, L. J. (2017). Local Anesthetics. In Z. H. Bajwa, R. J. Wooton, & C. A. Warfield (Eds.), *Principles and Practices of Pain Medicine, 3e.* New York, N.Y.: McGraw-Hill Education.

Lewis, S. R., Price, A., Walker, K. J., McGrattan, K., & Smith, A. F. (2015). Ultrasound guidance for upper and lower limb blocks. *Cochrane Database of Systematic Reviews, 9.* CD006459.

Lexicomp. (2018). *Caffeine and sodium benzoate: Drug information. Retrieved from UpToDate app.* Wolters Kluwer Health.

Lirk, P., Picardi, S., & Hollmann, M. W. (2014). Local anesthetics: 10 essentials. *European Journal of Anesthesiology, 31*(11), 575–585. https://doi.org/10.1097/EJA.0000000000000137.

Liu, S. S., & Wu, C. L. (2007). Effect of postoperative analgesia on major postoperative complications: a systemic update of the evidence. *Anesthesia & Analgesia, 104*(3), 689–702.

Liu, H., Tariq, R., Liu, G. L., Yan, H., & Kaye, A. D. (2017). Inadvertent intrathecal injections and best practice management. *Acta Anaesthesiologica Scandinavica, 61*(1), 11–22.

Lukof, A., Viscusi, E. R., Schechter, L., Lenart, S., Colfer, K., & Witkowski, T. (2017). Organization of an Acute Pain Management Service Incorporating Regional Anesthesia Techniques. In A. Hadzic (Ed.), *Hadzic's Textbook of Regional Anesthesia and Acute Pain Management, 2e.* New York, N.Y.: McGraw-Hill Education.

Maalouf, D. B., & Liu, S. S. (2009). Clinical application of epidural analgesia. In R. S. Sinatra, O. A. de Leon-Casasola, B. Ginsberg, & E. R. Viscusi (Eds.), *Acute Pain Management* (pp. 221–229). Cambridge, New York: Cambridge University Press.

Macfarlane, A. J., Brull, R., & Chan, V. W. (2018). In M. C. Pardo, & R. D. Miller (Eds.), *Spinal, Caudal, and Epidural Anesthesia* (pp. 273–303). Philadelphia, PA: Elsevier. *Basics of Anesthesia, 7th Ed.*

Macintyre, P. E., & Schug, S. A. (2015). *Acute pain management: A practical guide.* Boca Raton, FL: CRC Press.

Madison, S. J., & Ilfeld, B. M. (2018). Peripheral nerve blocks. In J. F. Butterworth IV,, D. C. Mackey, & J. D. Wasnick (Eds.), *Morgan & Mikhail's clinical anesthesiology, 6e.* New York, NY: McGraw-Hill.

Malik, K., & Nelson, A. (2018). Overview of low back pain disorders. In H. T. Benzon, S. N. Raja, S. S. Liu, S. M. Fishman, & S. P. Cohen (Eds.), *Essentials of Pain Medicine* (4th Ed., pp. 193–206). Philadelphia: Elsevier.

Malik, O., Kaye, A. D., Kaye, A., Belani, K., & Urman, R. D. (2017). Emerging roles of liposomal bupivacaine in anesthesia practice. *Journal of Anaesthesiology, Clinical Pharmacology*, 33(2), 151.

Mankowitz, S. L. (2017). Laceration management. *Journal of Emergency Management*, 53(3), 369–382.

Marroquin, B., Feng, C., Balofsky, A., Edwards, K., Iqbal, A., Kanel, J., … Wissler, R. (2017). Neuraxial opioids for post-cesarean delivery analgesia: can hydromorphone replace morphine? A retrospective study. *International Journal of Obstetric Anesthesia*, 30, 16–22.

McClymont, W., & Celnick, D. (2018). Techniques of epidural block. *Anaesthesia & Intensive Care Medicine.*, 19(11), 600–606.

Meier, A. W., Auyong, D. B., Yuan, S. C., Lin, S. E., Flaherty, J. M., & Hanson, N. A. (2018). Comparison of continuous proximal versus distal adductor canal blocks for total knee arthroplasty: a randomized, double-blind, noninferiority trial. *Regional Anesthesia and Pain Medicine*, 43(1), 36–42.

Merchea, A., Lovely, J. K., Jacob, A. K., Colibaseanu, D. T., Kelley, S. R., Mathis, K. L., … Larson, D. W. (2018). Efficacy and Outcomes of Intrathecal Analgesia as Part of an Enhanced Recovery Pathway in Colon and Rectal Surgical Patients. *Surgery Research and Practice*, 2018, 8174579.

Miller, T. E., & Moon, R. E. (2018). Anesthesia for gastrointestinal surgery. In D. E. Longnecker, S. C. Mackey, M. F. Newman, W. S. Sandberg, & W. M. Zapol (Eds.), *Anesthesiology, 3e*. New York: McGraw-Hill.

Monahan, A. M., & Ilfeld, M. M. (2017). Continuous peripheral nerve blocks. In A. Hadzic (Ed.), *Hadzic's Textbook of Regional Anesthesia and Acute Pain Management, 2e*. New York, N.Y.: McGraw-Hill Education.

Murray, A., & Hagen, N. A. (2005). Hydromorphone. *Journal of Pain and Symptom Management*, 29(5), 57–66.

Narouze, S., Benzon, H. T., Provenzano, D., Buvanendran, A., De Andres, J., Deer, T., … Huntoon, M. A. (2018). Interventional spine and pain procedures in patients on antiplatelet and anticoagulant medications: Guidelines from the American Society of Regional Anesthesia and Pain Medicine, the European Society of Regional Anaesthesia And Pain Therapy, The American Academy of Pain Medicine, The International Neuromodulation Society, The North American Neuromodulation Society, and the World Institute of Pain. *Regional Anesthesia and Pain Medicine*, 43(3), 225–262.

Nathan, N., & Wong, C. A. (2014). Spinal, epidural, and caudal anesthesia: anatomy, physiology, and technique. In D. Chestnut, C. Wong, L. Tsen, W. D. Ngan Kee, Y. Beilin, & J. Mhyre (Eds.), *Chestnut's Obstetric Anesthesia: Principles and Practice* (5th ed., pp. 229–261). Philadelphia, PA: Saunders.

Neal, J. M., Woodward, C. M., & Harrison, T. K. (2018). The American Society of Regional Anesthesia and Pain Medicine Checklist for Managing Local Anesthetic Systemic Toxicity: 2017 Version. *Regional Anesthesia and Pain Medicine*, 43(2), 150–153. https://doi.org/10.1097/AAP.0000000000000726.

Neal, J. M., Barrington, M. J., Fettiplace, M. R., Gitman, M., Memtsoudis, S. G., Mörwald, E. E., … Weinberg, G. (2018). The Third American Society of Regional Anesthesia and Pain Medicine Practice Advisory on Local Anesthetic Systemic Toxicity: Executive Summary 2017. *Regional Anesthesia and Pain Medicine*, 43(5), 113–123. https://doi.org/10.1097/AAP.0000000000000720.

Nelson, A., Benzon, H. T., & Jabri, R. S. (2017). Diagnosis and Management of Spinal and Peripheral Nerve Hematoma. In A. Hadzic (Ed.), *Hadzic's Textbook of Regional Anesthesia and Acute Pain Management, 2e*. New York, NY: McGraw-Hill.

Nicolotti, D., Iotti, E., Fanelli, G., & Compagnone, C. (2016). Perineural catheter infection: a systematic review of the literature. *Journal of Clinical Anesthesia*, 35, 123–128.

Noble, K. A. (2015). Local anesthesia toxicity and lipid rescue. *Journal of PeriAnesthesia Nursing*, 30(4), 321–335.

Nunes, J., Nunes, S., Viega, M., Cortez, M., & Seifert, I. (2015). A prospective, randomized blinded-endpoint, controlled study – continuous epidural infusion versus programmed intermittent epidural bolus in labor analgesia. *Revista Brasileira De Anestesiologia*, 66(5), 439–444. https://doi.org/10.1016/j.bjane.2014.12.006.

Odor, P. M., Bampoe, S., Hayward, J., Chis Ster, I., & Evans, E. (2016). Intrapartum epidural fixation methods: a randomised controlled trial of three different epidural catheter securement devices. *Anaesthesia*, 71(3), 298–305.

Ohashi, K., Dalleur, O., Dykes, P. C., & Bates, D. W. (2014). Benefits and risks of using smart pumps to reduce medication error rates: A systematic review. *Drug Safety*, 37(11), 1011–1020. https://doi.org/10.1007/s40264-014-0232-1.

Ona, X. B., Osorio, D., & Cosp, X. B. (2015). Drug therapy for treating post-dural puncture headache. *Cochrane Database of Systematic Reviews*, https://doi.org/10.1002/14651858.CD007887.pub3. Issue 7. Art. No.: CD007887. DOI:.

O'Neill, J., & Helwig, E. (2016). Postoperative management of the physiological effects of spinal anesthesia. *Journal of PeriAnesthesia Nursing*, 31(4), 330–339.

Orebaugh, S. L., & Cruz Eng, H. (2020). Neuraxial anatomy. *NYSORA*. Retrieved from https://www.nysora.com/techniques/neuraxial-and-perineuraxial-techniques/neuraxial-anatomy-anatomy-relevant-neuraxial-anesthesia/.

Orebaugh, S. L., & Kirkham, K. R. (2017). Introduction to ultrasound-guided regional anesthesia. In A. Hadzic (Ed.), *Hadzic's Textbook of Regional Anesthesia and Acute Pain Management, 2e*. New York, NY: McGraw-Hill.

Ottestad, E., & Gowda, A. (2017). Ultrasound in the Diagnosis and Treatment of Pain. In Z. H. Bajwa, R. Wootton, & C. A. Warfield (Eds.), *Principles and Practice of Pain Medicine, 3e*. New York, NY: McGraw-Hill.

Park, J. S., Choi, G. S., Kwak, K. H., Jung, H., Jeon, Y., Park, S., & Yeo, J. (2015). Effect of local wound infiltration and transversus abdominis plane block on morphine use after laparoscopic colectomy: a nonrandomized, single-blind prospective study. *Journal of Surgical Research*, 195(1), 61–66.

Pasero, C., Eksterowicz, N., Primeau, M., & Crowley, C. (2007). Registered nurse management and monitoring of analgesia by catheter techniques. *Pain Management Nursing*, 8(2), 48–54. https://doi.org/10.1016/j.pmn.2007.02.003.

Pasero, C., & M. McCaffery, M. (Eds.). (2011). *Pain Assessment and Pharmacologic Management*. St. Louis, MO: Mosby.

Patel, N., & Sadoughi, A. (2015). Pharmacology of Local Anesthetics. In A. D. Kaye, A. M. Kaye, & R. D. Urman (Eds.), *Essentials of Pharmacology for Anesthesia, Pain Medicine, and Critical Care* (pp. 179–194). New York: Springer.

Patel, V. B. (2015). Equipment Used in Pain Management. In S. Diwan, & P. S. Staats (Eds.), *Atlas of Pain Medicine Procedures*. New York, NY: McGraw-Hill.

Perlas, A., Chaparro, L. E., & Chin, D. J. (2016). Lumbar neuraxial ultrasound for spinal and epidural anesthesia: A systematic review and meta-analysis. *Regional Anesthesia & Pain Medicine*, 41(2), 251–260. https://doi.org/10.1097/AAP.0000000000000184.

Raeder, J., & Spreng, U. J. (2017). Intra-articular and periarticular infiltration of local anesthetics. In A. Hadzic (Ed.), *Hadzic's Textbook of Regional Anesthesia and Acute Pain Management, 2e*. New York, NY: McGraw-Hill.

Rahangdale, R., Tureanu, L., & Benzon, H. T. (2018). Truncal blocks: Paravertebral, intercostal, pectoral nerve, supra-capular, ilioinguinal, iliohypogastric nerve, and transversus abdominis plane blocks. In H. T. Benzon, S. N. Raja, S. S. Liu, S. M. Fishman, & S. P. Cohen (Eds.), *Essentials of Pain Medicine* (4th Ed., pp. 779–788). Philadelphia, PA: Elsevier.

Raman, S., Lin, M., & Krishnan, N. (2018). Systematic review and meta-analysis of the efficacy of liposomal bupivacaine in colorectal resections. *Journal of Drug Assessment*, 7(1), 43–50.

Ranasinghe, J. S., Davidson, F. E., & Birnbach, D. J. (2017). Combined Spinal–Epidural Anesthesia. In A. Hadzic (Ed.), *Hadzic's Textbook of Regional Anesthesia and Acute Pain Management, 2e*. New York, NY: McGraw-Hill.

Ray, N., Schmidt, P., & Ottestad, E. (2018). Management of Acute Postoperative Pain. In D. E. Longnecker, S. C. Mackey, M. F. Newman, W. S. Sandberg, & W. M. Zapol (Eds.), *Anesthesiology, 3e*. New York, NY: McGraw-Hill.

Rodriguez-Aldrete, D., Candiotti, K. A., Janakiraman, R., & Rodriguez-Blanco, Y. F. (2016). Trends and new evidence in the management of acute and chronic post-thoracotomy pain—an overview of the literature from 2005 to 2015. *Journal of Cardiothoracic and Vascular Anesthesia*, 30(3), 762–772.

Rosero, E. B., & Joshi, G. P. (2016). Nationwide incidence of serious complications of epidural analgesia in the United States. *Acta Anaesthesiologica Scandinavica*, 60(6), 810–820.

Satomi, S., Kakuta, N., Murakami, C., Sakai, Y., Tanaka, K., & Tsutsumi, Y. M. (2018). The Efficacy of Programmed Intermittent Epidural Bolus for Postoperative Analgesia after Open Gynecological Surgery: A Randomized Double-Blinded Study. *BioMed Research International*, 2018(6297247).

Sayed, D., & Diwan, S. (2015). Infection: Prevention, Diagnosis, and Management. In S. Diwan, & P. S. Staats (Eds.), *Atlas of Pain Medicine Procedures*. New York: McGraw-Hill.

Schulz-Stübner, S., Pottinger, J. M., Coffin, S. A., & Herwaldt, L. A. (2017). Infection Control in Regional Anesthesia. In A. Hadzic (Ed.), *Hadzic's Textbook of Regional Anesthesia and Acute Pain Management, 2e*. New York NY: McGraw-Hill.

Schulz-Stübner, S., Pottinger, J. M., Coffin, S. A., & Herwaldt, L. A. (2020). Infection control in regional anesthesia. *NYSORA*. Retrieved 8/20/20 from https://www.nysora.com/foundations-of-regional-anesthesia/complications/infection-control-regional-anesthesia/.

Shah, K., Lo, C., Babich, M., Tsao, N. W., & Bansback, N. J. (2016). Bar code medication administration technology: a systematic review of impact on patient safety when used with computerized prescriber order entry and automated dispensing devices. *The Canadian Journal of Hospital Pharmacy*, 69(5), 394.

Sharawi, N., Carvalho, B., Habib, A. S., Blake, L., Mhyre, J. M., & Sultan, P. (2018). A Systematic Review Evaluating Neuraxial Morphine and Diamorphine-Associated Respiratory Depression After Cesarean Delivery. *Anesthesia & Analgesia*, 127(6), 1385–1395.

Simmons, S. W., Taghizadeh, N., Dennis, A. T., Hughes, D., & Cyna, A. M. (2012). Combined spinal-epidural versus epidural analgesia in labour. *Cochrane Database of Systematic Reviews*, https://doi.org/10.1002/14651858.CD003401.pub3. Issue 10. Art. No.: CD003401. DOI:.

Singh, P. M., Borle, A., Kaur, M., Trikha, A., & Sinha, A. (2018). Opioid-sparing effects of the thoracic interfascial plane blocks: A meta-analysis of randomized controlled trials. *Saudi Journal of Anaesthesia*, 12(1), 103.

Singh, P. M., Borle, A., Trikha, A., Michos, L., Sinha, A., & Goudra, B. (2017). Role of periarticular liposomal bupivacaine infiltration in patients undergoing total knee arthroplasty—a meta-analysis of comparative trials. *The Journal of Arthroplasty*, 32(2), 675–688.

Sites, B. D., Taenzer, A. H., Herrick, M. D., Gilloon, C., Antonakakis, J., Richins, J., & Beach, M. L. (2012). Incidence of local anesthetic systemic toxicity and postoperative neurologic symptoms associated with 12,668 ultrasound-guided nerve blocks: an analysis from a prospective clinical registry. *Regional Anesthesia and Pain Medicine*, 37(5), 478–482.

Smith, D. I., & Anderson, R. (2016). Epidural Catheter Migration in a Patient with Severe Spinal Stenosis. *Case Reports in Anesthesiology*, 6124086.

Soffin, E. M., & Liu, S. S. (2018). Patient-Controlled Analgesia. In H. T. Benzon, S. N. Raja, S. S. Liu, S. M. Fishman, & S. P. Cohen (Eds.), *Essentials of Pain Medicine* (4th Ed., pp. 117–122e2.). Philadelphia, PA: Elsevier.

Solanki, A., & Akhouri, V. K. (2017). Acute Pain Management in Adults. In Z. H. Bajwa, R. Wootton, & C. A. Warfield (Eds.), *Principles and Practice of Pain Medicine, 3e*. New York, NY: McGraw-Hill.

Soliman, H. O. (2018). Comparative Study between Lidocaine 2% and Dexamethasone Local Wound Infiltration Effect on Postoperative Pain Post Mastectomy: A Randomized Controlled Study. *Advances in Breast Cancer Research*, 7(04), 243.

Suzuki, S., Gerner, P., & Lirk, P. (2019). Local anesthetics. In H. C. Hemmings, & T. D. Egan (Eds.), *Pharmacology and Physiology for Anesthesia* (pp. 390–411). Philadelphia: Elsevier.

Sviggum, H. P., Arendt, K. W., Jacob, A. K., Niesen, A. D., Johnson, R. L., Schroeder, D. R., ... Mantilla, C. B. (2016). Intrathecal hydromorphone and morphine for postcesarean delivery analgesia: determination of the ED90 using a sequential allocation biased-coin method. *Anesthesia & Analgesia*, 123(3), 690–697.

Svircevic, V., van Dijk, D., Nierich, A. P., Passier, M. P., Kalkman, C. J., Van der Heijden, G. J. M. G., & Bax, L. (2013). Meta-analysis of thoracic epidural anesthesia versus general anesthesia for cardiac surgery. *Anesthesiology*, 114(2), 271–282.

Tam, K. W., Chen, S. Y., Huang, T. W., Lin, C. C., Su, C. M., Li, C. L., ... Wu, C. H. (2015). Effect of wound infiltration with ropivacaine or bupivacaine analgesia in breast cancer surgery: a meta-analysis of randomized controlled trials. *International Journal of Surgery*, 22, 79–85.

Thiruvenkatarajan, V., Eng, H. C., & Adhikary, S. D. (2018). An update on regional analgesia for rib fractures. *Current Opinion in Anesthesiology*, 31(5), 601–607.

Toledano, R. D., & Van De Velde, M. (2017). Epidural anesthesia and analgesia. In A. Hadzic (Ed.), *Hadzic's Textbook of Regional and Acute Pain Management* (pp. 380–445). New York, N.Y.: McGraw-Hill Education.

Tran, D. Q., Elgueta, M. F., Aliste, J., & Finlayson, R. J. (2017). Diaphragm-Sparing Nerve Blocks for Shoulder Surgery. *Regional Anesthesia and Pain Medicine*, 42(1), 32–38.

Trissel, L. A., Ashworth, L. D., & Ashworth, J. (2018). *Trissel's Stability of Compounded Formulations* (6th Edition). American Pharmacists Association. https://doi.org/10.21019/9781582122960.fm.

Tsai, H. C., Yoshida, T., Chuang, T. Y., Yang, S. F., Chang, C. C., Yao, H. Y., ... Chen, K. Y. (2017). Transversus abdominis plane block: an updated review of anatomy and techniques. *BioMed Research International*, 8284363.

Tsui, B. C. H., Dryden, A. M., & Finucane, B. T. (2018). Management of Acute Postoperative Pain. In D. E. Longnecker, S. C. Mackey, M. F. Newman, W. S. Sandberg, & W. M. Zapol (Eds.), *Anesthesiology*, 3e. New York, NY: McGraw-Hill.

Tubog, T. D., Harenberg, J. L., Buszta, K., & Hestand, J. D. (2018). Prophylactic Nalbuphine to Prevent Neuraxial Opioid-Induced Pruritus: A Systematic Review and Meta-Analysis of Randomized Controlled Trials. *Journal of PeriAnesthesia Nursing.*, 34(3), 491–501.

Tummala, V., Rao, L. N., Vallury, M. K., & Sanapala, A. (2015). A comparative study-efficacy and safety of combined spinal epidural anesthesia versus spinal anesthesia in high-risk geriatric patients for surgeries around the hip joint. *Anesthesia, Essays and Researches*, 9(2), 185.

Uchino, T., Miura, M., Oyama, Y., Matsumoto, S., Shingu, C., & Kitano, T. (2016). Lateral deviation of four types of epidural catheters from the lumbar epidural space into the intervertebral foramen. *Journal of Anesthesia*, 30(4), 583–590.

Uskova, A., & O'Connor, J. E. (2015). Liposomal bupivacaine for regional anesthesia. *Current Opinion in Anaesthesiology*, 28(5), 593–597.

Vandepitte, C., Lopez, A. M., Van Boxstael, S., & Jalil, H. (2020). Ultrasound-guided ankle block. In *New York School of Regional Anesthesia [NYSORA] Based on Hadzic's textbook of RAPM* (2nd ed.). *2017*. Retrieved 8/20/20 from: https://www.nysora.com/ultrasound-guided-ankle-block-2.

Vandepitte, C., Lopez, A. M., & Jalil, H. (2020). Ultrasound-guided axillary block. In *New York School of Regional Anesthesia [NYSORA] Based on Hadzic's textbook of RAPM* (2nd ed.). *2017*. Retrieved 8/20/20 from https://www.nysora.com/ultrasound-guided-axillary-brachial-plexus-block-2.

Vecchione, A. (2014). *Errors continue to plague smart pumps. Health IT News.* Retrieved 8/20/20 from https://www.healthcareitnews.com/news/errors-continue-plague-smart-pumps.

Verlinde, M., Hollmann, M. W., Stevens, M. F., Hermanns, H., Wedehausen, R., & Lirk, P. (2016). Local anesthetic-induced neurotoxicity. *International Journal of Molecular Sciences*, 17(3), 339. https://doi.org/10.3390/ijms17030339.

Vineyard, J. C., Toohey, J. S., Neidre, A., Fogel, G., & Joyner, R. (2014). Evaluation of a single-dose, extended-release epidural morphine formulation for pain control after lumbar spine surgery. *Journal of Surgical Orthopaedic Advances*, 23(1), 9–12.

Vloka, J. D., Hadzic, A., & Gautier, P. (2017). Femoral Nerve Block. In A. Hadzic (Ed.), *Hadzic's Textbook of Regional and Acute Pain Management* (pp. 380–445). New York: McGraw-Hill Education.

Vyas, K. S., Rajendran, S., Morrison, S. D., Shakir, A., Mardini, S., Lemaine, V., ... Vasconez, H. C. (2016). Systematic review of liposomal bupivacaine (Exparel) for postoperative analgesia. *Plastic and Reconstructive Surgery*, 138(4), 748e–756e.

Wang, K., & Zhang, H. X. (2017). Liposomal bupivacaine versus interscalene nerve block for pain control after total shoulder arthroplasty: a systematic review and meta-analysis. *International Journal of Surgery*, 46, 61–70.

Warren, D. T., Nelson, K., & Neal, J. M. (2018). Neuraxial Anesthesia, Chapter 42. In D. E. Longnecker, S. C. Mackey, M. F. Newman, W. S. Sandberg, & W. M. Zapol (Eds.), *Anesthesiology*. New York, NY: McGraw-Hill.

Wasson, N. R., & Fisher, L. J. (2017). Ultrasound-Guided Peripheral Nerve Blockade. In Z. H. Bajwa, R. Wootton, & C. A. Warfield (Eds.), *Principles and Practice of Pain Medicine*, 3e. New York, NY: McGraw-Hill.

Wiesmann, T., Hoff, L., Prien, L., Torossian, A., Eberhart, L., Wulf, H., & Feldmann, C. (2018). Programmed intermittent epidural bolus versus continuous epidural infusion for postoperative analgesia after major abdominal and gynecological cancer surgery: a randomized, triple-blinded clinical trial. *BMC Anesthesiology*, 18(1), 154.

Woodworth, G. E., Ivie, R. M. J., Nelson, S. M., Walker, C. M., & Maniker, R. B. (2017). Perioperative breast analgesia: A qualitative review of anatomy and regional techniques. *Regional Anesthesia and Pain Medicine*, 42(5), 609–631.

Yaksh, T. & Wallace, M. (2017). Opioids, analgesia, and pain management. In L. L. Brunton, R. Hilal-Dandan, & B. C. Knollmann (Eds.), *Goodman & Gilman's: The Pharmacological Basis of Therapeutics*, 13e. McGraw-Hill.

Yalamuri, S., Klinger, R. Y., Bullock, W. M., Glower, D. D., Bottiger, B. A., & Gadsden, J. C. (2017). Pectoral fascial (PECS) I and II blocks as rescue analgesia in a patient undergoing minimally invasive cardiac surgery. *Regional Anesthesia and Pain Medicine*, 42(6), 764–766.

Yarwood, J., & Berrill, A. (2010). Nerve blocks of the anterior abdominal wall. *British Journal of Education*, 6(1), 182–186. https://doi.org/10.1093/bjaceaccp/mkq035.

Yeung, J. H. Y., Gates, S., Naidu, B. V., Wilson, M. J. A., & Gao Smith, F. (2016). Paravertebral block versus thoracic epidural for patients undergoing thoracotomy. *Cochrane Database of Systematic Reviews*. https://doi.org/10.1002/14651858.CD009121.pub2. Issue 2. Art. No: CD009121. doi:.

Zhang, S., Wu, X., Guo, H., & Ma, L. (2015). Thoracic epidural anesthesia improves outcomes in patients undergoing cardiac surgery: meta-analysis of randomized controlled trials. *European Journal of Medical Research*, 20(1), 25.

Zhang, S., Geng, F., Wang, J., Zhang, Z., & Du, C. (2018). Rapid Recovery of Spontaneous Spinal Epidural Hematoma without Surgical Treatment: Case Report and Literature Review. *World Neurosurgery*, 115, 216–219.

Chapter 19 Interventional Approaches

Nitin K. Sekhri, Emily Davis, Ann Quinlan-Colwell, Maureen F. Cooney

CHAPTER OUTLINE

Anatomy of the Central Nervous System, pg. 533

Spinal Pain, pg. 533

Diagnostic Imaging, pg. 537

Spinal Injections, pg. 538

    Epidural Corticosteroid Injections, pg. 538

    Facet Injections, pg. 539

    Vertebral Body Augmentation, pg. 541

Implantable Therapies, pg. 543

    Spinal Cord Stimulators, pg. 543

    Intrathecal Drug Delivery System, pg. 549

Key Points, pg. 554

Case Scenario, pg. 554

Acknowledgement, pg. 555

References, pg. 555

INTERVENTIONAL pain management is a pain management subspecialty in which conditions associated with pain are diagnosed and treated primarily with interventional techniques, either alone or in combination with other therapies, with the goal of intervening at specific nociceptive sites to relieve pain (Serrano et al., 2014). Patients living with chronic pain who have tried less invasive therapies yet have not attained improvement in their pain management and more importantly their functional ability may be candidates for interventional pain management approaches, including the use of advanced implantable therapies.

The interventional or invasive procedures discussed in this chapter include spinal injections, nerve blocks, radiofrequency ablation (RFA), neurostimulation, and intrathecal drug delivery systems (IDDSs). In addition to the procedures reviewed in this chapter, the field of interventional pain management is expanding and includes growth in neuromodulation and interventions such as peripheral nerve blocks and peripheral nerve stimulation. The growth in interventional options may in part be explained by improved imaging, increased skill level of practitioners, and research findings. The growth in interest in interventional pain management is also in response to efforts to reduce opioid prescribing in recognition of the growth of opioid abuse. Between 2000 and 2013, interventional procedures as treatment for pain among older adults increased by 236%, with a 417% increase in injections of the facet and sacroiliac joints, even though the number of Medicare beneficiaries only increased by 31% (Manchikanti, Pampati, Falco, & Hirsch, 2015a). The dramatic increase in procedures has led to the establishment of the American Society of Interventional Pain Physicians (ASIPP), the Spine Intervention Society, and the American Interventional Headache Society, all of which are relatively new organizations associated with clinicians who use interventional procedures.

The purpose of this chapter is to describe interventional pain procedures used to manage pain that is not readily responsive to less invasive methods, including pharmacologic, nonpharmacologic, and physical therapies. Interventional pain procedures can be incorporated into a multimodal analgesic plan of care to optimize pain relief while reducing reliance on analgesic medications (Brooks & Udoji, 2016). They are often used for patients in the outpatient setting to reduce chronic pain and pain originating from a spinal cause.

Anatomy of the Central Nervous System

Basic knowledge of the anatomy of the nervous system, along with the soft tissues and skeletal system related to the spine, is important for clinicians who are involved in the care of patients undergoing pain management interventions. Even when the cause of pain is not in the spine, the spine is a common focus of interventional pain management. Box 19.1 provides a brief review of the anatomy of the nervous system. Fig. 19.1 illustrates the anatomy of the spine.

Spinal Pain

Spinal pain, particularly low back pain, is a common chief complaint in the primary care setting and is often the chief complaint of patients who present for interventional pain

Box 19.1 | Anatomy of the Spine

- The spinal cord lies within the vertebral canal and extends from the foramen magnum to the first or second lumbar vertebra. The spinal cord is covered by three meninges: the outermost layer is the dura mater, the middle layer is the arachnoid mater, and the innermost layer is the pia mater. The pia mater rests on neural tissue and is typically separated from the other two layers by the cerebrospinal fluid (CSF).

- The spinal nerves are protected by vertebrae and a cavity created in the center of the bone, called the spinal canal, which originates in the cervical spine and ends in the sacrum. This canal encloses the spinal cord in the cervical, thoracic, and lumbar region, ending by the second lumbar vertebrae in adults and giving rise to nerve roots called the cauda equina.

- The spinal cord and the nerve roots are bathed in CSF, which is contained by the meninges. The canal contains crucial blood vessels along with ligaments for structural support. A crucial ligament for many pain management procedures is the ligamentum flavum, which runs in the posterior aspect of the canal.

- The epidural space lies just beyond the ligamentum flavum and before the first layer of the meninges (the dura mater). This is a potential space containing lymphatics, spinal nerve roots, connective tissue, fat, small arteries, and an extensive vertebral venous plexus. The epidural space is a common target for administration of corticosteroids or placement of leads for neuromodulation.

- The spinal canal is surrounded by the bones of the vertebrae. The 33 vertebrae include 7 cervical, 12 thoracic, 5 lumbar, 5 fused elements of the sacrum, and 4 or 5 fused elements of the coccyx. The bony components of the vertebra include a vertebral body that carries the body's weight, two pedicles that extend posteriorly and surround the spinal canal and epidural space and then join a pair of laminae.

- The vertebral bodies are separated by intervertebral discs.

- Intervertebral discs have two layers: The outermost layer is a fibrous tissue called the annulus, and the innermost layer is a gelatinous substance called the nucleus pulposus, which provides crucial cushioning to the spine and body.

- The laminae are fused at the midline and form the posterior-most part of the vertebrae, the spinous process, which is usually palpable on examination.

- The laminae are medial to the facet joints.

- Facet joints are located in the cervical, thoracic, and lumbar areas of the spine.

- The facet joints allow for movement in the spine and have a joint capsule similar to the knee or hip. The nerve supply to the facet joints is complex.

- Spinal nerve roots are divided into two segments, the ventral and the dorsal rami. The dorsal rami mostly provide sensory input from the periphery to the spinal cord, thus transmitting pain.

- The dorsal rami in the lumbar spine are split into two branches, the lateral and the medial branches.

- The medial branch supplies sensory input to the spinal cord from the facet joint to that level and possibly to the levels above and below.

- Because of the complex innervation of the facet joints, the medial branches at the level of interest, the level above, and the level below must be anesthetized to cause blockade of the facet joint.

Modified from Pino, C. A., & Rathmell, J. P. (2018). Interventional management of chronic pain. In D. E. Longnecker, S. C. Mackey, M. F. Newman, W. S. Sandberg, & W. M. Zapol (Eds.), *Anesthesiology* (3rd ed.). New York, NY: McGraw-Hill.

management. In a consensus study of pain in America, published by the Institute of Medicine (2011), back pain is frequently cited as a common source of chronic pain, disability, and high health care expenditures. There are many possible sources of back pain. Low back pain may be idiopathic and is frequently caused by internal disc disruption (IDD), which results from annular tears, intervertebral disc collapse, and mechanical failure; other sources of pain result from herniated nucleus pulposus (HNP), segmental instability, and degenerative disc disease (DDD) (Izzo, Popolizio, D'Aprile, & Muto, 2015). With HNP, the most common cause of low back pain, more than 95% of the protruded or extruded discs occur at L4-5 or L5-S1 levels (Lee, Cohen, & Abdi, 2017).

Radicular pain is pain that originates in the spine and radiates into a dermatome of a nerve root; it may or may not be associated with radiculopathy in which there is a block in the conduction of sensory or motor axons leading to numbness or weakness (Izzo et al., 2015). The most common cause of radicular pain is disc herniation; the inflammatory process with release of inflammatory mediators is the primary mechanism involved in the pathophysiology of pain associated with disc herniation (Izzo et al., 2015). Mechanical nerve root compression also can lead to radicular pain and radiculopathy (Keene, 2017).

Facet joint arthropathy or lumbar facet syndrome (LFS) is another source of back pain that is estimated to account for up to 40% of all back pain (Lee et al., 2017).

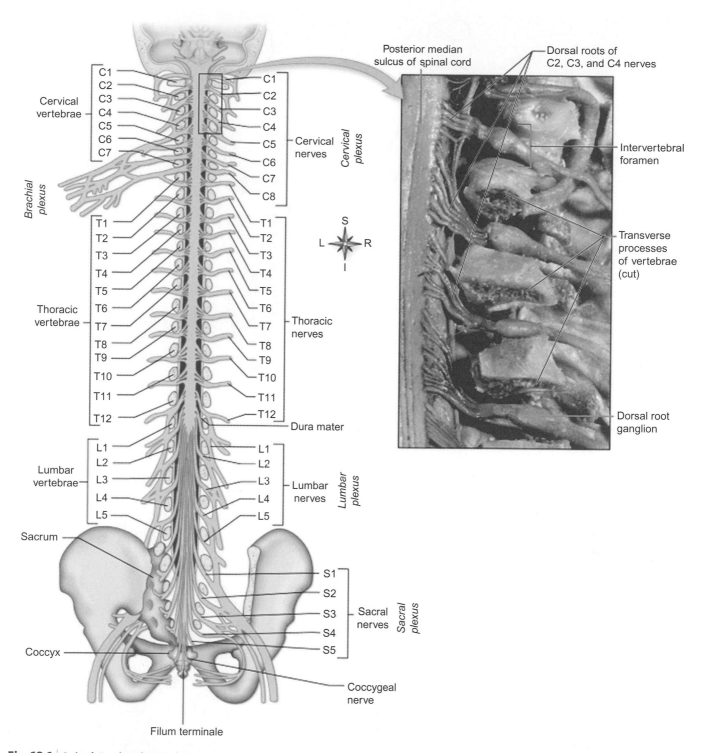

Fig. 19.1 | Spinal Cord and Spinal Nerves. The illustration shows spinal nerve names and location of spinal plexuses. *Inset* is a dissection of the cervical region of the spinal cord showing emerging cervical nerves. The spinal cord is viewed from behind (posterior aspect). (In Patton, K., & Thibodeau, G. [2020]. *Structure & function of the body* [16th ed.] St. Louis, MO: Mosby. From Vidic B Suarez FR. [1984]. *Photographic atlas of the human body.* St. Louis, MO: Mosby.)

LFS develops from degeneration of the lumbar zygapophyseal (facet) joint (Lopez, Navarro, Vargas, Alape, & Lopez, 2019; Manchikanti, Hirsch, Falco, & Boswell, 2016; Mimaroglu et al., 2017). It can lead to disc herniations, stenosis, and degenerative changes of the facet joint. The

diagnosis of facet joint arthropathy is challenging because the typical presentation is nonspecific low back pain with possible radiation to posterior thighs, hips, and buttocks in a nondermatomal pattern and unlike sciatic pain associated with disc herniations, it is not relieved by rest (Manchikanti

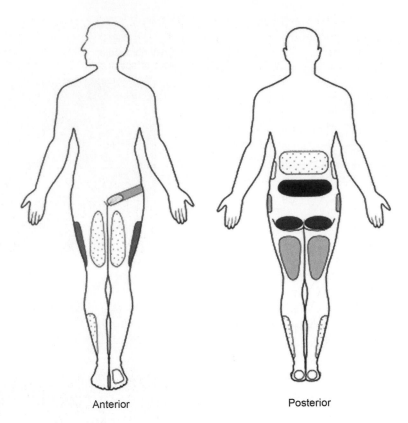

Anterior   Posterior

Fig. 19.2 | Lumbar Facet Referral Patterns. (From Benzon, H., Raja, S. N., Fishman, S. E., Liu, S. S., & Cohen, S. P. (2011). *Essentials of pain medicine.* Philadelphia, PA: Saunders.)

et al., 2016; Mimaroglu et al., 2017). Fig. 19.2 illustrates the referral pattern for pain arising from the lumbar facets. Radiographs may show degeneration and overgrowth of the facet joints, but false negative results are possible. The diagnosis of LFS is usually determined by a diagnostic block with an injection of a local anesthetic (Perolat et al., 2018; Vega & Acevedo-González, 2018).

Facet arthropathy is not limited to the lumbar region. Neck pain is very common in the United States and will likely increase because of cervical spine flexion associated with mobile device use and poor ergonomics, which lead to rapid degeneration of the cervical spine (Guan et al., 2016; Shan et al., 2013; Xie, Szeto, & Dai, 2017). Like the lumbar spine, the joints in the cervical spine can be affected, resulting in cervical facet syndrome, which is characterized by pain in the neck, shoulder, and occiput and headaches (Gutierrez & Wahezi, 2017). Fig. 19.3 illustrates the referral pattern for pain arising from the cervical facet joints. Common findings on physical examination include tenderness of the cervical facet joint when palpated and pain reproduced with extension, lateral flexion, or rotation of the neck in the absence of neurologic findings (Gutierrez & Wahezi, 2017). The diagnosis of cervical facet syndrome may be made by blockade of the nerves innervating the joints with local anesthetic (similar to the lumbar spine); however, authors of a recent systematic review concluded accurate diagnosis was best made with intersegmental mobility testing (Usunier et al., 2018).

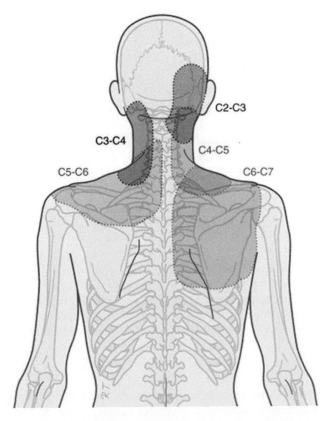

Fig. 19.3 | Cervical Facet Referral Patterns. (From Pico, T. C., Hamid, B., Burton, A. W., & Huntoon, M. A. [2012]. *Spinal injections and peripheral nerve blocks* [pp. 193–199]. Philadelphia, PA: Saunders.)

Spinal stenosis, another source of back pain, is a term that may refer to central canal narrowing, foraminal narrowing, or lateral recess stenosis and is associated with axial or radicular pain that may be provoked by hyperextension of the spine, walking, or descending movements. Spinal stenosis may be caused by other conditions such as disc protrusions, facet joint arthropathy, facet cysts, or spondylolisthesis (Lee et al., 2017). Clinical presentation may vary depending on the location and cause of narrowing but may include unilateral or bilateral radicular pain and radiculopathy extending to multiple dermatomes.

There are many other causes of spinal pain that may be considered for interventional pain procedures. Congenital or degenerative scoliosis may be associated with facet pain, discogenic pain, disc herniations, and stenosis, and treated based on the type of pathologic condition. Sacroiliac (SI) joint pain may manifest as unilateral buttock pain or pain that that radiates bilaterally to the lower extremities down to the feet. Like facet arthropathy, SI joint pain is not readily diagnosed by clinical examination or imaging but requires a diagnostic block.

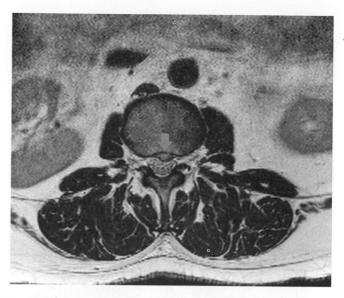

Fig. 19.4 | **T2 axial magnetic resonance image of the lumbar spine showing herniated nucleus pulposus** *(arrow)*. (Photo courtesy of Nitin K. Sekhri.)

Diagnostic Imaging

Diagnostic imaging is usually performed before interventional pain management approaches. The purpose of the imaging is to attempt to identify the source of pain and determine whether an interventional pain management approach is indicated and feasible. The main types of diagnostic imaging include plain film x rays, computed tomography (CT) scans and magnetic resonance imaging (MRI). Plain film x-rays may serve limited value as screening for osteoporosis in at-risk patients, and evaluation of hardware, but if abnormalities are seen on a radiograph, a follow-up CT scan is usually necessary. CT scans are easier to obtain, are less costly than MRI, and can provide good images of solid organs and bony structures, whereas MRI is superior in providing images of soft tissues such as nerves and ligaments (Peri, Jindal, & Hackney, 2017). For example, MRI can be useful in substantiating the need for epidural corticosteroid injections (ECSIs) for the treatment of herniations of intervertebral discs (Figs. 19.4 and 19.5). Each test has associated limitations; x-ray is not very useful in diagnosing significant pathologic conditions, CT scans expose the patient to radiation, whereas MRI does not, yet MRI involves a longer imaging duration, which may not be well tolerated by some. MRI is contraindicated for many safety reasons, including situations in which patients have implanted devices such as pacemakers, aneurysm clips, and spinal cord stimulators, because the MRI may cause damage to or dislodgement of the device; in such cases, CT scan with contrast can be a viable alternative (Peri et al., 2017).

Back pain is often difficult to correlate with imaging findings. Although some imaging studies such as MRI may demonstrate abnormalities that are more common in

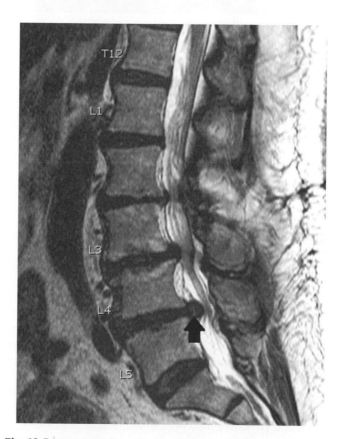

Fig. 19.5 | **T2 sagittal magnetic resonance image of the lumbar spine showing disc desiccation and herniated nucleus pulposus** *(arrow)*. (Photo courtesy of Nitin K. Sekhri.)

those with low back pain, especially in people younger than 50 years of age, the importance of imaging studies is sometimes of questionable value in the diagnosis of spinal pain (Hartvigsen et al., 2018). Approximately 50% of those with HNP noted on MRI are asymptomatic (Lee et al., 2017).

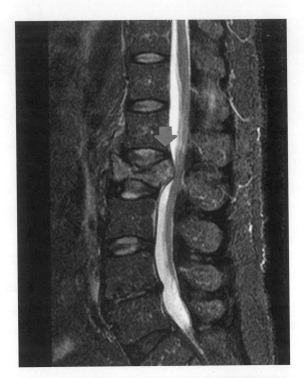

Fig. 19.6 | Short tau inversion recovery (STIR) magnetic resonance image with *arrow* **pointing to area of retropulsion into the spinal canal causing severe stenosis.** (Photo courtesy of Nitin K. Sekhri.)

Patients with radicular pain may lack evidence of nerve root compression on imaging, whereas those with myelographic and MRI evidence of nerve root abnormalities or spinal cord compression (Fig. 19.6) may be pain-free and otherwise asymptomatic (Hartvigsen et al., 2018; Keene, 2017).

Spinal Injections

Spinal interventional pain procedures are used to localize and identify the source of pain as well as to treat pain that has a spinal origin. The efficacy and safety of spinal injections have been extensively studied, and results are conflicting and controversial (Manchikanti & Benyamin, 2015; Manchikanti & Falco, 2015). Spinal injections are categorized by location (cervical, thoracic, lumbar, or sacral) and indication (diagnostic or therapeutic). ECSIs and facet joint injections are among the most common spinal injections, but other procedures such as medial branch blocks and RFAs are also performed (Keene, 2017).

Epidural Corticosteroid Injections

Indications

ECSIs are used in multimodal pain management for pain resulting from herniation of discs, spinal stenosis, discogenic pain unrelated to the facets or sacroiliac joints, and pain from postsurgery syndrome (Manchikanti et al., 2015b). The most common indication for ECSI is

herniated nucleus pulposus (Smith, Youn, Guay, Laufer, & Pilltsis, 2016). Using fluoroscopic guidance, ECSIs are administered using the interlaminar, transforaminal, or caudal approach (Smith et al., 2016).

Although ECSIs are common, it is important to note none of the glucocorticoids used for epidural administration are approved by the U.S. Federal Drug Administration (FDA) for this use (FDA, 2014). Use of glucocorticoids for epidural administration is considered an off-label use. In 2014 the FDA issued a warning about rare but serious neurologic risks associated with ECSIs after analysis of ECSI-related adverse events that were reported to the FDA between 1997 and 2014 (FDA, 2014). After the FDA issued the warning, a multisociety pain workgroup evaluated data and reported back to the FDA, after which the FDA upheld the warning (Racoosin, Seymour, Cascio, & Gill, 2015; Rathmell et al., 2015). Controversy arose in response to the FDA warning and multisociety pain workgroup report, with some experts reporting the warnings were issued despite insufficient assessment of the evidence and noting there are certain factors associated with greater risk than others, such as cervical transforaminal epidural injections.

Manchikanti and Falco (2015) recommend several measures to reduce ECSI-related risks for neurologic complications associated with inadvertent intraarterial injections and arachnoiditis. These recommendations include the need for careful assessment of medical necessity for ECSI, use of fluoroscopy for all ECSIs, avoidance of injections through scar tissue, use of alternative approaches to lumbar transforaminal ECSI with consideration of individual patient risks and awareness that local anesthetic may be as effective as a corticosteroid and avoidance of cervical transforaminal ECSI (Manchikanti & Falco, 2015). Rathmell et al. (2015) reported the use of sedation during cervical interlaminar or transforaminal ECSIs increases risks for spinal cord injuries because patients would be unable to communicate pain or other symptoms that would warn of impending spinal cord injury during the procedure. Therefore recommendations are to maintain communication with the patient throughout the procedure; sedation should be avoided, or, if necessary, only anxiolysis or minimal sedation is advised (Rathmell et al., 2015).

Contraindications

Coagulopathy, current anticoagulant therapy, infection, and poorly controlled diabetes are absolute contraindications for epidural injections (Brooks & Udoji, 2016). It is necessary to consider the vascularity of the spinal area and issues related to coagulopathy or use of anticoagulants because of risks for bleeding and potential epidural hematoma development (Narouze et al., 2018). (See Chapter 18 for more detail related to spinal injections and risks associated with coagulopathy and anticoagulation.) Professional associations have published guidelines that may be used to guide the performance of interventional spine and pain procedures when patients are receiving antiplatelet and anticoagulant medications (Narouze et al., 2018). Because of the vascularity of the epidural space, active local or systemic infections along with sepsis are absolute contraindications to ECSIs (Urbana-Champaign & Manchikanti, 2014). Patient refusal is always considered an absolute contraindication. Relative contraindications include congenital or surgical anatomy or anatomic changes that would compromise the safety of the procedure, allergic reactions to contrast or medication to be injected, and immunosuppression (Brooks & Udoji, 2016). Radiation exposure is usually contraindicated in pregnant women; therefore, pregnancy testing is necessary before procedures involving fluoroscopy or CT scan (Smith et al., 2016). Allergy to any of the medications or materials is a contraindication (Pountos, Panteli, Walters, Bush, & Giannoudis, 2016).

Research

Long-term outcomes of ECSIs have yet to be established. It is thought there is a short-term benefit to patients with lumbar radiculopathy or cervical radiculopathy. In a long-term follow-up study of 78 patients who were enrolled in an earlier randomized controlled trial and received lumbar transforaminal ECSIs for lumbar radicular pain resulting from intervertebral disc herniation, at 6 months after injections, more than 70% of the participants reported 80% or more reduction in pain; at 5- to 9-year follow-up, only 39 of the original patients were accessible, and, of these, 30 (76.9%) reported a history of recurrent pain (Kennedy et al., 2018). Given the catastrophic complications that can occur from infections, direct nerve trauma, direct spinal cord trauma, or ischemia, it is necessary to ensure all precautions are taken to ensure safety and efficacy for these procedures (Epstein, 2018; Kennedy et al., 2018; Singh, Cardozo, & Christolias, 2017). Particularly for cervical transforaminal epidurals, the use of ultrasound may provide a safety margin that is greater than provided with fluoroscopy (Zhang et al., 2019). Ultrasound allows for visualization of blood vessels, nerves, soft tissues, and spread of injected medication around nerves, whereas fluoroscopy allows for only identification of bony landmarks and real-time needle visualization. Further work needs to be done on the use of ultrasound for pain management procedures in the spine, particularly with ECSIs (Wang, 2018; Zhang et al., 2019).

Facet Injections

Facet injections are often used to treat patients with low back pain and are also used to treat neck pain. Fluoroscopy is used during injections of the facet joints to visualize the intraarticular location, which is thought to be responsible for pain. A combination of local anesthetic and glucocorticoid in a small volume is injected into the joint(s). Facet injections have not been well supported in longitudinal studies; more evidence is needed to determine if this relatively simple and safe procedure is as effective as more invasive procedures such as medial branch neurotomy.

Medial Branch Blocks

Medial branch block is another procedure used to treat LFS. The nerve supply to the facet joints is complex; the dorsal rami of the spinal nerve roots mostly provide sensory input from the periphery to the spinal cord, thus transmitting pain. The dorsal rami in the lumbar spine are split into two branches, the lateral and the medial branches. The medial branch supplies sensory input to the spinal cord from the facet joint to that level of the spinal cord and possibly to the level above and below and therefore becomes the target of this block. Box 19.2 presents a more detailed description of the medial branch block.

Similar to lumbar facet medial branch blocks, thoracic or cervical medial branch blocks may be performed to alleviate pain from an identified facet joint. The procedure involves injection of local anesthetic with or without glucocorticoid into the medial branches of the facet joint determined to be the source of pain and also into the levels above and below (Patel & Datta, 2015).

Neurotomy

Neurotomy, a procedure that results in destruction of the nerve involved in the patient's pain presentation, may be performed if the patient has a positive response to medial branch blockade for cervical or LFS. A positive response is identified by at least a 50% reduction in pain. In some cases, two or more medial branch blocks are performed before neurotomy to ensure the positive response is not related to a placebo response (Manchikanti et al., 2016).

Box 19.2 | Medial Branch Block for Facet Syndrome

Fluoroscopy is used to visualize the facet joint and the medial branch of the spinal nerve associated with this facet joint that corresponds to the source of the patient's pain syndrome (based on history, physical, and imaging).

Once the facet joint and nerve are identified, a small volume (usually <1 mL) of highly concentrated local anesthetic, with or without glucocorticoid, is injected into the medial branches at the level of interest, the level above, and the level below to effectively block pain arising from the facet joint.

For example, if the right L4-L5 facet joint was the likely cause of the patient's pain syndrome based on history, physical examination, and imaging, anesthetizing the L3 and L4 medial branch along with the L5 dorsal rami may be necessary.

Modified from Pino, C. A., & Rathmell, J. P. (2018). Interventional management of chronic pain. In D. E. Longnecker, S. C. Mackey, M. F. Newman, W. S. Sandberg, & W. M. Zapol (Eds.), *Anesthesiology* (3rd ed.). New York, NY: McGraw-Hill.

Radiofrequency is the preferred technique to create destruction of the nerves innervating the facets (Facchini, Spinnato, Guglielmi, Albisinni, & Bazzocchi, 2017; Holz & Sehgal, 2016). The nerves selected for neurotomy are those identified by prior blockade and are located for the neurotomy by fluoroscopic guidance. A radiofrequency needle is inserted along the beam of the fluoroscopy machine, and attempts are made to parallel the medial branch or dorsal rami (if L5 level) to facilitate a more efficacious neurotomy. Blockade is performed with a short-acting local anesthetic possibly mixed with long-acting local anesthetic and corticosteroid for flare symptoms that can occur afterward. Radiofrequency using a very high frequency is then applied to the selected location through the radiofrequency probe (Vrooman & Rosenquist, 2018).

Contraindications

There are several important contraindications to any procedures used to address facet syndromes. As with epidurals, it is necessary to consider the vascularity of the spinal area and issues related to bleeding disorders, coagulopathy, or use of anticoagulant must be considered because of the risks for bleeding and potential hematoma development (Narouze et al., 2018). As with epidural injections, the timing of antiplatelet therapy or anticoagulant medication administration must be considered, and facet joint procedures may be postponed until bleeding risks associated with these medications are reduced. In addition, active infections that can spread into the neuraxial space, patient refusal, pregnancy, and psychogenic pain are contraindications (Patel & Datta, 2015).

Complications

Overall complications related to procedures involving the facet joint are rare given the posterior position of the neuroanatomy. In one multicenter study, the complication rate was reported as 1.9% among more than 26,000 interventional pain procedures, including epidural, medial branch blocks, facet joint injections, and radiofrequency neurotomies (Carr et al., 2016). Vasovagal syncope, infections, and allergic reactions are the most common adverse effects (Carr et al, 2016; Perolat et al., 2018).

Facet Injections

Although complications related to injections of the facet joints are rare, intravascular injection of local anesthetic is possible; however, local anesthetic systemic toxicity would be unlikely because of the low volume of local anesthetic used. Another potential complication of procedures involving the facet joints is spread of local anesthetic into contiguous structures such as the epidural space, intervertebral foramen, or spinal axis; to reduce this risk, contrast is injected before local anesthetic injection to ensure the local anesthetic is injected into the desired area (Keel & Earle, 2017). When corticosteroids are administered, side effects, although unlikely given the small doses administered, may include Cushing syndrome, osteoporosis, bone necrosis, weight gain, fluid retention, and hyperglycemia (Patel & Datta, 2015).

Exacerbation of pain is a possible adverse effect of intraarticular facet injection. In the cervical facets, because the joint space is narrow, the advancement of the needle in the joint can cause abrasion of the surfaces of the joint and lead to increased pain, which is usually temporary (Pino & Rathmell, 2018). Intraarticular injection can result in rupture of the joint capsule if too large a volume of local anesthetic is used (Vrooman & Rosenquist, 2018). Other complications of intraarticular injections and medial branch blocks are related to the level of the procedure, placement of the needle, and potential damage to nearby structures. These complications are rare because imaging and radiopaque contrast are used before injection of local anesthetic but may include puncture of the dura, spinal cord trauma, subdural injection, neural trauma, and hematoma formation (Patel & Datta, 2018; Vrooman & Rosenquist, 2018).

Complications of Radiofrequency Ablation

The incidence of complications of RFA are less than 1% (Perolat et al., 2018). However, given its high energy and destructive nature, there is a risk for permanent complications. The proximity of the medial branch or dorsal ramus to the nerve root poses a rare but possible risk to ablation of the nerve root that could result in motor weakness and sensory deficits in a dermatomal fashion after the procedure is completed (Desai, 2015; Kim, Gilhool, & Furman, 2012). It is important for the patient to be able to communicate if severe pain develops during the procedure because it will warn the interventionalist that the nerve root is very near (Kim et al., 2012; Perolat et al., 2018). More common adverse effects involve neuropathic pain sensations (Perolat et al., 2018). Corticosteroids are sometimes administered through the radiofrequency cannula around the nerve during the time of ablation to alleviate this neuritic type of pain; however, there is controversy about the effectiveness of this practice and limited evidence to support it (Odonkor, Shin, & Cohen, 2017). In a retrospective review in which 87 patients did not receive a corticosteroid and 77 were treated with corticosteroid through the radiofrequency cannula, there was no statistically reported difference in the development of neuritis (Singh, Miccio, Modi, & Sein, 2019). Vigilance must be maintained if patients report increased pain, because a hematoma, neuritis, and/or infection may be present.

Postprocedure Care

Immediately after procedures to alleviate pain from facet joint syndrome, patients are monitored for signs of adverse effects. Vital signs are monitored until stable and returned to baseline, and if sedation was used during the procedure, monitoring continues until the effects of the sedation have resolved and the patient returns to a presedation level. The patient is assessed for development of any signs of local anesthetic toxicity. After the procedure, neurologic status is assessed to include monitoring for sensory and/or motor deficits, and, if unanticipated deficits are noted, the interventionalist is notified for further assessment and intervention.

When local anesthetic is used, patients are warned of potential sensory and motor block after the procedure, which may last 4 hours or longer depending on the type of local anesthetic and the need for caution to avoid injury and falls (Cohen & Soriano, 2018). The insertion site is assessed for bleeding, and the patient is instructed to call the interventionalist if signs of infection develop in the days after the procedure. Pain is also assessed, and if the patient experiences pain at the procedure access site(s), cold packs, acetaminophen, and nonsteroidal antiinflammatory medications (NSAIDs) may be used provided there are no contraindications (Kapoor & Shah, 2016). Patients can return home the day of the procedure but are cautioned not to drive and to avoid operating dangerous machinery, especially if sedated for the procedure.

Research

The use of ultrasound for facet procedures is an area of research interest. Ultrasound allows for better visualization of vascular structures and nerves and requires shorter administration duration and fewer needle passes than fluoroscopy, thus possibly decreasing the risk for intravascular injection, particularly for the cervical spine (Park, Lim, Lee, Ahn, & Park, 2017). Recent research in China indicates using sonography can improve accuracy of ultrasound-guided interventions (Chang et al., 2017). The innervation of the facet joints is complex and not well understood. Although it is known that the level above and below the involved joint provides significant sensory relay, research is needed to further expand understanding of the neuroanatomy. Additional studies are also needed to aid in determining the safest and most effective techniques for neurotomy. The long-term outcomes of a new technology using a cooled-tip RFA procedure over the traditional radiofrequency approach are yet to be determined (McCormick, Walker, Marshall, McCarthy, & Walega, 2014).

Vertebral Body Augmentation

Vertebral body augmentation (VBA) is most commonly done for vertebral body fractures occurring as sequelae of osteoporosis. Fig. 19.7 illustrates a vertebral compression fracture. Other indications include metastatic disease or primary illness (such as multiple myeloma), which may also weaken the vertebral body and cause a fracture. VBA may be considered after a trial of conservative therapy (usually 3 weeks), including NSAIDs or acetaminophen, opioids if pain is very severe, rest, and use of a brace to decreases the weight bearing of the affected vertebral body (Tsoumakidou et al., 2017). In a large retrospective study (n ≥ one million) of patients with osteoporotic vertebral body compression fractures, patients who received vertebroplasty or kyphoplasty had lower morbidity and mortality than groups who were treated

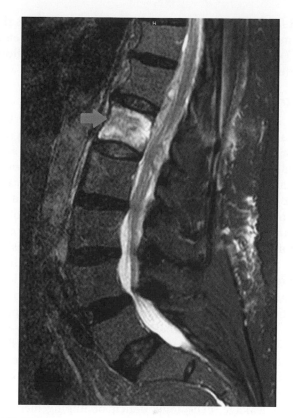

Fig. 19.7 | L1 Acute Vertebral Body Fracture *(arrow)*.

with conservative management alone (Edidin, Ong, Lau, & Kurtz, 2015). VBA augmentation is done most often by radiologists, followed by orthopedists and neurosurgeons (Degnan, Hemingway, & Hughes, 2017). During VBA, patients usually receive moderate sedation, deep sedation, or general anesthesia; however, simple vertebroplasty involving three levels or fewer in patients under 65 years of age may be done using only local anesthetic (Richmond, 2016).

Percutaneous vertebroplasty (PVP) and kyphoplasty are two fluoroscopically performed VBA procedures that involve placement of biomaterial, sometimes referred to as cement, to augment the fracture of the vertebral body (Choo et al., 2018). With PVP, a biomaterial, typically methyl methacrylate or polymethyl methacrylate (PMMA), is injected percutaneously into the vertebral body lesion (Amoretti et al., 2018; Frankl et al., 2016). Frequent imaging is necessary during the procedure to ensure there is only intraosseous spread. The biomaterial in the vertebral body reduces the compression, thus easing the pressure and lessening pain (McDonald, Lane, Diehn, & Wald, 2017). Kyphoplasty, another percutaneous procedure, also uses a biomaterial to augment the vertebral body fracture; however, before placement of the cement, a balloon device is inflated in the vertebral body to create a cavity in the bone for placement of the biomaterial (Chandra et al., 2017; Choo et al., 2018). Kyphoplasty may result in an increase in vertebral body height. The biomaterial used for kyphoplasty may be slightly more viscous than the material used with vertebroplasty (Chandra et al., 2017). After placement of the biomaterial, the balloons are deflated and removed.

Contraindications

VBA is contraindicated in patients with vertebral body fractures who are asymptomatic or improving with medical management (Tsoumakidou et al., 2017). Any active blood-borne or surgical infection is an absolute contraindication, and osteomyelitis is a strong contraindication to VBA (Hirsch et al., 2018). VBA is contraindicated for patients with unstable fractures, including three-column fractures (Tsoumakidou et al., 2017). Allergy to the materials used in VBA is a contraindication. Pregnancy is generally a contraindication, but if the benefit outweighs the risk, it is imperative to minimize exposure of radiation to the unborn child (Hirsch et al., 2018). Patients who have significant coagulopathy should not undergo the procedures and antiplatelet therapy, or anticoagulation must be held for an appropriate amount of time before VBA to reduce bleeding and risk for hematoma. Relative contraindications to VBA include unstable spine, fracture of the posterior spinal column because there is increased risk for cement leakage, neurologic deficit or impingement, and myelopathy related to the fracture (Hirsch et al., 2018; Tsoumakidou et al., 2017). The patient's underlying condition may pose a relative contraindication.

Complications

Complications associated with vertebral augmentation procedures are rare, but some risk exists. Careful patient selection is important to reduce risk for complications. Those with malignancy-related fractures, particularly fractures that are comminuted, involving the posterior wall of the vertebral body, or associated with epidural involvement would involve higher risk (Chandra et al., 2017). Complications of VBA include spinal cord compression, nerve root compression, venous embolism, and pulmonary embolism, which are related to migration of the biomaterial (cement) used in the procedure (Beall et al., 2017; Richmond, 2016; Tsoumakidou et. al., 2017). If cement migrates and compresses a nerve root, spinal cord, or cauda equina, it may be necessary to provide a nerve block or systemic corticosteroids and in rare circumstances, surgical decompression (Chandra et al., 2017). If intravascular embolization of cement occurs as a result of spread of the cement into vertebral or epidural veins, advanced medical management and critical care support may be necessary.

Kyphoplasty has been shown to be associated with an increased risk for fractures of adjacent vertebral bodies while vertebroplasty has been associated with a higher risk for cement leakage than kyphoplasty (Choo et al., 2018; Yaltirik, Ashour, Reis, Özdoğan, & Atalay, 2016). However, a meta-analysis of 12 studies that included a total of 1328 patients, of which 768 patients had undergone kyphoplasty or vertebroplasty and the remaining patients had conservative treatment, noted there was no increase in risk for additional vertebral body fractures with either procedure, including vertebral bodies adjacent to the VBA levels, compared with the group who had conservative therapy (Zhang, Xu, Zhang, Gao, & Zhang, 2017). VBA performed in the lumbar spine below the level of the spinal cord (usually L2) may result in nerve root injury. Potential dural injury and ensuing cerebrospinal fluid (CSF) leak is a risk; however, a study of a right-sided approach to VBA demonstrated reduced risk with this procedural approach (Liu, Tang, Zhang, Gu, & Yu, 2019). Other potential complications include respiratory issues and infection, which are rare but serious untoward consequences (Park et al., 2018).

Postprocedure Care

After VBA, activity restrictions for the first 3 hours are usually implemented: patients are usually kept supine in bed for 2 hours, followed by continued bed rest for another hour with the ability to raise the head of the bed to a 30-degree level (Chandra et al., 2017). During the postprocedural period, the patient's neurologic status is assessed, including assessment of pain and for signs and symptoms of sensory or motor deficits and assessment for other procedural complications. The development of radicular pain may indicate extravasation of the cement into the area of a nerve root and requires prompt notification of the interventionalist for further evaluation and treatment. If patients present with signs of pulmonary, cardiovascular, or cerebral embolization, prompt notification of the interventionalist and in some cases transfer to a critical care setting for further management may be necessary.

Pain assessment often reveals the compression fracture pain has resolved, but patients may report new acute pain related to the procedure. This procedural pain usually lasts only a short time, resolving in 1 to 3 days, and NSAIDs, acetaminophen, and nonpharmacologic measures may be used, unless contraindications exist (Chandra et al., 2017). Patients are often discharged the same evening or next day and are followed in the outpatient setting. Postprocedure follow-up includes assessment of pain, analgesic use, and functional assessment. Dietary or pharmacologic interventions (e.g., calcium, vitamin D, bisphosphonates) and physical therapies may be implemented after VBA to reduce risks for subsequent fractures. If new pain occurs, imaging is necessary to determine whether new fractures have developed.

Research

The optimal time frame for VBA after fracture is unclear because some studies included patients who had vertebral fracture within the year before VBA, whereas other studies limited use of VBA to patients who sustained fracture within a few months (Denoix et al., 2018; Kaliya-Perumal & Lin, 2018; Ruiz Santiago et al., 2014; Wang et al., 2015; Yang et al., 2016). Research is needed to clarify the optimal time for performance of VBA. Indications for the use of one type of VBA over another are not well established or supported by research. There is evidence to support lower complication rates with balloon kyphoplasty, including reduced risk for cement extravasation, but more head-to-head trials regarding outcomes and complications are needed (Edidin et al., 2015; Yaltirik et al., 2016).

Bone malignancies can cause compression fractures. There is growing interest in ablating localized tumors with RFA immediately before placement of the PMMA with percutaneous vertebroplasty in addition to chemotherapy and radiation, but more research is needed for definitive answers (Greenwood et al., 2015; Wallace, Greenwood, & Jennings, 2015; Wallace et al., 2016). Additional research is needed to more clearly ascertain patient-specific risk factors and to compare long-term outcomes of VBA with traditional spinal surgery (Choo et al., 2018).

Implantable Therapies

Patients living with chronic pain, not limited to spinal pain, who have tried less invasive therapies yet have not attained improvement in their pain management and more importantly their functional ability, may be candidates for more advanced implantable therapies. Implanted pain devices are advanced treatments for patients with refractory pain (Bolash et al., 2015; Geurts, Joosten, & van Kleef, 2017). Spinal cord stimulation (SCS; also referred to as dorsal column stimulation) and targeted drug delivery systems are well-established and accepted treatment options for chronic pain when less invasive therapies have not provided optimal improvement (Lamer, Deer, & Hayek, 2016). A referral to a pain specialist or spine surgeon for evaluation to identify and potentially implement these advanced therapies is necessary when treating patients with refractory pain (Lamer et al., 2016). These pain devices are usually implanted in a surgical center or hospital surgical setting, and patients are followed in the outpatient setting for evaluation of responses to the therapy, setting adjustments, and pump refills.

Spinal Cord Stimulators

Electrical stimulation has been described as treatment for pain for more than two thousand years since a physician in Rome used the electric discharge of torpedo fish to treat the pain of gout and headaches (Tsoucalas, Karamanou, Lymperi, Gennimata, & Androutsos, 2014). The therapy of electrical stimulation has evolved significantly over the past five decades since development and acceptance of the gate control theory (see Chapter 3). This theory provides the support for the development of spinal cord stimulators that activate large nerve fibers through electrical stimulation to provide analgesia (Melzack & Wall, 1967; Sdrulla, Guan, & Raja, 2019).

Spinal cord stimulators, which were first described by Dr. C.N. Shealy in 1967 (Shealy, Mortimer, & Reswick,

1967), are used in a multimodal approach to chronic pain management when pain has not responded to less invasive procedures or analgesic medications (Verrills, Sinclair, & Barnard, 2016). Different explanations have been provided to explain the mechanism of action of SCS. It is thought that SCS modulates nociceptive activity, and the experience of pain, by transmission of electric impulses to the dorsal aspect of the spinal cord, where these impulses inhibit dorsal horn neuronal activity caused by peripheral noxious stimuli (Malinowski, Kim, & Deer, 2018; Patel, Halpern, Shepherd, & Timpone, 2017; Peng, Min, Zejun, Wei, & Bennett, 2015). Other mechanisms may contribute to the beneficial effects of SCS. The efficacy of SCS may be related to inhibition of pain transmission by creation of a conduction block of the nociceptive fibers (Elliott & Simopoulos, 2017). Another possible explanation for the efficacy of SCS is that neurohormonal mechanisms that involve mediators such as endogenous opioids, γ-aminobutyric acid (GABA), adenosine, serotonin, and substance P, may contribute to the neuromodulatory effects of SCS (Elliott & Simopoulos, 2017). For example, GABA is thought to be released in the dorsal horn by electrical stimulation and GABA is involved in suppression of allodynia and hyperalgesia (Elliott & Simopoulos, 2017).

SCS was initially approved by the FDA for treatment of neuropathic extremity pain (Lempka & Patil, 2018; Verrills et al., 2016; Walsh, Machado, & Krishnaney, 2015). Over the years, the FDA approval has extended to include treatment of chronic pain associated with failed back surgery, complex regional pain syndrome (CRPS), peripheral neuropathy, amputation, multiple sclerosis, injuries to the spinal cord, postherpetic neuralgia, and other neuralgias (Raviv & Piltsis, 2018). Box 19.3 presents a list of indications for SCS.

Box 19.3 | Indications for Spinal Cord Stimulation

- Postlaminectomy pain syndrome: persistent radiculopathy and axial back pain
- Ilioinguinal neuralgia
- Phantom limb pain
- Brachial plexitis
- Complex regional pain syndrome type 1 (reflex sympathetic dystrophy) and type 2 (causalgia)
- Peripheral neuropathy
- Postherpetic neuralgia
- Stump pain
- Adhesive arachnoiditis
- Postthoracotomy pain or intercostal neuralgia
- Peripheral vascular disease
- Chronic angina

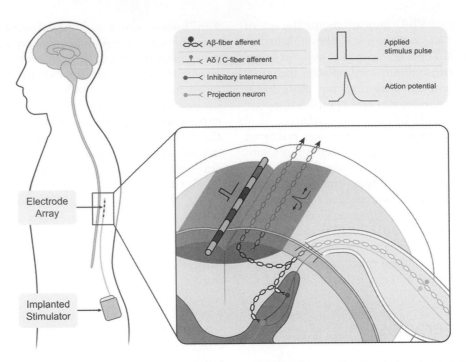

Aβ-fiber afferent

Aδ / C-fiber afferent

Inhibitory interneuron

Projection neuron

Applied stimulus pulse

Action potential

Electrode Array

Implanted Stimulator

Fig. 19.8 | **Spinal Cord Stimulator System.** (From Lempka, S. F., & Patil, P. G. [2018]. Innovations in spinal cord stimulation for pain. *Current Opinion in Biomedical Engineering, 8,* 51–60.)

Recognition of potential adverse effects associated with chronic opioid use and growth in awareness of opioid use disorder have resulted in consideration of nonopioid analgesic options for patients with chronic pain. SCS offers an important nonpharmacologic option for chronic pain treatment. With appropriate patient selection, SCS is considered a cost-effective intervention for chronic pain (Malinowski et al., 2018) with the rate of successful pain relief reaching as high as 85% (Patel et al., 2017).

Devices

Traditional, or classic, SCS is designed to create paresthesias over a specific region that replace the sensation of pain and result in analgesia within hours or sooner (Thomson et al., 2018; Verrills et al., 2016). Fig. 19.8 provides a schematic representation of a conventional SCS system. A conventional SCS device is described in Box 19.4. A recent SCS development is the dorsal root ganglion–SCS (DRG-SCS), which is designed to direct stimulation over areas of the spine not easily addressed by traditional SCS (Liem et al., 2015). DRG-SCS is capable of directly activating cell bodies of the neurons that innervate the area of pain (Liem et al., 2015). Box 19.5 provides a comparison of dorsal root ganglion stimulation to SCS. The dorsal root ganglion is a bundle of sensory nerve cell bodies (Vialle, Vialle, Contreras, & Junior, 2015) located at each nerve root of the spinal cord on the posterior aspect of the nerve in the neural foramina (Deer et al., 2017b). These nerve fibers are crucial for the transduction and transmission of the nociceptive pathway and are involved with neuropathic pain and pain sensitization (Deer et al., 2017b; Verrills et al., 2016). Benefits of DRG stimulation are illustrated

| Box 19.4 | Spinal Cord Stimulator Description |

A traditional spinal cord stimulation (SCS) system is composed of an external wireless control that regulates impulses from a subcutaneously placed pulse generator that transmits the impulses through connecting wires to the electrode leads, which are placed in the epidural space that innervates the targeted spinal dermatome (Patel, Halpern, Shepherd, & Timpone, 2017).

SCS leads are either percutaneous or paddle-type electrodes (see Fig. 19.10). Percutaneous leads are fed into the epidural space through the needle and guided to the appropriate level using fluoroscopic imaging. Paddle or laminotomy electrodes are placed during a laminotomy by spine surgeons under direct visualization at the desired level and confirmed by fluoroscopy.

The location of lead placement depends on the spinal dermatome, which corresponds to the region of pain. For example, upper extremity pain is treated with leads placed in the cervical epidural space, and lower extremity and back pain are treated with leads placed in the thoracic spine, because this is where the nerves in those spaces converge in the spinal cord.

by the fact that in February 2016 the FDA approved DRG stimulation for the treatment of pain from CRPS.

There have been many advances in SCS devices in recent years resulting in sub-perception SCS. These devices, which include the burst and kilohertz-frequency SCS (kHz-SCS),

| Box 19.5 | Comparison of Dorsal Route Ganglion Stimulation and Spinal Cord Stimulation |

SIMILARITIES OF DRG COMPARED TO SCS

* Psychological screening is obtained.
* MRI obtained and reviewed before the procedure.
* Trial is completed before permanent placement.
* Risks of the procedure are similar.

DIFFERENCES OF DRG COMPARED TO SCS

* DRG stimulation is subthreshold.
* DRG level of placement is at the dermatomal area of pain.
* DRG leads are not MRI compatible at this time; SCS leads have "conditional" compatibility.
* DRG is not currently used for neck and arm pain.

DRG, Dorsal root ganglion; *MRI*, magnetic resonance imaging; *SCS*, spinal cord stimulation.

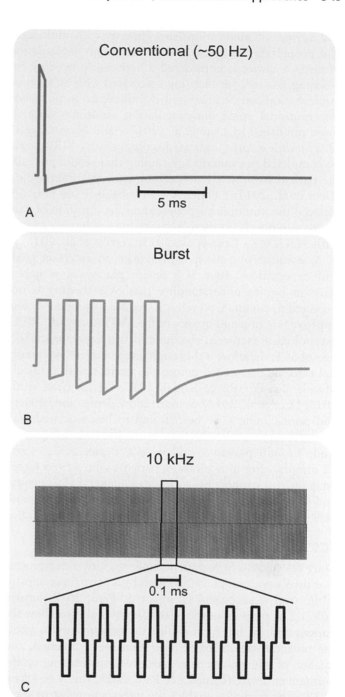

Fig. 19.9 | **Spinal Cord Stimulator Electrical Waveforms.** (From Lempka, S. F., & Patil, P. G. [2018]. Innovations in spinal cord stimulation for pain. *Current Opinion in Biomedical Engineering, 8*(12), 51–60.)

are considered sub-perception because they do not cause paresthesia, which occurs with conventional SCS, and can provide onset of analgesia over numerous hours or days (Thomson et al., 2018). The kHz-SCS device, which uses tonic pulse stimulation to rapidly block nerve conduction in models, was approved by the FDA in 2015 (Lempka & Patil, 2018). Such blocking can at least theoretically interrupt the transmission of pain messaging to cerebral locations. The kHz-SCS device delivers far more power than traditional SCS devices, and it is theorized that pain reduction is at least in part related to increased temperature of local tissues (Zannou et al., 2019). As with the traditional paresthesia SCS, there is Level 1 evidence to support use of the high-frequency sub-perception devices (Verrills et al., 2016).

Another important improvement is the development and implementation of high-frequency and burst wave-forms that are thought to have more action on the dorsal anterior cingulate cortex of the brain (De Ridder & Vanneste, 2016; Raviv & Piltsis, 2018). Appropriately named, burst SCS, which was FDA approved in 2016, is characterized by the delivery of closely spaced electrical pulses (five) in periodic bursts designed to simulate the biological thalamic bursts that naturally occur within the nervous system (De Ridder, Plazier, Kamerling, Menovsky, & Vanneste, 2013; Lempka & Patil, 2018; Verrills et al., 2016). The premise underlying burst SCS is that thalamic cells fire in a two-fold manner using both tonic and burst effort (De Ridder et al., 2013). The burst device is designed to provide analgesia with minimal or no paresthesia, but there is limited evidence to support effectiveness (Verrills et al., 2016). Fig. 19.9 provides a representation of different types of electrical waveforms available with some SCS devices.

Patient Selection

Careful patient selection is paramount to a successful stimulator implant (Deer et al., 2014). Patients who are considered for SCS must be thoroughly evaluated preoperatively with a detailed history of their pain, including previous and current treatments. A preprocedural medical screening includes a complete physical examination with strong neurologic focus, any physical contraindications to SCS, and review of medications/supplements with anticoagulant properties (Deer et al., 2014). Although implantation of an SCS device is considered a high-risk procedure for bleeding, the risk for bleeding associated with SCS device implantation can be mitigated by adherence to published interventional spine anticoagulation guidelines such as those published by Deer et al. (2017c) and Narouze et al. (2018). Unless contraindicated, a preoperative MRI should be completed to evaluate any finding that would preclude the patient from safely proceeding with this intervention (Deer et al., 2017a). Patients with substance use disorder, tobacco use, multiple surgeries, and long duration of pain are reported to be at increased risk for not having success with SCS (De La Cruz et al., 2015; Verrills et al., 2016).

Assessment of patient expectations to ascertain goals and expectations after SCS device placement is imperative to ensure understanding that SCS therapy is not expected to eliminate pain but to reduce pain intensity and improve function and quality of life (Atkinson et al., 2011). Psychological factors are recognized as influencing the success of SCS; therefore a thorough and complete psychological screening is needed before the stimulator trial (Block, Marek, Ben-Porath, & Kukal, 2017; De La Cruz et al., 2015; Deer et al., 2014). Somatization, depression, anxiety, and poor coping have been found to be associated with poor outcomes with SCS (Deer et al., 2014). In a follow-up study of 386 patients with an SCS device at 3, 6, and 12 months after implantation, patients who scored higher on pain catastrophizing scales had higher pain intensity and lower pain relief, quality of life, and satisfaction with SCS (Rosenberg, Schultz, Duarte, Rosen, & Raza, 2015).

SCS Trial

Once selected for SCS, patients undergo a two-step process that involves a trial phase followed by a permanent implant if the trial is successful (Lempka & Patil, 2018; Snyder, 2017). The purpose of the 3- to 10-day trial is to allow the patient and the interventionalist the opportunity to assess the potential benefit of SCS on pain relief, function, and quality of life enhancement before implantation of the permanent device (Lempka & Patil, 2018; Raviv & Piltsis, 2018). The trial also enables the interventionalist to select the optimal settings such as electrode placement, voltage, and pulse intervals (Lempka & Patil, 2018; Raviv & Piltsis, 2018). A successful trial is associated with at least a 50% decrease in pain intensity (Moore & McCrory, 2016).

For the trial, patients are usually brought to an ambulatory care interventional procedural setting where, under imaging and sterile conditions, a lead is temporarily placed in the epidural space and connected to an external programmable pulse generator (battery) (Lempka & Patil, 2018; Raviv & Piltsis, 2018). The patient is awake during the procedure. The lead is placed in the epidural space at the level that corresponds to the targeted area of pain relief. For example, if the upper extremity or hand is the area of neuropathic pain, the lead may be placed in the cervical epidural space, but if the pain is in the lower extremity,

the lead is usually placed in the thoracic epidural space (Veizi & Hayek, 2015). During the procedure, the patient provides feedback and is carefully assessed by the interventionalist and representative for the device company. Adjustments are made in the stimulator programming to ensure the electrodes provide paresthesias or sensations over the appropriate anatomic distribution of pain.

After the procedure and before discharge, further adjustments are made on the external programmable pulse generator to optimize the stimulation. Patients are thoroughly educated about the use and care of the programmable pulse generator and the plan for follow-up evaluation to determine effectiveness of SCS. In the days after the placement of the stimulator trial, as patients become more physically active, phone calls and/or office visits are necessary for reevaluation to determine if setting changes are needed to optimize pain relief. At the conclusion of the trial, the leads are removed in an office setting.

SCS Device Implantation

If a trial is successful, the patient returns to the ambulatory care interventional procedural setting for implantation of the pulse generator (implantable pulse generator [IPG]) into a pocket of subcutaneous tissue; the generator is connected to the percutaneously placed lead or paddle lead that was placed by a laminotomy, and the electrodes are placed in the epidural space that achieved successful stimulation during the trial (Veizi & Hayek, 2015; Verrills et al., 2016). Fig. 19.10 illustrates different types of per-

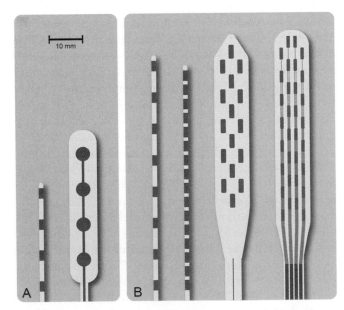

Fig. 19.10 | **Spinal Cord Lead Designs:** (A) Older-generation leads, with 4 electrodes; percutaneous on left, paddle on right. (B) Newer-generation lead,s with 8 to 16 electrodes on percutaneous leads (two leads on left) and 16-32 electrodes on paddle leads (two leads on right). (From Lempka, S. F., & Patil, P. G. [2018]. Innovations in spinal cord stimulation for pain. *Current Opinion in Biomedical Engineering, 8*(12), 51–60.)

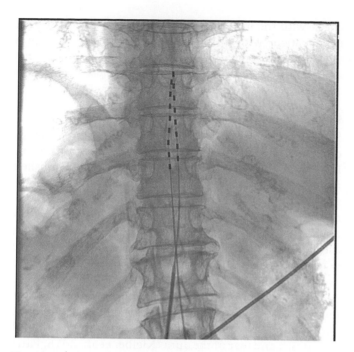

Fig. 19.11 | Two eight-contact percutaneous leads, staggered placed at superior endplate of T8.

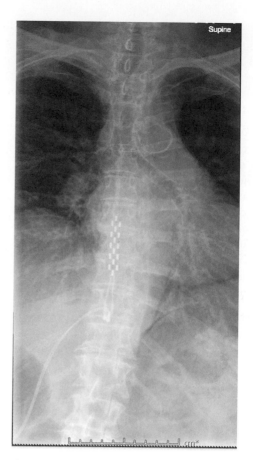

Fig. 19.12 | Permanent Paddle Lead Placed at T7-8.

cutaneous and paddle leads, Fig. 19.11 is an image of percutaneous lead placement, Fig. 19.12 is an implanted paddle lead image, and Fig. 19.13 is an image of DRG-SCS lead placement. Patient input into the site selection for the IPG is encouraged; the usual implantation site is in the gluteal region, although the abdomen is sometimes used, with avoidance of the belt line (Moore & McCrory, 2016). Optimization of electrode placement and energy during the procedure is the same as in the trial, with the patient providing feedback about the areas of distribution of the paresthesias or sensations and their correspondence to the pain distribution. After device placement, patients are given an external programming device, which enables them to turn the stimulator on or off, adjust the strength of the stimulation, change the programming and make other adjustments in the system to optimize pain relief. The programming device varies depending on the type of implanted system, with some appearing as handheld remote control devices similar to television remote controllers and others similar to smart phones or tablets. Box 19.6 summarizes the patient education that is provided for those who have had an implanted SCS device. The device companies provide detailed education to the patient related to the specific care, management, and maintenance of the SCS device.

After implantation of the SCS device, the patient maintains close contact with the interventionalist and representative from the device company to guide necessary setting adjustments and troubleshoot any problems with the SCS device. The life of the battery in the IPG varies depending on the type of SCS device; the interventionalist and device company representative monitor for signs of battery failure. Because the field of neuromodulation is

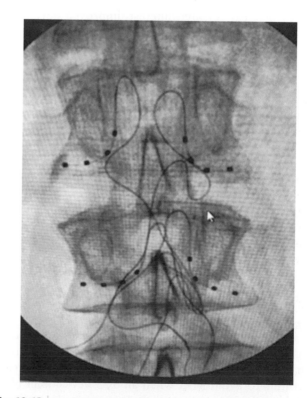

Fig. 19.13 | Lead Placement for Dorsal Root Ganglion Stimulation.

Box 19.6	Spinal Cord Stimulation Patient Education

TRIAL

- Risks of the procedure
- Expectation of trial
- Goals of trial
- Any medication changes during the trial
- Signs and symptoms of complications
- Contact physician and device representative if any signs of complications or concerns
- Use and care of the programmable pulse generator
- Restrictions during the trial:
  - Avoid deep bending or twisting at level of leads
  - Do not shower or get dressings wet

PERMANENT IMPLANTATION

- Reinforce same information as trial
- Restrictions following permanent placement
- Implantation site care
- Rechargeable versus primary cell battery
- Expectations of the permanent SCS surgery
- Medications after the SCS has been placed
- MRI compatibility

MRI, Magnetic resonance imaging; *SCS,* spinal cord stimulation.

an area of great research interest, improved devices are evolving; rechargeable batteries are relatively new, but their life span may be 9 years or longer (Eldabe, Buchser, & Duarte, 2015).

Contraindications

Contraindications for SCS include infection, anatomic issues (e.g., severe stenosis, spinal instability, epidural scars), neuropathy that is able to be treated conservatively, and any serious patient condition that prohibits SCS device implantation, such as total denervation (Raviv & Piltsis, 2018; Snyder, 2017). The inability to hold anticoagulation for the procedure or coagulopathy may be considered contraindications (Moore & McCrory, 2016). Consultation with the cardiology team is recommended if the patient has a pacemaker or defibrillator (Moore & McCrory, 2016).

Precautions

Patients who are likely to require future MRIs may not be considered appropriate candidates for SCS (Moore & McCrory, 2016). Because of the potential for thermal damage from MRI, it is generally advised by many manufacturers to avoid MRI when an SCS device is in place (Walsh et al., 2015). As new devices are made available, MRI compatibility may be possible, but it is necessary to

check with the manufacturer before performing an MRI on a patient with an SCS device. Likewise, many SCS devices are incompatible with the use of electrocautery, and the manufacturer also should be consulted before this technique (Walsh et al., 2015).

Complications

SCS is generally considered safe, with rare serious complications. Although generally considered safe, the International Neuromodulation Society has published recommendations to improve patient safety and reduce risks of injuries and complications associated with neurostimulation modalities (Deer et al., 2017a). Serious adverse events can be minimized or prevented through astute patient selection and procedural technique (Kleiber et al., 2016; Malinowski et al., 2018). Adverse events include those related to the mechanics of the device (e.g., malfunction, lead fracture, lead failure, or migration), premature battery depletion, infection, pain, and epidural or spinal cord injury, including epidural hematoma and tear of the dura (Kleiber et al., 2016; Patel et al., 2017; Raviv & Piltsis, 2018; Verrills et al., 2016). In some cases, the patient may become tolerant to SCS and will have less or no relief of pain (Malinowski et al., 2018). Minor side effects of headache and dizziness have been reported with burst stimulation (Hou, Kemp, & Grabois, 2016). Because the pulse generators in kilohertz devices require more charging, there is a risk for poor compliance related to the increased work needed by the patient (Thomson et al., 2018).

Other complications include dural puncture at the time of epidural needle placement, postdural puncture headache, pain related to components of the SCS device, and skin erosion over the leads or hardware (Eldabe et al., 2015; Deer et al., 2017a). Although rare, neurologic injury is possible as a result of direct trauma related to the needle puncture, percutaneous lead placement, or placement of paddle leads (Deer et al., 2017a). There are also risks for epidural hematoma formation and epidural abscess formation (Eldabe et al., 2015). Conditions such as persistent infection, failure to achieve adequate pain relief, increased pain, and skin erosion, or hardware failure may necessitate removal of the SCS device (Eldabe et al., 2015). Box 19.7 summarizes adverse effects associated with SCS.

Postimplantation Care

After placement of an SCS device, the patient is assessed for any neurologic deficits and any other complications related to the procedure. It is necessary to provide patient education about the device, activity restrictions, signs of SCS-related complications, and descriptions of emergency situations requiring prompt medical attention and ensure that instructions are understood. It is particularly important to instruct patients to avoid excessive bending and twisting at the waist for lumbar leads, or bending and twisting of the neck for cervical leads for a minimum of

Box 19.7 | Spinal Cord Stimulation Adverse Effects

DEVICE RELATED

- Pain at the site of the IPG and/or the battery
- Lead migration
- Lead fracture
- Painful stimulation
- Ineffective stimulation
- Motor stimulation
- IPG failure

SURGERY RELATED

- Infection and neuraxial abscess
- Bleeding
- CSF leak caused by inadvertent dural puncture
- Epidural hematoma
- Direct trauma to nervous system

CSF, Cerebrospinal fluid; *IPG,* implantable pulse generator.

4 weeks after implantation to reduce risks for lead fracture. Soft cervical collars are sometimes used to remind patients to restrict neck motion (Pino & Rathmell, 2018). Box 19.6 summarizes the content for patient education after SCS trial or permanent implantation.

Research

Although SCS is a generally safe and cost-effective intervention that may offer improved pain control and function, there is room for improvement. Between one-third and half of patients treated with SCS do not experience 50% less pain over a sustained time (Courtney et al., 2015). Advances in technology have resulted in newer forms of SCS that require additional research as well as research to determine if sub-perception devices can be used in conjunction with traditional paresthesia SCS devices (Thomson et al., 2018).

Intrathecal Drug Delivery System

IDDS, intrathecal therapy (ITT), and intrathecal drug delivery (ITDD) describe the process of delivering analgesic medication directly to the CSF located through a battery-operated pump that is surgically placed in the subarachnoid space (Bolash et al., 2015; Pope, Deer, Bruel, & Falowski, 2016). The advantages of intrathecal therapy are related to the ability to deliver medication directly into the central nervous system (CNS), avoiding the effects and adverse effects associated with systemic administration. Intrathecal delivery allows much lower doses to be used than when oral, intravenous, or systemic routes are used; for example, the oral dose of morphine is estimated to be 300 times higher than the intrathecal dose (Duarte, Lambe, Raphael, Eldabe, & Andronis, 2016). However, individual genetic variations result in variable oral to intrathecal conversion ratios. Advantages include increased potency, reduction of systemic exposure, reduction in required dosage, and reduction in side effects (Duarte et al., 2016).

Opioid receptors were discovered in 1971, and identification of opioid receptors on nerve tissue in 1973 led the way for development of intrathecal opioids that could provide selective analgesia while reducing side effects. The first human study demonstrating pain relief by use of intrathecal morphine was reported by Wang, Nauss, and Thomas in 1979 and in the following years, identification of GABA and glutamatergic and other receptors in the CNS led to the development of other medications for intrathecal delivery (Rizvi & Kumar, 2015). The first programmable IDDS was used in 1981, allowing providers to treat patients living with cancer pain with a small fixed infusion rate of morphine (Chandran, 2017; Duarte et al., 2016; Onofrio, Yaksh, & Arnold, 1982). Early systems were not reprogrammable, and changes in dose were achieved only by refilling the pump with a different concentration of medication. IDDS have developed and expanded over the years to include simple continuous infusion rates, flexible dosing with variable increases in volume of delivery, and patient-activated dosing features, and as these devices continue to evolve, there is an emphasis on miniaturization of the device, durability, dosing accuracy, and catheter design (Pope & Deer, 2017; Rizvi & Kumar, 2015).

Indications

Common indications for IDDS are intractable cancer and noncancer pain (Duarte et al., 2016). Very small amounts of medication are used with IDDS, and thus there are fewer side effects than with systemic medications; it is a viable option for patients with chronic pain who require opioids and find the side effects unbearable (Adler & Lotz, 2017; Chandran, 2017). IDDS is used in the treatment of nociceptive, neuropathic, visceral, or mixed type pain (Deer et al., 2016). This system is also effectively used for delivering baclofen as a treatment for painful spasticity (Chandran, 2017; Duarte et al., 2016). Although IDDS is used to treat the pain of CRPS, data do not support improvements in pain control or reductions in opioid use (Herring et al., 2018).

Patient Selection

Appropriate patient selection is essential for patient success with IDDS and includes a comprehensive, holistic assessment of the patient, including symptoms, diagnoses, current treatments, bleeding risk, past treatments, and psychological and social evaluation of the patient (Adler & Lotz, 2017; Deer et al., 2016; Duarte et al., 2016). Before placement of an IDDS, it is necessary to stop specific antiplatelet or anticoagulation medications in accordance with guidelines from the American Society of Regional Anesthesia and Pain Medicine and others (Narouze et al., 2018). If patients are not able to temporarily stop these medications to allow IDDS placement, they are not candidates for this therapy. Psychological evaluation is important to identify mental health conditions that would pose barriers to positive outcomes from IDDS (Deer et al., 2016) and to identify psychosis, schizophrenia, and severe anxiety/depression, which could contraindicate IDDS or use of some medications (Hadidi & Baranidharan, 2016). In patients with cancer who have a short life expectancy, the psychological screening may afford the opportunity for counseling related to death and dying (Deer et al., 2016). The financial status of the patient and insurance coverage are also important considerations (Pope et al., 2016,).

Devices

Although the specifics of manufactured IDDS are different, they all consist of a catheter that is surgically placed in the intrathecal space and tunneled to the implanted reservoir, which contains the infusion pump and medication to be infused (Adler & Lotz, 2017). Fig. 19.14 is an image of an implanted IDDS. Some have a feature that allows patient-controlled bolus doses of intrathecal medication within programmed limits. Others have a feature that permits the addition of scheduled bolus doses to the continuous infusion (Adler & Lotz, 2017). Like spinal cord stimulators, IDDS have particular restrictions and requirements related to MRI safety.

Intrathecal Medications

Two medications, morphine and ziconotide, are approved by the FDA for intrathecal administration for treatment of pain by an IDDS (Deer et al., 2016). The Polyanalgesic Consensus Conference (PACC) recommends the use of

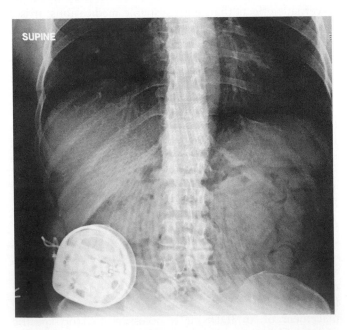

Fig. 19.14 | **Implanted Intrathecal Pump.**

Box 19.8 | Medications Used in Intrathecal Drug Delivery Systems

- Morphine (FDA approved)
- Ziconotide (FDA approved)
- Baclofen (FDA approved; for spasticity)
- HYDROmorphone (off label)
- FentaNYL (off label)
- SUFentanil (off label)
- Bupivacaine (off label)
- CloNIDine (off label)

Deer, T. R., Pope, J. E., Hayek, S. M., Bux, A., Buchser, E., Eldabe, S., . . . & Mekhail N. (2017). The Polyanalgesic Consensus Conference (PACC): Recommendations on intrathecal drug infusion systems best practices and guidelines. *Neuromodulation, 20*(2), 96–132.

these FDA-approved medications but recognizes that off-label intrathecal medication monotherapy and combination therapy are considered when the approved medications are contraindicated or ineffective; the use of fentaNYL or an admixture with bupivacaine is supported in the recommendations (Deer et al., 2016). Box 19.8 provides a list of FDA-approved and off-label medications used in intrathecal medication delivery (Deer et al., 2016). Baclofen is FDA approved for treatment of intractable spasticity (Lamer et al., 2016).

Preservative-free morphine is the most commonly used opioid in ITDD systems and is the only FDA-approved opioid for use by the intrathecal route (Deer et al., 2016). Many studies involving the use of preservative-free morphine in IDDS infusion systems have documented its efficacy as a first-line analgesic in the treatment of chronic pain and cancer pain (Deer et al., 2016). Intrathecal morphine produces analgesia primarily through its effect on spinal opioid receptors, but because of its hydrophilicity, it may spread rostrally by the CSF and bind to opioid receptors in the brainstem and upper areas of the brain and sometimes into systemic circulation (Webster, 2015). In the guidelines provided by the PACC, older studies are cited that demonstrate reductions in pain scores, reductions in oral opioid use, and improvements in quality of life (Deer et al., 2016).

It is important to consider the history of opioid use before use of opioid in an IDDS. Cross-tolerance has been shown between systemic and intrathecal morphine, and therefore the intrathecal starting morphine dose is calculated based on the usual daily systemic morphine dose (Deer et al., 2016). The starting dose of an opioid varies according to the patient's baseline opioid use, with conservative initial dosing and consideration of risks for cardiopulmonary depression (Deer et al., 2016). An intrathecal morphine bolus dose of 0.075 mg to 0.15 mg has been safely used in intrathecal trials, and the recommendation is to use the lowest dose estimated to provide pain relief. When used in a continuous infusion, the initial dose is suggested to be 50% of the effective trial bolus dose (Deer et al., 2016).

The opioid use history is also necessary to consider the potential efficacy of intrathecal morphine. If systemic opioid dose escalations did not provide analgesia, it is less likely that intrathecal opioids as monotherapy will be effective; it is recommended that systemic opioids be weaned or doses significantly reduced before initiation of intrathecal infusions, because inability to tolerate the wean and the continued requirement for high systemic doses of opioids suggest the likelihood that intrathecal monotherapy with an opioid will not be successful (Deer et al., 2016). In such cases, use of ziconotide or combination of intrathecal medications may be necessary. For example, in the treatment of cancer pain, a combination of opioid and local anesthetic (bupivacaine) may be used as first-line therapy (Deer et al., 2016).

Although systemic opioid side effects are reduced with intrathecal morphine, risk for respiratory depression must still be considered. The level of placement of the catheter affects the risk; catheters placed higher in the intrathecal space increase risk for rostral spread with greater risk for morphine reaching the respiratory centers in the brain, resulting in respiratory depression (Webster, 2015). In addition to the morphine-related side effects addressed in Chapters 11 through 13, the histamine release noted with intrathecal morphine may result in bradycardia and hypotension. Intrathecal morphine (and off-label intrathecal HYDROmorphone) may cause dependent and lower extremity peripheral edema as a result of vasodilatation (Pope, Deer, Amirdelfan, McRoberts, & Azeem, 2017), or it is hypothesized that rostral spread of hydrophilic opioids (morphine and HYDROmorphone) may lead to secretion of vasopressin from the posterior pituitary, resulting in water retention and peripheral edema (Deer et al., 2016). Urinary retention is another recognized side effect of intrathecal morphine infusion that may necessitate dose adjustments (Deer et al., 2016). (See Chapter 11 for more detailed information related to morphine pharmacology and Chapters 12 and 13 for details related to unwanted opioid effects.)

Ziconotide is a nonopioid intrathecal analgesic for patients with neuropathic or nociceptive pain (Deer et al., 2016). It was studied in randomized, placebo-controlled trials of patients with chronic cancer-related and non–cancer-related chronic refractory pain and was shown to provide significant pain relief compared to placebo for causes such as neuropathic, myelopathic, radiculopathic, and spinal pain and failed back surgery syndrome (McDowell & Pope, 2015). Ziconotide provides analgesia by blocking calcium-dependent channels along the nociceptive pathway responsible for action potential propagation and decreases release of pronociceptive (pain-promoting) neurotransmitters such as glutamate and substance P (Webster, 2015). It does not diffuse out of the CSF rapidly and, like morphine,

it spreads rostrally to sites in the CNS (Webster, 2015). The compound, which has low addiction potential (Rizvi & Kumar, 2015; Webster, 2015), was isolated from the venom of the marine snail, *Conus magus* (Webster, 2015).

Advantages of ziconotide over morphine include that it is not an opioid agonist and therefore does not have the endocrine side effects or tolerance effects associated with opioids. In addition to the absence of an opioid addiction risk, there are no risks for respiratory depression, withdrawal effects, opioid-induced hyperalgesia effects, and other systemic opioid effects (McDowell & Pope, 2016). A significant limitation of ziconotide is that it has a narrow therapeutic window and is often associated with extensive side effects (Deer et al., 2016; Rizvi & Kumar, 2015; Webster, 2015). Side effects reported in at least 25% of the 1254 patients in a trial of a continuous intrathecal ziconotide infusion include dizziness, nausea, confusion, and uncontrolled eye movement. Serious side effects of ziconotide include severe psychiatric symptoms, confusion, elevation of serum creatine kinase, meningitis, and reduced mental alertness (Drugs@FDA: Prialt, 2011).

It has been proposed that the tolerability of ziconotide may be related to the rate of dose increase rather than the actual ziconotide dose. Intrathecal trials with low doses and slow transition to continuous infusion at low initial doses followed by small, upward dose titrations based on pain relief and tolerability may prove beneficial (McDowell & Pope, 2016), but patients need to understand that it will take time to titrate to a dose that will provide pain relief (Brookes, Eldabe, & Batterham, 2017). Ziconotide is recommended to be tried alone before opioids (Adler & Lotz, 2017).

IDDS Trial

There are a number of ways to trial an IDDS (Duarte et al., 2016). For pain not related to malignancy an IDDS trial is warranted; however, for malignancy-associated pain, particularly in those with limited life expectancy, a decision may be made to forgo the trial and proceed straight to implantation (Bruel & Burton, 2016). An IDDS trial may involve administration of a bolus of the selected medication into either the epidural or the intrathecal space; another technique is to provide a continuous infusion trial with placement of a temporary epidural or intrathecal catheter (Adler & Lotz, 2017). The goal of the trial is to determine if the patient experiences adequate analgesia and potentially improved function and can tolerate the device and medication delivery that is consistent with patient expectations (Adler & Lotz, 2017). A trial is considered successful if there is a 50% reduction in pain and 50% functional improvement (Czernicki et al., 2015).

Permanent Implantation

After a successful trial with patients who experience a positive outcome during the trial with no significant side effects, a programmable IDDS, which houses the medication reservoir, is surgically implanted into a subcutaneous pocket and connected to a tunneled catheter that has its tip in the intrathecal space (Campos & Pope, 2018). To maximize analgesia and minimize side effects, the catheter level should be at the convergence of the nerves in the spinal cord associated with and in close proximity to the area of pain (Deer et al., 2016; Pope et al., 2016).

Contraindications

Contraindications for IDDS include systemic or local infections, bleeding disorders, spinal anatomy changes, psychosis, schizophrenia, and severe anxiety or depression (Hadidi & Baranidharan, 2016). Placement is contraindicated if the patient is on antiplatelet or anticoagulation therapy and those medications must be stopped in accordance with guidelines (Narouze et al., 2018). Additional contraindications include immune system compromise, inadequately controlled diabetes, substance use disorder, and mental health disorders that are not optimally controlled (Lamer et al., 2016).

Complications

Complications associated with IDDS are summarized in Box 19.9. Surgical complications, including infection, bleeding, nerve injury, dura puncture, and CSF fluid leaks are possible with both the IDSS trial and the permanent procedure (Czernicki et al., 2015; Hadidi & Baranidharan, 2016). Additional potential complications include catheter dislodgement, shredding, fractures, holes, and obstruction (Hadidi & Baranidharan, 2016). A catheter tip granuloma is a rare complication of an inflammatory mass at the intrathecal catheter tip typically associated with the chronic continuous infusion of high-concentration opioids at higher daily doses. Catheter tip granulomas are not associated with ziconotide use (McDowell & Pope, 2016). A seroma, a serous fluid collection in the pump pocket, can develop after pump placement and may persist for up

to 2 months. A similar collection, a hygroma, can occur when a CSF leak occurs around the dorsal incision or catheter insertion site and usually resolves spontaneously within 2 weeks (Czernicki et al., 2015).

In addition to complications related to the surgical implantation of the IDDS or catheter-related problems, adverse effects associated with IDDS may be related to the specific medication infused and the dose of medication. These adverse effects are addressed in previous sections. Medication adverse effects may be associated with complications related to the refilling of the IDDS. When refilling the intrathecal medication pump reservoir, it is possible to inadvertently inject the medication into the pump reservoir pocket, a subcutaneous injection, rather than into the pump port (Webster, 2015). The subcutaneous injection may result in a medication overdose or underdose. Overdose or underdose also can occur because of pump failure, and opioid overdose may lead to respiratory depression. Ziconotide overdose has been shown to possibly cause sedation for a short duration but is not associated with life-threatening outcomes (Webster, 2015). Box 19.10 lists signs and symptoms of ziconotide overdose.

Postprocedure Care

There is no consensus about the need for hospitalization for an intrathecal trial or after pump implantation because safety data are lacking. A benefit of inpatient hospitalization is that it offers the flexibility of trial of different intrathecal medications and doses with just one dural puncture (Deer et al., 2016). It is suggested that if the starting intrathecal opioid dose exceeds recommended guidelines, an overnight hospital stay is advised. If the plan is to discharge a patient after intrathecal pump implantation, the initial 24-hour intrathecal dose should be 50% of the successful trial dose, and if ziconotide is infused, in the absence of neurologic problems before the infusion, a 6-hour observation period after infusion initiation is recommended (Deer et al., 2016).

After implantation of an IDDS, the IDDS dose is titrated very slowly and patients are closely monitored for adverse effects, especially in the days immediately after

---

Box 19.9	Intrathecal Drug Delivery System Adverse Effects

Device and Procedure Related

- Pain at the site reservoir/pump
- Catheter migration
- Catheter fracture

IDDS Implantation Procedure Related

- Infection
- Bleeding
- CSF leak
- Epidural hematoma
- Epidural abscess
- Neurologic injury

CSF, Cerebrospinal fluid; *IDDS,* intrathecal drug delivery system.

Box 19.10	Signs of Ziconotide Overdose

- Extreme drowsiness
- Vision problems
- Confusion
- Speech problems
- Severe psychiatric symptoms
- Nausea and vomiting
- Dizziness
- Ataxia/abnormal gait
- Reduced consciousness
- Urinary retention

implantation (Adler & Lotz, 2017). It is advisable, especially during the pump trial and early days after implantation, to avoid administration of medications such as benzodiazepines and antihistamines that would confound an assessment for adverse effects, such as excessive sedation, related to the intrathecal medications (Adler & Lotz, 2017). After implant, frequent office visits may be necessary to assess the response to IDDS medications and titrate doses. At each visit, a pain assessment and physical examination for signs of complications are necessary (Adler & Lotz, 2017).

The intrathecal medication reservoir is refilled through a port that is identified by palpation over the skin. Medication refills take place in an outpatient practice setting or in some cases in the patient's home by trained clinicians on a regular basis (usually every 1–3 months) and with any change in medication or concentration (Lamer et al., 2016). When refilling pumps, the medication, dosing, and flow rate are checked for accuracy and adjustments are made using the external IDDS programmer (Adler & Lotz, 2017).

Patient education is essential to successful use of an IDDS. It is important to ensure that patients understand it is unrealistic to expect that an IDDS will eliminate pain or cure the underlying condition. It is intended to help manage pain (Adler & Lotz, 2017). Other important patient educational interventions include the following (Adler & Lotz, 2017):

- Patients should be shown the IDDS pump and encouraged to participate in selection of the site for creation of the pocket for pump placement (usually below the waist).
- It is necessary for patients to carry device identification cards to allow bypassing of airport and store security scanners that could alter pump settings.
- Hyperbaric chambers and air flights at more than 13,000 feet in an unpressurized cabin should be avoided.
- Activity should be paced to reduce injury risk as pain is controlled.

When a patient with an implanted IDDS is hospitalized and requires surgery, it is necessary for certain precautions to be taken. Ideally, contact should be made with the clinician who manages the patient's IDDS. Before a procedure the IDDS should be interrogated to determine the age of the device, the last time it was evaluated, current medication, dose, dosing regimen (fixed, flex, patient demand), and date for next refill (Nadherny, Anderson, & Abd-Elsayed, 2018). If the pump contains an opioid, it is necessary to consider risks for opioid-related adverse effects if additional systemic opioids are administered during the hospitalization or risks for withdrawal if the IDDS is inadvertently stopped (Nadherny et al., 2018). Alterations in the patient's body temperature may affect pump function; temperatures higher than 39 degrees Celsius may increase medication delivery rate and lead to overdose, and low body temperature may decrease the rate of pump delivery and lead to increased pain and possible withdrawal (Nadherny et al., 2018).

- Manufacturer recommendations for the use of MRI with specific pump types and models must be determined before an MRI is performed, because the MRI scanner can temporarily stall the pump motor (Adler & Lotz, 2017).
- If cardiac defibrillation is needed, efforts should be made to keep the path of current far away from the IDDS if possible.
- Diathermy (including shortwave, microwave, or ultrasound) may cause heating of the intrathecal pump and alter the infusion rate and is not recommended near the pump or catheter.
- Electroconvulsive therapy may cause alterations in pump operation and medication delivery.
- High-output ultrasound and lithotripsy are not recommended with an IDDS, but, if necessary, the beam should be focused away from the pump.
- Radiation therapy can damage the pump and, if possible, should be avoided over the pump, or the pump should be shielded with lead to avoid damage (Nadherny et al., 2018).

To optimize safety, it is recommended to interrogate the intrathecal infusion pump after procedures involving energy fields to ensure the IDDS is functioning properly and delivering medication at the desired rate. When patients are admitted to the inpatient setting with IDDS, all clinicians should be aware of the presence of the IDDS, its settings, and associated precautions to prevent inadvertent adverse outcomes. It is also necessary to recognize unanticipated changes in the patient's condition that could result from IDDS malfunction, resulting in overdose or withdrawal symptoms.

Research

Many areas of research related to intrathecal medication delivery in the management of chronic cancer and noncancer pain are underway, and others are needed. Researchers continue to examine cost-effectiveness of intrathecal therapy, especially in noncancer pain (Campos & Pope, 2018). Studies to examine the complication of intrathecal granuloma development, including identification of risks and risk reduction strategies are needed (Veizi et al., 2016b). The complication of peripheral edema related to intrathecal drug delivery is an area of research interest as investigators attempt to identify risks and risk reduction strategies. For example, the benefits of rotation from intrathecal morphine or HYDROmorphone to intrathecal fentaNYL and determination of whether opioid choice affects peripheral edema development is an area of research interest (Veizi, Tornero-Bold, & Hayek, 2016a).

Research and development efforts continue to develop intrathecal pumps with longer life spans and fewer device malfunctions (Bolash et al., 2015). There is interest in the potential for development of smaller and more sophisticated IDDSs. Engineering efforts to improve hardware of the pump and intrathecal catheter and infusion strategies are expected to yield improvements in IDDS therapies (Campos & Pope, 2018). In addition to product development, systematic collection of data to examine the quality, efficacy, and safety of IDDS is necessary to understand IDDS product performance, adverse effects, device events, and overall risks to patients (Konrad et al., 2016). Studies are needed to determine the long-term outcomes of IDDS use in a variety of pain conditions.

Key Points

- Interventional pain procedures may be used in a multimodal analgesic plan of care to optimize pain relief while reducing reliance on systemic analgesic medications.
- Chronic back pain is often an indication for spinal interventional pain procedures, including injections and implantable therapies.
- Diagnostic imaging is usually necessary to determine the cause of chronic pain conditions before interventional pain procedures.
- Computed tomography (CT) scans are fairly easy to obtain and can provide good images of solid organs and bony structures. Magnetic resonance imaging is preferred over CT scans when soft tissue images, such as imaging of nerves and ligaments, are needed.
- Consensus is lacking related to the efficacy and safety of spinal injections in the treatment of back pain.
- Epidural corticosteroid injections, facet joint injections, medial branch blocks, and radiofrequency ablation are interventional pain procedures used to treat chronic back pain of different causes.
- Interventional pain injections often involve injection of local anesthetic and/or glucocorticoids.
- Vertebral body augmentation, including percutaneous vertebroplasty and kyphoplasty, involves placement of biomaterial into the vertebral body to reduce compression of the vertebral body and alleviate the pain associated with acute compression fractures.
- Implantable pain therapies include placement of spinal cord stimulators and intrathecal drug delivery systems (IDDSs).
- Appropriate patient selection for placement of implantable pain therapies is necessary to optimize successful outcomes and minimize adverse effects.
- The efficacy of spinal cord stimulation (SCS) is supported by the gate control theory; SCS is theorized to provide pain relief by transmission of electric impulses to the dorsal aspect of the spinal cord to block dorsal horn neuronal activity.
- Advanced SCS techniques such as dorsal root ganglion stimulation and more complex devices such as sub-perception devices have been developed and

provide improved pain relief. These advances continue to evolve as SCS research continues.
- IDDSs allow delivery of medication directly into the central nervous system, thereby optimizing analgesic effectiveness and reducing adverse effects associated with systemic medication administration.
- The U.S. Food and Drug Administration–approved IDDS analgesics are morphine and ziconotide. Intrathecal baclofen is approved for treatment of spasticity. Other medications are administered off-label when approved medications are ineffective or contraindicated.
- IDDS adverse effects are associated with procedure-related complications, device malfunction, intrathecal catheter, or IDDS medication.
- Patient education, particularly with placement of implantable pain therapies, is necessary to ensure patients have realistic expectations related to effectiveness of the therapy in alleviating pain and improving function. Patient education is also necessary to ensure safe functioning of the device and prompt recognition and attention in the event of a complication or adverse effect.

Case Scenario

Mr. V. has had chronic back pain for the past 15 years after a work-related injury in which he sustained thoracic vertebral compression fractures. He has not had imaging of his spine in at least 5 years, but reports that at that time he had several levels of herniated discs. Mr. V. has a history of atrial fibrillation and takes an oral anticoagulant to reduce his stroke risk. He is overweight but has no other medical problems. His primary care provider has been writing prescriptions for oxyCODONE (oxycodone controlled-release) 30 mg orally (PO) bid, and oxyCODONE 15 mg PO qid as needed, for which he usually takes four doses daily. Mr. V. was informed by his primary care provider that he is going to wean him off opioids over the next 2 months because he has concerns about oversight of prescribing practices by regulatory agencies. Mr. V. has been trying to locate another clinician who will continue to write opioid prescriptions but has been unable to find anyone. He recently visited an outpatient pain specialist, who informed him he would not write opioid prescriptions, but if imaging shows a pathologic condition in his spine, he would be willing to offer Mr. V. several interventional options. You are Mr. V.'s cousin and a registered nurse. Mr. V. comes to you with the following questions he hopes you can answer:

1. The clinician wants Mr. V. to have an MRI. Mr. V. had a CT scan 5 years ago. Why is an MRI necessary, and why can't he have another CT scan, because it is a faster and easier test?

2. Mr. V. has heard from his friends that perhaps an epidural corticosteroid would be a good way to control his pain. He wants to know why an epidural corticosteroid would be used, what does the procedure involve, and what are the risks and benefits? Does he have any special consideration that would need to be addressed for him to have an epidural corticosteroid injection?

3. Mr. V. has been reading about other ways to manage back pain, such as a kyphoplasty. He wants to know your opinion about a kyphoplasty. What pathologic condition would he need to have for a kyphoplasty to be considered? What does the procedure entail?

4. Mr. V. has also been reading about implanted devices and would like you to explain how a spinal cord stimulator works to alleviate pain.

5. Mr. V. has been comfortable taking opioids for his back pain and thinks the best option for him might be an intrathecal drug delivery system (IDDS). He does not know anything about it, but he has heard that the pump could be filled with morphine and he would need to get it refilled at certain intervals. Can you explain what an IDDS involves? What medications could he receive? How is the pump implanted? How is his dose calculated? Are there any contraindications? How does the pump get refilled? What if his pain worsens—can he get the dose increased?

Acknowledgement

The authors of this chapter acknowledge the contributions of Shalvi B. Parikh to this work.

References

Adler, J. A., & Lotz, N. M. (2017). Intrathecal pain management: a team-based approach. *Journal of Pain Research, 10,* 2565–2575.

Amoretti, N., Diego, P., Amélie, P., Andreani, O., Foti, P., Antomarchi, H., … Boileau, P. (2018). Percutaneous vertebroplasty in tumoral spinal fractures with posterior vertebral wall involvement: Feasibility and safety. *European Journal of Radiology, 104,* 38–42.

Atkinson, L., Sundaraj, S. R., Brooker, C., O'Callaghan, J., Teddy, P., Salmon, J., … Majedi, P. M. (2011). Recommendations for patient selection in spinal cord stimulation. *Journal of Clinical Neuroscience, 18*(10), 1295–1302.

Beall, D. P., Coe, J. D., McIlduff, M., Bloch, D., Hornberger, J., Warner, C., & Tutton, S. M. (2017). Serious Adverse Events Associated with Readmission Through One Year After Vertebral Augmentation with Either a Polyetheretherketone Implant or Balloon Kyphoplasty. *Pain Physician, 20,* 521–528.

Block, A. R., Marek, R. J., Ben-Porath, Y. S., & Kukal, D. (2017). Associations between pre-implant psychosocial factors and spinal cord stimulation outcome: Evaluation using the MMPI-2-RF. *Assessment, 24*(1), 60–70.

Bolash, R., Udeh, B., Saweris, Y., Guirguis, M., Dalton, J. E., Makarova, N., & Mekhail, N. (2015). Longevity and cost of implantable intrathecal drug delivery systems for chronic pain management: a retrospective analysis of 365 patients. *Neuromodulation: Technology at the Neural Interface, 18*(2), 150–156.

Brooks, A. K., & Udoji, M. A. (2016). Interventional techniques for management of pain in older adults. *Clinics in Geriatric Medicine, 32*(4), 773–785.

Brookes, M. E., Eldabe, S., & Batterham, A. (2017). Ziconotide monotherapy: a systematic review of randomised controlled trials. *Current Neuropharmacology, 15*(2), 217–231.

Bruel, B. M., & Burton, A. W. (2016). Intrathecal therapy for cancer-related pain. *Pain Medicine, 17*(12), 2404–2421.

Campos, L. W., & Pope, J. E. (2018). Intrathecal Drug Delivery: Implantation. In *Advanced Procedures for Pain Management* (pp. 393–403). Cham, Switzerland: Springer.

Carr, C. M., Plastaras, C. T., Pingree, M. J., Smuck, M., Maus, T. P., Geske, J. R., … Kennedy, D. J. (2016). Immediate adverse events in interventional pain procedures: a multi-institutional study. *Pain Medicine, 17*(12), 2155–2161.

Chandra, R. V., Shah, V., Leslie-Mazwi, T. M., Rabinov, J. D., Yoo, A. J., & Hirsch, J. A. (2017). Vertebral Augmentation. In Z. H. Bajwa, R. Wootton, & C. A. Warfield (Eds.), *Principles and Practice of Pain Medicine* (3rd ed.). New York, NY: McGraw-Hill.

Chandran, S. (2017). Intrathecal Drug Delivery. In *Drug Delivery* (pp. 401–410). Boca Raton, FL: CRC Press.

Chang, K. V., Lin, C. P., Lin, C. S., Wu, W. T., Karmakar, M. K., & Özçakar, L. (2017). Sonographic tracking of trunk nerves: essential for ultrasound-guided pain management and research. *Journal of Pain Research, 10,* 79.

Choo, S., Malik, A. T., Jain, N., Yu, E., Kim, J., & Khan, S. N. (2018). 30-day adverse outcomes, re-admissions and mortality following vertebroplasty/kyphoplasty. *Clinical Neurology and Neurosurgery, 174,* 129–133.

Cohen, B. R., & Soriano, E. T. (2018). Pulsed radiofrequency neuromodulation in interventional pain management: A growing technology. *Journal of Radiology Nursing, 37*(3), 181–187.

Courtney, P., Espinet, A., Mitchell, B., Russo, M., Muir, A., Verrills, P., & Davis, K. (2015). Improved pain relief with burst spinal cord stimulation for two weeks in patients using tonic stimulation: results from a small clinical study. *Neuromodulation: Technology at the Neural Interface, 18*(5), 361–366.

Czernicki, M., Sinovich, G., Mihaylov, I., Nejad, B., Kunnumpurath, S., Kodumudi, G., & Vadivelu, N. (2015). Intrathecal drug delivery for chronic pain management-scope, limitations and future. *Journal of Clinical Monitoring and Computing, 29*(2), 241–249.

De La Cruz, P., Fama, C., Roth, S., Haller, J., Wilock, M., Lange, S., & Pilitsis, J. (2015). Predictors of spinal cord stimulation success. *Neuromodulation: Technology at the Neural Interface, 18*(7), 599–602.

Deer, T. R., Pope, J. E., Hayek, S., Bux, A., Buchser, E., Eldabe, S., & Grider, J. S. (2016). The polyanalgesic consensus conference (PACC): Recommendations on intrathecal drug infusion systems best practices and guidelines. *Neuromodulation: Technology at the Neural Interface, 20*(2), 96–132.

Deer, T. R., Lamer, T. J., Pope, J. E., Falowski, S. M., Provenzano, D. A., Slavin, K., … Williams, K. (2017a). The neurostimulation appropriateness consensus committee (NACC) safety guidelines for the reduction of severe neurological injury. *Neuromodulation: Technology at the Neural Interface, 20*(1), 15–30.

Deer, T. R., Levy, R. M., Kramer, J., Poree, L., Amirdelfan, K., Grigsby, E., ... Mekhail, N. (2017b). Dorsal root ganglion stimulation yielded higher treatment success rate for complex regional pain syndrome and causalgia at 3 and 12 months: A randomized comparative trial. *Pain*, 158(4), 669–681. https://doi.org/10.1097/j.pain.0000000000000814.

Deer, T. R., Mekhail, N., Provenzano, D., Pope, J., Krames, E., Thomson, S., ... Buvanendran, A. (2014). The appropriate use of neurostimulation: avoidance and treatment of complications of neurostimulation therapies for the treatment of chronic pain. *Neuromodulation: Technology at the Neural Interface*, 17(6), 571–598.

Deer, T. R., Narouze, S., Provenzano, D. A., Pope, J. E., Falowski, S. M., Russo, M. A., ... Carlson, J. D. (2017c). The Neurostimulation Appropriateness Consensus Committee (NACC): recommendations on bleeding and coagulation management in neurostimulation devices. *Neuromodulation: Technology at the Neural Interface*, 20(1), 51–62.

Degnan, A. J., Hemingway, J., & Hughes, D. R. (2017). Medicare Utilization of Vertebral Augmentation 2001 to 2014: Effects of Randomized Clinical Trials and Guidelines on Vertebroplasty and Kyphoplasty. *Journal of the American College of Radiology*, 14(8), 1001–1006.

De La Cruz, P., Fama, C., Roth, S., Haller, J., Wilock, M., Lange, S., & Pilitsis, J. (2015). Predictors of spinal cord stimulation success. *Neuromodulation: Technology at the Neural Interface*, 18(7), 599–602.

Denoix, E., Viry, F., Ostertag, A., Parlier-Cuau, C., Laredo, J. D., Cohen-Solal, M., ... Funck-Brentano, T. (2018). What are the predictors of clinical success after percutaneous vertebroplasty for osteoporotic vertebral fractures? *European Radiology*, 28(7), 2735–2742.

De Ridder, D., & Vanneste, S. (2016). Burst and tonic spinal cord stimulation: different and common brain mechanisms. *Neuromodulation: Technology at the Neural Interface*, 19(1), 47–59.

De Ridder, D., Plazier, M., Kamerling, N., Menovsky, T., & Vanneste, S. (2013). Burst spinal cord stimulation for limb and back pain. *World Neurosurgery*, 80(5), 642–649.

Desai, M. J., Hargens, L. M., Breitenfeldt, M. D., Doth, A. H., Ryan, M. P., Gunnarsson, C., & Safriel, Y. (2015). The rate of magnetic resonance imaging in patients with spinal cord stimulation. *Spine*, 40(9), E531.

Drugs@FDA. (2011). *Prialt (ziconotide)solution, intrathecal infusion. [Highlights of prescribing information]*. Retrieved 8/29/20 from https://www.accessdata.fda.gov/drugsatfda_docs/label/2011/021060s006lbl.pdf.

Duarte, R. V., Lambe, T., Raphael, J. H., Eldabe, S., & Andronis, L. (2016). Intrathecal drug delivery systems for the management of chronic non-cancer pain: protocol for a systematic review of economic evaluations. *BMJ Open*, 6(7), e012285.

Edidin, A. A., Ong, K. L., Lau, E., & Kurtz, S. M. (2015). Morbidity and mortality after vertebral fractures: Comparison of vertebral augmentation and nonoperative management in the Medicare population. *Spine*, 40(15), 1228–1241. https://doi.org/10.1097/BRS.0000000000000992.

Eldabe, S., Buchser, E., & Duarte, R. V. (2015). Complications of spinal cord stimulation and peripheral nerve stimulation techniques: a review of the literature. *Pain Medicine*, 17(2), 325–336.

Elliott, J. A., & Simopoulos, T. T. (2017). Neuromodulation for Pain. In Z. H. Bajwa, R. Wootton, & C. A. Warfield (Eds.), *Principles and Practice of Pain Medicine* (3rd ed.). New York, NY: McGraw-Hill.

Epstein, N. E. (2018). Major risks and complications of cervical epidural steroid injections: An updated review. *Surgical Neurology International*, 9, 86. https://doi.org/10.4103/sni.sni_85_18.

Facchini, G., Spinnato, P., Guglielmi, G., Albisinni, U., & Bazzocchi, A. (2017). A comprehensive review of pulsed radiofrequency in the treatment of pain associated with different spinal conditions. *The British Journal of Radiology*, 90(1073), 20150406.

Frankl, J., Sakata, M. P., Choudhary, G., Hur, S., Peterson, A., & Hennemeyer, C. T. (2016). A Classification System for the Spread of Polymethyl Methacrylate in Vertebral Bodies Treated with Vertebral Augmentation. *Tomography: A Journal for Imaging Research*, 2(3), 197–202.

Geurts, J. W., Joosten, E. A., & van Kleef, M. (2017). Current status and future perspectives of spinal cord stimulation in treatment of chronic pain. *Pain*, 158(5), 771–774.

Gómez Vega, J. C., & Acevedo-González, J. C. (2018). Clinical diagnosis scale for pain lumbar of facet origin: Systematic review of literature and pilot study. *Neurocirugía (English Edition)*, 30(3), 133–143.

Greenwood, T. J., Wallace, A., Friedman, M. V., Hillen, T. J., Robinson, C. G., & Jennings, J. W. (2015). Combined ablation and radiation therapy of spinal metastases: A novel multimodality treatment approach. *Pain Physician*, 18(6), 573–581.

Guan, X., Fan, G., Chen, Z., Zeng, Y., Zhang, H., Hu, A., ... He, S. (2016). Gender difference in mobile phone use and the impact of digital device exposure on neck posture. *Ergonomics*, 59(11), 1453–1461.

Gutierrez, D. E., & Wahezi, S. E. (2017). Zygapophyseal (Facet) Pain Syndrome. In *Musculoskeletal Sports and Spine Disorders* (pp. 349–351). Cham, Switzerland: Springer.

Hadidi, S., & Baranidharan, G. (2016). Implantable technology for pain management. *Anaesthesia & Intensive Care Medicine*, 17(11), 536–542.

Hartvigsen, J., Hancock, M. J., Kongsted, A., Louw, Q., Ferreira, M. L., Genevay, S., ... Smeets, R. J. (2018). What low back pain is and why we need to pay attention. *The Lancet*, 391(10137), 2356–2367.

Herring, E. Z., Frizon, L. A., Hogue, O., Mejia, J. U., Rosenquist, R., Bolash, R. B., ... Nagel, S. J. (2018). Long-term outcomes using intrathecal drug delivery systems in complex regional pain syndrome. *Pain Medicine*, 20(3), 515–520.

Hirsch, J. A., Beall, D. P., Chambers, M. R., Andreshak, T. G., Brook, A. L., Bruel, B. M., ... Tutton, S. M. (2018). Management of vertebral fragility fractures: a clinical care pathway developed by a multispecialty panel using the RAND/UCLA Appropriateness Method. *The Spine Journal*, 18(11), 2152–2161.

Holz, S. C., & Sehgal, N. (2016). What is the correlation between facet joint radiofrequency outcome and response to comparative medial branch blocks? *Pain Physician*, 19(3), 163–172.

Hou, S., Kemp, K., & Grabois, M. (2016). A systemic evaluation of burst spinal cord stimulation for chronic back and limb pain. *Neuromodulation*, 19(4), 398–405.

Institute of Medicine. (2011). *Relieving pain in America: a blueprint for transforming prevention, care, education, and research*. Washington, DC: The National Academies Press. Retrieved 8/29/2020 from https://doi.org/10.17226/13172.

Izzo, R., Popolizio, T., D'Aprile, P., & Muto, M. (2015). Spinal pain. *European Journal of Radiology*, 84(5), 746–756.

Kaliya-Perumal, A. K., & Lin, T. Y. (2018). Clinical outcomes of percutaneous vertebroplasty for selective single segment dorsolumbar vertebral compression fractures. *Journal of Clinical Orthopaedics and Trauma, 9,* S140–S144.

Kapoor, S. G., & Shah, S. N. (2016). Cervical medial branch blocks and radiofrequency neurotomy. In D. K. Baheti, S. Bakshi, R. P. Gehdoo, & S. Gupta (Eds.), *Interventional Pain Management: A Practical Approach.* Philadelphia, PA: Jaypee Medical, Inc.

Keel, J. C., & Earle, J. (2017). Intraarticular Injections. In Z. H. Bajwa, R. Wootton, & C. A. Warfield (Eds.), *Principles and Practice of Pain Medicine (3rd Ed.).* New York, NY: McGraw-Hill.

Keene, D. (2017). Spinal Injections (Including Epidural Steroids and Medial Branch Blocks). In Z. H. Bajwa, R. Wootton, & C. A. Warfield (Eds.), *Principles and Practice of Pain Medicine (3rd Ed.).* New York, NY: McGraw-Hill.

Kennedy, D. J., Zheng, P. Z., Smuck, M., McCormick, Z. L., Huynh, L., & Schneider, B. J. (2018). A minimum of 5-year follow-up after lumbar transforaminal epidural steroid injections in patients with lumbar radicular pain due to intervertebral disc herniation. *The Spine Journal, 18*(1), 29–35.

Kim, R. E., Gilhool, J. J., & Furman, M. B. (2012). Lumbar zygapophysial joint nerve (medial branch) radiofrequency neurotomy, posterior approach. In M. B. Furman, T. S. Lee, & L. Berkwits (Eds.), *141. Atlas of Image-Guided Spinal Procedures E-Book.* Philadelphia, PA: Saunders.

Kleiber, J. C., Marlier, B., Bannwarth, M., Theret, E., Peruzzi, P., & Litre, F. (2016). Is spinal cord stimulation safe? A review of 13 years of implantations and complications. *Revue Neurologique, 172*(11), 689–695.

Konrad, P. E., Huffman, J. M., Stearns, L. M., Plunkett, R. J., Grigsby, E. J., Stromberg, E. K., … Weaver, T. W. (2016). Intrathecal drug delivery systems (IDDS): the implantable systems performance registry (ISPR). *Neuromodulation: Technology at the Neural Interface, 19*(8), 848–856.

Lamer, T. J., Deer, T. R., & Hayek, S. M. (2016). Advanced innovations for pain. *Paper presented at the Mayo Clinic Proceedings, 91*(2), 246–258.

Lee, A. C., Cohen, S. P., & Abdi, S. (2017). Low Back Pain. In Z. H. Bajwa, R. Wootton, & C. A. Warfield (Eds.), *Principles and Practice of Pain Medicine (3rd Ed.).* New York, NY: McGraw-Hill.

Lempka, S. F., & Patil, P. G. (2018). Innovations in spinal cord stimulation for pain. *Current Opinion in Biomedical Engineering, 8*(12), 51–60.

Liem, L., Russo, M., Huygen, F. J., Van Buyten, J. P., Smet, I., Verrills, P., … Kramer, J. (2015). One-year outcomes of spinal cord stimulation of the dorsal root ganglion in the treatment of chronic neuropathic pain. *Neuromodulation: Technology at the Neural Interface, 18*(1), 41–49.

Liu, J., Tang, J., Zhang, Y., Gu, Z. C., & Yu, S. H. (2019). Percutaneous Vertebral Augmentation for Osteoporotic Vertebral Compression Fracture in the Midthoracic Vertebrae (T5-8): A Retrospective Study of 101 Patients with 111 Fractured Segments. *World Neurosurgery, 122*(2), e1381–e1387.

Lopez, W. O. C., Navarro, P. A., Vargas, M. D., Alape, E., & Lopez, P. A. C. (2019). Pulsed Radiofrequency Versus Continuous Radiofrequency for Facet Joint Low Back Pain: A Systematic Review. *World Neurosurgery, 122*(2), 390–396.

Malinowski, M. N., Kim, C. H., & Deer, T. R. (2018). Complications of Spinal Cord Stimulation. In *Neuromodulation* (pp. 657–668). St. Louis, MO: Academic Press.

Manchikanti, L., & Benyamin, R. M. (2015). Key safety considerations when administering epidural steroid injections. *Pain Management, 5*(4), 261–272.

Manchikanti, L., & Falco, F. J. (2015). Safeguards to prevent neurologic complications after epidural steroid injections: analysis of evidence and lack of applicability of controversial policies. *Pain Physician, 18*(2), E129–E138.

Manchikanti, L., Hirsch, J. A., Falco, F. J., & Boswell, M. V. (2016). Management of lumbar zygapophysial (facet) joint pain. *World Journal of Orthopedics, 7*(5), 315–337. https://doi.org/10.5312/wjo.v7.i5.315.

Manchikanti, L., Pampati, V., Falco, F. J., & Hirsch, J. A. (2015a). An updated assessment of utilization of interventional pain management techniques in the Medicare population: 2000–2013. *Pain Physician, 18*(2), E115–E127.

Manchikanti, L., Nampiaparampil, D. E., Manchikanti, K. N., Falco, F. J., Singh, V., Benyamin, R. M., … Hirsch, J. A. (2015b). Comparison of the efficacy of saline, local anesthetics, and steroids in epidural and facet joint injections for the management of spinal pain: A systematic review of randomized controlled trials. *SNI Spine, a supplement to Surgical Neurology International, 6*(S4), S194–S235.

McCormick, Z. L., Walker, J., Marshall, B., McCarthy, R., & Walega, D. R. (2014). A novel modality for facet joint denervation: Cooled radiofrequency ablation for lumbar facet syndrome. A case series. *Physical Medicine and Rehabilitation International, 1*(5), 5.

McDonald, R. J., Lane, J. I., Diehn, F. E., & Wald, J. T. (2017). Percutaneous vertebroplasty: Overview, clinical applications, and current state. *Applied Radiology, 46*(1), 24–30.

McDowell, G. C., & Pope, J. E. (2016). Intrathecal ziconotide: dosing and administration strategies in patients with refractory chronic pain. *Neuromodulation: Technology at the Neural Interface, 19*(5), 522–532.

Melzack, R., & Wall, P. D. (1967). Pain mechanisms: A new theory. *Survey of Anesthesiology, 11*(2), 89–90.

Mimaroglu, C., Altinay, B. M., Duger, C., Isbir, A. C., Gursoy, S., Kaygusuz, K., & Kol, I. O. (2017). The evaluation of radiofrequency facet nerve denervation in the patients with lumbar facet syndrome: experience with 493 patients. *Anaesthesia Pain & Intensive Care, 21*(4), 438–441.

Moore, D. M., & McCrory, C. (2016). Spinal cord stimulation. *British Journal of Anesthesia Education, 16*(8), 258–263.

Nadherny, W., Anderson, B., & Abd-Elsayed, A. (2018). Perioperative and Periprocedural Care of Patients with Intrathecal Pump Therapy. *Neuromodulation: Technology at the Neural Interface., 22*(7), 775–780. https://doi.org/10.1111/ner.12880.

Narouze, S., Benzon, H. T., Provenzano, D., Buvanendran, A., De Andres, J., Deer, T., … Huntoon, M. A. (2018). Interventional spine and pain procedures in patients on antiplatelet and anticoagulant medications: Guidelines from the American Society of Regional Anesthesia and Pain Medicine, the European Society of Regional Anaesthesia and Pain Therapy, the American Academy of Pain Medicine, the International Neuromodulation Society, the North American Neuromodulation Society, and the World Institute of Pain. *Regional Anesthesia and Pain Medicine, 43*(3), 225–262.

Odonkor, C. A., Shin, B. C., & Cohen, S. P. (2017). The Effect and Role of Steroids in Facet Joint Radiofrequency Denervation: A Narrative Review. *Current Physical Medicine and Rehabilitation Reports, 5*(4), 180–185.

Onofrio, B. M., Yaksh, T. L., & Arnold, P. G. (1982). Continuous low-dose intrathecal morphine administration in the treatment of chronic pain of malignant origin. *Obstetrical & Gynecological Survey, 37*(4), 270–271.

Park, K. D., Lim, D. J., Lee, W. Y., Ahn, J., & Park, Y. (2017). Ultrasound versus fluoroscopy-guided cervical medial branch block for the treatment of chronic cervical facet joint pain: a retrospective comparative study. *Skeletal Radiology*, 46(1), 81–91.

Park, J. W., Park, S. M., Lee, H. J., Lee, C. K., Chang, B. S., & Kim, H. (2018). Infection following percutaneous vertebral augmentation with polymethylmethacrylate. *Archives of Osteoporosis*, 13, 1–10.

Patel, S. H., Halpern, C. H., Shepherd, T. M., & Timpone, V. M. (2017). Electrical stimulation and monitoring devices of the CNS: An imaging review. *Journal of Neuroradiology*, 44(3), 175–184.

Patel, V. B., & Datta, S. (2015). Facet Joint Interventions: Intra-Articular Injections, Medial Branch Blocks, and Radiofrequency Ablations. In S. Diwan, & P. S. Staats (Eds.), *Atlas of Pain Medicine Procedures* (p. 2015). New York, NY: McGraw-Hill.

Peng, L., Min, S., Zejun, Z., Wei, K., & Bennett, M. I. (2015). Spinal cord stimulation for cancer-related pain in adults. *Cochrane Database of Systematic Reviews*, (6), CD009389.

Peri, N., Jindal, G., & Hackney, D. B. (2017). Radiologic Evaluation of Spinal Disease. In Z. H. Bajwa, R. Wootton, & C. A. Warfield (Eds.), *Principles and Practice of Pain Medicine* (3rd ed.). New York, NY: McGraw-Hill.

Perolat, R., Kastler, A., Nicot, B., Pellat, J. M., Tahon, F., Attye, A., ... Krainik, A. (2018). Facet joint syndrome: from diagnosis to interventional management. *Insights into Imaging*, 9(5), 773.

Pino, C. A., & Rathmell, J. P. (2018). Interventional Management of Chronic Pain. In D. E. Longnecker, S. C. Mackey, M. F. Newman, W. S. Sandberg, & W. M. Zapol (Eds.), *Anesthesiology* (3rd Ed.). New York, NY: McGraw-Hill.

Pope, J. E., & Deer, T. R. (2017). Intrathecal Drug Delivery: An Overview of Modern Concepts in Advanced Pain Care. In Z. H. Bajwa, R. Wootton, & C. A. Warfield (Eds.), *Principles and Practice of Pain Medicine* (3rd Ed.). New York, NY: McGraw-Hill.

Pope, J. E., Deer, T. R., Amirdelfan, K., McRoberts, W. P., & Azeem, N. (2017). The pharmacology of spinal opioids and ziconotide for the treatment of non-cancer pain. *Current Neuropharmacology*, 15(2), 206–216.

Pope, J. E., Deer, T. R., Bruel, B. M., & Falowski, S. (2016). Clinical uses of intrathecal therapy and its placement in the pain care algorithm. *Pain Practice*, 16(8), 1092–1106.

Pountos, I., Panteli, M., Walters, G., Bush, D., & Giannoudis, P. V. (2016). Safety of Epidural Corticosteroid Injections. *Drugs in R&D*, 16(1), 19–34. https://doi.org/10.1007/s40268-015-0119-3.

Racoosin, J. A., Seymour, S. M., Cascio, L., & Gill, R. (2015). Serious neurologic events after epidural glucocorticoid injection: the FDA's risk assessment. *New England Journal of Medicine*, 373(24), 2299–2301.

Rathmell, J. P., Benzon, H. T., Dreyfuss, P., Huntoon, M., Wallace, M., Baker, R., ... Buvanendran, A. (2015). Safeguards to prevent neurologic complications after epidural steroid injections consensus opinions from a multidisciplinary working group and national organizations. *Anesthesiology: The Journal of the American Society of Anesthesiologists*, 122(5), 974–984.

Raviv, N., & Piltsis, J. G. (2018). Spinal cord stimulation. In K. J. Burchiel, & A. M. Rasain (Eds.), *Functional Neurosurgery & Neuromodulation* (pp. 44–48). St. Louis, MO: Elsevier.

Richmond, B. J. (2016). Vertebral augmentation for osteoporotic compression fractures. *Journal of Clinical Densitometry*, 19(1), 89–96.

Rizvi, S., & Kumar, K. (2015). History and present state of targeted intrathecal drug delivery. *Current pain and headache reports*, 19(2), 1.

Rosenberg, J. C., Schultz, D. M., Duarte, L. E., Rosen, S. M., & Raza, A. (2015). Increased pain catastrophizing associated with lower pain relief during spinal cord stimulation: results from a large post-market study. *Neuromodulation: Technology at the Neural Interface*, 18(4), 277–284.

Ruiz Santiago, F., Santiago Chinchilla, A., Guzmán Álvarez, L., Pérez Abela, A. L., del Castellano Garcia, M. M., & Pajares López, M. (2014). Comparative review of vertebroplasty and kyphoplasty. *World Journal of Radiology*, 6(6), 329–343. https://doi.org/10.4329/wjr.v6.i6.329.

Sdrulla, A. D., Guan, Y., & Raja, S. N. (2019). Spinal Cord Stimulation: Clinical Efficacy and Potential Mechanisms. *Pain Practice*, 18(8), 1048–1067.

Serrano, B. M., Cuenca, E. C., Higuera, E. G., Esplá, A. F., Díaz, E. G., de Andrés Ares, J., & Rodríguez, F. G. (2014). Anticoagulation and interventional pain management. *Techniques in Regional Anesthesia and Pain Management*, 18(1-2), 58–64.

Shan, Z., Deng, G., Li, J., Li, Y., Zhang, Y., & Zhao, Q. (2013). Correlational analysis of neck/shoulder pain and low back pain with the use of digital products, physical activity and psychological status among adolescents in Shanghai. *Plos One*, 8(10), e78109.

Shealy, C. N., Mortimer, J. T., & Reswick, J. B. (1967). Electrical inhibition of pain by stimulation of the dorsal columns: Preliminary clinical report. *Anesthesia & Analgesia*, 46(4), 489–491.

Singh, J. R., Cardozo, E., & Christolias, G. C. (2017). The clinical efficacy for two-level transforaminal epidural steroid injections. *PM and R*, 9(4), 392–397.

Singh, J. R., Miccio, J. V., Modi, D. J., & Sein, M. T. (2019). The Impact of Local Steroid Administration on the Incidence of Neuritis following Lumbar Facet Radiofrequency Neurotomy. *Pain Physician*, 22(1), 69–74.

Smith, H., Youn, Y., Guay, R. C., Laufer, A., & Pilitsis, J. G. (2016). The Role of Invasive Pain Management Modalities in the Treatment of Chronic Pain. *The Medical Clinics of North America*, 100(1), 103–115.

Snyder, R. (2017). Spinal cord stimulation trial, patient and device selection, and implantation technique. In *Seminars in Spine Surgery: Vol. 29* (pp. 150–152). Philadelphia, PA: WB Saunders. No. 3.

Thomson, S. J., Tavakkolizadeh, M., Love-Jones, S., Patel, N. K., Gu, J. W., Bains, A., ... Moffitt, M. (2018). Effects of rate on analgesia in kilohertz frequency spinal cord stimulation: results of the PROCO randomized controlled trial. *Neuromodulation: Technology at the Neural Interface*, 21(1), 67–76.

Tsoucalas, G., Karamanou, M., Lymperi, M., Gennimata, V., & Androutsos, G. (2014). The "torpedo" effect in medicine. *International Maritime Health*, 65(2), 65–67.

Tsoumakidou, G., Too, C. W., Koch, G., Caudrelier, J., Cazzato, R. L., Garnon, J., & Gangi, A. (2017). CIRSE guidelines on percutaneous vertebral augmentation. *Cardiovascular and Interventional Radiology*, 40(3), 331–342.

Urbana-Champaign, I., & Manchikanti, L. (2014). Epidural steroid injections safety recommendations by the multi-society pain workgroup (MPW): More regulations without evidence or clarification. *Pain Physician*, 17, E575–E588.

U.S. Food and Drug Administration. (2014). FDA Drug Safety Communication: FDA requires label changes to warn of rare but serious neurologic problems after epidural corticosteroid injections for pain. Published April 23. https://www.fda.gov/drugs/drug-safety-and-availability/fda-drug-safety-communication-fda-requires-label-changes-warn-rare-serious-neurologic-problems-after#:~:text=%5B04%2D23%2D2014%5D,stroke%2C%20paralysis%2C%20and%20death.

Usunier, K., Hynes, M., Schuster, J. M., Cornelio-Jin Suen, A., Sadi, J., & Walton, D. (2018). Clinical Diagnostic Tests versus Medial Branch Blocks for Adults with Persisting Cervical Zygapophyseal Joint Pain: A Systematic Review and Meta-Analysis. *Physiotherapy Canada, 70*(2), 179–187.

Veizi, E., & Hayek, S. M. (2015). Spinal Cord Stimulation: Implantation Techniques. In S. Diwan, & P. S. Staats (Eds.), *Atlas of Pain Medicine Procedures*. New York, NY: McGraw-Hill.

Veizi, E., Tornero-Bold, M., & Hayek, S. M. (2016a). Resolution of intrathecal hydromorphone or morphine-induced peripheral edema by opioid rotation to fentanyl: a case series. *Pain Practice, 16*(6), E94–E98.

Veizi, I. E., Hayek, S. M., Hanes, M., Galica, R., Katta, S., & Yaksh, T. (2016b). Primary hydromorphone-related intrathecal catheter tip granulomas: is there a role for dose and concentration? *Neuromodulation: Technology at the Neural Interface, 19*(7), 760–769.

Verrills, P., Sinclair, C., & Barnard, A. (2016). A review of spinal cord stimulation systems for chronic pain. *Journal of Pain Research, 9*, 481–492.

Vialle, E., Vialle, L. R., Contreras, W., & Junior, C. J. (2015). Anatomical study on the relationship between the dorsal root ganglion and the intervertebral disc in the lumbar spine. *Revista Brasileira de Ortopedia (English Edition), 50*(4), 450–454.

Vrooman, B. M., & Rosenquist, R. W. (2018). Chronic Pain Management. In J. F. Butterworth IV, D. C. Mackey, & J. D. Wasnick (Eds.), *Morgan & Mikhail's Clinical Anesthesiology (6th Ed.)*. New York, NY: McGraw-Hill.

Wallace, A. N., Greenwood, T. J., & Jennings, J. W. (2015). Radiofrequency ablation and vertebral augmentation for palliation of painful spinal metastases. *Journal of Neuro-Oncology, 124*(1), 111–118.

Wallace, A. N., Tomasian, A., Vaswani, D., Vyhmeister, R., Chang, R. O., & Jennings, J. W. (2016). Radiographic local control of spinal metastases with percutaneous radiofrequency ablation and vertebral augmentation. *American Journal of Neuroradiology, 37*(4), 759–765.

Walsh, K. M., Machado, A. G., & Krishnaney, A. A. (2015). Spinal cord stimulation: a review of the safety literature and proposal for perioperative evaluation and management. *The Spine Journal, 15*(8), 1864–1869.

Wang, D. (2018). Image guidance technologies for interventional pain procedures: ultrasound, fluoroscopy, and CT. *Current Pain and Headache Reports, 22*(1), 6.

Wang, H., Sribastav, S. S., Ye, F., Yang, C., Wang, J., Liu, H., & Zheng, Z. (2015). Comparison of percutaneous vertebroplasty and balloon kyphoplasty for the treatment of single level vertebral compression fractures: A meta-analysis of the literature. *Pain Physician, 18*(3), 209–222.

Wang, J. K., Nauss, L. A., & Thomas, J. E. (1979). Pain relief by intrathecally applied morphine in man. *Survey of Anesthesiology, 23*(6), 384.

Webster, L. R. (2015). The relationship between the mechanisms of action and safety profiles of intrathecal morphine and ziconotide: A review of the literature. *Pain Medicine, 16*(7), 1265–1277.

Xie, Y., Szeto, G., & Dai, J. (2017). Prevalence and risk factors associated with musculoskeletal complaints among users of mobile handheld devices: A systematic review. *Applied Ergonomics, 59*, 132–142.

Yaltirik, K., Ashour, A. M., Reis, C. R., Özdoğan, S., & Atalay, B. (2016). Vertebral augmentation by kyphoplasty and vertebroplasty: 8 years experience outcomes and complications. *Journal of Craniovertebral Junction & Spine, 7*(3), 153.

Yang, E. Z., Xu, J. G., Huang, G. Z., Xiao, W. Z., Liu, X. K., Zeng, B. F., & Lian, X. F. (2016). Percutaneous Vertebroplasty Versus Conservative Treatment in Aged Patients With Acute Osteoporotic Vertebral Compression Fractures: A Prospective Randomized Controlled Clinical Study. *Spine, 41*(8), 653.

Zannou, A. L., Khadka, N., Truong, D. Q., Zhang, T., Esteller, R., Hershey, B., & Bikson, M. (2019). Temperature increases by kilohertz frequency spinal cord stimulation. *Brain Stimulation, 12*(1), 62–72.

Zhang, H., Xu, C., Zhang, T., Gao, Z., & Zhang, T. (2017). Does percutaneous vertebroplasty or balloon kyphoplasty for osteoporotic vertebral compression fractures increase the incidence of new vertebral fractures? A meta-analysis. *Pain Physician, 20*(1), E13–E28.

Zhang, X., Shi, H., Zhou, J., Xu, Y., Pu, S., Lv, Y., ... Du, D. (2019). The effectiveness of ultrasound-guided cervical transforaminal epidural steroid injections in cervical radiculopathy: a prospective pilot study. *Journal of Pain Research, 12*, 171.

Chapter 20 Exercise and Movement

Ann Quinlan-Colwell

CHAPTER OUTLINE

Fear of Pain With Movement, pg. 561

    Fear of Pain, pg. 561

    Fear-Avoidance Model, pg. 561

    Assessment of Fear of Pain With Movement, pg. 562

    Treatment of Fear of Pain With Movement, pg. 563

Exercise-Induced Hypoalgesia, pg. 564

Movement, pg. 564

    Movement When Recovering With Acute Pain, pg. 565

    Paleo Movement, pg. 565

    Movement With Chronic Pain, pg. 565

    The Feldenkrais Method, pg. 565

Dance Movement Therapy, pg. 565

    Connection Dance, pg. 566

    Biodanza, pg. 566

Exercise, pg. 566

    Isometric Exercise, pg. 566

    Pilates Exercise, pg. 567

    Land Aerobic Exercise, pg. 568

    Aquatic Exercise, pg. 568

    Strengthening Exercises, pg. 569

    Goldfish Exercise, pg. 569

Tai Chi, pg. 569

Yoga, pg. 570

Physical Therapy, pg. 571

    Therapeutic Exercise, pg. 572

    Mechanical Modalities, pg. 573

    Passive Therapies, pg. 573

    Electrotherapeutic Modalities, pg. 574

Patient Education for All Exercise and Movement, pg. 576

Key Points, pg. 576

Case Scenario, pg. 576

References, pg. 578

THE hazards of not moving are frequently seen among people who live with chronic low back pain (CLBP), which is thought to have a lifetime prevalence rate of up to 80%, with as many as 20% of those individuals experiencing permanently reduced activity (Mostagi, et al., 2015; Patrick, Ermanski, & Knaub, 2014). Reduction in activity is particularly concerning because movement and exercise are critically important to overall good health (Chaput, Carson, Gray, & Tremblay, 2014). Having a sedentary lifestyle can either contribute to or exacerbate pain and increase the risk for reinjury or sustaining a new injury.

In addition to improving activity and function, exercise has a specific analgesic benefit. *Exercise-induced hypoalgesia (EIH)* provides a type of endogenous modulation of pain (Koltyn, Brellenthin, Cook, Sehgal, & Hillard, 2014). (See Chapter 3 for detailed discussion of pain modulation.) Exercise can be effective as an intervention both in preventing pain (e.g., aerobic exercise to prevent migraine headaches) and as part of a multimodal plan in treating pain (e.g., neck and shoulder exercises to treat tension headaches) (Daenen, Varkey, Kellmann & Nijs, 2015). Unfortunately, fear of moving or being active is a barrier for many people living with chronic pain. That fear of moving with the resulting avoidance of activity are correlated with impaired function, greater chronicity, and compensatory changes in lifestyle, such as reducing or eliminating enjoyable activities and potentially increased pain (Dawson, Schlutter, Hodges, Stewart, & Turner, 2011; Hanney, Kolber, & Beekhuizen, 2009).

This chapter will explore the fear of movement and how it is related to pain and effective pain management, the positive analgesic effects of exercise, EIH, and a variety of activities that can be used by people living with chronic pain. Specifically, movement, exercise, tai chi, yoga, dance, and physical therapy used as therapies within a multimodal approach to alleviate or treat a variety of painful conditions will be discussed. Although these activities are presented individually, they often can be combined with the person using more than one activity at any given time period. Determining if it is appropriate to participate in and to combine activities needs to be discussed with the clinician coordinating pain management for the person and the various movement instructors. Before beginning any movement or exercise program, it is important for the person living with pain to discuss the proposed activity or activities with a clinician, who needs to assess the ability of the person, consider the safety of the activity for the individual, and address any modifications of the activity that may be necessary for the individual.

At least initial instruction for each of the techniques should be done by an expert in the therapy; thus the reader is advised to identify local qualified instructors. When attending classes or groups is not feasible because of financial, location, or transportation barriers, many of the interventions can be accessed through electronic format such as the internet and smartphones. Although the electronic venue is a good option for many people who have barriers that prohibit in-person classes, there is a caution with doing so. When no instructor observes the person, there is no opportunity for feedback or correction regarding form or activity. Poor form or incorrectly performing exercises could lead to further injury. For that reason, it is prudent to encourage patients to receive initial instruction with at least periodic in-person follow-up with an experienced instructor.

Fear of Pain With Movement

Fear of Pain

Fear of pain is related to the survival attribute of withdrawing from and avoiding the unconditioned stimulus of pain; however, rather than just being the reflex of withdrawing from a painful stimulus, sometimes deeper fear develops and results in avoiding movements or activities that potentially will cause pain (Meulders, Karsdorp, Claes, & Vlaeyen, 2015). One theory for fear of pain is that people who perceive pain as very threatening develop fear of movements that they think will increase pain or cause additional injury (Biggs, Meulders, & Vlaeyen, 2016). Another layer of the fear of movement is *perceptual pain–related fear generalization,* which occurs when fear of pain is extended to subsequent movements that are different from but are perceived by the person as being similar to the original movement that caused pain (Meulders, Vandael, & Vlaeyen, 2017). This can be maladaptive and counterproductive if it results in the person unnecessarily avoiding additional movements and activities, resulting in a cycle of disuse and maladaptive behaviors that results in continuation with possible intensification of pain (Dawson et al., 2011). A second cycle can develop as the cycle of fear of pain leads to limiting activity that then leads to weight gain that leads to less activity and more weight gain (Amy & Kozak, 2012; Arranz, 2017).

Fear-Avoidance Model

The fear-avoidance model (Fig. 20.1) provides a framework for understanding the relationships between fear of pain, further disability, and developing chronic pain (Lethem, Slade, Troup, & Bentley, 1983). The model suggests that a cycle starts with a fear of pain, which can be addressed in one of two ways. It is important to understand the person does not choose one way versus the other and it is not known specifically what leads to one path versus the other. Through a desire to return to normal activities, the pain can be met with effective interventions resulting in a positive restoration of activity. Alternatively, the fear of pain can be met with avoidance, which can evolve into increased fear and a debilitating spiral of physical limitations and amplifying the perception of pain or catastrophizing, which is "an exaggerated negative mental set about real or anticipated pain and is often considered a precursor to pain-related fear of movement" (Combs & Thorn, 2015, p. 161). With avoidance comes negative imaging, which leads to further fear of moving, then avoiding activities, which leads to disuse and more pain. This all reinforces the initial negative feelings about pain (Lethem et al., 1983; Werti, 2014). There is more discussion of this in Chapter 22.

The authors of a large systematic review of patients with CLBP reported within 6 months of injury fear of pain and fear of the possibility of injury can complicate and delay recovery (Werti et al., 2014). In a prospective cohort study, Archer, Seebach, Mathis, Riley, and Wegener (2014) described a group of patients (n = 120) after spinal surgery who feared movement 6 weeks postoperatively. In that study, the participants who reported increased intensity of pain had greater pain interference and disability and poorer physical health in general at 6 months follow-up. These findings indicate a need for early identification of patients at risk and for intervention to optimize activity, recovery, and function. This is consistent with a large meta-analysis (n = 118 studies) that reported a positive association between greater fear avoidance and higher pain intensity reports, meaning that people who had more fear or pain with more avoidance of activities that could potentially be painful, also perceived pain with greater intensity (Kroska, 2016). The authors of another large meta-analysis (n = 46 studies) reported a strong positive relationship between disability and pain-related fear (Zale, Lange, Fields, & Ditre, 2013). Unfortunately, this fear of moving may cause people to be reluctant to participate in therapies that involve physical movement (Combs & Thorn, 2015). This was demonstrated by Combs and Thorn, who conducted an interesting study with people with CLBP investigating the relationships among attitudes about yoga, kinesiophobia, and pain catastrophizing. They reported that fear of movement and pain catastrophizing were strongly correlated with negative attitudes about yoga and about willingness to try it to improve pain, function, and quality of life. When the fear of movement or activity occurs, it is unfortunate because physical movement can be supportive of rehabilitation and ease

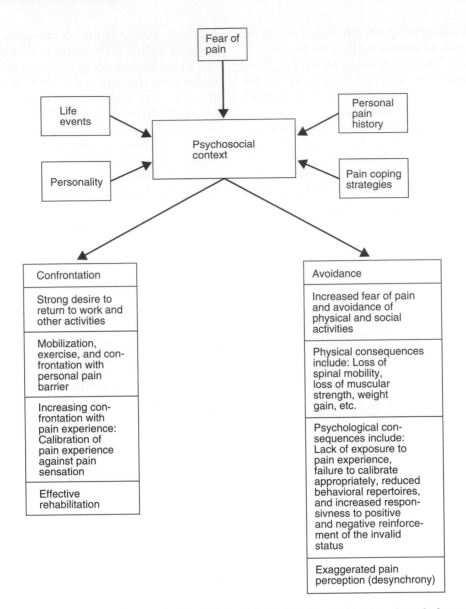

Fig. 20.1 | **Fear Avoidance Model.** (From Lethem, J., Slade, P. D., Troup, J. D. G., & Bentley, G. [1983]. Outline of a fear-avoidance model of exaggerated pain perception—1. *Behavior Research Therapy*, 21[4], 401–408.)

pain. (See Chapters 8 and 22 for more discussion of the fear avoidance.)

Movement and exercise instructors can be instrumental in educating and supporting people who are fearful. The importance of education and support can be seen in the example of a young man who is referred for yoga to help manage back pain. He may be reluctant to try yoga. However, if after basic introductions and education about yoga, the yoga instructor asks him if he has any reservations, it may encourage him to share concerns. Rather than just resisting exercise, he may be afraid he will lose his balance with some postures and look foolish or he may be afraid of falling and causing more pain. The instructor can not only alleviate his concerns but tailor postures to address his needs and concerns.

Assessment of Fear of Pain With Movement

The *Tampa Scale for Kinesiophobia (TSK)* is a tool designed to measure fear of movement. It consists of 17 items that are rated on a 4-point Likert scale ranging from strongly agree to strongly disagree, with scores ranging between 17 and 68. It is validated in a number of different countries to assess fear of movement in people with CLBP, upper extremity pain, fibromyalgia syndrome (FMS), and osteoarthritis (OA) (Archer et al., 2014; Roelofs et al., 2011). The *TSK-11* (Fig. 20.2) is a shorter version with 11 of the original 17 questions that was also determined to be valid and reliable (Perry & Francis, 2013; Tkachuk & Harris, 2012; Woby, Roach, Urmston, & Watson, 2005). Although it is generally used as a baseline evaluation

Tampa Scale-11 (TSK-11)   Name: _____   Date: _____

This is a list of phrases that other patients have used to express how they view their condition. Please circle the number that best describes how you feel about each statement.

	Strongly Disagree	Somewhat Disagree	Somewhat Agree	Strongly Agree
1. I'm afraid I might injure myself if I exercise.	1	2	3	4
2. If I were to try to overcome it, my pain would increase.	1	2	3	4
3. My body is telling me I have something dangerously wrong.	1	2	3	4
4. People aren't taking my medical condition seriously enough.	1	2	3	4
5. My accident/problem has put my body at risk for the rest of my life.	1	2	3	4
6. Pain always means I have injured my body.	1	2	3	4
7. Simply being careful that I do not make any unnecessary movements is the safest thing I can do to prevent my pain from worsening.	1	2	3	4
8. I wouldn't have this much pain if there wasn't something potentially dangerous going on in my body.	1	2	3	4
9. Pain lets me know when to stop exercising so that I don't injure myself.	1	2	3	4
10. I can't do all the things normal people do because it's too easy for me to get injured.	1	2	3	4
11. No one should have to exercise when he/she is in pain.	1	2	3	4

Fig. 20.2 | TSK- 11: A Shortened Version of the Tampa Scale for Kinesiophobia. (From Woby, S. R., Roach, N. K., Urmston, M., & Watson, P. J. [2005]. Psychometric properties of the TSK- 11: A shortened version of the Tampa Scale for Kinesiophobia. *Pain, 117*[1–2], 137–144.)

before starting an exercise or movement program, it also can be used for reassessment before modifying a movement or exercise program.

Treatment of Fear of Pain With Movement

Treatment or interventions for fear of pain most frequently involve cognitive-behavioral techniques (Meulders et al., 2015). This often has been approached through sensitization techniques that involve altering how pain is experienced as a way to modify perception of the noxious stimuli (Guck, Burke, Rainville, Hill-Taylor, & Wallace, 2015; Lederman, 2014). One technique is to work with the person to alter personal memories of pain and painful activities and then exposing the person to these or similar activities in a very safe environment (Nijs, Girbés, Lundberg, Malfliet, & Sterling, 2015). A recent feasibility study assessed the benefit of using motion-capture software, avatars, and virtual technologies among patients with CLBP with fear of movement (Springer, George, & Robinson, 2016). The researchers of that study concluded that technology could be used for desensitization of movement and fear of pain by arranging individual video clips in a hierarchical manner from most anxiety-producing activities to least anxiety-producing activities. (See Chapter 22 for additional discussion of desensitization and exposure.)

Self-efficacy and expectations for recovery are correlated with less fear of movement and positive outcomes. Self-efficacy is the confidence the person has regarding ability to accomplish a certain activity to achieve a desired outcome (Carriere, Thibault, Milioto, & Sullivan, 2015; Costa, Maher, McAuley, & Hancock, 2011). Perry and Francis (2013) reported self-efficacy was correlated with less pain catastrophizing and less negative pain behaviors but did not mediate fear of movement related to pain. However, Costa et al. (2011) found self-efficacy was a stronger mediator than fear of movement as an influencing factor among people with CLBP developing or not developing pain and disability. Another study from Canada assessed fear of movement among people with whiplash injuries and reported patients who had expectations of returning to work had less fear of movement and were more successful than those who did not expect to return to work (Carriere et al., 2015). In other studies, it was found that inducing a positive attitude and learning safety measures among participants were effective in attenuating pain related to fear of movement (Geschwind, Meulders, Peters, Vlaeyen, & Meulders, 2015; Meulders, Meulders, & Vlaeyen, 2014). Interestingly, the authors of a more recent study reported that among study participants, even when positive cues were associated with rewards, negative cues associated with fear of pain were so strong that the negative cues possibly reduced the positive effect achieved through positive cues for moving (Claes, Vlaeyen, & Crombez, 2016).

Mirror therapy (see Chapter 27) has been reported to be effective in reducing fear of pain (Louw et al., 2017). Recent studies have also reported overcoming fear of pain with activity programs, including isometric exercise (Smith et al., 2017), Pilates exercise (Cruz-Díaz, Bergamin, Gobbo, Martínez-Amat, & Hita-Conreras, 2017; Oksuz & Unal, 2017), stretching in water (Keane, 2017), and while using interactive activity games (Voon et al., 2016). A commonality among these interventions is that generally they are not perceived as activities associated with painful movements and generally they are not expected to cause pain. The results of these studies are consistent with the important role of expectation in the experiences of fear of pain and fear avoidance. It is important to help people manage fear of exercise, not only to help control pain but also to improve function and quality of life.

Exercise-Induced Hypoalgesia

EIH is a type of endogenous modulation of pain resulting from exercise that manifests in a reduction in pain sensitivity and increases in pain threshold and pain tolerance (Koltyn et al., 2014). The classic explanation of EIH is that it is the result of the effect of endorphins that are released as a consequence of exercise activating the central opioid system (Thoren, Floras, Hoffman, & Seals, 1990). More recently, there is support for the involvement of nonopioid factors in EIH. Previously, much of the research regarding nonopioid factors involved with EIH was done in rats (Galidinao et al., 2014). Recent research has shown activity of the intricate neuromodulatory endocannabinoid system alone and in combination with endorphins contributes to EIH in humans (Crombie, Brellenthin, Hillard, & Koltyn, 2017; Koltyn et al., 2014). Interestingly, research to date indicates that EIH is reported with patellar tendinopathy (Rio et al., 2015), OA, rheumatoid arthritis (RA) (Koltyn et al., 2014), and heat-induced pain (Brellenthin, Cook, Sehgal, & Koltyn, 2012) but not with the neuropathic pain conditions such as FMS or diabetic neuropathies (Knauf & Koltyn, 2014; Koltyn et al., 2014).

At least in chronic arthritic pain conditions, the absence of EIH is another undesirable component of the cycle that occurs when activity is limited by pain. In addition to the physiologic process involved in EIH, recent research indicates that EIH is also affected by psychosocial factors, including mood and positive environments (Brellenthin, Crombie, Cook, Sehgal, & Koltyn, 2016) as well as age and gender (Naugle, Naugle, & Riley, 2016; Naugle, Naugle, Fillingim, & Riley, 2014). Younger adults, both males and females, tend to achieve greater EIH compared to older adults (Naugle et al., 2016).

Movement

Movement is individually experienced by all people with various abilities and ranges. When movement is not optimal, symptoms such as pain can develop, increasing and limiting activities and quality of life (Comerford & Mottram, 2012). In contrast, good movement is finding ways to best move in an efficient manner (McNeil & Blandford, 2015) while avoiding undesirable symptoms. McNeil and Blandford described movement health from the perspective of a wellness model as "a desired state that is not only injury free and absent of the presence of uncontrolled movement but also a state that allows the exerciser to choose how to move" (McNeil & Blandford, 2015, p. 151). Blandford (2014a, b) recommends *awareness, control, intensity,* and *variability* as necessary to achieve and maintain good movement health:

- Be *aware* of body, how the body moves/functions, and the quality of body movement.
- Have *control* over what he calls the *software* of the central nervous system and the *hardware* of the musculoskeletal system.
- Use different and appropriate *intensity* for different tasks required (e.g., maintaining good posture requires low intensity; strength conditioning requires high intensity).
- Employ *variability* using a variety of approaches for any given movement.

Movement When Recovering With Acute Pain

When patients are recovering from an acute pain experience, it is important for them to move as often and as much as possible consistent with clinician advice. Education about the most effective way to move using good body mechanics and the short-term use of prescribed assistive devices are important aspects of postoperative care and recovery. Physical therapy may be a necessary and important component in this process of moving to prevent dis-use and complications of inactivity. It is also important to pace activities with rest. (See Chapter 22 for discussion of pacing activities with rest.)

Paleo Movement

Current education about movement health is very timely. In mid-2016 *The Lancet* published a second series of articles identifying the risks of sedentary behavior (Ekelund et al., 2016). Bowman (2014) described how from birth there are differences in the way people moved when humans were members of a hunter and gatherer society compared with the way people move in Western societies today. She purports that the appliances and devices of modern Western society have severely curtailed not only activity (i.e., exercise) but also movement. She encourages *paleo movement* or a *movement-rich* life that includes interrupting sitting with a variety of small tasks and movement breaks (McNeil, 2017).

Setting goals of increasing activities with short periods of activity that are consistent with the expectations of the person throughout the day often facilitates greater adherence with the plan of activity and reaching goals. Once initial goals are achieved they can be stretched to include longer duration, increased frequency, or greater effort. These can include planning activities by keeping the remote control in a room different from where the television is located, storing root vegetables in the garage or cellar, selecting distant parking places, biking or walking rather than driving a vehicle, climbing stairs rather than riding an elevator, and having walking meetings rather than sitting meetings. Although these activities are primarily designed to promote good health and prevent complications of sedentary lifestyle, the concepts can be used to help people with pain increase movement and improve their lifestyle as well.

Movement With Chronic Pain

For people with chronic pain to incorporate more movement will likely require time, education, encouragement, and taking small steps. There are at least three reasons taking small steps is important. First, the small steps, or even baby steps, are less likely to cause a significant increase in pain. Second, taking small steps will not be overwhelming to the person physically or psychologically. Third, small steps for short periods can be a reasonable expectation and can be easily incorporated into daily life and then built upon. The steps can be increased to include more movement done for a longer period and done more frequently. Using this method incorporates the activity into daily life with continual positive reenforcement of achieving goals (i.e., "I was able to do more today than yesterday") with improvement in self-efficacy.

The author has used this method with patients for years with positive results. One woman started by walking on a treadmill at 1/2 mile per hour for 5 minutes per day. She increased it by 1 minute per week and gradually increased the speed. At the end of 1 year she was walking on the treadmill for nearly 1 hour per day at 3 miles per hour. She had lost nearly 100 lb and had minimized the discomfort from her chronic back pain.

The Feldenkrais Method

The *Feldenkrais method (FM)* has been used worldwide for many years to educate people about movement. This is accomplished through development of sensory motor and cognitive awareness of how the body moves, and how it is moving at any given time. To achieve that, Feldenkrais developed the *awareness through movement (ATM)* technique, which involves several lessons in which structured movements are taught (Henry, Paungmali, Mohan, & Ramli, 2016). Through FM education, patients with chronic pain are taught to be aware of the different parts of their bodies through the sensory proprioceptors in muscles and joints *(kinesthetic awareness)* and the relationship of those body parts to other parts of the body *(proprioception)* (Wu, Meleger, Witkower, Mondale, & Borg-Stein, 2015). The FM is reported to be effective among people with chronic musculoskeletal, neck, scapular, and back pain (Mohan, Paungmali, Sitilertpisan, Henry, & Mohamad, 2017; Wu et al., 2015). It also is used to improve function (Wu et al., 2015) and balance (Mohan et al., 2017). The authors of a recent systematic review concluded that FM is effective in controlling neck and back pain, but that better designed research is needed to further explore benefit (Mohan et al., 2017).

Dance Movement Therapy

Dance movement therapy (DMT) is classified within the creative arts therapy field and is defined as "the psychotherapeutic use of movement and dance to support intellectual, emotional, and motor functions of the body. As a modality of the creative arts therapies, DMT looks at the correlation between movement and emotion" (American Dance Therapy Association [ADTA], ND). At least part of the benefit of DMT is due to the release of endorphins, which help reduce pain (Stringer, 2015). Dance movement therapists are prepared at the master's or doctoral level of education (ADTA, ND). As members of a multidisciplinary care team, they assess patients and create plans for intervention using DMT (Welling, 2015). Although DMT is most often associated with behavioral health issues, including anxiety and depression, it is also used as a therapeutic intervention to help people living with Parkinson's disease, cancer, multiple sclerosis, FMS, and other conditions characterized with chronic pain (Bräuninger, 2014; Shanahan, Morris, Bhriain, Saunders, & Clifford, 2015; Welling, 2015). Applying ballroom dance techniques, DMT has been used successfully in therapy to resume movement, increase function, and reduce pain after hand trauma (Tartaglia, 2014).

Shim et al. (2017) conducted a group DMT study (n = 22) to assess the effect of a 10-week DMT group program on resilience-building in people living with chronic pain with pain intensity scores of 4 or greater on a scale of 0 to 10. Participants were adults living in inner-city Philadelphia. The results were significant for improvements in resilience and reduction in kinesiophobia and pain intensity. Equally as impressive as the statistical results were the participant comments of feeling more alive and wanting to be more active. These results may be due to the participants enjoying the activity, which can be an important factor for increasing participation.

In a small feasibility study (n = 31) involving older adults with OA, half participated in 12 weeks of dance-based therapy while continuing regular exercise and the second half only continued regular exercise. Although the results were not statistically significant, they were promising. Participants in the dance therapy group reported somewhat less pain, needing to take less pain medicine, and having greater gait speed with activity compared to their nondancing counterparts (Krampe et al., 2014). Although these studies consisted of small samples, they are encouraging and supportive of DMT as a potentially enjoyable intervention to improve mobility, balance, physical strength, and pain control in patients living with chronic pain. Additional research is needed with larger samples and rigorous methodology.

Connection Dance

Connection dance is a choreographed series of movements based on the movement principles of Bartenieff, who proposed that there are rudimentary coordination patterns within the human body (Shim, 2015). Bartenieff, whose work was based on the teachings of the choreographer and philosopher Rudolf Laban, identified the differences among active, passive, and neutral body weight (Bartenieff, 2002). Active body weight resists gravity, whereas passive body weight does not. In comparison, neutral body weight is when the body is supported by muscles (deTord & Bräuninger, 2015). Connection dance has been used effectively with patients living with chronic pain (Shim et al., 2017). People living with chronic pain who participated in a research study reported that connection dance helped them better manage their pain, feel

in control of their pain, comfort themselves, and have fun (Shim, 2015).

Biodanza

Biodanza is a particular type of DMT. It is described as "a therapeutic strategy that combines music, movement, and emotions to induce integrative living experience or *vivencias* (vivid, intensely felt moment in the 'here and now') in group participants" (Segura-Jiménez et al., 2017, p. 319). In one small study involving 27 women with FMS, participants reported their acute pain was reduced and the reduction was sustained after the Biodanza sessions. Improvement in pain control was greatest among women who had higher pain intensity before the intervention, and women who reported greater satisfaction with the program also had better acute pain control (Segura-Jiménez et al., 2017). Again, research is warranted to further investigate the benefit of Biodanza as part of a multimodal approach to pain management.

Exercise

Exercise is often limited or totally avoided by people living with pain, but the opposite is advised by professional organizations, including the American Geriatric Society and the American College of Sports Medicine (Laubenstein & Beissner, 2016). In addition, the American Physical Therapy Association (APTA) has a campaign, *#ChoosePT Opioid Awareness Campaign,* that encourages activity and exercise as part of a multimodal approach of pain management (APTA, 2019). Exercise leads to greater muscular strength and improved balance. Thus, exercise can be effective in helping people with chronic pain function more effectively and more safely while helping to control pain. A large meta-analysis of studies involving more than 4000 participants concluded that exercise is beneficial for helping to control pain in people with knee OA (Juhl, Christensen, Roos, Zhang, & Lund, 2014). The authors of that meta-analysis advised that it is more beneficial to identify one type of exercise (e.g., aerobic or strength training) done three times per week under supervision with focus on achieving benefits from it rather than mixing different types of exercise (e.g., aerobic and strength training) (Juhl et al., 2014). This focused approach facilitates a manageable program that is not overwhelming to patients who are working to control pain and improve function. There are a variety of exercises from which the person living with pain can choose.

Isometric Exercise

Isometric exercises consist of a static contraction during which the muscle length and joint position remain unchanged (Anwer & Alghadir, 2014; Koltyn et al., 2014). Isometric exercises have been predominantly associated with EIH, with analgesia occurring in as little as 3 minutes of isometric activity as seen in people with neck pain from whiplash injury doing wall squat exercises and quickly reducing pain, but those in a control group with 30 minutes of aerobic bicycling did not reduce pain (Smith et al., 2017; Vaegter, 2017). This is an interesting phenomenon, particularly because the hypoalgesia occurred in an area of the body with chronic pain (neck), but the isometric exercise involved a distant area of the body (legs) (Smith et al., 2017). In an Egyptian study, isometric exercise was taught to women (n = 90) with OA, who reported benefits of reduction in stiffness and improvement in physical ability (Sorour, Ayoub, & Abd El Aziz, 2014). A similar study with people with knee OA in India reported improvement in muscle function and decreases in disability and pain after a 5-week isometric quadricep exercise program (Anwer & Alghadir, 2014). Finally, in a small study (n = 36), isometric exercise was used to maintain muscle strength for older adults who had injured an extremity (Safa'ah & Srimurayani, 2017). Rio et al. (2015) suggested that isometric exercise may be useful at the beginning of a rehabilitation exercise program for people with painful tendon conditions. Isometric exercises also have the benefit of being able to be done in a variety of positions (standing, sitting, lying).

As with all movement and exercise programs, each participant needs to be evaluated by a clinician and approved for the activity. Traditionally, isometric exercises are considered contraindicated in people with cardiac artery disease and those participating in cardiac rehabilitation because of the potential for dramatic increase in blood pressure resulting in myocardial injury (Lin et al., 2012). Isometric exercises are also considered contraindicated for patients with Marfan's syndrome, in others who have aortopathy or aortic root dilatation (Chaddha et al., 2015), and in patients with chronic aortic dissection (Bossone, Ferrara, & Citro, 2015). The effect of a sustained isometric muscle contraction was compared in women with FMS and those without FMS. The women with FMS had increased muscle pain with isometric contractions and less physical activity (Umeda et al., 2015). Considering those results, women with FMS may need to avoid isometric exercises or use them with caution, starting very slowly and assessing the effect.

Pilates Exercise

Pilates is an exercise method performed either on a mat or with a special apparatus with the intention of improving muscle control, movement, strength, and flexibility, based on principles of "centering, concentration, control, precision, breath, and flow" (Wells, Kolt, & Bialocerkoski, 2012, p. 254) (Table 20.1). In a recent study comparing people with CLBP who used floor mats or apparatus-facilitated Pilates, those using the apparatus seemed to progress faster, but both groups had reduced pain, less functional impairment, and less kinesiophobia with the exercises (Cruz-Díaz et al., 2017). In another study in which people doing floor mat Pilates

Table 20.1 | Traditional Pilates Principles

Traditional Principle	Definition
1. Centering	Tightening of the muscular center of the body or "powerhouse," located between the pelvic floor and the ribcage during exercises
2. Concentration	Cognitive attention required to perform exercise
3. Control	Close management of posture and movement during exercise
4. Precision	Accuracy of exercise technique
5. Flow	Smooth transition of movements within the exercise sequence
6. Breathing	Moving air into and out of lungs in coordination with exercise

From Wells, C., Kolt, G. S., & Bialocerkoski, A. (2012). Defining Pilates exercise: A systematic review. *Complementary Therapies in Medicine*, 20(4), 253–262.

exercises were compared with those using equipment-based exercise, it was found that the participants using the floor mats reported less pain and may have had more increase in amplitude of muscle (de Oliveira et al., 2017).

Pilates also has been used effectively to reduce pain and increase function in patients with shoulder pain (Atilgan et al., 2017). After a 14-week Pilates program, researchers reported improvement in pain control and balance among the participants (n = 13) compared to the control group (n = 11) (Patti et al., 2016). In another study, in which women with osteoporosis (n = 60) participated, half of the participants were randomized to a Pilates group and half to a home exercise group (Küçükçakır, Altan, & Korkmaz, 2013). The women in the Pilates group reported improvement in function with less pain intensity. In one systematic review, Pilates was reported as superior to other exercise for people living with CLBP (Wells, Kolt, Marshall, Hill, & Bialocerkowski, 2014). However, in other studies, when Pilates was compared to generic types of exercise, the results were contradictory among studies regarding which was superior with regard to flexibility and function among people living with chronic pain, but the consensus was that Pilates was at least as effective as others in helping to manage pain (Marshall, Kennedy, Brooks, & Lonsdale, 2013; Mostagi et al., 2015).

Similarly, the authors of a Cochrane review concluded there was insufficient evidence to determine superiority of Pilates versus other exercise and that determinations about what exercise type is best for a person needs to be based on individual patient factors (Yamato et al., 2015). One factor that may be important to consider is kinesiophobia (Cruz-Díaz et al., 2017). In a recent small study of patients with osteoporosis (n = 40), the researchers concluded Pilates was effective in improving function while reducing both pain and kinesiophobia (Oksuz & Unal, 2017). A related benefit of Pilates is that in addition to pain control it has been correlated with reductions in fear of falling and fall prevention (Küçükçakır et al., 2013) in older adults with CLBP (Cruz-Díaz et al., 2015). Similar results were found among a sample (n = 39) of community-dwelling older adults with no specific endorsement of location of pain (Josephs, Pratt, Meadows, Thurmond, & Wagner, 2016).

Land Aerobic Exercise

Land aerobic exercise can be undertaken in a variety of ways. The most available and inexpensive, except for the cost of supportive footwear, is walking (Browne, Diersing, & Hilliard, 2017). It also is the aerobic exercise most frequently encouraged for older adults (Laubenstein & Beissner, 2016). In a review of research studies involving walking programs, despite significant differences in design, walking was noted to have a positive impact on older adults with complaints of pain (Laubenstein & Beissner, 2016). Compliance and pain control among one group of Irish adults living with CLBP (n = 246) was greater with a supervised walking program (n = 82) compared with fitness training exercise classes (n = 83) or with physical therapy (n = 81) (Hurley et al., 2015). The authors of a systematic review and meta-analysis of studies involving adults with chronic musculoskeletal pain who exercised by walking, compared to exercise other than walking and no exercise, found similar results (O'Connor, Tully, Ryan, Bleakley, & McDonough, 2015). The authors of that review concluded that when using the U.S. Preventive Services Task Force system, walking is an appropriate and beneficial exercise for people with chronic pain of a musculoskeletal nature. Information on the U.S. Preventive Services Task Force can be located at https://search.uspreventiveservicestaskforce.org. In a small study with people with OA of the knee, the researchers concluded walking several times for less than a 30-minute duration could be helpful but walking for 30 minutes or longer could have negative effects (Farrokhi et al., 2017).

As with all exercise programs, it is recommended that each patient be assessed by a clinician to determine if a walking program is an appropriate exercise for the individual and then follow up with any pain that seems to develop as a result of the walking program (Browne et al., 2017). High-intensity aerobic exercise is contraindicated for patients with comorbid aortopathy, aortic dilatation, or Marfan's syndrome (Chaddha et al., 2015).

Aquatic Exercise

Aquatic exercise consists of exercise done while the person is immersed in a water environment that is commonly within a temperature range of 32° to 36° C (Bartels et al., 2016). People with painful conditions often can participate in more strenuous exercise programs for longer duration when done in water because there is less joint loading (the amount of force on a weight bearing joint when active) with less joint pain (Roper, Bressel, & Tillman, 2013). When available, aquatic exercise is a positive option for people who cannot participate fully in land exercises or for whom land exercises are contraindicated because of the potential aggravation of pain or other reasons (Hale, Waters, & Henderson, 2012). Two additional benefits of water aerobics are that they do not stress joints the way land exercises do and there is less risk for falling, which may be a concern or fear of people with painful conditions (Hale et al., 2012). In one study (n = 29) using AquaStretch, which is a type of stretching the back in water, the researchers reported significant reductions in pain, kinesiophobia, and self-perception of disability compared to those doing a similar back stretch on land (Keane, 2017). Aquatic exercises are a good option for obese individuals who have pain and for whom land exercises are painful (Zdziarski, Wasser, & Vincent, 2015). The authors of a recent review of 16 studies (n = 1351 subjects) investigating various exercise programs with obese individuals with CLBP reported greatest adherence rates with aquatic and resistance exercises (Wasser, Vasilopoulos, Zdziarski, & Vincent, 2017).

A systematic review of randomized controlled trials (RCTs) of people with low back pain who participated in aquatic exercises reported the aquatic exercise was effective in reducing pain and improving function among the participants but was not necessarily better than land-based exercise (Olson, Kolber, Patel, Pabian, & Hanney, 2013). The authors of two meta-analyses concluded among people with musculoskeletal conditions, aquatic exercise was at least moderately helpful in reducing pain and improving function and quality of life (Barker et al., 2014; Waller et al., 2014). In a Cochrane review, people from 13 different trials with lower extremity OA who participated in aquatic exercise programs reported pain intensity scores reduced an average of 5 points with a range of 3 to 8 on a numeric scale of 0 to 100 (Bartels et al., 2016). Those who completed the program reported pain intensity of approximately 41 points and quality of life of approximately 57 compared with those who did not participate who rated pain an average of 46 points and quality of life 50 on the same scale of 0 to 100. Although those results are lower than what is often accepted as clinically meaningful, the authors of that review concluded there was moderate evidence to support aquatic exercise to reduce pain while increasing quality of life. A second Cochrane review evaluated 16 studies (n = 881 subjects) in which participants were people living with FMS who participated in water aerobic exercises (Bidonde et al., 2014). The authors of that review reported there were statistically significant reductions in stiffness and low to moderate evidence of improvement in other symptoms, including pain.

Two innovative types of water exercises involve aquatic treadmills (Lambert et al., 2015; Roper et al., 2013; Zdziarski et al., 2015) and aquatic cycles (Rewald et al., 2017). Aquatic treadmills are increasingly used to train and rehabilitate humans, dogs, and horses (Tranquille, Nankervis, Walker, Tacey, & Murray, 2016). Aquatic treadmills decrease the stress of impact on lower extremity structure and improve cardiovascular effort (Macdermid, Fink, & Stannard, 2015). When combined with resistance exercises, aquatic treadmill exercise reportedly helped with increasing skeletal muscle mass and strength (Lambert et al., 2015). A small study (n = 14) found that at least immediately after exercise people with OA of the knee had dramatically less pain (100% less) after using an aquatic treadmill compared to when the same participants used a land treadmill (Roper et al., 2013).

Aquatic cycling is a water exercise; about which there is little research, particularly regarding the effect on pain (Rewald et al., 2017). When participating in aquatic cycling, the person is underwater to the chest level with the water supporting the joints during cycling, which theoretically avoids pain during cycling (Rewald et al., 2017). However aquatic cycling was not found to reduce pain sensation in one study (Wahl et al., 2017). These interventions need further research to assess the potential benefit of EIH and possible benefit as vehicles for improving function and quality of life for people living with chronic pain. Box 20.1 presents the precautions and contraindications for aquatic therapy.

Strengthening Exercises

Strengthening exercises have not been used for pain control as much as other types of exercise, however there is some evidence that it may be beneficial and needs further research. One study with wheelchair-dependent participants (n = 16) who used videoconferencing to follow a 12-week home-based, telerehabilitation program to strengthen the muscles of their painful shoulders reported improvement in function and a reduction in pain (Van Straaten, Cloud, Morrow, Ludewig, & Zhao, 2014). Results of a meta-analysis of studies using strengthening and aerobic exercise with people awaiting hip and knee replacement surgeries showed that people awaiting hip but not knee surgery benefited from exercise programs by increasing function and decreasing pain (Gill & McBurney, 2013). As with all exercise types, additional studies are needed to assess the benefit of strengthening exercise among people living with chronic pain.

Goldfish Exercise

Goldfish exercise is a novel type of exercise developed in Japan for use by people living with oral submucous fibrosis (OSMF) and temporomandibular joint (TMJ) pain. It is based on the swimming movement of goldfish (Jain & Shukla, 2017). When it was used in a small RCT (n = 16) with people with OSMF, the benefits among those who used goldfish exercise (n = 8) had significant improvement ($P < .05$) in the ability to open their mouths and less TMJ-related disability compared to those who did not use the goldfish exercise (n = 8) (Jain & Shukla, 2017). Despite the benefits in function in that study there was no statistical difference in pain between the two groups. Because the groups were small, all results need to be considered from that perspective. Additional research is needed, with larger groups for longer duration, to evaluate the potential benefit regarding pain and function of goldfish exercise among people with TMJ with and without OSMF. It could potentially be an important component of a multimodal approach of pain management for people living with the pain of TMJ.

Tai Chi

Tai chi, or the traditional Chinese term *Tai Ji Quan*, is a component of traditional Chinese martial arts that in addition to self-defense is used for improving the mind and body and general well-being (Guo, Qiu, & Liu, 2014). It is a holistic modality that coordinates physical and mental relaxation using slow, gentle, intentional movements that at times are synchronized with breathing and sometimes imagery (Laubenstein & Beissner, 2016; Wayne et al., 2013; Zhang, 2012). The simplicity and the ability for tai chi to be practiced almost anywhere with no special equipment are advantages for using it (Field, 2016). In addition, a systematic review of 18 RCTs found tai chi to be associated only with minor aches and pains and no serious injuries or adverse events (Wayne, Berkowitz, Litrownick, Buring, & Yeh, 2014).

In a study (n = 503) of community-dwelling adults who were all older than 70 years, with no major medical disorders, knee pain worsened after tai chi (Day, Hill, Stathakis, Flicker, & Jolley, 2015). However, in another

---

Box 20.1	Precautions and Contraindications for Aquatic Therapy

- Fevers, infections, rashes
- Cardiac history
- Incontinence without protection
- Open wounds without appropriate dressings
- Fear of water
- Limited lung capacity
- Unstable cardiac condition

From Pagliarulo, M. (2012). *Introduction to physical therapy* (4th ed.). St. Louis: Mosby.

year-long study (n = 204) the researchers concluded that participants with knee OA who practiced tai chi had outcomes similar to those with standard physical therapy (Wang et al., 2015). The authors of a systematic review and meta-analysis with 5 RCTs (n = 252 subjects) concluded that tai chi was effective in reducing pain and stiffness and improving physical function (Lauche, Langhorst, Dobos, & Cramer, 2013). Similarly, in another systematic review and meta-analysis of 18 RCTs, tai chi was effective in reducing pain among participants with OA in approximately 5 weeks and was also effective in reducing pain with CLBP and osteoporosis (Kong et al., 2016). The rigorous Jadad scale scored results of a meta-analysis of 7 RCTs (n = 348 subjects) were statistically significant with pain intensity decreased and physical function increased among participants with OA who participate in tai chi (Yan et al., 2013).

An interesting study with older adults (n = 55) with knee OA and cognitive impairment assessed the benefit of a 20-week tai chi program. At the end of the study, participants in the tai chi group reported significantly lower pain by verbal descriptive scores, their video-taped pain behavior scores were lower, and there was a trend of lower analgesic need. Since the participants had cognitive impairment, this study is particularly interesting because the results are more likely related to the physiologic experience of tai chi rather than any cognitive or emotional response (Tsai et al., 2015).

Reports of pain reduction from studies using tai chi interventions with people with FMS are mixed (Kong, 2016). A 12-week intervention of tai chi compared with education for people with FMS was effective in statistically reducing pain intensity and pain interference and improved function/mobility (Jones et al., 2012). An Italian study using Tai Ji Quan with patients with FMS reported statistically significant improvement in widespread pain ($P < .01$) and pain per tender point scoring ($P < .001$) and improvement in sleep, activity, and mood (Bongi et al., 2016). Although tai chi is most often associated with community participation and chronic pain, it is used successfully as an intervention in at least one acute care hospital for patients recovering from illness and surgery (Erich & Quinlan-Colwell, 2017). The tai chi instructor in that setting modifies instructions for people who are only able to sit or remain in bed.

Additional research is needed to assess the benefit of tai chi for people living with a variety of chronic pain conditions. One challenge with comparing results of existing tai chi studies is that the study protocols are highly variable (Field, 2016; Laubenstein & Beissner, 2016). At times, the lack of strong research methodology has contributed to reluctance in recommending tai chi for health promotion and pain management (Harmer, 2014). Replication of a rigorous study protocol with different populations would help with comparing results and improving the base of evidence regarding the role of tai chi in managing pain.

Yoga

Yoga is a practice with ancient origins in Indian philosophy that combines spiritual and physical features (Goode et al., 2016). Yoga focuses on breathing techniques *(pranayama)*, physical movement or postures *(asana)*, meditation *(dyana)*, relaxation, and lifestyle adjustment (Cramer, Lauche, Haller, & Dobos, 2013). Although there are other forms of yoga (e.g., Dru, Iyengar, Viniyoga, Pranayama, integrated approach), the most commonly known form of yoga in Western countries is Hatha yoga, which is also among the most commonly practiced of all nonpharmacologic interventions (Cho, Moon, & Kim, 2015; Cramer, Lauche, Langhorst, & Dobos, 2016). Despite the popularity of Hatha yoga, some clinicians think that Viniyoga has a more therapeutic focus and thus could be more beneficial for managing chronic pain conditions (Hillinger, Wolever, McKernan, & Elam, 2017). However, a systematic review of the effect of various yoga styles on pain management showed no difference in effectiveness or benefit and the authors concluded that individual preference and accessibility can be the basis for selecting a type of yoga (Cramer et al., 2016).

Of the estimated 15 million adults in the United States who have used yoga at least once, it is estimated that 20% of them use it for managing CLBP (Cramer et al., 2013). In fact, much of the research involving yoga as an intervention for pain is with people living with CLBP, and reports indicate that it is effective relieving pain in people with moderate to severe CLBP (Stein, Weinberg, Sherman, Lemaster, & Saper, 2014). The results of a systematic review of six RCTs from three countries were supportive of yoga for people with CLBP with strong evidence for short-term benefit of pain relief and moderate-evidence for pain relief over longer periods with no association with any serious adverse effects (Cramer et al., 2013). Through evidence mapping, which "uses descriptive epidemiology to characterize information for a broad area of medicine and identify gaps in the research" (Goode et al., 2016, p. 171), yoga was found to be potentially beneficial for people with nonspecific CLBP of either short or long duration and is most likely reasonable when part of a multimodal treatment plan (Goode et al., 2016). It is suggested that the positive effects of yoga are the result of improved flexibility, improved coordination/strength, and decreases in stress and anxiety (Büssing, Ostermann, Lüdtke, & Michalsen, 2012).

Two studies yielded insight into possible physiologic reasons why yoga has analgesic benefit. Fourteen average-weight premenopausal women with CLBP who completed a 12-week Hatha yoga program reported improvement in pain related to physical functioning, which the investigators hypothesized may be related to the effect of yoga on inflammatory markers (Cho et al., 2015). In another 12-week yoga program with a similar sample in Korea, the women who participated in yoga reported statistically significant less pain by a visual analogue scale ($P < .001$) and improved back flexibility ($P < .01$) (Lee, Moon, & Kim, 2014). In that study the women who practiced yoga also demonstrated increased brain-derived neurotrophic factor (BDNF) ($P < .01$) compared to controls who had increased pain and a decrease in BDNF. The change and difference in BDNF is interesting because BDNF is thought to modulate nociception (see Chapter 3), which may provide insight into the physiologic mechanism through which yoga provides pain relief (Lee, Moon, & Kim, 2014).

When looking at demographic characteristics of people who used yoga to manage pain (n = 92) the participants were more likely to be generally healthy, well-educated women of a higher socioeconomic group (Stein et al., 2014). However, the authors of that review concluded that benefit to participants is not adversely affected by socioeconomic and demographic characteristics other than education. The absence of negative impact associated with most demographic factors regarding yoga was supported by two qualitative studies. Researchers in Maryland looked at the acceptability of yoga that consisted of classes and home practice as an intervention with Hispanic and African-American people with RA (Middleton et al., 2017). In that study, not only did the participants actively take part in the yoga classes and home practice but they continued to do so after conclusion of the formal study. Researchers in Boston explored the benefit of yoga among low-income minority people living with CLBP. The investigators concluded yoga was perceived by those in the sample as being a way to relieve pain, relax, and better manage stress. Not surprisingly, the participants identified time constraints, motivation, and fear of injury as barriers, and confidence in the yoga instructor was reported as a facilitator for attendance (Keosaian et al., 2016). Akin to these findings, a qualitative study conducted with clinicians regarding the feasibility of using yoga with patients identified allocating space, transportation, leadership support, and staff perceptions and attitudes as factors that could affect the success or failure of a yoga program (Waddington et al., 2017).

In addition to CLBP, yoga has been helpful with other types of pain, including OA, RA, FMS (Hillinger et al., 2017), and migraine headaches (Büssing et al., 2012). The authors of a systematic review and meta-analysis of 7 RCTs (n = 362 subjects) reported that when compared to other movement therapies (i.e., qigong and tai chi) used by people living with FMS, yoga was the only one that was significant in reducing pain, as well as fatigue and depression, with an increase in quality of life (Langhorst, Klose, Dobos, Bernardy, & Häuser, 2013). The authors of a large systematic review and meta-analysis of 17 studies (n = 1626 subjects) reported significant improvement among people living with OA, RA, and CLBP and concluded yoga is a safe intervention for people living with chronic pain related to those conditions (Ward, Stebbings, Cherkin, & Baxter, 2013). Like tai chi, yoga is most often

associated with community participation and chronic pain. However, it also is used successfully as an intervention in at least one acute care hospital for patients recovering from illness and surgery, where it is also modified for those who are limited to chair or bed activities (Erich & Quinlan-Colwell, 2017).

Similar to research issues with tai chi, not only do yoga studies have different protocols and diverse samples, but, in addition, there are several types of yoga with different types often being taught and used in research studies (Cho et al., 2015; Cramer et al., 2013). Further research with rigorous methods with consideration for potential bias and comparing yoga to established interventions is needed (Cramer et al., 2013). Additional research is needed to identify how best to bring yoga to groups who may benefit but who have had limited exposure to it (Middleton et al., 2017). Exploration of using yoga with patients who have acute pain and are immobile during acute medical conditions or after surgical procedures is needed. Waddington et al. (2017) identified the need to also conduct research into the perceptions and attitudes of health care staff about complementary interventions such as yoga and the effect the staff attitudes have on patients with whom they work regarding the modalities. Finally, Eaves et al. (2015) recommended that research is needed to discover how clinicians can work with people to achieve realistic expectations and encourage self-care and empowerment using modalities such as yoga.

Physical Therapy

Physical therapy is the health care profession with a focus on maintenance, improvement, or restoration of movement and activity to improve quality of life and optimize function (APTA, 2011). Although physical therapists use a wide variety of techniques when working with patients with pain, the topic of physical therapy is included in this chapter because a major focus of their work is on function and movement. The profession dramatically evolved during the last 100 years since the origins of working to improve the functional ability of wounded soldiers and later children recovering from polio to the current profession, which requires completion of graduate education (Furze, Tichenor, Fisher, Jensen, & Rapport, 2016). Similar to the nursing process, physical therapists use a process for patient care that includes the following (APTA, 2011):

- Assessment and evaluation of the person, beginning with a history of the current condition
- Physical examination, including appropriate testing and measurement
- Development of a physical therapy diagnosis
- Estimation of a prognosis
- Development of a plan of care with specified interventions that is done in partnership with the patient

- Use of patient-specific interventions within the physical therapy scope of practice
- Education of patients
- Reassessment, reevaluation, and measurement of outcomes

The scope of practice for physical therapists includes a variety of treatments that can be used to help control pain and improve function and quality of life. The particular interventions used by physical therapists differ slightly by the scope of practice defined by the state where the practice is located (APTA, 2011). Related to the primary focus of physical therapy being restoration and movement, increasingly physical therapists are involved as clinicians in multimodal approaches of pain management using interventions that include therapeutic exercise, mechanical modalities, passive therapies, and electrotherapeutic modalities (Ginnerup-Nielsen, Christensen, Thorborg, Tarp, & Henriksen, 2016). It is important to note that individual physical therapists may have expertise with additional interventions they can use to help patients manage pain and improve function (Box 20.2).

Therapeutic Exercise

The therapeutic exercises used by physical therapists include physical movements and activities that are specifically designed to improve physical function and health (APTA, 2017). Intentional exercises of this type are used by physical therapists who work with patients across the health care continuum. Stretching, strengthening, and aerobic exercise are central to recovery of many acute painful conditions such as patellofemoral pain (Capin & Snyder-Mackler, 2018) and femoroacetabular impingement (Mansell, Rhon, Marchant, Slevin, & Meyer, 2016). They are an important component of postoperative recovery, particularly after spinal (Louw, Puentedura, & Diener, 2016) and orthopedic surgeries (Szuba, Markowska, Czamara, & Noga, 2016). Box 20.3 presents the various therapeutic exercises used by physical therapists.

Box 20.2 | Physical Therapy Interventions Beneficial for Painful Conditions

Assistive and adaptive devices, including:
- Canes
- Crutches
- Walkers
- Hospital beds

Balance and agility training

Electrotherapeutic modalities, including:
- Biofeedback
- Electrical muscle stimulation (EMS)
- High-voltage pulsed current (HVPC)
- Neuromuscular electrical stimulation (NEMS)
- Transcutaneous electrical nerve stimulation (TENS)

Gait training

Manual therapies including:
- Soft tissue mobilization
- Therapeutic massage

Mechanical interventions, including:
- Compression therapy
- Mechanical motion devices (e.g., continuous passive motion)
- Taping
- Traction
- Vasopneumatic compression devices

Physical agents, including:
- Cryotherapy (see Chapter 27)
- Thermotherapy (see Chapter 27)
- Ultrasound

Neuromuscular training

Devices, including:
- Orthotic
- Prosthetic

- Protective devices
- Braces

Education, including:
- Patient education
- Family education

Relaxation training, including relaxation breathing

Sound agents including:
- Phonophoresis
- Ultrasound

Supportive devices, including:
- Compression clothing
- Elastic wraps
- Slings
- Soft neck collars

Therapeutic exercise, including:
- Active
- Aerobic
- Endurance
- Flexibility passive
- Range of motion
- Strengthening

Home evaluation

Modified from American Physical Therapy Association (APTA). (2009). *Minimum required skills of physical therapist graduates at entry-level.* Alexandria, VA: The Association; American Physical Therapy Association (APTA). (2011). *Today's physical therapist: A comprehensive review of a 21st-century health care profession.* Alexandria, VA: The Association; and Pagliarulo, M. A. (2012). Physical therapy for musculoskeletal conditions. In *Introduction to physical therapy* (pp. 170–112, 4th ed.). St. Louis, MO: Mosby.

Box 20.3	Therapeutic Exercises Used by Physical Therapists

- Range-of-motion exercises
  - Active
  - Passive
- Resistance exercises
  - Isometric
  - Isotonic concentric
  - Isotonic eccentric
  - Isokinetic
- Core strengthening
- Flexibility
- Balance and coordination exercises
- Functional exercises
- Aquatic exercises
- Cardiovascular exercises
- Home exercise programs

From Pagliarulo, M. (2012). *Introduction to physical therapy* (4th ed.). St. Louis, MO: Mosby.

Therapeutic exercises are commonly used when physical therapists work with patients who are living with chronic pain involving the low back (Bernet, Peskura, Meyer, Bauch, & Donaldson, 2019), neck (Pangarkar & Lee, 2011), pelvis (Bradley, Rawlins, & Brinker, 2017), shoulders (Marinko, Chacko, Dalton, & Chacko, 2011), and other painful musculoskeletal areas of the body (Søgaard & Jull, 2015). In fact, therapeutic exercise is recommended as the basic intervention for CLBP in Brazil (Ferreira et al., 2019). Exercise is a critical component of functional restoration programs designed to help people return to more normal functioning (Mayer, Gatchel, Brede, & Theodore, 2014). An innovative use of therapeutic exercise was reported in recent work in Denmark, where restorative exercise was used as part of physical therapy rehabilitation working with patients living with complex regional pain syndrome (GalveVilla, Rittig-Rasmussen, Mikkelsen, & Poulsen, 2016).

Therapeutic exercises are frequently combined with manual therapy as intervention for painful situations. The authors of a systematic review and meta-analysis of such a combined therapeutic approach used with people with TMJ disorders concluded the evidence was of low quality, but that was primarily because of methodologic issues of the studies (Armijo-Olivo et al., 2016).

Mechanical Modalities

Mechanical modalities used by physical therapists to help control pain include compression therapies and traction devices (APTA, 2009).

Compression therapy used by physical therapists is traditionally associated with lymphatic compression therapy for women who develop painful lymphedema after mastectomy, which can be accomplished by using stretch bandages or compression sleeves (Ochalek, Gradalski, & Szygula, 2015). However, this form of therapy is currently being researched in a number of innovative ways for a variety of painful conditions. A newer version of traditional lymphatic compression is intermittent pneumatic compression, which uses pump devices (Rockson, 2018). The researchers of a small study in Egypt (n = 28) reported that when sequential pneumatic compression therapy was used among women with painful varicose veins, compared with those women who only had exercise (n = 13), those who had the sequential pneumatic compression (n = 15) reported significantly improved pain control (Yamany & Hamdy, 2016).

The differences among materials and mechanisms used for compression is being studied to better understand and improve compression textiles (Liu, Guo, Lao, & Little, 2017). Compression therapy is also being looked at as part of a multimodal approach to managing pain with other types of painful conditions. American researchers are investigating the potential benefit of compression lymphedema therapy as a treatment for complex regional pain syndrome (Armstrong, Look, Christie, & Allen, 2016). Physical therapy researchers in Poland are investigating the benefit of using compression therapy combined with exercise as measures to prevent and treat leg edema and venous thrombosis (Ochalek, Pacyga, Curyło, Frydrych-Szymonik, & Szygula, 2017).

Traction is defined as "manual or mechanically assisted application of an intermittent or continuous distractive force" (Sutton et al., 2016, p. 1546). Traction devices have traditionally been used by physical therapists as interventions for pain, muscle spasms, and protruding intervertebral discs; however, the benefit has been questioned by researchers, including the authors of two systematic reviews (Madson & Hollman, 2015; Thackeray, Fritz, Childs, & Brennan, 2016). Despite that, intermittent mechanical traction of the cervical spine continues to be recommended for neck pain in the 2017 clinical practice guidelines from the Orthopaedic Section of the APTA (Blandpied et al., 2017).

Passive Therapies

Passive therapies used by physical therapists working with patients with pain include spinal massage, manipulation therapy, thermal agents, hydrotherapy, and low-level laser (Ferreira et al., 2019; Sutton et al., 2016). Passive exercises with thermal therapy (heat or cold) are also used by the physical therapist as therapy for painful conditions. Recently, those combined therapies have been specifically included in the plan of postoperative care of patients after TMJ surgery (De Meurechy, Loos, Mommaerts, 2019).

Thermal agents are used by physical therapists for a variety of reasons, including pain management (Pagliarulo,

2012). In general cryotherapy (cold) is used during the acute phase after injury with the intention for pain and to reduce inflammation (Hanks, Levine, & Bockstahler, 2015). The authors of an extensive systematic review (n = 40 studies) of physical therapy interventions after total knee arthroplasty procedures concluded there is low level evidence to support cryotherapy to prevent and improve range of motion postoperatively (Curry, Goehring, Bell, & Jette, 2018). The authors of that systematic review did note that additional rigorous research is needed. Heat is used to reduce muscle spasms and pain while increasing the pliability of surrounding tissue (Hanks et al., 2015). *Fluid therapy* is a specific type of thermal therapy used by physical therapists to promote healing by immersing the affected part of the body of the patient in a device that is filled with a sawdust-like substance and circulating water controlled at a therapeutic temperature (Pagliarulo, 2012). (See Chapter 27 for more information on thermal therapies.)

Manual therapy involves specialized techniques that involve the physical therapist using his or her hands as therapeutic tools to manipulate or mobilize affected tissues or joints (Bishop et al., 2015). Manual therapies can be considered in two groups. The first type of manual therapy is *soft tissue mobilization,* which includes massage and myofascial release to relax and improve metabolism with tissues that are tense and painful (Pagliarula, 2012). The second type of manual therapy is *joint mobilization,* which is used with joints that are inflexible with limited mobility (Pagliarula, 2012). The authors of a systematic review (n = 13) reported that study results were inconsistent and did not clearly support the benefit of manual therapy for pain management (Voogt et al., 2015). Again, methodology may have been a factor in at least some of the studies.

These techniques are used either alone or in conjunction with other physical therapy modalities to reduce pain with a variety of painful musculoskeletal conditions, including the back (Ju, Choi, Yang, & Lee, 2015), neck (Blandpied et al., 2017), knees related to osteoarthritis (Fitzgerald, 2016), hip and knee pain conditions (Hinman, 2014), elbow (Frydman, Johnston, Smidt, Green, & Buchbinder, 2018), Achilles tendinopathy (Jayaseelan, Kecman, Alcorn, & Sault, 2017), TMJ (Armijo-Olivo et al., 2016), and pelvic floor pain (Hartmann, 2016). (See Chapter 24 for more information on manual therapies used for pain.)

Dry needling is used by some physical therapists as a therapeutic component of a multimodal approach when treating myofascial pain (APTA, 2012). The skin is penetrated with a fine filiform needle to stimulate underlying myofascial trigger points and tissues (APTA, 2012; Koppenhaver, et al., 2017). Dry needling is used to treat a wide variety of pain myofascial conditions affecting the low back (Koppenhaver et al., 2017), shoulder (Hando, Rhon, Cleland, & Snodgrass, 2018), trapezius muscles (Ziaeifar, Arab, Mosallanezhad, & Nourbakhsh, 2018), face related to TMJ issues (Vier, de Almeida, Neves, dos Santos, & Bracht, 2019), abdomen (with uncertain cause)

(Rajkannan & Vijayaraghavan, 2018), and carpal tunnel (Gascon-Garcia, Bagur-Calafat, Girabent-Farrés, & Balius, 2018). Physical therapists are not allowed to use dry needling in every state, so it is important to ascertain where it is allowed (Espejo-Antúnez et al., 2017; Hall, Mackie, & Ribeiro 2018; Morihisa, Eskew, McNamara, & Young, 2016). This is another intervention in which rigorous research is needed.

Taping has long been used by physical therapists using athletic tape to protect, support, and stabilize injured joints while allowing normal movement (Bandyopadhyay & Mahapatra, 2012). Data and support are inconsistent for using taping of injured joints, including the knee (Collins, et al., 2018) and ankle (Bandyopadhyay & Mahapatra, 2012; Halim-Kertanegara, Raymond, Hiller, Kilbreath, & Refshauge, 2017). It is possible that taping provides a sense of security that in turn reduces anxiety and fear related to moving the injured area (Halim-Kertanegara et al., 2017). A second and more recent form of taping is Kinesio Taping, developed in Japan during the 1970s, which uses a tape that is thinner and has greater elasticity to apply tension and maintain extension of the muscle (Parreira, Costa, Junior, Lopes, & Costa, 2014).

The authors of individual studies and systematic reviews report inconsistent benefit with taping of joints (Araujo et al., 2018; Beneciuk, Bishop, & George, 2016), including patellofemoral (Collins et al., 2018) and shoulder (Bhashyam, Logan, Rider, Schurko, & Provenher, 2018) joints. The results of a systematic review of the effectiveness of taping spinal areas yielded no clear support that taping is effective for spinal pain (Vanti et al., 2015). Similarly, when Kinesio Taping was added to exercise and manual therapy with people with CLBP (n = 148), no additional benefit was reported (Added et al., 2016). The authors of another systematic review noted the use of Kinesio Taping may have benefit as part of a multimodal plan of care, but additional research is needed (Nelson, 2016).

Table 20.2 presents a summary of common physical agents used by physical therapists.

Electrotherapeutic Modalities

Electrical stimulation is a noninvasive, counter-irritant intervention that promotes analgesia through activation of the endogenous nociception network (Coutaux, 2017; Zeng et al., 2015). It has been used for analgesia for thousands of years, beginning with the use of Nile catfish and later torpedo fish (Coutaux, 2017; North & Prager, 2018). Today, physical therapists use several types of electrical nerve stimulation, including *electrical muscle stimulation (EMS), neuromuscular electrical stimulation (NMES), high-voltage pulsed current (HVPC), and transcutaneous electrical nerve stimulation (TENS)* (APTA, 2009). In addition, *iontophoresis* is a therapy in which medication is administered to a specific area using a transcutaneous process using electrical current (Brickman, 2018).

Table 20.2 | Summary of Common Biophysical Agents Used in Physical Therapy

Physical Effect	Biophysical Agents	Physiologic Effects	Clinical Indications
Superficial heat	Hot packs Paraffin Fluid therapy Whirlpool	Increases blood flow Increases metabolism: Promotes healing and removal of waste products Decreases pain Decreases stiffness	Pain Joint stiffness
Deep heat	Ultrasound Short-wave diathermy	Increases blood flow Increases metabolism: Promotes healing and removal of waste products Decreases pain Decreases stiffness	Muscle spasm Pain Joint stiffness
Cold	Ice packs Ice massage Cold whirlpool Cold compression	Decreases blood flow Decreases metabolism Decreases edema Decreases pain	Acute injury Swelling Pain Muscle spasm After exercise
Electrical stimulation	Transcutaneous electrical nerve stimulation (TENS) Iontophoresis Electrical stimulation for wound healing Neuromuscular electrical stimulation	Decreases pain Decreases inflammation Promotes wound healing Reeducates muscles Decreases spasticity	Pain Inflammation Wounds Nerve regeneration Muscle weakness and imbalance

From Pagliarulo, M. (2012). *Introduction to physical therapy* (4th ed.). St. Louis, MO: Mosby.

EMS is a passive intervention in which electrodes are used transcutaneously to generate an isometric contraction of muscle tissue with minimal movement of the associated joints (Hodgson & Tipping, 2016). In a systematic review by the American College of Physicians, when used for low back pain, EMS was not found to have more than minimal support for benefit (Chou et al., 2017). Similarly, the authors of a clinical practice guideline from the American College of Physicians reported insufficient evidence to support the use of EMS (Qaseem, Wilt, McLean, & Forciea, 2017).

NMES is used in physical therapy primarily to improve muscle function and strength rather than for pain control; however, because muscle strength and function support improved ability to manage pain, it can be relevant in a multimodal plan of analgesia. A systematic review of 11 studies, with 6 of the studies in a meta-analysis, was done to assess the benefit of NMES and standard of care with the outcome measure of anterior cruciate ligament strength postoperatively (Hauger et al., 2018). The authors of that review concluded that when NMES was added to standard of care physical therapy there was significant improvement in function and strength of quadricep muscles postoperatively. In another systematic review assessing the benefit of using NMES with people living with cancer, the authors concluded that NMES was correlated with significant improvement in muscle strength and quality of life function and is an area needing additional research

(O'Connor, Caulfield, & Lennon, 2018). The authors of that review noted that there is a need for additional research.

TENS, which was first reported in 1967 by Wall and Sweet, uses electrical currents by cutaneous electrodes to achieve analgesia (Coutaux, 2017; Wall & Sweet, 1967). With TENS, painless but strong electrical sensation is used to stimulate low-threshold cutaneous afferent pain receptors, thereby interrupting nociceptive transmission (Johnson, Claydon, Herbison, Paley, & Jones, 2017). Today TENS is commercially available in devices called units that are inexpensive and simple to use (de Almeida, da Silva, Júnior, Liebano, & Durigan, 2018).

Although research results are inconclusive, internationally TENS is used for analgesia with a variety of painful chronic conditions, including low back pain and other musculoskeletal disorders (Coutaux, 2017; Sluka, Bjordal, Marchand, & Rakel, 2013). The authors of one systematic review with meta-analysis reported patients who used TENS reported improved pain control and functional ability (de Almeida et al., 2018). Despite widespread use, research results supporting benefits of TENS continue to be inconclusive, which again at least in part is related to research methodology (Sluka et al., 2013). The inconsistent results may also speak to the need for better education of patients using TENS units (Gladwell, Badlan, Cramp, & Palmer,

2016). Increasingly, TENS is being studied as an intervention for acute pain, including labor pain (Santana et al., 2016) and postoperative pain (Bjersá, Jildenstaal, Jakobsson, Egardt, & Olsén, 2015; Yılmaz, Karakaya, Baydur, & Tekin, 2018). It is important for patients and clinicians to know that manufacturers of TENS units note that they are contraindicated for use by people who live with epilepsy, are pregnant, or who have cardiac pacemakers, and the United Kingdom Chartered Society of Physiotherapy also lists bleeding disorders as a contraindication (Jones & Johnson, 2009).

Physical therapists provide education and consultation for all aspects of health care ranging from individual patients and families to health care agencies (APTA, 2011). An important contribution of physical therapy consultation is home assessment to evaluate how well patients living with pain are able to function within their homes and to recommend what they can do to improve safety. A growing option for people with transportation issues is to receive ongoing physical therapy via telerehabilitation programs in their own homes (Levy, Silverman, Jia, Geiss, & Omura, 2015).

Patient Education for All Exercise and Movement

It is not reasonable to expect every clinician to have expertise on every exercise and movement therapy available. However, it is important for clinicians to know what exercise and movement therapies are available and what resources are available for them as clinicians and for the person in pain. The information in this chapter, the references provided, national organizations, and local instructors are all resources to use when assessing and educating patients regarding movement and exercise activities. It is imperative to remember that not all activities are appropriate for all people, patients need to be assessed for ability to participate, they need to be educated regarding any individual cautions to be taken during exercise, and they need to be followed to reassess the effect of the activity.

The clinician can position the person living with pain to be successful in movement and activities by being aware of some basic concepts (Bacon, 2017) (Table 20.3). An initial step is to guide the person to select a movement or activity he or she will most be able to enjoy and to feel successful when undertaking. Educate patients that most if not all activities can be adapted for their particular levels of ability and endurance. Teaching patients how to minimize muscle soreness can be done by encouraging them to start low and gradually increase participation and by using stretching techniques on a regular basis to improve muscle function (Medeiros & Lima, 2017). Teaching patients to use analgesic medications before movement and exercise programs to achieve greatest analgesic benefit during activities may help them be successful (see Chapters 10, 11, 15, and 16). Reassessing the person to identify what has worked and what has been problematic enables the clinician to help the person redesign movements/activities to best lead to success, better pain management, and greater function.

Key Points

- Fear of movement can limit activity and negatively affect quality of life.
- Exercise-induced hypoalgesia is a process of reducing pain through movement and exercise.
- Several movements and exercises are shown to be beneficial for controlling pain and improving function and quality of life.
- Selection of a particular movement or exercise depends on the condition of the person, any comorbidities, availability of the activity, and patient preference.
- Movements and activities can be modified to meet the needs of the individual participant.
- It is best to encourage each person to select a movement or exercise that he or she finds enjoyable.
- Patients need to know it is not only acceptable but is also advised to modify movements and activities to adjust to any physical limitations they may have.
- Before starting a movement or exercise program, it should be reviewed with the clinician overseeing care.
- Clinicians have a responsibility to learn about movement and exercise options for pain management as part of a multimodal analgesic plan of care.
- Clinicians need to educate patients about movement and exercise therapies and how they can benefit the person to control pain and improve function and quality of life.
- Physical therapy is an important component in a plan of multimodal analgesia.

Case Scenario

Ralph is a 52-year-old man who is married and has four teenage children. He has had chronic lower back pain for 3 years since he fell out of a tree while trimming it at his mothers-in-law's house. It is hard for him to control his pain while working as a police officer because he cannot use most pain medications. He is thinking about retiring early but does not want to do that because he really likes his work and likes to be active. In addition, he cannot really afford to retire. His wife keeps trying to talk him into taking lessons in tai chi or yoga, but he does not want to get involved with that "sissy stuff." He comes to the clinic today telling you that he feels really stressed and asking about what he can do to "get rid of this pain so that I can continue working."

1. What things do you need to consider in sharing options for treatment with Ralph?
2. What movement or exercise options might Ralph try?
3. What information/education can you share with him about the options?

Table 20.3 | Talking Points for Patient Teaching About Movement and Exercise

Barriers to Beginning an Exercise or Movement Program	Clinician Role
Attempting to increase activities can be frightening. Fears of increasing pain and of failure may prevent a person from participating in physical activities.	It is important to assess and listen to concerns of the person, then address them to alleviate fears, modify participation in the activity, or identify a different activity.
Some people may think of movement or exercise as boring or taking up too much time.	Clinicians can work with the person to identify how movement or exercise can be incorporated into daily routines. For example, recruiting family members to join in group activities (e.g., walking, dance, yoga, tai chi) or coordinating movement or exercise with other activities (e.g., watching television, praying).
Patients may think they are not able to do certain movements or activities because of pain or other limitations.	Most movements and activities can be modified to meet the functional ability of each individual, but patients may not know and need to be educated and reassured. Patients need to be assessed to identify individual needs for modification and educated how these can be implemented.
Patients may resist an exercise program because they do not like to exercise.	Participating in movements or activities that are enjoyable for the person will lead to greater participation and success. Assess what activities are pleasurable but may not be considered exercise (e.g., dancing, walking, bicycling).

Patients Need Preparation for Movement and Activities	Clinician Role
People living with pain may not be familiar with the idea of exercise and do not know what is safe.	Clinicians need to know what movements and exercises are reasonable and educate the person while encouraging the person to choose what is personally the most reasonable.
Patients may have very specific questions about movements or activities.	It is important for clinicians to have experts, organizations, and literature to consult for specific information.
Lack of flexibility can lead to muscle soreness, pain, and reluctance to continue with the activity.	Patients need to be instructed in how to improve muscle flexibility with gentle stretching movements.
People may not know what cautions or safety measures are needed.	Clinicians need to educate patients about any cautions there are concerning the activity with the physical condition of the individual and what safety measures the patient may need to take regarding the physical condition.
Pain can be frightening and a significant barrier to activity.	Patients need to be educated how to best coordinate activities with their schedule of multimodal analgesic medications.

Patients Need Support to Continue With Movement and Exercise	Clinician Role
After initially trying an activity, patients may become discouraged that they are not very quickly becoming good at it.	Clinicians need to reassure patients that proficiency takes time and needs to be assessed depending on the abilities of each person.
People who are not experienced with movement therapies or exercise may not think they are benefitting from the activities.	Listening to concerns and reassuring the person that being active is a process and doing well with the activity is progress and beneficial.
People may not know if it is all right to remain with the level of movement or exercise or if they can safely increase their activities.	Reassessing the person to identify what has worked and what has been problematic enables the clinician to help the person to be reassured and redesign their movements/activities as necessary to best lead to success, better pain management and greater function.

Primarily based on Bacon, J. L. (2017). Building a bridge to the nonexerciser. *ACSM's Health & Fitness Journal, 21*(1), 41–43; and Medeiros, D. M., & Lima, C. S. (2017). Influence of chronic stretching on muscle performance: Systematic review. *Human Movement Science, 54*, 220–229.

4. What considerations are important for him to think about when deciding on what to try?

5. What forms of movement or exercise could be helpful in supporting Ralph in his goal to return to work?

6. What concerns or fears may Ralph have about trying movement therapies or exercise?

7. Once Ralph decides on a movement or exercise to try, how will you assess the benefit for him?

8. What other clinicians could be consulted to help Ralph?

9. What education do you need to provide to Ralph about his decision?

10. As a clinician what is/are your obligation/s to Ralph?

References

Added, M. A. N., Costa, L. O. P., De Freitas, D. G., Fukuda, T. Y., Monteiro, R. L., Salomão, E. C., … Costa, L. D. C. M. (2016). Kinesio Taping does not provide additional benefits in patients with chronic low back pain who receive exercise and manual therapy: a randomized controlled trial. *Journal of Orthopaedic & Sports Physical Therapy*, 46(7), 506–513.

American Dance Therapy Association (ADTA). (ND). What is dance/movement therapy? *American Dance Therapy Association*. http://adta.org/wp-content/uploads/2015/12/What-is-DanceMovement-Therapy.pdfdta.org Accessed 07/17/2020.

American Physical Therapy Association (APTA). (2009). *Minimum Required Skills of Physical Therapist Graduates at Entry-level*. Alexandria, VA: American Physical Therapy Association.

American Physical Therapy Association (APTA). (2011). *Today's Physical Therapist: A comprehensive review of a 21st century health care profession*. Alexandria, VA: American Physical Therapy Association.

American Physical Therapy Association (APTA). (2012). *Physical Therapists & The Performance of Dry Needling: An Educational Resource Paper*. Alexandria, VA: American Physical Therapy Association.

American Physical Therapy Association (APTA). (2017). *Guide to Physical Therapist Practice*. Alexandria, VA: American Physical Therapy Association. doi:https://doi.org/10.2522/ptguide3.0_978-1-931369-85-5.

American Physical Therapy Association (APTA). (2019). *Move Forward: Physical Therapy Brings Motion to Live*. https://www.moveforwardpt.com/ChoosePT/Toolkit. (Accessed 4 July 2019).

Amy, E. A., & Kozak, A. T. (2012). "The more pain I have, the more I want to eat": obesity in the context of chronic pain. *Obesity*, 20(10), 2027–2034.

Anwer, S., & Alghadir, A. (2014). Effect of isometric quadriceps exercise on muscle strength, pain, and function in patients with knee osteoarthritis: a randomized controlled study. *Journal of Physical Therapy Science*, 26(5), 745–748.

Araujo, A. C., Parreira, P. D. C. S., Junior, L. C. H., da Silva, T. M., da Luz Junior, M. A., Costa, L. D. C. M., & Costa, L. O. P. (2018). Medium term effects of Kinesio Taping in patients with chronic non-specific low back pain: a randomized controlled trial. *Physiotherapy*, 104(1), 149–151.

Archer, K. R., Seebach, C. L., Mathis, S. L., Riley, L. H., & Wegener, S. T. (2014). Early postoperative fear of movement predicts pain, disability, and physical health six months after spinal surgery for degenerative conditions. *The Spine Journal*, 14(5), 759–767.

Armijo-Olivo, S., Pitance, L., Singh, V., Neto, F., Thie, N., & Michelotti, A. (2016). Effectiveness of manual therapy and therapeutic exercise for temporomandibular disorders: systematic review and meta-analysis. *Physical Therapy*, 96(1), 9–25.

Armstrong, S., Look, J., Christie, L. F., & Allen, R. (2016). *Lymphedema Therapy for the Treatment of Complex Regional Pain Syndrome*. Tacoma, WA: University of Puget Sound. Sound Ideas Physical Therapy Research Symposium.

Arranz, L. I. (2017). Effects of obesity on function and quality of life in chronic pain. pp. 151–170. In R. R. Watson, & S. Zibadi (Eds.), *Nutritional Modulators of Pain in the Aging Population*. London: Elseveier Inc.

Atilgan, E., Aytar, A., Çağlar, A., Aytar, A., Arin, G., & Űnal, E. (2017). The effects of clinical Pilates exercises on patients with shoulder pain: A randomized clinical trial. *Journal of Bodywork & Movement Therapies*, 21(4), 847–851.

Bacon, J. L. (2017). Building a Bridge to the Nonexerciser. *ACSM's Health & Fitness Journal*, 21(1), 41–43.

Bandyopadhyay, A., & Mahapatra, D. (2012). Taping in sports: a brief update. *Journal of Human Sport & Exercise*, 7(2), 544–552.

Barker, A. L., Talevski, J., Morello, R. T., Brand, C. A., Rahmann, A. E., & Urquhart, D. M. (2014). Effectiveness of aquatic exercise for musculoskeletal conditions: a meta-analysis. *Archives of Physical Medicine and Rehabilitation*, 95(9), 1776–1786.

Bartenieff, I. (2002). *Body Movement: Coping with the Environment*. New York, NY: Routledge.

Bartels, E. M., Juhl, C. B., Christensen, R., Hagen, K. B., Danneskiold-Samsøe, B., Dagfinrud, H., & Lund, H. (2016). Aquatic exercise for the treatment of knee and hip osteoarthritis. *The Cochrane Library.*, 3, CD005523.

Beneciuk, J. M., Bishop, M. D., & George, S. Z. (2016). Clinical prediction rules for physical therapy interventions: a systematic review. *Physical Therapy*, 89(2), 114–124.

Bernet, B. A., Peskura, E. T., Meyer, S. T., Bauch, P. C., & Donaldson, M. B. (2019). The effects of hip-targeted physical therapy interventions on low back pain: A systematic review and meta-analysis. *Musculoskeletal Science and Practice.*, 39, 91–100.

Bhashyam, A. R., Logan, C. A., Rider, S. M., Schurko, B., & Provenher, M. T. (2018). A Systematic Review of Taping for Pain Management in Shoulder Impingement. *The Orthopaedic Journal at Harvard Medical School*, 19, 18–23.

Bidonde, J., Busch, A. J., Webber, S. C., Schachter, C. L., Danyliw, A., Overend, T. J., … Rader, T. (2014). Aquatic exercise training for fibromyalgia. *The Cochrane Library.*, (10), CD011336.

Biggs, E. E., Meulders, A., & Vlaeyen, J. W. S. (2016). The neuroscience of pain and fear. In M. A. Flaten, & M. al'Absi (Eds.), *Neuroscience of Pain, Stress, and Emotion: Psychological and Clinical Implications* (pp. 133–157). St. Louis, MO: Elsevier.

Bishop, M. D., Torres-Cueco, R., Gay, C. W., Lluch-Girbés, E., Beneciuk, J. M., & Bialosky, J. E. (2015). What effect can manual therapy have on a patient's pain experience? *Pain Management*, 5(6), 455–464.

Bjerså, K., Jildenstaal, P., Jakobsson, J., Egardt, M., & Olsén, M. F. (2015). Adjunct high frequency transcutaneous electric stimulation (TENS) for postoperative pain management during weaning from epidural analgesia following colon surgery: results from a controlled pilot study. *Pain Management Nursing, 16*(6), 944–950.

Blandford, L. (2014a). Injury Prevention and Movement Control. In *Vol 1. Core Values and Posture*. London: YMCAed.

Blandford, L. (2014b). Injury Prevention and Movement Control. In *Vol 2. Core Values and Posture*. London: YMCAed.

Blandpied, P. R., Gross, A. R., Elliott, J. M., Devaney, L. L., Clewley, D., Walton, D. M., ... Boeglin, E. (2017). Neck pain: revision 2017: clinical practice guidelines linked to the international classification of functioning, disability and health from the orthopaedic section of the American Physical Therapy Association. *Journal of Orthopaedic & Sports Physical Therapy, 47*(7), A1–A83.

Bongi, S. M., Paoletti, G., Calà, M., Del Rosso, A., El Aoufy, K., & Mikhaylova, S. (2016). Efficacy of rehabilitation with Tai Ji Quan in an Italian cohort of patients with fibromyalgia syndrome. *Complementary Therapies in Clinical Practice, 24*, 109–115.

Bossone, E., Ferrara, F., & Citro, R. (2015). Medical Treatment in Chronic Aortic Dissection. In A. Evangelista, & C. Nienaber (Eds.), *Vol. 7. Pharmacotherapy in Aortic Disease* (pp. 239–262). Cham, Switzerland: Springer.

Bowman, K. (2014). *Move Your DNA Restore Your Health through Natural Movement*. Propriometrics Press.

Bradley, M. H., Rawlins, A., & Brinker, C. A. (2017). Physical therapy treatment of pelvic pain. *Physical Medicine and Rehabilitation Clinics, 28*(3), 589–601.

Bräuninger, I. (2014). Specific dance movement therapy interventions – Which are successful? An intervention and correlation study. *The Arts in Psychotherapy, 41*(5), 445–457.

Brellenthin, A., Cook, D., Sehgal, N., & Koltyn, K. (2012). The influence of submaximal isometric exercise on temporal summation of heat pain. *The Journal of Pain, 13*(4 Supplement), S49.

Brellenthin, A. G., Crombie, K. M., Cook, D. B., Sehgal, N., & Koltyn, K. (2016). Psychosocial influences on exercise-induced hypoalgesia. *Pain Medicine, 18*(3), 538–550.

Brickman, K. A., Zaciewski, T. G., Bahl, R., Fink, B. N., Gibbons, M. P., Sidani, R. S., ... Wellock, A. R. (2018). Iontophoresis: as a new treatment modality in the management of acute soft tissue injuries in the emergency department. *Translation: The University of Toledo Journal of Medical Sciences, 2*, 1–3.

Browne, K. L., Diersing, D., & Hilliard, T. (2017). Musculoskeletal Assessment and Management of Patients Participating in a Walking Program. *The Journal for Nurse Practitioners, 13*(1), 26–33.

Büssing, A., Ostermann, T., Lüdtke, R., & Michalsen, A. (2012). Effects of yoga interventions on pain and pain-associated disability: a meta-analysis. *The Journal of Pain, 13*(1), 1–9.

Capin, J. J., & Snyder-Mackler, L. (2018). The current management of patients with patellofemoral pain from the physical therapist's perspective. *Annals of Joint, 3*(5), 40.

Carriere, J. S., Thibault, P., Milioto, M., & Sullivan, M. (2015). Expectancies mediate the relations among pain catastrophizing, fear of movement, and return to work outcomes after whiplash injury. *The Journal of Pain, 16*(12), 1280–1287.

Chaddha, A., Eagle, K. A., Braverman, A. C., Kline-Rogers, E., Hirsch, A. T., Brook, R., & Franklin, B. A. (2015). Exercise and Physical Activity for the Post–Aortic Dissection Patient: The Clinician's Conundrum. *Clinical Cardiology, 38*(11), 647–651.

Chaput, J. P., Carson, V., Gray, C. E., & Tremblay, M. S. (2014). Importance of all movement behaviors in a 24 hour period for overall health. *International Journal of Environmental Research and Public Health, 11*(12), 12575–12581.

Cho, H. K., Moon, W., & Kim, J. (2015). Effects of yoga on stress and inflammatory factors in patients with chronic low back pain: A non-randomized controlled study. *European Journal of Integrative Medicine, 7*(2), 118–123.

Chou, R., Deyo, R., Friedly, J., Skelly, A., Hashimoto, R., Weimer, M., & Grusing, S. (2017). Nonpharmacologic therapies for low back pain: a systematic review for an American College of Physicians clinical practice guideline. *Annals of Internal Medicine, 166*(7), 493–505.

Claes, N., Vlaeyen, J. W. S., & Crombez, G. (2016). Pain in context: cues predicting a reward decrease fear of movement related pain and avoidance behavior. *Behaviour Research and Therapy, 84*(1), 35–44.

Collins, N. J., Barton, C. J., Van Middelkoop, M., Callaghan, M. J., Rathleff, M. S., Vicenzino, B. T., ... de Oliveira Silva, D. (2018). 2018 Consensus statement on exercise therapy and physical interventions (orthoses, taping and manual therapy) to treat patellofemoral pain: recommendations from the 5th International Patellofemoral Pain Research Retreat, Gold Coast, Australia, 2017. *British Journal of Sports Medicine, 52*(18), 1170–1178.

Combs, M. A., & Thorn, B. E. (2015). Yoga attitudes in chronic low back pain: roles of catastrophizing and fear of movement. *Complementary Therapies in Clinical Practice, 21*(3), 160–165.

Comerford, M., & Mottram, S. (2012). Uncontrolled pain pp. 3–22. *Kinetic control-e-book: The management of uncontrolled movement*. In Elsevier Health Sciences. Australia: Elsevier Australia.

Costa, L.d. M., Maher, C. G., McAuley, J. H., & Hancock, M. J. (2011). Self-efficacy is more important than fear of movement in mediating the relationship between pain and disability in chronic low back pain. *European Journal of Pain, 15*(2), 213–219.

Coutaux, A. (2017). Non-pharmacological treatments for pain relief: TENS and acupuncture. *Joint Bone Spine, 84*(6), 657–661.

Cramer, H., Lauche, R., Haller, H., & Dobos, G. (2013). A systematic review and meta-analysis of yoga for low back pain. *The Clinical Journal of Pain, 29*(5), 450–460.

Cramer, H., Lauche, R., Langhorst, J., & Dobos, G. (2016). Is one yoga style better than another? A systematic review of associations of yoga style and conclusions in randomized yoga trials. *Complementary Therapies in Medicine, 25*, 178–187.

Crombie, K. M., Brellenthin, A. G., Hillard, C. J., & Koltyn, K. F. (2017). Endocannabinoid and opioid system interactions in exercise-induced hyperalgesia. *Pain Medicine, 19*(1), 118–123. https://doi.org/10.1093/pm/pnx058.

Cruz-Díaz, D., Bergamin, M., Gobbo, B. S., Martínez-Amat, A., & Hita-Conreras, F. (2017). Comparative effects of 12 weeks of equipment based and mat Pilates in patients with chronic low back pain on pain, function and transversus abdominis activation. A randomized controlled trial. *Complementary Therapies in Medicine, 33*(1), 72–77. https://doi.org/10.1016/j.ctim.2017.06.004.

Cruz-Díaz, D., Martínez-Amat, A., De la Torre-Cruz, M. J., Casuso, R. A., de Guevara, & Hita-Conreras, F. (2015).

Effects of a six-week Pilates intervention on balance and fear of falling in women aged over 65 with chronic low-back pain: A randomized controlled trial. *Maturitas, 82*(4), 371–376.

Curry, A. L., Goehring, M. T., Bell, J., & Jette, D. U. (2018). Effect of Physical Therapy Interventions in the Acute Care Setting on Function, Activity, and Participation After Total Knee Arthroplasty: A Systematic Review. *Journal of Acute Care Physical Therapy, 9*(3), 93–106.

Daenen, L., Varkey, E., Kellmann, M., & Nijs, J. (2015). Exercise, not to exercise, or how to exercise in patients with chronic pain? Applying science to practice. *The Clinical Journal of Pain, 31*(2), 108–114.

Dawson, A. P., Schlutter, P. J., Hodges, P. W., Stewart, S., & Turner, C. (2011). Fear of movement, passive coping, manual handling, and severe or radiating pain increase the likelihood of sick leave due to low back pain. *Pain, 152*(7), 1517–1524.

Day, L., Hill, K. D., Stathakis, V. Z., Flicker, L., & Jolley, D. (2015). Impact of Tai-Chi on falls among preclinically disabled older people. A randomized controlled trial. *Journal of the American Medical Directors Association, 6*(5), 42–426.

de Almeida, C. C., da Silva, V. Z. M., Júnior, G. C., Liebano, R. E., & Durigan, J. L. Q. (2018). Transcutaneous electrical nerve stimulation and interferential current demonstrate similar effects in relieving acute and chronic pain: a systematic review with meta-analysis. *Brazilian Journal of Physical Therapy, 22*(5), 347–354.

De Meurechy, N. K., Loos, P.-J., & Mommaerts, M. Y. (2019). Postoperative physiotherapy after open temporomandibular joint surgery: A three-step program. *Journal of Oral and Maxillofacial Surgery., 77*(5), 932–950.

de Oliveira, N. T. B., Freitas, S. M. S. F., Fuhro, F. F., da Luz, M. A., Amorim, C. F., & Cabral, C. M. N. (2017). Muscle activation during Pilates exercises in participants with chronic nonspecific low back pain: A cross-sectional case-control study. *Archives of Physical Medicine and Rehabilitation, 98*(1), 88–95.

deTord, P., & Bräuninger, I. (2015). Grounding: Theoretical application and practice in dance movement therapy. *The Arts in Psychotherapy, 43*(1), 16–22.

Eaves, E. R., Sherman, K. J., Ritenbaugh, C., Hsu, C., Nichter, M., Turner, J. A., & Cherkin, D. C. (2015). A qualitative study of changes in expectations over time among patients with chronic low back pain seeking four CAM therapies. *BMC Complementary and Alternative Medicine, 15*(1), 12.

Ekelund, U., Steene-Johnanessen, J., Brown, W. J., Wang, M., Owen, N., & Lee, I.-M. (2016). Does physical activity attenuate, or even eliminate, the detrimental association of sitting time with mortality? A harmonized meta-analysis of data from more than 1 million men and women. *Lancet, 388*(10051), 1302–1310.

Erich, M., & Quinlan-Colwell, A. (2017). Celebrating 20 years of the Healing Arts Network. *Southern Pain Society Newsletter.* Summer, 3-4.

Espejo-Antúnez, L., Tejeda, J. F. H., Albornoz-Cabello, M., & Rodriguez-Mansilla, J. (2017). Dry needling in the management of myofascial trigger points: A systematic review of randomized controlled trials. *Complementary Therapies in Medicine, 33*, 46–57.

Farrokhi, S., Jayabalan, P., Gustafson, J. A., Klatt, B. A., Sowa, G. A., & Piva, S. R. (2017). The influence of continuous versus interval walking exercise on knee joint loading and pain in patients with knee osteoarthritis. *Gait & Posture, 56*, 129–133.

Ferreira, G., Costa, L. M., Stein, A., Hartvigsen, J., Buchbinder, R., & Maher, C. G. (2019). Tackling low back pain in Brazil: a wake-up call. *Brazilian Journal of Physical Therapy., 23*(3), 189–195.

Field, T. (2016). Knee osteoarthritis pain in the elderly can be reduced by massage therapy, yoga and tai chi: a review. *Complementary Therapies in Clinical Practice, 22*, 87–92.

Fitzgerald, G. K., Fritz, J. M., Childs, J. D., Brennan, G. P., Talisa, V., Gil, A. B., … Abbott, J. H. (2016). Exercise, manual therapy, and use of booster sessions in physical therapy for knee osteoarthritis: a multi-center, factorial randomized clinical trial. *Osteoarthritis and Cartilage, 24*(8), 1340–1349.

Frydman, A., Johnston, R. V., Smidt, N., Green, S., & Buchbinder, R. (2018). Manual therapy and exercise for lateral elbow pain. *Cochrane Database of Systematic Reviews, 6*, CD013042.

Furze, J. A., Tichenor, C. J., Fisher, B. E., Jensen, G. M., & Rapport, M. J. (2016). Physical therapy residency and fellowship education: reflections on the past, present, and future. *Physical therapy, 96*(7), 949–960.

Galidinao, G., Romero, T., da Silva, J. F. P., Aguiar, D., de Paula, A. M., & Perez, A. (2014). Acute resistance exercise induces antinociception by activation of the endocannabinoid system in rats. *Anesthesia and Analgesia, 119*(3), 702–715.

GalveVilla, M., Rittig-Rasmussen, B., Mikkelsen, L. M. S., & Poulsen, A. G. (2016). Complex regional pain syndrome. *Manual Therapy, 26*, 223–230.

Gascon-Garcia, J., Bagur-Calafat, C., Girabent-Farrés, M., & Balius, R. (2018). Validation of the range of dry needling with the fascial winding technique in the carpal tunnel using ultrasound. *Journal of Bodywork and Movement Therapies, 22*(2), 348–353.

Geschwind, N., Meulders, M., Peters, M. L., Vlaeyen, J. W. S., & Meulders, A. (2015). Can experimentally induced positive affect attenuate generalization of fear of movement-related pain? *The Journal of Pain, 16*(3), 258–269.

Gill, S. D., & McBurney, H. (2013). Does exercise reduce pain and improve physical function before hip or knee replacement surgery? A systematic review and meta-analysis of randomized controlled trials. *Archives of Physical Medicine and Rehabilitation, 94*(1), 164–176.

Ginnerup-Nielsen, E., Christensen, R., Thorborg, K., Tarp, S., & Henriksen, M. (2016). Physiotherapy for pain: a meta-epidemiological study of randomised trials. *British Journal of Sports Medicine, 50*(16), 965–971.

Gladwell, P., Badlan, K., Cramp, F. A., & Palmer, S. (2016). Problems, solutions, and strategies reported by users of TENS for chronic musculoskeletal pain: A qualitative exploration using patient interviews. *Physical Therapy, 96*(7), 1039–1048.

Goode, A. P., Coeytaux, R. R., McDuffie, J., Duan-Porter, W., Sharma, P., Mennella, H., … Williams, J. W. (2016). An evidence map of yoga for low back pain. *Complementary Therapies in Medicine, 25*(2), 170–177.

Guck, T. P., Burke, R. V., Rainville, C., Hill-Taylor, D., & Wallace, D. P. (2015). A brief primary care intervention to reduce fear of movement in chronic low back pain patients. *Translational Behavioral Medicine, 5*(1), 113–121.

Guo, Y., Qiu, P., & Liu, T. (2014). Tai Ji Quan: an overview of its history, health benefits, and cultural value. *Journal of Sport and Health Science, 3*(1), 3–8.

Hale, L. A., Waters, D., & Herbison, P. (2012). A randomized controlled trial to investigate the effects of water-based exercise to improve falls risk and physical function in older adults with lower-extremity osteoarthritis. *Archives of Physical Medicine and Rehabilitation, 93*(1), 27–34.

Halim-Kertanegara, S., Raymond, J., Hiller, C. E., Kilbreath, S. L., & Refshauge, K. M. (2017). The effect of ankle taping on functional performance in participants with functional ankle instability. *Physical Therapy in Sport, 23,* 162–167.

Hall, M. L., Mackie, A. C., & Ribeiro, D. C. (2018). Effects of dry needling trigger point therapy in the shoulder region on patients with upper extremity pain and dysfunction: a systematic review with meta-analysis. *Physiotherapy, 104*(2), 167–177.

Hando, B. R., Rhon, D. I., Cleland, J. A., & Snodgrass, S. J. (2019). Dry needling in addition to standard physical therapy treatment for sub-acromial pain syndrome: a randomized controlled trial protocol. *Brazilian Journal of Physical Therapy., 23*(4), 355–363.

Hanks, J., Levine, D., & Bockstahler, B. (2015). Physical agent modalities in physical therapy and rehabilitation of small animals. *Veterinary Clinics of North America: Small Animal Practice, 45,* 29–44.

Hanney, W. J., Kolber, M. J., & Beekhuizen, K. S. (2009). Implications for physical activity in the population with low back pain. *American Journal of Lifestyle Medicine, 3*(1), 63–70.

Harmer, P. A. (2014). So much research, so little application: Barriers to dissemination and practical implementation of Tai Ji Quan. *Journal of Sport and Health Science, 3*(1), 16–20.

Hartmann, D. (2016). An Alternative Physical Therapy Approach to the Overactive Pelvic Floor. In *The Overactive Pelvic Floor* (pp. 275–283). Cham, Switzerland: Springer.

Hauger, A. V., Reiman, M. P., Bjordal, J. M., Sheets, C., Ledbetter, L., & Goode, A. P. (2018). Neuromuscular electrical stimulation is effective in strengthening the quadriceps muscle after anterior cruciate ligament surgery. *Knee Surgery, Sports Traumatology, Arthroscopy, 26*(2), 399–410.

Henry, L. J., Paungmali, A., Mohan, V., & Ramli, A. (2016). Feldenkrais method and movement education – an alternate therapy in musculoskeletal rehabilitation. *Polish Annals of Medicine, 23*(1), 68–74.

Hillinger, M. G., Wolever, R. Q., McKernan, L. C., & Elam, R. (2017). Integrative Medicine for the Treatment of Persistent Pain. *Primary Care: Clinics in Office Practice, 44*(2), 247–264.

Hinman, R. (2014). Manual physiotherapy or exercise leads to sustained reductions in pain and physical disability in people with hip and knee osteoarthritis. *Journal of Physiotherapy, 60*(1), 56.

Hodgson, C. L., & Tipping, C. J. (2017). Physiotherapy management of intensive care unit-acquired weakness. *Journal of Physiotherapy, 63*(1), 4–10.

Hurley, D. A., Tully, M. A., Lonsdale, C., Boreham, C. A., van Mechelen, W., & Mc Donough, S. M. (2015). Supervised walking in comparison with fitness training for chronic back pain in physiotherapy: results of the SWIFT single blinded randomized controlled trial. *Pain, 156*(1), 131–147.

Jain, S. N., & Shukla, Y. U. (2017). Effect of goldfish exercise on pain, mouth opening and temporomandibular joint disability in oral submucous fibrosis: A randomized controlled trial. *International Journal of Therapies and Rehabilitation Research, 6*(2), 205–210.

Jayaseelan, D. J., Kecman, M., Alcorn, D., & Sault, J. D. (2017). Manual therapy and eccentric exercise in the management of Achilles tendinopathy. *Journal of Manual & Manipulative Therapy, 25*(2), 106–114.

Johnson, M. I., Claydon, L. S., Herbison, G. P., Paley, C. A., & Jones, G. (2017). Transcutaneous electrical nerve stimulation (TENS) for fibromyalgia in adults. *Cochrane Database of Systematic Reviews, 10*(10), CD012172.

Jones, I., & Johnson, M. I. (2009). Transcutaneous electrical nerve stimulation. *Continuing Education in Anaesthesia, Critical Care & Pain, 9*(4), 130–135.

Jones, K. D., Sherman, C. A., Mist, S. D., Carson, J. W., Bennett, R. M., & Li, F. (2012). A randomized controlled trial of 8-form Tai chi improves symptoms and functional mobility in fibromyalgia patients. *Clinical Rheumatology, 31*(8), 1205–1214.

Josephs, S., Pratt, M. L., Meadows, E. C., Thurmond, S., & Wagner, A. (2016). The effectiveness of Pilates on balance and falls in community dwelling older adults. *Journal of Bodywork and Movement Therapies, 20*(4), 815–823.

Ju, T., Choi, W., Yang, Y., & Lee, S. (2015). Effects of Hip Mobilization on Pain and Function for Chronic Low Back Pain Individuals with Limited Range of Hip Joint Motion. *Indian Journal of Science and Technology, 8*(26), 1–6.

Juhl, C., Christensen, R., Roos, E. M., Zhang, W., & Lund, H. (2014). Impact of Exercise Type and Dose on Pain and Disability in Knee Osteoarthritis: A Systematic Review and Meta-Regression Analysis of Randomized Controlled Trials. *Arthritis & Rheumatology, 66*(3), 622–636.

Keane, L. G. (2017). Comparing AquaStretch with supervised land based stretching for chronic back pain. *Journal of Bodywork & Movement Therapies, 21*(2), 297–305.

Keosaian, J. E., Lemaster, C. M., Dresner, D., Godersky, M. E., Paris, R., Sherman, K. J., & Saper, R. B. (2016). "We're all in this together": A qualitative study of predominantly low income minority participants in a yoga trial for chronic low back pain. *Complementary Therapies in Medicine, 24*(1), 34–39.

Knauf, M., & Koltyn, K. F. (2014). Exercise-induced modulation of pain in adults with and without painful diabetic neuropathy. *The Journal of Pain, 15*(6), 656–663.

Koltyn, K. F., Brellenthin, A. G., Cook, D. B., Sehgal, N., & Hillard, C. (2014). Mechanisms of exercise-induced hypoalgesia. *The Journal of Pain, 15*(12), 1294–1304.

Kong, L. J., Lauche, R., Klose, P., Bu, J. H., Yang, X. C., Guo, C. Q., ... Cheng, Y. W. (2016). Tai chi for chronic pain conditions: a systematic review and meta-analysis of randomized controlled trials. *Scientific Reports, 6.* https://doi.org/10.1038/srep25325.

Koppenhaver, S. L., Walker, M. J., Rettig, C., Davis, J., Nelson, C., Su, J., ... Hebert, J. J. (2017). The association between dry needling-induced twitch response and change in pain and muscle function in patients with low back pain: a quasi-experimental study. *Physiotherapy, 103*(2), 131–137.

Krampe, J., Wagner, J. M., Hawthorne, K., Sanazaro, D., Wong-Anuchit, C., & Raaf, S. (2014). Does dance-based therapy increase gait speed in older adults with chronic lower extremity pain: A feasibility study. *Geriatric Nursing, 35*(5), 339–344.

Kroska, E. B. (2016). A meta-analysis of fear-avoidance and pain intensity: the paradox of chronic pain. *Scandinavian Journal of Pain, 13*(1), 43–58.

Küçükçakır, N., Altan, L., & Korkmaz, N. (2013). Effects of Pilates exercises on pain, functional status and quality of life in women with postmenopausal osteoporosis. *Journal of Bodywork and Movement Therapies, 17*(2), 204–211.

Lambert, B. S., Shimkus, K. L., Fluckey, J. D., Riechman, S. E., Greene, N. P., Cardin, J. M., & Crouse, S. F. (2015). Anabolic responses to acute and chronic resistance exercise are enhanced when combined with aquatic treadmill exercise. *American Journal of Physiology-Endocrinology and Metabolism*, 308(3), E192–E200.

Langhorst, J., Klose, P., Dobos, G. J., Bernardy, K., & Häuser, W. (2013). Efficacy and safety of meditative movement therapies in fibromyalgia syndrome: a systematic review and meta-analysis of randomized controlled trials. *Rheumatology International*, 33(1), 193–207.

Laubenstein, S., & Beissner, K. (2016). Exercise and movement-based therapies in geriatric pain management. *Clinics Geriatric Medicine*, 32(4), 737–762.

Lauche, R., Langhorst, J., Dobos, G., & Cramer, H. (2013). A systematic review and meta-analysis of Tai Chi for osteoarthritis of the knee. *Complementary Therapies in Medicine*, 21(4), 396–406.

Lederman, E. (2014). Pain management and ROM desensitization. In *Therapeutic Stretching* (pp. 127–151). London: Churchill Livingston.

Lee, M., Moon, W., & Kim, J. (2014). Effect of yoga on pain, brain-derived neurotrophic factor, and serotonin in premenopausal women with chronic low back pain. *Evidence-Based Complementary and Alternative Medicine*. https://doi.org/10.1155/2014/203173.

Lethem, J., Slade, P. D., Troup, J. D. G., & Bentley, G. (1983). Outline of a fear-avoidance model of exaggerated pain perception – 1. *Behaviour Research Therapy*, 21(4), 401–408.

Levy, C. E., Silverman, E., Jia, H., Geiss, M., David Omura, D. P. T., & A, M. H. (2015). Effects of physical therapy delivery via home video telerehabilitation on functional and health-related quality of life outcomes. *Journal of Rehabilitation Research and Development*, 52(3), 361–370.

Lin, S., Lu, X., Chen, S., Ye, F., Zhang, J., Ma, Y., & Li, J. (2012). Human coronary collateral recruitment is facilitated by isometric exercise during acute coronary occlusion. *Journal of Rehabilitation Medicine*, 44(8), 691–695.

Liu, R., Guo, X., Lao, T. T., & Little, T. (2017). A critical review on compression textiles for compression therapy: Textile-based compression interventions for chronic venous insufficiency. *Textile Research Journal*, 87(9), 1121–1141.

Louw, A., Puentedura, E. J., & Diener, I. (2016). A descriptive study of the utilization of physical therapy for postoperative rehabilitation in patients undergoing surgery for lumbar radiculopathy. *European Spine Journal*, 25(11), 3550–3559.

Louw, A., Puentedura, E. J., Reese, D., Parker, P., Miller, T., & Mintken, P. E. (2017). Immediate effects of mirror therapy in patients with shoulder pain and decreased range of motion. *Archives of Physical Medicine and Rehabilitation*, 98(10), 1941–1947. https://doi.org/10.1016/j.apmr.2017.03.031.

Macdermid, P. W., Fink, P. W., & Stannard, S. R. (2015). Shock attenuation, spatio-temporal and physiological parameter comparisons between land treadmill and water treadmill running. *Journal of Sport and Health Science*, 6(4), 482–488.

Madson, T. J., & Hollman, J. H. (2015). Lumbar traction for managing low back pain: a survey of physical therapists in the United States. *Journal of Orthopaedic & Sports Physical Therapy*, 45(8), 586–595.

Mansell, N. S., Rhon, D. I., Marchant, B. G., Slevin, J. M., & Meyer, J. L. (2016). Two-year outcomes after arthroscopic surgery compared to physical therapy for femoroacetabular impingement: a protocol for a randomized clinical trial. *BMC Musculoskeletal Disorders*, 17(1), 60–69.

Marinko, L. N., Chacko, J. M., Dalton, D., & Chacko, C. C. (2011). The effectiveness of therapeutic exercise for painful shoulder conditions: a meta-analysis. *Journal of Shoulder and Elbow Surgery*, 20(8), 1351–1359.

Marshall, P. W., Kennedy, S., Brooks, C., & Lonsdale, C. (2013). Pilates exercise or stationary cycling for chronic nonspecific low back pain: does it matter? A randomized controlled trial with 6-month follow-up. *Spine*, 38(15), E952–E959.

Mayer, T. G., Gatchel, R. J., Brede, E., & Theodore, B. R. (2014). Lumbar surgery in work-related chronic low back pain: can a continuum of care enhance outcomes? *The Spine Journal*, 14(2), 263–273.

Morihisa, R., Eskew, J., McNamara, A., & Young, J. (2016). Dry needling in subjects with muscular trigger points in the lower quarter: a systematic review. *International Journal of Sports Physical Therapy*, 11(1), 1.

Mostagi, F. Q. R. C., Dias, J. M., Pereira, L. M., Obara, K., Mazuquin, B. F., Silva, M. F., ... Lima, T. B. (2015). Pilates versus general exercise effectiveness on pain and functionality in non-specific chronic low back pain subjects. *Journal of Bodywork and Movement Therapies*, 19(4), 636–645.

McNeil, W. (2017). The movement. *Journal of Bodywork & Movement Therapies*, 21(3), 725–730.

McNeil, W., & Blandford, L. (2015). Movement health. *Journal of Bodywork & Movement*, 19(1), 150–159.

Medeiros, D. M., & Lima, C. S. (2017). Influence of chronic stretching on muscle performance: Systematic review. *Human Movement Science*, 54, 220–229.

Meulders, A., Meulders, M., & Vlaeyen, J. W. S. (2014). Positive effect protects against deficient safety learning during extinction of fear of movement-related pain in healthy individuals scoring relatively high on trait anxiety. *The Journal of Pain*, 15(6), 632–644.

Meulders, A., Vandael, K., & Vlaeyen, J. W. S. (2017). Generalization of pain-related fear based on conceptual knowledge. *Behavior Therapy*, 48(3), 295–310.

Meulders, A., Karsdorp, P. A., Claes, N., & Vlaeyen, J. W. S. (2015). Comparing counterconditioning and extinction as methods to reduce fear of movement-related pain. *The Journal of Pain*, 16(12), 1353–1365.

Middleton, K. R., López, M. M., Moonaz, S. H., Tataw-Ayuketah, G., Ward, M. M., & Wallen, G. R. (2017). A qualitative approach exploring the acceptability of yoga for minorities living with arthritis: 'Where are the people who look like me?'. *Complementary Therapies in Medicine*, 31, 82–89.

Mohan, V., Paungmali, A., Sitilertpisan, P., Henry, L. J., & Mohamad, N. B. (2017). Feldenkrais method on neck and low back pain to the type of exercises and outcome measurement tools: A systematic review. *Polish Annals of Medicine*, 24(1), 77–83.

Naugle, K. M., Naugle, K. E., & Riley, J. L. (2016). Reduced Modulation of Pain in Older Adults After Isometric and Aerobic Exercise. *The Journal of Pain*, 17(6), 719–728.

Naugle, K. M., Naugle, K. E., Fillingim, R. B., & Riley, J. L., 3rd. (2014). Isometric exercise as a test of pain modulation: effects of experimental pain test, psychological variables, and sex. *Pain Medicine*, 15(4), 692–701.

Nelson, N. L. (2016). Kinesio taping for chronic low back pain: A systematic review. *Journal of Bodywork and Movement Therapies*, 20(3), 672–681.

Nijs, J., Girbés, E. L., Lundberg, M., Malfliet, A., & Sterling, M. (2015). Exercise therapy for chronic musculoskeletal pain: innovation by altering pain memories. *Manual Therapy, 20*(1), 216–220.

North, R. B., & Prager, J. P. (2018). History of spinal cord stimulation. In E. S. Krames, P. H. Peckham, & A. R. Rezai (Eds.), *Neuromodulation: Comprehensive Textbook of Principles, Technologies, and Therapies* (2nd Ed, pp. 587–596). London: Elsevier.

O'Connor, D., Caulfield, B., & Lennon, O. (2018). The efficacy and prescription of neuromuscular electrical stimulation (NMES) in adult cancer survivors: a systematic review and meta-analysis. *Supportive Care in Cancer*, 1–16.

O'Connor, S. R., Tully, M. A., Ryan, B., Bleakley, C. M., Baxter, G. D., & McDonough. (2015). Walking exercise for chronic musculoskeletal pain: systematic review and meta-analysis. *Archives of Physical Medicine and Rehabilitation, 96*(4), 724–734.e3.

Oksuz, S., & Unal, E. (2017). The effects of the clinical Pilates exercises on kinesiophobia and other symptoms related to osteoporosis: randomized control trial. *Complementary Therapies in Clinical Practice, 26*(1), 68–72.

Olson, D. A., Kolber, M. J., Patel, C., Pabian, P., & Hanney, W. J. (2013). Aquatic exercise for treatment of low-back pain: a systematic review of randomized controlled trials. *American Journal of Lifestyle Medicine, 7*(2), 154–160.

Ochalek, K., Gradalski, T., & Szygula, Z. (2015). Five-year assessment of maintenance combined physical therapy in postmastectomy lymphedema. *Lymphatic Research and Biology, 13*(1), 54–58.

Ochalek, K., Pacyga, K., Curyło, M., Frydrych-Szymonik, A., & Szygula, Z. (2017). Risk Factors Related to Lower Limb Edema, Compression, and Physical Activity During Pregnancy: A Retrospective Study. *Lymphatic Research and Biology, 15*(2), 166–171.

Pagliarulo, M. A. (2012). Physical therapy for musculoskeletal conditions. In *Introduction to Physical Therapy* (4th Ed, pp. 170–212). St. Louis, MO: Mosby.

Pangarkar, S., & Lee, P. C. (2011). Conservative treatment for neck pain: medications, physical therapy, and exercise. *Physical Medicine and Rehabilitation Clinics, 22*(3), 503–520.

Parreira, P. D. C. S., Costa, L. D. C. M., Junior, L. C. H., Lopes, A. D., & Costa, L. O. P. (2014). Current evidence does not support the use of Kinesio Taping in clinical practice: a systematic review. *Journal of Physiotherapy, 60*(1), 31–39.

Patrick, N., Emanski, E., & Knaub, M. A. (2014). Acute and chronic low back pain. *Medical Clinics, 98*(4), 777–789.

Patti, A., Bianco, A., Paoli, A., Messina, G., Montalto, M. A., Bellafiore, M., ... Palma, A. (2016). Pain perception and stabilometric parameters in people with chronic low back pain after a Pilates exercise program: a randomized controlled trial. *Medicine, 95*(2), e2414.

Perry, E. V., & Francis, A. J. P. (2013). Self-efficacy, pain-related fear, and disability in a heterogeneous pain sample. *Pain Management Nursing, 14*(14), e124–e134.

Qaseem, A., Wilt, T. J., McLean, R. M., & Forciea, M. A. (2017). Noninvasive treatments for acute, subacute, and chronic low back pain: a clinical practice guideline from the American College of Physicians. *Annals of Internal Medicine, 166*(7), 514–530.

Rajkannan, P., & Vijayaraghavan, R. (2019). Dry needling in chronic abdominal wall pain of uncertain origin. *Journal of Bodywork and Movement Therapies, 23*(1), 94–98.

Rewald, S., Mesters, I., Lenssen, A. F., Bansi, J., Lambeck, J., de Bie, R. A., & Waller, B. (2017). Aquatic cycling—What do we know? A scoping review on head-out aquatic cycling. *PloS One, 12*(5), e0177704.

Rio, E., Kidgell, D., Purdam, C., Gaida, J., Moseley, G. M., & Cook, J. (2015). Isometric exercise induces analgesia and reduces inhibition in patellar tendinopathy. *British Journal of Sports Medicine, 49*(5), 1277–1283.

Rockson, S. G. (2018). Intermittent Pneumatic Compression Therapy. In *Lymphedema* (pp. 443–448). Cham, Switzerland: Springer.

Roelofs, J., van Breukelen, G., Sluiter, J., Frings-Dresen, M. H. W., Gossens, M., & Vlaeyen, J. W. S. (2011). Norming of the Tampa Scale for Kinesiophobia across pain diagnosis and various countries. *Pain, 152*(5), 1090–1095.

Roper, J. A., Bressel, E., & Tillman, M. D. (2013). Acute aquatic treadmill exercise improves gait and pain in people with knee osteoarthritis. *Archives of Physical Medicine and Rehabilitation, 94*(3), 419–425.

Safa'ah, N., & Srimurayani, I. D. (2017). Effectiveness of Isometric and Range of Motion (ROM) Exercise Toward Elderly Muscle Strength in Pasuruan Integrated Service Unit, Elderly Social Services in Lamongan. *Biomedical Engineering, 3*(1), 7–15.

Santana, L. S., Gallo, R. B. S., Ferreira, C. H. J., Duarte, G., Quintana, S. M., & Marcolin, A. C. (2016). Transcutaneous electrical nerve stimulation (TENS) reduces pain and postpones the need for pharmacological analgesia during labour: a randomised trial. *Journal of Physiotherapy, 62*(1), 29–34.

Segura-Jiménez, V., Gatto-Cardia, C. M., Martins-Pereira, C. M., Delgado-Ferández, M., Aparicio, V. A., & Carbonell-Baeza, A. (2017). Biodanza reduces acute pain severity in women with fibromyalgia. *Pain Management Nursing, 18*(5), 318–327.

Shanahan, J., Morris, M. E., Bhriain, O. N., Saunders, J., & Clifford, A. M. (2015). Dance for people with Parkinson disease: What is the evidence telling us? *Archives of Physical Medicine and Rehabilitation, 96*(2), 141–153.

Shim, M. (2015). *A Model of Dance/Movement for Resilience-building in People Living with Chronic Pain: A Mixed Methods Grounded Theory Study*. Philadelphia, PA: Dissertation Submitted to Drexel University.

Shim, M., Johnson, R. B., Gasson, S., Goodill, S., Jermyn, R., & Bradt, J. (2017). A model of dance/movement therapy for resilience-building in people living with chronic pain. *European Journal of Integrative Medicine, 9*(1), 27–40.

Sluka, K. A., Bjordal, J. M., Marchand, S., & Rakel, B. A. (2013). What makes transcutaneous electrical nerve stimulation work? Making sense of the mixed results in the clinical literature. *Physical Therapy, 93*(10), 1397–1402.

Smith, A., Ritchie, C., Pedler, A., McCamley, K., Roberts, K., & Sterling, M. (2017). Exercise induced hypoalgesia is elicited by isometric, but not aerobic exercise in individuals with chronic whiplash associated disorders. *Scandinavian Journal of Pain, 15*(1), 14–21.

Søgaard, K., & Jull, G. (2015). Therapeutic exercise for prevention, treatment and rehabilitation of musculoskeletal pain and function. *Manual Therapy, 20*(5), 631–632.

Sorour, A. S., Ayoub, A. S., & Abd El Aziz, E. M. (2014). Effectiveness of acupressure versus isometric exercise on pain, stiffness, and physical function in knee osteoarthritis female patients. *Journal of Advanced Research, 5*(2), 193–200.

Springer, K. S., George, S. Z., & Robinson, M. E. (2016). The development of a technology-based hierarchy to assess chronic low back pain and pain-related anxiety from a fear-avoidance model. *The Journal of Pain*, 17(8), 904–910.

Stein, K. M., Weinberg, J., Sherman, K. J., Lemaster, C. M., & Saper, R. (2014). Participant Characteristics Associated with Symptomatic Improvement from Yoga for Chronic Low Back Pain. *Journal of Yoga & Physical Therapy*, 4(1), 151. https://doi.org/10.4172/2157-7595.1000151.

Stringer, M. (2015). Structured dance as a healing modality for women. *Journal of Obstetrics and Gynecological & Neonatal Nursing*, 44(4), 459–461.

Sutton, D. A., Côté, P., Wong, J. J., Varatharajan, S., Randhawa, K. A., Yu, H., ... Carroll, L. J. (2016). Is multimodal care effective for the management of patients with whiplash-associated disorders or neck pain and associated disorders? A systematic review by the Ontario Protocol for Traffic Injury Management (OPTIMa) Collaboration. *The Spine Journal*, 16(12), 1541–1565.

Szuba, Ł., Markowska, I., Czamara, A., & Noga, H. (2016). Quantitative analysis of peak torque and power–velocity characteristics of shoulder rotator muscles after arthroscopic labral repair. *Journal of Science and Medicine in Sport*, 19(10), 805–809.

Tartaglia, M. (2014). Using dance in hand therapy. In *Fundamentals of Hand Therapy* (2nd Edition, pp. 189–191). St. Louis, MO: Elsevier.

Thackeray, A., Fritz, J. M., Childs, J. D., & Brennan, G. P. (2016). The effectiveness of mechanical traction among subgroups of patients with low back pain and leg pain: a randomized trial. *Journal of Orthopaedic & Sports Physical Therapy*, 46(3), 144–154.

Thoren, P., Floras, J. S., Hoffman, P., & Seals, D. R. (1990). Endorphins and exercise: Physiological mechanisms and clinical implications. *Medicine & Science in Sports & Exercise*, 22(4), 417-428.

Tkachuk, G. A., & Harris, C. A. (2012). Psychometric properties of the Tampa Scale for Kinesiophobia-11. *The Journal of Pain*, 13(10), 970–977.

Tranquille, C. A., Nankervis, K. J., Walker, V. A., Tacey, J. B., & Murray, R. C. (2016). Current knowledge of equine water treadmill exercise: what can we learn from human and canine studies. *Journal of Equine Veterinary Science*, 50(1), 76–83.

Tsai, P. F., Chang, J. Y., Beck, C., Kuo, Y. F., Keefe, F. J., & Rosengren, K. (2015). A supplemental report to a randomized cluster trial of a 20-week Sun-style Tai Chi for osteoarthritic knee pain in elders with cognitive impairment. *Complementary Therapies in Medicine*, 23(4), 570–576.

Umeda, M., Corbin, L. W., & Maluf, K. S. (2015). Examination of contraction-induced muscle pain as a behavioral correlate of physical activity in women with and without fibromyalgia. *Disability and Rehabilitation*, 37(20), 1864–1869.

Vaegter, H. B. (2017). Exercising non-painful muscles can induce hypoalgesia in individuals with chronic pain. *Scandinavian Journal of Pain*, 15(1), 60–61.

Van Straaten, M. G., Cloud, B. A., Morrow, M. M., Ludewig, P. M., & Zhao, K. D. (2014). Effectiveness of home exercise on pain, function, and strength of manual wheelchair users with spinal cord injury: a high-dose shoulder program with telerehabilitation. *Archives of Physical Medicine and Rehabilitation*, 95(10), 1810–1817.

Vanti, C., Bertozzi, L., Gardenghi, I., Turoni, F., Guccione, A. A., & Pillastrini, P. (2015). Effect of taping on spinal pain and disability: systematic review and meta-analysis of randomized trials. *Physical Therapy*, 95(4), 493–506.

Vier, C., de Almeida, M. B., Neves, M. L., dos Santos, A. R. S., & Bracht, M. A. (2019). The effectiveness of dry needling for patients with orofacial pain associated with temporomandibular dysfunction: a systematic review and meta-analysis. *Brazilian Journal of Physical Therapy.*, 23(10), 3–11.

Voogt, L., de Vries, J., Meeus, M., Struyf, F., Meuffels, D., & Nijs, J. (2015). Analgesic effects of manual therapy in patients with musculoskeletal pain: a systematic review. *Manual Therapy*, 20(2), 250–256.

Voon, K., Silberstein, I., Eranki, A., Phillips, M., Wood, F. M., & Edgar, D. W. (2016). Xbox Kinect ™ based rehabilitation as a feasible adjunct for minor upper limb burns rehabilitation: a pilot RCT. *Burns*, 42(8), 1797–1804.

Waddington, E. A., Fuller, R. K. R., Barloon, R. C., Comiskey, G. H., Portz, J. D., Holmquist-Johnson, H., & Schmid, A. A. (2017). Staff perspectives regarding the implementation of a yoga intervention with chronic pain self-management in a clinical setting. *Complementary Therapies in Clinical Practice*, 26, 12–20.

Wahl, P., Sanno, M., Ellenberg, K., Frick, H., Böhm, E., Haiduck, B., ... Bloch, W. (2017). Aqua Cycling Does Not Affect Recovery of Performance, Damage Markers, and Sensation of Pain. *The Journal of Strength & Conditioning Research*, 31(1), 162–170.

Wall, P. D., & Sweet, W. H. (1967). Temporary abolition of pain in man. *Science*, 155(3758), 108–109.

Waller, B., Ogonowska-Slodownik, A., Vitor, M., Lambeck, J., Daly, D., Kujala, U. M., & Heinonen, A. (2014). Effect of therapeutic aquatic exercise on symptoms and function associated with lower limb osteoarthritis: systematic review with meta-analysis. *Physical Therapy*, 94(10), 1383–1395.

Wang, C., Schmid, C. H., Iversen, M. D., Harvey, W. F., Fielding, R. A., Driban, J. B., ... McAlindon, T. (2015). Comparative Effectiveness of Tai Chi Versus Physical Therapy for Knee Osteoarthritis. *Annals of Internal Medicine*, 165(2), 77–86.

Ward, L., Stebbings, S., Cherkin, D., & Baxter, G. D. (2013). Yoga for Functional Ability, Pain and Psychosocial Outcomes in Musculoskeletal Conditions: A Systematic Review and Meta-Analysis. *Musculoskeletal Care*, 11(4), 203–217.

Wasser, J. G., Vasilopoulos, T., Zdziarski, L. A., & Vincent, H. K. (2017). Exercise Benefits for Chronic Low Back Pain in Overweight and Obese Individuals. *PM&R*, 9(2), 181–192.

Wayne, P. M., Berkowitz, D. L., Litrownik, D. E., Buring, J. E., & Yeh, G. Y. (2014). What do we really know about the safety of tai chi? A systematic review of adverse event reports in randomized trials. *Archives of Physical Medicine and Rehabilitation*, 95(12), 2470–2483.

Wayne, P. M., Manor, B., Novak, V., Costa, M. D., Hausdorff, J. M., Goldberger, A. L., ... Davis, R. B. (2013). A systems biology approach to studying Tai Chi, physiological complexity and healthy aging: design and rationale of a pragmatic randomized controlled trial. *Contemporary Clinical Trials*, 34(1), 21–34.

Welling, A. (2015). *Where do dance/movement therapists work? What do they do? American Dance Therapy Association.* https://adta.org/2015/01/13/where-do-dancemovement-therapists-work-what-do-they-do/. Retrieved 07/16/2017.

Wells, C., Kolt, G. S., & Bialocerkoski, A. (2012). Defining Pilates exercise: A systematic review. *Complementary Therapies in Medicine, 20*(4), 253–262.

Wells, C., Kolt, G. S., Marshall, P., Hill, B., & Bialocerkowski, A. (2014). The effectiveness of Pilates exercise in people with chronic low back pain: a systematic review. *Plos One, 9*(7), e100402.

Werti, M. M. (2014). *Prognosis of clinical pain conditions: The example of complex regional pain syndrome1 and low back pain.* Datawyse | Universitaire Pers Maastricht: Amsterdam Production.

Werti, M. M., Rasmussen-Barr, E., Held, U., Weiser, S., Bachmann, L. M., & Brunner, F. (2014). Fear avoidance beliefs-a moderator of treatment efficacy in patients with low back pain: A systematic review. *The Spine Journal, 14*(11), 2658–2678.

Woby, S. R., Roach, N. K., Urmston, M., & Watson, P. J. (2005). Psychometric properties of the TSK- 11: A shortened version of the Tampa Scale for Kinesiophobia. *Pain, 117*(1–2), 137–144. https://doi.org/10.1016/j.pain.2005.05.029.

Wu, P. I.-K., Meleger, A., Witkower, A., Mondale, T., & Borg-Stein, J. (2015). Nonpharmacologic options for treating acute and chronic pain. *Physical Medicine & Rehabilitation, 7*(11), S278–S294.

Yamany, A., & Hamdy, B. (2016). Effect of sequential pneumatic compression therapy on venous blood velocity, refilling time, pain and quality of life in women with varicose veins: a randomized control study. *Journal of Physical Therapy Science, 28*(7), 1981–1987.

Yamato, T. P., Maher, C. G., Saragiotto, B. T., Hancock, M. J., Ostelo, R. W., Cabral, C. M., ... Costa, L. O. (2015). Pilates for low back pain. *Cochrane Database of Systematic Reviews,* (7).

Yan, J. H., Gu, W. J., Sun, J., Zhang, W. X., Li, B. W., & Pan, L. (2013). Efficacy of Tai Chi on pain, stiffness and function in patients with osteoarthritis: a meta-analysis. *PloS One, 8*(4), e61672.

Yılmaz, E., Karakaya, E., Baydur, H., & Tekin, İ. (2018). Effect of Transcutaneous Electrical Nerve Stimulation on Postoperative Pain and Patient Satisfaction. *Pain Management Nursing., 25*(4), 276–280.

Zale, E. L., Lange, K. L., Fields, S. A., & Ditre, J. W. (2013). The relation between pain-related fear and disability a meta-analysis. *The Journal of Pain, 14*(10), 1019–1030.

Zeng, C., Yang, T., Deng, Z. H., Yang, Y., Zhang, Y., & Lei, G. H. (2015). Electrical stimulation for pain relief in knee osteoarthritis: systematic review and network meta-analysis. *Osteoarthritis and Cartilage, 23*(2), 189–202.

Zdziarski, L. A., Wasser, J. G., & Vincent, H. K. (2015). Chronic pain management in the obese patient: a focused review of key challenges and potential exercise solutions. *Journal of Pain Research, 8*(1), 63.

Zhang, F. (2014). Tai chi as a potentially effective treatment for neck pain. *Journal of the Formosan Medical Association, 113*(4), 199–200.

Ziaeifar, M., Arab, A. M., Mosallanezhad, Z., & Nourbakhsh, M. R. (2018). Dry needling versus trigger point compression of the upper trapezius: a randomized clinical trial with two-week and three-month follow-up. *Journal of Manual & Manipulative Therapy,* 1–10.

Chapter 21 Distraction and Relaxation

Michele Erich, Ann Quinlan-Colwell, Susan O'Conner-Von

CHAPTER OUTLINE

Distraction, pg. 586

Types of Distraction, pg. 587

Humor, pg. 587

Art, Coloring, Drawing, and Doodling, pg. 588

Electronic Games, pg. 589

Virtual Reality and Immersion or Immersive Virtual Reality, pg. 589

Relaxation, pg. 591

Breathing Activities, pg. 592

Types of Relaxation Breathing, pg. 592

Evidence and Indications for Pain Management, pg. 593

Cautions, pg. 593

Progressive Muscle Relaxation, pg. 594

Evidence and Indications for Pain Management, pg. 595

Cautions, pg. 596

Music Therapy, pg. 596

Music Therapy as a Profession, pg. 597

Music Therapy and Multimodal Pain Management, pg. 598

Indications Using Music for Pain Control, pg. 598

Evidence and Indications for Pain Management, pg. 599

Concerns, Cautions, and Contraindications, pg. 600

Animal-Assisted Therapy, pg. 600

Definitions, pg. 600

Indications for Animal-Assisted Therapy and Animal-Assisted Activity, pg. 600

Evidence and Indications for Pain Management, pg. 601

Cautions, pg. 603

Guided Imagery, pg. 603

Evidence and Indications for Pain Management, pg. 603

Cautions and Contraindications, pg. 604

Autogenic Training, pg. 604

Evidence and Indications for Pain Management, pg. 604

Contraindications, pg. 605

Key Points, pg. 605

Case Scenario, pg. 605

References, pg. 606

IN this chapter the use of distraction and relaxation as ways to manage or control pain will be explored. The strong interrelationship of the cognitive, emotional, and physical aspects of a person are the foundation supporting the use of these techniques as one component of a multimodal approach to managing acute and chronic pain (Foji, Tadayonfar, Mohsenpour, & Rakhshani, 2015). By using various techniques and interventions, patients can actively participate in controlling acute or chronic pain both during hospitalization and when at home. In situations in which it is available, information about the relationship between the technique and nociception will be discussed. From a pain management perspective, it is difficult to separate techniques into distraction and relaxation because the two conditions often overlap. Because relaxation is often considered to be a method of distraction (McBain, Mulligan, & Newman, 2015), it will be discussed as such in this chapter. Although the interventions are described in isolation, the techniques can often be combined with each other, with other nonpharmacologic interventions, and with medications in a multimodal approach to optimally manage pain.

Distraction

Distraction is a pain management coping strategy that works by shifting conscious attention or focus in a direction different from the noxious stimuli (i.e., perception of pain), and by doing so the impact of pain is perceived to be less (Moore, Stewart, Barnes-Holmes, Barnes-Holmes, & McGuire, 2015; Subnis, Starkweather, & Menzies, 2016). Attention can be focused either internally (e.g., tensing and relaxing muscles) or externally (e.g., concentrating on a picture or sound). Distraction techniques facilitate analgesia by reducing perception of pain and decreasing cerebral pain-related stimulation through the release of endogenous opioids and other electrophysiologic changes (Subnis et al., 2016). The immediate benefit of distraction is better documented in the literature than what may be the potential benefit over time (Armfield & Marek, 2017). An interesting quality of distraction and relaxation therapies is that in addition to helping control pain, they can simultaneously benefit an assortment of other symptoms that are often related to pain, such as anxiety, fatigue, insomnia, and nausea, and can achieve the benefit with no untoward side effects (Kwekkeboom, 2016).

Types of Distraction

Distraction is a nonpharmacologic pain intervention that can be undertaken either actively or passively. *Active distraction* involves interaction by the participant in an activity such as art, puzzles, electronic devices, games, virtual reality, or relaxation measures (Czarnecki et al., 2011; Elmali & Akpinar, 2017). A simple example of active distraction is the "cough trick" used for venipuncture or cannulation. The person is instructed to inhale deeply and cough twice while keeping arms motionless, causing a Valsalva maneuver, with the venous insertion occurring during the second cough (Boerner et al., 2015) (see Chapter 27 for more discussion on this technique). *Passive distraction* involves less active participation, such as occurs with watching television, viewing movies, listening to the radio, or listening to music (Czarnecki et al., 2011; Elmali & Akpinar, 2017).

Evidence and Indications for Pain Management

Although most of the literature and research regarding distraction to control pain is done with children rather than with adults, researchers conducted a phenomenologic study with seven adults receiving wound care for burns (Boluda et al., 2016). In that study, the participants reported distraction was the most consistent method of pain control they used. The researchers of that study added that it was possible an additional component of the overall positive effect of distraction was the caring relationship the nurses shared with the patients. The importance of interpersonal involvement with distraction was also seen in findings reported from a Canadian study (n = 98) involving patients who underwent minor surgery with regional analgesia who were randomized into four groups: standard of care (SOC), distraction with a mobile phone game, text messaging a companion, and text massaging a stranger (Guillory, Hancock, Woodruff, & Keilman, 2015). Those participants who text messaged a stranger used more positive words and were nearly seven times (6.77) less likely to use as much analgesia as those in the SOC group. Those who text messaged a companion used more anatomic words and were a little more than

four times (4.39) less likely to use as much analgesia as those in the SOC group. The patients who used the mobile phone for a game were nearly twice (1.96) as likely to use less analgesia as those in the SOC group. All distraction methods were to some degree effective, but the methods involving interpersonal interaction were more effective, and, interestingly, those in which there was positive language with strangers were most effective. Further research with distraction and distraction in combination with interpersonal involvement with family, friends, professionals, and strangers is warranted.

Humor

Humor as a coping skill is also called *coping humor* and is the attribute of having the inclination to use humor as a technique to cope with situations that are challenging, difficult, or stressful (Sliter, Kale, & Yuan, 2014). Several humor styles can be used in a variety of ways ranging from positive and helpful to hostile (i.e., sarcasm or ridiculing others), self-defeating, and maladaptive (Rnic, Dozois, & Martin, 2016). Humor is an emotion-oriented coping technique that can be used to normalize emotional or stressful situations by altering and reconsidering stressors but can also be used to avoid dealing with stressors (Ito & Matsushima, 2017).

Using humor as a positive coping technique to help control and deal with pain is not a new concept. In the 14th century a French physician named Henri de Mondeville distracted his patients during surgery by using humor and later used it as method to facilitate recovery (Savage, Lujan, Thipparthi, & DiCarlo, 2017). Freud suggested humor may be the most effective of all coping techniques (Freud, 1960; Sliter et al., 2014). Perhaps the most well-known use of humor was immortalized by Norman Cousins. While hospitalized with intractable pain, Cousins wrote:

"I made the joyous discovery that ten minutes of genuine belly laughter had an anesthetic effect and would give me at least two hours of pain-free sleep. When the pain-killing effect of the laughter wore off, we would switch on the motion picture projector again, and, not infrequently, it would lead to another pain-free sleep interval." (Cousins, 1979, p. 39).

Evidence and Indications for Pain Management

It is thought that physiologic processes, including reduction of cortisol and catecholamines combined with the increase in endorphins, support the analgesic benefit of humor as a buffer to stress and promote relaxation (Savage et al., 2017; Sliter et al., 2014). In addition, exposure to humor as well as a keen appreciation of humor are correlated with having increased thresholds and tolerance of pain (Proyer & Wolf, 2017). Through six experimental studies, during which participants either watched comedic videos in a laboratory setting or watched comedic theater performances, researchers concluded that pain thresholds and pain tolerance are significantly higher after laughter (Dunbar et al., 2011). Those researchers attributed the increased ability to manage pain to the release of endorphins. In addition, laughter comprises an involuntary neuroanatomic pathway that includes the amygdala, thalamus, and hypothalamus parts of the brain (Woodbury-Fariña & Antongiorgi, 2014), which are also involved in pain perception and modulation.

Cautions

Caution cannot be thrown to the wind when considering humor as a distraction for pain. There are at least two important pitfalls to consider. First, it is important to remember many people use humor to cope with various stressful situations, including challenges of aging (Berk, 2015), work-related stress (Berk, 2015; Sliter et al., 2014), and pain (Cousins, 1979). As a result, patients may be using humor as a coping mechanism while experiencing significant pain. When doing so, the self-report of pain intensity should not be disbelieved because the body language and behavior of the person are inconsistent with the report of pain by the person. It is important to remember that pain-related behaviors and use of coping mechanisms are unique for each person. As described in Chapters 2, 4, and 8, behaviors may be influenced by the type of pain, previous experiences with pain, cultural background, and a variety of other factors, including using humor to cope with pain. Second, when using humor with patients it is important to remember humor is perceived both individually and culturally; therefore it is important to use humor that will not offend the person, the person's family, or others who may be exposed to it.

Art, Coloring, Drawing, and Doodling

Art, drawing, and coloring are anecdotally encouraged by clinicians to help distract and soothe patients with pain (Pritham & McKay, 2014). Little information is available on how often artistic techniques are used to control pain or their effectiveness. However, in recent years, the use of adult coloring books has grown dramatically, with more than 12 million adult coloring books sold in 2015. This interest is what most likely led to *coloring meet-up groups* forming in some communities (Halzack, 2016). One art therapy group dedicated to people living with chronic pain was successfully piloted and could be replicated (O'Neill & Moss, 2015). In that group, participants created self-expression art drawings and paintings. The authors of that study reported results indicated substantial benefits for the participants but acknowledged the sample was too small to establish statistical significance.

Evidence and Indications for Pain Management

Unfortunately, there has been very little research to support art, coloring, drawing, or doodling as distraction techniques for pain control, however the studies done

are quite diverse, yet promising. An older study (n = 50) investigated how a 1-hour art therapy session affected nine symptoms, including pain, among adults living with cancer (Nainis et al., 2006). Except for nausea, the results showed significant improvement in all symptoms, including pain. Another study evaluated the effect of reducing anxiety comparing coloring plaid forms, coloring a mandala, or drawing/coloring on blank paper (Curry & Kasser, 2005). The participants in that study had less anxiety when coloring either the mandala or plaid form compared to coloring on the blank paper, which may have been due to the degree of attention required in coloring complex patterns. In a subsequent study replicating the Curry and Kasser study, the investigators reported when compared to coloring a blank page, coloring a mandala was significantly more effective in reducing anxiety (van der Vennet & Serice, 2012). Comparison of the effect of these same three art activities on anxiety was subsequently assessed among undergraduate college students (Drake, Searight, & Olson-Pupek, 2014). In that study, the investigators reported all of the activities were significantly effective, but that coloring the plaid pattern also resulted in reduced depression and tension (Drake et al., 2014). Although none of these studies assessed the effect of coloring, drawing, or doodling on pain per se, anxiety is a symptom that often coexists with pain and is known to affect the ability of the person to manage pain. (See Chapters 8 and 22 for more information about the relationship between anxiety and pain.)

A recent small study (n = 24) compared the cerebral activation of participants during coloring, doodling, and free drawing (Kaimal et al., 2017). With all three activities, there was activation of the prefrontal cortex of the brain, which is involved with the perception of reward, with the greatest activation of that area seen when doodling. The participants in that study associated activities with greater self-perception with formulating good ideas and solving problems. A randomized controlled trial (RCT) in Korea used mindfulness-based art therapy among women with breast cancer (Jang, Kang, Lee, & Lee, 2016). In that research, a mental health therapist used mindfulness principles during a 12-session program that encouraged participants to express their physical and emotional pain through drawing and coloring. Although the results were promising, the group was small (n = 24) and further research is needed. (See Chapter 22 for discussion of mindfulness-based therapy.) The authors of a systematic review of studies using art as an intervention for pain among people living with cancer, reported that because the quality of the studies was not rigorous, there needs to be additional research with improved methodology, control, and enlarged sample sizes (Kim, Loring, & Kwekkeboom, 2017).

Art is not only used by patients as part of a multimodal approach to manage pain but also can be used by clinicians to improve understanding and empathy of patients who are experiencing pain. Nurse researchers in Ireland found nursing students who participated in an art program more fully understood how patients felt and experienced pain when they visualized the pain through the personal artistry of the person experiencing pain (McCabe, Neill, Granville, & Grace, 2013). Those results not only speak to how profound communication through art is but also to the different ways clinicians can work with patients to improve understanding and empathy. One U.S. medical school used excursions to art museums to help clinicians explore their perceptions about pain and their abilities to communicate with patients living with pain (Marr & Baruch, 2016). The authors of that work concluded the experience highlighted the ability for clinicians to change how they felt and behaved about patients in pain.

An easy way to help patients use art therapy is to print blank generic coloring pages for them to color using crayons or coloring pencils. The rhythmic action of coloring is both soothing and distracting. An alternative is for the person to use plain paper and pencil or crayon to free draw or doodle.

Research to assess the effect of coloring among adult patients experiencing pain is needed. The aspects of art that have been researched need further exploration and replication in new and expanded populations. Additional ways to use art and coloring to help control pain needs to be investigated.

Electronic Games

Electronic games can be used as distraction by most people without prolonged education or preparation. The person playing the game can improve skill while enjoying the activity and receiving immediate positive reinforcement (Horne-Moyer, Moyer, Messer, & Messer, 2014; Hudlicka, 2016; Ingadottir et al., 2017). Electronic games are a form of active distraction and are associated with greater pain tolerance, lower perceived pain intensity, less anxiety, and greater pleasure than passive forms of distraction such as watching a movie (Jameson, Trevena, & Swain, 2011). It is possible the interactive aspect of electronic games, which requires a greater degree of attention and focus than passive mediums, enhances the distraction and subsequent benefit of pain relief. Although most of the research involving electronic games was reported as being done with children, the games are successfully used by people along the age spectrum from small children in the hospital or at home to older adults in long-term care to promote relaxation, control pain, reduce anxiety, improve physical and cognitive function, and treat fear and disability related to chronic pain (Horne-Moyer et al., 2014). Because many of the games and social media are available on smart phones, it is advantageous for clinicians to have wireless access and recharging stations available for patients and families in health care settings such as waiting rooms and emergency departments (EDs). This could be particularly helpful in EDs, because patients and family members are rarely prepared for needing to be there and thus most likely do not have a charging device with them. Because they may be concerned about saving their battery for making needed phone calls, they may not be able to use their phone to participate in distracting activities.

Evidence and Indications for Pain Management

Using electronic games for pain control based on the concept of distraction has been designed to help children and adults control both acute and chronic pain and to better endure painful procedures (Hudlicka, 2016; Ingadottir et al., 2017). Serious games based on electroencephalography are specifically designed for patients with chronic pain and can be used by patients in a home setting (Sourina, Wang, & Nguyen, 2011). The authors of a systematic review of the various therapeutic uses of active videogames reported that they are a distraction technique effective to reduce anxiety and pain intensity while increasing pain tolerance during painful burn treatments in teens and young adults (Staiano & Flynn, 2014). They were also effective in reducing pain intensity among women with chronic pain involved with systemic lupus (Staiano & Flynn, 2014).

Research is needed to explore the potential benefits, ascertain true advantages, and identify any potential problems or adverse effects. In addition, active electronic games based on established theories and concepts of health promotion and symptom management are needed to both improve effect and facilitate better research (Orji, Mandryk, Vassileva, & Gerling, 2013). Another area in which distraction research is needed is to determine if there is a greater analgesic benefit with interactive distraction, including electronic games, compared with more passive forms of distraction such as watching television or movies.

Cautions

Cautions include concerns for possible seizure and potential muscle strain particularly with overuse (e.g., neck, arm, thumb) (Horne-Moyer et al., 2014).

Virtual Reality and Immersion or Immersive Virtual Reality

Virtual reality (VR) and immersion virtual reality or immersive virtual reality (IVR) as techniques to attenuate pain are the result of rapidly advancing technology that enables participants to actively remove themselves from a painful situation and submerge themselves in an alternative virtual environment (Gold, Belmont, & Thomas, 2007; Li, et al., 2017). The rudimentary groundwork for using VR with pain control was the *virtual reality mirror box* used to help people manage the distress experienced in conjunction with phantom limb sensations (Ramachandran & Rogers-Ramachandran, 1996). (See Chapters 20 and 27 for more discussion of mirror box therapy.)

VR uses combinations of interactive devices and systems to provide a multisensory simulated three-dimensional (3D) environment in which the participating person interacts within the virtual setting through visual, auditory, and at times tactile stimuli conveyed via a computer (Botella, Baños, García-Palacios, & Quero, 2017; Garrett et al., 2014; Trost et al., 2015). At least in part, the actions of the participating person controls what occurs within the artificial environment (Trost et al., 2015). Although VR is considered a new technique to help manage pain, it has a long history. VR dates to the first flight simulator called the Link Trainer, created in 1929 by Edward Link to instruct airplane pilots how to fly planes while remaining in a fixed position on the ground (Kim, 2016).

With acute pain management VR is used as a distraction technique to relieve pain during experimental and painful situations such as physical therapy, venipunctures, burns, and care of wounds (Botella et al., 2017; Gold et al., 2007; Maani et al., 2017). The basis of how and why VR can be effective in controlling pain is that the VR experience actively entices conscious attention into the virtual reality environment, resulting in less attention being given to painful stimuli (Keefe et al., 2012).

IVR occurs when stimuli simulate real-world 3D prompts through the use of head-mounted displays that then convey stereoscopic 3D illusions through computer-generated imagery, which is done while tracking head movements (Fig. 21.1). It provides a total experience in which the participant has a feeling of being naturally present within and moving through the artificial surroundings (Garrett et al., 2014). In some instances, IVR uses olfactory and tactile displays in addition to visual and auditory stimuli (Keefe et al., 2012). The resulting sense of immersion allows for more fully and actively participating in the experience rather than just observing. The degree to which attention is distracted is significant.

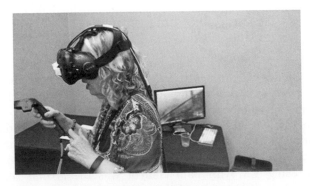

Fig. 21.1 | Immersive Virtual Reality. (Courtesy Ann Quinlan-Colwell.)

Evidence and Indications for Pain Management

On a basic level, the effectiveness of VR in controlling pain is based on the VR experience enticing the attention and then immersing the participant into the 3D virtual reality environment, which results in less attention being given to painful stimuli (Keefe et al., 2012; Malloy & Milling, 2010). Although more research is needed to determine the effects of VR and IVR on the nociceptive process, it is hypothesized that in addition to being in competition with pain sensations for the attention of the person, there is interaction with the anterior cingulate cortex that can result in potentially ignoring pain and creating analgesia (Gold et al., 2007) (see Chapter 3). An early systematic review noted that participants had increased pain relief when the VR had enhanced sophistication resulting in a more complete immersion experience (Malloy & Milling, 2010).

VR has been used for the last two decades as a distraction intervention for acute pain (Gold et al., 2007; Malloy & Milling, 2010). Although research has generally been positive, investigators of a small study (n = 45) with enlisted men in the U.S. military who underwent a flexible cystoscopy for the first time, reported no difference in the mitigation of pain among those who used VR compared to those who did not use VR (Walker et al., 2014). However, the researchers of another study in which VR was used with U.S. soldiers with serious combat wounds reported pain reduction when the soldiers used a custom-made VR goggle system (Maani et al., 2011). Of particular interest in that study was that the soldiers who had the greatest benefit with pain reduction using the VR were those who previously (with no VR) had the greatest pain intensity. The report of a systematic review of 17 studies concluded that distraction through VR is effective for immediate but short-duration relief of pain and pain anxiety in situations with acute pain (Garrett et al., 2014). The authors of another systematic review of 11 studies concluded that the greater the degree of participant presence (being engaged with the VR process) and enjoyment experienced by the person experience during the VR, the greater is the degree of distraction and analgesia (Triberti, Repetto, & Riva, 2014). However, in that review, coexisting anxiety and positive feelings were noted as factors affecting the experience. Additional rigorous research with diverse populations is needed in this area, which has potential to help manage pain with distraction and potentially facilitate relaxation.

Indications for VR and IVR are clearest for acute pain, including pain associated with physical therapy, and for procedural pain, including venipunctures, burns, and care of wounds (Botella et al., 2017; Gold et al., 2007). In a study (n = 36) assessing the benefit of VR during debridement of burn wounds in children, adolescents, and adults, the researchers reported pain was significantly less during the first 3 days using VR and then remained consistent at the lower level on days 4 through 6, indicating pain control with VR continues with repetition (Faber, Patterson, & Bremer, 2013). The Veterans Administration is investigating

VR as an intervention for painful procedures, including treatment of burns, because in one report pain associated with burn care was relieved between 30% and 50% when VR was used (Litwack, 2015). VR has also been used with dental procedures to relieve pain and anxiety (Wiederhold, Gao, & Wiederhold, 2014) during a variety of painful interventions (Armfield & Heaton, 2013) with patients exhibiting increased pain thresholds and greater pain tolerance with VR (Loreto-Quijada et al., 2014).

VR has less frequently been used as an intervention for people living with chronic pain. In one small (n = 20) randomized controlled crossover clinical study a specifically designed VR game was used with the people who used the VR game reporting less perceived pain intensity during the VR game session (Jin, Choo, Gromala, Shaw, & Squire, 2016). It is conceivable that VR can be as effective with chronic pain as a more intense distraction technique than the commonly used distraction techniques. It also can be used for people with pain to gain confidence with using distraction for pain control and with increasing mobility (Keefe et al., 2012). A small open-label case series study (n = 5) of nonimmersive VR used mirror visual feedback weekly for 1 to 2 months (Sato et al., 2010). At the end of that time, four of the patients reported more than 50% less pain intensity after the sessions. Similar equipment was used in a proof-of-concept study with two patients with facial pain (Won & Collins, 2012). After four sessions, one patient with allodynia reported improvement in pain intensity and slight increase in facial movement that persisted after the conclusion of the four sessions. Impressively, she continued to use less medication during the 6 months after the intervention. At baseline, the second patient had hyperesthesia but did not have allodynia. Although she reported no improvement in pain intensity, she reported willingness to continue with the intervention if available. Despite being small studies, those reviewed demonstrate that the potential benefits of using VR with chronic pain are promising. Particularly encouraging are the reports of the analgesic effects persisting for periods after conclusion of the interventions. Again, more research with more diverse populations of people living with chronic pain is needed.

In addition to distracting from pain, graded exposure through VR has been used with people who have pain-related fear with chronic pain and disability. (See Chapters 3, 8, 20, and 22 for more about fear of pain.) In one review, the authors reported that *virtual reality graded exposure therapy (VRGET)* using the principle of gradually exposing or confronting a person with progressively more intense activities the person finds frightening with the intention of mitigating the fearful beliefs. In that review, the authors concluded that VRGET offers potential as an intervention for modifying the pain-related fear that can be involved with chronic pain and disability (Trost & Parsons, 2014). VRGET offers a potential option for people living with chronic pain who do not have easy access (e.g., financial, insurance, transportation) to providers of traditional CBT. (Also see Chapter 22 for more about graded exposure and CBT.)

Relaxation

Relaxation is commonly used as a distraction technique to help manage pain (McBain et al., 2015). Data from the 2007 *National Health Interview Survey Alternative Medicine Supplement* revealed characteristics of people in the United States who use relaxation practices as individuals who are more likely to be younger or middle age, female, and non-Hispanic, with low to middle income and a college education, with no active insurance, and more likely to participate in a health-focused lifestyle (Lee & Yeo, 2013).

Relaxation is most frequently associated with the *relaxation response*, which is explained as a hypometabolic state of quiet that can be brought about through conscious effort while awake (Benson & Klipper, 1975; Park, Traeger, Vranceanu, Scult, Lerner, Benson, Denninger, & Fricchione, 2013; Wallace, Benson, & Wilson, 1971). Benson stressed a critical component of the relaxation response is that it is a state of being, not a particular method (Park, Traeger, Vranceanu, Scult, Lerner, Benson, Denninger, & Fricchione, 2013). This state of relaxation or relaxation response or *loosening* (Romas & Sharma, 2017) can be elicited through a variety of activities or techniques involving breathing, yoga (Romas & Sharma, 2017), imagery, meditation, mindfulness (Table 21.1) (Traeger et al., 2013), biofeedback, and autogenic training (McBain et al., 2015) (Table 21.1). Breathing, progressive muscle relaxation, and imagery are discussed later. Yoga is discussed in Chapters 20 and 25. Biofeedback is discussed in Chapter 22. Mindfulness and meditation are discussed in Chapters 22 and 25.

Table 21.1	**New Hanover Regional Medical Center Healing Arts Network, Wilmington, N.C.**	
Pet Therapy Program Participants	**Quotes**
A patient with neuropathic pain in fingers and toes	"The dog helped last time I was here, and I think it will help again."
A patient's family member	"She may not get as much out of this as I do. I know she likes dogs, but I love seeing the dogs."
Pharmacist	"This does as much for me as the patients."
Several medical residents	"This does as much good for us."
Intensive care nurse	"We really need this."
Intensive care nurse	"Now my day is good."

These activities have important benefits. Once they are learned, they can be mastered and used independently whenever the person needs or wants to do so. They do not require another person to be involved and do not involve any special equipment. They also can be used alone or as part of a multimodal approach to pain management in combination with other pharmacologic and nonpharmacologic interventions. They are extremely cost effective and in many instances without any charge.

Breathing Activities

Breathing and, in particular, the conscious control of breathing, is an important component of relaxation, emotional regulation, and pain management (Armfield & Mark, 2017; Arsenault, Ladouceur, Lehmann, Rainville, & Piché, 2013). In addition, it is among the top three complementary modalities used in the United States (Chiramonte, D'Adamo, & Morrison, 2014). When breathing is inadvertently held or is inadequate, as occurs with anxiety or fear, there is inadequate aeration of the lungs resulting in blood not being well oxygenated, which can result in or increase anxiety and fatigue, making it more difficult for the person to deal with pain.

Focusing on and consciously slowing respirations is basic in many relaxation practices such as yoga and meditation (Arsenault et al., 2013). Organized breathing exercises affect cerebral function, neuroendocrine activity, and functions of the autonomic nervous system (Patwardhan, Mutalik, & Tillu, 2015). Intentionally slowing breathing has been correlated with less pain intensity (Jafari, Vlaeyen, Van den Bergh, & Van Diest, 2017b). By breathing more fully, the person can reduce anxiety, feel more in control, and be better able to manage pain (Armfield & Marek, 2017).

Respiratory-induced hypoalgesia (RIH) is the term used to describe the modulation of pain that occurs when breathing is slowed and controlled (Martin et al., 2012). Although to date, the precise mechanisms involved with RIH have not been isolated, it is conceivable there is an interplay of physiologic along with psychologic factors contributing to the effect (Jafari et al., 2017). Certainly, additional research is needed to learn more about this phenomenon. The importance of this research was highlighted in the PubMed abstract of one Cochrane review in which the need for research into the relationship between controlled breathing and pain reduction was described as being an "urgent need for well designed trials in this area" (Barker, Jones, O'Connell, & Everard, 2013).

Types of Relaxation Breathing

Diaphragmatic Breathing

Diaphragmatic breathing is simple to do and involves directing consciousness to the process of breathing (Busch et al., 2012), with increasing diaphragmatic excursion (Morrow, Brink, Grace, Pritchard, & Lupton-Smith, 2016),

slowing of inhalation, and exhalation of air while decreasing the effort expanded by the axillary muscles of the shoulders, neck, and chest (Morrow et al., 2016; Park, Oh, & Kim, 2013a). Another way to describe diaphragmatic breathing is that it is an exercise to expand the descent of the diaphragm when inhaling and to expand the ascent of the diaphragm when exhaling (Alaparthi, Augustine, Anand, & Mahale, 2016). Although some practitioners teach participants to monitor the expansion of the abdomen during diaphragmatic breathing, that is not necessarily relevant because the abdomen can expand without any associated movement of the diaphragm (Morrow et al., 2016).

Abdominal Breathing

Abdominal breathing, as it suggests, focuses attention on the abdomen and is designed to relax and distract by being attentive to the activity and progress. The person lies supine with hands on the abdomen (or alternately the chest) and is encouraged to breathe normally without anxiety. Next the person is told to inhale through the nose without raising the chest but while making effort to raise or expand the abdomen. Finally, the person is instructed to exhale while contracting the abdomen again with minimum chest activity (Song, Xu, Zhang, Ma, & Zhao, 2013).

Yogic Breathing or Pranayama

Yogic breathing, or *pranayama,* is an important component of the practice of yoga in general, aiming not only to help facilitate relaxation and relieve stress but also to improve the flow of energy (Hakked, Balakrishnan, & Krishnamurthy, 2017), increase pulmonary vital capacity, and increase oxygen in the blood (Romas & Sharma, 2017). (See Chapter 20 and 25 for a more detailed discussion of yoga.) Traditionally *pranayama* has four distinct facets consisting of inhaling breath *(puraka),* pausing or internal retention of breath *(antar kumbhaka),* exhaling breath *(reclama),* and an external retention of breath *(bahir kumbhaka)* (Hakked, Balakrishnan, & Krishnamurthy, 2017; Romas & Sharma, 2017).

Alternate Nostril Breathing

Another form of yogic breathing is alternative nostril breathing. With this technique, (1) a full breath is exhaled; (2) with the right nostril closed, inhalation is through the left nostril; (3) then the breath is held with both nostrils closed; (4) the breath is fully exhaled; and (5) with the left nostril closed inhalation is through the right nostril, and the cycle continues (Hakked, Balakrishnan, & Krishnamurthy, 2017).

Square Breathing

Square breathing is a technique similar to traditional *pranayama* (yogic breathing) that involves intention, control, and regulation of respiration with four distinct phases. Specifically, the person (1) breathes in to the count of 4,

Square Breathing

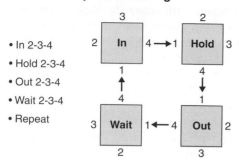

- In 2-3-4
- Hold 2-3-4
- Out 2-3-4
- Wait 2-3-4
- Repeat

Fig. 21.2 | Square Breathing Diagram. (Courtesy © 2008 Ann Quinlan-Colwell.)

(2) holds the breath for a count of 4, (3) breathes out to the count of 4, and (4) waits for the count 4 (El Korh & Giuliani, 2016; Quinlan-Colwell, 2012) (Fig. 21.2). The cycle can be repeated for as long as desired or needed and used whenever needed or desired. The technique is used clinically with patients with anxiety disorders (El Korh & Giuliani, 2016) and pain by helping to control anxious breathing, diverting attention, and promoting relaxation (Quinlan-Colwell, 2012). When working with a patient who is anxious or afraid and hyperventilating, the clinician can guide the person in the four aspects of the square starting at a pace consistent with the speed the patient is breathing and gradually guide them to breathe more slowly. This technique can be helpful when patients who are experiencing acute pain are moving for the first time such as a patient who has had abdominal surgery getting out of bed for the first time postoperatively. Square breathing not only distracts from the activity but also helps prevent hyperventilation and ease anxiety. One author (AQC) has successfully used this technique for many years with patients who experience both acute and chronic pain. Many nurses who have learned it also use it to manage stressful situations.

Lamaze Breathing

The Lamaze technique of controlled breathing has been used for decades as a basis for women preparing for childbirth to learn to reduce the perception of pain related to contractions, labor, and childbirth while increasing relaxation (Lothian, 2011). Promoting relaxation is important because the pelvic muscles tense with anxiety, which leads to increased pain (Cicek & Basar, 2017). In addition, it is suggested relaxation eases labor and the pain of contractions by increasing blood flow and the response of catecholamines with increased efficiency of contractions (Brown, Douglas, & Flood, 2001; Cicek & Basar, 2017). During the last few decades in the United States, Lamaze breathing has evolved from the woman and her partner needing to follow a very precise pattern of quick breathing to a slower rhythm of breathing, which is individualized for each patient (Lothian & DeVries, 2010).

Evidence and Indications for Pain Management

Although the exact mechanism by which slow deep breathing is beneficial with pain management is not yet known, it is known that there is increased stimulation of vagal afferents in the bronchopulmonary tract when respirations are slowed (Zautra, Fasman, Davis, & Arthur, 2010). It is also thought that during inspiration there is some inhibition of cerebral and/or spinal nociception (Arsenault et al., 2013). Specifically, using controlled breathing during labor and childbirth has been suggested as being effective by facilitating a greater amount of available oxygen, which enhances maternal energy during contractions of childbirth labor (Gupta, Raddi, & Gupta, 2016). In a systematic review of 31 studies, the reviewers concluded that controlled breathing was correlated with reduced pain intensity in some studies reviewed, but physiologic data supporting it were insufficient and additional research is needed (Jafari, Courtois, Van den Bergh, Vlaeyen, & Van Diest, 2017a).

Internationally, results have been somewhat variable involving research in which various breathing techniques were used with people experiencing different types of pain. Two studies reviewing the effect of using breathing exercises during chest tube removal were inconsistent; with one finding no benefit for analgesia and the other finding positive analgesic effect (Gelinas, Arbour, Michaud, Robar, & Côté, 2013). The investigator of a study done in India with women during the first stage of labor (n = 48) noted the women who used the breathing exercises (n = 24) reported less pain intensity ($P = .05$) than those who did not use breathing (n = 24) (Dengsangluri, 2015). Similarly, a study in Korea (n = 64) used relaxation breathing to assist with pain and anxiety during care of burns. The authors reported that pain at the time of care ($P = .01$) and then over time ($P = .001$) and anxiety at the time of care ($P = .01$) and then over time ($P = .02$) were significantly reduced using relaxation breathing (Park, Oh, & Kim, 2013). An interesting small study (n = 16) compared measured attentive deep slow breathing in which participants were instructed to concentrate and be attentive to breathing with deep slow relaxation breathing. The investigators found pain thresholds were significantly increased only in the participants who did the deep slow relaxation breathing (Busch et al., 2012). In an innovative study reviewing 57 applications (apps) (electronic applications for phones or computers) that could be used for pediatric patients to manage pain using breathing, diaphragmatic breathing, yoga, and other CBT interventions were reviewed, and 19 of the apps were reported to have clinical usefulness in a variety of settings (Smith et al., 2015).

The various breathing techniques are interventions that need further research using rigorous methodology with people with a variety of painful conditions and situations.

Cautions

Cautions were not discussed in any of the literature reviewed, and none have been anecdotally reported to the authors. Breathing techniques are simple to learn and teach, inexpensive, and generally effective as an intervention for pain, anxiety, and stress. It is a technique that clinicians can use to help patients control pain and relieve anxiety and for themselves during stressful situations.

Progressive Muscle Relaxation

Progressive muscle relaxation (PMR) is a method used to achieve relaxation of body and mind (Armfield & Marek, 2017), thus eliciting the relaxation response described previously (Chiramonte et al., 2014). Traditionally, PMR calls for the person to tense muscles while inhaling and relax muscles while exhaling in a coordinated rhythm sequentially throughout the body (Armfield & Mareck, 2017;

Chiramonte et al., 2014) (Box 21.1). Most often the sequence begins with either the head or the feet and progresses to the opposite body area. It was developed by Edmund Jacobson, whose intention was for the person to tense and then relax the same muscle with the intention to learn the difference between those two states or feelings (Crane & Ward, 2016). Sometimes the person is encouraged to hold the tension for a certain period, followed by assuming a state of relaxation, which is retained for a certain time (e.g., 30 seconds) (Song et al., 2013). Initially, the person is guided in the process. Box 21.2 presents a sample script that can be used to guide patients in PMR (Chiramonte et al., 2014). Such a script can be used as a guide until the person learns the sequence and can do it without the

---

Box 21.1 | Muscle Relaxation Procedures

The following script can be used with patients for muscle relation:

"The tension and anxiety that you tell me you feel when you think about receiving dental treatment may be caused by the tensing of your muscles, even if you don't realize that your muscles are tense. If you like, I'd be happy to teach you a way to relax your muscles that may help you feel calm. As a result, the dental treatment may feel more comfortable for you. Relaxation is the opposite of anxiety. It's impossible to feel both relaxed and tense at the same time. The exercise involves relaxing your muscles systematically throughout your body. Would you like to try that?

"Begin by putting all of your consciousness in your feet. Don't worry if your attention drifts away. For many patients, it takes a little practice to be able to move your attention to a specific part of your body (momentary hesitation). Feel your feet. Your feet may feel either warm or cool at this moment. Imagine the muscles in your feet. Make them tense and hold for a count of four … 1, 2, 3, 4. Now relax those muscles and notice how they feel while I count to four (momentary hesitation) … 1, 2, 3, 4. Make those muscles tense again as I count slowly to four … 1, 2, 3, 4. Notice how your muscles feel. Breathe in and feel the tension, and breathe out to feel the relaxation. Perhaps you'd like to try it again … breathe in and feel your muscles tighten, and breathe out to feel the relaxation (momentary hesitation).

"When you're ready, move your attention to your calves (momentary hesitation). Notice how the muscles in your calves feel. Those muscles may feel warm or cool. Imagine those muscles for a moment. Now, inhale and make those muscles tense while holding your breath for a count of four (momentary hesitation) … 1, 2, 3, 4. Now exhale and relax those muscles and notice how they feel while I slowly count to four … 1, 2, 3, 4. I suggest that we repeat that. Breathe in and make those muscles tense as I count to four (momentary hesitation) … 1, 2, 3, 4. Hold the tension. Now slowly exhale while relaxing those muscles as I count to four (momentary hesitation) … 1, 2, 3, 4."

After reading this script, the clinician might suggest that the patient try on his or her own to breathe in and feel tension in the calves and breathe out, feeling the calf muscles relax. Use the same technique to alternately tense and relax the thigh and buttocks muscles.

After completing the procedures for the feet, calves, thighs, and buttocks, move on to the next three major muscle groups: (1) hands, forearms, and biceps; (2) chest, stomach, and lower back; and (3) head, face, throat, and shoulders. The technique is often most effective when the clinician moves slowly from one muscle group to the next. One approach is to suggest that the patient move all of his or her attention to the hands, forearms, and biceps and then to move the attention to the individual set of muscles in, for instance, the hands. It is helpful to talk slowly and softly and to provide suggestions after the relaxation phase, such as your muscles may feel loose, limp, or calm. Using rhythmic breathing to coordinate the muscle tightening and relaxing is frequently a good way to help the patient fully participate in this exercise. Make suggestions such as the sound of your breath exhaling will help remind you to relax your muscles. Some patients find it helpful for the dentist to make a tape of the entire procedure so the patient can take it home and practice.

For most people, relaxing quickly and effectively requires a great deal of practice. It is a good idea for the dentist to remind the patient that it may take several practice sessions before he or she is able to feel relaxed in the dental chair. Above all, the dentist should not become impatient if the patient cannot relax immediately after beginning the relaxation procedures.

From Armfield, J., & Marek, C. L. (2017). Patients who are anxious and fearful. In S. Stefanac, & S. Nesbit. *Diagnosis and treatment planning in dentistry* (3rd ed., pp. 323–341). St. Louis, MO: Elsevier.

Box 21.2 | Sample Script for Progressive Muscle Relaxation Guidance

Find a comfortable position in a location where you will not be interrupted. You may sit up or lie down, however you are most comfortable.

You will be focusing your attention on your body for the next few minutes. If your mind wanders, simply bring your attention back to your body.

Take a deep breath into your abdomen while trying to push your belly button out as you breathe in. Hold your breath for a few seconds, and then slowly breathe out. Take another deep breath while trying to push out your belly button as you take in a healing breath.... Hold for a few seconds ... then slowly release your breath.

As you exhale, imagine the tension in your body being released and flowing out of your body. And again inhale ... hold ... and exhale. Feel your body beginning to relax.

Now tighten the muscles in your forehead by raising your eyebrows as high as you can. Hold for about 5 seconds. And abruptly release and feel that tension fall away.

Pause for about 10 seconds. Now smile widely and feel your mouth and cheeks tense. Hold for about 5 seconds and release; noticing the softness in your face. Now just breathe slowly for about 10 seconds while feeling your face relax more and more with each breath.

Next, tighten your eye muscles by squinting your eyelids tightly shut. Hold for about 5 seconds and release.

Pause for about 10 seconds while breathing slow, relaxing breaths.

Now lift your shoulders up as though they could touch your ears. Hold for about 5 seconds and release quickly while feeling their heaviness. Pause for about 10 seconds; feel your arms getting heavy and warm as you continue to breathe slow, relaxing breaths.

Tense your upper back by pulling your shoulders back while trying to make your shoulder blades touch. Hold for about 5 seconds and release.

Pause for about 10 seconds while breathing slow, relaxing breaths.

Tighten your chest by taking a deep breath in, hold it for about 5 seconds, and exhale to blow out all the tension.

Breath in ... and out. In ... and out. Let go of all the stress. In ... and out.

Now, tightly but without straining, clench your fists. Hold for about 5 seconds and release.

Pause for about 10 seconds. Now, flex your biceps. Feel that buildup of tension. You may even visualize that muscle tightening. Hold for about 5 seconds, release, and enjoy that feeling of limpness. Breath slowly in ... and out.

Now tighten your triceps by extending your arms out and locking your elbows. Hold for about 5 seconds and release. Pause for about 10 seconds while imagining that all your stress and tension are leaving your body through your fingertips.

Now tighten the muscles in your abdomen by sucking in your abdomen. Hold for about 5 seconds and release. Pause for about 10 seconds while breathing slowly deep into your abdomen and notice your belly button moving away from your body with each inhalation.

Gently arch your lower back. Hold for about 5 seconds and relax. Pause for about 10 seconds.

Feel the limpness in your upper body letting go of the tension and stress, hold for about 5 seconds, and relax. Your arms are heavy and warm ... the tension is leaving your body through your fingertips.

Tighten your buttocks. Hold for about 5 seconds ..., release, and imagine your hips falling loose. Pause for about 10 seconds while breathing slow, relaxing breaths.

Tighten your thighs by pressing your knees together. Hold for about 5 seconds ... and release.

Pause for about 10 seconds. Now flex your feet, pull your toes toward you, and feel the tension in your calves. Hold for about 5 seconds and relax; feel the weight of your legs sinking down. Pause for about 10 seconds.

Curl your toes and tense your feet. Hold for about 5 seconds and release. Pause for about 10 seconds.

Now imagine a wave of relaxation slowly spreading through your body beginning at your head and going all the way down to your feet.

Breathe in ... and out ... in ... out ... in ... out.

From Chiramonte, D., D'Adamo, C., & Morrison, B. (2014). Integrative approaches to pain management. In H. Benzon et al., *Practical management of pain* (5th ed., pp. 658–668). St. Louis, MO: Mosby.

external prompting. The PMR technique incorporates not only breathing but also distraction because the person needs to focus on the part of the body for either tension or relaxation and in focusing on inhalation or exhalation. As the person is able to relax muscles and reduce tension in the body, anxious responses are interrupted and the person is able to feel more at ease (Park, Traeger, Vranceanu, Scult, Lerner, Benson, Denninger, & Fricchione, 2013).

Evidence and Indications for Pain Management

PMR is a skill often taught to patients to help them self-manage pain and other symptoms of chronic illnesses (Perlman, Rosenberger, & Ali, 2018), including musculoskeletal pain (Blödt, Pach, Roll, & Witt, 2014; Lauche, et al., 2013), cancer pain (Somers, et al., 2015), and pain of sickle cell disease (Dampier, 2014). PMR is used effectively to manage headache pain (Meyer, et al., 2016; Park, Traeger, Vranceanu, Scult, Lerner, Benson, Denninger, & Fricchione, 2013). Much of the research has been with small groups and the results are mixed. In one small study (n = 30) PMR was significantly more effective in reducing both stress and pain related to tension headaches when compared with transcutaneous electrical nerve stimulation (TENS) (see Chapter 20), which was significant only for reducing stress (Kumar & Raje, 2014). Reports from systematic reviews have been inconsistent regarding the benefit of PMR in relieving chronic pain. One review involving patients living with rheumatoid arthritis reported some analgesic benefit from PMR, and another reported analgesic benefit when PMR was used in combination with other nonpharmacologic interventions (McBain et al., 2015). An innovative use of PMR was studied in Italy with people with amputated lower extremities who suffered with phantom limb pain and/or phantom sensations in the limbs (Brunelli et al., 2015). Over a 4-week time span, the participants in that study (n = 51) were either in a twice per week group using mental imagery, PMR, and phantom exercise or in a control group who only had physical therapy on the intact lower extremities. The participants in the PMR group reported significantly less intensity and disturbance of the phantom pain and sensations after PMR compared with those in the control group.

One author of this chapter (AQC) has taught PMR to patients before surgery for them to learn, practice, and then use postoperatively to manage pain. Unpublished data from that work supports the intervention used in that way for patients to effectively manage postoperative pain. She also uses it with patients with acute pain and teaches it to patients with chronic pain for the same reason with positive reports of improved pain control.

Two recent research studies evaluated the effect of PMR on the human brain. A small Japanese study (n = 11) compared functional magnetic resonance imaging (fMRI) during a control session and then during a PMR session (Kobayashi & Koitabashi, 2016). With structured breathing the researchers in that study found activity in several portions of the brain, including the insula, which is involved with pain control and emotional responses. Another group of investigators in Spain compared distribution of glucose in the brains of subjects who had received sublingual diazePAM (n = 28) with those undergoing PMR (n = 28) and with controls (n = 28) (Pifarré et al., 2015). The findings in that study were that a statistically significant reduction in cortical metabolism occurred in both the diazePAM and PMR groups compared to the control group, but importantly there was no significant difference between the PMR and diazePAM groups. This is a noteworthy finding considering the concerns of coadministering benzodiazepine medications with opioids (Dowell, Haegerich, & Chou, 2016). The investigators of a third study of students (n = 101) consisting of six different groups over a 4-year period, reported cortisol secretion was significantly less when

participants used an abbreviated PMR program (Chellew, Evans, Fornes-Vives, Pérez, & Garcia-Banda, 2015).

Because PMR does not require any particular equipment, it is frequently incorporated in self-care and self-management of pain programs (Blödt et al., 2014; Perlman et al., 2018). Smart phone program applications or apps can guide people in PMR to manage pain, including musculoskeletal pain (Alexander & Joshi, 2016; Blödt et al., 2014; McKay, Przeworski, & O'Neill, 2016). This is promising because this technology was used successfully to help people working in offices in Korea reduce intensity of pain (Lee et al., 2017). PMR was used as part of a feasibility study that concluded mobile health can be an effective method for patients with cancer to use pain coping skills (Somers et al., 2015). This is yet another area in need of further research with strong methodology.

Considering the results of studies on the effect of PMR on the human brain indicate that it has the potential to be an effective first-line intervention for anxiety and relaxing muscles. Replication of these studies with larger and more diverse samples is warranted. PMR is an intervention that needs further research, including replication of studies that have been conducted involving subjects with the same and different types of painful conditions. Rigorous research designed to evaluate the use of PMR with patients in the different situations described in this section and before painful procedures is needed.

Cautions

No specific cautions were found regarding PMR; however, it may be prudent to avoid the component of tensing of muscles in painful areas of the body. In those areas, the relaxation of muscles alone may be helpful.

Music Therapy

"Music hath charms to soothe a savage beast." This is the more familiar version of the full quote: "Music hath charms to soothe a savage breast, to soften rocks, or bend a knotted oak" from the *Mourning Bride* by William Congreve (Congreve, 1697). To most this means music can have a calming effect on mankind. The impact of music on humans has been understood on some level for centuries. In Biblical times, it was reported that music was used to calm and soothe emotions as illustrated by David playing his harp to calm Saul whenever Saul was troubled, and Saul would feel better (Hauck, Metzner, Rohlffs, Lorenz & Engel, 2013; Samuel 16:14–23; Thaut, 2015). In ancient Greece priests used music to restore balance with the body and soul and to evoke emotions, and the philosophers thought music had a therapeutic purpose (Pretorius, 2017). People dealing with mania were prescribed listening to flute music and those with depression were prescribed listening to dulcimer music (Dobrztnska,

Cesarz, & Rymaszewska, 2006). Plato was quoted as saying "music is medicine to the soul" (Pretorius, 2017, p. 4).

More recent reports about the therapeutic benefit of music came from veteran's hospitals after World Wars I and II when nurses and doctors noticed the positive effects in patients when musicians were playing. The music helped the hospitalized veterans cope with the emotional and physical trauma from the war. That is where the profession of *music therapy* originated. These basic understandings of the therapeutic impact and benefit of music on people resulted in the need for further research resulting ultimately in the development of a college curriculum and the profession of music therapy (American Music Therapy Association [AMTA], 2014; Spencer, 2013).

Music Therapy as a Profession

The American Music Therapy Association (AMTA) defines music therapy as "the clinical and evidence-based use of music interventions to accomplish individualized goals within a therapeutic relationship by a credentialed professional who has completed an approved music therapy program" (AMTA, ND). The profession of music therapy has evolved and grown over time. Music therapists now work with a wide range of clients of all ages in a variety of settings, including medical hospitals, schools, nursing homes, wellness centers, behavioral health hospitals, and correctional facilities, among other settings. Cognitive, neuropsychological, and sensory processes are involved in the experience of hearing and listening to music with effects on learning, emotions, and therapeutic benefit with reductions in stress and pain (Pretorius, 2017; Strauss, Van Heerden, & Joubert, 2016). Benefits of music therapy include helping with pain management, stress relief, expression of feelings, memory, communication, physical rehabilitation, and promoting wellness and relaxation (AMTA, ND; Kobylański, Walczak, Stępień, Bereziewicz, & Pytko-Polończyk, 2015; Pretorius 2017; Spencer, 2013).

Music therapists conduct individualized assessments to develop patient-centered treatment plans. Patient objectives and goals are addressed through music interventions that facilitate nonmusical changes resulting in improvement for the patient. Music therapy sessions include passively listening to music, actively playing music and/or singing, and creation of original music to express oneself. Bonde (2017) noted that when music therapy is used in a hospital setting (music therapy in medicine) it is the therapeutic use of music by a professional therapist who develops a vital relationship with patients with the intention to achieve goals. Bonde contrasted this description of the music therapy professional with a nonclinical musician or volunteer who brings music to the ill person or the hospitalized patient.

The systematic use of music facilitates anxiety reduction, positive changes in mood (Thoma et al., 2015), and active participation in one's own treatment (AMTA, ND; Patterson et al., 2015). The investigators of an interesting study (n = 160) in South Africa reported clinical significance in the ability of patients with inhibited symptoms of psychosis to be attentive and to follow instructions when the music tempo (i.e., the speed of music and changes in harmony) was increased. Conversely patients with agitated symptoms of psychosis demonstrated clinically significant improvement in following directions when the music tempo was slowed (Strauss et al., 2016). Although this is not directly applicable to people being able to manage pain, it does speak to the strong cognitive effect of music on behavior. Additional research is warranted.

Music therapy interventions must be coordinated and conducted by a nationally board-certified music therapist. The education is extensive, involving 4 years of academic work along with 1200 hours of extensive clinical training under the supervision of a board-certified music therapist. After completion of this training the therapist candidate is eligible to take the national board certification examination to become a music therapist board certified (MT-BC). The certification must be renewed every 5 years by completing continuing education or retaking the examination. Music therapists design interventions based on data collected in a patient assessment, collaboration with the patient health care team, and identification of goals and interventions to best meet the needs of the patient (AMTA, ND, 2014). Pain management programs seeking to incorporate music into their multimodal treatment protocols will bring a broader spectrum to the services offered to their patients by adding a nationally board-certified music therapist (Box 21.3).

Box 21.3 | Distinguishing Music Interventions and Music Therapy

It is important to note the difference between music interventions and music therapy when designing a pain management program.

- Well-intentioned volunteer musicians can offer entertainment, which may be enjoyable and provide distraction and relief of stress, but they are not providing music therapy.
- Trained bedside musicians can offer live musical experiences that enhance the environment and support the healing process but are not music therapy.
- Listening to music on your own can offer relaxation and enjoyment but is also not music therapy

Music Therapy and Multimodal Pain Management

Using music therapy as a component of a multimodal approach to pain control is based in the concept that pain is multifaceted and uniquely experienced by each person (Quinlan-Colwell, 2012). Several theories explain the ways pain can be managed or controlled. One of these is the gate control theory (GCT), which describes the theoretical interplay among connections (i.e., *gates*) in the spinal cord and brain through which painful stimuli are perceived then subsequently through which the painful stimuli are modulated (Melzack & Wall 1965). Through the lens of the GCT, feelings, thoughts, and activities affect whether and to what degree the gates are opened or closed to achieve modulation of pain (Melzak & Wall, 1965). Thus, identifying ways to influence or control these feelings, thoughts, and activities is an important aspect of pain control (Hauck et al., 2013).

Music is a beneficial tool in controlling pain because music provides a sensory experience that is familiar, safe, and predictable. Physiologically music can help reduce cardiac and respiratory rates and help reduce anxiety and promote relaxation (Vaajoki, Pietilä, Kankkunen, & Vehviläinen-Julkunen, 2012). Also, as seen in the South African study, the musical experience can refocus attention (Strauss et al., 2016), which can provide distraction and help modify the pain experience and perception of pain (Hauck et al., 2013). Music therapists work to help patients find the most successful ways to use music to deal with pain and work toward achieving individual goals (Hauck et al., 2013).

For example, a patient experiencing pain may benefit from singing a song or playing an instrument as well as from using music, imagery, and breathing techniques. This is possible because the music and activity stimulate normal somatosensory input to the brain and reduces the perception of pain (Hauck et al., 2013). In addition, relaxation techniques rely on the mind and emotions to control pain so when paired with music the experience enables individuals to control their pain level as they strive to reach their pain management goals (Hauck et al., 2013).

Indications Using Music for Pain Control

When music therapy interventions are designed to decrease pain and reduce anxiety and depression, positive outcomes are possible. The outcomes are guided by the patient goals, individual emotional and cognitive responses to the music, and the therapeutic relationship (Bonde, 2017). Music therapy sessions involve active music (e.g., singing or playing instruments) and passive music (e.g., listening to music), which can be paired with breathing, imagery, and a variety of relaxation techniques. Music therapy sessions can be with either an individual or groups. Active music playing/singing sessions provide a focus on the act of making music, which redirects the attention away from pain. This helps the person modify the pain experience and perception of pain.

Creating music within the framework of music therapy involves the use of a variety of hand drums, rhythm instruments, guitar, ukulele, and piano among other instruments, as well as voice. The music therapist structures and facilitates the session, allowing for high success and ease in creative expression on the instruments for all patients no matter what their musical background. It is not required for patients to have any prior musical experience to be successful in creating music as a positive focus or outlet for self-expression in music therapy sessions.

An example of using music therapy with a patient trying to control pain after surgery may involve engaging the person to improvise on an alto xylophone. The music therapy goals could include refocusing attention away from the recent surgery and pain being experienced and providing a positive outlet for self-expression to help the person begin to process the change in health or recent surgery by refocusing on creating music. The patient may be alert and interactive but initially hesitant to play the xylophone. When the therapist introduces the instrument and asks if the person would like to try to play, the person may initially decline and ask the therapist to play something. To encourage the patient to participate, the therapist may demonstrate how easy it is to play by tapping out a few notes and then again ask the person to play the instrument. If willing to try, the patient could learn that tapping on the xylophone and creating music can be distracting with at least temporary relief from pain (Fig. 21.3).

In music therapy, passive music listening sessions can be done individually or in a group setting. The sessions are multimodal, including breathing, imagery, and progressive muscle relaxation with music to aid in pain management by refocusing attention away from pain and more on other parts of the body or on positive images or memories. Live or specifically selected recorded music is played while the music therapist leads the patient through a breathing exercise to refocus attention and calm the mind. Once the patient is calmer the music therapist will lead the patient through predetermined imagery scenes to

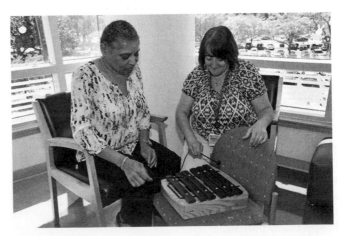

Fig. 21.3 | Music Therapy. (Courtesy Michele Erich author and Theresa White.)

facilitate greater relaxation and decreased physical and emotional tension and stress. Because live music played or provided by a music therapist has a more interactive quality, it can be personalized during the session to adjust to the patient, and thus it generally has a more profound effect than recorded music (Standley & Walworth, 2010).

The importance of the role of the music therapist is seen in helping patients select music to which they can most significantly relate. As part of the therapeutic process, music therapists generally guide patients to focus on finding instrumental music with consistent dynamics and slower tempos and help patients create or design their personal relaxation imagery. The phrases *find your happy place* or *go to your happy place* are simple statements that can profoundly affect the person with pain. Being able to find a place in your mind that makes you feel happy, relaxed, peaceful, or safe is powerful. Guided imagery techniques can also help reduce the pain signals being sent to the brain, enhance pain tolerance, and develop relaxation skills (Bresler, 2016).

Another example of a music therapy session involves the use of music to help decrease pain, stress, and anxiety. The music therapist uses music and breathing exercises to help patients focus their attention on their bodies and the present moment. Music, either recorded or live, is played throughout the session to help patients focus. One type of session includes progressive muscle relaxation exercises with the music and breathing. Another involves music and imagery with breathing exercises. Patients are often asked to report how they are feeling, both physically and emotionally, when entering the music therapy group and then again after the relaxation session. During many years of clinical experience, one author (ME) has found many patients report a decrease in pain, tension, and anxiety. Some generic examples of patient reports, to the author, after music therapy relaxation sessions are "I feel peaceful," "I feel better,"

"My (back, head, leg) doesn't hurt as much," "I feel calmer," and "we should do this every day."

Evidence and Indications for Pain Management

During at least the last 30 years, researchers have reported decreases in pain perception among patients who have participated in music therapy sessions involving music listening (Davis & Thaut 1989; Kane et al., 2004; Özer, Özlü, Arslan, & Günes,2013; Voss et al., 2004; Zimmerman, Nieveen, Barnason, & Schmaderer, 1996). Although much of the early research in music therapy was anecdotal and qualitative, the research produced over the past 25 to 30 years has been more quantitative. That research has allowed music therapy to be measured against similar standards for other pain management interventions. The author of a meta-analysis on the effect of music with pain in the medical setting reported music interventions may help relieve procedural

pain and different types of pain such as cancer pain, acute pain, and chronic pain (Lee, 2016).

There are many examples in the international literature demonstrating positive effects of music and music therapy on various types of pain. Patients in a study on recovering from spine surgery (n = 60) who received music therapy demonstrated a significant change in pain perception as reported on the visual analog pain scale, with pain ratings decreasing by more than 1 point in the music group but ratings increasing in the control group (Mondanaro et al., 2017). An innovative study in Taiwan (n = 38) with patients undergoing craniotomy surgery while awake demonstrated the effect of music on anxiety, heart rate, and blood pressure (Wu, Huang, Lee, Wang, & Shih, 2017). In that study each of those parameters was reduced in the patients who listened to music, which contributed to a more positive surgical experience for those patients. Oncology patients who received music therapy in a small study in India (n = 14) reported statistically significant reduction in pain scores (Krishnaswamy & Nair 2016). Women with unrelieved pain after gynecologic surgeries often report distress during the recovery period. Researchers who used music with that group of patients reported music helped decrease intensity of pain, anxiety, and fatigue and decreased the amount of analgesic medication required (Sin, Man, Wai, & Chow, 2015). Perhaps the most challenging pain to manage is pain with burn injuries. Music listening has also been shown to decrease anxiety in a study (n = 46) looking at the use of patient-preferred music with patients receiving wound care for burns (Ghezeljeh, Ardebili, Rafii, & Haghani, 2017). The patients who listened to their preferred music along with usual medication showed a statistically significant decrease in pain and anxiety along with an increase in relaxation levels while the painful procedures were performed.

Several studies involving patients with pain while undergoing cancer treatments reported music therapy as a positive intervention, with a Cochrane review (n = 52) concluding that music therapy may improve anxiety and pain (Wieland & Santesso, 2017); however, the quality of the research needs to be improved. Studies with rigorous methodology with precautions to minimize or eliminate researcher bias need to be done. Music and imagery experiences are multidimensional and difficult to evaluate. Measurement instruments designed to account for this will help effectively evaluate the music and imagery experiences and benefits. Meadows, Burns, and Perkins (2015) (n = 76) reported on the development and evaluation of the Music Therapy Self-Rating Scale used with patients undergoing cancer care. The patients participated in supportive music and imagery sessions. The results concluded the Music Therapy Self-Rating Scale is psychometrically sound and effectively measures the patient experience during music and imagery sessions. Using it in future studies may improve methodology and comparison of results among studies.

Concerns, Cautions, and Contraindications

Music therapy complements the medical model of treatment for pain and is an important component of multimodal pain management. Overall music therapy is a positive intervention for pain management when conducted by a trained music therapy professional; however, there are four cautions. First, although music therapy is a noninvasive intervention with many positive outcomes, one positive outcome also involves a caution. Because music elicits emotions and can assist patients in recognizing feelings, it can help in coping with the emotions related to pain. However, the response to music and elicited emotions can have a physiologic impact on the person, so heart rate, respiration rate, and blood pressure may need to be monitored. The physiologic changes can bring a greater awareness to the patient's body and potentially can result in an increased awareness or perception of pain. Another caution involves the emotional impact of music. The feelings elicited may cause patients to feel vulnerable and need professional support to begin coping with what they are experiencing and processing emotions. A third caution involves patients dealing with pain who are medically unstable. For example, any type of music, no matter how soothing, is contraindicated in a patient with high intracranial pressure. The final caution is to ensure the person providing music therapy is a trained music therapy professional. Music therapy interventions cannot be implemented by a volunteer musician, a health care professional who is also an amateur musician, or an iPod/MP3 player music listening program with recorded music. Although all music therapists are musicians, not all musicians are music therapists (see Box 21.3).

Animal-Assisted Therapy

The therapeutic value of the human-animal bond has been explored for centuries as a variety of animals have been domesticated to provide companionship and psychological support (Arkow, 2015). Florence Nightingale was one of the first to record the health benefits of connecting with animals. She noted that a small pet could be an excellent companion for patients, especially those with chronic conditions (Nightingale, 1992). The first recorded use of animals for therapy in the United States was in 1942 at an Army Convalescent Hospital in New York, where injured service personnel worked with farm animals as part of their therapeutic recovery and relaxation (Arkow, 2015). The father of modern pet therapy was Boris Levinson, a New York child psychotherapist who used his dog Jingles to gain the trust of his patients. His extensive documentation about the therapeutic value of the human-animal bond brought recognition to the health care community. Levinson (1962) was the first to coin the term *pet therapy*. Since that time, there has been

a proliferation of therapy teams, advances in animal-human research, and an evolution in terminology.

Definitions

Currently, there are over 20 different definitions of animal-assisted therapy (AAT) and 12 different terms for the same human-animal activity (Fine, 2015). In an effort to provide consistency of terminology and guidelines for practice and research, a white paper was created by the International Association of Human-Animal Interaction Organizations (IAHAIO), a global association of 60 interprofessional organizations that engage in education, practice, and research in AAT, animal-assisted activity (AAA), and service animal training (IAHAIO, 2018). The white paper includes the following internationally accepted definitions.

Animal-Assisted Therapy

"Animal-assisted therapy (AAT) is a goal-oriented, planned and structured therapeutic intervention directed and/or delivered by health, education and human service professionals" (IAHAIO, 2018, p. 5). Key features of AAT are (1) specific goals are set for each patient, (2) progress is measured, and (3) interactions are documented. The goals are designed by any health care professional who uses AAT in the treatment process (American Veterinary Medical Association [AVMA], 2017a). A physical goal could include, for example, walking a dog to improve mobility and function. A cognitive goal could include distraction from pain by interacting with the animal or improved verbal expression about the person's pain experience. An illustration of an emotional goal could be the motivation shown by walking the animal. Although a variety of animals, such as cats, rabbits, horses, and dolphins, provide AAT, dogs account for the highest percentage of animals used for AAT (Grandin et al., 2015).

Animal-Assisted Activity

"Animal-assisted activity (AAA) is a planned informal interaction and visitation conducted by the human-animal team for motivational, educational, and recreational purposes" (IAHAIO, 2018, p. 5). Key features of AAA are (1) specific goals are not planned for each patient, (2) visit activities are spontaneous, and (3) interactions are not documented. AAAs are less structured and provide human and animal contact for recreation, education, or pleasure. Examples include a visit by an animal to a hospital, hospice, long-term care center, school, or prison with the intent to bring comfort and companionship to the residents (Rivera, 2010).

Indications for Animal-Assisted Therapy and Animal-Assisted Activity

The variety of uses and settings in which AAT and AAA can be used are limitless, because they can be a great diversion from pain and can aid in relaxation. Bringing animal therapy teams into health care settings can bring the benefits of having pets in our lives to those who are dealing with health issues, physical pain, emotional issues, and/or stressful situations. AAT and AAA visits can help improve vital signs, decrease perception of pain levels, decrease anxiety, improve coping skills, and increase socialization (Arkow, 2015; Hart & Yamamoto, 2015). All of which promote increased relaxation and diversion from pain.

When a patient with pain gently reaches out to pet a dog and then smiles it is clear in that moment the pain is no longer the focus; rather, the dog is the focus along with the owner, who often talks with the patient about his or her interest in animals and personal pets the patient may have had in the past or has currently. Along with the smile, patients often demonstrate a decrease in body tension as they begin to relax. Moreover, patients who are cared for at the health care facility long term or who return often look forward to the visits from the therapy dogs. Patients who experience the benefit of an AAA or AAT visit may ask for pet therapy on subsequent hospitalizations to help them better control and cope with pain.

These visits can also help health care professionals relax during a stressful day (Stevens, Kepros, & Mosher, 2017). When staff members are less stressed they can be more effective in assisting patients who are struggling with pain issues. When therapy dogs are present in a hospital or extended care facility, the dogs and their owners are often stopped by family members and staff as they pass through the hallways on their way to see patients. At one medical center, requests for therapy dog visits have come from staff in nursing, respiratory, mental health, environmental services, physicians, and the business department. Therapy dog visits offer a healthy diversion from the stress these professionals encounter throughout the day (M. Erich, personal communication, June 12, 2017) (Table 21.2). The importance of the therapy dog visits at that medical center was witnessed during the COVID-19 pandemic when the therapy dogs were not allowed in the buildings. To ease the daily stress, one author (M.E.) facilitated "virtual pet therapy" with the therapy dogs visiting with clinicians virtually on a phone. The smiles in the eyes of the staff attested to how much they appreciated this novel intervention.

Evidence and Indications for Pain Management

An abundance of evidence from studies demonstrates the physical and/or psychological benefits gained from the human-animal bond. Most of these studies examined the animal's ability to attenuate a person's stress response. Stress-reduction strategies, such as petting an animal, can help reduce the buildup of stress hormones, including aldosterone, adrenaline, and cortisol (Wolff & Frishman, 2005). In addition, the hormone oxytocin can lower cortisol levels, lower blood pressure, decrease anxiety, and increase the pain threshold. Petting an animal is one of the best ways to increase oxytocin levels through physical touch (Chandler, 2017).

A number of studies have examined the use of AAT for patients dealing with pain, for example, adults with chronic pain (Marcus et al., 2012), adults with fibromyalgia (Marcus et al., 2013), adults after joint replacement surgery (Havey, Vlasses, Vlasses, Ludwig-Beymer, & Hackbarth, 2014), children undergoing dental procedures (Havener et al., 2001), and hospitalized children (Barker, Knisely, Schubert, Green, & Ameringer, 2015; Braun, Stangler, Narveson, & Pettingell, 2009; Sobo, Eng, & Kassity-Krich, 2006). "Pleasure experienced from interacting with a therapy animal may actually help to counteract some of the physical pain or discomfort resulting from patients' illness." (Chandler, 2017, p. 290).

Marcus et al. (2012) investigated whether therapy dog visits could counteract the physical pain or distress for adults in an outpatient chronic pain clinic waiting room and compared these effects to time spent in a waiting room without a therapy dog visit. The sample consisted of a total of 295 therapy dog visits: 235 visits with patients, 34 visits with family/friends, and 26 visits with staff. The study participants could choose to spend clinic waiting time with a certified therapy dog or in the clinic waiting room without a therapy dog. Statistically significant improvements were reported on pain, mood, and other measures of distress among those patients who spent time with the therapy dog compared to those who remained in the clinic waiting room. Significant improvements were also reported by family/friends and staff after therapy dog visits. For this sample, results revealed that therapy dog visits can significantly improve the feelings of well-being.

Havey et al. (2014) conducted a retrospective study examining the impact of AAT on the use of oral pain medication by patients (mean age of 66 years) after total joint replacement surgery. Subjects in the intervention group (n = 46) were matched with the control group (n = 46) on gender, age, length of stay, ethnicity, and diagnosis code for type of joint replacement. Patients in the intervention group received AAT every day for 5 to 15 minutes after surgery, patients in the control group received no AAT. Results revealed that patients who received AAT after surgery had statistically significant less pain medication use than the control group.

Sobo, Eng, and Kassity-Krich (2006) conducted one of the first studies to examine the effectiveness of therapy dog visits for children with postsurgical pain. These researchers used a convenience sample of 25 children (ages 5–18 years) who underwent surgery during their hospitalization. After surgery, each child received a one-time visit by Lizzy, a West Highland terrier. Of interest, each child could choose the level of interaction with Lizzy. In passive interaction, Lizzy would sit quietly with the child, in low interaction Lizzy would do an occasional trick, and in high interaction the child could actively play with and walk Lizzy. Despite the small sample size, there was a statistically significant decrease in pain levels

Table 21.2 | Example Techniques for Eliciting the Relaxation Response

Technique	Concept	Mechanism
Breath awareness	Shift from shallow breathing to abdominal breathing. Draw air deep into lungs using even breath.	Improve ability of respiratory system to produce energy from oxygen and remove waste.
Self-hypnosis	Narrow consciousness without completely losing awareness, to allow suspension of disbelief and experience of thoughts and images as real.	Facilitates both focused, intense mental activity and state of relaxation simultaneously.
Guided imagery	Use imagination to refocus mind on positive, healing images.	Negative thoughts influence feelings and behavior and exacerbate physical symptoms. Thoughts become reality (i.e., you are what you think you are). Therefore imagination is used to reduce subjective stress and treat physical symptoms.
Autogenic training	Use verbal commands that suggest bodily warmth and heaviness in limbs.	Word phrases suggest relaxation to the unconscious mind, which manifests the desired responses in the body. Aims to reverse "fight or flight" response during physical or emotional stress by promoting relaxation of the voluntary arm and leg muscles, inducing peripheral vasodilation, and normalizing cardiac activity.
Progressive muscle relaxation	Alternately tense and relax different muscle groups, to better distinguish between these two states.	Based on premise that the body responds to anxiety-provoking phenomena with muscle tension that increases subjective anxiety. Muscle relaxation reduces physiologic tension and therefore blocks the subjective anxious response.
Transcendental meditation	Engage in attempting to anchor attention nonjudgmentally on a silent mantra.	Negative emotion cannot persist when focusing on something other than the target of the emotion. Habitual thought patterns lose influence when brought to conscious awareness. Present focus reduces emotional extremes. Meditation also slows sympathetic nervous system activity.
Mindful awareness	Observation or attention to phenomena in the moment nonjudgmentally as they enter awareness	Strong emotions become manageable by focusing on sensations rather than the content of emotional thoughts.
Yoga	Movement meditation correlated with the breath.	Yoga is a comprehensive system of practices for physical and psychological health and well-being and incorporates multiple techniques, including physical postures/exercises, breathing exercises, and meditation/concentration techniques. As an integrative discipline, yoga takes advantage of the simultaneous application of its component techniques, all of which contribute to eliciting the relaxation response.

From Park, E. R., Traeger, L., Vranceanu, A. M., Scult, M., Lerner, J. A., Benson, H., ... & Fricchione, G. L. (2013). The development of a patient-centered program based on the relaxation response: The Relaxation Response Resiliency Program (3RP). *Psychosomatics, 54*(2), 165–174.

after each dog visit. In addition, interview data revealed 8 themes regarding the dog visits: (1) was a distraction from the pain, (2) eased the pain, (3) was calming, (4) reminded them of home, (5) provided company, (6) was nice to cuddle with, (7) was fun, and (8) brought happiness.

Although there has been a great increase in AAT research over the past three decades, Kazdin (2011) notes that many of the studies have methodologic flaws, such as small sample size, use of a single group without a control group, use of a single measurement, pretest to posttest design only, and lack of randomization of intervention. Future research on AAT is needed that includes examining the efficacy of AAT for various pain conditions, random assignment to the AAT group and standard care group, examination of the frequency and duration of the AAT, and appropriate uses of AAT across cultural and ethnic groups.

Cautions

A number of potential risks are involved in having animals in health care settings, including allergies, transmission of infectious diseases, and injuries (Fine, 2015). However, Brodie, Biley, and Shewring (2002) conducted a comprehensive review examining the potential risks of animals in health care settings and found a low incidence of such occurrences and concluded that the potential benefits far outweighed the minor risks. Moreover, these potential risks can be greatly decreased by using registered AAT teams who have been adequately trained, along with consistently using standard hand hygiene before and after every visit and having anyone who pets the animal use hand hygiene (IAHAIO 2018; Murthy et al., 2015). Guidelines from the Centers for Disease Control and Prevention (2003) require that AAT animals be bathed, groomed, fully vaccinated, and free of parasites. In addition, most AAT organizations require annual examinations and preventive care by a veterinarian to assess the physical and behavioral health and well-being of the animal (AVMA, 2017b; IAHAIO, 2018; Pet Partners, 2016).

Guided Imagery

The nervous systems of humans use *imagery* as a means through which impressions, ideas, conceptions, recollections, and dreams are chronicled for retrieval whenever access is needed or desired (Rossman, 2018). *Guided imagery* is a relaxation technique, with the goal of achieving a desired positive outcome, in which the participating person uses one or more of the five senses to deliberately focus attention to invoke soothing images of a non-real environment (Hadjibalassi, Lambrinou, Papastavrou, & Papathanassoglou, 2018; Tsitsi, Charalambous, Papastavrou, & Raftopoulos, 2017; Wesch, Callow, Hall, & Pope, 2016). The outcomes of guided imagery can be designed to meet the needs of each patient, including relaxation, pain relief, healing, positive results of surgery, and security with the care of clinicians (Charette, et al., 2016; Hamlin & Robertson, 2017; Jacobson et al., 2016; Kwekkeboom & Bratzke, 2016). The imagery can be guided by a clinician who is present with the person in a clinical setting or through video or audio recordings the person uses when convenient at their location of choice (Hamlin & Roberston, 2017). The participating person is encouraged by the guide to become calm through a relaxation technique such as breathing. Then by triggering the senses to elicit images the person is led to a soothing location where the person can be encouraged to feel relaxed, comfortable, and without pain, anxiety, or distress (dos Santos Felix et al., 2019;

Foji et al., 2015). The fullest guided imagery experience is achieved when the person is guided to use all five senses to fully experience being in the imagined location of his or her choice (Hamlin & Robertson, 2017).

Evidence and Indications for Pain Management

At least one way in which guided imagery is effective as part of a multimodal approach to pain management is by distracting attention away from acute and chronic pain, while moving the focus of the person toward a pleasant experience, and thus lessening the sensory component of pain (Hamlin & Robertson, 2017). Current literature is replete with research studies and systematic reviews of guided imagery used for management of pain and other symptoms. Through one systematic review of studies (n = 10 studies) in which guided imagery was used with critically ill patients (n = 1391 total subjects), the authors concluded guided imagery "is a promising patient-centered approach for the improvement of a number of patient outcomes," including pain and anxiety (Hadjibalassi et al., 2018, p. 73). The authors of an integrated review of guided imagery used in conjunction with other relaxation interventions supported use of guided imagery among postoperative patients (dos Santos Felix et al., 2019). The authors of that review also called for the establishment of guidelines and support for clinical use of guided imagery and additional research to further guide and support use. When guided imagery was considered in a systematic review of RCTs (n = 7 studies) involving people who were diagnosed with arthritis and other rheumatic diseases, the authors reported guided imagery conveyed by listening to an audio taping was a safe and cost-effective component of a multimodal analgesic plan of care (Giacobbi et al., 2015). The authors of a recent meta-analysis evaluating the effect of imagery on function, mobility, pain, and self-efficacy with people after injuries (n = 10 studies) reported a nonsignificant but large negative effect of imagery on perceived pain, small nonsignificant positive effect of imagery on function, and a large positive nonsignificant effect on self-efficacy (Zach, Dobersek, Inglis, & Tenenbaum, 2018). The lack of significance in that analysis may have been related to the heterogeneity of the various studies.

More recent studies include guided imagery done with a variety of groups involving people with pain for whom dealing with pain control was particularly challenging; however, most of the studies involved small samples. In a quasi-experimental study, when people living with fibromyalgia who participated in a guided imagery group (n = 30) were compared with those in a control group (n = 30), those in the guided imagery intervention group reported markedly less pain than those in the control group (Onieva-Zafra, García, & Del Valle, 2015). In another study with patients with fibromyalgia, those in the intervention group in which guided imagery was used with patients in addition to usual care (n = 36) compared to usual care alone (n = 36), those who received guided imagery reported significantly less pain intensity after 10 weeks of guided imagery (Menzies, Lyon, Elswick, McCain, & Gray, 2014). Guided imagery was used effectively with children living with sickle cell disease (n = 20) with reductions in both pain intensity and pain frequency (Dobson & Byrne, 2014). Imagery was used in a very small study (n = 5) with athletes who had experienced malleolar fractures (Wesch, Callow, Hall, & Pope, 2016). In that study, two of the five athletes reported considerable improvement in ability to participate in physical therapy and all five reported positive experiences using imagery.

Not all research has yielded positive benefits for pain control. In a very small study with older adults who were living with pain and cancer, guided imagery (n = 5) was compared with planned rest (n = 4) (Adeola et al., 2015). The investigators in that study reported the participants who received guided imagery reported greater pain levels than those in the planned rest group. The authors acknowledge the sample size was very small and also note there may have been differences in disease progression among the participants. The results of this study may also speak to the importance of rest (see Chapters 8 and 22). Finally, researchers of an interesting study with patients who underwent total knee replacement did not find a specific reduction in patient reports of pain; however, 6 months after surgery the participants in the guided imagery group (n = 29 of 58) did have significantly lower concentrations of cortisol in their hair, which is suggestive of lower levels of stress (Jacobson et al., 2016).

In at least two research studies, coincidental data have supported beneficial effects of clinicians who are exposed to patients receiving guided imagery. The researchers of one interesting study reported that during surgery to excise facial carcinomas, neither recorded guided imagery nor relaxing music with excisional surgery was associated with reductions in either pain or anxiety among the patients (music, n = 54; guided imagery, n = 50; and control, n = 51); however, there was a correlation with the degree of anxiety reported by surgeons when patients were participating in one of those therapies (Alam et al., 2016). Similar benefits for clinicians were reported by Burhenn, Olausson, Villegas, and Kravits (2014), who reported that nurses who led patients with guided imagery reported personally feeling increased senses of calm and relaxation. Additional research with replication of existing work and rigorous methodology in larger samples is needed.

Cautions and Contraindications

Although there are no reported side effects with guided imagery and it is generally considered safe, there are cautions and contraindications. Guided imagery should be used cautiously and only by clinicians experienced with guided imagery in patients who are not able to communicate with the clinician, those with fragile medical conditions (e.g., cardiac, respiratory), and those with mental health disorders or histories of such disorders, including histories of abuse (Hamlin & Robertson, 2017; Rossman, 2018; Tick et al., 2018). Guided imagery is considered contraindicated in people with dementia, altered mental status, inability to concentrate, or psychiatric disorders (e.g., psychosis) or among those who have cultural or religious beliefs that are in opposition with guided imagery (Hamlin & Robertson, 2017; Rossman, 2018).

Autogenic Training

Autogenic training (AT) was developed in Germany between 1920 and 1930 by Johannes Heinrich Schultz (1953) as a structured process of autosuggestion (Irnich, 2013). Schultz considered AT to be a type of self-hypnosis in which the body learns to respond to instructions spoken by the person participating in AT (Crane & Ward, 2016) (see Chapter 22 for discussion of hypnosis). It has subsequently been described as "psychophysiological self-control therapy" (Romas & Sharma, 2017, p. 54), which is consistent with the literal meaning of *self origin*, indicating the individual is in control of his or her personal being. The person who participates in AT initially is encouraged to passively be attentive to sensations in the body, particularly warmth and heaviness, without trying to change them (Romas & Sharma, 2017) (Box 21.4). With experience, images and situations uniquely important for the person are incorporated in the AT process (Irnich, 2013).

Evidence and Indications for Pain Management

Evidence regarding the effectiveness of AT for pain control is inconsistent. Researchers of a large study in Spain (n = 484) reported that a psychoeducational intervention including AT resulted in reduced pain intensity and greater functional ability (Luciano et al., 2011). In a subsequent smaller study in Spain (n = 93) AT was used as part of a CBT intervention with women with fibromyalgia (Castel, Cascón, Padrol, Sala, & Rull, 2012). It was reported that the women in the study who participated in CBT had lower pain intensity and catastrophizing scores both immediately and at 6 months follow-up than those in the AT group. In a small study (n = 21) in Japan, AT was helpful in reducing symptoms of the painful condition irritable bowel syndrome (Shinozaki et al., 2010). Yet a systematic review of seven controlled trials reported no consistent evidence to support the use of autogenic training to relieve pain of tension headaches (Ernst, 2014). Similarly, from a review of studies using AT for people with chronic nonspecific neck pain it was reported there was no effect on pain intensity (Shearer et al., 2015).

In addition to being used for pain, AT is widely used for managing stress, particularly in Europe and Japan (Romas & Sharma, 2017). It is also used for managing insomnia (Pinheiro, Mendes, Pais, Carvalho, & Cabral, 2015). Internationally, it has been used by clinicians as

Box 21.4 | Autogenic Training

Autogenic training (AT) owes its origin to the work of German neurologist Johannes Heinrich Schultz. He described it as a self-hypnotic procedure. Autogenic therapy is a derivative of hypnosis and also has been described as psychophysiologic self-control therapy.

Since its origin in Germany, it has remained quite popular in European countries and Japan. This technique became known in North America when one of Schultz's followers, Wolfgang Luthe, a physician, immigrated to Canada and translated much of this work into English. Ample evidence shows that it is a useful stress-reduction technique. It is also useful as a curative approach in dealing with anxiety and related disorders.

The term *autogenic* is derived from the Greek words *autos,* meaning "self," and *genos,* meaning "origin." Therefore, in this technique, the self-regulation and self-healing powers of the mind are channeled in a positive manner. The practitioner of AT concentrates on his or her body sensations in a passive manner without directly or volitionally bringing about any change. The key sensations on which the mind is focused include those of heaviness and warmth. Focusing on these sensations provides the body with a feeling of relaxation because these sensations are normally associated with the relaxation process.

Modified from Romas, J. A., & Sharma, J. (2017). Relaxation. In J. Romas, & M. Sharma. *Practical Stress Management: A Comprehensive Workbook* (7th ed., pp. 47–67). St. Louis, MO: Academic Press.

---

a self-care technique by nurses (Crane & Ward, 2016), for stress management for new surgeons (Mache, Danzer, Klapp, & Groneberg, 2015), and by nursing students (Lim & Kim, 2014).

Contraindications

Contraindications listed for using AT are people with severe anxiety, depression, or delusions (Irnich, 2013).

Key Points

- Distraction and relaxation are interventions that can be used by patients as one aspect of a multimodal approach to control acute and chronic pain.
- Distraction and relaxation techniques can be used alone or in combination with each other and other components of multimodal pain management.
- Breathing is an important self-care strategy to help manage pain and anxiety.
- Advancing technology is enabling improvement in some distraction and relaxation techniques and increasing the availability to patients who may not have easy access.
- Animal-assisted activities provide a sense of normalcy and fun into the health care setting.
- Animal-assisted therapy can provide motivation for patients during difficult therapies and treatments.
- Music therapy involves much more than just listening to music. It is a specialized profession facilitated by credentialed professionals.
- The power of music paired with a therapeutic relationship makes music therapy a valuable tool for pain management.

- Distraction, relaxation, animal, and music therapy can be important components in a plan for multimodal analgesia.
- Distraction, relaxation, animal, and music therapy can be used by patients during hospitalization and at home for patients to be actively involved and empowered in their management of pain.
- Many of the relaxation and distraction techniques are portable and inexpensive or without cost.
- Internationally, relaxation and distraction techniques are used effectively as part of a multimodal approach to pain management.
- Additional research is needed to better understand the benefit of distraction, relaxation, animal, and music therapy in multimodal pain management.
- Additional rigorous research is needed to replicate studies and expand the evidence to support use of relaxation and distraction as components of multimodal pain management.

Case Scenario

Melissa is a 38-year-old woman who was admitted to the hospital last week after a motor vehicle collision (MVC) in which she was the restrained driver. The driver side window was open, and Melissa sustained a degloving of the distal portion of her left upper extremity, fractures of the third through sixth ribs (left), and assorted abrasions and contusions. She is generally healthy apart from chronic low back pain (CLBP), which she attributes to three pregnancies and difficult labors. She is 5 ft 6 inches and weighs 225 lb. Before the MVC she was using oxyCODONE 10 mg qid as needed for pain. She expresses concerns about needing to take more opioids because she says her mother and two of her three siblings "are addicted to pain medicine." She wants to know what she can do to help the pain during the painful wound care of her left arm and then use to help her manage her CLBP and take fewer oxyCODONE pills. She tells you that there are not many resources where she lives; she does not have much money and has only basic insurance.

1. What distraction options can you offer to Melissa?
2. How do you explain to her how these options can be helpful for her?
3. What relaxation techniques can you offer to Melissa?
4. How do you explain to her how these options can be helpful for her?
5. What resources can Melissa access to use these pain management options at home?

References

Adeola, M. T., Baird, C. L., Prouty Sands, L., Longoria, N., Henry, U., Nielsen, J., & Shields, C. G. (2015). Active Despite Pain: Patient Experiences with Guided Imagery with Relaxation Compared to Planned Rest. *Clinical Journal of Oncology Nursing, 19*(6), 649–652.

Alam, M., Roongpisuthipong, W., Kim, N. A., Goyal, A., Swary, J. H., Brindise, R. T., ... Yoo, S. (2016). Utility of recorded guided imagery and relaxing music in reducing patient pain and anxiety, and surgeon anxiety, during cutaneous surgical procedures: A single-blinded randomized controlled trial. *Journal of the American Academy of Dermatology, 75*(3), 585–589.

Alaparthi, G. K., Augustine, A. J., Anand, R., & Mahale, A. (2016). Comparison of Diaphragmatic Breathing Exercise, Volume and Flow Incentive Spirometry, on Diaphragm Excursion and Pulmonary Function in Patients Undergoing Laparoscopic Surgery: A Randomized Controlled Trial. *Minimally Invasive Surgery, 2016*. Article ID I967532.

Alexander, J. C., & Joshi, G. P. (2016). Smartphone applications for chronic pain management: Critical appraisal. *Journal of Pain Research, 9*(9), 731–734.

American Music Therapy Association (AMTA). (ND). *Music Therapy and Music Based Interventions in the Treatment and Management of Pain: Selected References and Key Findings.* http://www.musictherapy.org/assets/1/7/MT_Pain_2010.pdf.

American Music Therapy Association (AMTA). (2014). Setting the record straight: What music therapy is and is not. http://www.musictherapy.org/amta_press_release_on_music_therapy_-_jan_2014/.

American Veterinary Medical Association. (2017a). *Animal-assisted interventions: Definitions.* Retrieved from https://www.avma.org/KB/Policies/Pages/Animal-Assisted-Interventions-Definitions.aspx.

American Veterinary Medical Association. (2017b). *Wellness guidelines for animals in animal-assisted activity, animal-assisted therapy, and resident animal programs.* Retrieved from https://ebusiness.avma.org/files/productdownloads/wellness_AAA.pdf.

Arkow, P. (2015). *Animal-assisted therapy and activities: A study and research resource guide for the use of companion animals in animal-assisted interventions* (11th ed.). Stratford, NJ: AnimalTherapy.net.

Armfield, J. M., & Heaton, L. J. (2013). Management of fear and anxiety in the dental clinic: A review. *Australian Dental Journal, 58*(4), 390–407.

Armfield, J., & Marek, C. L. (2017). Patients who are anxious and fearful. In *Diagnosis and Treatment Planning in Dentistry* (3rd Ed., pp. 323–341). St. Louis: Elsevier.

Arsenault, M., Ladouceur, A., Lehmann, A., Rainville, P., & Piché, M. (2013). Pain modulation induced by respiration: phase and frequency effects. *Neuroscience, 252*, 501–511.

Barker, N. J., Jones, M., O'Connell, N. E., & Everard, M. L. (2013). Breathing exercises for dysfunctional breathing/hyperventilation syndrome in children. *Cochrane Database Systematic Reviews, 12*. https://doi.org/10.1002/14651858.CD010376.pub2. Available at https://www.ncbi.nlm.nih.gov/pubmed/24347088. Accessed 02/14/2018.

Barker, S., Knisely, J., Schubert, C., Green, J., & Ameringer, S. (2015). The effect of an animal-assisted intervention on anxiety and pain in hospitalized children. *Anthrozoos, 28*(1), 101–112.

Benson, H., & Klipper, M. Z. (1975). *The Relaxation Response.* New York, NY: Morrow.

Berk, R. A. (2015). The greatest veneration: Humor as a coping strategy for the challenges of aging. *Social Work in Mental Health, 13*(1), 30–47.

Blödt, S., Pach, D., Roll, S., & Witt, C. M. (2014). Effectiveness of app-based relaxation for patients with chronic low back pain (Relaxback) and chronic neck pain (Relaxneck): study protocol for two randomized pragmatic trials. *Trials, 15*(1), 490.

Boerner, K. E., Birnie, K. A., Chambers, C. T., Taddio, A., McMurtry, C. M., Noel, M., ... Riddell, R. P. (2015). Simple psychological interventions for reducing pain from common needle procedures in adults: systematic review of randomized and quasi-randomized controlled trials. *The Clinical Journal of Pain, 31*(Supp 10), S90–S98.

Boluda, M. P., Asencio, J. M., Vela, A. C., Mayor, S. G., Campos, A. L., Leiva, I. L., ... Kaknani-Uttumchandani, S. (2016). The dynamic experience of pain in burn patients: A phenomenological study. *Burns, 42*(5), 1097–1104.

Bonde, L. O. (2017). If music be the food of life - play on? *European Journal of Integrative Medicine, 9*(1), 41–43.

Botella, C., Baños, R. M., García-Palacios, A., & Quero, S. (2017). Virtual reality and other realities. In S. G. Hofmann, & J. G. Gordon (Eds.), *The Science of Cognitive Behavioral Therapy* (pp. 551–590). New York, NY: Academic Press.

Braun, C., Stangler, T., Narveson, J., & Pettingell, S. (2009). Animal-assisted therapy as a pain relief intervention for children. *Complementary Therapies in Clinical Practice, 15*(2), 105–109.

Bresler, D. E. (2016). Guided imagery: A multipurpose technique for helping people in pain. In R. A. Bonakdar, & A. W. Sukiennik (Eds.), *Integrative Pain Management* (pp. 399–413). New York, NY: Oxford University Press.

Brodie, S. J., Biley, F. C., & Shewring, M. (2002). An exploration of the potential risks associated with using pet therapy in healthcare settings. *Journal of Clinical Nursing, 11*(4), 444–456.

Brown, S. T., Douglas, C., & Flood, L. P. (2001). Women's Evaluation of Intrapartum Nonpharmacologic Pain Relief Methods Used in Labor. *The Journal of Perinatal Education, 10*(3), 1–8.

Brunelli, S., Morone, G., Iosa, M., Ciotti, C., De Giorgi, R., Foti, C., & Traballesi, M. (2015). Efficacy of progressive muscle relaxation, mental imagery, and phantom exercise training on phantom limb: a randomized controlled trial. *Archives of Physical Medicine and Rehabilitation*, 96(2), 181–218.

Burhenn, P., Olausson, J., Villegas, G., & Kravits, K. (2014). Guided imagery for pain control. *Clinical Journal of Oncology Nursing*, 18(5), 501–503.

Busch, V., Magerl, W., Kern, U., Haas, J., Hajak, G., & Eichhammer, P. (2012). The effect of deep and slow breathing on pain perception, autonomic activity, and mood processing—an experimental study. *Pain Medicine*, 13(2), 215–228.

Castel, A., Cascón, R., Padrol, A., Sala, J., & Rull, M. (2012). Multicomponent cognitive-behavioral group therapy with hypnosis for the treatment of fibromyalgia: long-term outcome. *The Journal of Pain*, 13(3), 255–265.

Centers for Disease Control and Prevention. (2003). Guidelines for environmental infection control in healthcare facilities. *MMWR Recommendations & Reports*, 52(RR-10), 1–2.

Chandler, C. (2017). *Animal-assisted therapy in counseling.* New York, N.Y.: Routledge.

Charette, S., Fiola, J. L., Charest, M. C., Villeneuve, E., Théroux, J., Joncas, J., … Le May, S. (2015). Guided imagery for adolescent post-spinal fusion pain management: A pilot study. *Pain Management Nursing*, 16(3), 211–220.

Chellew, K., Evans, P., Fornes-Vives, J., Pérez, G., & Garcia-Banda, G. (2015). The effect of progressive muscle relaxation on daily cortisol secretion. *Stress*, 18(5), 538–544.

Chiramonte, D., D'Adamo, C., & Morrison, B. (2014). Integrative approaches to pain management. In H. Benzon, J. Rathmell, C. L. Wu, D. C. Turk, C. E. Argoff, & R. W. Hurley (Eds.), *Practical Management of Pain* (5th Ed.) (pp. 658–668. e3). St. Louis: Mosby.

Cicek, S., & Basar, F. (2017). The effects of breathing techniques training on the duration of labor and anxiety levels of pregnant women. *Complementary Therapies in Clinical Practice*, 29, 213–219.

Congreve, W. (1697). *The Mourning Bride.* www.enotes.com/topics/mourning-bride.

Cousins, N. (1979). *Anatomy of an Illness as Perceived by the Patient.* NY, NY: Bantom Books.

Crane, P. J., & Ward, S. F. (2016). Self-healing and self-care for nurses. *AORN Journal*, 104(5), 386–400.

Curry, N. A., & Kasser, T. (2005). Can coloring mandalas reduce anxiety? *Art Therapy*, 22(2), 81–85.

Czarnecki, M. L., Turner, H. N., Collins, P. M., Doellman, D., Wrona, S., & Reynolds, J. (2011). Procedural pain management: A position statement with clinical practice recommendations. *Pain Management Nursing*, 12(2), 95–111.

Dampier, C. (2014). The management of pain from Sickle Cell Disease. In H. T. Benzon, J. P. Rathmell, C. L. Wu, D. Turk, C. E. Argoff, & R. W. Hurley (Eds.), In: *Practical Management of Pain* (5th Ed.) (pp. 997–1002.e2). Philadelphia: Mosby.

Davis, W. B., & Thaut, M. H. (1989). The Influence of Preferred Relaxing Music on Measures of State Anxiety, Relaxation and Physiological Responses. *Journal of Music Therapy*, 26(4), 168–187.

Dengsangluri, J. A. (2015). Effect of breathing exercise in reduction of pain during first stage of labour among primigravidas. *International Journal of Health Science Research IJHSR*, 5(6), 390–398.

Dobrztnska, E., Cesarz, H., & Rymaszewska, A. K. (2006). Music therapy- history, definitions and application. *Archives of Psychiatry and Psychotherapy*, 8(1), 47–52.

Dobson, C. E., & Byrne, M. W. (2014). Using guided imagery to manage pain in young children with sickle cell disease. *AJN The American Journal of Nursing*, 114(4), 26–36.

dos Santos Felix, M. M., Ferreira, M. B. G., da Cruz, L. F., & Barbosa, M. H. (2019). Relaxation Therapy with Guided Imagery for Postoperative Pain Management: An Integrative Review. *Pain Management Nursing*, 20(1), 3–9.

Dowell, D., Haegerich, T. M., & Chou, R. (2016). CDC Guideline for prescribing opioids for chronic pain – United States, 2016. *Journal of the American Medical Association*, 315(15), 1624–1645.

Drake, C. R., Searight, H. R., & Olson-Pupek, K. (2014). The influence of art-making on negative mood states in university students. *American Journal of Applied Psychology*, 2(3), 69–72.

Dunbar, R. I., Baron, R., Frangou, A., Pearce, E., van Leeuwin, E. J., Stow, J., … Van Vugt, M. (2011). Social laughter is correlated with an elevated pain threshold. *Proceedings of the Royal Society of London B: Biological Sciences*, 279(1731), 1161–1167.

El Korh, P., & Giuliani, F. (2016). CBT of a person living in a situation of mental handicap and presenting an anxiety disorder coupled with a specific phobia. *Clinical Psychiatry*, 2(2), 1–5.

Elmali, H., & Akpinar, R. B. (2017). The effect of watching funny and unfunny videos on post-surgical pain levels. *Complementary Therapies in Clinical Practice*, 26(1), 36–41.

Ernst, E. (2014). Reference Module in Neuroscience & Biobehavioral Psychology. In R. Daroff, & M. J. Aminoff (Eds.), *Encyclopedia of Neurological Science* (2nd Ed). (pp. 738–742) New York, NY: Academic Press.

Faber, A. W., Patterson, D. R., & Bremer, M. (2013). Repeated use of immersive virtual reality therapy to control pain during wound dressing changes in pediatric and adult burn patients. *Journal of Burn Care & Research*, 34(5), 563–568.

Fine, A. (2015). *Handbook on animal-assisted therapy: Foundations and guidelines for animal-assisted interventions* (4th ed.). New York, NY: Academic Press.

Foji, S., Tadayonfar, M. A., Mohsenpour, M., & Rakhshani, M. H. (2015). The study of the effect of guided imagery on pain, anxiety and some other hemodynamic factors in patients undergoing coronary angiography. *Complementary Therapies in Clinical Practice*, 21(2), 119–123.

Freud, S. (1960). *Jokes and Their Relation to the Unconscious.* New York, NY: Norton.

Garrett, B., Taverner, T., Masinde, W., Gromala, D., Shaw, C., & Negraeff, M. (2014). A rapid evidence assessment of immersive virtual reality as an adjunct therapy in acute pain management in clinical practice. *The Clinical Journal of Pain*, 30(12), 1089–1098.

Gelinas, C., Arbour, C., Michaud, C., Robar, L., & Côté, J. (2013). Patients and ICU nurses' perspectives of non-pharmacological interventions for pain management. *Nursing in Critical Care*, 18(6), 307–318.

Ghezeljeh, T. N., Ardebili, F. M., Rafii, F., & Haghani, H. (2017). The effects of patient-preferred music on anticipatory anxiety, post-procedural burn pain and relaxation level. *European Journal of Integrative Medicine*, 9, 141–147.

Giacobbi, P. R., Stabler, M. E., Stewart, J., Jaeschke, A. M., Siebert, J. L., & Kelley, G. A. (2015). Guided imagery for arthritis and other rheumatic diseases: A systematic review of randomized controlled trials. *Pain Management Nursing, 16*(5), 792–803.

Gold, J. I., Belmont, K. A., & Thomas, D. A. (2007). The neurobiology of virtual reality pain attenuation. *CyberPsychology & Behavior, 10*(4), 536–544.

Grandin, T., Fine, A., O'Haire, M., Carlisle, G., & Bowers, C. (2015). The roles of animals for individuals with Autism Spectrum Disorder. In A. Fine (Ed.), *Handbook on animal-assisted therapy: Foundations and guidelines for animal-assisted interventions* (pp. 225–236). New York, NY: Academic Press.

Guillory, J. E., Hancock, J. T., Woodruff, C., & Keilman, J. (2015). Text messaging reduces analgesic requirements during surgery. *Pain Medicine, 16*(4), 667–672.

Gupta, B., Raddi, S. A., & Gupta, R. S. (2016). Effectiveness of Slow Paced Breathing on Labour Pain Perception among Primigravida Mothers Admitted in Maternity Unit of Selected Hospital Of Belgaum, Karnataka. *Imperial Journal of Interdisciplinary Research, 3*(3), 1621–1625.

Hadjibalassi, M., Lambrinou, E., Papastavrou, E., & Papathanassoglou, E. (2018). The effect of guided imagery on physiological and psychological outcomes of adult ICU patients: A systematic literature review and methodological implications. *Australian Critical Care, 31*(1), 73–86.

Hakked, C. S., Balakrishnan, R., & Krishnamurthy, M. N. (2017). Yogic breathing practices improve lung functions of competitive young swimmers. *Journal of Ayurveda and Integrative Medicine, 8*(2), 99–104.

Halzack, S. (2016). The big business behind the adult coloring book craze. *The Washington Post*, Business Section. March 12, 2016.

Hamlin, A. S., & Robertson, T. M. (2017). Pain and Complementary Therapies. *Critical Care Nursing Clinics, 29*(4), 449–460.

Hart, L., & Yamamoto, M. (2015). Recruiting psychosocial health effects of animals for families and communities: Transition to practice. In A. Fine (Ed.), *Handbook on animal-assisted therapy: Foundations and guidelines for animal-assisted interventions* (pp. 53–72). New York, NY: Academic Press.

Havener, L., Gentes, L., Thaler, B., Megel, M., Baun, M., Driscoll, F., … Agrawal, S. (2001). The effects of a companion animal on distress in children undergoing dental procedures. *Issues in Comprehensive Pediatric Nursing, 24*(2), 137–152.

Havey, J., Vlasses, F., Vlasses, P., Ludwig-Beymer, P., & Hackbarth, D. (2014). The effect of animal-assisted therapy on pain management use after joint replacement. *Anthrozoos, 27*(3), 361–369.

Hauck, M., Metzner, S., Rohlffs, F., Lorenz, J., & Engel, A. K. (2013). The influence of music and music therapy on pain-induced neuronal oscillations measured by magnetencephalography. *Pain, 154*(4), 539–547.

Horne-Moyer, H. L., Moyer, B. H., Messer, D. C., & Messer, E. S. (2014). The use of electronic games in therapy: a review with clinical implications. *Current Psychiatry Reports, 16*(12), 520.

Hudlicka, E. (2016). Virtual affective agents and therapeutic games. In D. D. Luxton (Ed.), *Artificial Intelligence in Behavioral and Mental Health Care.* (pp. 81–115). St. Louis: Elsevier.

Ingadottir, B., Blondal, K., Thue, D., Zoega, S., Thylen, I., & Jaarsma, T. (2017). Development, usability, and efficacy of serious game to help patients learn about pain management after surgery: An evaluation study. *JMIR Serious Games, 5*(2), e10.

International Association of Human-Animal Interaction Organizations [IAHAIO]. (2018). *IAHAIO White Paper: The IAHAIO Definitions for Animal-Assisted Intervention and Guidelines for Wellness of Animals Involved.* Retrieved from http://www.iahaio.org.

Irnich, C. (2013). Relaxation techniques: body and mind. pp. 245-252. In D. Irnich (Ed.), *Myofascial Trigger Points.* London: Churchill Livingstone.

Ito, M., & Matsushima, E. (2017). Presentation of coping strategies associated with physical and mental health during health check-ups. *Community Mental Health Journal, 53*(3), 297–305.

Jacobson, A. F., Umberger, W. A., Palmieri, P. A., Alexander, T. S., Myerscough, R. P., Draucker, C. B., … Kirschbaum, C. (2016). Guided imagery for total knee replacement: A randomized, placebo-controlled pilot study. *The Journal of Alternative and Complementary Medicine, 22*(7), 563–575.

Jafari, H., Courtois, I., Van den Bergh, O., Vlaeyen, J. W., & Van Diest, I. (2017a). Pain and respiration: a systematic review. *Pain, 158*(6), 995–1006.

Jafari, H., Vlaeyen, J., Van den Bergh, O., & Van Diest, I. (2017, Octoer). Beyond distraction? The effect of slow deep breathing on pain. *Biological Psychology, 129*, 381.

Jameson, E., Trevena, J., & Swain, N. (2011). Electronic gaming as pain distraction. *Pain Research and Management, 16*(1), 27–32.

Jang, S. H., Kang, S. Y., Lee, H. J., & Lee, S. Y. (2016). Beneficial effect of mindfulness-based art therapy in patients with breast cancer – a randomized controlled trial. *Explore, 12*(5), 333–340.

Jin, W., Choo, A., Gromala, D., Shaw, C., & Squire, P. (2016). A virtual reality game for chronic pain management: A randomized, controlled clinical study. In J. D. Westwood, S. W. Westwood, & L. Felländer-Tsai (Eds.), *Medicine Meets Virtual Reality 22: NextMed MMVR22.* https://doi.org/10.3233/978-1-61499-625-154.

Kaimal, G., Ayaz, H., Herres, J., Dieterich-Hartwell, R., Makwana, B., Kaiser, D. H., & Nasser, J. A. (2017). Functional near-infrared spectroscopy assessment of reward perception based on visual self-expression: Coloring, doodling, and free drawing. *The Arts in Psychotherapy, 55*(1), 85–92.

Kane, F. M., Brodie, E. E., Coull, A., Coyne, L., Howd, A., Milne, A., … Robbins, R. (2004). The Analgesic Effect of Odour and Music Upon Dressing Change. *The British Journal of Nursing, 13*(Supp 4), S4–S12.

Kazdin, A. (2011). Establishing the effectiveness of animal-assisted therapies: Methodological standards, issues, and strategies. In P. McCardle, S. McCune, J. Griffin, & V. Maholmes (Eds.), *How animals affect us: Examining the influence of human-animal interaction on child development and human health* (pp. 35–51). Washington, D.C.: American Psychological Association.

Keefe, F. J., Huling, D. A., Coggins, M. J., Keefe, D. F., Rosenthal, M. Z., Herr, N. R., & Hoffman, H. G. (2012). Virtual reality for persistent pain: a new direction for behavioral pain management. *Pain, 153*(11), 2163–2166.

Kim, B. (2016). Virtual reality as an artistic medium: A study on creative projects using contemporary head-mounted displays. Master's Thesis Media Lab Helsinki Department of Media School of Arts, Design and Architecture Aalto University, Espoo, Finland.

Kim, K. S., Loring, S., & Kwekkeboom, K. (2017). Use of Art-Making Intervention for Pain and Quality of Life Among Cancer Patients: A Systematic Review. *Journal of Holistic Nursing*, 36(14), 341–353.

Kobayashi, S., & Koitabashi, K. (2016). Effects of progressive muscle relaxation on cerebral activity: An fMRI investigation. *Complementary Therapies in Medicine*, 26(1), 33–39.

Kobylański, J., Walczak, M., Stępień, K., Bereziewicz, W., & Pytko-Polończyk, J. (2015). Music therapy–history of development (part 2). *MEDtube Science: The use of smart glasses in healthcare*, 3(4), 27–30.

Krishnaswamy, P., & Nair, S. (2016). Effect of music therapy on pain and anxiety levels of cancer patients: A pilot study. *Indian Journal of Palliative Care*, 22(3), 307.

Kumar, S., & Raje, A. (2014). Effect of progressive muscular relaxation exercises versus transcutaneous electrical nerve stimulation on tension headache: A comparative study. *Hong Kong Physiotherapy Journal*, 32(2), 86–91.

Kwekkeboom, K. L. (2016). Cancer symptom cluster management. *Seminars in Oncology Nursing*, 32(4), 373–382.

Kwekkeboom, K. L., & Bratzke, L. C. (2016). A systematic review of relaxation, meditation, and guided imagery strategies for symptom management in heart failure. *The Journal of Cardiovascular Nursing*, 31(5), 457–468.

Lauche, R., Materdey, S., Cramer, H., Haller, H., Stange, R., Dobos, G., & Rampp, T. (2013). Effectiveness of home-based cupping massage compared to progressive muscle relaxation in patients with chronic neck pain: a randomized controlled trial. *PloS one*, 8(6), e65378.

Lee, E. K. O., & Yeo, Y. (2013). Relaxation practice for health in the United States: Findings from the national health interview survey. *Journal of Holistic Nursing*, 31(2), 139–148.

Lee, J. H. (2016). The Effects of Music on Pain: A Meta-Analysis. *Journal of Music Therapy*, 53(4), 430–477.

Lee, M., Lee, S. H., Kim, T., Yoo, H. J., Kim, S. H., Suh, D. W., ... Yoon, B. (2017). Feasibility of a smartphone-based exercise program for office workers with neck pain: An individualized approach using a self-classification algorithm. *Archives of Physical Medicine and Rehabilitation*, 98(1), 80–87.

Levinson, B. (1962). The dog as co-therapist. *Mental Hygiene*, 46(1), 59–65.

Li, L., Yu, F., Shi, D., Shi, J., Tian, Z., Yang, J., ... Jiang, Q. (2017). Application of virtual reality technology in clinical medicine. *American Journal of Translational Research*, 9(9), 3867.

Lim, S. J., & Kim, C. (2014). Effects of autogenic training on stress response and heart rate variability in nursing students. *Asian Nursing Research*, 8(4), 286–292.

Litwack, K. (2015). Pain management in military trauma. *Critical Care Nursing Clinics of North America*, 27(2), 235–246.

Loreto-Quijada, D., Gutiérrez-Maldonado, J., Nieto, R., Gutiérrez-Martínez, O., Ferrer-García, M., Saldana, C., ... Liutsko, L. (2014). Differential effects of two virtual reality interventions: distraction versus pain control. *Cyberpsychology, Behavior, and Social Networking*, 17(6), 353–358.

Lothian, J. A. (2011). Lamaze breathing. *The Journal of Perinatal Education*, 20(2), 118–120.

Lothian, J. A., & DeVries, C. (2010). *The official Lamaze guide: Giving birth with confidence* (2nd ed.). Minnetonka, MN: Meadowbrook Press.

Luciano, J. V., Martínez, N., Peñarrubia-María, M. T., Fernandez-Vergel, R., García-Campayo, J., Verduras, C., ... Serrano-Blanco, A. (2011). Effectiveness of a psychoeducational treatment program implemented in general practice for fibromyalgia patients: a randomized controlled trial. *The Clinical Journal of Pain*, 27(5), 383–391.

Maani, C. V., Hoffman, H. G., Morrow, M., Maiers, A., Gaylord, K., McGhee, L. L., & DeSocio, P. A. (2017). Virtual reality pain control during burn wound debridement of combat-related burn injuries using robot-like arm mounted VR goggles. *Journal of TRAUMA*, 71(1). https://doi.org/10.1097/TA.0b013e31822192e2. (Suppl), S125–30.

Mache, S., Danzer, G., Klapp, B., & Groneberg, D. A. (2015). An Evaluation of a Multicomponent Mental Competency and Stress Management Training for Entrants in Surgery Medicine. *Journal of Surgical Education*, 72(6), 1102–1108.

Malloy, K. M., & Milling, L. S. (2010). The effectiveness of virtual reality distraction for pain reduction: a systematic review. *Clinical Psychology Review*, 30(8), 1011–1018.

Marcus, D., Bernstein, C., Constantin, J., Kunkel, F., Breuer, P., & Hanlon, R. (2012). Animal-assisted therapy at an outpatient pain management clinic. *Pain Medicine*, 13(1), 45–57.

Marcus, D., Bernstein, C., Constantin, J., Kunkel, F., Breuer, P., & Hanlon, R. (2013). Impact of animal-assisted therapy for outpatients with fibromyalgia. *Pain Medicine*, 14(1), 43–51.

Marr, B., & Baruch, J. (2016). The weight of pain: What does a 10 on the pain scale mean? An innovative use of art in medical education to enhance pain management (FR482A). *Journal of Pain and Symptom Management*, 51(2), 381–382.

Martin, S. L., Kerr, K. L., Bartley, E. J., Kuhn, B. L., Palit, S., Terry, E. L., ... Rhudy, J. L. (2012). Respiration-induced hypoalgesia: exploration of potential mechanisms. *The Journal of Pain*, 13(8), 755–763.

McBain, H., Mulligan, K., & Newman, S. P. (2015). Nonpharmacologic pain management. In M. C. Hochberg, A. J. Silman, J. S. Smolen, M. E. Weinblatt, & M. H. Weismann (Eds.), *Rheumatology 6th Ed (Vol 1)* pp. 401–405. Philadelphia, PA: Elsevier.

McCabe, C., Neill, F., Granville, G., & Grace, S. (2013). Evaluation of an art in health care elective module–A nurse education initiative. *Nurse Education in Practice*, 13(2), 113–117.

McKay, D., Przeworski, A., & O'Neill, S. (2016). Emerging technologies for clinical practice. pp. 365–378. In D. McKay, A. Przeworski, & S. O'Neill (Eds.), *Computer-Assisted and Web-based Innovations in Psychology, Special Education, and Health*. New York, NY: Academic Press.

Meadows, A., Burns, D., & Perkins, S. (2015). Measuring Supportive Music and Imagery Interventions: The Development of the Music Therapy Self-Rating Scale. *Journal of Music Therapy*, 52(3), 353–375.

Melzack, R., & Wall, P. D. (1965). Pain mechanisms: a new theory. *Science*, 150(3699), 971–979.

Menzies, V., Lyon, D. E., Elswick, R. K., McCain, N. L., & Gray, D. P. (2014). Effects of guided imagery on biobehavioral factors in women with fibromyalgia. *Journal of Behavioral Medicine*, 37(1), 70–80.

Meyer, B., Keller, A., Wöhlbier, H. G., Overath, C. H., Müller, B., & Kropp, P. (2016). Progressive muscle relaxation reduces migraine frequency and normalizes amplitudes of contingent negative variation (CNV). *The Journal of Headache and Pain*, 17(1), 37.

Mondanaro, J. F., Homel, P., Lonner, B., Shepp, J., Lichtensztein, M., & Loewy, J. V. (2017). Music therapy increases comfort and reduces pain in patients recovering from spine surgery. *American Journal of Orthopedics*, 46(1), E13–E22.

Moore, H., Stewart, I., Barnes-Holmes, D., Barnes-Holmes, Y., & McGuire, B. E. (2015). Comparison of acceptance and distraction strategies in coping with experimentally induced pain. *Journal of Pain Research*, 8, 139.

Morrow, B., Brink, J., Grace, S., Pritchard, L., & Lupton-Smith, A. (2016). The effect of positioning and diaphragmatic breathing exercises on respiratory muscle activity in people with chronic obstructive pulmonary disease. *South African Journal of Physiotherapy*, 72(1), 1–6.

Murthy, R., Bearman, G., Brown, S., Bryant, K., Chinn, R., Hewlett, A., ... Weber, D. (2015). Animals in healthcare facilities: Recommendations to minimize potential risks. *Infection Control & Hospital Epidemiology*, 36(5), 495–516.

Nainis, N., Paice, J. A., Ratner, J., Wirth, J. H., Lai, J., & Shott, S. (2006). Relieving symptoms in cancer: innovative use of art therapy. *Journal of Pain and Symptom Management*, 31(2), 162–169.

Nightingale, F. (1992). *Notes on nursing*. Philadelphia, PA: J. B. Lippincott. (Original work published 1859).

O'Neill, A., & Moss, H. (2015). A community art therapy group for adults with chronic pain. *Art Therapy*, 32(4), 158–167.

Onieva-Zafra, M. D., García, L. H., & Del Valle, M. G. (2015). Effectiveness of guided imagery relaxation on levels of pain and depression in patients diagnosed with fibromyalgia. *Holistic Nursing Practice*, 29(1), 13–21.

Orji, R., Mandryk, R. L., Vassileva, J., & Gerling, K. M. (2013, April). Tailoring persuasive health games to gamer type. In *Proceedings of the SIGCHI Conference on Human Factors in Computing Systems* (pp. 2467–2476) ACM.

Özer, N., Özlü, Z. K., Arslan, S., & Günes, N. (2013). Effect of music on postoperative pain and physiologic parameters of patients after open heart surgery. *Pain Management Nursing*, 14(1), 20–28.

Park, E., Oh, H., & Kim, T. (2013). The effects of relaxation breathing on procedural pain and anxiety during burn care. *Burns*, 39(6), 1101–1106.

Park, E. R., Traeger, L., Vranceanu, A. M., Scult, M., Lerner, J. A., Benson, H., ... Fricchione, G. L. (2013). The development of a patient-centered program based on the relaxation response: The Relaxation Response Resiliency Program (3RP). *Psychosomatics*, 54(2), 165–174.

Patwardhan, B., Mutalik, G., & Tillu, G. (2015). Lifestyle and behavior pp. 141-172. In B. Patwardhan, G. Mutalik, & G. Tillu (Eds.), *Integrative Approaches for Health: Biomedical Research, Ayurveda and Yoga*. St. Louis: Academic Press.

Patterson, S., Duhig, M., Darbyshire, C., Counsel, R., Higgins, N., & Williams, I. (2015). Implementing music therapy on an adolescent inpatient unit: A mixed-methods evaluation of acceptability, experience of participation and perceived impact. *Australasian Psychiatry*, 23(5), 556–560.

Perlman, A., I, Rosenberger, L., & Ali, A. (2018). Osteoarthritis, pp 639-650.e3. In D. Rakel (Ed.), *Integrative Medicine* (4th Edition). St. Louis: Elsevier.

Partners, Pet. (2016). *Position Statement on Animal Health and Welfare*. Retrieved from https://petpartners.org.

Pifarré, P., Simó, M., Gispert, J. D., Plaza, P., Fernández, A., & Pujol, J. (2015). Diazepam and Jacobson's progressive relaxation show similar attenuating short-term effects on stress-related brain glucose consumption. *European Psychiatry*, 30(2), 187–192.

Pinheiro, M., Mendes, D., Pais, J., Carvalho, N., & Cabral, T. (2015). Sleep quality – impact of relaxation techniques and autogenic training in patients diagnosed with insomnia. *European Psychiatry*, 30(Suppl 1), 28–31. March 2015, 1781.

Pretorius, M. (2017). A metaphysical and neuropsychological assessment of musical tones to affect the brain, relax the mind and heal the body. *Verbum et Ecclesia*, 38(1), 1–9.

Pritham, U. A., & McKay, L. (2014). Safe management of chronic pain in pregnancy in an era of opioid misuse and abuse. *Journal of Obstetric, Gynecologic & Neonatal Nursing*, 43(5), 554–567.

Proyer, R.T., & Wolf, A. (2017). Humor and well-being. In *Reference Module in Neuroscience and Biobehavioral Psychology*. https://doi.org/10.1016/B978-0-12-809324-5.05590-5.

Quinlan-Colwell, A. (2012). *Pain Management for Older Adults: A Clinical Guide for Nurses*. New York, NY: Springer.

Ramachandran, V. S., & Rogers-Ramachandran, D. (1996). Synaesthesia in phantom limbs induced with mirrors. *Proceedings of the Royal Society of Biological Sciences*, 263(1369), 377–386.

Rivera, M. (2010). *On dogs and dying: Inspirational stories from hospice hounds*. West Lafayette, IN: Purdue University Press.

Rnic, K., Dozois, D. J., & Martin, R. A. (2016). Cognitive distortions, humor styles, and depression. *Europe's Journal of Psychology*, 12(3), 348.

Romas, J. A., & Sharma, J. (2017). Relaxation. pp. 47–67. In J. Romas, & M. Sharma (Eds.), *Practical Stress Management: A Comprehensive Workbook* (7th Edition). St. Louis: Academic Press.

Rossman, M. L. (2018). Osteoarthritis, pp. 930–936.e1. In D. Rakel (Ed.), *Integrative Medicine* (4th Edition). St. Louis: Elsevier.

Sato, K., Fukumori, S., Matsusaki, T., Maruo, T., Ishikawa, S., Nishie, H., ... Matsumi, M. (2010). Nonimmersive virtual reality mirror visual feedback therapy and its application for the treatment of complex regional pain syndrome: an open-label pilot study. *Pain Medicine*, 11(4), 622–629.

Savage, B. M., Lujan, H. L., Thipparthi, R. R., & DiCarlo, S. E. (2017). Humor, laughter, learning, and health! A brief review. *Advances in Physiology Education*, 41(3), 341–347.

Schultz, J. (1953). *Das Autogene Training*. Stuttgart, Germany: Geerg-Thieme Vertag.

Shearer, H. M., Carroll, L. J., Wong, J. J., Côté, P., Varatharajan, S., Southerst, D., ... van der Velde, G. M. (2015). Are psychological interventions effective for the management of neck pain and whiplash-associated disorders? A systematic review by the Ontario Protocol for Traffic Injury Management (OPTIMa) Collaboration. *The Spine Journal*, 16(12), 1566–1581.

Shinozaki, M., Kanazawa, M., Kano, M., Endo, Y., Nakaya, N., Hongo, M., & Fukudo, S. (2010). Effect of autogenic training on general improvement in patients with irritable bowel syndrome: A randomized controlled trial. *Applied Psychophysiology and Biofeedback*, 35(3), 189–198. https://doi.org/10.1007/s10484-009-9125-y.

Sin, Man, Wai, & Chow. (2015). Ka Ming Effect of Music Therapy in Postoperative Pain Management in Gynecological Patients. *A Literature Review Pain Management Nursing*, 16(6), 978–987 (December).

Sliter, M., Kale, A., & Yuan, Z. (2014). Is humor the best medicine? The buffering effect of coping humor on traumatic stressors in firefighters. *Journal of Organizational Behavior*, 35(2), 257–272.

Smith, K., Iversen, C., Kossowsky, J., O'Dell, S., Gambhir, R., & Coakley, R. (2015). Apple apps for the management of pediatric pain and pain-related stress. *Clinical Practice in Pediatric Psychology*, 3(2), 93–107.

Sobo, E., Eng, B., & Kassity-Krich, N. (2006). Canine visitation (pet) therapy: Pilot data on decreases in child pain perception. *Journal of Holistic Nursing*, 24(1), 51–57.

Somers, T. J., Abernethy, A. P., Edmond, S. N., Kelleher, S. A., Wren, A. A., Samsa, G. P., & Keefe, F. J. (2015). A pilot study of a mobile health pain coping skills training protocol for patients with persistent cancer pain. *Journal of Pain and Symptom Management*, 50(4), 553–558.

Song, Q. H., Xu, R. M., Zhang, Q. H., Ma, M., & Zhao, X. P. (2013). Relaxation training during chemotherapy for breast cancer improves mental health and lessens adverse events. *International Journal of Clinical and Experimental Medicine*, 6(10), 979–984.

Sourina, O., Wang, Q., & Nguyen, M. K. (2011). EEG-based "serious" games and monitoring tools for pain management. *Studies in Health Technology and Informatics*, 163(1), 606–610. PubMed: 21335865.

Spencer, J. (2013). *"A Historical Review of Music Therapy and the Department of Veterans Affairs."* PhD diss. Molloy College.

Staiano, A. E., & Flynn, R. (2014). Therapeutic uses of active videogames: a systematic review. *Games for Health Journal*, 3(6), 351–365.

Standley, J. M., & Walworth, D. (2010). *Music Therapy with Premature Infants Research and Developmental Interventions* (2nd edition) (pp. 55). Silver Spring, MD: The American Music Therapy Association.

Stevens, P., Kepros, J., & Mosher, B. (2017). Use of a dog visitation program to improve patient satisfaction in trauma patients. *Journal of Trauma Nursing*, 24(2), 97–101.

Strauss, M., Van Heerden, S. M., & Joubert, G. (2016). Occupational therapy and the use of music tempo in the treatment of the mental health care user with psychosis. *South African Journal of Occupational Therapy*, 46(1), 21–26.

Subnis, U. B., Starkweather, A., & Menzies, V. (2016). A current review of distraction-based interventions for chronic pain management. *European Journal of Integrative Medicine*, 8(5), 715–722.

Thaut, M. H. (2015). Music as therapy in early history. In *217. Progress in Brain Research* (pp. 143–158). St. Louis: Elsevier.

Thoma, M. V., Zemp, M., Kreienbühl, L., Hofer, D., Schmidlin, P. R., Attin, T., ... Nater, U. M. (2015). Effects of music listening on pre-treatment anxiety and stress levels in a dental hygiene recall population. *International Journal of Behavioral Medicine*, 22(4), 498–505.

Tick, H., Nielsen, A., Pelletier, K., Bonakdar, R., Simmons, S., Glick, R., ... Saper, R. B. (2018). Evidence-Based Nonpharmacologic Strategies for Comprehensive Pain Care the Consortium Pain Task Force Whit`1`e Paper. *Explore (NY)*, 14(3), 177–211.

Traeger, L., Park, E. R., Sporn, N., Repper-DeLisi, J., Convery, M. S., Jacobo, M., & Pirl, W. F. (2013, July). Development and Evaluation of Targeted Psychological Skills Training for Oncology Nurses in Managing Stressful Patient and Family Encounters. In *Oncology Nursing Forum*, 40(4), E328–E336.

Triberti, S., Repetto, C., & Riva, G. (2014). Psychological Factors Influencing the Effectiveness of Virtual Reality–Based Analgesia: A Systematic Review. *Cyberpsychology, Behavior, and Social Networking*, 17(6), 335–345.

Trost, Z., & Parsons, T. D. (2014). Beyond Distraction: Virtual Reality Graded Exposure Therapy as Treatment for Pain-Related Fear and Disability in Chronic Pain. *Journal of Applied Biobehavioral Research*, 19(2), 106–126.

Trost, Z., Zielke, M., Guck, A., Nowlin, L., Zakhidov, D., France, C. R., & Keefe, F. (2015). The promise and challenge of virtual gaming technologies for chronic pain: the case of graded exposure for low back pain. *Pain Management*, 5(3), 197–206.

Tsitsi, T., Charalambous, A., Papastavrou, E., & Raftopoulos, V. (2017). Effectiveness of a relaxation intervention (progressive muscle relaxation and guided imagery techniques) to reduce anxiety and improve mood of parents of hospitalized children with malignancies: A randomized controlled trial in Republic of Cyprus and Greece. *European Journal of Oncology Nursing*, 26, 9–18.

Vaajoki, A., Pietilä, A. M., Kankkunen, P., & Vehviläinen-Julkunen, K. (2012). Effects of listening to music on pain intensity and pain distress after surgery: an intervention. *Journal of Clinical Nursing*, 21(5-6), 708–717.

van der Vennet, R., & Serice, S. (2012). Can coloring mandalas reduce anxiety? A replication study. *Art Therapy*, 29(2), 87–92.

Voss, J. A., Good, M., Yates, B., Baun, M. M., Thompson, A., & Hertzog, M. (2004). Sedative Music Reduces Anxiety and Pain During Chair Rest after Open-Heart Surgery. *Pain*, 112, 197–203.

Walker, M. R., Kallingal, G. J., Musser, J. E., Folen, R., Stetz, M. C., & Clark, J. Y. (2014). Treatment efficacy of virtual reality distraction in the reduction of pain and anxiety during cystoscopy. *Military Medicine*, 179(8), 891–896.

Wallace, R. K., Benson, H., & Wilson, A. F. (1971). A wakeful hypometabolic physiologic state. *American Journal of Physiology*, 221(3), 795–799.

Wesch, N., Callow, N., Hall, C., & Pope, J. P. (2016). Imagery and self-efficacy in the injury context. *Psychology of Sport and Exercise*, 24(1), 72–81.

Wiederhold, M. D., Gao, K., & Wiederhold, B. K. (2014). Clinical use of virtual reality distraction system to reduce anxiety and pain in dental procedures. *Cyberpsychology, Behavior, and Social Networking*, 17(6), 359–365.

Wieland, L. S., & Santesso, N. (2017). A summary of a Cochrane review: Music interventions for improving psychological and physical outcomes in cancer patients. *European Journal of Integrative Medicine*, 9(1), 50–51.

Wolff, A., & Frishman, W. (2005). Animal-assisted therapy and cardiovascular disease. In W. Frishman, M. Weintraub, & M. Micozzi (Eds.), *Complementary and Integrative Therapies for Cardiovascular Disease* (pp. 362–368). St. Louis, MO: Mosby.

Won, A. S., & Collins, T. A. (2012). Non-immersive, virtual reality mirror visual feedback for treatment of persistent idiopathic facial pain. *Pain Medicine, 13*(9), 1257–1258.

Woodbury-Fariña, M. A., & Antongiorgi, J. L. (2014). Humor. *Psychiatric Clinics of North America, 37*(4), 561–578.

Wu, P.-Y., Huang, M.-L., Lee, W.-P., Wan, C., & Sih, W.-M. (2017). Effects of Music Listening on Anxiety and Physiological Responses in Patients Undergoing Awake Craniotomy Patients. *Complementary Therapies in Medicine, 32*(1), 56–60.

Zach, S., Dobersek, U., Inglis, V., & Tenenbaum, G. (2018). A meta-analysis of mental imagery effects on post-injury functional mobility, perceived pain, and self-efficacy. *Psychology of Sport and Exercise, 34*(1), 79–87.

Zautra, A. J., Fasman, R., Davis, M. C., & Arthur, D. (2010). The effects of slow breathing on affective responses to pain stimuli: an experimental study. *Pain, 149*(1), 12–18.

Zimmerman, L., Nieveen, J., Barnason, S., & Schmaderer, M. (1996). The effects of music interventions on postoperative pain and sleep in coronary artery bypass graft (CABG) patients. *Scholarly Inquiry for Nursing Practice, 10*(2), 153–170.

Chapter 22 Cognitive-Behavioral and Psychotherapeutic Interventions as Components of Multimodal Analgesic Pain Management

Geralyn Datz, Ann Quinlan-Colwell

CHAPTER OUTLINE

Integrative, Interdisciplinary, and Multimodal Pain Treatment, pg. 613

Interdisciplinary Pain Rehabilitation or Functional Restoration Programs, pg. 615

Cognitive-Behavioral Therapy, pg. 617

Goal Setting, pg. 617

Identifying Maladaptive Thinking, pg. 619

Cognitive Restructuring, pg. 620

Problem-Solving, pg. 620

Behavioral Activation (Graded Behavioral Activation), pg. 621

Exposure Therapy (Graded Exposure Therapy), pg. 621

Coping Skill Development, pg. 621

Coping With Trigger Factors, pg. 622

Relapse Prevention and Maintenance of Skills, pg. 622

Evidence Supporting Cognitive-Behavioral Therapy for Pain Management, pg. 622

Cautions and Contraindications, pg. 624

The Activating Event Belief Consequence Model, pg. 624

Evidence for Pain Management, pg. 624

Acceptance and Commitment Therapy, pg. 625

Evidence for Pain Management, pg. 625

Biofeedback (Applied Psychophysiology), pg. 626

Evidence for Pain Management, pg. 626

Mindfulness-Based Stress Management and Mindfulness-Based Cognitive Therapy, pg. 627

Evidence for Pain Management, pg. 628

Psychoeducation, pg. 630

Evidence for Pain Management, pg. 631

Key Points, pg. 631

Case Scenario, pg. 631

References, pg. 631

Integrative, Interdisciplinary, and Multimodal Pain Treatment

The biopsychosocial approach to pain acknowledges there are multiple influences that shape the experience of pain and determine its clinical presentation. Pain emerges as a complex interplay of physiologic emotional and societal factors. The biopsychosocial model provides a foundation for multimodal pain management. Providers are invited and challenged to go beyond pure biomedical approaches to address and manage pain, particularly chronic pain in the context of the various areas in which a patient with pain may be struggling. We know that not all pains are created equal. Pain is not only experienced in different ways by different people, but it can be experienced in diverse ways by each person at different times (Pasero, Quinlan-Colwell, Rae, Broglio, & Drew, 2016). From a biopsychosocial perspective, the experience of pain and the degree of compliance with

Table 22.1 | Biopsychosocial Factors Affecting Pain

Biological or physical factors	Cause and pathologic processes of pain Genetics: Including neurochemistry, pain threshold, pain tolerance, metabolism Medications: Including polymorphisms, comorbidities, side effects Immune response
Psychological	Comorbid disorders: Depression, anxiety, trauma Emotions: Including anger and fear Attitudes Memories: Including adverse childhood experiences (ACEs) Understanding and learning Beliefs Behavioral health: Including anxiety, depression, catastrophizing, hypervigilance, symptom magnification
Social factors	Culture: Including traditions, beliefs about pain, medication, nonpharmacologic interventions Family support or lack of support Socioeconomic status Access and barriers to care

an analgesic plan of care are influenced by biological or physical, psychological and emotional, and social factors (Schubiner, 2018) (Table 22.1). In this chapter a variety of cognitive-behavioral and psychotherapeutic interventions for pain management will be reviewed as part of a multimodal approach. (See Chapter 8 for discussion addressing assessment of psychological factors affecting pain.)

Incorporating cognitive-behavioral therapy (CBT) as part of a multimodal approach to pain management in adults was recommended, with moderate-quality evidence, by the clinical practice committee representing the American Pain Society, the American Society of Regional Anesthesia and Pain Medicine, and the American Society of Anesthesiologists (Chou et al., 2016). The CBT approach to pain management has a long history. The psychologist Wilbert Fordyce was a pioneer in implementing learning concepts and operant behavioral based psychological and physical interventions with people living with chronic pain (Fordyce, 1976). At the time of his practice, his method was considered radical. He approached patients by accepting without question the patient's report of pain in conjunction with a focus on pain-related behav-

iors and a belief that the behaviors and consequently the pain experience could be modified with positive operant conditioning techniques (Main, Keefe, Jensen, Vlaeyen, & Vowles, 2015). Along with John Loesser, Dr. Fordyce established the first interdisciplinary pain management program at the University of Washington Department of Physical Medicine and Rehabilitation in which he encouraged patients to gradually increase participation in exercise, which is the basis of current functional restoration programs (Gatchel, McGeary, McGeary, & Lippe, 2014). Simultaneously at the University of Washington, anesthesiologist John Bonica proposed that chronic pain management needed to be provided from a multidisciplinary approach addressing physical, psychological, and social needs with providers located in a central location (Loeser, 2017) (see Chapter 1 for more information on John Bonica). Since that time, a number of prominent researchers have contributed to the modern understanding of pain as a product of the interplay of subjective experience, brain signaling, environmental factors, co-occurring psychological conditions, and learned behavioral and thinking patterns (Table 22.2).

Table 22.2 | Important Early Contributors to CBT and Pain Management

Selected Early Contributor(s)	Contribution(s)
Melzack & Wall (1965)	Gate Control Theory of Pain
Melzack (1990)	Neuromatrix Theory of Pain
Turk, Miechenbuam, & Genest (1983)	Integrating cognitive behavioral techniques
Keefe & Gil (1986)	Cognitive Behavioral Therapy and Pain, Psychosocial aspects of chronic pain
Sullivan, Bishop, & Pivik (1995)	Pain Catastrophizing

Table 22.2	Important Early Contributors to CBT and Pain Management—Cont'd	
Selected Early Contributor(s)	**Contribution(s)**
Thorn (2004); Turner & Romano (2001)	Cognitive Therapy for Chronic Pain
Gatchel & Okifuji (2006); Gatchel, Peng, Peters, Fuchs, & Turk (2007); Turk & Monarch (2002)	Biopsychosocial nature of pain, demise of biomedical model; CBT
Jensen Turner & Romano (2007)	Pain beliefs & Pain coping
Gatchel & Mayer (2008); Gatchel & Okifuji (2006); Turk & Swanson (2007)	Role and value of interdisciplinary pain programs
Gatchel et al. (2007); Vlayen & Linton (2000)	Fear-avoidance

Melzack, R., & Wal, P. D. (1965). Pain Mechanisms: A New Theory. Science.; Melzack, R. (1990). Phantom limbs and the concept of a neuromatrix. *Trends in Neurosciences, 13*(3), 88-92; Turk, D. C., Meichenbaum, D., & Genest, M. (1983). *Pain and behavioral medicine: A cognitive-behavioral perspective.* New York, NY: Guilford Press; Keefe, F. J., & Gil, K. M. (1986). Behavioral concepts in the analysis of chronic pain syndromes. *J Consult Clin Psychol., 54*(6), 776–83; Sullivan, M.J., Bishop, S. R., & Pivik, J. (1995). The Pain Catastrophizing Scale: Development and validation. *Psychological Assessment, 7* (4), 524–532; Thorn B. (2004). *Cognitive Therapy for Chronic Pain: a step by step guide.* 1st Ed. Guilford Press; Turner, J. A., & Romano, J. M. (2001). Cognitive-behavioral therapy for chronic pain. In J. D. Loeser & J. J. Bonica (Eds.), *Bonica's management of pain* (3rd ed., pp. 1751–1758.). Philadelphia, PA: Lippincott Williams & Wilkins; Gatchel, R. J., & Okifuji, A. (2006). Evidence-based scientific data documenting the treatment and cost-effectiveness of comprehensive pain programs for chronic nonmalignant pain. *The Journal of Pain, 7*(11), 779–793; Gatchel, R. J., Peng, Y., Peters, M. L., Fuchs, P. N., & Turk, D. C. (2007). The biopsychosocial approach to chronic pain: Scientific advances and future directions. *Psychological Bulletin,* 133, 581–624. doi:10.1037/ 0033-2909.133.4.581; Turk, D. C., & Monarch, E. S. (2002). Biopsychosocial perspective on chronic pain. In D. C. Turk & R. J. Gatchel (Eds.), *Psychological approaches to pain management: A practitioner's handbook* (2nd ed., pp. 3–29). New York, NY: Guilford Press; Jensen, M. P., Turner, J. A., & Romano, J. M. Changes after multidisciplinary pain treatment in patient pain beliefs and coping are associated with concurrent changes in patient functioning. *Pain.* 2007 Sep;131(1-2):38-47; Gatchel, R. J., & Mayer, T. G. (2008). Evidence-based review of the effectiveness of functional restoration for the management of chronic low back pain. *The Spine Journal,* 8, 65–69; Gatchel, R. J., & Okifuji, A. (2006). Evidence-based scientific data documenting the treatment and cost-effectiveness of comprehensive pain programs for chronic nonmalignant pain. *The Journal of Pain, 7*(11), 779–793; Turk, D. C., & Swanson, K. (2007). Efficacy and cost-effectiveness treatment of chronic pain: An analysis and evidence-based synthesis. In M. E. Schatman & A. Campbell (Eds.), *Chronic pain management: Guidelines for multidisciplinary program development* (pp. 15–38). New York, NY: Informa Healthcare; Gatchel et al., 2007 (previously cited); Vlaeyen, J. W., & Linton S. J. (2000). Fear-avoidance and its consequences in chronic musculoskeletal pain: a state of the art. *Pain, 85*(3), 317–332.

Interdisciplinary Pain Rehabilitation or Functional Restoration Programs

The interdisciplinary pain rehabilitation programs (IPRPs) or functional restoration programs (FRPs) begun by Drs. Loesser and Fordyce are still operational internationally and continue to function from a strong evidence base (Caby, Olivier, Janik, Vanvelcenaher, & Pelayo, 2016; Fore et al., 2015; Gatchel et al., 2014; Mathews & Davin, 2014; Pujol et al., 2015). These programs are hallmarks of multimodal and integrative approaches for teaching people how to effectively manage pain, reduce the impact of pain on their lives, and increase the functional ability level of the individuals in pain. Interdisciplinary programs are characterized by involvement of clinicians from a variety of specialized areas (e.g., pain clinicians, nurses, psychologists, physical therapists, occupational therapists, addictionologists, vocational rehabilitation specialists, social workers, and other health care providers) who interact with the person in pain in a collaborative manner (Mathews & Davin, 2014; Pujol et al., 2015; Sussman et al., 2015) (Box 22.1). These programs have two important goals. First is to interrupt and reverse the deconditioning process. Second is to teach the person to manage pain actively rather than passively by introducing the participant to new, healthy lifestyle behaviors and practices as preparation for returning to work (Caby et al., 2016). There is strong evidence that FRP programs have positive effects on restoration of function with moderate evidence for reduction in pain (Pujol et al., 2015). For people living with chronic low back pain (CLBP), Weiner and Nordin (2010) found interdisciplinary care demonstrated greater overall effectiveness than many other common pain management interventions, including medication and CBT alone (Weiner & Nordin, 2010).

Functional restoration programs are widely accepted nationally and internationally (Peterson, Smith, Khan, & Arnold, 2013) and were adopted by both the U.S. Army and the U.S. Air Force (Pujol et al., 2015). The Functional Occupational Restoration Treatment (FORT) program was designed to decrease chronic pain, increase functioning, and retain military members on active duty using an interdisciplinary functional restoration model adapted to address the occurrence of pain in the military (Gatchel et al., 2009). The initial participants in the FORT program (n = 30) reported significant improvements for functional capacity, health-related quality of life, and military retention at 6-month and 1-year follow-up, compared to those in the group who received the usual treatment (n = 36), who showed no significant change in physical or psychosocial outcomes over the 1-year assessment span. In addition, participants who completed treatment as usual were three times more likely than FORT participants to receive

---

Box 22.1 | Components of Functional Restoration Programs

- The premise is that pain is multidimensional and real and perceived impairments in function can be improved through learning structured activity and improving mental and physical health.
- The program in an interdisciplinary approach with a variety of collaborating clinicians to guide and support participating people living with chronic pain to improve activity and functional ability.
- Clinicians collaborate, learn from each other, and support consistent messages and education.
- Physical therapists educate participants in core skill building and strength stabilization.
- Psychologists work with participants using cognitive-behavioral therapy, acceptance therapy, mindfulness-based stress reduction, and relapse prevention skills.

- Participants are educated in recognizing pain signals and understanding the pathophysiology of pain and how the brain processes pain information.
- Participants are taught about the relationship of the body with the mind in the perception, processing, experience, and control of pain.
- Progress of participants is recorded and measured.
- Potential participants may be enrolled in a program in an effort to avoid surgery (e.g., spine surgery).
- The programs are cost effective (particularly when started early in the recovery process), with a high percentage of participants returning to work with reduced health care utilization.

---

a medical discharge from active duty service. Those in the group who received the usual treatment were also more likely to seek increased levels of pain-related health care and used more medications than those in the FORT group. The success of this research project supports the efficacy of the interdisciplinary/functional restoration approach even when modified for special populations such as the military, in which several effective interdisciplinary pain management models continue (Schoneboom et al., 2016). Despite successful outcomes with functional restoration, FRPs remain underused within the United States (Malladi, 2015). This is true for many reasons, with inadequate health coverage being a primary limitation (Box 22.2).

Box 22.2 | Clinical Application[a]

The Pain Rehabilitation Program, which has been functioning since 2014 in Hattiesburg, Mississippi, is a 20-day intensive outpatient program geared to the recovery of patients with pain that consists of a multidisciplinary team delivering interventions to treat the whole person who is living with pain. The team teaches the participants to understand chronic pain is not only a physical sensation but also an experience that affects the entire individual, including moods, sleep, relationships, ability to work, and engagement in social and pleasurable activity. The team thinks this understanding is the key to recovering from the consuming process of chronic pain. The multidisciplinary team is supervised and led by the clinical director, a pain psychologist (PhD). The pain psychologist directs the programming and meets with each patient 1 hour weekly for cognitive-behavioral therapy (CBT), coaching, and tracking of progress.

A physical medicine and rehabilitation physician (DO) also meets with patients weekly to monitor progress, educate about injury/disease processes and recovery, and adjust medications. A doctor of physical therapy (DPT) and a physi-

cal therapy assistant (PTA) work with patients for 3 hours per day, gradually teaching attendees how to safely increase activity, providing ergonomic education, and working on strength and conditioning training.

For 3 hours per day, patients participate in cognitive-behavioral group psychotherapy for chronic pain. The CBT class topics include chronic pain psychoeducation, the transmission of pain signals, coping skills, instruction on pain medications, medication side effects, problem-solving, understanding anxiety and depression, sleep restoration, and relapse prevention, including planning for pain flare-ups.

For 1 hour daily, patients are educated by a registered yoga therapist (RYT) in yoga, meditation, or mindfulness training. Yoga and meditation help teach attendees how to build attention skills, directing attention away from the sensations of pain, calming their central nervous system, and achieving a greater sense of subjective peace.

Nutritional needs of patients living with pain are often overlooked; therefore each day there is at least 1 hour dedicated to nutritional education. Patients living with chronic

Box 22.2 | Clinical Application—Continued

pain may become overweight or underweight, eat foods that make their inflammatory response more active, and often have little understanding of macronutrients. Data suggest that high-protein eating plans may be favorable for patients living with pain. All participants enrolled in the program are encouraged to track their eating habits and daily macronutrient and water intake. This one intervention often has profound effects for the patients.

Finally, program patients are also taught self-massage and given instruction and treatment by a licensed massage therapist on several occasions. Throughout all 4 weeks of the program there are many interactive activities designed to teach attendees about how to recover their lost identity and claim a new identity despite the experience of having chronic pain. The attendees often have homework assignments and other written activities during the program to assist in their understanding of the new material and implementing it in their daily lives. Each week progress is tracked on a number of domains, including physical therapy progress, emotional responses, pain acceptance, depression, anxiety, and other measures of psychological adjustment. At the end of the program a graduation ceremony is held that recognizes each patient as an individual, and each attendee is given detailed feedback from all of the members of the treatment team. This is often an emotional and cathartic experience

for all present. At graduation, the attendees are given a written summary and informed of their exact progress over the 4 weeks. Often the progress is quite dramatic from week 1 to week 4. Some enrollees have gone from "severe" to "no" depression, "severe" panic attacks to "none." Participants had as much as a 2500% improvement in physical abilities. The Pain Rehabilitation Program also has a 75% return to work rate. Even for those who are not electing to work there are significant improvements in physical activity, walking ability, sleep, strength, and weight tolerance.

The Pain Rehabilitation Program primarily serves the residents of Louisiana, Alabama, and Mississippi; however, any resident is welcome. This program serves a tremendous need for an underserved area for individuals who live with chronic pain. Individuals who attend the program stay overnight during the 4 weeks at an extended stay hotel and travel about a quarter of a mile to the facility each day. Financially, the Pain Rehabilitation Program is covered by Workers' Compensation insurance and some private insurance carriers and also has a self-pay option.

Geralyn Datz, PhD

---

[a]See chapters 10, 11, 15, 16 (medications), 20 (physical therapy and yoga), 24 (self massage), 25 (meditation), and 27 (diet and weight management).

Cognitive-Behavioral Therapy

CBT is best understood as a conceptual framework and philosophy based on theoretical premises (Waltman & Sokol, 2017). From that framework, with an empathetic and confirming approach, focused goal-oriented therapy is designed to help the person modify cognition and behavior (Hardy, 2014; McCracken, Sato, & Taylor, 2013; Waltman & Sokol, 2017). This can be done during individual sessions or in group sessions (Ehde, Dillworth, & Turner, 2014; Wooton & Warfield, 2009). CBT is a present-focused, interactive therapist-led intervention that explores how the patient thinks about himself or herself, the world, and other people. It addresses how behaviors affect thoughts and feelings and how thoughts and feelings address behaviors with the intention to help patients change cognitions (how they think) and behaviors (what they do) (Hardy, 2014). In a deliberate manner in collaboration with the patient, the therapist coordinates interventions that address the current clinical condition of the patient. These goal-focused interventions are planned with forward momentum. Thus they are undertaken and then continue through goal attainment, evaluation, and outcome gathering (Wenzel, 2017). Numerous strategies

are used by CBT therapists, but goal setting, identifying maladaptive thinking, cognitive restructuring, behavioral activation, exposure, and problem-solving are basic (Wenzel, 2017) (Table 22.3).

CBT is used in the treatment of a plethora of conditions, including pain, anxiety, and depression (Hardy, 2014; Tang, Waltman, & Sokol, 2017). A critical concept when considering CBT as part of a multimodal approach for pain management is that pain may not have a psychological cause, but the response to pain and how the aspects of pain (intensity, quality, duration) are perceived are affected by many psychosocial influences (Okifuji & Skinner, 2009; Wooton & Warfield, 2009) (Box 22.3). The large majority of people experience pain as a form of suffering. Thus another way of understanding this is that chronic pain is not imaginal (imagined), but it is interpreted, understood, and reacted to, within the brain.

Goal Setting

SMART Goal setting with *specific, measurable, attainable, realistic, and timely* ways of evaluating a spoken goal is an important part of CBT (Box 22.4). When working with people living with chronic pain, goals of CBT are generally developed to lessen pain avoidance, ease the pain

Table 22.3 | Common Treatment Components of Interdisciplinary Pain Management Program and Their Respective Aims and Methods.

Component	Aim	Method
Psycho-education	To improve knowledge and understanding of chronic pain and to explain treatment rationale for improving subsequent adherence to the treatment process	Can be didactic, interactive, or a combination of both. Topics of discussion may include: pain causes and mechanisms; distinction between acute and chronic pain; psychology of chronic pain; pros and cons of available treatment strategies for chronic pain; lifestyle factors (e.g., work, stress, diet, weight, smoking, alcohol, exercise, physical activity, use of medications) affecting chronic pain
Physical exercise [a]	To increase the amount of physical activity for improving fitness, strength, stamina, flexibility, and overall physical health	May take the form of walking, gym circuit exercise, aerobic, tai chi, yoga, pilates, etc. implemented by prescribing, demonstrating, and facilitating the execution of simple repetitive exercise according to personal goals or agreed upon quotas; by altering the rate and amount of exercise over time as per ability; by purposeful activity scheduling; by signing up to gym classes
Relaxation	To identify the state of tension and to recognize the role of physiological tension and emotional distress in worsening pain experience; a self-regulatory strategy for improving control	May take the form of breathing exercise; progressive muscle relaxation; guided imagery
Graded activation [a]	To re-engage and to improve the amount of healthy activity as per the patient's goal	May involve goal-setting; identification and management of barriers to valued activity; activity scheduling, pacing, and continuous practice
Graded exposure [a]	To confront and disconfirm pain-related fear of movement and catastrophic thinking that promotes avoidance behavior	May involve structured and gradual reintroduction to feared movement and activity in the form of a behavioral experiment
Cognitive restructuring	To identify and challenge maladaptive thoughts and beliefs that promote distress and suffering	May involve discussion; challenging and replacing automatic thoughts; behavioral experiments
Mindfulness	To promote awareness, acceptance of pain experience, nonjudgemental thinking; a self-regulatory attention training strategy	May take the form of mindfulness breathing exercises and meditation
Communication skills training	To improve communication with family, friends, colleagues, employers, and health care providers for strengthening social support and minimizing unnecessary misunderstandings and conflicts	May involve reflective listening; assertiveness training; perspective taking; education about the role of health care providers and the organization and co-ordination between different service units.
Self management and relapse prevention	To integrate new coping skills and behavioral patterns into real day-to-day life outside of treatment settings, for generalizing and maintaining treatment gain	May involve making medium to long-term plans; self-monitoring techniques; discussions on setback management and appropriate goal adjustment

[a] These components are best delivered with support from physiotherapists and/or physicians.
Tang, N. K. (2018). Cognitive behavioural therapy in pain and psychological disorders: Towards a hybrid future. *Progress in Neuro-Psychopharmacology and Biological Psychiatry, 87*(Pt.b), 281–289.

Box 22.3	Components of Cognitive-Behavioral Therapy

- Provide education about pain and particular syndrome.
- Encourage acceptance of some level of pain.
- Discuss appropriate uses of medications, exercise, and physical modalities (e.g., heat, cold).
- Foster a self-management perspective.
- Focus on function rather than cure.
- Assist in goal setting.
- Teach relaxation.
- Provide information and guidance about pacing and increasing activities.
- Provide guidance on ways in which to improve sleep.
- Emphasize identifying and eliminating maladaptive thoughts.
- Provide strategies to help cope with relapse.
- Provide skills and skills training for ways in which to cope with interpersonal problems.

From Turk, D. C. (2017). Pain management. In *Reference module in neuroscience and biobehavioral psychology* (pp. 785–791). New York, NY: Elsevier.

Box 22.4	SMART Goals (Using the Example of Wanting to Increase Exercise)

Specific: Walk 15 minutes every day before breakfast (avoid generic goals such as "exercise more").
Measurable: Track time on kitchen calendar spent walking for the next month.
Attainable: I currently am able to walk 15 minutes but do so sporadically. Physically I am able to do this, and it is realistic to wake up 15 minutes earlier.
Relevant: Increasing exercise or adjusting is a vital part of my pain treatment plan.
Time-sensitive: I will find my tennis shoes today and start walking tomorrow.

From Lemmon, R., & Roseen, E. J. (2018). Chronic low back pain. In D. Rakel. *Integrative medicine* (4th ed., pp. 662–675e). St. Louis, MO: Elsevier.

experience through modifiable factors, and decrease associated distress from pain while improving function. These goals are accomplished by helping the person identify, correct, or decrease maladaptive thoughts and behaviors while increasing self-efficacy (Ehde et al., 2014). They also can be a point of discussion and measurement during future visits with the clinician (Lemmon & Rosen, 2018).

Self-efficacy is an important component of CBT because it is the belief by the person that he or she can effectively accomplish required activities and behaviors to achieve the desired goal (Okifuji & Skinner, 2009). In CBT the therapist works with the person to transform goals that are not realistic, such as always being pain free or resuming activities that are no longer feasible, into goals that are reasonable and attainable within a specific time frame. For example, rather than having a goal of working out at a fitness center, which the person currently cannot afford, the person can be encouraged to do stretching exercises for 5 minutes each day for 1 week at home, then increase to 10 minutes each day for a second week, and so on. These instructions can be followed by initiating a walking routine with gradual increments in time and intensity as pain is better controlled and endurance is developed. This system of goal setting can be used over time to achieve progressively more challenging goals, while the patient and clinician are able to track and monitor progress over time. SMART goals can be applied to many other areas of life to ease depression, improve socialization, and facilitate return to work or activities the person previously enjoyed.

Identifying Maladaptive Thinking

Maladaptive thinking includes perceptions and thoughts that are not helpful and may be destructive for the person (Wenzel, 2017). Such thinking, which may be inaccurate or dysfunctional, can occur when a person lives with distressed situations such as living with chronic pain (Crofford, 2015) (Box 22.5). Distorted perceptions along with automatic thoughts of a negative nature are associated with increased risk for depression (Dozios & Beck, 2008; Hardy, 2014). Identifying automatic thoughts is essential to the CBT process (Wooton & Warfield, 2009), and this is achieved by asking the patient what was being thought during a particular situation or during a pain flare or pain episode. Initially, the therapist works with the patient to identify negative and possibly inaccurate thoughts, such as "This pain will never end" or "This pain will surely kill me." The patient is encouraged to write down the negative thoughts, to learn about common thinking errors, such as overgeneralizing, polarizing (all or nothing thinking), and catastrophizing. Common thinking errors were first discussed by psychologist Aaron Beck (1976). These errors were later expanded upon by his student, psychiatrist David Burns (2012).

Subsequently, the therapist uses open-ended questions to help the person evaluate the automatic thoughts and determine if there is a factual basis for them (Hardy, 2014; Wenzel, 2017). As with other conditions, maladaptive thinking among people living with pain includes thoughts such as punitiveness, pessimism, incompetence, impaired self-control, defectiveness, mistrust, vulnerability, and isolation (Dozois & Beck, 2008). This may be seen in

Box 22.5 | Examples of Negative Cognitive Patterns

Polarizing pattern: Black-and-white thinking. If a patient's performance falls short of perfect, he or she sees himself or herself as a total failure, leading to a high expectation that is often unattainable.

Overgeneralization pattern: A patient generalizes beyond the specific facts of a situation and sees a single negative experience as a never-ending pattern of defeat.

Catastrophizing pattern: A patient consistently assumes the worst possible outcomes. Her or his understanding of her or his own plight is extremely negative, and she or he tends to interpret relatively minor problems as major catastrophes.

Filtering pattern: A patient focuses on a single negative detail, rather than a whole picture, of the event and lets the single detail characterize the entire experience.

Emotional reasoning pattern: A patient assumes that his or her negative emotions reflect the reality. "I really feel it; therefore this must be true."

From Okifuji, A., & Skinner, M. (2009). Psychological aspects of pain. In H. S. Smith (Ed.), *Current therapy in pain* (pp. 513–518). Philadelphia, PA: Saunders.

statements such as "I'm worthless because of pain," "My pain will never go away," "My pain will never get better," or "Everyone thinks I'm lying about my pain."

Cognitive Restructuring

After maladaptive thoughts are identified, cognitive restructuring is used to alter the thoughts to help the person better cope with painful sensations and even modify behaviors related to disability caused by pain (Kohl, Rief, & Glombiewski, 2013). During the process of cognitive restructuring, maladaptive thoughts are challenged and replaced (Tang, 2017). It involves monitoring thoughts, maintaining thought logs, challenging thoughts, and replacing automatic thoughts. The patient is taught to link the negative thinking with the common thinking errors they have learned to identify. In this way, they begin the process of restructuring thought processes. The patient is then taught to record the negative thoughts, continue to identify the thinking errors that are occurring, and appropriately challenge them with a rational coping statement. This is called the *triple column technique or the three-column technique* (Burns, 1999). Cognitive restructuring is considered an essential step in learning to better manage painful conditions (Kohl, Rief, & Glombiewski, 2014). An example of cognitive restructuring is to replace thoughts such as "My pain will never go away" with the restructure thought "When I am in pain, I remind myself

how much I appreciate it when I am not in pain" (Kohl et al., 2014) or "I will use my exercises and remember that my severe pain eases and that I have control."

The concept of cognitive restructuring can involve working with the person in pain to consider new or different ways of functioning through changing maladaptive patterns of thinking (Rini et al., 2015). Part of this is helping the person identify cognitive barriers, including fear of pain, fear of judgement, self-deprecation, all or nothing thinking, and resistance to change. The person can be encouraged to replace "I've always done it this way, and I don't want to change" with "I can learn new ways that will help me be able to accomplish the tasks I want to do with less pain." By removing resistance to change and allowing for problem-solving, the person with pain can begin making modifications to their lifestyle and accommodate new adaptive behaviors.

Activity pacing is an important skill to help conserve energy and work in more efficient ways to reduce or eliminate exhaustion and flare ups of pain. It involves planning for and adhering to designated periods of rest to avoid exhaustion and exacerbation of pain. An example is rather than washing dishes for 20 minutes, wash the dishes for 10 minutes, then rest for 10 minutes, and then resume washing for 10 minutes. Related to this is the technique of *adapting*, which involves using new methods to do usual tasks such as laundry, housekeeping, cooking, and interacting with children. An example is rather than to stand at a counter, sit on a high stool when preparing food for meals.

Problem-Solving

Problem-solving is most effectively used by creating an environment in which the person can identify different ways (Gauntlett-Gilbert & Brook, 2018) to accomplish needed or desired activities such as driving, working, grocery shopping, or leisure activities. It may involve modifying activities or using supportive devices. For some people living with chronic pain, problem-solving often becomes very difficult due to the presence of constant fear and worry. Some people living with chronic pain can be thought of as trapped in a "perseverance loop," actively and repeatedly engaged in effortful attempts to solve the wrong problem (Eccleston & Crombez, 2007). It is therefore necessary to teach them ways to focus productively on the problems in living and quality of life that pain presents. One principle used is thought restructuring to encourage the person to be willing to accept help and share responsibility or delegate tasks to others. Although conceptually challenging for many people, delegating is often a realistic option for people living in families or those who have other social supports. To encourage people to delegate and accept help, it may be helpful to ask the person living with pain how it makes him or her feel to help other people. Most often, the person relays that helping others generates a positive feeling within, making him or her feel good. The therapist can then encourage the person living in pain to *allow* others to feel those positive feelings by *allowing* others to be of help to the person living with pain.

Behavioral Activation (Graded Behavioral Activation)

Behavioral activation (BA) is a CBT technique in which activities identified as supportive of long-term goals for pain management are identified and enacted (Kim, Crouch, & Olatunji, 2017). The basis for this lies in the theory that cues in the environment activate the *approach and avoidance systems* to be alert for either a punishment or a reward. There are two processes that occur. *Behavioral inhibition (BI)* is activated by cues that signal potential danger, harm, or distress specific to the person, resulting in a reluctance or avoidance behavior. Through a separate process, when the person-specific cues are associated with rewards, thoughts, feelings, and behaviors are encouraged and supported through a dynamic complex process known as the *behavioral activation system (BAS)* (Jensen, Ehde, & Day, 2016). Although they are related in concept, it is thought that BIS and BAS are independently involved with two discrete neurophysiologic networks (Jensen, Tan, & Chua, 2015). From an *operant conditioning* perspective (the probability of a behavior is increased when it is associated with receiving a positive consequence and/or avoided when experiencing an adverse consequence), it is reasonable that sensations or activities that elicit negative sensations, emotions, or consequences will be avoided, whereas those that result in positive sensations, emotions, or consequences will be sought (Okifuji & Skinner, 2009; Simons, Elman, & Borsook, 2014).

In *graded behavioral activation (GBA)* people living with chronic pain learn to increase participation in healthy activities of their own design through a process that involves goal setting, identifying any obstacles, dealing with the obstacles, managing time, pacing involvement, and continuing to increase and improve this progression (Tang, 2017). Through this process it is possible to interrupt counterproductive cycles of avoidance, fear, and pain by gradually increasing participation in activities that were previously avoided (Kim et al., 2017). This is related to the concept of *exposure* or *graded exposure therapy* (Fig. 22.1).

Exposure Therapy (Graded Exposure Therapy)

Exposure therapy arose as a CBT treatment from studying avoidance behavior that is based in fear and anxiety related to an initial trauma (e.g., falling and sustaining a serious injury) (Foa, 2011; Jayasinghe et al., 2014). It is a technique used to confront and disconfirm pain-related fear of movement and catastrophic thinking that promotes avoidance behavior and to provide new experiences that

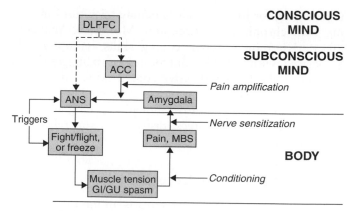

Fig. 22.1 | The Neurology of Psychophysiologic Disorders (thick solid line, activating; dashed line, deactivating). *ACC,* Anterior cingulate cortex; *ANS,* autonomic nervous system; *DLPFC,* dorsolateral prefrontal cortex; *GI,* gastrointestinal; *GU,* genitourinary; *MBS,* mind-body syndrome. (Schubiner, H. [2018]. Emotional awareness of pain. In D. Rakel [Ed.], *Integrative medicine* [4th ed., pp. 945–953.e2]. Philadelphia, PA: Elsevier.)

afford mastery and success. In exposure therapy, specific techniques to support the person are used in progressively confronting the fearful or anxiety-provoking situation. The intent is to lessen the fear or anxiety perceived by the person as related, but less threatening and innocuous, stimuli are repeatedly introduced in a systematic manner (Difede et al., 2014; Foa, 2011; Ljótsson et al., 2014). These techniques can be *in vivo* (reality), *imaginal* (cognitively based), or *interoceptive* (creating physiologic responses) (Craske et al., 2011; Foa, 2011). They can be presented with graduating intensity or strong (flooding therapy) intensity or of brief or prolonged duration (Craske, Treanor, Conway, Zbozinek, & Vervliet, 2014).

Prolonged exposure therapy evolved from work with people with posttraumatic stress disorder (PTSD) (Foa, 2011). As the process is repeated with increasing exposure to the feared stimulus, inhibition or even long-term extinction occurs (Ljótsson et al., 2014). Exposure therapy is established as being effective for working with people with anxiety and fear disorders (Craske et al., 2014). This therapy also can be an important CBT intervention when working with patients who live with chronic pain who are fearful of movement, wound care, or other activities perceived to provoke anxiety or fear because of the anticipated pain involved. (See Chapter 20 for discussion of fear avoidance with movement.)

Coping Skill Development

CBT is designed to empower the patient to self-manage symptoms and develop different ways of thinking about and perceiving pain and discomfort while learning and improving coping skills to self-manage pain symptoms. In some instances, the coping strategies people have developed to manage other aspects of their lives are not possible for them to use (e.g., running) or are counterproductive (e.g., sitting for long periods watching television) in coping with chronic pain (Eccleston, Morley, & Williams, 2013). Learning effective coping skills is consistently associated with positive outcomes for managing pain (Kroon et al., 2014). Effective coping skills can include but are not limited to setting goals, stretching perspective, identifying/changing negative thoughts, pacing activities, using good body mechanics, distraction, and relaxation (Edmond et al., 2017).

Coping With Trigger Factors

Learning to manage *trigger factors* is an important component of relapse prevention and management. Trigger factors are "measurable precipitants associated with an increased probability of an attack" or exacerbation (Lipton et al., 2014, p. 1395). When considering pain management from a multimodal preventive perspective the goal is to identify, adapt to, control, or in some cases, avoid trigger factors. These are commonly seen with diet, sleep, lighting, odors, or stress-related trigger factors among people who have migraine headaches, whereas head and neck movements are more frequently seen as triggers of tension type headaches (Gantenbein, Afra, Jenni, & Sándor, 2012; Martin et al., 2014). Although traditionally total avoidance of triggers has been taught and encouraged, that may actually result in greater sensitivity to the triggers (Martin, 2010). Rather, it may be more effective to learn to cope with or manage the triggers (Martin et al., 2014). Learning to manage trigger factors is an important aspect of relapse prevention and management (Lipton et al., 2014).

Relapse Prevention and Maintenance of Skills

Relapse prevention and maintenance of skills that involves incorporating learned techniques (i.e., coping skills, new behaviors) into daily life (Hardy, 2014; Tang, 2017) is an important focus of cognitive-behavioral treatment for chronic pain. Through a multimodal approach, a plan for daily management of pain can include techniques such as appropriately using medications, meditating, stretching, exercising, distraction, relaxation, and other nonpharmacologic interventions. Plans can be made for mild to moderate pain increases to be managed using heat, ice, supportive devices, TENS units, increasing distraction, or other effective techniques. Plans for managing severe pain can include calling others for support; taking time to rest; warm salt baths; modifying, postponing or cancelling a scheduled activity; or other appropriate adaptations. (See Chapters 20 through 27 for more detailed discussion of nonpharmacologic interventions to include in a multimodal pain management plan of therapy.)

Patients learn to pace activities and rest to enable them to participate in family obligations and work, social, leisure, and other enjoyable activities (also see Chapter 20). An important part of relapse prevention is for the people living with chronic pain to continually monitor and evaluate the effectiveness of new coping skills, develop awareness of early indicators of an exacerbation or relapse, and acknowledge challenges and successes when dealing with pain management challenges (Naylor, Keefe, Brigidi, Naud, & Helzer, 2008).

Finally, patients are taught how to have an individualized mind-body-spirit oriented *panic plan* to implement during mild, moderate, or severe exacerbations of pain. Such events are normal and expected, but patients often are continually surprised by their presence, particularly severe flare ups. Designing a personalized plan in advance of a flare-up enables the patient with pain to know how to respond to different types of increases in pain. It also reduces anxiety about what to do when pain changes unexpectedly. Panic plans need to be individualized for each person based on individual preferences, what works to manage the pain, available resources, and the environment. For example, mild pain increases can be addressed by distraction, active meditation, and movement. Moderate pain increases are often attended to with stretching, massage, guided imagery, heat, ice, or a TENS unit. Severe pain increases can be dealt with by coping statements (e.g., "I have been through this before") rest, use of music, changing plans, active breathing, guided imagery, social or spiritual support, baths or showers, and rescue medication if indicated. For clients with severe emotional distress during active pain flares, calling or texting a crisis hotline also can be a coping strategy.

Evidence Supporting Cognitive-Behavioral Therapy for Pain Management

For more than three decades, there has been established value for using CBT as part of a multimodal approach to pain management. Research generally is supportive of positive benefits and effects from CBT and supports CBT as an important process in helping patients learn to live better with chronic pain (Crofford, 2015; Ehde et al., 2014; McCracken et al., 2013). CBT allows for tailoring to patient needs, preferences, and medical circumstances. Efficacy for using CBT is reported with a variety of painful conditions (Hardy, 2014), including musculoskeletal pain, arthritis, CLBP, fibromyalgia syndrome (FMS), sickle cell disease, temporomandibular joint (TMJ) pain, and lupus (Cheatle, 2016). It is also effective as part of a multimodal approach, including physical therapy, medications (Mathews, 2014), and other nonpharmacologic interventions. (See Chapters 10 through 19 for discussion of medication, Chapter 21 for discussion of physical therapy, and Chapters 20 through 27 for nonpharmacologic interventions.)

A Cochrane review of studies in which CBT was used with people living with FMS (n = 23 studies, n = 2301 participants) reported slight incremental reductions in pain and disability with low-grade evidence (Bernardy, Klose,

Busch, Choy, & Häuser, 2012). The authors of another systematic review (n = 35 studies, n = 4788 participants) concluded CBT is beneficial in relieving pain but is more effective in helping people living with chronic pain reduce disability and markedly improve quality of life (Eccleston et al., 2013). Those are particularly important benefits because physical ability and quality of life are often impaired among people living with chronic pain. Benefits such as these are why it is advised to implement CBT intervention with people early in the course of chronic pain situations (Hanscom, Brox, & Bunnage, 2015).

An important outcome variable in CBT research with chronic pain is *pain catastrophizing* which is "an exaggerated negative cognitive-affective orientation toward pain" and is a strong predictor of pain-related outcomes (Schütze et al., 2017). CBT was evaluated among patients with FMS who were categorized as high-catastrophizing (n = 16) (Lazaridou et al., 2017). In that study, compared with those who received pain-related education but no CBT, the participants in the CBT group reported less pain and demonstrated less catastrophizing at the conclusion of treatment and at the 6-month follow-up. In another study in which CBT was provided for 11 weeks, the participants (n = 13) had comparison testing done at baseline and after the CBT program (Seminowicz et al., 2013). From a physiologic perspective, the effect of CBT on gray matter of the human cerebral cortex was evaluated through magnetic resonance imaging (MRI) scans. The gray matter of those participants living with chronic pain who received CBT was increased in areas of the prefrontal cerebral cortex and hippocampus. Those findings were correlated with decreased pain catastrophizing.

Adaptive coping with trigger factors has been studied in people living with headaches. In a study comparing avoidance behavior with no treatment and learning to cope with triggers of migraine headaches (n = 127), the participants who were taught to effectively cope with the triggers reported markedly fewer headaches (50%) and required less medication (Martin et al., 2014). In another study with people with migraine headaches (n = 62 subjects, n = 4579 days) who maintained smartphone diaries, the most common headache triggers were stress (58%), sleep deprivation (55%), and fatigue (47%) (Park, Chu, Kim, Park, & Cho, 2016). In addition, the participants who reported triggers were more likely to have significantly greater pain (P < .001) and pain-related disability (P < .001).

An interesting study was conducted among college students (n = 563), comparing BIS with BAS (Jensen et al., 2015). In that study, BIS was associated with greater pain intensity and frequency of headaches and BAS was not associated with pain intensity but was associated with fewer headaches. These results warrant additional research to explore the roles of the BIS and BAS with relation to pain intensity, frequency of pain episodes, and opportunities for pain management using BAS-guided interventions.

Technology can be used to support CBT efforts with people living with chronic pain. These efforts and advances are proving not only to be effective but also to be important options for people who have limited insurance or who have other barriers to participating in CBT in person (Vallury, Jones, & Oosterbroek, 2015) (Table 22.4). In the Cooperative Pain Education and Self-management (COPES) trial, investigators compared the benefit of in-person CBT with CBT that was prompted by an *interactive voice response-based CBT (IVR-CBT)* among military veterans with chronic back pain (n = 104) (Heapy et al., 2017). Those researchers concluded the IVR-CBT (n = 54) is equally as effective as the in-person CBT (n = 50) and there was less attrition in the IVR-CBT group. The results of that study are encouraging for the future use of IVR-CBT.

The development and honing of coping skills are an important aspect of CBT. The benefit of coping skill development and management of chronic pain was seen in a study in which the data of 113 of the COPES participants was subsequently analyzed (Edmond et al., 2017). The authors of that work reported that regardless of CBT method there was a negative correlation between practicing coping skills and pain intensity, pain interference, and depression. Although not specific to pain, the authors of a systematic review of research using *computerized CBT (CCBT)* (n = 11 studies) reported CCBT can be effective as an intervention for people with anxiety and depression (Vallury et al., 2015). In the Netherlands, the internet was used for people living with cancer (n = 31) to participate in a 9-week Mindfulness-Based Cognitive Therapy (MBCT) program that was designed to address fatigue, fear of recurrence of cancer, effect of cancer on communication, movement exercise, and pain (Compen et al., 2017). Evaluation of the *PainCOACH* assessed the use of pain coping skill training via the internet program by that name, to teach coping skills to patients with chronic pain (n = 113) (Rini et al., 2016). The participants in that study reported significant reductions in pain with positive effect

Table 22.4	Barriers Specific to Cognitive Behavioral Interventions	
Patient	Lack of insurance
	Lack of financial support
	Perceived stigma of psychological or mental health care
	Inadequate knowledge of benefit
Environmental	Lack of providers in area
	Lack of transportation
System	Inadequate or absent referral system
	Inadequate knowledge of benefit

Based upon Cheatle, M. D. (2016). Biopsychosocial approach to assessing and managing patients with chronic pain. *Medical Clinics, 100*(1), 43–53.

on self-efficacy, with 91% of participants completing the eight training modules.

The previously discussed study exploring triggers among people with migraine headaches who maintained smart phone diaries was accomplished with smartphone technology (Park et al., 2016). An automated telephone-based system called *Telephone Interactive Voice Response (TIVR)* was used to support people living with chronic pain in maintaining advances made with CBT and minimizing relapse (Naylor et al., 2008). When that system was studied (n = 51), the participants who used the TIVR demonstrated significant improvement (P ≤ .001) in reducing pain, improving coping, and reducing relapse. *Telephonic CBT (tCBT)* was used with people living with chronic widespread pain (n = 442) with 82% continuing for follow-up at the end of 2 years (Beasley et al., 2015). In that study, participants were involved with a 6-month tCBT program and those in an exercise program had modest and sustained improvement over 2 years compared to those in the usual care cohort. Additional benefits of a program such as this is that it is very cost-effective, and the participants learn skills they can continue to use and incorporate into their daily lives.

Exposure therapy incorporated with virtual reality (see Chapter 21) was used in a study with patients with PTSD with promising results in managing depression, sleep disturbances, and anger (Difede et al., 2014). Although virtual reality has been used for a number of years with acute pain, it is now being considered as a potential intervention for chronic pain (Keefe et al., 2012). Increased interest is being garnered in using virtual reality graded for use specifically with patients with chronic pain, disability, and fear related to pain (Parsons & Trost, 2014).

Further research is needed to evaluate the effectiveness of using technology as a delivery mode through which people can participate in CBT (Vallury et al., 2015), particularly among people living with chronic pain conditions. Although technologic advances are promising, a concern is that many of the commercially available computer applications (apps) to help people self-manage pain are not supported by research and have rarely had health care provider involvement during development (Lalloo, Jibb, Rivera, Agarwal, & Stinson, 2015). Telephone-delivered CBT is an area in need of further investigation to determine what types of CBT and what methods of delivery are most effective (Beasley, 2015). These are areas in which clinician involvement in development and research is sorely needed.

Cautions and Contraindications

Working to make lifestyle changes and controlling trigger factors can be discouraging (Gantenbein et al., 2012). It is recommended that CBT interventions are coordinated with and supervised by a licensed clinician who has expertise working with CBT with people living with pain.

The Activating Event Belief Consequence Model

The learning/behavior paradigm uses the ABC Model of CBT, which consists of the (A) *analysis* of *antecedent* or *activating* events, (B) *beliefs* of the person, and (C) *consequences* arising without conscious awareness while living with (C) chronic pain (Conti, Kraus-Schulman, & Stanley, 2017; Montgomery et al., 2014). This model arose from *rational-emotive therapy*, which posits that rather than the events per se being disturbing to people, it is the individual perception of events that becomes disturbing (Dryden, 1990). For example, through this model an (A) activating event might be a flare of chronic pain, which might be experienced followed by the belief (B), "My pain is getting worse." The consequence (C) would then be the person feeling depressed thoughts, anxiety over pain worsening, and helpless, with perception of even greater pain intensity. This may become a vicious circle, with beliefs such as, "I am worthless," or "I am no good to anyone," or "I cannot provide for my family." Psychological consequences of feeling rejected, sad, and shamed may develop with ensuing consequences of isolation, overmedication, fear of pain with avoidance of activities, and sedentary behaviors, resulting in deconditioning. This contributes to a self-fulfilling prophecy of physical weakness, proneness to injury, depression, irritability, anger, and anxiety that fuels more self-deprecating beliefs in a vicious cycle. By acknowledging the physical pain and encouraging the person to change the undesirable beliefs, replacing the negative thoughts with positive ones, such as "I am worthwhile," and "I am valuable," and "I can to do stretching exercises without pain," the cycle can be interrupted. By interrupting the cycle, the person can be in a better position to control pain (Fig. 22.2).

Evidence for Pain Management

The ABC model was tested among people who had low back pain (LBP) that was sustained related to their occupation (n = 241) (Besen, Young, & Shaw, 2015). The researchers of that study reported support of the ABC model with two interesting findings. First, they found the outcome of return to work was not particularly related to the intensity of pain; however, the likelihood of returning to work was less among those participants whose behavior involved pain catastrophizing and fear avoidance. They also reported that support of the person from the employing organization was correlated with positive outcomes, particularly with the person developing confidence regarding ability to return to work. The authors concluded CBT can be effective in assisting people living with LBP to change thoughts of maladaptive thinking (e.g., pain catastrophizing, fear-avoidance). In a small pilot study (n = 20), the

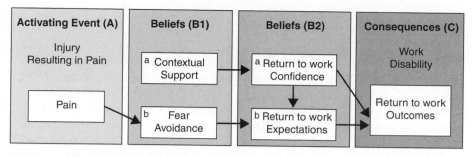

Fig. 22.2 | AB(B)C model of work disability showing the conceptual model of constructs and pathways amongst them. (From Besen, E., Young, A. E., & Shaw, W. S. [2015]. Returning to work following low back pain: Towards a model of individual psychosocial factors. *Journal of Occupational Rehabilitation, 25*[1], 25–37.)

ABC model was used as part of a CBT educational self-management program with women in Iran who were living with chronic pain (Salayani et al., 2016). The women in that study reported significant reductions in anxiety and depression; ironically, however, the effect on pain was not reported.

Acceptance and Commitment Therapy

Acceptance and commitment therapy (ACT) is a relatively new cognitive-behavioral process approach based on rational frame theory with the intent of living mindfully and changing behavior using *psychological flexibility* (Cheatle, 2016). Psychological flexibility is the ability to consistently participate in a pattern of behavior or to change the pattern of behavior contingent upon the benefits of the situation consistent with personal goals and values and to continue to do so despite adverse thoughts or physical sensations (i.e., pain) (Herbert et al., 2017; McCracken et al., 2013). Psychological flexibility uses a process known as *self-as-context* (Yu, Norton, & McCracken, 2017). In ACT, there are six main tenets or processes, as follows (Cheatle, 2016; Herbert et al., 2017; McCracken et al., 2013):

- Awareness and nonjudgmentally accepting situations
- Discovering and identifying what is valued
- Being present and aware of the current time
- Using cognitive diffusion strategies (observing thoughts without being controlled by the thoughts)
- Using self as the observer
- Having committed action (with willingness to experience difficult thoughts)

With psychological flexibility, the intention of ACT is for people with chronic pain to learn to behave congruent with individual goals and values while living in the current moment despite feeling painful sensations (Herbert et al., 2017; Simpson, Mars, & Esteves, 2017). By using this self-management technique, it is possible for the person with chronic pain to feel greater control over both pain and desired activities.

Evidence for Pain Management

In one pilot study (n = 73) at 3-month follow-up, the participants with chronic pain who were in the ACT cohort reported significantly greater pain acceptance with less disability depression, compared to those who received treatment as usual (McCracken et al., 2013). The results of a systematic review of randomized controlled trials (RCTs) in which ACT was evaluated (n = 10 trials, n = 623 participants) noted ACT seemed to be effective as an intervention for chronic pain, especially in the context of improving function both physically and emotionally (Hann & McCracken, 2014). The authors of that review did make the qualification that the individual studies were small and had important potential bias risks. Similar conclusions and qualifications were made in a more recent systematic review (French, Golijani-Moghaddam, & Schröder, 2017). In a larger study (n = 213) *self-as-context* was used with people in chronic pain (Yu et al., 2017). The researchers of that study reported that there were significant improvement in pain acceptance and reductions in pain intensity with small and medium effect sizes and those results continued at the 9-month follow-up.

When cognitive restructuring, acceptance (ACT), and distraction were compared (n = 109), acceptance was more effective than cognitive restructuring for increasing tolerance of pain, but distraction was superior to acceptance in reports of reduced pain intensity (Kohl et al., 2013). However, when patients with FMS (n = 60) who participated in ACT or cognitive restructuring were compared with controls, cognitive restructuring correlated with greater tolerance of cold pain (Kohl et al., 2014).

Interoceptive exposure therapy (paying attention to body sensations) was compared to attention control (monitoring symptoms, reading educational material, and discussions with therapist) and stress management in people living with irritable bowel syndrome (IBS) (n = 110) (Craske et al., 2011). Among other beneficial effects, the results of that study showed significantly less pain vigilance among those in the interoceptive exposure group compared to the other two groups.

Although ACT is most frequently used in a professional setting either individually or with groups (Herbert et al.,

2017; McCracken et al., 2013; Simpson et al., 2017), there are books (Dahl, Luciano, & Wilson, 2005) that can support use of ACT, and most recently it has been used in a telehealth format (Herbert et al., 2017). From a study comparing a telehealth version of ACT with in-person therapy (n = 128) among American veterans with chronic pain, the researchers concluded the telehealth version had results and benefits similar to those with in-person therapy (Herbert et al., 2017). This is an important finding because treatment availability, location, transportation, and cost are potential barriers for patients living with chronic pain who could benefit from ACT.

Even though different aspects of CBT have established benefit with many conditions, including chronic pain, further research is needed. Research is particularly needed to clarify the effectiveness of different techniques in clinical care and from a public health perspective (Hanscom et al., 2015). Additional rigorous research with larger samples is needed to expand on the benefit of ACT with a variety of chronic pain diagnoses (Barban, 2016) and to compare in-person therapy with telehealth therapy.

Biofeedback (Applied Psychophysiology)

Biofeedback is primarily a behavioral therapy (Eccleston et al., 2013) through which patients learn, in real time, to be more aware of what is occurring within their bodies, particularly physiologic activities that are generally considered under involuntary control (Hillinger, Wolever, McKernan, & Elam, 2017; Mathews, 2014; Vögele, 2015). The information gained during the biofeedback session is used to regulate either physiologic or psychological processes or both (Gevirtz, 2017), with the intention of managing symptoms and improving health (Frank, Khorshid, Kiffer, Moravec, & McKee, 2010). Initially, the patient learns to pay attention through equipment or instruments that provide measurements of body functions, such as heart rate, respiratory rate, cerebral activity, and surface muscle tension (Mathews, 2014; Turk, 2017). Gradually the person is able to gain control without needing the equipment (Jung, Yang, & Myung, 2017). Frequently, the cues for monitoring the response to pain are either visual or auditory (Hillinger et al., 2017).

The premise for using biofeedback is that various functional disorders result from sustained excess levels of sympathetic nervous system and hypothalamic-pituitary-adrenal (HPA) system activity (Gevirtz, 2017) and painful muscular conditions often involve hyperactivity that is stress induced (Turk, 2017). By learning to become aware of and then controlling physiologic cues or stimuli, through principles of operant conditioning, the painful activity can be lessened (Gevirtz, 2017; Jung et al., 2017). Through use of feedback about neuromuscular activity, people with various types of pain (e.g.,

musculoskeletal pain, headache, irritable bowel pain, TMJ pain, orofacial pain; phantom limb pain, and other chronic pains) can potentially reduce muscle tension and pain sensations (Frank et al., 2010; Gevirtz, 2017; Tan, Glaros, Sherman, & Wong, 2017; Vögele, 2015; Yoo, Keszler, & Petrin, 2018) (Table 22.5). Using biofeedback encourages incremental positive changes to occur with awareness from the patient, thus reinforcing behavior, encouraging greater engagement, evolving into more substantial benefits while empowering the person with control over painful sensations and increasing self-efficacy (Jung et al., 2017). Biofeedback is used internationally and is one of the most commonly used complementary inventions among people with CLBP in Turkey (Aktaş & Karabulut, 2017).

Evidence for Pain Management

Reports of functional MRIs (fMRIs) done during a type of biofeedback (neurofeedback) included information showing a downregulation of the oxygen in the blood, which lends support to benefit with managing chronic pain (Guan et al., 2015). Biofeedback used with people with pelvic floor pain is reported to be effective approximately 50% of the time (Bonder & Rispoli, 2017). When biofeedback was combined with electrostimulation and compared with electromagnetic stimulation in treatment of refractory chronic pelvic pain in men (n = 45), pain was significantly less and quality of life was improved ($P < .05$) with the benefit of the combination of electrostimulation and biofeedback greater than electrostimulation alone (Yang, Huang, Lai, Zeng, & Chen, 2017).

Earlier studies were inconsistent regarding the evidence of biofeedback with LBP, with one report of low-quality

Table 22.5	Requirements for Biofeedback
Necessary Condition	**Example**
1. There must be an obvious and quantifiable response.	Muscle tension causing neck or back pain.
2. The response must be variable with observable change.	Muscles have the ability to tense and relax.
3. There needs to be noticeable stimulus or cue.	Discomfort, soreness, pain are stimuli that can be easily identified.
4. Active involvement of a motivated person is needed.	A person who lives with chronic pain may be motivated to actively participate in this therapy.

Based upon Jung, K. W., Yang, D.-H., & Myung, S.-J. (2017). Biofeedback therapy. In *Reference module in neuroscience and biobehavioral psychology* (pp. 1–5). New York, NY: Elsevier.

evidence for effectiveness with LBP (Henschke et al., 2010) and the authors of another reporting that it was efficacious for LBP, headaches in adults, and TMJ pain (Frank et al., 2010). More recently, the authors of a pilot study (n = 20) described less pain intensity and fear avoidance with improvement at the 3-month follow-up (Weeks, Whitney, Tindall, & Carter, 2015). The authors of an even more recent meta-analysis from Germany concluded biofeedback is effective for LBP both when used alone and when used in conjunction with other therapies in a multimodal approach (Sielski, Rief, & Glombiewski, 2017).

Although biofeedback is generally associated with chronic conditions, visual biofeedback was used in a small study (n = 12) to improve participation in therapy with people recovering from acute lower extremity fractures (Raaben, Holtslag, Leenen, Augustine, & Blokhuis, 2018). Visual biofeedback was successfully used with people who had undergone total knee arthroplasties (n = 20) to improve their gait during high-demand walking (Christensen et al., 2018). Additional research is needed to evaluate the use of biofeedback in a variety of chronic pain conditions such as postthoracotomy pain syndrome (Khelemsky & Neckman, 2018). Although biofeedback is considered successful treatment for pain, additional research, clinical practice guidelines, and standards of quality assurance are needed (Vögele, 2015).

Mindfulness-Based Stress Management and Mindfulness-Based Cognitive Therapy

Mindfulness meditation arose from the Buddhist tradition; however, mindfulness meditation is more commonly known today as a secular cognitive type of meditation (Day, Jensen, Ehde, & Thorn, 2014b) and for that reason is discussed from a multimodal analgesic perspective with CBT. Several other forms of meditation that are more closely aligned with a spiritual focus are discussed in Chapter 25. Mindfulness meditation is a central aspect of Mindfulness-Based Stress Reduction (MBSR) program founded by Jon Kabat-Zinn. In his book *Full Catastrophe Living: How to Cope with Stress, Pain and Illness Using Mindfulness Meditation,* Kabat-Zinn described mindfulness as "paying attention on purpose, in the present moment, and nonjudgmentally, to the unfolding experience moment to moment" (Kabat-Zinn, 1990, p. 145) (Table 22.6 and Box 22.6). Mindfulness meditation is considered to be a method for achieving mindfulness, which is often perceived as being an integral aspect of human consciousness (Black, 2011). The specific process of mindfulness meditation is differentiated from *mindful awareness,* which is described as the process of living in

Table 22.6 | Kabat-Zinn Attitudes and Behaviors Helpful in Developing Mindfulness

Attitude	Behavior
Being nonjudgmental	Witnessing personal experiences impartially without making hasty conclusions
Being patient	Allowing events to occur without expediting them
Having a beginner's mind	Being open and receptive to new opportunities and possibilities, avoiding being attached to personal experiences or proficiency
Being trusting	Developing a confidence and trust in self and private feelings
Avoiding striving	Being attentive to what is happening at the current time and what is the current experience without trying to change it
Being accepting	Being aware of how things actually are here and now
Letting go	Allowing what is happening to do so without trying to change it, letting things be

From Kabat-Zinn, J. (1990). Full catastrophe living: How to cope with stress, pain and illness using mindfulness meditation. London, UK: Piatkus Books; and Grecucci, A., Pappaianni, E., Siugzdaite, R., Theuninck, A., & Job, R. (2015). Mindful emotion regulation: Exploring the neurocognitive mechanisms behind mindfulness. *BioMed Research International,* 1–9. Article ID 670724.

the present with continually being attentive to what is occurring (Shapiro, Brown, Thoresen, & Plante, 2011)

A variant of MBSR is the integration of the mindfulness concepts with traditional CBT principles, which evolved into MBCT. In MBCT, established CBT techniques are used to bring awareness of the interactions of thoughts, feelings, sensations, and behaviors and using mindfulness techniques to develop a mindful awareness of those interactions in a nonjudgmental way (Day & Thorn, 2016; Day et al., 2014b). Day et al. (2014b) developed a model specifically using MBSR and MBCT concepts with people living with chronic pain (Fig. 22.3).

When MBCT is used with people in pain, instead of focusing on how badly they want pain to stop, they are taught to pay attention to chronic pain with curiosity and without judgment. This approach is very different from what the brain of a patient experiencing pain would naturally do when the physiologic experience of pain occurs, because typically the mind of a person experiencing pain will create multiple negative judgements and negative thoughts about chronic pain. It is now understood, when working with people in pain, an important component of MBCT is for the person to gain the ability to accept pain and in the face of pain participate in activities that

STOP

- Find a quiet place where you will not be interrupted for the next several minutes.
- Set your cell phone alarm to vibrate for 5 or more minutes, and then forget about time altogether. You can adjust the length of your meditation time as you feel is appropriate.
- Sit comfortably in an alert position with a straight and relaxed back. With eyes open or closed, position your hands as you like.
- Allow an intention for this time, such as, "May I allow myself to be present to the simplicity of movements in the body as breathing, feeling, and sensing. May I enjoy the benefits of silence and stillness."

OBSERVE

- Notice the sensations of the body such as posture, feet on the floor, and hips on the chair.
- Allow the breath to flow in and out of the nose at a natural and unforced rate. Avoid manipulating either a slower or faster rate. Just let the body breathe and simply notice the sensations of breathing.
- Moment by moment, allow yourself to take *pause, breathe,* and *feel.*

LET IT BE

- For this time now, *let everything be as it is* without reacting to or trying to change anything. Like a watchful bystander, just witness your experience moment by moment as it happens, whether pleasant or unpleasant.
- If your thoughts drift into stories, fantasies, daydreams, ruminations, or other distractions, simply stop, drop into the sensations of breathing, and allow all sensations and thoughts to roll past the screen of your awareness like moving frames on a filmstrip.

And . . .

RETURN

- Let the breath be your anchor in the present moment. If you become distracted or caught up in any particular *thought, image, emotion,* or *sensation (TIES mnemonic),* just bring your attention back to the breath and *return again and again* to the experience of breathing in a nonjudgmental and self-forgiving way.
- At the end of your meditation period, remain still for a few more moments. Notice how you feel. Be present by taking a moment to *pause, breathe,* and *feel* whatever is happening in any experience at any point in the day.

From Fortney, L. (2018). Recommending meditation. In D. Rakel (Ed.), *Integrative medicine* (4th ed., pp. 945–953.e2). Philadelphia, PA: Elsevier.

are important to them (Day & Thorn, 2016). Advantages of mindfulness meditation are that it is a simple to learn, portable, self-induced strategy that is cost effective and can be used in conjunction with other components of a multimodal approach to pain management, including medications. In addition, there are few side effects with mindfulness meditation (Fig. 22.4) and rarely are any of them serious (Gotink et al., 2015).

Evidence for Pain Management

For centuries the effectiveness of mindfulness meditation to control pain by changing attention to pain and expectations about pain through mindfulness meditation was reported by contemplatives (Zeidan, Grant, Brown, McHaffie, & Coghill, 2012). Now, there is evidence mindfulness meditation causes physiologic changes in the brain. Meditation is reported to affect areas of the brain (e.g., anterior cingulate cortex, ventrolateral prefrontal cortex, and amygdala) that are involved with the process of cognitively modulating pain (Grecucci, Pappaianni, Siugzdaite, Theuninck, & Job, 2015; Zeidan et al., 2011).

Mindfulness meditation is specifically associated with lower frontal lobe theta wave activity, which increases with long-term practice (Tanaka et al., 2014). Increased activity in the prefrontal and cingulate cortexes, insula, and hippocampus was demonstrated on fMRI studies of the brains of people participating in MBSR and MBCT (Gotink, Meijboom, Vernooij, Smits, & Hunink, 2016). The fMRI of those participants also demonstrated less activity of the amygdala with improved connectivity with the prefrontal cortex and quicker deactivation after contact to emotional stimuli. The developers of one model propose that there are neural circuits through which intimate detachment occurs and it is through that detachment that mindfulness is effective for pain control (Grecucci et al., 2015).

Mindfulness meditation has been used by people living with headaches and chronic pain and those with behavioral health and substance use disorders (Fortney, 2018). Some of the chronic pain situations in which mindfulness has been effective are irritable bowel, FMS, and LBP (Zeidan et al., 2012). The authors of a 2015 meta-analysis of RCTs (n = 115 RCTs, n = 8683 subjects)

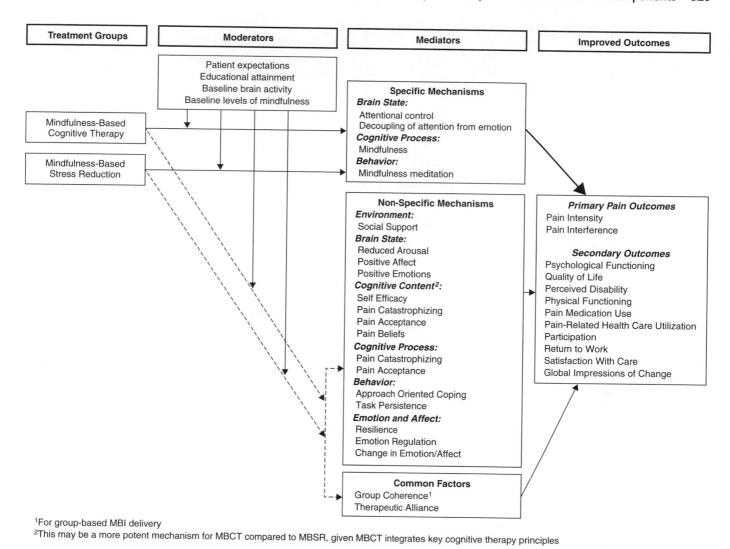

[2]This may be a more potent mechanism for MBCT compared to MBSR, given MBCT integrates key cognitive therapy principles

Fig. 22.3 | An evidence-based, specific, testable model of the mechanisms of MBIs for chronic pain management. *MBI,* Mindfulness-Based Interventions; *MBCT,* Mindfulness-Based Cognitive Therapy; *MBSR,* Mindfulness-Based Stress Reduction. (From Day, M. A., Jensen, M. P., Ehde, D. M., & Thorn, B. E. [2014]. Toward a theoretical model for mindfulness-based pain management. *The Journal of Pain, 15*[7], 691–703.

concluded MBSR and MBCT are effective in alleviating symptoms of chronic pain and the frequently comorbid diagnoses of cancer, anxiety, depression, and cardiovascular disorders (Gotink et al., 2015). The authors of that meta-analysis also reported that mindful interventions are effective in maintaining health and preventing illness in both children and adults. When used with people living with chronic headaches (n = 21), those responding to the intervention reported less pain, less use of analgesic medications, and a difference in their relationship to pain (Day, Thorn, & Rubin, 2014a). In another study in which MBCT was used with people living with chronic headaches (n = 24), pain acceptance with participation in valued activities was found to be a significant mediator (Day & Thorn, 2016). Similar results were reported when mindfulness as used with people with nonspecific chronic pain (n = 109) (la Cour & Petersen, 2015). Interestingly, when MBSR was compared with CBT and usual care (n = 342), there were no meaningful differences

between those in the CBT and MBSR groups, but both of those groups had significantly less pain catastrophizing (P = .001) compared to those in the usual care group (Turner et al., 2016).

Mindfulness interventions have been studied for many years in patients with chronic pain situations (Day et al., 2014a; Fortney, 2018; Gotink et al., 2015). An innovative study evaluated the effect of a brief mindfulness training (n = 86), hypnotic suggestion (n = 73), and education (n = 85) with people experiencing acute pain while hospitalized (Garland et al., 2017). In that study, participants in all three groups reported significantly less anxiety and pain intensity (hypnotic suggestion = 29%, mindfulness meditation = 23%, and psychoeducation = 9% less). The use of mindfulness for acute pain is supported by studies in which mindfulness meditation was successfully taught to people, with only 4 days of training achieving significant reductions in pain intensity (40%) and pain unpleasantness (57%) (Zeidan et al., 2011).

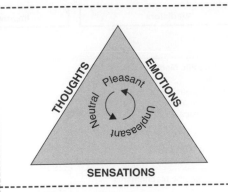

Mindfulness practice (SOAP):

- **Stop:** Pause, notice your breathing, settle into the present moment just as it is...
- **Observe:** Drop into the body, being aware of and feeling whatever is happening in this moment (sensations/feelings/thinking)...
- **Assess:** Without judgment, recognize the pleasant/unpleasant/neutral nature of this experience and let it go...
- **Proceed:** Take a deep breath, and move on...

Triangle of mindful experience:

- **Mental thoughts:** Rumination, thinking, storylines, narratives, mental images, internal conversations, and so on...
- **Emotional feelings:** Love, hate, fear, guilt, anger, joy, sadness, anxiety, and so on...
- **Physical sensations:** Sound, touch, taste, smell, vibration, pressure, and so on...

Intentional kindness practice:

- May I/you/we be well
- May I/you/we be at ease
- May I/you/we be safe and protected
- May I/you/we understand and be understood

Fig. 22.4 | Mindfulness "Practice as You Go" Cards (a Cutout Handout for Patients). (Fortney, L. [2018]. Recommending Meditation. In D. Rakel [Ed.], *Integrative medicine* (4th ed., pp. 945–953.e2]. Philadelphia, PA: Elsevier.

Although evidence indicates MBSM and MBCT are important interventions for helping people living with pain learn to manage pain and optimize their quality of life, additional research is needed to assess the benefit of mindfulness meditation with a variety of acute and chronic painful conditions. The MBCT model for use with patients living with chronic pain needs to be tested with a variety of conditions using strong methodology (Day et al., 2014b). Research is also needed to determine if a formal 8-week education program and daily practice is necessary (Day et al., 2014a; Zeidan et al., 2011). The role of mindfulness interventions in the acute care setting and with acute pain is a new vista with promising results that needs further research (Garland et al., 2017). From an innovative perspective, research into the potential role for electronic applications for teaching and supporting mindfulness activities is needed.

Psychoeducation

Psychoeducation is intended to teach patients techniques they can use or adapt to personally manage symptoms (e.g., pain) while learning coping skills with a goal of empowering the person to actively participate in treatment (pain management) (Vanhaudenhuyse et al., 2018). Education is a primary and crucial element of CBT interventions (Agoston & Sieberg, 2016; Tang, 2017). The World Health Organization underscored the importance of patient education by advising that patient education, including coping skills, needs to be the first step of non-

pharmacologic management of arthritis and rheumatism and is an important component of tertiary prevention (minimizing disease complications) (Wittenauer, Smith, & Aden, 2013). Psychoeducation can be didactive, a discussion, or a combination and is designed to enhance what is known and understood by the person about pain and what are reasonable expectations regarding managing pain (Tang, 2017).

The use of education as a prevention strategy is an extremely important but often underestimated aspect of multimodal pain management. During the last 20 years it has become increasingly evident that chronic pain can result from inadequately managed acute pain (see Chapter 2). *Preparation*, or preparatory education, consists of sharing information about procedures and surgeries before the event so the person is prepared for what will occur, what equipment will be used (Agoston & Sieberg, 2016), and what pain can be expected and how it will be controlled. This is the type of education provided at many hospitals known as *pre-op classes* or *pre-op education*. In the United Kingdom, preoperative education of patients before undergoing an amputation is standard of care (Niraj & Niraj, 2014). Patients who receive individually tailored education before surgery usually have positive postoperative outcomes, including less opioid use and shorter lengths of stay (Chou et al., 2016).

One focus of psychoeducation among people living with chronic pain is to help them change the meaning of their pain (Harvie, Moseley, Hillier, & Meulders, 2017). Another important focus of psychoeducation among people living with chronic pain is to deal with fear-avoidance beliefs and behaviors, which can severely limit function;

however, current evidence supports that education be done by patient-centered cognitive-behavioral therapists rather than rehabilitation specialists (Baez, Hoch, & Hoch, 2017).

Using a holistic view including the pathophysiology of chronic pain is a good way to convey education as an intervention to the family and the person living with pain. (Agoston & Sieberg, 2016). Frequently, psychoeducation occurs in groups that are supportive and nondirective (Vanhaudenhuyse et al., 2018). As with many other interventions, the education is also available by technology, including computer-based programs and mobile phone applications (Wurm et al., 2017).

Evidence for Pain Management

In a study comparing online pain management psychoeducation with online MBCT, both interventions were effective for reducing pain interference and pain catastrophizing with improving pain acceptance with no difference between the two groups; however, participants in the MBCT group reported greater improvement in satisfaction with quality of life (Dowd et al., 2015). In a study comparing psychoeducation plus physiotherapy (PT) (n = 169) compared with self-hypnosis plus self-care learning and controls (n = 157), those subjects in the psychoeducation plus PT reported improved control over pain, less belief that hurt means harm is being done, and less attachment to the need for a physician to find a cure for the pain (Vanhaudenhuyse et al., 2018). There were large treatment effects in reduced pain catastrophizing for patients who received education through a brief intervention project (n = 57) that addressed pain, pain catastrophizing, and skills to improve self-regulation (Darnall, 2016).

As with other interventions, additional research with rigorous methodologies among a variety of acute and chronic pain situations, including the emergency department is needed (Block, Thorn, Kapoor, & White, 2017). Research comparing psychoeducation provided by cognitive-behavioral therapists compared with other clinicians is warranted (Baez et al., 2017). Additional research is needed to compare the effectiveness of technologically provided education.

Key Points

- Pain is perceived and understood in the brain, but that does not mean it is not real.
- Pain is a multidimensional experience that requires multimodal and integrative interventions.
- Integrative and multidisciplinary approaches to pain management support the entire person, including the various dimensions of the pain experience.
- Coping skill development is crucial for people to learn how to live most effectively with pain.

- Cognitive-behavioral therapy (CBT) interventions are an important component of a multimodal approach to pain management.
- CBT is a modality that can be self-empowering to help the person more effectively manage the experience of pain.

Case Scenario

Stuart is a 37-year-old roofer who injured his back when he fell after another worker driving a bulldozer hit the ladder Stuart was descending. He now has constant pain radiating down both legs that sometimes feels like needles. He has not been able to work for the last 9 months since his injury. He tells you "it wasn't an accident it was negligence." He also tells you that he just wants "the pain to go away" so that he "can get back to a normal life and work to pay bills." He admits that the constant pain has changed his relationship with his wife because "I don't feel like a real man now." As he tells you about his constant pain and how it has affected his entire life, his muscles become more tense, his face furrows, and his voice tone escalates. You also notice that his eyes begin to swell with tears.

1. What types of negative thoughts do you think Stuart has?
2. What emotions do you think upset Stuart?
3. How can you introduce CBT to Stuart?
4. What types of CBT interventions could be of help to Stuart?
5. What other clinicians could be consulted?

References

Agoston, A. M., & Sieberg, C. B. (2016). Nonpharmacologic treatment of pain. *Seminars in Pediatric Neurology, 23*(3), 220–223.

Aktaş, Y. Y., & Karabulut, N. (2017). A cross sectional study on complementary and alternative medicine use among a sample of Turkish hospital outpatients with chronic lower back pain. *European Journal of Integrative Medicine, 16,* 33–38.

Baez, S., Hoch, M. C., & Hoch, J. M. (2018). Evaluation of Cognitive Behavioral Interventions and Psychoeducation Implemented by Rehabilitation Specialists to Treat Fear-Avoidance Beliefs in Patients with Low Back Pain: A Systematic Review. *Archives of Physical Medicine and Rehabilitation., 99*(11), 2287–2298.

Barban, K. (2016). Acceptance and commitment therapy: an appropriate treatment option for older adults with chronic pain. *Evidence-based Nursing, 19*(4), 123.

Beasley, M., Prescott, G. J., Scotland, G., McBeth, J., Lovell, K., Keeley, P., ... & Macfarlane, G. J. (2015). Patient-reported improvements in health are maintained 2 years after completing a short course of cognitive behaviour therapy, exercise or both treatments for chronic widespread pain: long-term results from the MUSICIAN randomised controlled trial. *RMD Open, 1*(1), 1–13.

Beck, A. T. (1976). *Cognitive Therapy and Emotional Disorders*. New York, NY: New American Library.

Bernardy, K., Klose, P., Busch, A. J., Choy, E. H., & Häuser, W. (2012). Cognitive behavioural therapies for fibromyalgia syndrome. *The Cochrane Database of Systematic reviews*, (9), CD009796. Online. Available from: http://www.the-healthwell.info/node/579792. (Accessed 3 January 2018).

Besen, E., Young, A. E., & Shaw, W. S. (2015). Returning to work following low back pain: towards a model of individual psychosocial factors. *Journal of Occupational Rehabilitation*, 25(1), 25–37.

Black, D. S. (2011). A brief definition of mindfulness. *Behavioral Neuroscience*, 7(2), 109–110.

Block, P. R., Thorn, B. E., Kapoor, S., & White, J. (2017). Pain Catastrophizing, rather than Vital Signs, Associated with Pain Intensity in Patients Presenting to the Emergency Department for Pain. *Pain Management Nursing*, 18(2), 102–109.

Bonder, J. H., Chi, M., & Rispoli, L. (2017). Myofascial Pelvic Pain and Related Disorders. *Physical Medicine and Rehabilitation Clinics*, 28(3), 501–515.

Burns, D. D. (1999). *Feeling good: The new mood therapy*. New York, NY: Harper Collins.

Burns, D. D. (2012). *Feeling good: The new mood therapy*. New York: New American Library.

Caby, I., Olivier, N., Janik, F., Vanvelcenaher, J., & Pelayo, P. (2016). A controlled and retrospective study of 144 chronic low back pain patients to evaluate the effectiveness of an intensive functional restoration program in France. *Healthcare*, 4(2), 23. https://doi.org/10.3390/healthcare4020023.

Cheatle, M. D. (2016). Biopsychosocial approach to assessing and managing patients with chronic pain. *Medical Clinics*, 100(1), 43–53.

Chou, R., Gordon, D. B., de Leon-Casasola, O. A., Rosenberg, J. M., Bickler, S., Brennan, T., & Wu, C. L. (2016). Management of Postoperative Pain: A Clinical Practice Guideline From the American Pain Society, the American Society of Regional Anesthesia and Pain Medicine, and the American Society of Anesthesiologists' Committee on Regional Anesthesia, Executive Committee, and Administrative Council. *Journal of Pain*, 17(2), 131–157. https://doi.org/10.1016/j.jpain.2015.12.008.

Christensen, J. C., LaStayo, P. C., Marcus, R. L., Stoddard, G. J., Foreman, K. B., Mizner, R. L., ... Pelt, C. E. (2018). Visual knee-kinetic biofeedback technique normalizes gait abnormalities during high-demand mobility after total knee arthroplasty. *The Knee.*, 25(1), 73–82.

Compen, F. R., Bisseling, E. M., Schellekens, M. P., Jansen, E. T., van der Lee, M. L., & Speckens, A. E. (2017). Mindfulness-Based Cognitive Therapy for Cancer Patients Delivered via Internet: Qualitative Study of Patient and Therapist Barriers and Facilitators. *Journal of Medical Internet Research*, 19(12), e407.

Conti, E. C., Kraus-Schulman, C., & Stanley, M. A. (2017). Cognitive-Behavioral Therapy in Older Adults. In S. G. Hofman, & G. J. G. Asmundson (Eds.), *The Science of Cognitive Behavioral Therapy* (pp. 223–256). San Diego, CA: Elsevier Academic Press.

Craske, M. G., Treanor, M., Conway, C. C., Zbozinek, T., & Vervliet, B. (2014). Maximizing exposure therapy: an inhibitory learning approach. *Behaviour Research and Therapy*, 58, 10–23.

Craske, M. G., Wolitzky-Taylor, K. B., Labus, J., Wu, S., Frese, M., Mayer, E. A., & Naliboff, B. D. (2011). A cognitive-behavioral treatment for irritable bowel syndrome using interoceptive exposure to visceral sensations. *Behaviour Research and Therapy*, 49(6), 413–421.

Crofford, L. J. (2015). Psychological aspects of chronic musculoskeletal pain. *Best Practice & Research in. Clinical Rheumatology*, 29(1), 147–155.

Dahl, J., Luciano, C., & Wilson, K. (2005). *Acceptance and commitment therapy for chronic pain*. Oakland, CA: New Harbinger Publications.

Darnall, B. D. (2016). Pain psychology and pain catastrophizing in the perioperative setting: A review of impacts, interventions and unmet needs. *Hand Clinics*, 32(1), 33–39.

Day, M. A., & Thorn, B. E. (2016). The mediating role of pain acceptance during mindfulness-based cognitive therapy for headache. *Complementary Therapies in Medicine*, 25, 51–54.

Day, M. A., Thorn, B. E., & Rubin, N. J. (2014a). Mindfulness-based cognitive therapy for the treatment of headache pain: A mixed-methods analysis comparing treatment responders and treatment non-responders. *Complementary Therapies in Medicine*, 22(2), 278–285.

Day, M. A., Jensen, M. P., Ehde, D. M., & Thorn, B. E. (2014b). Toward a theoretical model for mindfulness-based pain management. *The Journal of Pain*, 15(7), 691–703.

Difede, J., Cukor, J., Wyka, K., Olden, M., Hoffman, H., Lee, F. S., & Altemus, M. (2014). D-cycloserine augmentation of exposure therapy for post-traumatic stress disorder: a pilot randomized clinical trial. *Neuropsychopharmacology*, 39(5), 1052–1058.

Dowd, H., Hogan, M. J., McGuire, B. E., Davis, M. C., Sarma, K. M., Fish, R. A., & Zautra, A. J. (2015). Comparison of an online mindfulness-based cognitive therapy intervention with online pain management psychoeducation: a randomized controlled study. *The Clinical Journal of Pain*, 31(6), 517–527.

Dozios, D. J. A., & Beck, A. T. (2008). Cognitive schemas, beliefs and assumptions. In D. S. Dobson, & D. J. A. Dozios (Eds.), *Risk Factors in Depression* (pp. 119–143). St. Louis, MO: Elsevier.

Dryden, W. (1990). Self-disclosure in rational emotive therapy. In M. Fisher, & S. A. Shueman (Eds.), *Self-Disclosure in the Therapeutic Relationship* (pp. 61–74). New York, NY: Springer Science + Business Media.

Eccleston, C., & Crombez, G. (2007). Worry and chronic pain: a misdirected problem solving model. *Pain*, 132(3), 233–236.

Eccleston, C., Morley, S. J., & Williams, A. D. C. (2013). Psychological approaches to chronic pain management: evidence and challenges. *British Journal of Anaesthesia*, 111(1), 59-63.

Edmond, S., Driscoll, M., Higgins, D., LaChappelle, K., Cervone, D., Goulet, J., ... Heapy, A. (2017). (301) Process of change in CBT for chronic pain: Examining skill practice and knowledge. *The Journal of Pain*, 18(4), S50–S51.

Ehde, D. M., Dillworth, T. M., & Turner, J. A. (2014). Cognitive-behavioral therapy for individuals with chronic pain: Efficacy, innovations, and directions for research. *American Psychologist*, 69(2), 153–166.

Foa, E. B. (2011). Prolonged exposure therapy: past, present, and future. *Depression and Anxiety*, 28(12), 1043–1047.

Fordyce, W. E. (1976). *Behavioral methods for chronic pain and illness*. St. Louis, MO: Mosby.

Fore, L., Perez, Y., Neblett, R., Asih, S., Mayer, T. G., & Gatchel, R. J. (2015). Improved functional capacity evaluation performance predicts successful return to work one year after completing a functional restoration rehabilitation program. *PM&R*, 7(4), 365–375.

Fortney, L. (2018). Recommending Meditation. In D. Rakel (Ed.), *Integrative Medicine* (4th Ed, pp. 945–953.e2). Philadelphia, PA: Elsevier.

Frank, D. L., Khorshid, L., Kiffer, J. F., Moravec, C. S., & McKee, M. G. (2010). Biofeedback in medicine: who, when, why and how? *Mental Health in Family Medicine*, 7(2), 85–91.

French, K., Golijani-Moghaddam, N., & Schröder, T. (2017). What is the evidence for the efficacy of self-help acceptance and commitment therapy? A systematic review and meta-analysis. *Journal of Contextual Behavioral Science.*, 6(4), 360–374.

Gantenbein, A. R., Afra, J., Jenni, W., & Sándor, P. S. (2012). Complementary and alternative treatments for migraine. *Techniques in Regional Anesthesia and Pain Management*, 16(1), 76–81.

Garland, E. L., Baker, A. K., Larsen, P., Riquino, M. R., Priddy, S. E., Thomas, E., & Nakamura, Y. (2017). Randomized Controlled Trial of Brief Mindfulness Training and Hypnotic Suggestion for Acute Pain Relief in the Hospital Setting. *Journal of General Internal Medicine*, 32(10), 1106–1113.

Gatchel, R. J., McGeary, D. D., McGeary, C. A., & Lippe, B. (2014). Interdisciplinary chronic pain management: past, present, and future. *American Psychologist*, 69(2), 119–130.

Gatchel, R. J., McGeary, D. D., Peterson, A., Moore, M., LeRoy, K., Isler, W. C., ... Edell, T. (2009). Preliminary findings of a randomized controlled trial of an interdisciplinary military pain program. *Military Medicine*, 174(3), 270–277.

Gauntlett-Gilbert, J., & Brook, P. (2018). Living well with chronic pain: the role of pain-management programmes. *BJA Education*, 18(1), 3–7.

Gevirtz, R. (2017). Biofeedback. In *Reference Module in Neuroscience and Biobehavioral Psychology* (pp. 1–6). New York, NY: Elsevier.

Gotink, R. A., Meijboom, R., Vernooij, M. W., Smits, M., & Hunink, M. M. (2016). 8-week mindfulness based stress reduction induces brain changes similar to traditional long-term meditation practice–a systematic review. *Brain and Cognition*, 108, 32–41.

Gotink, R. A., Chu, P., Busschbach, J. J., Benson, H., Fricchione, G. L., & Hunink, M. M. (2015). Standardised mindfulness-based interventions in healthcare: an overview of systematic reviews and meta-analyses of RCTs. *PLoS One*, 10(4), e0124344.

Grecucci, A., Pappaianni, E., Siugzdaite, R., Theuninck, A., & Job, R. (2015). Mindful emotion regulation: exploring the neurocognitive mechanisms behind mindfulness. *BioMed Research International*, 2015, 1–9. Article ID 670724.

Guan, M., Ma, L., Li, L., Yan, B., Zhao, L., Tong, L., ... Shi, D. (2015). Self-regulation of brain activity in patients with postherpetic neuralgia: a double-blind randomized study using real-time FMRI neurofeedback. *PLoS One*, 10(4), e0123675.

Hann, K. E., & McCracken, L. M. (2014). A systematic review of randomized controlled trials of Acceptance and Commitment Therapy for adults with chronic pain: Outcome domains, design quality, and efficacy. *Journal of Contextual Behavioral Science*, 3(4), 217–227.

Hanscom, D. A., Brox, J. I., & Bunnage, R. (2015). Defining the role of cognitive behavioral therapy in treating chronic low back pain: an overview. *Global Spine Journal*, 5(06), 496–504.

Hardy, K. V. (2014). Cognitive behavioral therapy. In *Reference Module in Neuroscience and Behavioral Psychology - Encyclopedia of the Neurological Sciences* (2nd Ed, pp. 822–823). New York, NY: Elsevier.

Harvie, D. S., Moseley, G. L., Hillier, S. L., & Meulders, A. (2017). Classical conditioning differences associated with chronic pain: a systematic review. *The Journal of Pain*, 18(8), 889–898.

Heapy, A. A., Higgins, D. M., Goulet, J. L., LaChappelle, K. M., Driscoll, M. A., Czlapinski, R. A., ... Kerns, R. D. (2017). Interactive Voice Response–Based Self-management for Chronic Back Pain: The COPES Noninferiority Randomized Trial. *JAMA Internal Medicine*, 177(6), 765–773.

Henschke, N., Ostelo, R. W., van Tulder, M. W., Vlaeyen, J. W., Morley, S., Assendelft, W. J., & Main, C. J. (2010). Behavioural treatment for chronic low-back pain. *The Cochrane Database of Systematic Reviews*, 2010(7). doi:https://doi.org/10.1002/14651858.CD002014.pub3.

Herbert, M. S., Afari, N., Liu, L., Heppner, P., Rutledge, T., Williams, K., ... Atkinson, J. H. (2017). Telehealth Versus In-Person Acceptance and Commitment Therapy for Chronic Pain: A Randomized Noninferiority Trial. *The Journal of Pain*, 18(2), 200–211.

Hillinger, M. G., Wolever, R. Q., McKernan, L. C., & Elam, R. (2017). Integrative Medicine for the Treatment of Persistent Pain. *Primary Care: Clinics in Office Practice*, 44(2), 247–264.

Jayasinghe, N., Sparks, M. A., Kato, K., Wilbur, K., Ganz, S. B., Chiaramonte, G. R., & Evans, A. T. (2014). Exposure-based CBT for older adults after fall injury: Description of a manualized, time-limited intervention for anxiety. *Cognitive and Behavioral Practice*, 21(4), 432–445. https://doi.org/10.1080/00029157.2008.10401654.

Jensen, M. P., Ehde, D. M., & Day, M. A. (2016). The behavioral activation and inhibition systems: implications for understanding and treating chronic pain. *The Journal of Pain*, 17(5), 529–e1.

Jensen, M. P., Tan, G., & Chua, S. M. (2015). Pain intensity, headache frequency, and the behavioral activation and inhibition systems. *The Clinical Journal of Pain*, 31(12), 1068–1074.

Jung, K. W., Yang, D.-H., & Myung, S.-J. (2017). Biofeedback therapy. In *Reference Module in Neuroscience and Biobehavioral Psychology* (pp. 1–5). New York, NY: Elsevier.

Kabat-Zinn, J. (1990). *Full Catastrophe Living: How to Cope with Stress, Pain and Illness Using Mindfulness Meditation*. London, UK: Piatkus Books.

Keefe, F. J., Huling, D. A., Coggins, M. J., Keefe, D. F., Rosenthal, M. Z., Herr, N. R., & Hoffman, H. G. (2012). Virtual reality for persistent pain: a new direction for behavioral pain management. *PAIN®*, 153(11), 2163–2166.

Khelemsky, Y., & Neckman, D. (2018). Postthoracotomy pain syndrome. In M. Freedman, J. Gehret, G. Young, & L. Kamen (Eds.), *Challenging Neuropathic Pain Syndromes* (pp. 129–134). St. Louis, MO: Elsevier.

Kim, E. H., Crouch, T. B., & Olatunji, B. O. (2017). Adaptation of behavioral activation in the treatment of chronic pain. *Psychotherapy*, 54(3), 237–244.

Kohl, A., Rief, W., & Glombiewski, J. A. (2013). Acceptance, cognitive restructuring, and distraction as coping strategies for acute pain. *The Journal of Pain, 14*(3), 305–315.

Kohl, A., Rief, W., & Glombiewski, J. A. (2014). Do fibromyalgia patients benefit from cognitive restructuring and acceptance? An experimental study. *Journal of Behavior Therapy and Experimental Psychiatry, 45*(4), 467–474.

Kroon, F. P., van der Burg, L. R., Buchbinder, R., Osborne, R. H., Johnston, R. V., & Pitt, V. (2014). Self-management education programmes for osteoarthritis. *The Cochrane Database of Systematic Reviews, 1*, CD008963.

la Cour, P., & Petersen, M. (2015). Effects of mindfulness meditation on chronic pain: a randomized controlled trial. *Pain Medicine, 16*(4), 641–652.

Lalloo, C., Jibb, L. A., Rivera, J., Agarwal, A., & Stinson, J. N. (2015). "There's a pain app for that": Review of patient-targeted smartphone applications for pain management. *The Clinical Journal of Pain, 31*(6), 557–563.

Lazaridou, A., Kim, J., Cahalan, C. M., Loggia, M. L., Franceschelli, O., Berna, C., & Edwards, R. R. (2017). Effects of Cognitive-Behavioral Therapy (CBT) on brain connectivity supporting catastrophizing in fibromyalgia. *The Clinical Journal of Pain, 33*(3), 215–221.

Lemmon, R., & Roseen, E. J. (2018). Chronic low back pain. In D. Rakel (Ed.), *Integrative Medicine* (4th Ed, pp. 662–675e). St. Louis, MO: Elsevier.

Lipton, R. B., Buse, D. C., Hall, C. B., Tennen, H., DeFreitas, T. A., Borkowski, T. M., ... Haut, S. R. (2014). Reduction in perceived stress as a migraine trigger: Testing the "let-down headache" hypothesis. *Neurology, 82*(16), 1395–1401.

Ljótsson, B., Hesser, H., Andersson, E., Lackner, J. M., El Alaoui, S., Falk, L., ... Nowinski, S. (2014). Provoking symptoms to relieve symptoms: a randomized controlled dismantling study of exposure therapy in irritable bowel syndrome. *Behaviour Research and Therapy, 55*, 27–39.

Loeser, J. D. (2017). John J. Bonica: born 100 years ago. *Pain, 158*(10), 1845–1846.

Main, C. J., Keefe, F. J., Jensen, M. P., Vlaeyen, J. W., & Vowles, K. E. (2015). *Fordyce's Behavioral Methods for Chronic Pain and Illness: Republished with Invited commentaries.* Philadelphia, PA: Lippincott Williams & Wilkins.

Malladi, N. (2015). Interdisciplinary rehabilitation. *Physical Medicine and Rehabilitation Clinics, 26*(2), 349–358.

Martin, P. R. (2010). Managing headache triggers: Think 'coping' not 'avoidance'. *Cephalalgia, 30*(5), 634–637.

Martin, P. R., Reece, J., Callan, M., MacLeod, C., Kaur, A., Gregg, K., & Goadsby, P. J. (2014). Behavioral management of the triggers of recurrent headache: a randomized controlled trial. *Behaviour Research and Therapy, 61*, 1–11.

Mathews, M. (2014). Multimodal treatment of pain. *Neurosurgery Clinics of North America, 25*(4), 803–808.

Mathews, M., & Davin, S. (2014). Chronic pain rehabilitation. *Neurosurgery Clinics, 25*(4), 799–802.

McCracken, L. M., Sato, A., & Taylor, G. J. (2013). A trial of a brief group-based form of acceptance and commitment therapy (ACT) for chronic pain in general practice: pilot outcome and process results. *The Journal of Pain, 14*(11), 1398–1406.

Meyer, W. J., Martyn, Jeevendra Martyn, J. A., Wiechman, S., Thomas, C. R. & Woodson, L. (2017). Management of pain and other discomforts in burned patients. In: D. Herndon (Ed). Total Burn Care (5th Ed.) (pp. 679-699 e.6). Philadelphia, PA: Elsevier.

Montgomery, G. H., David, D., Kangas, M., Green, S., Sucala, M., Bovbjerg, D. H., ... Schnur, J. B. (2014). Randomized controlled trial of a cognitive-behavioral therapy plus hypnosis intervention to control fatigue in patients undergoing radiotherapy for breast cancer. *Journal of Clinical Oncology, 32*(6), 557–563.

Naylor, M. R., Keefe, F. J., Brigidi, B., Naud, S., & Helzer, J. E. (2008). Therapeutic interactive voice response for chronic pain reduction and relapse prevention. *Pain, 134*(3), 335–345.

Niraj, S., & Niraj, G. (2014). Phantom limb pain and its psychologic management: a critical review. *Pain Management Nursing, 15*(1), 349–364.

Okifuji, A., & Skinner, M. (2009). Psychological aspects of pain. In H. S. Smith (Ed.), *Current Therapy in Pain* (pp. 513–518). Philadelphia, PA: Saunders.

Park, J. W., Chu, M. K., Kim, J. M., Park, S. G., & Cho, S. J. (2016). Analysis of trigger factors in episodic migraineurs using a smartphone headache diary applications. *PLoS One, 11*(2), e0149577.

Parsons, T. D., & Trost, Z. (2014). Virtual reality graded exposure therapy as treatment for pain-related fear and disability in chronic pain. In *Virtual, Augmented Reality and Serious Games for Healthcare 1* (pp. 523–546). Berlin, Germany: Springer.

Pasero, C., Quinlan-Colwell, A., Rae, D., Broglio, K., & Drew, D. (2016). American Society for Pain Management Nursing position statement: Prescribing and administering opioid doses based solely on pain intensity. *Pain Management Nursing, 17*(3), 170–180.

Peterson, J. C., Smith, K. A., Khan, T., & Arnold, P. M. (2013). The interdisciplinary management of spinal disorders: A review of outcomes. *Techniques in Regional Anesthesia and Pain Management, 17*(4), 157–162.

Pujol, L. A., Sussman, L., Clapp, J., Nilson, R., Gill, H., Boge, J., & Goff, B. (2015). Functional restoration for chronic pain patients in the military: Early results of the San Antonio Military Medical Center functional restoration program. *US Army Medical Department Journal*, 1–7.

Raaben, M., Holtslag, H. R., Leenen, L. P., Augustine, R., & Blokhuis, T. J. (2018). Real-time visual biofeedback during weight bearing improves therapy compliance in patients following lower extremity fractures. *Gait & Posture, 59*, 206–210.

Rini, C., Porter, L. S., Somers, T. J., McKee, D. C., DeVellis, R. F., Smith, M., ... Mariani, C. (2015). Automated, Internet-based Pain Coping Skills Training to Manage Osteoarthritis Pain: A Randomized Controlled Trial. *Pain, 156*(5), 837.

Salayani, F., EbrahimAbad, M. A., Mashhadi, A., Hoseini, R. A., Ghavidel, R. A., & Nejad, H. M. (2016). Effect of Cognitive Pain Self-Management Program on Depression, Anxiety, and Stress in Women with Chronic Musculoskeletal Pain: A Pilot Study. *Evidence Based Care, 6*(2), 39–48.

Schoneboom, B. A., Perry, S. M., Barnhill, W. K., Giordano, N. A., Nicely, K. L. W., & Polomano, R. C. (2016). Answering the call to address chronic pain in military service members and veterans: Progress in improving pain care and restoring health. *Nursing Outlook, 64*(5), 459–484.

Schubiner, H. (2018). Emotional awareness of pain. In D. Rakel (Ed.), *Integrative Medicine* (4th Ed, pp. 963–970.e2). Philadelphia, PA: Elsevier.

Seminowicz, D. A., Shpaner, M., Keaser, M. L., Krauthamer, G. M., Mantegna, J., Dumas, J. A., ... & Naylor, M. R. (2013). Cognitive-behavioral therapy increases prefrontal cortex gray matter in patients with chronic pain. *The Journal of Pain, 14*(12), 1573–1584.

Shapiro, S. L., Brown, K. W., Thoresen, C., & Plante, T. G. (2011). The moderation of mindfulness-based stress reduction effects by trait mindfulness: results from a randomized controlled trial. *Journal of Clinical Psychology*, 67(3), 267–277.

Sielski, R., Rief, W., & Glombiewski, J. A. (2017). Efficacy of biofeedback in chronic back pain: a meta-analysis. *International Journal of Behavioral Medicine*, 24(1), 25–41.

Simons, L. E., Elman, I., & Borsook, D. (2014). Psychological processing in chronic pain: a neural systems approach. *Neuroscience & Biobehavioral Reviews*, 39, 61–78.

Simpson, P. A., Mars, T., & Esteves, J. E. (2017). A systematic review of randomised controlled trials using Acceptance and commitment therapy as an intervention in the management of non-malignant, chronic pain in adults. *International Journal of Osteopathic Medicine*, 24, 18–31.

Sussman, L., Clapp, J., Keizer, B., Gill, H., Boge, J., & Goff, B. (2015). (533) Functional restoration in a military chronic pain population: first year outcomes from the SAMMC Functional Restoration Program. *The Journal of Pain*, 16(4), S109.

Tan, G., Glaros, A., Sherman, R., & Wong, C. Y. (2017). Integrative Approaches to Orofacial Pain: Role of Biofeedback and Hypnosis. In *Orofacial Disorders* (pp. 317–324). Cham, Switzerland: Springer.

Tanaka, G. K., Peressutti, C., Teixeira, S., Cagy, M., Piedade, R., Nardi, A. E., ... & Velasques, B. (2014). Lower trait frontal theta activity in mindfulness meditators. *Arquivos de Neuropsiquiatria*, 72(9), 687–693.

Tang, N. K. (2017). Cognitive behavioural therapy in pain and psychological disorders: Towards a hybrid future. *Progress in Neuro-Psychopharmacology and Biological Psychiatry.*, 87(Pt B), 281–289.

Turk, D. C. (2017). Pain management. In *Reference Module in Neuroscience and Biobehavioral Psychology* (pp. 1–5). New York, NY: Elsevier.

Turner, J. A., Anderson, M. L., Balderson, B. H., Cook, A. J., Sherman, K. J., & Cherkin, D. C. (2016). Mindfulness-based stress reduction and cognitive behavioral therapy for chronic low back pain: similar effects on mindfulness, catastrophizing, self-efficacy, and acceptance in a randomized controlled trial. *Pain*, 157(11), 2434–2444.

Vallury, K. D., Jones, M., & Oosterbroek, C. (2015). Computerized cognitive behavior therapy for anxiety and depression in rural areas: a systematic review. *Journal of Medical Internet Research*, 17(6), e139. doi:https://doi.org/10.2196/jmr.4145.

Vanhaudenhuyse, A., Gillet, A., Malaise, N., Salamun, I., Grosdent, S., Maquet, D., ... Faymonville, M. E. (2018). Psychological interventions influence patients' attitudes and beliefs about their chronic pain. *Journal of Traditional and Complementary Medicine.*, 8(2), 296–302.

Vögele, C. (2015). Behavioral Medicine. In *International Encyclopedia of the Social & Behavioral Sciences* (2nd Ed., pp. 463–469). New York, NY: Elsevier.

Waltman, S. H., & Sokol, L. (2017). The generic model of cognitive behavioral therapy: a case conceptualization-driven approach. In S. G. Hofmann, & G. J. G. Asmundson (Eds.), *The Science of Cognitive Behavioral Therapy* (pp. 3–17). London: Academic Press.

Weeks, D. L., Whitney, A. A., Tindall, A. G., & Carter, G. T. (2015). Pilot randomized trial comparing intersession scheduling of biofeedback results to individuals with chronic pain: influence on psychologic function and pain intensity. *American Journal of Physical Medicine & Rehabilitation*, 94(10S), 869–878.

Weiner, S. S., & Nordin, M. (2010). Prevention and management of chronic back pain. *Best Practice & Research Clinical Rheumatology*, 24(2), 267–279.

Wenzel, A. (2017). Basic Strategies of Cognitive Behavioral Therapy. *Psychiatric Clinics*, 40(4), 597–609.

Wittenauer, R., Smith, L., & Aden, K. (2013). Background paper 6.12 osteoarthritis. In *Priority Medicines for Europe and the World: "A Public Health Approach to Innovation."* World Health Organization.

Wooton, J., & Warfield, C. (2009). Cognitive therapy for chronic pain. In H. S. Smith (Ed.), *Current Therapy in Pain* (pp. 521–525). Philadelphia, PA: Saunders.

Wurm, M., Strandberg, E. K., Lorenz, C., Tillfors, M., Buhrman, M., Holländare, F., & Boersma, K. (2017). Internet delivered transdiagnostic treatment with telephone support for pain patients with emotional comorbidity: a replicated single case study. *Internet Interventions*, 10, 54–64.

Yang, M. H., Huang, Y. H., Lai, Y. F., Zeng, S. W., & Chen, S. L. (2017). Comparing electromagnetic stimulation with electrostimulation plus biofeedback in treating male refractory chronic pelvic pain syndrome. *Urological Science*, 28(3), 156–161.

Yoo, S., Kenzler, M., & Petrin, Z. (2018). Amputation-related pain. In M. Freedman, J. Gehret, G. Young, & L. Kamen (Eds.), *Challenging Neuropathic Pain Syndromes* (pp. 119–127). St. Louis, MO: Elsevier.

Yu, L., Norton, S., & McCracken, L. M. (2017). Change in "Self-as-Context" ("Perspective-Taking") Occurs in Acceptance and Commitment Therapy for People With Chronic Pain and Is Associated With Improved Functioning. *The Journal of Pain*, 18(6), 664–672.

Zeidan, F., Grant, J. A., Brown, C. A., McHaffie, J. G., & Coghill, R. C. (2012). Mindfulness meditation-related pain relief: evidence for unique brain mechanisms in the regulation of pain. *Neuroscience Letters*, 520(2), 165–173.

Zeidan, F., Martucci, K. T., Kraft, R. A., Gordon, N. S., McHaffie, J. G., & Coghill, R. C. (2011). Brain mechanisms supporting the modulation of pain by mindfulness meditation. *Journal of Neuroscience*, 31(14), 5540–5548.

Chapter 23 Energy Healing Therapies or Biofield Therapies as Components of Multimodal Analgesic Pain Management

Ann Quinlan-Colwell, Susan O'Conner-Von

CHAPTER OUTLINE

Reiki, pg. 637

Indications, pg. 637

Evidence for Pain Management, pg. 637

Cautions, pg. 638

Therapeutic Touch, pg. 638

Evidence for Pain Management, pg. 639

Cautions, pg. 641

Healing Touch, pg. 642

Evidence for Pain Management, pg. 642

Cautions, pg. 642

Acupuncture, pg. 642

Evidence for Pain Management, pg. 643

Caution, pg. 644

Auricular Acupuncture, pg. 644

Evidence for Pain Management, pg. 645

Caution, pg. 647

Acupressure, pg. 647

Evidence for Pain Management, pg. 647

Caution, pg. 647

Key Points, pg. 648

Case Scenario, pg. 648

References, pg. 648

ENERGY modalities, or biofield therapies as they are also called, have ancient roots (Fontaine, 2015; Jain & Mills, 2010). The specific therapies discussed in this chapter are Therapeutic Touch (TT), Reiki, Healing Touch (HT), acupuncture, auricular acupuncture, and acupressure. Modern science supports the concept that various systems in the human body accept, process, store, conduct, and in other ways utilize a variety of types of energy (Oschman, 2016a; Oschman, 2016c). A commonality among them is that they all arose from the awareness that the mind and body are influenced by subtle energies (Hillinger, Wolever, McKernan, & Elam, 2017). TT and HT are specifically associated with the unitary energy field concepts from the work of Martha Rogers (Hanley, Coppa, & Shields, 2017; Krieger, 1973; Krieger, 1979; Krieger, 2017; Lincoln, Nowak, Schommer, Briggs, Fehrer, & Wax, 2014). The human energy field is a dynamic, continuous whole of energy that encompasses a person, extends beyond the actual body in a distinct pattern, and intertwines in a continuous mutual process with the environmental energy field (Shields, Fuller, Resnicoff, Butcher, & Frisch, 2016).

The conclusions derived from one systematic review (n = 66 clinical studies) were that there is strong evidence for these therapies reducing pain intensity in people living with chronic pain and moderate evidence for reducing pain among acute care hospitalized patients and people with a cancer diagnosis (Jain & Mills, 2010). A reduction in the need for pain medications has been reported, and although there is equivocal evidence about the effectiveness of these interventions with effective measures of pain, that could be related to findings that the degree of improvement is associated with the degree of experience of the clinician using the therapy (Hillinger et al., 2017).

Reiki

The word Reiki (pronounced ray-kee) is composed of two Japanese words; rei means universal and *ki* means life force (Jackson & Latini, 2016). Many think the origin of Reiki can be traced to ancient Tibet and that it was rediscovered by Dr. Mikao Usui, a Japanese physician and monk (Fontaine, 2015). One of the 21 students Dr. Usui trained to be a Reiki Master was Dr. Chujiro Hayashi, a medical physician and retired naval captain who opened a Reiki clinic in Tokyo. Reiki was eventually introduced outside of Japan by Hawayo Takata, who was born in 1900 in the Hawaiian territory. While traveling to Japan, she became a patient of Dr. Usui and within months of arriving at his clinic, her health was restored from severe asthma. She was eventually accepted as Dr. Usui's student and became a Reiki master before returning to Hawaii in 1937. Takata moved to Honolulu and for the next four decades practiced and taught Reiki in the United States and Canada until she died in 1980 (Miles, 2008).

As a result of these early Reiki masters, Reiki is practiced around the world and used by many patients to complement conventional Western medicine. A Reiki treatment supports the whole person—physically, emotionally, mentally, and spiritually. According to the National Center for Complementary and Integrative Health (NCCIH, 2018), Reiki is a complementary health approach in which Reiki practitioners place their hands lightly on or just above a person with the goal of facilitating the person's own healing response. When a Reiki practitioner places his or her hands on an area of a person's clothed body, Reiki flows through the practitioner into the person receiving the treatment. This flow may be felt as any type of sensation: heat, cold, vibration, tingling, or heaviness or no sensation at all. A full Reiki treatment takes about 60 to 90 minutes (Reiki Alliance, 2017).

Reiki is based on an Eastern belief in an energy that supports the body's natural healing abilities. The practitioner is not the source of energy; instead the practitioner is the conduit for the flow of energy. Reiki does not treat diseases, but instead helps to restore a person's balance and promote relaxation (Miles, 2008). To become a Reiki practitioner, there are three levels of training and no requirement to be a health care professional (Wagner & Thompson, 2014). Through Reiki training the practitioner learns the importance of presence and centering for being the conduit for the flow of energy (Shields & Wilson, 2016).

Indications

According to the NCCIH (2018), Reiki is used for a variety of conditions, including pain, anxiety, fatigue,

stress, and depression. Energy modalities such as Reiki are assumed to function in a manner similar to that of relaxation, "shifting autonomic nervous system function to improve health and reduce inflammation" (Chiasson, 2016, p. 566). The emphasis of the use of Reiki is on healing, not cure, "which is believed to occur by Reiki energy connecting individuals to their own innate spiritual wisdom and highest good" (Ringdahl, 2018, p. 413). Reiki has been used for the purpose of acting as a catalyst to healing in a variety of populations dealing with pain, for example, persons with fibromyalgia (Assefi, Bogart, Goldberg, & Buchwald, 2008), patients with cancer (Bossi, Ott, & DeChristofaro, 2008; Coakley & Barron, 2012; Jain & Mills, 2010), community-dwelling older adults with chronic pain (Richeson, Spross, Lutz, & Peng, 2010), women with cesarean section incisional pain (Midilli & Gunduzoglu, 2016), patients with total knee arthroplasty (Notte, Fazzini, & Mooney, 2016), and women after hysterectomy (Vitale & O'Connor, 2006).

Evidence for Pain Management

Research evidence is emerging on the positive effects of Reiki on pain and anxiety, as revealed in an in-depth literature review of 12 randomized controlled trials (RCTs) (Thrane & Cohen, 2014). However, more rigorous, large-scale studies are needed to develop appropriate biofield measurement tools and examine mechanisms of action to provide solid evidence for practice (Hennegahan & Schnyer, 2015). In preparation for a large-scale multisite study, Baldwin, Vitale, Brownell, Kryak, and Rand (2017) conducted a pilot study to examine the use of Reiki on pain, stress, and anxiety in adults (ages 50–85 years) undergoing total knee replacement surgery. This three-armed RCT (n = 45) consisted of a group of subjects (n = 15) receiving three or four 30-minute Reiki sessions plus the usual standard of care, another group of subjects (n = 15) receiving three or four 30-minute sham Reiki sessions plus standard of care, and a third group of subjects (n = 15) receiving three or four sessions of "quiet time" plus standard of care. The sessions were held 1 hour before surgery, then 24, 48, and 72 hours after surgery (Baldwin, et al., 2017). Results revealed that Reiki significantly decreased pain, stress, and anxiety in adult patients undergoing total knee replacement surgery. In addition, patients in the Reiki group used less opioid pain medication postoperatively than the other two study groups. Critical to this study design was the use of sham Reiki as a placebo, which in this study "indicates that Reiki goes above and beyond a placebo effect" (Baldwin et al., 2017, p. 86).

Reiki also has been tested in the pediatric population. Kundu, Lin, Oron, and Doorenbos (2014) conducted a double-blind RCT with children (N = 38, ages 9 months to 4 years, 42% male) undergoing dental procedures. Before surgery, each of the study subjects was randomly assigned to a Reiki treatment or sham Reiki treatment, which was provided in an examination room in the surgical area. On the patient's arrival to the recovery room after surgery, data collected included pain scores, analgesic use, and side effects related to treatment. These data were again collected at 30, 60, 120, and 180 minutes later. Family satisfaction with perioperative care was assessed 24 hours after surgery (Kundu et al., 2014). The effect of Reiki on the outcome measures was analyzed using a multiple linear regression model. Results revealed there was no statistically significant differences between the Reiki group and the sham Reiki (control) group for this single session of Reiki for young children before dental surgery. These investigators noted the limitations of a small, heterogeneous sample and lack of measures to examine any immune or neuroendocrine changes as a result of Reiki (Kundu et al., 2014).

Cautions

Despite the long clinical use, the body of research examining the effects of Reiki is in the early stages, yet many patients with chronic pain reportedly find relief while using Reiki (Chiasson, 2016). Of importance to note, Reiki is considered to be safe because no negative or harmful effects on study subjects have been found in any Reiki studies (NCCIH, 2015).

Therapeutic Touch

TT is a transpersonal, holistic therapy that grew from the work of Dolores Krieger, PhD, RN, and Dora Kunz (Fig. 23.1) at the Theosophical Society retreat center at Pumpkin Hollow Farm in upstate New York. It was there, during the early 1970s, when they considered the early work of TT as a present-day interpretation of ancient healing (Hanley et al., 2017; Krieger, 1979; Oschman, 2016b).

Since that time, it has evolved into an evidence-based therapy and transpersonal healing therapy that is used internationally and taught in more than 80 college curricula and 90 different countries (Hanley et al., 2017; Krieger, 2017; Therapeutic Touch International Association [TTIA], 2016).

The concept supporting TT is that humans are composed of energy in the form of an intricate energy field and each person has the natural ability to augment healing in others (Oschman, 2016b; TTIA, 2016) through an energy process that includes humans and their environment (Bultemeier, 2014; Hanley et al., 2017). Although the nursing theoretical basis of TT was originally closely aligned with Rogers' Science of Unitary Human Beings theory (Rogers, 1994), a more recent practice-based Theory of Healing has evolved from the work of longtime TT practitioners (Hanley et al., 2017).

In healthy people, energy is balanced and flows without interruption, but when there is illness, trauma, or disease, the energy becomes imbalanced. TT is a focused, intentional compassionate process by which the practitioner works to rebalance and restore the energy field to a balanced state (Krieger, 2017; TTIA, 2016). Krieger (2017) stressed that in addition to having a conscious intention to help the person, compassion is a central intrinsic component of TT and without compassion TT is not occurring.

TT is a bit of a misnomer because generally the practitioner often does not actually touch the person but rather works in the energy field surrounding the physical body of the person (Erich & Quinlan-Colwell, 2017). TT is the intentional use of the hands of the practitioner to attune the practitioner with the energy field that surrounds the person with the intent of helping the person through modulation of the person's energy field. Generally, the

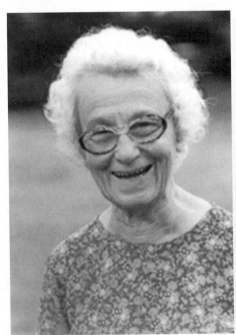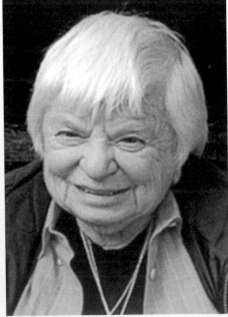

Fig. 23.1 | Dolores Krieger and Dora Kunz. (From Oschman, J. L. [2016]. *Energy medicine* [2nd ed.]. London: Churchill Livingstone.)

practitioner's hands work in an area that is between 2 and 6 inches above the skin (Quinlan-Colwell, 2012; TTIA, 2016). For patients dealing with intense pain who can tolerate very little touch or movement, TT can be an important option that can often help them tolerate painful treatments such as wound care (see Clinical Application). It is used with patients in a variety of arenas, including homes, hospitals, long-term care facilities, and clinics. It is used with people of all ages, ranging from neonates in neonatal intensive care units to older adults in palliative care (Erich & Quinlan-Colwell, 2017; Hanley et al., 2017; TTIA, 2016).

It is important to note that TT can be learned and used by anyone, not just clinicians; however, it is a discipline and practice is necessary (TTIA, 2016). The TT process begins with the TT practitioner centering self with a *call for compassion* for the person or healing partner (Hp). As the TT practitioner draws closer to the Hp, *in the approach* there is awareness of the energy interactions. During *the outreach* the TT practitioner seeks indications of subtle energy imbalances, which leads to *the search* with a focus of assessing the energy field of the patient for imbalances, stress, discomfort, or anxiety. Using the information from the search, there is a purposeful and individualized intervention during the *rebalancing phase*. This rebalancing phase is designed to support the person, promote balance of the energy field, and promote healing. This is followed by a reassessment or evaluation and closure, or the *done* phase (Hanley et al., 2017; Krieger, 2002, 2017; Quinlan-Colwell, 2012; Tabatabaee, Tafreshi, Rasouli, Aledavood, Alavi Majd, & Farahmand, 2016a; TTIA, 2016) (Fig. 23.2).

Evidence for Pain Management

The most common initial response to TT is a feeling of relaxation. TT has been used to help manage many symptoms (Box 23.1), including the alleviation of pain and anxiety. TT has been researched extensively with positive reports of effectiveness for relieving anxiety, promoting relaxation, alleviating pain, promoting healing of wounds, and assisting with the death process

(Jain & Mills, 2010; Oschman, 2016b; Potter, 2013; Quinlan-Colwell, 2012; Tabatabaee et al., 2016b). TT has been used to help manage many symptoms, including the alleviation of pain and anxiety. When compared to control and placebo (sham TT), TT significantly reduced anxiety in men living with cancer (n = 60) (Tabatabaee, Tafreshi, Rasouli, Aledavood, Majd, & Farahmand, 2015). TT has been used with patients with phantom limb pain, with the patients anecdotally reporting a sensation of the phantom limb being gently touched (Leskowitz, 2014).

TT is relatively unique among nonpharmacologic interventions because, in addition to clinical research, the physiologic effect of TT has been studied for many years (Gronowicz, Jhaveri, Clarke, Aronow, & Smith, 2008; Jain & Mills, 2010; Krieger, 1973; Jhaveri, Walsh, Wang, McCarthy, & Gronowicz, 2008). The bio-effect of TT was first investigated by Krieger in 1972, when hemoglobin levels were found to be significantly improved in those who received TT compared to those in a control group (Krieger, 1973). Later investigators reported that in culture fibroblasts, osteoblasts and tenocytes showed increased proliferation when treated with TT (Gronowicz et al., 2008) as well as in human osteoblast DNA synthesis (Jhaveri et al., 2008). A more recent study compared TT with sham TT with mice injected with aggressive breast cancer cells (666c14) (Gronowicz, Secor, Flynn, Jellison, & Kuhn, 2015). In that study, after 26 days, there was no identified effect on the primary tumor but the mice receiving TT had significantly reduced metastasis, reduced specific splenic lymphocyte subsets, and some reduction of macrophages and lymphocytes. In another recent study (n = 24), researchers in Brazil reported that after 1 week the fibroblast counts of rats who received TT were significantly higher and the wounds had shrunk in size (de Souza, Rosa, Blanco, Passaglia, & Stabile, 2017).

For many years, TT has been used with patients with acute and chronic pain, and much of the research in this area consists of older studies. Table 23.1 presents a synopsis of those studies. A Cochrane review reported a moderate effect on pain with a relationship between effectiveness with the level of experience of the practitioner (So, Jiang, & Qin, 2008). The author of another literature review concluded that TT is safe to recommend as part of a multimodal approach for pain control (Monroe, 2009). When TT was used with surgical patients, pain was well controlled with TT. In another study (n = 90) the majority (73%) of those who received TT had significant reductions in pain and improved function (McCormack, 2009). Among patients who underwent percutaneous laser disk decompression (n = 91), the patients who received TT had significantly (P < .05) less pain than those who did not (Xu, Sun, & Wu, 2009).

With literature support, TT was used as a protocol in burn units (Gamst-Jensen, Vedel, Lindberg-Larsen, & Egerod, 2014). Analysis of data regarding TT when used with patients with burns, showed those who received TT reported less pain, used less morphine, and after 10 days of receiving TT described less pain anxiety as

Therapeutic Touch Process

Shifts in Consciousness

- A Call of Compassion
- The Approach

o The Outreach
o The Search

❖ The Rebalancing

➤ Done
➤ Recall

Krieger, 2015

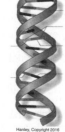

Hanley, Copyright 2016

Elements/Actions

- Centering–intention preparation/grounding

o Assessment/Planning

❖ Rebalancing Actions-reassessment

➤ Evaluation/Finishing
➤ Reflective Practice

Fig. 23.2 | **Helix LOC TT Elements.** (Courtesy © Mary Anne Hanley.)

Table 23.1 | Sampling of Publications in Which Therapeutic Touch Was Used with People with Pain

Date	Author	Title	Reference
1980	Boguslawski, M.	Therapeutic Touch: A facilitator of pain relief.	Topics in Clinical Nursing, 2(1), 27–37.
1986	Keller, E. & Bzdek, V. M.	The use of Therapeutic Touch in the management of pain.	The Nursing Clinics of North America, 22(3), 705–714.
1987	Wright, S. M.	Effects of Therapeutic Touch on tension headache pain.	Nursing Research, 35(2), 101–106.
1993	Meehan, T. C.	Therapeutic Touch and postoperative pain: A Rogerian research study.	Nursing Science Quarterly, 6(2), 69–78.
1996	Apostle-Mitchell, M., & MacDonald, G.	An innovative approach to pain management in critical care: Therapeutic Touch.	Official journal of the Canadian Association of Critical Care Nurses/ CACCN, 8(3), 19–22.
1997	Peck, S.D. (Eckes) (1997).	The effectiveness of Therapeutic Touch for decreasing pain in elders with degenerative arthritis.	Journal of Holistic Nursing, 15(2), 176–198.
1998	Turner, J.G., Clark, A.J., Gauthier, D.K., & Williams, M.	The effect of Therapeutic Touch on pain and anxiety in burn patients.	Journal of Advanced Nursing, 28(1), 10–20.
1998	Lin, Y. & Taylor, A. G.	Effects of Therapeutic Touch in reducing pain and anxiety in an elderly population.	Integrative Medicine, 1(4), 155–162.
2000	Leskowitz, E. D.	Phantom limb pain treated with Therapeutic Touch: A Case Report.	Archives of Physical Rehabilitation Medicine, 81(4), 522–24.
2002	Philcox, P., Rawlins, L., & Rodgers, L.	Therapeutic Touch and its effect on phantom limb and stump pain.	Australian Rehabilitation Nurses' Association, 5(1), 17–21.
2004	Denison, B.	Touch the pain away: New research on Therapeutic Touch and persons with fibromyalgia syndrome.	Holistic Nursing Practice, 18(3), 142–151.
2004	O'Mathuna, D. P.	Therapeutic Touch for pain.	Alternative Therapies in Women's Health, 6(3), 17–20.
2006	MacNeil, M.S.	Therapeutic Touch, pain, and caring: Implications for nursing practice.	International Journal for Human Caring, 10(1): 40–48.
2007	Frank, L. S., Frank, J. L., March, D., Makari-Judson, G., Barham, R. B., & Mertens, W. C.	Does Therapeutic Touch ease the discomfort of distress of patients undergoing stereotactic core breast biopsy, a randomized clinical trial.	Pain Medicine, 8(5), 419–424.
2009	McCormack, G. L.	Using non-contact Therapeutic Touch to manage post-surgical pain in the elderly.	Occupational Therapy International, 16(1), 44–56. doi:10.1002/oti.264
2010	Aghabati, N., Mohammadi, E., Esmaiel, Z.	The effect of Therapeutic Touch on pain and fatigue of cancer patients undergoing chemotherapy	*Evidence-Based Complementary and Alternative Medicine* 7, (3),375–381.
2010	Marta, I. R., Baldan, S. S., Berton, A. F., Pavam, M., & da Silva, M. P.	The effectiveness of Therapeutic Touch on pain, depression and sleep in patients with chronic pain: clinical trial.	Revista Da Escola De Enfermagem Da USP, 44(4), 1100–1106. doi:10.1590/ S0080-62342010000400035 [Portuguese].
2010	Smith, A., Kimmel, S., & Milz, S.	Effects of Therapeutic Touch on pain, function and well being in persons with osteo-arthritis of the knee: a pilot study.	The Internet Journal of Advanced Nursing Practice, 10(2). Full Text Available at: https://ispub.com/IJANP/10/2/10007
2011	Sahawneh, L. J. F.	Effectiveness of Therapeutic Touch on pain management among patients with cancer: Literature Review.	Middle East Journal of Nursing, 5(4), 21–24.

Table 23.1 | Sampling of Publications in Which Therapeutic Touch Was Used with People with Pain—cont'd

Date	Author	Title	Reference
2012	Busch, M., Visser, A., Eybrechts, M., van Komen, R., Oen, I., Olff, M., Dokter, J., & Boxma, H.	The implementation and evaluation of Therapeutic Touch in burn patients: An instructive experience of conducting a scientific study within a non-academic nursing setting.	Patient Education and Counseling, 89(3), 439–446.
2014	Dorri, S. & Bahrami, M.	The effect of Therapeutic Touch on pain relief in patients with cancer	Journal of Urmia Nursing & Midwifery Faculty, 12(8), 767–776. [Persian].
2016	Tabatabaee, A., Tafreshi, M., Rassouli, M., Aledavood, S., AlaviMajd, H., & Farahmand, S	Effect of Therapeutic Touch on pain related parameters of patients with cancer: A randomized clinical trial.	*Materia Socio-Medica,* 28(3), 220–223.
2018	Mueller, G., Palli, C., & Schumacher, P.	The effect of Therapeutic Touch on back pain in adults on a neurological unit: An experimental pilot study	*Pain Management Nursing,* 20(1), 75–81.

Aghabati, Nahid, Eesa Mohammadi, and Zahra Pour Esmaiel. (2010). "The effect of therapeutic touch on pain and fatigue of cancer patients undergoing chemotherapy." *Evidence-Based Complementary and Alternative Medicine, 7,* (3),375–381; Apostle-Mitchell, M., & MacDonald, G. (1996). An innovative approach to pain management in critical care: Therapeutic Touch. *Official journal of the Canadian Association of Critical Care Nurses/ CACCN, 8*(3), 19–22; Boguslawski, M. (1980). Therapeutic Touch: A facilitator of pain relief. *Topics in Clinical Nursing, 2*(1), 27–37; Busch, M., Visser, A., Eybrechts, M., van Komen, R., Oen, I., Olff, M., Dokter, J., & Boxma, H. (2012). The implementation and evaluation of Therapeutic Touch in burn patients: An instructive experience of conducting a scientific study within a non-academic nursing setting. *Patient Education and Counseling, 89*(3), 439–446. doi:10.1016/j.pec.2012.08.012; Denison, B. (2004). Touch the pain away: New research on Therapeutic Touch and persons with fibromyalgia syndrome. *Holistic Nursing Practice, 18*(3), 142–151; Dorri, S. & Bahrami, M. (2014). The effect of Therapeutic Touch on pain relief in patients with cancer [Persian]. *Journal of Urmia Nursing & Midwifery Faculty, 12*(8), 767–776; Frank, L. S., Frank, J. L., March, D., Makari-Judson, G., Barham, R. B., & Mertens, W. C. (2007). Does Therapeutic Touch ease the discomfort or distress of patients undergoing stereotactic core breast biopsy, a randomized clinical trial. *Pain Medicine, 8*(5), 419–424; Keller, E. & Bzdek, V. M. (1986). Effects of Therapeutic Touch on tension headache pain. *Nursing Research, 35*(2), 101–106; Leskowitz, E. D. (2000). Phantom limb pain treated with Therapeutic Touch: A case report. *Archives of Physical Rehabilitation Medicine, 81*(4), 522–24; Lin, Y. & Taylor, A. G. (1998). Effects of Therapeutic Touch in reducing pain and anxiety in an elderly population. *Integrative Medicine, 1*(4), 155–162; MacNeil, M.S. (2006). Therapeutic Touch, pain, and caring: Implications for nursing practice. *International Journal for Human Caring, 10*(1): 40–48; Marta, I. R., Baldan, S. S., Berton, A. F., Pavam, M., & da Silva, M. P. (2010). [The effectiveness of Therapeutic Touch on pain, depression and sleep in patients with chronic pain: clinical trial] [Portuguese]. *Revista Da Escola De Enfermagem Da USP, 44*(4), 1100–1106. doi:10.1590/S0080-62342010000400035; McCormack, G. L. (2009). Using non-contact Therapeutic Touch to manage post-surgical pain in the elderly. *Occupational Therapy International, 16*(1), 44–56. doi:10.1002/oti.264; Meehan, T. C. (1993). Therapeutic Touch and postoperative pain: A Rogerian research study. *Nursing Science Quarterly, 6*(2), 69–78; Mueller, G., Palli, C., & Schumacher, P. (2019). The effect of therapeutic touch on back pain in adults on a neurological unit: An experimental pilot study. *Pain Management Nursing, 20*(1), 75–81; O'Mathuna, D. P. (2004). Therapeutic Touch for pain. *Alternative Therapies in Women's Health, 6*(3), 17–20; Peck, S.D. (Eckes) (1997). The effectiveness of Therapeutic Touch for decreasing pain in elders with degenerative arthritis. *Journal of Holistic Nursing, 15*(2), 176–198; Philcox, P., Rawlins, L., & Rodgers, L. (2002). Therapeutic Touch and its effect on phantom limb and stump pain. *Australian Rehabilitation Nurses' Association, 5*(1), 17–21; Sahawneh, L. J. F. (2011). Effectiveness of Therapeutic Touch on pain management among patients with cancer: Literature review. *Middle East Journal of Nursing, 5*(4), 21–24; Smith, A., Kimmel, S., & Milz, S. (2010). Effects of Therapeutic Touch on pain, function and well being in persons with osteo-arthritis of the knee: a pilot study. *The Internet Journal of Advanced Nursing Practice, 10*(2). https://ispub.com/IJANP/10/2/10007 Accessed 8/13/2020; Tabatabaee, A., Tafreshi, M. Z., Rassouli, M., Aledavood, S. A., AlaviMajd, H., & Farahmand, S. K. (2016). Effect of therapeutic touch on pain related parameters in patients with cancer: a randomized clinical trial. *Materia Socio-Medica, 28*(3), 220–223; Turner, J.G., Clark, A.J., Gauthier, D.K., & Williams, M. (1998). The effect of Therapeutic Touch on pain and anxiety in burn patients. *Journal of Advanced Nursing, 28*(1), 10–20; Wright, S. M. (1987). The use of Therapeutic Touch in the management of pain. *The Nursing Clinics of North America, 22*(3), 705–714.

well (Busch et al., 2012). In a trial with people living with chronic pain, those who received TT in addition to cognitive-behavioral therapy (CBT) (see Chapter 22) reported more self-efficacy and were more willing to continue with the program (Simpson, 2015). The authors of a systematic review of TT reported TT was used successfully with patients with dementia, particularly in reducing behavioral symptoms (Cabrera et al., 2015) that could be indicative of pain (see Chapter 7). The investigators of a small but encouraging study with neonates (N = 10) concluded TT was effective in reducing brain activation, which induces sensory punctuate stimulation as measured by oxyhemoglobin (Honda et al., 2013). That study is important because it provides preliminary information on how TT may be involved in hypoalgesia. It also provides information on an opportunity to better manage pain in neonates, thus preventing negative long-term sequelae that could evolve from opioid monotherapy.

Despite clinical efficacy and significant research over the years, additional current research is needed (Monroe, 2009; Newshan & Staats, 2013; Tabatabaee et al., 2016a). As with most complementary and integrative health approaches, the established evidence-based efficacy of TT is limited by the lack of RCTs (Anderson & Taylor, 2012; Monzillo & Gronowicz, 2011). Research is needed with more rigorous methodology (Jain & Mills, 2010; Potter, 2013; Senderovich et al., 2016) involving staff who are experienced with both TT and research (Busch et al., 2012).

Cautions

Numerous researchers have reported that no adverse effects were noted or reported with TT and that it is a safe therapy as part of a multimodal approach to care of people with pain (Monroe, 2009; Newhan & Staats, 2013).

The Therapeutic Touch (TT) practitioner was consulted by the wound care nurse (WCRN) to work with her during wound care of a man with Fournier gangrene. He consistently rated the intensity of his pain as 10 on a scale of 0 to 10. In addition, he had great anxiety about the wound care, reapplication of the wound vac and dressing changes and even with very high doses of medications of conscious sedation, he was in great pain during the procedures. The WCRN hoped TT would help him to relax so that the medications used for conscious sedation could be more effective. The TT clinician met with him the day before the next scheduled wound care and explained TT. He agreed, saying, "I'll try anything." He agreed to trying TT at that time, so he would know what to expect the next day. He reported that it was relaxing and "seems to help with the pain." The next day, TT was used during the wound care and he tolerated the procedure much better and with less medication than used previously. The following day he was very grateful, and requested TT daily, in addition to wound care, to help manage pain and anxiety. He continued to do well with good healing and appreciation for the TT he received.

For additional information on TT, including education, resources, and clinicians, the reader is referred to http://therapeutictouch.org/.

Healing Touch

HT developed in 1989 by Janet Mentgen, BSN, RN, is discussed as a specific form of energy healing that induces relaxation and is designed to restore a natural flow of energy and direct healing in the body through the clinician using hands on or above the body (Anderson & Taylor, 2011; Oschman, 2016b). Mentgen clarified that HT was "defined since its beginnings as a program of study of various energy-linked approaches, including the many full body and more localized techniques . . . which provides multidimensional healing to restore balance in the dynamic human being" (Mentgen & Hover-Kramer, 2002, p. 5). Although HT has been compared with TT in that restoring balance and harmony in the energy system is a goal (Foley, Anderson, Mallea, Morrison, & Downey, 2016; Lincoln et al., 2014), it is different in many ways, including the attention to spirituality and intuition with balancing of chakras, which are the energy centers of the body (Rao, Hickman, Sibbritt, Newton, & Phillips, 2016). A variety of interventions are used (Anderson, Friesen, Swengros, Herbst, & Mangione, 2017). There are six levels of hands-on skill training with certification (Oschman, 2016b).

Evidence for Pain Management

In the last decade, the amount of research with HT has markedly increased. In a small pilot study (N = 19), people with osteoarthritis of the knee who for 6 weeks received at home HT (n = 12) reported substantial improvements in pain intensity and interference compared with those who received a friendly visit (n = 7) (Lu, Hart, Lutgendorf, & Perkhounkova, 2013). When used with patients with sickle cell disease the effect of HT was not significant but did trend toward lower pain scores (Thomas, Stephenson, Swanson, Jesse, & Brown, 2013). When used with patients who underwent laparoscopic bariatric surgery (n = 46) the patients who received a modified HT technique reported significant improvement in postoperative pain control, nausea, and anxiety (Anderson et al., 2015). When used with a variety of outpatient surgical patients, HT did not have a meaningful difference in pain scores when compared to usual care but there was a trend in lower opioid use (Foley et al., 2016). When HT was used in multimodal combination with a healing harp those participants who receive both HT and healing harp (n = 37) had greater average relief of pain and anxiety than those who received only HT (n = 1978) (Lincoln et al., 2014).

As with the other biofield modalities, HT needs additional research with strong methodologies and designs (Anderson & Taylor, 2011). A challenge specific in conducting research with HT is that there is often individual modification of the original teachings by the clinicians involved with the research (Anderson et al., 2015), which makes comparison or replication of studies challenging.

Cautions

No specific cautions were identified in the literature regarding the use of HT. Reporting of any adverse events or the lack of them is needed in future research.

For additional information on Healing Touch, the reader is referred to https://www.healingtouchprogram.com/ or Healing Touch International.

Acupuncture

Acupuncture is one of the treatment techniques that has origins in ancient Traditional Chinese Medicine dating more than 3000 years. The basic tenet is that it is necessary to have the vital energy of the body, or qi, to flow in a balanced manner to achieve and maintain health. From this perspective, qi (chi) flows through 12 main and 8 extraordinary meridians (channels) located throughout the bodies of all living beings. Along the meridians are acupuncture points (acupoints) where the meridians interconnect, bringing the total number of acupoints to 561, of which only 200 are used routinely (Chiaramonte, D'Adamo, & Morrison, 2013; Yap, 2016). Although the acupoints are not anatomically visible, some believe they at times match with depressions or other qualities in the musculoskeletal or neurologic systems (Chiaramonte, D'Adamo, & Morrison, 2013), but there is no strong evidence for these relationships (Yap, 2016).

Vickers and Linde (2014) noted that despite being widely used the use and effectiveness of acupuncture remains largely debated, and this is mostly related to not being able to identify a specific mechanism of action. Although the exact mechanism of action is not clear, there are many theories of how acupuncture works, including through stimulation of the immune, circulatory, endocrine, and nervous systems, but the strongest support is through the release of endorphins, which have been identified as being higher in cerebrospinal fluid after treatment with acupuncture (Chiaramonte et al., 2013; Yap, 2016). Clinicians must be appropriately licensed in the individual state or country to practice acupuncture, and preparation is extensive (World Health Organization [WHO], 2013).

Acupuncture is used internationally as treatment for many conditions, including pain, and is recognized as an intervention in at least 103 countries (Chiaramonte et al., 2013; Lauche, Cramer, Häuser, Dobos, & Langhorst, 2015; Vernooij & Marcelissen, 2017; Yap, 2016; WHO, 2013). Although the practice of acupuncture has increased during the last 20 years, unfortunately, the cost is still only covered fully or partially by insurance benefit in a small number of countries (18/103) (WHO, 2013). Acupuncture is listed with an open recommendation in the German guideline for treatment of fibromyalgia (Lauche et al., 2015) and is reported as the most popular of the nonpharmacologic interventions in the Netherlands, where it was studied with people with a variety of painful conditions (Vernooij & Marcelissen, 2017). In that study (N = 110) it was found that both primary and secondary pain intensity scores, functional ability, and general well-being and health significantly improved ($P < .001$) and continued during the 16 weeks of follow-up. In addition, participants reduced use of analgesic medications by 44.5% during the 4-week trial.

The World Health Organization (WHO) has identified numerous conditions that are appropriate for treatment with acupuncture and has categorized them according to acupuncture being an effective treatment (category 1), effective further evidence is needed (category 2), individual reports of benefit and may be helpful (category 3), and it may be helpful under certain conditions (category 4). Painful conditions are listed in only the first and second categories (Table 23.2) (Yap, 2016).

Evidence for Pain Management

Results of research studies have been inconsistent; however, some studies reported strong evidence for pain relief (Lauche et al., 2015). One area of confusion and concern with acupuncture research has been the positive results that are often reported with sham acupuncture or

Table 23.2	Pain-Related Conditions That Can Be Treated With Acupuncture as Listed by the World Health Organization
Category 1	Biliary colic, primary dysmenorrhea, acute epigastralgia, postoperative pain, renal colic, sprain, pain in dentistry (dental pain, temporomandibular dysfunction), facial pain, headache, knee pain, low back pain, neck pain, periarthritis of shoulder, rheumatoid arthritis, sciatica, tennis elbow
Category 2	Abdominal pain (acute gastroenteritis or gastrointestinal spasm), acute exacerbation of chronic cholecystitis, earache, eye pain due to subconjunctival injection, herpes zoster, labor pain, endoscopic examination pain, pain in thromboangiitis obliterans, sore throat (including tonsillitis), acute spinal pain, stiff neck, cancer pain, fibromyalgia and fasciitis, gouty arthritis, postherpetic neuralgia, osteoarthritis, chronic prostatitis, radicular and pseudoradicular pain syndrome, complex regional pain syndrome

From Yap, S. H. (2016). Acupuncture in pain management. *Anaesthesia & Intensive Care Medicine, 17*(9), 448–450.

treatment with needles or tapping on parts of that body that are not acupoints (Chen et al., 2016; Lai, 2016). The concern was underscored by the National Institutes for Health and Care Excellence in the United Kingdom when they noted in their 2016 guidelines for treatment of low back pain (LBP) and sciatica that there was insufficient proof of a treatment effect from acupuncture that was more effective than a placebo effect of sham acupuncture (NICE, 2016). This decision resulted in disagreement and subsequent refute (Lai, 2016; Trinh, Diep, & Dorsher, 2017). One challenge to the decision posed was regardless of the effect of sham acupuncture if it is clinically effective by patient perception and patient report in relieving pain it can be argued to be an effective treatment (Alper, Shah, Malone-Moses, Manheimer, & Ehrlich, 2016). This is an interesting and important consideration, not just with acupuncture but with many of the integrative therapies.

Several meta-analyses have addressed the effect of sham acupuncture in research studies. The difference in acupuncture versus sham acupuncture was noted in a meta-analysis (n = 14 studies; n = 3835 subjects) of the comparison among people with chronic knee pain from osteoarthritis with those receiving real acupuncture reporting significantly more pain relief ($P < .002$), better function ($P < .01$), and the effects lasting over time ($P < .06$) for both variables (Cao, Zhang, Gao, & Jiang, 2012). The authors of another meta-analysis (n = 29 studies, n = 17,922 subjects) of studies using acupuncture for a variety of musculoskeletal and headache conditions concluded acupuncture is effective, and the important differences between acupuncture and sham acupuncture support the premise that effects of acupuncture are more than those of placebo. They also noted that the effect of sham acupuncture indicates acupuncture is more than just the effects resulting from needle placement (Vickers et al., 2012). However, the authors of a very large review of acupuncture studies (n = 139) with 166 intervention and control pairs, reported stronger treatment effects when acupuncture was compared with no treatment rather than with sham acupuncture, which may have unintentionally produced a placebo effect. In that review, studies included traditional acupuncture, medical acupuncture, and electro-acupuncture (Chen et al., 2016).

There has been other research using acupuncture in relation with pain with interesting results. In three studies, when acupuncture was used in women to treat endometriosis, acupuncture was reported to be effective in reducing the intensity of pain. In addition to reducing pain, of the three studies, one in which analgesic medication use by the participants was measured, less medication was used. Of the three studies, the one that tracked return to usual activities reported faster return to those activities after acupuncture (Lund & Lundeberg, 2015).

From a physiologic perspective a review was done of seven studies (n = 163) in which acupuncture was used with people with arthritis, LBP, carpal tunnel syndrome, and fibromyalgia and brain imaging (functional magnetic resonance imaging in five and positron emission tomography in two studies) assessed central nervous system (CNS) connectivity. Through that review the authors concluded that despite heterogeneity of the samples and studies, as well as methodologic flaws, the studies supported the belief that acupuncture can change CNS pain-related functional connectivity (Santiago, Tumilty, Mącznik, & Mani, 2016). Through a qualitative study in which participants were asked about their experience and expectations with complementary modalities, those experiencing acupuncture reported that as time passed, their expectations and subsequent predictions about the results became stronger predictors of the results (Eaves et al., 2015). It could be argued that this is another placebo effect, but it also can be argued that this is reinforcement of positive effects attained through acupuncture treatments.

Despite the amount of research done, there is still a need to establish evidence for use of acupuncture. This is challenged by the scarce amount of financial support for research (WHO, 2013). Future research with attention to methodology, rigor, design, use of appropriate controls, blinding, and outcome measurement is needed (Chen et al., 2016; Ning & Lao, 2015; Santiago et al., 2016; Zeng & Chung, 2015).

Caution

Acupuncture is generally considered safe, but reported adverse effects range from fatigue, mild bleeding, bruising, or pain at the insertion site to vasovagal reflex, loss

Table 23.3 | Cautions and Contraindications to Acupuncture

Cautions	Points near arteries and veins
	Localized skin lesions (infection, tumor, burns, ulcer)
	Anticoagulants/antiplatelet therapy
	Deep puncture in back, chest, nape, and periorbital regions
Contraindications	Acupuncture in the lower abdomen, lumbar, and sacral regions of pregnant women within the first trimester
	Acupuncture to LI4, BL60, SP6 in pregnant women
	Points over fontanelle of infants
	Fasted/starving patients
	Severe fatigue/exhaustion
	Metal allergy
	Needle phobia
	Electro-acupuncture in those with a pacemaker or implanted devices
	Sepsis
	Coagulopathy

From Yap, S. H. (2016). Acupuncture in pain management. *Anaesthesia & Intensive Care Medicine, 17*(9), 448–450.

of consciousness, pneumothorax, neurovascular trauma, trapped or retained needle/needle fragment, and injury of solid organs (Yap, 2016). As with other interventions, adverse events are more likely to occur with less experienced clinicians. As listed in Table 23.3, there are a number of conditions for which there is contraindication or there needs to be caution used (Yap, 2016).

Auricular Acupuncture

Auricular acupuncture (AA) is a particular type of acupuncture that dates back to ancient Chinese medicine and particularly the classic medical text *Yellow Emperor's Canon of Medicine* (Huang et al., 2016). It also has a long history of use throughout the Mediterranean countries (Walker, Pock, Ling, Kwon, & Vaughan, 2016). Despite this history, AA is often associated with Paul Nogier, a French physician, who in 1950, created the pictorial concept of the homunculus as an inverted fetal mapping on the external ear (Walker et al., 2016) (Fig. 23.3; Table 23.4). Acupoints corresponding to various body structures and organs, are located on the pinna portion of the ear (Huang et al., 2016; Yap, 2016) (Fig. 23.4). It is not known exactly how AA works. One suggestion is that since the majority (15/20) of AA points used to manage pain are located in parts of the pinna innervated by the auricular branch of the vagal nerve, the pain-relieving effects may be due to stimulation of that nerve (Usichenko, Hacker, & Lotze, 2017).

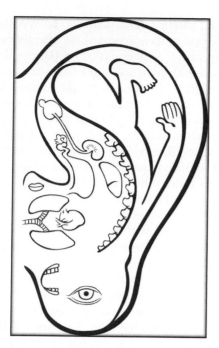

Fig. 23.3 | Representation of "homunculus in the ear." (From Walker, P. H., Pock, A., Ling, C. G., Kwon, K. N., & Vaughan, M. [2016]. Battlefield acupuncture: Opening the door for acupuncture in Department of Defense/Veteran's Administration health care. *Nursing Outlook, 64*(5), 491–498.)

Evidence for Pain Management

AA is used extensively by the Veterans Administration and Department of Defense, with several thousand of their clinicians having learned the modality, which they call *battlefield acupuncture,* that is a unique type of AA (Gallagher, 2016; Niemzow, 2020; Walker et al., 2016). In one study in which active duty military were functioning in an emergency setting (n = 87), those who received AA plus standard of care reported a 23% decrease in pain compared to those who only received standard of care (Walker et al., 2016). From a different perspective, a review was done of medical records of patients (n = 147) at the Atlanta Veterans Affairs Medical Center who received AA treatments, noting reductions in pain averaged 60% with more than 83% of the patients reporting some degree of positive benefit (Huang et al., 2016). The authors of a large systematic review (n = 13 studies, n = 806 subjects) concluded that AA was second only to acupressure in pain relief (Yeh et al., 2014).

The analgesic benefit of AA has been reported with people living with a variety of different types of painful conditions. A large multicenter study (n = 212) investigating the effect of AA on low back and pelvic pain in pregnant women (Vas et al., 2014). AA was also effective in reducing pain in 92% of women with dysmenorrhea (Leong, 2014). Among patients with migraine-type headaches (n = 46), 83.7% reported of that group reported positive effect when treated with AA, with almost half (21/46) reporting that AA was markedly effective (Hou et al., 2016). AA is promising

Nr.	AA Points	Number of RCTs, Where the AA Point was Used	Source of Afferent Innervation
1	Shenmen	12	ABVN, GAN
2	Lung	7	ABVN, GAN
3	Thalamus	5	ABVN, GAN
4	Cushion	4	GAN
5	Hip	3	ABVN, GAN
6	Knee	3	ABVN, GAN
7	Lumbar spine	1	ABVN, GAN
8	Toe	1	ABVN, GAN
9	Ankle	1	ABVN, GAN
10	Finger	1	GAN
11	Uterus	1	ABVN
12	Wrist	1	GAN
13	Elbow	1	GAN
14	Heart	1	ABVN, GAN
15	Tooth	1	ABVN, GAN
16	Mouth	1	ABVN, GAN
17	Valium	1	ATN, ABVN
18	Cingulate gyrus	1	ATN, ABVN
19	Point zero	1	ABVN, ATN
20	Cervical spine	1	GAN

Table 23.4 | Features of Auricular Acupuncture (AA) Points in 17 Randomized Controlled Trials Included into Systematic Review on Analgesic Effects of AA

AA, auricular acupuncture; *RCT*, randomized controlled trial; *ATN*, auriculotemporal nerve (from trigeminal nerve); *ABVN*, auricular branch of vagal nerve; *GAN*, great auricular nerve (from cervical plexus).
From Usichenko, T., Hacker, H., & Lotze, M. [2017]. Transcutaneous auricular vagal nerve stimulation (taVNS) might be a mechanism behind the analgesic effects of auricular acupuncture. *Brain Stimulation, 10*(6), 1042–1044.

as an effective treatment for chronic pain. The authors of a review of the literature (n = 15 studies) concluded that it was particularly promising for chronic LBP and tension headaches, with results lasting up to 3 months after treatment (Zhao, Tan, Wang, & Jin, 2015). Additional research is needed to assess benefit, need for follow-up treatments, effect on quality of life, and cost-effectiveness of using AA to treat chronic pain.

AA is being used with increasing frequency in the postoperative setting. For several years, AA has been considered to be an effective way to manage postoperative pain

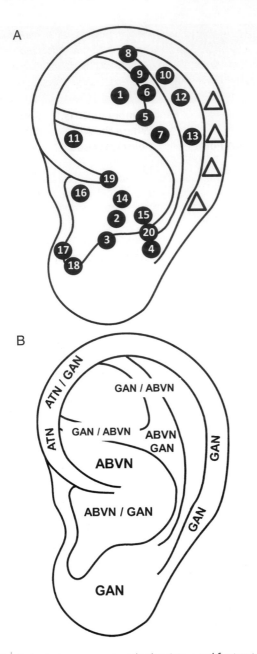

Fig. 23.4 | A, Auricular acupuncture (AA) points, used for treatment of patients with acute and chronic pain in randomized controlled trials (RCTs) included into meta-analysis of Asher et al., 2010. Black circles with numbers: various specific AA, the nomenclature is given in Table 23.4; triangles: non-acupuncture points for sham acupuncture on the helix of the auricle as a control condition in several RCTs from the meta-analysis. B, Anatomic map of afferent nerve supply according to Peuker and Filler, 2002, where cymba conchae is exclusively supplied by the auricular branch of the vagal nerve (ABVN); cavity of conchae is exclusively supplied by ABVN in 45% of cases and by ABVN and the great auricular nerve (GAN) from the cervical plexus in 55%; tail of helix is exclusively supplied GAN; antihelix is exclusively supplied by ABVN in 73%, exclusively supplied by GAN in 18%, and supplied by ABVN and GAN in 9%; the crura of antihelix are supplied by GAN in 91% and ABVN in only 9%. ATN: auriculotemporal nerve (from trigeminal nerve). (From Usichenko, T., Hacker, H., & Lotze, M. [2017]. Transcutaneous auricular vagal nerve stimulation (taVNS) might be a mechanism behind the analgesic effects of auricular acupuncture. *Brain Stimulation, 10*[6], 1042–1044.)

(Asher et al., 2010; Gliedt, Daniels, & Wuollet, 2015). Systematic reviews have reported the effectiveness of AA as a postoperative analgesic method (Usichenko, 2017). AA was used with patients who had laparoscopic cholecystectomies (n = 46) who were randomized to receive either AA or standard of care analgesia postoperatively (Toca-Villegas et al., 2017). In that study, during the first six hours postoperatively, the majority of patients who received AA (20/23, or 87%) reported pain intensity scores less than 4 in 10 compared with reductions reported by only 48% of those who received standard of care analgesia (P < .004). The participants in the AA group also used significantly less analgesic medications (P < .0001). In one study using AA with postoperative patients (n = 34) after total knee arthroplasty, compared to the controls (n = 16), the patients who received AA (n = 18) had similar pain control immediately postoperatively, but required less opioids and had fewer side effects, participated in rehabilitation activities sooner, and had less pain during postoperative days 3 through 7 (He, Tong, Li, Jing, & Yao, 2013). AA also has been effectively used to manage postoperative nausea and vomiting (Moore & Hickey, 2017). Another acute pain situation in which AA is demonstrated as effective is with procedural burn care and dressings (Cuignet, Pirlot, Ortiz, & Rose, 2015).

Use of AA is also reported in unusual and interesting situations. Physicians in New York City emergency departments (EDs) reported positive results when they used AA, which they called battlefield acupuncture, with ED patients for whom it was not appropriate to use opioids. Two of the patients had severe muscle spasms, and a third had painful carpal tunnel syndrome. Not only did they all experience significant pain reduction in the EDs, they also reported continued pain relief during telephone follow-up several days later (Tsai, Fox, Murakami, & Tsung, 2016). Physicians in a Greek hospital reported that when a man with chronic obstructive pulmonary disease sustained multiple rib fractures and pneumothorax with pulmonary contusions was unable to effectively breathe, he was treated with AA, resulting in nearly immediate pain relief and ability to take deep breaths with analgesia lasting several hours with subsequent resolution of pain for 5 days after a second AA treatment (Papadopoulos, Tzimas, Liarmakopoulou, & Petrou, 2017). The effectiveness of AA for pain management is not surprising considering that AA has been for years the most frequently used form of acupuncture with people in treatment for opioid substance use disorder to relieve withdrawal symptoms and alleviate cravings (Kailasam, Anand, & Melyan, 2016). (See Chapter 14 for extensive discussion of opioid use disorder.)

As with other energy therapies, additional research with more rigorous methodology and homogeneous samples is needed (Zhao et al., 2015). It is also important to work to identify how AA can best be used as part of a multimodal approach to management of both acute and chronic pain (Gliedt et al., 2015).

Caution

Adverse effects of AA are minor, including dizziness, diaphoresis, and irritation or pain at the insertion site (Huang et al., 2016). Precautions to prevent adverse effects include strict adherence to sterilization and avoiding robust stimulation with elderly, weakened patients or those with known hypertension (Zhao et al., 2016).

Acupressure

Acupressure is another complementary modality that has roots in ancient China (Mehta, Dhapte, Kadam, & Dhapte, 2017). It is a modality in which the therapist applies pressure to stimulate acupoints (the same points used with acupuncture) by using pressure exerted by fingers and hands with the intention to balance energy and achieve a therapeutic result (Chen & Wang, 2014; Raddadi, Adib-Hajbaghery, Ghadirzadeh, & Kheirkhah, 2017). Although the precise mechanism of action is not known, it is suggested that through pressure on the acupoints occurring along the meridians there is a compensation of any imbalance in the vital energy field (*qi* or *chi*) (Mehta et al., 2017; Raddadi et al., 2017). One suggestion of how acupressure is involved in analgesia is that it may increase the release of serotonin and modulate pain through the descending pain pathways (Pak, Micalos, Maria, & Lord, 2015).

As with auricular acupuncture, auricular acupressure is the use of acupressure on acupoints on the auricle of the ear with the understanding that the body is represented on the external ear. Auricular acupressure is more popular in China, where it is often used as a self-care technique. This category of acupressure involves stimulation of the acupoints by using plant seeds or magnetic pellets that are adhered with tape to both sides of the external ear (Yeh et al., 2014).

Evidence for Pain Management

Acupressure is used to relieve pain in the area where pressure is applied and in distant areas of the body to which the acupoints correspond (Mehta et al., 2017). It has been used with patients with LBP, chronic headaches, trauma, dysmenorrhea, labor pain, procedural pain, lumbar hernia, postoperative pain, and acute pain (Chen & Wang, 2014; Chung, Tsou, Chen, Lin, & Yeh, 2014; Levett, Smith, Dahlen, & Bensoussan, 2014; Rizi, Shamsalinia, Ghaffari, Keyhanian, & Nabi, 2017; Romoli, Greco, & Giommi, 2016). The authors of two large systematic reviews (n = 15) (Chen & Wang, 2014); (n = 13) (Yeh et al., 2014) concluded that acupressure reduces pain in a number of painful conditions in a variety of populations. The authors of one of those systematic reviews added that acupressure had the greatest amount of evidence for pain relief (Yeh et al., 2014). In a review of acupressure used

for dysmenorrhea, it was reported as being effective in reducing pain (Abaraogu & Tabansi-Ochuogu, 2015). Acupressure was also found to be helpful in controlling dysmenorrhea and LBP in a in study with students (n = 129) during a year-long follow-up study (Chen, Wang, Chiu, & Hu, 2015).

Acupressure is effectively used to ease pain and discomfort associated with labor and childbirth and offers the additional benefit of empowering the mother and partner who can learn to use the acupressure techniques (Levett et al., 2014). Compared to placebo and to standard of care control in one study with patients (n = 90) undergoing bone marrow biopsy, the patients (n = 30) who received acupressure reported significantly (P < .001) less pain (Rizi et al., 2017). An interesting use of acupressure was with athletes (n = 79) with acute injuries (Macznik, Schneiders, Athens, & Sullivan, 2017). In that study, the athletes who received acupressure reported statistically significant (P < .05) less pain than the control and sham groups. Because the ear is generally accessible and rarely injured, it is suggested that auricular acupressure can be an effective intervention to control pain in trauma situations both before arriving and after arrival in an ED (Pak et al., 2015).

Acupressure is increasingly combined with electric stimulation, which at times is referred to as *integrative acupoint stimulation* (Chung et al., 2014). Auricular acupressure was evaluated in conjunction with transcutaneous electric acupoint stimulation (TEAS) in postoperative patients after back surgery (n = 135) (Chung et al., 2014). In that study the patients who received the auricular acupressure and TEAS at the real acupoint (n = 45) reported significantly less pain and used significantly less morphine by patient-controlled analgesia (PCA) compared to the control (n = 45) or sham acupressure/TEAS group (n = 45).

In another systematic review (n = 15 studies) to determine the effectiveness of acupressure with people living with chronic pain, the authors concluded that it is effective for reducing the intensity of chronic pain, but additional research is needed (Zhao et al., 2015). It is generally noted that additional research is needed to identify evidence-based treatment techniques, to expand the research to other populations (Chen & Wang, 2014; Chen et al., 2015; Zhao et al., 2015) and to replicate studies that have been completed. A potential use of acupressure that needs additional research is self-acupressure to enable people to self-manage symptoms, including pain, stress, anxiety, and insomnia (Ing, 2017; Song et al., 2015).

Caution

Auricular acupuncture and acupressure is considered a safe intervention with no connection with infection, bleeding, or hepatitis, which are at times associated with acupuncture (Raddadi et al., 2017; Rizi et al., 2017). As with all complementary modalities, it is advised for patients to consult with their clinicians to ascertain the modality is safe for them.

Key Points

- Biofield therapies are a reasonable and safe option to include in multimodal pain management.
- Adverse effects of these interventions when used for pain control are mild to nonexistent.
- There is at least moderate support for the use of the biofield modalities with patients suffering with pain.
- Further research of the biofield modalities is needed, with rigorous methodology, larger samples, and possible expansion and replication of earlier studies.

Case Scenario

Tarah is a young nurse who works in the emergency department (ED) and often floats to the postoperative units. She is concerned about safely helping her patients manage their pain and is interested in integrative therapies, especially energy work. She started a clinical ladder project to bring integrative therapies to the ED to help patients better manage their pain. Tarah asks you about biofields and energy work. She wants to know what recommendations she should make.

1. How do you explain biofields and energy work to her?
2. What biofield modalities do you suggest to her for use in the ED?
3. What do you tell her about the evidence for each of these therapies?
4. What cautions do you need to share with her?
5. What resources would you recommend to Tarah if she wants to learn more about and use the different therapies herself?

References

Abaraogu, U. O., & Tabansi-Ochuogu, C. S. (2015). As acupressure decreases pain, acupuncture may improve some aspects of quality of life for women with primary dysmenorrhea: a systematic review with meta-analysis. *Journal of Acupuncture and Meridian Studies, 8*(5), 220–228.

Alper, B. S., Shah, A., Malone-Moses, M., Manheimer, E. W., & Ehrlich, A. (2016). Point-of-care application of guidelines and evidence on acupuncture for chronic low back pain. *European Journal of Integrative Medicine, 8*(4), 326–328.

Anderson, J. G., Friesen, M. A., Swengros, D., Herbst, A., & Mangione, L. (2017). Examination of the use of healing touch by registered nurses in the acute care setting. *Journal of Holistic Nursing, 35*(1), 97–107.

Anderson, J. G., & Taylor, A. G. (2011). Effects of Healing Touch in clinical practice: a systematic review of randomized clinical trials. *Journal of Holistic Nursing, 29*(3), 221–228.

Anderson, J. G., & Taylor, A. G. (2012). Biofield therapies and cancer pain. *Clinical Journal of Oncology Nursing, 16*(1), 43–48.

Anderson, J. G., Suchicital, L., Lang, M., Kukic, A., Mangione, L., Swengros, D., & Friesen, M. A. (2015). The effects of Healing Touch on pain, nausea, and anxiety following bariatric surgery: a pilot study. *EXPLORE: The Journal of Science and Healing, 11*(3), 208–216.

Asher, G. N., Jonas, D. E., Coeytaux, R. R., Reilly, A. C., Loh, Y. L., Motsinger-Reif, A. A., & Winham, S. J. (2010). Auriculotherapy for pain management: a systematic review and meta-analysis of randomized controlled trials. *The Journal of Alternative and Complementary Medicine, 16*(10), 1097–1108.

Assefi, N., Bogart, A., Goldberg, J., & Buchwald, D. (2008). Reiki for the treatment of fibromyalgia: A randomized controlled trial. *The Journal of Alternative and Complementary Medicine, 14*(9), 1115–1122.

Baldwin, A., Vitale, A., Brownell, E., Kryak, E., & Rand, W. (2017). Effects of Reiki on pain, anxiety, and blood pressure in patients undergoing knee replacement. *Holistic Nursing Practice, 31*(2), 80–89.

Bossi, L., Ott, M., & DeCristofaro, S. (2008). Reiki as a clinical intervention in oncology nursing practice. *Clinical Journal of Oncology Nursing, 12*(3), 489–494.

Bultemeier, K. (2014). Rogers' Science of Unitary Human Beings in Nursing Practice. In M. R. Aligood (Ed.), *Nursing Theory: Utilization & Application* (5th Ed). St. Louis: Elsevier.

Busch, M., Visser, A., Eybrechts, M., van Komen, R., Oen, I., Olff, M., ... Boxma, H. (2012). The implementation and evaluation of Therapeutic Touch in burn patients: an instructive experience of conducting a scientific study within a non-academic nursing setting. *Patient Education and Counseling, 89*(3), 439–446.

Cabrera, E., Sutcliffe, C., Verbeek, H., Saks, K., Soto-Martin, M., Meyer, G., ... RightTimePlaceCare Consortium. (2015). Non-pharmacological interventions as a best practice strategy in people with dementia living in nursing homes. A systematic review. *European Geriatric Medicine, 6*(2), 134–150.

Cao, L., Zhang, X. L., Gao, Y. S., & Jing, Y. (2012). Needle acupuncture for osteoarthritis of the knee. A systematic review and updated meta-analysis. *Saudi Medical Journal, 33*(5), 526–532.

Chen, H., Ning, Z., Lam, W. L., Lam, W. Y., Zhao, Y. K., Yeung, J. W. F., ... Lao, L. (2016). Types of Control in Acupuncture Clinical Trials Might Affect the Conclusion of the Trials: A Review of Acupuncture on Pain Management. *Journal of Acupuncture and Meridian Studies, 9*(5), 227–233.

Chen, H. M., Wang, H. H., Chiu, M. H., & Hu, H. M. (2015). Effects of acupressure on menstrual distress and low back pain in dysmenorrheic young adult women: an experimental study. *Pain Management Nursing, 16*(3), 188–197.

Chen, Y. W., & Wang, H. H. (2014). The effectiveness of acupressure on relieving pain: a systematic review. *Pain Management Nursing, 15*(2), 539–550.

Chiaramonte, D., D'Adamo, C., & Morrison, B. (2013). Integrative approaches to pain management. In H. T. Benzon, J. P. Rathmell, C. L. Wu, D. C. Turk, C. E. Argoff, & R. W. Hurley (Eds.), *Practical Management of Pain* (5th Ed., pp. 658–668.e3). St. Louis: Mosby.

Chiasson, A. (2016). Energy medicine and pain management. In R. Bonakdar, & A. Sukiennik (Eds.), *Integrative pain management* (pp. 560–575). New York: Oxford University Press.

Chung, Y. C., Tsou, M. Y., Chen, H. H., Lin, J. G., & Yeh, M. L. (2014). Integrative acupoint stimulation to alleviate postoperative pain and morphine-related side effects: a sham-controlled study. *International Journal of Nursing Studies, 51*(3), 370–378.

Coakley, A., & Barron, A. (2012). Energy therapies in oncology nursing. *Seminars in Oncology Nursing, 28*(1), 55–63.

Cuignet, O., Pirlot, A., Ortiz, S., & Rose, T. (2015). The effects of electroacupuncture on analgesia and peripheral sensory thresholds in patients with burn scar pain. *Burns, 41*(6), 1298–1305.

de Souza, A. L. T., Rosa, D. P. C., Blanco, B. A., Passaglia, P., & Stabile, A. M. (2017). Effects of Therapeutic Touch on healing of the skin in rats. *Explore: The Journal of Science and Healing, 13*(5), 333–338.

Eaves, E. R., Sherman, K. J., Ritenbaugh, C., Hsu, C., Nichter, M., Turner, J. A., & Cherkin, D. C. (2015). A qualitative study of changes in expectations over time among patients with chronic low back pain seeking four CAM therapies. *BMC Complementary and Alternative Medicine, 15*(1), 12.

Erich, M., & Quinlan-Colwell, A. (2017). Celebrating 20 years of the integrative healing arts network. *Southern Pain Society Newsletter.* July, 2017.

Foley, M. K. H., Anderson, J., Mallea, L., Morrison, K., & Downey, M. (2016). Effects of Healing Touch on postsurgical adult outpatients. *Journal of Holistic Nursing, 34*(3), 271–279.

Fontaine, K. (2015). *Complementary & alternative therapies for nursing practice.* New York: Pearson.

Gallagher, R. M. (2016). Advancing the pain agenda in the veteran population. *Anesthesiology Clinics, 34*(2), 357–378.

Gamst-Jensen, H., Vedel, P. N., Lindberg-Larsen, V. O., & Egerod, I. (2014). Acute pain management in burn patients: appraisal and thematic analysis of four clinical guidelines. *Burns, 40*(8), 1463–1469.

Gliedt, J. A., Daniels, C. J., & Wuollet, A. (2015). Narrative review of perioperative acupuncture for clinicians. *Journal of Acupuncture and Meridian Studies, 8*(5), 264–269.

Gronowicz, G., Secor, E. R., Flynn, J. R., Jellison, E. R., & Kuhn, L. T. (2015). Therapeutic touch has significant effects on mouse breast cancer metastasis and immune responses but not primary tumor size. *Evidence-Based Complementary and Alternative Medicine, 2015.* Article ID 926565 https://doi.org/10.1155/2015/926565.

Gronowicz, G. A., Jhaveri, A., Clarke, L. W., Aronow, M. S., & Smith, T. H. (2008). Therapeutic Touch stimulates the proliferation of human cells in culture. *The Journal of Alternative and Complementary Medicine, 14*(3), 233–239.

Hanley, M. A., Coppa, D., & Shields, D. (2017). A Practice-Based Theory of Healing Through Therapeutic Touch: Advancing Holistic Nursing Practice. *Journal of Holistic Nursing, 35*(4), 369–381.

He, B. J., Tong, P. J., Li, J., Jing, H. T., & Yao, X. M. (2013). Auricular acupressure for analgesia in perioperative period of total knee arthroplasty. *Pain Medicine, 14*(10), 1608–1613.

Hennegahan, A., & Schnyer, R. (2015). Biofield therapies for symptom management in palliative and end-of-life care. *American Journal of Hospice & Palliative Medicine, 32*(1), 90–100.

Hillinger, M. G., Wolever, R. Q., McKernan, L. C., & Elam, R. (2017). Integrative Medicine for the Treatment of Persistent Pain. *Primary Care: Clinics in Office Practice, 44*(2), 247–264.

Honda, N., Han, S., Wada, N., Loo, K. K., Higashimoto, Y., & Fukuda, K. (2013). Effect of therapeutic touch on brain activation of preterm infants in response to sensory punctate stimulus: a near-infrared spectroscopy-based study. *Archives of Disease in Childhood-Fetal and Neonatal Edition, 98*(3), F244–F248.

Hou, X. B., Ying, S. U. N., Zhao, R. Z., Hui, Z. H. A. O., Wang, H. Z., & Jia, C. S. (2016). Experience of professor Jia Chun-sheng in rapid analgesia by subcutaneous pene-tration needling of auricular acupuncture. *World Journal of Acupuncture-Moxibustion, 26*(1), 49–52.

Huang, W., Halpin, S. N., & Perkins, M. M. (2016). A case series of auricular acupuncture in a veteran's population using a revised auricular mapping-diagnostic paradigm (RAMP-uP). *Complementary Therapies in Medicine, 27*, 130–136.

Ing, J. W. (2017). Head and Neck Cancer Pain. *Otolaryngologic Clinics of North America, 50*(4), 793–806.

Jackson, C., & Latini, C. (2016). Touch and hand-mediated therapies. In B. Dossey, & L. Keegan (Eds.), *Holistic nursing: A handbook for practice* (pp. 299–319). Burlington, MA: Jones & Bartlett Learning.

Jain, S., & Mills, P. (2010). Biofield therapies: Helpful or full of hype? A best evidence synthesis. *International Journal of Behavioral Medicine, 17*(1), 1–16.

Jhaveri, A., Walsh, S. J., Wang, Y., McCarthy, M., & Gronowicz, G. (2008). Therapeutic touch affects DNA synthesis and mineralization of human osteoblasts in culture. *Journal of Orthopaedic Research, 26*(11), 1541–1546.

Kailasam, V. K., Anand, P., & Melyan, Z. (2016). Establishing an animal model for National Acupuncture Detoxification Association (NADA) auricular acupuncture protocol. *Neuroscience Letters, 624*, 29–33.

Krieger, D. (1973). The relationship of touch with intent to help or heal subjects: In-vivo hemoglobin values: A study of personalized interaction. *Nursing Research Conference, 9*, 39–58.

Krieger, D. (1979). *Therapeutic Touch: How to use your hands to help or heal.* New York: Simon & Schuster.

Krieger, D. (2002). *Therapeutic Touch as Transpersonal Healing.* New York: Lantern Books.

Krieger, D. (2017). Compassion as power in the transpersonal healing practices of therapeutic touch: a highly human function. Keynote delivered at the Therapeutic Touch International Association's Fourth International Congress, April 21–23, 2017, Chicago, IL. https://therapeutictouch.org/wp-content/uploads/2017/01/Dees-Chicago-Paper-COMPASSION-AS-POWER.pdf Accessed 8/13/2020.

Kundu, A., Lin, Y., Oron, A., & Doorenbos, A. (2014). Reiki therapy for postoperative oral pain in pediatric patients: Pilot data from a double-blind, randomized clinical trial. *Complementary Therapies in Clinical Practice, 20*, 21–25.

Lai, L. (2016). NICE should reconsider its recommendation to withdraw acupuncture from its 2016 guidelines on low back pain and sciatica. *European Journal of Integrative Medicine, 8*(4), 329–331.

Lauche, R., Cramer, H., Häuser, W., Dobos, G., & Langhorst, J. (2015). A systematic overview of reviews for complementary and alternative therapies in the treatment of the fibromyalgia syndrome. *Evidence-Based Complementary and Alternative Medicine, 2015.* Article ID 610615, 13 pages https://doi.org/10.1155/2015/610615.

Leong, F. C. (2014). Complementary and alternative medications for chronic pelvic pain. *Obstetrics and Gynecology Clinics, 41*(3), 503–510.

Leskowitz, E. (2014). Phantom limb pain: An energy/trauma model. *Explore: The Journal of Science and Healing, 10*(6), 389–397.

Levett, K. M., Smith, C. A., Dahlen, H. G., & Bensoussan, A. (2014). Acupuncture and acupressure for pain management in labour and birth: a critical narrative review of current systematic review evidence. *Complementary Therapies in Medicine, 22*(3), 523–540.

Lincoln, V., Nowak, E. W., Schommer, B., Briggs, T., Fehrer, A., & Wax, G. (2014). Impact of Healing Touch with Healing Harp on Inpatient Acute Care Pain: A Retrospective Analysis. *Holistic Nursing Practice*, 28(3), 164–170.

Lu, D. F., Hart, L. K., Lutgendorf, S. K., & Perkhounkova, Y. (2013). The effect of Healing Touch on the pain and mobility of persons with osteoarthritis: A feasibility study. *Geriatric Nursing*, 34(4), 314–322.

Lund, I., & Lundeberg, T. (2015). Endometriosis pain and acupuncture. *Acupuncture and Related Therapies*, 3(2), 19–23.

Macznik, A. K., Schneiders, A. G., Athens, J., & Sullivan, S. J. (2017). Does Acupressure Hit the Mark? A Three-Arm Randomized Placebo-Controlled Trial of Acupressure for Pain and Anxiety Relief in Athletes with Acute Musculoskeletal Sports Injuries. *Clinical Journal of Sport Medicine*, 27(4), 338–343.

McCormack, G. L. (2009). Using non-contact therapeutic touch to manage post-surgical pain in the elderly. *Occupational Therapy International*, 16(1), 44–56.

Mehta, P., Dhapte, V., Kadam, S., & Dhapte, V. (2017). Contemporary acupressure therapy: Adroit cure for painless recovery of therapeutic ailments. *Journal of Traditional and Complementary Medicine*, 7(2), 251–263.

Mentgen, J., & Hover-Kramer, D. (2002). The development of Healing Touch as a major force in energy-ordered healing practices. In D. Hover-Kramer, & J. Mentgen (Eds.), *Healing Touch: Guidebook for Practitioners* (2nd Ed., pp. 3–7). Albany, NY: Delmar–Thomson Learning Inc.

Midilli, T., & Gunduzoglu, N. (2016). Effects of Reiki on pain and vital signs when applied to the incision area of the body after cesarean section surgery. *Holistic Nursing Practice*, 30(6), 368–378.

Miles, P. (2008). *Reiki: A comprehensive guide*. New York: Penguin.

Monroe, C. M. (2009). The effects of Therapeutic Touch on pain. *Journal of Holistic Nursing*, 27(2), 85–92.

Monzillo, E., & Gronowicz, G. (2011). New insights on Therapeutic Touch: a discussion of experimental methodology and design that resulted in significant effects on normal human cells and osteosarcoma. *EXPLORE: The Journal of Science and Healing*, 7(1), 44–51.

Moore, C. B., & Hickey, A. H. (2017). Increasing Access to Auricular Acupuncture for Postoperative Nausea and Vomiting. *Journal of PeriAnesthesia Nursing*, 32(2), 96–105.

National Center for Complementary and Integrative Health (NCCIH). (2015). *Reiki: In depth*. (Publication No. D315). Retrieved from https://nccih.nih.gov/sites/nccam.nih.gov/files/Reiki_11-30-2015.pdf.

National Center for Complementary and Integrative Health (NCCIH). (2018). Reiki. Retrieved from https://www.nccih.nih.gov/health/reiki August 13, 2020.

Newshan, G., & Staats, J. A. (2013). Evidence-based pain guidelines in HIV care. *Journal of the Association of Nurses in AIDS Care*, 24(1), S112–S126.

NICE. (2016). Low back pain and sciatica: management of non-specific low back pain and sciatica: Assessment and non-invasive treatments. In N. C. G. Centre (Ed.), *Draft for Consultation, NICE*.

Niemzow, R. (2020). Battlefield acupuncture seminars. Retrieved from: https://www.battlefieldacupuncture.net/home/battlefieldacupuncture/ August 13, 2020.

Ning, Z., & Lao, L. (2015). Acupuncture for pain management in evidence-based medicine. *Journal of Acupuncture and Meridian Studies*, 8(5), 270–273.

Notte, B., Fazzini, C., & Mooney, R. (2016). Reiki's effect on patients with total knee arthroplasty: A pilot study. *Nursing*, 46(2), 17–23.

Oschman, J. L. (2016a). Introducing and Defining Energy and Energy Medicine. In *Energy Medicine: The Scientific Basis* (2nd Ed, pp. 1–10). St. Louis: Elsevier.

Oschman, J. L. (2016b). Bodywork, Energetic and Movement Therapies. In *Energy Medicine: The Scientific Basis* (2nd Ed, pp. 101–112). St. Louis: Elsevier.

Oschman, J. L. (2016c). Energy 'Circuits in the Body' In: *Energy Medicine: The Scientific Basis*. (2nd Ed., pp. 145–168). St. Louis: Elsevier.

Pak, S. C., Micalos, P. S., Maria, S. J., & Lord, B. (2015). *Nonpharmacological interventions for pain management in paramedicine and the emergency setting: a review of the literature Evidence-Based Complementary and Alternative Medicine*, 2015. ID873039 https://doi.org/10.1155/2015/87/3039.

Papadopoulos, G. S., Tzimas, P., Liarmakopoulou, A., & Petrou, A. M. (2017). Auricular acupuncture analgesia in thoracic trauma: a case report. *Journal of Acupuncture and Meridian Studies*, 10(1), 49–52.

Peuker, E. T., & Filler, T. J. (2002). The nerve supply of the human auricle. *Clinical Anatomy*, 15(1), 35–37.

Potter, P. J. (2013). Energy therapies in advanced practice oncology: an evidence-informed practice approach. *Journal of the Advanced Practitioner in Oncology*, 4(3), 139.

Quinlan-Colwell, A. (2012). Complementary interventions for pain management in older adults. In *Compact Clinical Guide to Geriatric Pain Management*. New York: Springer Publishing.

Raddadi, Y., Adib-Hajbaghery, M., Ghadirzadeh, Z., & Kheirkhah, D. (2017). Comparing the effects of acupressure at LI4 and BL32 points on intramuscular injection pain. *European Journal of Integrative Medicine*, 11(1), 63–68.

Rao, A., Hickman, L. D., Sibbritt, D., Newton, P. J., & Phillips, J. L. (2016). Is energy healing an effective non-pharmacological therapy for improving symptom management of chronic illnesses? A systematic review. *Complementary therapies in clinical practice*, 25, 26–41.

Reiki Alliance. (2017). Our organization. Retrieved from http://www.reikialliance.com/en/article/our-organization.

Richeson, N., Spross, J., Lutz, K., & Peng, C. (2010). Effects of Reiki on anxiety, depression, pain, and physiological factors on community-dwelling older adults. *Research in Gerontological Nursing*, 3(3), 187–199.

Ringdahl, D. (2018). Reiki. In R. Lindquist, M. Tracy, & M. Snyder (Eds.), *Complementary and Alternative Therapies in Nursing* (pp. 411–430). New York: Springer Publishing.

Rizi, M. S., Shamsalinia, A., Ghaffari, F., Keyhanian, S., & Nabi, B. N. (2017). The effect of acupressure on pain, anxiety, and the physiological indexes of patients with cancer undergoing bone marrow biopsy. *Complementary Therapies in Clinical Practice*, 29, 136–141.

Rogers, M. E. (1994). The science of unitary human beings: Current perspectives. *Nursing Science Quarterly*, 7(1), 33–35.

Romoli, M., Greco, F., & Giommi, A. (2016). Auricular acupuncture diagnosis in patients with lumbar hernia. *Complementary Therapies in Medicine*, 26, 61–65.

Santiago, M. V., Tumilty, S., Mącznik, A., & Mani, R. (2016). Does acupuncture alter pain-related functional connectivity of the central nervous system? A systematic review. *Journal of Acupuncture and Meridian Studies*, 9(4), 167–177.

Senderovich, H., Ip, M. L., Berall, A., Karuza, J., Gordon, M., Binns, M., ... Dunal, L. (2016). Therapeutic Touch® in a geriatric Palliative Care Unit: A retrospective review. *Complementary Therapies in Clinical Practice*, 24, 134–138.

Shields, D., & Wilson, D. (2016). Energy healing. In B. Dossey, & L. Keegan (Eds.), *Holistic nursing: A handbook for practice* (pp. 187–220). Burlington, MA: Jones & Bartlett Learning.

Shields, D., Fuller, A., Resnicoff, M., Butcher, H. K., & Frisch, N. (2016). Human Energy Field: A Concept Analysis. *Journal of Holistic Nursing*, 35(4), 352–368.

Simpson, C. A. (2015). Complementary medicine in chronic pain treatment. *Physical Medicine and Rehabilitation Clinics*, 26(2), 321–347.

So, P. S., Jiang, Y., & Qin, Y. (2008). Touch therapies for pain relief in adults. *Cochrane Database Syst Rev*. 2008;4:CD006535.

Song, H. J., Seo, H. J., Lee, H., Son, H., Choi, S. M., & Lee, S. (2015). Effect of self-acupressure for symptom management: a systematic review. *Complementary Therapies in Medicine*, 23(1), 68–78.

Tabatabaee, A., Tafreshi, M. Z., Rasouli, M., Aledavood, S. A., Majd, H. A., & Farahmand, S. K. (2015). Effects of therapeutic touch on anxiety in patients with cancer. *Avicenna Journal of Phytomedicine*, 5, 150–151.

Tabatabaee, A., Tafreshi, M. Z., Rassouli, M., Aledavood, S. A., AlaviMajd, H., & Farahmand, S. K. (2016a). Effect of therapeutic touch on pain related parameters in patients with cancer: a randomized clinical trial. *Materia Socio-medica*, 28(3), 220–223.

Tabatabaee, A., Tafreshi, M. Z., Rassouli, M., Aledavood, S. A., AlaviMajd, H., & Farahmand, S. K. (2016b). Effect of therapeutic touch in patients with cancer: a literature review. *Medical Archives*, 70(2), 142–147.

Therapeutic Touch International Association (TTIA) (2016). http://therapeutic-touch.org/ Accessed 10/09/2017.

Thomas, L. S., Stephenson, N., Swanson, M., Jesse, D. E., & Brown, S. (2013). A pilot study: the effect of Healing Touch on anxiety, stress, pain, pain medication usage, and physiological measures in hospitalized sickle cell disease adults experiencing a vaso-occlusive pain episode. *Journal of Holistic Nursing*, 31(4), 234–247.

Thrane, S., & Cohen, S. (2014). Effect of Reiki therapy on pain and anxiety in adults: An in-depth literature review of randomized trials with effect size calculations. *Pain Management Nursing*, 15(4), 897–908.

Toca-Villegas, J., Esmer-Sánchez, D., García-Narváez, J., Sánchez-Aguilar, M., & Hernández-Sierra, J. F. (2017). Efficacy of modified auriculotherapy for post-operative pain control in patients subjected to laparoscopic cholecystectomy. *Cirugía y Cirujanos (English Edition)*, 85(3), 220–224.

Trinh, K. V., Diep, D., & Dorsher, P. (2017). A Critical Look into the 2016 NICE Guidelines: Acupuncture for Low-Back Pain and Sciatica. *Medical Acupuncture*, 29(1), 20–24.

Tsai, S. L., Fox, L. M., Murakami, M., & Tsung, J. W. (2016). Auricular acupuncture in emergency department treatment of acute pain. *Annals of Emergency Medicine*, 68(5), 583–585.

Usichenko, T. (2017). From auricular acupuncture to transcutaneous auricular vagal nerve stimulation (taVNS). *Abstracts/Brain Stimulation*, 10(2), 346–540.

Usichenko, T., Hacker, H., & Lotze, M. (2017). Transcutaneous auricular vagal nerve stimulation (taVNS) might be a mechanism behind the analgesic effects of auricular acupuncture. *Brain Stimulation*, 10(6), 1042–1044.

Vas, J., Aranda-Regules, J. M., Modesto, M., Aguilar, I., Barón-Crespo, M., Ramos-Monserrat, M., ... Rivas-Ruiz, F. (2014). Auricular acupuncture for primary care treatment of low back pain and posterior pelvic pain in pregnancy: study protocol for a multicentre randomised placebo-controlled trial. *Trials*, 15(1), 288.

Vernooij, M., & Marcelissen, F. (2017). Measuring patient reported outcomes of acupuncture treatment on pain patients' health status. *Complementary Therapies in Clinical Practice*, 28, 192–199.

Vickers, A. J., & Linde, K. (2014). Acupuncture for chronic pain. *JAMA*, 311(9), 955–956.

Vickers, A. J., Cronin, A. M., Maschino, A. C., Lewith, G., MacPherson, H., Foster, N. E., ... Acupuncture Trialists' Collaboration. (2012). Acupuncture for chronic pain: individual patient data meta-analysis. *Archives of Internal Medicine*, 172(19), 1444–1453.

Vitale, A., & O'Connor, P. (2006). The effect of Reiki on pain and anxiety in women with abdominal hysterectomies: A quasi-experimental pilot study. *Holistic Nursing Practice*, 20(6), 263–272.

Wagner, J., & Thompson, S. (2014). Integrative nursing management of pain. In M. Kreitzer, & M. Koithan (Eds.), *Integrative nursing* (pp. 286–299). New York: Oxford University Press.

Walker, P. H., Pock, A., Ling, C. G., Kwon, K. N., & Vaughan, M. (2016). Battlefield acupuncture: Opening the door for acupuncture in Department of Defense/Veteran's Administration health care. *Nursing Outlook*, 64(5), 491–498.

World Health Organization (WHO). (2013). *WHO Traditional Medicine Strategy 2014–2023*. Geneva, Switzerland: World Health Organization.

Xu, S. H., Sun, Y. A., & Wu, H. Y. (2009). Effects of therapeutic touch on the intraoperative pain in patients undergoing percutaneous laser disk decompression [J]. *Chinese Journal of Nursing*, 8, 033.

Yap, S. H. (2016). Acupuncture in pain management. *Anaesthesia & Intensive Care Medicine*, 17(9), 448–450.

Yeh, C. H., Chiang, Y. C., Hoffman, S. L., Liang, Z., Klem, M. L., Tam, W. W., ... Suen, L. K. P. (2014). Efficacy of auricular therapy for pain management: a systematic review and meta-analysis. *Evidence-based Complementary and Alternative Medicine*, 2014. 934670.

Zeng, Y., & Chung, J. W. Y. (2015). Acupuncture for chronic nonspecific low back pain: an overview of systematic reviews. *European Journal of Integrative Medicine*, 7(2), 94–107.

Zhao, H., Liu, B. Y., Liu, Z. S., Xie, L. M., Fang, Y. G., Zhu, Y., ... Han, M. J. (2016). Clinical practice guidelines of using acupuncture for low back pain. *World Journal of Acupuncture-Moxibustion*, 26(4), 1–13.

Zhao, H. J., Tan, J. Y., Wang, T., & Jin, L. (2015). Auricular therapy for chronic pain management in adults: A synthesis of evidence. *Complementary Therapies in Clinical Practice*, 21(2), 68–78.

Chapter 24 Manual Therapies for Pain Management

Ann Quinlan-Colwell

CHAPTER OUTLINE

Manual Therapy, pg. 652

Osteopathy, Osteopathy Manual Medicine, or Osteopathic Manipulative Therapy, pg. 653

    Evidence for Pain Management, pg. 653

    Research, pg. 654

Craniosacral Therapy, pg. 654

    Evidence for Pain Management, pg. 654

    Cautions, pg. 655

Massage Therapy, pg. 655

    Evidence for Pain Management, pg. 656

    Cautions, pg. 658

Reflexology, pg. 659

    Evidence for Pain Management, pg. 660

    Cautions, pg. 663

Chiropractic Practice, pg. 664

    Evidence for Pain Management, pg. 664

    Cautions, pg. 665

Myofascial Trigger Point Therapy, pg. 666

    Evidence for Pain Management, pg. 666

    Cautions, pg. 667

Muscle Energy Technique, pg. 667

    Evidence for Pain Management, pg. 667

    Cautions, pg. 667

Fascial Distortion Model, pg. 667

    Evidence for Pain Management, pg. 668

    Cautions, pg. 668

Key Points, pg. 668

Case Scenario, pg. 668

Acknowledgments, pg. 668

References, pg. 668

Manual Therapy

Manual therapy is a term that is used frequently but is often poorly defined. Included within the umbrella of manual therapy are a variety of interventions used by therapists in different specialty areas, including physical therapists, osteopath physicians, chiropractors, massage therapists, craniosacral therapists (Harper, Jagger, Aron, Steinbeck, & Stecco, 2017), and orthopedic manual therapists (Bise, Piva & Erhard, 2017) (Table 24.1). The International Federation of Orthopedic Manual Therapists explains manual therapy as clinicians using expert hand movements "to improve tissue extensibility, increase range of motion, induce relaxation, mobilize or manipulate soft tissue and joints, modulate pain and reduce soft tissue swelling, inflammation or restriction" (Bise et al., 2017 p. 85). The authors of an extensive systematic review (n = 35 studies) concluded there is fair evidence to support use of manual and manipulative therapy alone and in conjunction with multimodal therapies for treatment of the painful conditions epicondylopathy, carpal tunnel syndrome, and temporomandibular joint disorders (Brantingham et al., 2013). Osteopathy manual medicine (OMM), craniosacral therapy (CST), massage, reflexology, chiropractic spinal manipulative therapies, trigger point therapies, muscle energy technique, and fascial distortion model are explored in this chapter. Manual interventions used by physical therapists are discussed in Chapter 20.

Education and credentialing, including licensure or certification, are available for clinicians who use these techniques. It is imperative to advise patients to ascertain that the manual therapist from whom they seek treatment is appropriately educated and credentialed. It is also important to interview the manual therapist to ensure the person has experience working with patients with pain and with any comorbidities the individual seeking treatment may have, including extremes in age.

Table 24.1 | Types of Therapy and Practitioners

Type of Therapy	Practitioner
Massage	
Osteopathy manual medicine (OMM)	Doctors of osteopathy
Craniosacral therapy	Osteopaths, craniosacral therapists
Spinal manipulative therapy (SMT)	Osteopaths, physical therapists, and chiropractors
Chiropractic manipulative therapy	Chiropractors
Dry needling	Physical therapists
Instrument-assisted soft tissue mobilization	Physical therapists
Myofascial release	Physical therapists
High velocity, low amplitude (HVLA)	Physical therapists

Harper, B., Jagger, K., Aron, A., Steinbeck, L., & Stecco, A. (2017). A commentary review of the cost effectiveness of manual therapies for neck and low back pain. *Journal of Bodywork and Movement Therapies, 21*(3), 684–691.

Osteopathy, Osteopathy Manual Medicine, or Osteopathic Manipulative Therapy

Although Andrew Taylor Still is considered the founder of osteopathy, comparable precepts were put forth much earlier in ancient Greece by Plato (Tyreman, 2013). Traditionally, osteopathy has been used as a holistic approach in the treatment of people with a variety of musculoskeletal conditions (e.g., neck, back, and shoulder pains) (Steel, Blaich, Sundberg, & Adams, 2017). That concise limiting description is no longer appropriate because osteopathy has evolved into a more intricate discipline with numerous characteristics and scopes of practice used internationally (Vogel, 2016).

Recently, in the United States, osteopathic manipulative therapy (OMT) is increasingly used with obstetric and gynecologic conditions. In fact, specialty certifications from the American Osteopathic Association are the fifth highest for obstetrics and gynecology (1359), with only orthopedic surgery (1380), emergency medicine (3208), primary internal medicine (4923), and family practitioners (12,519) having more certifications (Wieting, Weaver, Kramer & Morales-Egizi, 2017). This increase most probably is related to osteopathy being practiced differently in the United States, where osteopaths are licensed to practice medicine the same as those who have completed traditional medical education, whereas in other countries

osteopathy is still limited to manual therapy with musculoskeletal conditions (Steel et al., 2017).

Evidence for Pain Management

With an estimated 632 million people throughout the world with low back pain (LBP) (Licciardone, Gatchel, & Aryal, 2016) multimodal and nonsurgical interventions for LBP are needed and important. The investigators of a large study at the University of North Texas with people with LBP (n = 455) compared OMT (n = 230) with sham OMT (n = 225) (Licciardone, Minotti, Gatchel, Kearns, & Singh, 2013). Those investigators reported positive benefits of a moderate effect among people in the OMT group. In addition, the participants in the OMT group were more satisfied with care and used fewer prescription medications. Interestingly, there was no difference between the two groups in function or work ability. A follow-up secondary analysis was done assessing information of the 230 patients in that study who received OMT (Licciardone, Kearns, & Crow, 2014). During that work, the researchers found there was baseline prevalence of 51% for psoas syndrome (i.e., an imbalance of the muscle with point tenderness of the psoas muscle on palpation), which was found to be the only baseline dysfunction to predict improvement of the LBP. Subsequent analysis concluded that between 20% and 25% of subjects with LBP who received OMT had results consistent with clinical recovery or resolution of the LBP (Licciardone et al., 2016). In a separate randomized double blind study, OMT was compared with sham OMT among people living with chronic LBP (CLBP) (n = 186) (Licciardone & Aryal, 2014). In that study, compared to those who received sham OMT (n = 91), participants who received OMT (n = 95) were more than twice (52% versus 25%) as likely to demonstrate clinical response at or by the 12th week (Licciardone & Aryal, 2014). The authors of a systematic review of 15 studies, of which 12 studies involved pregnant or postpartum women who received OMT for LBP, reported pain was rated as clinically less and function was increased with OMT (Franke, Franke, & Fryer, 2014). Those authors qualified that additional research is needed.

OMT is used with a variety of other health care conditions with inconsistent support of effectiveness. Positive effects were seen among participants with a variety of musculoskeletal disorders in a large prospective study (n = 988) in Italy (Cerritelli, Verzella, & Barlafante, 2014). Improvements in general health and use of medications, with the greatest effect size seen in reports of pain, were reported with OMT. Similarly, people with chronic migraine headaches had significant improvement in headache impact test scores after OMT (Cerritelli et al., 2015). However, the evidence in a systematic review of six studies for the benefit of using OMT for migraine headaches was found to be low level (Cerritelli, Lacorte, Ruffini, & Vanacore, 2017). In another systematic review of OMT used with neurologic disorders, the authors reported there were few studies and they were diverse with low methodologic merit (Cerritelli, Ruffini, Lacorte, & Vanacore, 2016). An interesting use of OMT was in a small crossover placebo-controlled study (n = 31) with people living with refractory irritable bowel syndrome (IBS) (Attali, Bouchoucha, & Benamouzig, 2013). The authors of that study reported reduction of diarrhea, abdominal distention, and pain at the time of OMT and continuation of the reduction of those symptoms at 1 year follow-up (P < .05).

Research

Research using OMT involving women with gynecologic and obstetric disorders and pain has increased in recent years. A positive use of OMT was the reduction of pain intensity (P < .005) among women with dysmenorrhea (Schwerla, Wirthwein, Rütz, & Resch, 2014). The investigators of a large study with pregnant women (n = 400) compared OMT with standard of care compared with placebo ultrasound (Hensel, Carnes, & Stoll, 2016). The results of that study were unusual in that OMT was significantly more effective than standard of care for reducing pain and preventing deterioration of function, but OMT was not significantly different from the placebo ultrasound that was also more effective in those areas than was standard of care. In a phenomenologic study in Australia, women reported relief from back and pelvic pain and they thought OMT helped them ready their bodies for birthing (Sheraton, Streckfuss, & Grace, 2018).

Doctors of osteopathy clearly have much to offer in a multimodal approach of pain management. Additional research is needed with good methodology and including any reports of adverse events. Areas in need of research using OMT include obstetrics and gynecology (Ruffini, D'Alessandro, Cardinali, Frondaroli, & Cerritelli, 2016) including dysmenorrhea (Schwerla et al., 2014), patients with IBS (Attali et al., 2013), headaches (Cerritelli et al., 2015; Cerritelli et al., 2017), neurologic diseases (Cerritelli et al., 2016), LBP in general, and among pregnant women (Franke et al., 2014). International research is also needed to determine best practice measures, comparative effectiveness, and cost-to-benefit ratio of OMT (Steel et al., 2017).

Craniosacral Therapy

CST is a very gentle, nonthrusting manipulation technique developed by osteopath John Upledger, who created the term to distinguish the technique he developed from other interventions that involved manipulation of the cranium (Brough, Lindenmeyer, Thistlethwaite, Lewith, & Stewart-Brown, 2015). CST involves systematic assessment and treatment of the entire body by intervening with the central nervous system from the cranium to the sacrum (Haller, Cramer, Werner, & Dobos, 2015; Thomas

& Wahezi, 2012; Upledger, Grossinger, Ash, & Cohen, 2008). Specifically involved are the bones and sutures of the skull, spinal canal, dura mater, and related fascia and membranes (Arnadottir & Sigurdardottir, 2013; Irnich, 2013). The very gentle manipulation is done with the intent of achieving a sense of balance and healing by releasing restrictions in the sutures of the cranium, membranes of the brain and spine, and associated connective tissues (Brough et al., 2015; Haller et al., 2015) (Fig. 24.1). CST is generally used by trained professionals, including CST therapists, osteopaths, chiropractors, and other clinicians, who have pursued professional education and training in CST and are licensed to touch patients (Jäkel & von Hauenschild, 2012). It is important to ensure clinicians are appropriately educated and licensed (Box 24.1).

Evidence for Pain Management

Evidence from recent studies suggests that CST can be an effective component in multimodal pain management with a variety of conditions. The beneficial effect of CST on pain was reported from studies with people living with musculoskeletal pain (Brough et al., 2015), including persistent neck pain (Brough et al., 2015; Haller, Ostermann, Lauche, Cramer, & Dobos, 2014), and LBP (Białoszewski, Bebelski, Lewandowska, & Słupik, 2014; Castro-Sánchez, et al, 2016). It was also effectively used with headaches (Brough et al., 2015), including migraine headaches (Arnadottir & Sigurdardottir, 2013), and psychological-emotional pain (Brough et al., 2015). Rigorous research investigating the effect of CST on pain is not abundant. The authors of a 2012 systematic review reported finding only seven studies of CST, which were either randomized controlled trials (RCTs) or observationally designed (Jäkel & von Hauenschild, 2012). Of those, three studies specifically investigated the effect of CST on pain and all reported significant reductions

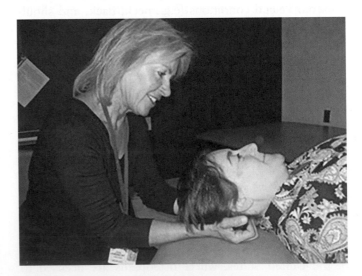

Fig. 24.1 | Craniosacral Therapy. Tissue release of the occipital base of the cranium. Photo courtesy of Joan Farrenkopf and Michele Erich.

Clinical Application of Cranial Sacral Therapy

A woman living with cancer explained how difficult it can be to remain positive when undergoing radiation therapy. She said that trying to remain "positive is really difficult, especially when you have the diagnosis I had." Before beginning radiation, she had a large tumor removed from her stomach. The treatments she received challenged her both physically, because she was constantly feeling nauseous, and mentally, because she was feeling rather defeated by the process. "Staying positive really helps with your energy level. It helps you focus, it helps you get through it," she explained. For this woman, craniosacral therapy helped ease the pain in her stomach, and ultimately she thought it changed her life by helping her feel positive again.

Modified From Turner, J. (2015). NHRMC offers patients integrative therapies. *WECT News*. Original Broadcast August 6, 2015. Retrieved October 9, 2017, from http://www.publicfile@wect.com

in pain among subjects who received CST compared to control groups. People living with LBP (n = 64) participated in a randomized study, and the participants who received 10 sessions of CST (n = 32) had statistically significant reductions in pain intensity compared to those who received 10 sessions of traditional massage (n = 32) (Castro-Sánchez et al., 2016). In one group of patients with nonspecific lumbosacral back pain, a benefit of CST was that the resting tension of the multifidus muscle was reduced (Białoszewski et al., 2014). There is also support that CST has some positive associations with increased mobility, reduced tension, enhanced breathing, reduced anxiety, improvements in sleep disorders, and enhanced quality of life (Brough et al., 2015; Haller et al., 2015). In one case report, a woman with traumatic brain injury and refractory headache pain reported pain scores decreasing from the 6- to 9-cm range to the 2- to 4-cm range on a 10-cm visual analogue scale (Haller et al., 2015).

Like osteopathy, CST is being used with increased frequency among pregnant women, and was the intervention used in a study with pregnant women with pelvic girdle pain (n = 123) (Elden et al., 2013). The investigators of that study reported that the participants who received CST (n = 63) reported significantly less pain in the morning and better function after CST. However, the effects were considered questionable by the researchers because there was no improvement seen in evening symptoms or in the use of sick leave. In a follow-up qualitative study, pregnant women with pelvic girdle pain were interviewed after receiving three CST treatments (Elden, Lundgren, & Robertson, 2014). The women in that study reported being distracted from pain, feeling relaxed, feeling secure

and optimistic, and having an increased awareness of their bodies

Well-designed rigorous research is needed to gain stronger evidence to guide the use of CST (Haller et al., 2014; Jäkel & von Hauenschild, 2012). Additional strong research will enable clinicians to educate patients and provide them with information to make the most judicious decisions (Zegarra-Parodi & Cerritelli, 2016) regarding CST as a component of a plan for multimodal management of pain.

Cautions

CST is generally considered to be a safe intervention with few reported adverse events. In one study (n = 20) using CST in patients who have migraine headaches, when CST was used on areas where cranial bone sutures were immobile, migraine pain was elicited (Arnadottir & Sigurdardottir, 2013). Because only gentle pressure is used in CST, this may not occur when CST is used by clinicians who are properly educated in the therapy. Replication studies are warranted to ascertain contributing factors. The only reported serious adverse event resulted in the death of an infant who received CST from a therapist who reportedly used incorrect technique (Todd, Carroll, Robinson, & Mitchell, 2015). This adverse event speaks to the importance of working with CST therapists who are certified and have experience treating people with characteristics and conditions similar to those of the person seeking treatment.

Massage Therapy

Massage is one of the oldest healing modalities, with ancient roots dating to 2700 BCE in China, where writings mentioned the use of massage to relieve muscle distress (Wolf & Brault, 2016). Later in Greece, Hippocrates advised "the physician must be experienced in many things, but most assuredly in rubbing" (Pearlman, 2016, p. 183). Massage therapy is a frequently used intervention for musculoskeletal pain, and those who employ it as a treatment report physical and psychological benefit (Field, 2018; Kennedy, Cambron, Sharpe, Travillian, & Saunders, 2016). It is widely used internationally, with approximately 18 million adults in the United States reportedly having received therapeutic massages during 2007 (Pearlman, 2016).

Although it is not certain precisely how massage works, there are numerous hypotheses with some supportive information. It is thought the therapeutic effects of massage occur as a result of changes in blood flow and relaxing tissues while facilitating modulation of pain. The underlying mechanisms are thought to be through stimulating drainage of the venous and lymphatic systems; releasing the intensity of adhesions (Field, 2014; Thomas &

Wahezi, 2012); improving muscle tone (Pearlman, 2016); and stimulating pressure receptors, which increases vagal activity, reduces cortisol (Field, 2016), increases serotonin in the body (Field, Diego, & Solien-Wolfe, 2014), and improves immune system function (Field, 2014). It is also thought that massage enables muscle cells to more effectively create new mitochondria, which then enables the muscles to recover quicker (Crane, 2012). There are several different forms/types/schools of massage therapy. These include Swedish, Shiatsu, connective tissue massage, myofascial release (Yuan, Matsutani, & Marques, 2015), traditional Thai (Keeratitanont, Jensen, Chatchawan, & Auvichayapat, 2015), Thai self-massage (Wamontree, Kanchanakhan, & Eungpinichpong, 2015), Japanese

Anma massage (Donoyama, Suoh, & Ohkoshi, 2014), hand massage (Field, 2016), and traditional Chinese *Tui Na* (Wei, Wang, Li, & Zhu, 2017). See Table 24.2 for the more common types of massage.

Evidence for Pain Management

With regard to the effect of massage on pain, reports from functional magnetic resonance imaging (fMRI) studies have associated moderate-pressure massage with increased circulation to the amygdala and hypothalamus with activity in the anterior cingulate cortex (Field, 2014), which are areas of the brain involved with pain perception (see Chapter 3). A long-held belief is that

Table 24.2 | Common Types of Massage

Type of Massage	Involves	Examples of Intentions	Comments
Effleurage	Gentle gliding of the fingers and hands in a circular rhythmic manner	Stimulates circulation and lymphatic drainage; relieves vascular congestion, muscle strains, and joint pain	
Pétrissage	Kneading-like movements with compression of skin between thumbs and fingers	Promotes relaxation, improve vascular and fluid circulation, increase suppleness of tissues, reduce adhesions	
Tapotement	Alternates contact with skin, including clapping, pounding, tapping, vibrating, hacking, or striking tissue with ulnar aspect of hand	Loosens secretions, especially of lungs	
Friction massage	Pressure applied perpendicular to muscle fibers in circular, long or transverse manner by fingers or hand massaging from superficial to deep	Split up adhesions of scar tissue, relax ligaments, and deactivate trigger points	Can be uncomfortable and cause bruising
Rolfing structural integration	Progressively deeper friction massage attempts to stretch the fascia	Through stretching fascia, improve body alignment and movement	Can be painful
Myofascial release	Gentle massage and stretching of muscles and fascia	Restore or improve range of motion and relieve pain	
Manual lymphatic drainage	Following massage of proximal area of extremity and then using gentle and superficial rhythmic movements guide lymph away from areas of damaged lymphatic vessels from distal to proximal portion of extremity	Relieve lymphedema	
Acupressure	Using finger and thumb pressure in circular movements with areas that are usually treated with acupuncture needles	Reestablish homeostasis or balance of the person's energy; used to relieve pain (including temporomandibular joint and headaches) and nausea	Can be performed on self

Table 24.2 | Common Types of Massage—cont'd

Type of Massage	Involves	Examples of Intentions	Comments
Shiatsu	Pressure is applied using fingers to effect change similar to acupuncture action on meridians	Promotes relaxation	
Japanese *Anma* massage	A full-body massage with kneading, pressing, and stroking of muscles and some joint exercise	Disease treatment, prevention, and rehabilitation	Is administered through clothing
Traditional Thai massage	Pressure applied to specific muscle areas for 5–10 seconds followed by stretching	Promote relaxation and relieve pain	Administered through clothing
Thai self-massage	Wilai massage stick used to apply pressure to particular areas of the back	Relieve back pain	Self-administered massage is possible whenever the individual desires without need for clinician or transportation
Tui Na	From ancient Chinese healing. Uses hands and feet, elbows, and knees to manipulate muscles and tissue using acupuncture principles	Used to treat pain, substance use disorder, and psychological disorders, among other conditions	Generally considered safe but at least one serious adverse event has been reported

Data from Donoyama, N., Suoh, S., & Ohkoshi, N. (2014). Effectiveness of Anma massage therapy in alleviating physical symptoms in outpatients with Parkinson's disease: A before-after study. *Complementary Therapies in Clinical Practice, 20*(4), 251–261; Keeratitanont, K., Jensen, M. P., Chatchawan, U., & Auvichayapat, P. (2015). The efficacy of traditional Thai massage for the treatment of chronic pain: A systematic review. *Complementary Therapies in Clinical Practice, 21*(1), 26–32; Mackawan, S., Eungpinichpong, W., Pantumethakul, R., Chatchawan, U., Hunsawong, T., & Arayawichanon, P. (2007). Effects of traditional Thai massage versus joint mobilization on substance P and pain perception in patients with non-specific low back pain. *Journal of Bodywork and Movement Therapies, 11*(1), 9-16; Wamontree, P., Kanchanakhan, N., & Eungpinichpong, W. (2015), Effects of traditional Thai self-massage using a massage stick versus ibuprofen on upper back pain associated with myofascial trigger points: A pilot study. *Journal of Health Research, 29*(6), 403–408; Wolf, C. J., & Brault, J. S. (2016). Manipulation, traction and massage. In D. X. Cifu (Ed.), *Braddom's physical medicine and rehabilitation* (5th ed., pp. 347–367. e3). Philadelphia, PA: Elsevier; Yuan, S. L. K., Matsutani, L. A., & Marques, A. P. (2015). Effectiveness of different styles of massage therapy in fibromyalgia: a systematic review and meta-analysis. *Manual Therapy, 20*(2), 257-264; and Zou, G., Wang, G., Li, J., Wu, G., Huang, J., & Huang, S. (2017). Danger of injudicious use of Tui-Na therapy in ankylosing spondylitis. *European Spine Journal, 26*(1), 178–180.

massage is effective by increasing circulation or blood flow, although repeated studies have not supported that concept (Tiidus, 2015). However, it is thought that stiffness of tissues and inflammation are reduced with massage (Crane, 2012).

Massage therapy has been researched in a variety of painful conditions, including pain resulting from arthritis, fibromyalgia (FMS), carpal tunnel syndrome, labor of childbirth, cardiac surgery, muscle disorders, pelvis, LBP, and assorted joint conditions (Field, 2016). When compared to no intervention, the results of a large systematic review of 26 randomized trials (n = 2565 total subjects) reported low-level to moderate-level evidence for short-term positive benefit of massage among people with knee osteoarthritis, shoulder pain, and some back pain (Bervoets, Luijsterburg, Alessie, Buijs, & Verhagen, 2015). However, in that review the authors concluded there was low-level to very low–level evidence when massage was compared with other interventions, including acupuncture (see Chapter 23), relaxation therapy (see Chapter 21), manipulation, and joint mobilization in people with musculoskeletal pains, LBP, and FMS. One of the challenges comparing the different studies is the

divergent diagnoses that underline the painful conditions of the participants in different studies. Another challenge when comparing massage research is that studies used different styles of massage. A systematic review and meta-analysis of massage therapy used with people living with FMS included a variety of types of massage and found different outcomes with each of them (Yuan et al., 2015). In that review, the studies in which Shiatsu massage was used reported improvements in pain and sleep. The studies in which myofascial release was used reported less pain, fatigue, and stiffness. The studies using connective tissue massage reported improved quality of life, including less depression. No specific positive outcomes were associated with Swedish massage when used with people with FMS in the studies included in that systematic review.

Massage therapy is not commonly used with hospitalized postoperative patients; however, it is potentially an important component of postoperative multimodal analgesia. Massage therapy was used postoperatively among patients after colorectal surgery (n = 127) (Dreyer et al., 2015). In that study patients either received massage for 20 minutes (n = 61) or relaxation and socialization (n

= 66). General satisfaction was not different between the two groups, but pain perception, anxiety, and tension were less among those who received massage. A systematic review (n = 6 studies) using massage with patients recovering from surgery revealed the authors of the majority of studies (n = 5) reported benefit and positive outcomes, including reduced pain (Ramesh et al., 2015). A subsequent systematic review and meta-analysis (n = 10 studies) involving patients receiving massage therapy after cardiac surgery (n = 888 total subjects) had similar findings (Miozzo, Stein, Bozzetto, & Plentz, 2016). In that review, patients had less anxiety and reduced pain. Use of massage as part of a multimodal approach to managing pain among hospitalized patients is an area that needs greater exploration, funding, and research.

Supporting the benefit of a multimodal approach to pain management is a small study (n = 20) that compared hand massage therapy (Table 24.3) with hand massage therapy plus topical analgesic (Field et al., 2014). Although both groups immediately after hand massage had less pain and improvements in grip strength and perception of grip strength, those who received both hand massage and the topical analgesic had greater

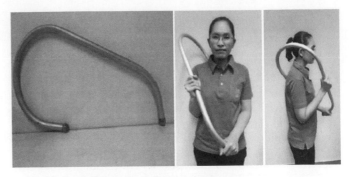

Fig. 24.2 | Holding a Wilai Massage Stick. (From Wamontree, P., Kanchanakhan, N., & Eungpinichpong, W. [2015]. Effects of traditional Thai self-massage using a massage stick versus ibuprofen on upper back pain associated with myofascial trigger points: A pilot study. *Journal of Health Research, 29*[6], 403–408.)

improvement in all areas. Hand massage is an easy-to-learn technique that does not take much time to use and could be beneficial in many different patient settings. An interesting self-care method of massage is Thai self-massage using the Wilai massage stick, which is reported to be effective for back pain (Wamontree et al., 2015) (Fig. 24.2). It is an intervention that patients could learn to use and that could be particularly helpful to patients with access barriers such as finances or transportation (see Chapter 4).

Internationally, research of massage therapy has been extensively done, but it has not been as robust in the United States, where it is used with increasing frequency even in allopathic medical locations (Field, 2016). Research with rigorous methodology and design to assess the benefit of massage in these settings is needed (Field, 2016). Research to identify occurrence of adverse event (Crawford et al., 2016) is needed. Research to determine the differences in benefit and adverse events with different types of massage is also needed. Studies are needed to identify and quantify outcomes when massage is used, including in the postoperative setting (Ramesh et al., 2015). Such research will provide information to guide massage being used as a component of multimodal pain management for acute and chronic pain.

Cautions

Massage therapy is generally considered a safe intervention for pain management with few adverse events, which include increase in pain, stiffness, and sore muscles (Crawford et al., 2016). Caution is advised when massage is used with people with bleeding disorders and should be avoided in areas of skin irritations, fractures, wounds, hematomas, and growths and possibly in people with lymphatic malignancies (Pearlman, 2016). As with other therapies, it is important to ascertain the clinical qualifications and licensure of the massage therapist and experience with treating similar patient populations.

Table 24.3 | Means for Premassage and Postmassage Plus Topical Analgesia Session Measures (Massage Alone Group Means in Parentheses)

Measures	First day		Last day	
	Pre	Post	Pre	Post
Grip strength	32	41[a]	41[a]	49[a]
	(31)	(38)[b]	(37)[b]	(42)[b]
Perceived grip strength	6	8[a]	8[a]	9[b]
	(5)	(6)[b]	(7)[b]	(8)[b]
Hand pain	4	2[a]	2[a]	1[b]
	(5)	(4)[b]	(4)[b]	(3)[b]
Depressed mood	8	6[a]	5[c]	3[a]
	(7)	(6)[b]	(6)[b]	(5)[b]
Sleep disturbance	29		22[c]	
	(26)		(21)[a]	

Superscripts in column 2 indicate significance levels for premassage and postmassage session changes for the first day, and those in column 4 indicate significance levels for premassage and postmassage session changes for the last day. Superscripts in column 3 indicate significance levels for changes from the first day to the last day.

[a] *P* < .01.
[b] *P* < .05.
[c] *P* < .005.

From Field, T., Diego, M., & Solien-Wolfe, L. (2014). Massage therapy plus topical analgesic is more effective than massage alone for hand arthritis pain. *Journal of Bodywork and Movement Therapies, 18*(3), 322–325.

Reflexology

Reflexology is another modality with ancient roots, in this case dating back to the Egyptians from approximately 2330 BCE, and the Chinese (Dahiya & Banerjee, 2016; Wolf & Brault, 2016). Today many consider modern reflexology advanced from the work of Dr. William Fitzgerald in Zone Therapy (Embong, Soh, Ming, & Wong, 2015; Fitzgerald, Bowers, & White, 1994). However, perhaps because she wrote about the benefits of reflexology, others consider Eunice Ingham a founder (Embong et al., 2015; Jones, Thomson, Lauder, Howie, & Leslie, 2012). Reflexology is considered a type of massage in northern European countries, where it is very popular (Jones et al., 2012). However, in the United States it is often considered a distinct discipline separate from massage (Wolf & Brault, 2016).

Reflexology is based on the *homuncular map* (Thomas & Wahezi, 2012; Wolf & Brault, 2016), which provides a representation or atlas in the brain of the connection of the central nervous system with various organs and structures of the body (Miller, 2015; Won, Bailenson, Lee, & Lanier, 2015). The homuncular map also has been described as a representation of the body that is denoted on hands and more frequently feet, with the left and right appendages corresponding with the appropriate organs and structures on the appropriate side of the body (Jones et al., 2012; Rollinson, Jones, Scott, Megson, & Leslie, 2016). This map forms the schemata illustrating how the various reflex points on the foot or hand correspond to different organs or structures (Samuel & Ebenezer, 2013) (Figs. 24.3 through 24.10).

The reflexology practitioner uses small deep circular movements with pressure or friction on specific points of the hands or soles of the feet combined with periodic

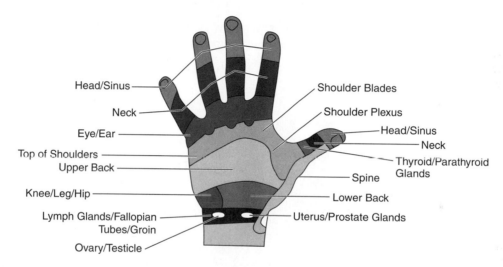

Fig. 24.3 | **Top of Left Hand.** (From Embong, N. H., Soh, Y. C., Ming, L. C., & Wong, T. W. [2015]. Revisiting reflexology: Concept, evidence, current practice, and practitioner training. *Journal of Traditional and Complementary Medicine, 5*[4], 197–206.)

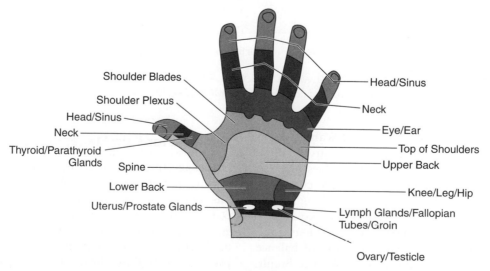

Fig. 24.4 | **Top Right Hand.** (From Embong, N. H., Soh, Y. C., Ming, L. C., & Wong, T. W. [2015]. Revisiting reflexology: Concept, evidence, current practice, and practitioner training. *Journal of Traditional and Complementary Medicine, 5*[4], 197–206.)

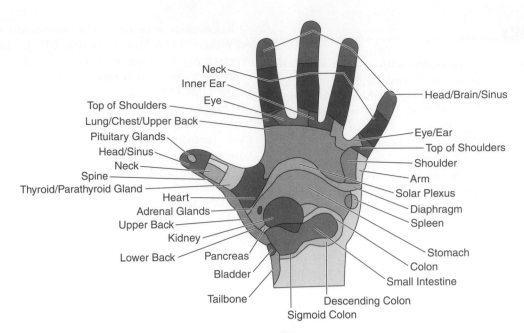

Fig. 24.5 | Left Palm. (From Embong, N. H., Soh, Y. C., Ming, L. C., & Wong, T. W. [2015]. Revisiting reflexology: Concept, evidence, current practice, and practitioner training. *Journal of Traditional and Complementary Medicine, 5*[4], 197–206.)

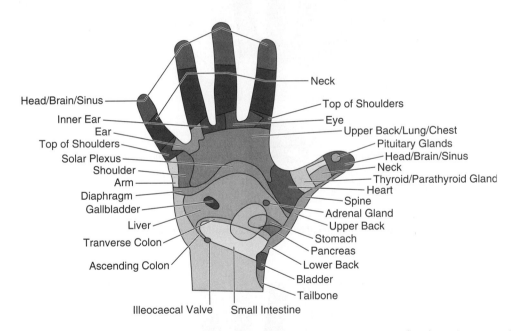

Fig. 24.6 | Right Palm. (From Embong, N. H., Soh, Y. C., Ming, L. C., & Wong, T. W. [2015]. Revisiting reflexology: Concept, evidence, current practice, and practitioner training. *Journal of Traditional and Complementary Medicine, 5*[4], 197–206.)

long movements with pressure (Thomas & Wahezi, 2012; Wolf & Brault, 2016). A maneuver particular to reflexology is called *thumb walking*, which involves bending the first thumb joint and placing the outside corner on the plantar surface of the foot and with a rocking motion moving the thumb forward in a caterpillar like motion (Jones et al., 2012). The objective of reflexology is to stimulate and help the body regain the sense of balance or equilibrium (Thomas & Wahezi, 2012; Wolf & Brault, 2016). See Fig. 24.11 for a sample protocol for a reflexology treatment.

Evidence for Pain Management

One suggestion of how reflexology is effective with controlling pain is that it stimulates the release of enkephalins and endorphins (Mobini-Bidgoli, Taghadosi, Gilasi, & Farokhian, 2017). Those substances have natural analgesic properties (Ellison, 2017). Foot reflexology has been used with a variety of painful conditions, including in people with migraine headaches (Kobza, Lizis, & Zięba, 2017), rheumatoid arthritis (Metin & Ozdemir, 2016), FMS (Korhan, Uyar, Eyigör, Yönt, & Khorshid, 2016),

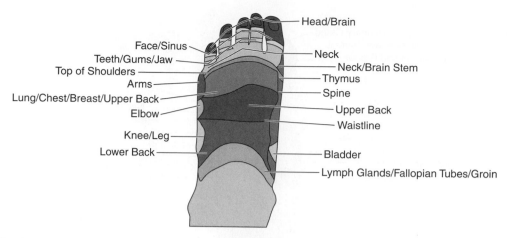

Fig. 24.7 | Top of Left Foot. (From Embong, N. H., Soh, Y. C., Ming, L. C., & Wong, T. W. [2015]. Revisiting reflexology: Concept, evidence, current practice, and practitioner training. *Journal of Traditional and Complementary Medicine, 5*[4], 197–206.)

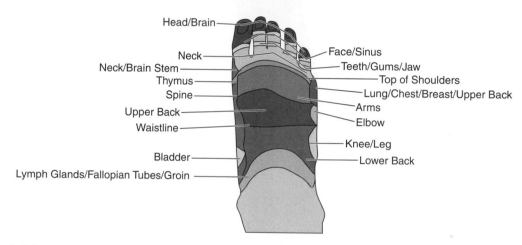

Fig. 24.8 | Top of Right Foot. (From Embong, N. H., Soh, Y. C., Ming, L. C., & Wong, T. W. [2015]. Revisiting reflexology: Concept, evidence, current practice, and practitioner training. *Journal of Traditional and Complementary Medicine, 5*[4], 197–206.)

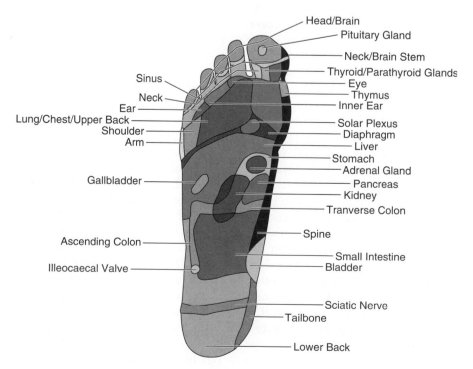

Fig. 24.9 | Right Sole. (From Embong, N. H., Soh, Y. C., Ming, L. C., & Wong, T. W. [2015]. Revisiting reflexology: Concept, evidence, current practice, and practitioner training. *Journal of Traditional and Complementary Medicine, 5*[4], 197–206.)

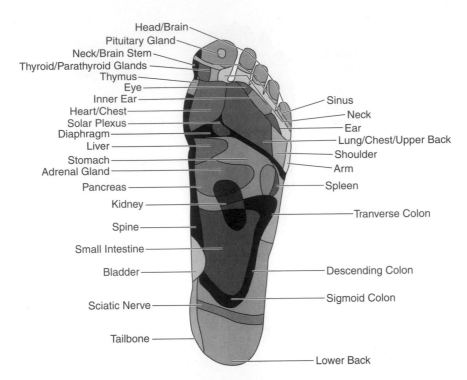

Fig. 24.10 | **Left Sole.** (From Embong, N. H., Soh, Y. C., Ming, L. C., & Wong, T. W. [2015]. Revisiting reflexology: Concept, evidence, current practice, and practitioner training. *Journal of Traditional and Complementary Medicine, 5*[4], 197–206.)

removal of chest tubes (Babajani, Babatabar, Ebadi, Mahmoudi, & Nasiri, 2014), and infants receiving vaccinations (Koç & Gözen, 2015). In a review of studies (n = 5) in which reflexology was used postoperatively (cesarean section, cancer, coronary bypass graft surgeries) the authors concluded that it was an effective intervention with that population to manage pain and anxiety (Ray & Natha, 2017). In a small controlled experimental study designed to discover the efficacy of reflexology to relieve pain compared with a control group using sham TENS the investigators found that reflexology increased both the threshold and the tolerance of acute pain (Samuel & Ebenezer, 2013).

The effectiveness of reflexology is often compared to the effectiveness of other nonpharmacologic interventions to control pain. One study (n = 51) compared the benefit of reflexology with aromatherapy and with a control group with no intervention (Metin & Ozdemir, 2016). The investigators of that study reported that during the 6-week trial, although subjects in both intervention groups had significantly less pain than the control group (P < .001), those in the reflexology group (n = 17) consistently had the lowest pain scores throughout the duration of the trial compared to either the aromatherapy (n = 17) or the control (n =17) group. In another study (n = 40), reflexology was compared to segmental massage of the entire body (Kobza et al., 2017). In that study, reflexology (n = 20) was found to be as effective in relieving migraine headache as segmental massage (n = 20), with no statistical difference between the two

groups. In a larger study (n = 90) participants were randomized to receive reflexology (n = 30), simple massage (n = 30), and control (n = 30) (Zarchi, Hosseini, Khankeh, Roghani, & Biglarian, 2016). In that study, the researchers concluded the patients who received reflexology had significantly lower pain scores (1.96 ± 1.6) compared with those who received simple massage (3.3 ± 1.64) and those in the control group (3.8 ± 0.02). Reflexology (n = 77) was compared with relaxation (n = 82) and standard of care (n = 76) among a group of patients living with CLBP in Great Britain (Poole, Gleen, & Murphy, 2007). In that study, there was no statistical difference in pain scores between the two groups but there was a greater trend in lower pain scores after the interventions among the participants who received reflexology. In a study with patients in an intensive care unit in Iran (n = 90), music therapy and reflexology were compared with standard of care (Yaghoubinia, Navidian, Sheikh, Safarzai, & Tabatabaei, 2016). In that study pain, which was rated using the Behavioral Pain Scale (see Chapter 7), was significantly lower (P < .0001) among the patients who received music therapy (n = 30) (see Chapter 21) and those who received reflexology (n = 30) compared with the control group (n = 30). However, there was no significant difference between the two intervention groups.

Hand reflexology offers an opportunity for ease of use in diverse settings. When hand reflexology was used in a study with people undergoing minimally invasive vascular surgery (n = 100), those who received the hand reflexology (n = 50) had significantly less intraoperative anxiety

Right Foot	Left Foot
1. Greet both feet simultaneously by cupping around forefoot, locate solar plexus reflex with thumbs and press and release while participant inhales and exhales until participant relaxes.	1. Greet both feet simultaneously by cupping around forefoot, locate solar plexus reflex with thumbs and press and release while participant inhales and exhales until participant relaxes.
2. Thoracic area (ball of foot). Diaphragm – thumb walk, push up and under metatarsal bones. Thyroid, parathyroid, shoulder – thumb walk up 5 zones and medial to lateral. Ileocecal valve thumb press for a few seconds.	2. Thoracic area (ball of foot). Diaphragm – thumb walk, push up and under metatarsal bones. Bronchi, lungs, heart, thyroid, parathyroid, shoulder – thumb walk up 5 zones and medial to lateral. Sigmoid thumb press for a few seconds.
3. Abdominal area (arch of foot). Kidney + adrenal – thumb walk across kidney, medial to lateral, adrenal thumb rotate and lift.	3. Abdominal area (arch of foot). Kidney + adrenal – thumb walk across kidney, medial to lateral, adrenal thumb rotate and lift.
4. Head and neck area (toes). Pituitary gland, brain, neck (big toe) – thumb walk around base, dorsal and plantar, thumb walk down brain. Locate pituitary reflex with tip of thumb, rotate and lift. (between big and second toe) pinch webbing with thumb and forefinger ×3.	4. Head and neck area (toes). Pituitary gland, brain, neck (big toe) – thumb walk around base, dorsal and plantar, thumb walk down brain. Locate pituitary reflex with tip of thumb, rotate and lift. (between big and second toe) pinch webbing with thumb and forefinger ×3.
5. Spine. Spinal twist, thumb walk up and down, massage whole foot.	5. Spine. Spinal twist, thumb walk up and down, massage whole foot.
6. Reproductive area (ankle). Uterus/prostate (inner foot below ankle bone) thumb walk. Ovaries/testes (outside foot below ankle bone) thumb walk.	6. Reproductive area (ankle). Uterus/prostate (inner foot below ankle bone) thumb walk. Ovaries/testes (outside foot below ankle bone) thumb walk.
7. Place palm of hands on soles of feet for a few seconds to finish.	7. Place palm of hands on soles of feet for a few seconds to finish.

Fig. 24.11 | **Reflexology Protocol.** (From Rollinson, K., Jones, J., Scott, N., Megson, I. L., & Leslie, S. J. [2016]. The acute (immediate) effects of reflexology on arterial compliance in healthy volunteers: A randomised study. *Complementary Therapies in Clinical Practice, 22,* 16–20.)

(3.24 versus 5.0 on an 11-point scale) and pain (3.44 versus 4.22), with pain being experienced for a shorter duration (Hudson, Davidson, & Whiteley, 2015). Similar results with a statistically significant reduction in anxiety were reported from a study using hand reflexology with patients having coronary angiography (Mobini-Bidgoli et al., 2017).

Despite positive results from small studies, there is little evidence in systematic reviews that reflexology has any demonstrated benefit for analgesia (Embong et al., 2015). The quality of research, including poor methodology and inconsistent design, limits the generalizability and evidence. Fully powered trials with appropriate sham control is needed (Close, Sinclair, McCullough, Liddle, & Hughes, 2016). Research is needed to assess the benefit of reflexology as part of a multimodal approach to pain management among people with a number of painful conditions. Such research has particularly been called for among pregnant women with LBP (Close et al., 2016). Analgesic medication use during pregnancy is a concern, and research of safe nonpharmacologic interventions for pain management during pregnancy is needed. It is also important to replicate and expand upon existing studies (Samuel & Ebenezer, 2013).

Cautions

Reflexology is generally considered safe, but there are cautions. It is imperative to connect with practitioners of reflexology who have appropriate education and experience in using the modality. Situations in which reflexology should be avoided include during the first trimester of pregnancy; in the presence of diarrhea or emesis; in the presence of infectious process or fever; with any localized inflammations or skin disorders of the hands, feet, or ears; and when there has been a negative reaction to reflexology in the past (Embong et al., 2015).

Chiropractic Practice

The chiropractic practice and manipulation approach involve the regular associations or connections of the spinal column with the nervous system and soft tissues of the body. When there is an impairment, the practice includes realigning the spinal column (Thomas & Wahezi, 2012). The formal history of chiropractic is relatively short, beginning in 1895 with D. D. Palmer (Cohen, 2016). From a holistic perspective, Palmer considered the body an active system, with positive impact being exerted on the combination of body, mind, and spirit of the person through adjustment of the spine and vertebral subluxation (Senzon, 2014). At the same time, Palmer spoke of the body in mechanical terms as similar to a machine (Kimura, Russell, & Scaringe, 2016).

There is no one definitive identity held by the chiropractic profession. Rather, there are a variety of philosophical thoughts, beliefs, professional practices, and concepts of what is scope of practice within the chiropractic profession. The lack of cohesion has resulted in division within the profession and confusion amongst other professionals and potential patients (Good, 2016; Triano & McGregor, 2016). The practice of the individual doctor of chiropractic (DC) is largely defined by the practice style and certification achieved by that person (Good, 2016) (Box 24.2). At the same time, Triano and McGregor (2016) separately suggested that there are some core tenets or practices within the chiropractic profession that primarily include diagnosing and treating patients with musculoskeletal complaints, especially affecting the spine. They think DCs use core chiropractic treatments, including methods that manually affect joints with the intention of affecting symptoms and/or function. The authors of the 2016 guidelines of the Council on Chiropractic Guidelines and Practice Parameters expanded on this belief by saying that DCs can work either independently or as members of multidisciplinary teams to restore function among patients with acute and chronic LBP and to educate patients to independently be responsible for their personal health (Globe et al., 2016). Evidence-based guidelines for chiropractic treatment were published by a Canadian group of DCs for intervention with adults with neck pain (Bryans et al., 2014).

One example of a specific chiropractic method is *active release techniques (ARTs)* in which the hand of the clinician is used to exert force on soft tissues that have been repeatedly traumatized or strained (Gliedt & Daniels, 2014; Robb & Pajaczkowski, 2011). Stretches and massage of the affected area are incorporated (Berbrayer &

BOX 24.2 Examples of Chiropractic Subgroups

CERTIFICATION BASED

- Advanced practice
- Diagnostic imaging
- Internal medicine
- Nutrition
- Neurology
- Orthopedics
- Pediatrics
- Rehabilitation
- Sports practitioner
- Wellness

PRACTICE STYLE BASED

- Alternative medicine practitioner (Neovitalists)
- Neuromusculoskeletal specialist
- Primary care physician
- Spinal care specialist (condition based)
- Subluxation-based family practitioner

TECHNIQUE BASED

- Activator methods
- Active release techniques
- Applied kinesiology
- Chiropractic biophysics
- Diversified
- Gonstead
- Network
- Sacro-occipital technique
- Thompson technique
- Upper cervical specific

From Good, C. J. (2016). Chiropractic identity in the United States: Wisdom, courage, and strength. *Journal of Chiropractic Humanities*, 23(1), 29–34.

Fredericson, 2014). It is theorized that ART causes analgesia as a result of the release of endocannabinoids that modulate pain (Robb & Pajaczkowski, 2011). Another example generally considered safe is *activator treatment* in which the DC uses a device that "produces a high-velocity, low-amplitude impact to the spine" (Cohen 2016, p. e162).

Evidence for Pain Management

The effect of chiropractic treatment on pain has mixed reports in the literature (Hawk et al, 2017). Although there is a large body of literature regarding chiropractic interventions, many of the publications are case reports. In one small retrospective case series study (n = 14) that involved patients with temporomandibular joint dysfunction (TMD), symptoms improved after an average of 13.6 chiropractic treatments and pain intensity scores decreased by 80.9% (from 8.3 ± 1.6 to 1.4 ± 1.1 on a numeric zero to ten scale) (Pavia, Fischer, & Roy, 2015). Less impressive was the conclusion of the authors of a systematic review (n = 8 studies) who found chiropractic care was somewhat effective when used with pregnant women (Alcantara, Alcantara, & Alcantara, 2015). In one small study (n = 9) with ice hockey athletes who experienced strains of the adductor muscles, pain thresholds increased after an ART intervention (Robb & Pajaczkowski, 2011). Two recent systematic reviews evaluated the benefit of spinal manipulative therapy (SMT). The authors of the first systematic review (n = 15 RCTs; 1711 patients) concluded there was moderate evidence that SMT is statistically associated with reductions in pain intensity and function (Paige et al., 2017). The other large systematic review, undertaken for the U.S. Department of Veterans Affairs Veterans Health Administration (n = 26 studies), concluded there was inadequate information to make recommendations regarding the use of SMT for LBP or neck pain usually administered by a DC (Shekelle, 2017). An innovative intervention was done at a free chiropractic clinic within a university health clinic with students seeking care primarily for LBP (Stevens, Campeanu, Sorrento, Ryu, & Burke, 2016). Unfortunately, although more than 300 students sought treatment for an average of six treatments, no report was issued about pain outcomes.

Based on the literature, recurrence of pain after chiropractic therapy, at least in Switzerland, appears to be low. In one large Swiss study (n = 722) people with LBP were followed for up to 1 year after chiropractic care and the recurrence rate of 13.4% was low, with duration of LBP before treatment being a strong indicator of recurrence (Knecht, Humphreys, & Wirth, 2017). In a similar Swiss study with people who received chiropractic intervention for neck pain (n = 642) the recurrence at 1 year was 11%, with older age and previous neck pain being risk factors for recurrence (Langenfeld, Humphreys, Swanenburg, & Peterson, 2015).

As with the other manual therapies, additional rigorous research with good methodology and generalizability is needed. An additional criticism of research in the area of chiropractic care is the heterogeneity of the studies (Paige et al., 2017; Shekelle, 2017).

Cautions

Although serious adverse events are reported as infrequently as one per million, minor and moderate adverse events include stiffness and soreness (Globe et al., 2016). The most common adverse effect is soreness (Paige et al., 2017). Fig. 24.12 presents contraindications for

Contraindications for Chiropractic Intervention

Conditions
• Severe osteoporosis
• Multiple myeloma
• Osteomyelitis
• Local primary bone tumors where osseous integrity is in question
• Local metastatic bone tumors
• Pagets disease

Neurologic conditions
• Progressive or sudden (i.e., cauda equina syndrome) neurologic deficit
• Spinal cord tumors that clinically demonstrate neurologic compromise or require specialty referral. In cases where the neoplasm has been properly assessed and is considered to be clinically quiescent and/or perhaps distant to therapeutic target site, then chiropractic manipulative therapy may be utilized.

Inflammatory conditions
• Rheumatoid arthritis in the active systemic stage, or locally in the presence of inflammation or atlantoaxial instability
• Inflammatory phase of ankylosing spondylitis
• Inflammatory phase of psoriatic arthritis
• Reactive arthritis (Reiter's syndrome)

Bleeding disorder
• Unstable congenital bleeding disorders, typically requiring specialty co management
• Unstable acquired bleeding disorders, typically requiring specialty co management
• Unstable abdominal aortic aneurysm

Other
• Structural instability (e.g., unstable spondylolithesis)
• Inadequate physical examination
• Inadequate manipulative training and skills

[a]In some cases, soft tissue, low velocity, low amplitude, or mobilization procedures may still be clinically reasonable and safe.

Fig. 24.12 | Contraindications. (From Globe, G., Farabaugh, R. J., Hawk, C., Morris, C. E., Baker, G., Whalen, W. M., . . . & Augat, T. [2016]. Clinical practice guideline: Chiropractic care for low back pain. *Journal of Manipulative and Physiological Therapeutics, 39*[1], 1–22.)

high-velocity manipulation (Globe et al., 2016). Stroke has been associated with chiropractic manipulation of the neck. One older woman who received chiropractic activator treatment suffered a cerebral hemorrhage after a treatment with the device used on the upper cervical spine (Cohen, 2016). A statement from the American Heart Association suggested that because clinical reports indicate mechanical force is involved in an unidentified number of cervical arterial dissections leading to strokes, before undergoing chiropractic care, potential patients should be informed of the potential risk for cervical arterial dissection (Biller et al., 2014). However, in a large case-crossover study (n = 15,523 cases) (n = 62,092 controls) there was no significant difference between the correlation of stroke after DC appointment and a primary care physician appointment (Cassidy et al., 2017).

An important nonphysiologic caution is that Medicare requirements of chiropractic practice and documentation are from the viewpoint of functional disability related to spinal pain resulting from subluxation, which is not consistent with traditional chiropractic tenets or viewpoint. Medicare also does not reimburse for chiropractic care that can be considered maintenance therapy (Seaman & Soltys, 2013).

Myofascial Trigger Point Therapy

Myofascial trigger points (MTrPs) are highly sensitive or hyperirritable, firm, distinct areas within tight bands of muscle that can be palpated (Shah et al., 2015). MTrPs can either be active or latent. Active MTrPs are characterized by unprompted pain that is local and referred, whereas local and referred pain occurs only with latent MTrPs when pressure is applied on them (Gerwin, 2014). Although latent MTrPs may sound innocuous, it is suggested that their presence is associated with muscle dysfunction that can negatively affect quality of life (Dommerholt, Grieve, Hooks, & Finnegan, 2017). It is important to note that these concepts in large are theoretical, and scientific evidence to support the underlying pathology has not been established (Quintner, Bove, & Cohen, 2014). It is theorized that *myofascial pain syndrome (MPS)* occurs when a number of active MTrPs are found in one particular area of the body (Grieve, Barnett, Coghill, & Cramp, 2013; Oh et al., 2016; Shah et al., 2015). MPS is considered common and limited to older adults because muscle atrophy increases with aging (Oh et al., 2016).

MTrP therapy is undertaken from a variety of perspectives, including the invasive interventions of dry needling (see Chapter 20), acupuncture (see Chapter 23), and trigger point injections, and the noninvasive interventions of ultrasound, laser, transcutaneous electrical nerve stimulation (see Chapter 20), and manual therapy with spray, stretch, and ischemic compression,

also called *trigger point pressure release (TrP)* (Dejung, Lewit, Irnich, & Schleip, 2013; Dommerholt et al., 2017; Grieve et al., 2013; Iverson, 2017; Schmitt & Irnich, 2013). *Ischemic compression (IC)* is described as "applying tolerably painful, persistent manual pressure (usually the thumb) against the tissue barrier of the MTrP" (Behrangrad & Kamali, 2017, p. 558). Although the term is still seen in the literature, ischemic compression is now considered an inaccurate and outdated term, with the preferred terms being *trigger point compression* (Dommerholt et al., 2017) or *trigger point pressure release (TrP)* (Grieve et al., 2013).

Evidence for Pain Management

MTrP therapy has not been researched as extensively as some of the other manual therapies, but the studies that were located are promising. MTrP is thought to play an important role in tension headaches and the associated treatment (Moraska et al., 2015). Treatment of MTrP was evaluated with people with chronic tension headaches (n = 62) (Moraska, Schmiege, Mann, Butryn, & Krutsch, 2017). In that study, pain pressure threshold was significantly improved in the IC group compared to the sham ultrasound or wait list groups and the improvements continued with subsequent treatments (Moraska et al., 2017). Other investigators compared trigger point compression with lumbopelvic manipulation among people living with patellofemoral pain syndrome (n = 40) (Behrangrad & Kamali, 2017). They reported pain intensity and the pain pressure threshold (lowest intensity at which pain is perceived) improved during the study and remained so at 3-month follow-up with trigger point compression (Behrangrad & Kamali, 2017).

Manual pressure of a therapist has been compared with pressure from an algometer, which is an instrument that measures the pressure exerted on the trigger point (Dommerholt et al., 2017; Taleb, Youssef, & Saleh, 2016). In one study the authors concluded that pain and range of motion were significantly improved among the participants who received treatment with algometer plus sham ultrasound (n = 15), compared with those who received manual treatment and sham ultrasound (n = 15) and those who received just sham ultrasound (n = 15) (Dommerholt et al., 2017).

An interesting application of MTrP therapy was done in a small Korean study (n = 11) in which the older adult participants were taught to use an inflatable therapy ball to exert pressure on trigger spots of the back (Oh et al., 2016). Using an air pump, the participants adjusted the pressure in the ball for maximal tolerability of pressure for a 10-minute session. All participants had increases in their pain pressure thresholds, and all but one had reduction in pain intensity. This is a very promising, inexpensive, and reasonable self-care intervention for people living with chronic back pain.

Replication of the described studies along with additional research with strong methodology and clear verbiage is needed.

Cautions

The only reported adverse events of MTrP therapy are soreness, bruising, and stiffness.

Muscle Energy Technique

Muscle energy technique (MET) is a nonthrust myofascial technique used in manual therapy and osteopathy that uses the voluntary isotonic and isometric muscle contractions of the patient against the counter-force exerted by a therapist in an exactly controlled direction that seems to enable smoother movement to a new obstacle (Bise et al., 2017; Cole, 2017; Franke, Fryer, Ostelo, & Kamper, 2016). It is practiced by a variety of clinicians who have manual-therapy licensure, including osteopaths, physicians, chiropractors, physical therapists, occupational therapists, and licensed massage therapists (Cole, 2017). A primary goal of MET is to promote muscle relaxation through contraction and stretching of the muscle with subsequent increase in range of motion (Cole, 2017). Indications for using MET include lengthening, strengthening, and mobilizing muscles and reducing edema and congestion in instances of muscle dysfunction of the back, pelvis, and legs (Franke et al., 2016). One hypothesis of why MET is effective with alleviating pain is that hypoalgesia is achieved through activation of descending inhibitory pain pathways in conjunction with increasing clearance of inflammatory neuropeptides by encouraging drainage of tissue fluids (Fryer & Fossum, 2010).

More recent insight was obtained with asymptomatic subjects (n = 12) when MET was used while magnetic and electrical stimulation of the brain measured corticospinal and spinal reflex excitability, which were significantly decreased with MET (Fryer & Pearce, 2013). When this was stimulation was done with a controlled repeated measure design with MET, medium effect (d = 0.52) was found but only a small effect (d = 0.19) with the control (Fryer, Glynn, Masin, Wroe, & Pearce, 2013).

Evidence for Pain Management

MET is the most frequently researched of the myofascial techniques (Webb, Rajendran, & Hyp, 2016). When MET was compared with positional release therapy among people with acute back pain, there was no difference in reports of pain (Naik, Anand, & Khatri, 2010). However, compared with corticosteroid injections, patients receiving MET not only had comparable improvements in function and reductions in pain inten-

sity at the time of the interventions but those receiving MET continued to have reductions in pain intensity during the following year (Küçükşen, Yilmaz, Sallı, & Uğurlu, 2013). In a study (n = 60) with women with trapezius muscle latent MTrPs, MET (n = 20) was compared with dry needling (n = 20) and with MET plus dry needling (n = 2) (Lari, Okhovatian, sadat Naimi, & Baghban, 2016). (See Chapter 20 for more about dry needling.) In that study all three groups had significantly reduced pain, increases in pain pressure threshold ($P < .001$), and increased function ($P < .001$), but the effects were greater in the group that received both interventions. In another study, MET was compared with another manual intervention, ART (Sadria et al., 2017). That study was done with workers and students (n = 64) with musculoskeletal distress and pain in the trapezius muscles, and both interventions, MET (n = 32) and ART (n = 32), were effective. Results were comparable, with participants in both groups having significant improvements in range of motion ($P < .001$) and reduction in pain intensity scores ($P < .05$) (Sadria et al., 2017). Finally, MET was often used clinically in combination with other interventions in a multimodal approach and the combinations proved effective in reducing pain in clinical trials (Fryer, 2011).

As with other nonpharmacologic therapies, there is a need for high-quality research in MET. The authors of a Cochrane systematic review concluded the research for MET is of poor quality (Franke et al., 2016). Criticisms of that review were that the research was characterized by small studies, poor methodology, and high risk for bias as a result of some of the methods. As with most nonpharmacologic interventions, the authors recommended larger studies with more rigorous methodology and protocols so they can be generalized and replicated.

Cautions

MET is generally considered a safe intervention because patients are essentially exerting their own muscle power in isotonic movement or resistance to the therapist.

Fascial Distortion Model

The fascial distortion model (FDM) was proposed by Stephen Typaldos, DO, in response to frustration with patients not being more fully involved in assessment and treatment and thinking that patients have a subconscious understanding of what is occurring in their bodies (Harrer, 2012). Initially Typaldos (1994) identified four subtypes of fascial distortion: trigger points, trigger bands, folding distortions, and continuum distortions. Subsequently, cylinder distortion and tectonic distortion have been added as subtypes (Harrer, 2012). With FDM, treatment consists of strong pressure held on the particular fascial subtype (Schulze, Finze, Bader, & Lison, 2014).

Evidence for Pain Management

Although FDM has gained some popularity among manual therapists, at the time of this writing, the only research involving FDM was found in three German studies. The first study (n = 60) compared FDM (n = 30) with traditional manual therapy (n = 30) in subjects with a diagnosis of frozen shoulder (Fink, Schiller & Buhick, 2012). In that study, those who received treatment in conjunction with FDM initially reported greater improvement in function and less pain, but function declined after treatments. Also, those in the FDM group reported pain during treatment twice as frequently as those in the control group. The second study in which FDM was used was a prospective case control study with German subjects with medial tibial stress syndrome that reported good results in pain and function (Schulze et al., 2014). The most recent study compared the use of FDM (n = 39) with guideline standard of care in people (n = 38) with acute, nonspecific LBP and reported quicker improvement and less medication use in the FDM group (Richter, Karst, Buhck, & Fink, 2017).

Aside from the studies discussed here, no other research could be found in which FDM was used or studied (Thalhamer, 2017). As with other modalities, clearly additional research with good methodology and reports of adverse events is needed.

Cautions

The caution for FDM is that there is little evidence and few studies. An important concern is the allegation that the painful stimulation that occurs with FDM may result in central sensitization and persistent pain (Thalhamer, 2017).

Key Points

- It is of critical importance that patients receive manual therapy only from a clinician who is appropriately credentialed with experience in treating patients with similar conditions.
- It is always recommended for patients to consult with their health care provider before initiating manual therapy interventions.
- There are different schools of thought and techniques with many of the manual therapies.
- Manual therapies are one complementary therapy within a multimodal approach to pain management.
- Additional rigorous research is needed to establish stronger evidence for the use of manual therapies to help people manage pain.

Case Scenario

Margaret is 63 years old and reports pain in her neck, shoulder, and back. She will only use acetaminophen for pain, and although it helps, the pain is persisting. She is still employed as a cook in a diner and spends most of each day standing and lifting heavy pots. She is resistant to taking other medications and participating in physical therapy (PT) because she previously had a negative experience with a PT office. She is interested in manual therapy and asks you to guide her in finding someone to give her some kind of manual therapy.

1. What types of manual therapy could be helpful for Margaret?
2. What strengths and weaknesses of each would you advise her?
3. When she asks you where she should start, how do you advise her?
4. What advice do you give to Margaret regarding selecting a manual therapist?
5. What important cautions about therapies do you share with Margaret?

Acknowledgments

The author appreciates the review and advice from Dr. Rajavi Parikh regarding osteopathy; Joan Farrenkopf regarding craniosacral therapy; and Susan Beam regarding massage.

References

Alcantara, J., Alcantara, J. D., & Alcantara, J. (2015). The use of validated outcome measures in the chiropractic care of pregnant patients: a systematic review of the literature. *Complementary Therapies in Clinical Practice*, 21(2), 131–136.

Arnadottir, T. S., & Sigurdardottir, A. K. (2013). Is craniosacral therapy effective for migraine? Tested with HIT-6 Questionnaire. *Complementary Therapies in Clinical Practice*, 19(1), 11–14.

Attali, T. V., Bouchoucha, M., & Benamouzig, R. (2013). Treatment of refractory irritable bowel syndrome with visceral osteopathy: Short-term and long-term results of a randomized trial. *Journal of Digestive Diseases*, 14(12), 654–661.

Babajani, S., Babatabar, H., Ebadi, A., Mahmoudi, H., & Nasiri, E. (2014). The effect of foot reflexology massage on the level of pain during chest tube removal after open heart surgery. *Journal of Critical Care Nursing*, 7(1), 15–22.

Behrangrad, S., & Kamali, F. (2017). Comparison of ischemic compression and lumbopelvic manipulation as trigger point therapy for patellofemoral pain syndrome in young adults: A double-blind randomized clinical trial. *Journal of Bodywork and Movement Therapies*, 21(3), 554–564.

Berbrayer, D., & Fredericson, M. (2014). Update on evidence-based treatments for plantar fasciopathy. *Physical Medicine & Rehabilitation*, 6(2), 159–169.

Bervoets, D. C., Luijsterburg, P. A., Alessie, J. J., Buijs, M. J., & Verhagen, A. P. (2015). Massage therapy has short-term benefits for people with common musculoskeletal disorders compared to no treatment: a systematic review. *Journal of Physiotherapy*, 61(3), 106–116.

Białoszewski, D., Bebelski, M., Lewandowska, M., & Słupik, A. (2014). Utility of craniosacral therapy in treatment of patients with non-specific low back pain. Preliminary report. *Ortopedia, Traumatologia, Rehabilitacja, 16*(6), 605–615.

Biller, J., Sacco, R. L., Albuquerque, F. C., Demaerschalk, B. M., Fayad, P., Long, P. H., & Shuaib, A. (2014). Cervical arterial dissections and association with cervical manipulative therapy. *Stroke, 45*(10), 3155–3174.

Bise, C. G., Piva, S. R., & Erhard, R. (2017). Manual Therapy. In J. D. Placzek, & D. A. Boyce (Eds.), *Orthopaedic Physical Therapy Secrets* (3rd Ed). St. Louis, MO: Elsevier.

Brantingham, J. W., Cassa, T. K., Bonnefin, D., Pribicevic, M., Robb, A., Pollard, H., … Korporaal, C. (2013). Manipulative and multimodal therapy for upper extremity and temporomandibular disorders: a systematic review. *Journal of Manipulative and Physiological Therapeutics, 36*(3), 143–201.

Brough, N., Lindenmeyer, A., Thistlethwaite, J., Lewith, G., & Stewart-Brown, S. (2015). Perspectives on the effects and mechanisms of craniosacral therapy: A qualitative study of users' views. *European Journal of Integrative Medicine, 7*(2), 172–183.

Bryans, R., Decina, P., Descarreaux, M., Duranleau, M., Marcoux, H., Potter, B., … White, E. (2014). Evidence-based guidelines for the chiropractic treatment of adults with neck pain. *Journal of Manipulative and Physiological Therapeutics, 37*(1), 42–63.

Cassidy, J. D., Boyle, E., Côté, P., Hogg-Johnson, S., Bondy, S. J., & Haldeman, S. (2017). Risk of carotid stroke after chiropractic care: a population-based case-crossover study. *Journal of Stroke and Cerebrovascular Diseases, 26*(4), 842–850.

Castro-Sánchez, A. M., Lara-Palomo, I. C., Matarán-Penarrocha, G. A., Saavedra-Hernández, M., Pérez-Mármol, J. M., & Aguilar-Ferrándiz, M. E. (2016). Benefits of Craniosacral Therapy in Patients with Chronic Low Back Pain: A Randomized Controlled Trial. *The Journal of Alternative and Complementary Medicine, 22*(8), 650–657.

Cerritelli, F., Verzella, M., & Barlafante, G. (2014). Quality of life in patients referring to private osteopathic clinical practice: A prospective observational study. *Complementary Therapies in Medicine, 22*(4), 625–631.

Cerritelli, F., Lacorte, E., Ruffini, N., & Vanacore, N. (2017). Osteopathy for primary headache patients: a systematic review. *Journal of Pain Research, 10*, 601.

Cerritelli, F., Ruffini, N., Lacorte, E., & Vanacore, N. (2016). Osteopathic manipulative treatment in neurological diseases: systematic review of the literature. *Journal of the Neurological Sciences, 369*, 333–341.

Cerritelli, F., Ginevri, L., Messi, G., Caprari, E., Di Vincenzo, M., Renzetti, C., … Provinciali, L. (2015). Clinical effectiveness of osteopathic treatment in chronic migraine: 3-Armed randomized controlled trial. *Complementary Therapies in Medicine, 23*(2), 149–156.

Close, C., Sinclair, M., Mc Cullough, J., Liddle, D., & Hughes, C. (2016). A pilot randomised controlled trial (RCT) investigating the effectiveness of reflexology for managing pregnancy low back and/or pelvic pain. *Complementary Therapies in Clinical Practice, 23*, 117–124.

Cohen, F. L. (2016). Cerebral hemorrhage following chiropractic activator treatment–case report and review of literature. *Journal of Neurological Surgery Reports, 77*(4), e162–e167.

Cole, J. (2017). A Comparison of Three Manipulative Therapy Techniques: CranioSacral Therapy, Muscle Energy Technique, and Fascial Distortion Model. In *Thesis*. Laramie, WY: University of Wyoming.

Crane, J. D. (2012). Massage therapy attenuates inflammatory signaling after exercise-induced muscle damage. *Science Translational Medicine, 4*(119), 119ra13. https://doi.org/10.1126/scitranslmed.3002882.

Crawford, C., Boyd, C., Paat, C. F., Price, A., Xenakis, L., Yang, E., & Evidence for Massage Therapy (EMT) Working Group. (2016). The impact of massage therapy on function in pain populations—A systematic review and meta-analysis of randomized controlled trials: Part I, patients experiencing pain in the general population. *Pain Medicine, 17*(7), 1353–1375.

Dahiya, S., & Banerjee, D. N. (2016). Complementary and alternative medicine: What is it good for? *Bulletin of Pharmaceutical Research, 6*(3), 83–92.

Dejung, B., Lewit, K., Irnich, D., & Schlip, R. (2013). Manual therapy and physiotherapy. In D. Irnich (Ed.), *Myofascial Trigger Points* (pp. 133–147). St. Louis, MO: Elsevier.

Dommerholt, J. (2017). A critical overview of the current myofascial pain literature–January 2017. *Journal of Bodywork and Movement Therapies, 21*(1), 141–147.

Dommerholt, J., Grieve, R., Hooks, T., & Finnegan, M. (2017). A critical overview of the current myofascial pain literature–March 2017. *Journal of Bodywork and Movement Therapies, 21*(2), 378–385.

Donoyama, N., Suoh, S., & Ohkoshi, N. (2014). Effectiveness of Anma massage therapy in alleviating physical symptoms in outpatients with Parkinson's disease: a before-after study. *Complementary Therapies in Clinical Practice, 20*(4), 251–261.

Dreyer, N. E., Cutshall, S. M., Huebner, M., Foss, D. M., Lovely, J. K., Bauer, B. A., & Cima, R. R. (2015). Effect of massage therapy on pain, anxiety, relaxation, and tension after colorectal surgery: A randomized study. *Complementary therapies in clinical practice, 21*(3), 154–159.

Elden, H., Lundgren, I., & Robertson, E. (2014). Effects of craniosacral therapy as experienced by pregnant women with severe pelvic girdle pain: an interview study. *Clinical Nursing Studies, 2*(3), 140.

Elden, H., Östgaard, H. C., Glantz, A., Marciniak, P., Linnér, A. C., & Olsén, M. F. (2013). Effects of craniosacral therapy as adjunct to standard treatment for pelvic girdle pain in pregnant women: a multicenter, single blind, randomized controlled trial. *Acta Obstetricia et Gynecologica Scandinavica, 92*(7), 775–782.

Ellison, D. L. (2017). Physiology of Pain. *Critical Care Nursing Clinics, 29*(4), 397–406.

Embong, N. H., Soh, Y. C., Ming, L. C., & Wong, T. W. (2015). Revisiting reflexology: Concept, evidence, current practice, and practitioner training. *Journal of Traditional and Complementary Medicine, 5*(4), 197–206.

Field, T. (2014). Massage therapy research review. *Complementary Therapies in Clinical Practice, 20*(4), 224–229.

Field, T. (2016). Massage therapy research review. *Complementary Therapies in Clinical Practice, 24*(8), 19–31.

Field, T. (2018). Pain and Massage Therapy: A Narrative Review. *Current Research in Complementary & Alternative Medicine,2018,* (1). CRCAM-125. DOI: 10.29011. CRCAM-125/100025.

Field, T., Diego, M., & Solien-Wolfe, L. (2014). Massage therapy plus topical analgesic is more effective than massage alone for hand arthritis pain. *Journal of Bodywork and Movement Therapies, 18*(3), 322–325.

Fink, M., Schiller, J., & Buhck, H. (2012). Efficacy of a manual treatment method according to the fascial distortion model in the management of contracted ("frozen") shoulder. *Zeitschrift fur Orthopadie und Unfallchirurgie, 150*(4), 420–427.

Fitzgerald, W. H., Bowers, E. F., & White, G. S. (1994). *Zone therapy*. Health Research Books.

Franke, H., Franke, J. D., & Fryer, G. (2014). Osteopathic manipulative treatment for nonspecific low back pain: a systematic review and meta-analysis. *BMC Musculoskeletal Disorders, 15*(1), 286.

Franke, H., Fryer, G., Ostelo, R. W., & Kamper, S. J. (2016). Muscle energy technique for non-specific low-back pain. A Cochrane systematic review. *International Journal of Osteopathic Medicine, 20*, 41–52.

Fryer, G. (2011). Muscle energy technique: An evidence-informed approach. *International Journal of Osteopathic Medicine, 14*(1), 3–9.

Fryer, G., & Fossum, C. (2010). Therapeutic mechanisms underlying muscle energy approaches. In C. Fernández-de-las-Peñas, L. Arendt-Nielsen, & R. D. Gerwin (Eds.), *Tension-type and Cervicogenic Headache: Pathophysiology, Diagnosis, and Management* (pp. 221–229). Sudbury, MA: Jones and Bartlett Publishers.

Fryer, G., & Pearce, A. J. (2013). The effect of muscle energy technique on corticospinal and spinal reflex excitability in asymptomatic participants. *Journal of Bodywork and Movement Therapies, 17*(4), 440–447.

Fryer, G., Glynn, B., Masin, K., Wroe, M., & Pearce, A. J. (2013). Lumbosacral Muscle Energy Technique produces immediate decreases in corticospinal and spinal reflex excitability in asymptomatic participants. *International Journal of Osteopathic Medicine, 16*(1), e5–e6.

Gerwin, R. D. (2014). Diagnosis of myofascial pain syndrome. *Physical Medicine and Rehabilitation Clinics, 25*(2), 341–355.

Gliedt, J. A., & Daniels, C. J. (2014). Chiropractic treatment of lateral epicondylitis: a case report utilizing active release techniques. *Journal of Chiropractic Medicine, 13*(2), 104–109.

Globe, G., Farabaugh, R. J., Hawk, C., Morris, C. E., Baker, G., Whalen, W. M., ... Augat, T. (2016). Clinical practice guideline: chiropractic care for low back pain. *Journal of Manipulative and Physiological Therapeutics, 39*(1), 1–22.

Good, C. J. (2016). Chiropractic Identity in the United States: Wisdom, Courage, and Strength. *Journal of Chiropractic Humanities, 23*(1), 29–34.

Grieve, R., Barnett, S., Coghill, N., & Cramp, F. (2013). Myofascial trigger point therapy for triceps surae dysfunction: a case series. *Manual Therapy, 18*(6), 519–525.

Haller, H., Cramer, H., Werner, M., & Dobos, G. (2015). Treating the sequelae of postoperative meningioma and traumatic brain injury: a case of implementation of craniosacral therapy in integrative inpatient care. *The Journal of Alternative and Complementary Medicine, 21*(2), 110–112.

Haller, H., Ostermann, T., Lauche, R., Cramer, H., & Dobos, G. (2014). Credibility of a comparative sham control intervention for Craniosacral Therapy in patients with chronic neck pain. *Complementary Therapies in Medicine, 22*(6), 1053–1059.

Harper, B., Jagger, K., Aron, A., Steinbeck, L., & Stecco, A. (2017). A commentary review of the cost effectiveness of manual therapies for neck and low back pain. *Journal of Bodywork and Movement Therapies, 21*(3), 684–691.

Harrer, G. (2012). The fascial distortion model. In R. Schliep, T. W. Findley, L. Chaitow, & P. A. Huijing (Eds.), *Fascia: The Tensional Network of the Human Body* (pp. 397–403). London: Churchill Livingstone.

Hawk, C., Schneider, M. J., Haas, M., Katz, P., Dougherty, P., Gleberzon, B., ... Weeks, J. (2017). Best Practices for Chiropractic Care for Older Adults: A Systematic Review and Consensus Update. *Journal of Manipulative and Physiological Therapeutics, 40*(4), 217–229.

Hensel, K. L., Carnes, M. S., & Stoll, S. T. (2016). Pregnancy Research on Osteopathic Manipulation Optimizing Treatment Effects: The PROMOTE Study Protocol. *The Journal of the American Osteopathic Association, 116*(11), 716–724.

Hudson, B. F., Davidson, J., & Whiteley, M. S. (2015). The impact of hand reflexology on pain, anxiety and satisfaction during minimally invasive surgery under local anaesthetic: A randomised controlled trial. *International Journal of Nursing Studies, 52*(12), 1789–1797.

Irnich, D. (2013). Complementary and alternative therapies and naturopathic treatments. In D. Irnich (Ed.), *Myofascial Trigger Points* (pp. 233–244). St. Louis, MO: Elsevier.

Iverson, M. D. (2017). Introduction to physical medicine, physical therapy and rehabilitation. In G. S. Firestein, R. C. Budd, S. E. Gabriel, I. B. McInnes, & J. R. O'Dell (Eds.), *Kelley and Firestein's Textbook of Rheumatology* (10th Ed., pp. 560–571). Philadelphia, PA: Elsevier.

Jäkel, A., & von Hauenshcild, P. (2012). A systematic review to evaluate the clinical benefits of craniosacral therapy. *Complementary Therapies in Medicine, 20*(6), 456–465.

Jones, J., Thomson, P., Lauder, W., Howie, K., & Leslie, S. J. (2012). Reflexology has an acute (immediate) haemodynamic effect in healthy volunteers: a double-blind randomised controlled trial. *Complementary Therapies in Clinical Practice, 18*(4), 204–211.

Keeratitanont, K., Jensen, M. P., Chatchawan, U., & Auvichayapat, P. (2015). The efficacy of traditional Thai massage for the treatment of chronic pain: a systematic review. *Complementary Therapies in Clinical Practice, 21*(1), 26–32.

Kennedy, A. B., Cambron, J. A., Sharpe, P. A., Travillian, R. S., & Saunders, R. P. (2016). Process for massage therapy practice and essential assessment. *Journal of Bodywork and Movement Therapies, 20*(3), 484–496.

Kobza, W., Lizis, P., & Zięba, H. R. (2017). Effects of feet reflexology versus segmental massage in reducing pain and its intensity, frequency and duration of the attacks in females with migraine: a pilot study. *Journal of Traditional Chinese Medicine, 37*(2), 214–219.

Koç, T., & Gözen, D. (2015). The effect of foot reflexology on acute pain in infants: A randomized controlled trial. *Worldviews on Evidence-Based Nursing, 12*(5), 289–296.

Korhan, E. A., Uyar, M., Eyigör, C., Yönt, G. H., & Khorshid, L. (2016). Effects of reflexology on pain in patients with fibromyalgia. *Holistic Nursing Practice, 30*(6), 351–359.

Kimura, M. N., Russell, R., & Scaringe, J. (2016). Professional Identity at Los Angeles College of Chiropractic. *Journal of Chiropractic Humanities, 23*(1), 61–67.

Knecht, C., Humphreys, B. K., & Wirth, B. (2017). An Observational Study on Recurrences of Low Back Pain During the First 12 Months After Chiropractic Treatment. *Journal of Manipulative and Physiological Therapeutics*, 40(6), 427–433.

Küçükşen, S., Yilmaz, H., Sallı, A., & Uğurlu, H. (2013). Muscle energy technique versus corticosteroid injection for management of chronic lateral epicondylitis: randomized controlled trial with 1-year follow-up. *Archives of Physical Medicine and Rehabilitation*, 94(11), 2068–2074.

Langenfeld, A., Humphreys, B. K., Swanenburg, J., & Peterson, C. K. (2015). Prognostic factors for recurrences in neck pain patients up to 1 year after chiropractic care. *Journal of Manipulative and Physiological Therapeutics*, 38(7), 458–464.

Lari, A. Y., Okhovatian, F., sadat Naimi, S., & Baghban, A. A. (2016). The effect of the combination of dry needling and MET on latent trigger point upper trapezius in females. *Manual Therapy*, 21, 204–209.

Licciardone, J. C., & Aryal, S. (2014). Clinical response and relapse in patients with chronic low back pain following osteopathic manual treatment: Results from the OSTEOPATHIC Trial. *Manual Therapy*, 19(6), 541–548.

Licciardone, J. C., Gatchel, R. J., & Aryal, S. (2016). Recovery from chronic low back pain after osteopathic manipulative treatment: a randomized controlled trial. *Journal of the American Osteopathic Association*, 116(3), 144–155.

Licciardone, J. C., Kearns, C. M., & Crow, W. T. (2014). Changes in biomechanical dysfunction and low back pain reduction with osteopathic manual treatment: Results from the OSTEOPARHIC Trial. *Manual Therapy*, 19(4), 324–330.

Licciardone, J. C., Minotti, D. E., Gatchel, R. J., Kearns, C. M., & Singh, K. P. (2013). Osteopathic manual treatment and ultrasound therapy for chronic low back pain: a randomized controlled trial. *The Annals of Family Medicine*, 11(2), 122–129.

Metin, Z. G., & Ozdemir, L. (2016). The effects of aromatherapy massage and reflexology on pain and fatigue in patients with rheumatoid arthritis: a randomized controlled trial. *Pain Management Nursing*, 17(2), 140–149.

Miller, D. W. (2015). Integrative Perspectives on Human Growth and Development: Insights into Acupuncture-Point Function from Developmental and Evolutionary Viewpoints. *Medical Acupuncture*, 27(2), 95–101.

Miozzo, A. P., Stein, C., Bozzetto, C. B., & Plentz, R. D. M. (2016). Massage therapy reduces pain and anxiety after cardiac surgery: A systematic review and meta-analysis of randomized clinical trials. *Clinical Trials and Regulatory Science in Cardiology*, 23, 1–8.

Mobini-Bidgoli, M., Taghadosi, M., Gilasi, H., & Farokhian, A. (2017). The effect of hand reflexology on anxiety in patients undergoing coronary angiography: A single-blind randomized controlled trial. *Complementary Therapies in Clinical Practice*, 27, 31–36.

Moraska, A. F., Schmiege, S. J., Mann, J. D., Butryn, N., & Krutsch, J. P. (2017). Responsiveness of myofascial trigger points to single and multiple trigger point release massages: a randomized, placebo controlled trial. *American Journal of Physical Medicine & Rehabilitation*, 96(9), 639–645.

Moraska, A. F., Stenerson, L., Butryn, N., Krutsch, J. P., Schmiege, S. J., & Mann, J. D. (2015). Myofascial trigger point-focused head and neck massage for recurrent

tension-type headache: a randomized, placebo-controlled clinical trial. *The Clinical Journal of Pain*, 31(2), 159.

Naik, P. P., Anand, H., & Khatri, S. M. (2010). Comparison of muscle energy technique and positional release therapy in acute low back pain–RCT. *Indian Journal of Physiotherapy and Occupational Therapy*, 4(2), 32–36.

Oh, S., Kim, M., Lee, M., Lee, D., Kim, T., & Yoon, B. (2016). Self-Management of Myofascial Trigger Point Release by using an Inflatable Ball among Elderly Patients with Chronic Low Back Pain: A Case Series. *Annals of Yoga Physical Therapy*, 1(3), 1013.

Paige, N. M., Miake-Lye, I. M., Booth, M. S., Beroes, J. M., Mardian, A. S., Dougherty, P., ... Shekelle, P. G. (2017). Association of Spinal Manipulative Therapy with Clinical Benefit and Harm for Acute Low Back Pain: Systematic Review and Meta-analysis. *JAMA*, 317(14), 1451–1460.

Pavia, S., Fischer, R., & Roy, R. (2015). Chiropractic Treatment of Temporomandibular Dysfunction: A Retrospective Case Series. *Journal of Chiropractic Medicine*, 14(4), 279–284.

Pearlman, A. (2016). Complementary and alternative medicine. In L. Goldman, & A. Schafer (Eds.), *Goldman Cecil Medicine* (25th Ed, pp. 181–184.e1). NY, NY: Elsevier Inc.

Poole, H., Glenn, S., & Murphy, P. (2007). A randomised controlled study of reflexology for the management of chronic low back pain. *European Journal of Pain*, 11(8), 878–887.

Quintner, J. L., Bove, G. M., & Cohen, M. L. (2014). A critical evaluation of the trigger point phenomenon. *Rheumatology*, 54(3), 392–399.

Ramesh, C., Pai, V. B., Patil, N., Nayak, B. S., George, A., George, L. S., & Devi, E. S. (2015). Effectiveness of massage therapy on post-operative outcomes among patients undergoing cardiac surgery: A systematic review. *International Journal of Nursing Sciences*, 2(3), 304–312.

Ray, M. B. S., & Natha, M. H. (2017). Foot reflexology: Effect on pain and anxiety in post operative patient. *International Education and Research Journal*, 3(5), 49–51.

Richter, D., Karst, M., Buhck, H., & Fink, M. G. (2017). Efficacy of Fascial Distortion Model Treatment for Acute, Nonspecific Low-Back Pain in Primary Care: A Prospective Controlled Trial. *Alternative Therapies in Health and Medicine.*, 23(5), AT5522.

Robb, A., & Pajaczkowski, J. (2011). Immediate effect on pain thresholds using active release technique on adductor strains: pilot study. *Journal of Bodywork and Movement Therapies*, 15(1), 57–62.

Rollinson, K., Jones, J., Scott, N., Megson, I. L., & Leslie, S. J. (2016). The acute (immediate) effects of reflexology on arterial compliance in healthy volunteers: A randomised study. *Complementary Therapies in Clinical Practice*, 22, 16–20.

Ruffini, N., D'Alessandro, G., Cardinali, L., Frondaroli, F., & Cerritelli, F. (2016). Osteopathic manipulative treatment in gynecology and obstetrics: a systematic review. *Complementary Therapies in Medicine*, 26, 72–78.

Sadria, G., Hosseini, M., Rezasoltani, A., Bagheban, A. A., Davari, A., & Seifolahi, A. (2017). A comparison of the effect of the active release and muscle energy techniques on the latent trigger points of the upper trapezius. *Journal of Bodywork and Movement Therapies.*, 21(4), 920–925.

Samuel, C. A., & Ebenezer, I. S. (2013). Exploratory study on the efficacy of reflexology for pain threshold and tolerance using an ice-pain experiment and sham TENS control. *Complementary Therapies in Clinical Practice*, 19(2), 57–62.

Schmitt, H. J., & Irnich, D. (2013). Trigger point infiltration. In D. Irnich. *Myofascial Trigger Points* (pp. 171–177). St. Louis, MO: Elsevier.

Schulze, C., Finze, S., Bader, R., & Lison, A. (2014). Treatment of medial tibial stress syndrome according to the fascial distortion model: a prospective case control study. *The Scientific World Journal, 2014.* ID 790626. In *6 pages.* https://doi.org/10.1155/2014/790626.

Schwerla, F., Wirthwein, P., Rütz, M., & Resch, K. L. (2014). Osteopathic treatment in patients with primary dysmenorrhea: A randomised controlled trial. *International Journal of Osteopathic Medicine, 17*(4), 222–231.

Seaman, D. R., & Soltys, J. R. (2013). Straight chiropractic philosophy as a barrier to Medicare compliance: a discussion of 5 incongruent issues. *Journal of Chiropractic Humanities, 20*(1), 19–26.

Senzon, S. A. (2014). Chiropractic Professionalization and Accreditation: An Exploration of the History of Conflict Between Worldviews Through the Lens of Developmental Structuralism. *Journal of Chiropractic Humanities, 21*(1), 25–48.

Shah, J. P., Thaker, N., Heimur, J., Aredo, J. V., Sikdar, S., & Gerber, L. (2015). Myofascial trigger points then and now: a historical and scientific perspective. *Physical Medicine &Rehabilitation, 7*(7), 746–761.

Shekelle, P. G., Paige, N. M., Miake-Lye, I. M., Beroes, J. M., Booth, M. S., & Shanman, R. (2017). The Effectiveness and Harms of Chiropractic Care for the Treatment of Acute Neck and Lower Back Pain: A Systematic Review. *Washington (DC): Department of Veterans Affairs (US).* 2017 Apr. Available from: https://www.ncbi.nlm.nih.gov/books/NBK441754/.

Sheraton, A., Streckfuss, J., & Grace, S. (2018). Experiences of pregnant women receiving osteopathic care. *Journal of Bodywork and Movement Therapies, 22*(2), 321–327.

Steel, A., Blaich, R., Sundberg, T., & Adams, J. (2017). The role of osteopathy in clinical care: Broadening the evidence-base. *International Journal of Osteopathic Medicine, 24*(2017), 32–36.

Steel, A., Sundberg, T., Reid, R., Ward, L., Bishop, F. L., Leach, M., & Adams, J. (2017). Osteopathic manipulative treatment: A systematic review and critical appraisal of comparative effectiveness and health economics research. *Musculoskeletal Science and Practice, 27*, 165–175.

Stevens, G., Campeanu, M., Sorrento, A. T., Ryu, J., & Burke, J. (2016). Retrospective Demographic Analysis of Patients Seeking Care at a Free University Chiropractic Clinic. *Journal of Chiropractic Medicine, 15*(1), 19–26.

Taleb, W. A., Youssef, A. R., & Saleh, A. (2016). The effectiveness of manual versus algometer pressure release techniques for treating active myofascial trigger points of the upper trapezius. *Journal of Bodywork and Movement Therapies, 20*(4), 863–869.

Thalhamer, M. C. (2017). A fundamental critique of the fascial distortion model and its application in clinical practice. *Journal of Bodywork and Movement Therapies, 22*(1), 112–117.

Thomas, M. A., & Wahezi, S. E. (2012). Complementary and alternative medicine treatments for back pain. In D. Vincent (Ed.), *Spine Secrets Plus* (2nd Ed, pp. 146–150). St. Louis: Mosby.

Tiidus, P. M. (2015). Alternative treatments for muscle injury: massage, cryotherapy, and hyperbaric oxygen. *Current Reviews in Musculoskeletal Medicine, 8*(2), 162–167.

Todd, A. J., Carroll, M. T., Robinson, A., & Mitchell, E. K. (2015). Adverse events due to chiropractic and other manual therapies for infants and children: a review of the literature. *Journal of Manipulative and Physiological Therapeutics, 38*(9), 699–712.

Triano, J. J., & McGregor, M. (2016). Core and Complementary Chiropractic: Lowering Barriers to Patient Utilization of Services. *Journal of Chiropractic Humanities, 23*(1), 1–13.

Typaldos, S. (1994). Introducing the fascial distortion model. *AAO Journal, 4*, 14–18.

Tyreman, S. (2013). Re-evaluating 'osteopathic principles'. *International Journal of Osteopathic Medicine, 16*(1), 38–45.

Upledger, J., Gossinger, R., Ash, D., & Cohen, D. (2008). *CarnioSacral Therapy What it is How it works.* Berkley, CA: North Atlantic Books.

Vogel, S. (2016). Osteopathy – a complex business. *International Journal of Osteopathic Medicine, 19*(1), 1–2.

Wamontree, P., Kanchanakhan, N., & Eungpinichpong, W. (2015). Effects of traditional Thai self-massage using a massage stick versus Ibuprofen on upper back pain associated with myofascial trigger points: a pilot study. *Journal of Health Research, 29*(6), 403–408.

Webb, T. R., & Rajendran, D. (2016). Myofascial techniques: what are their effects on joint range of motion and pain? a systematic review and meta-analysis of randomised controlled trials. *Journal of Bodywork and Movement Therapies, 20*(3), 682–699.

Wei, X., Wang, S., Li, L., & Zhu, L. (2017). Clinical evidence of Chinese massage therapy (Tui Na) for cervical radiculopathy: a systematic review and meta-analysis. *Evidence-Based Complementary and Alternative Medicine, 2017.* https://doi.org/10.1155/2017/9519285.

Wieting, J. M., Weaver, J. L., Kramer, J. A., & Morales-Egizi, L. (2017). Appendix 2: American Osteopathic Association Specialty Board Certification. *The Journal of the American Osteopathic Association, 117*(4), 268.

Wolf, C. J., & Brault, J. S. (2016). Manipulation, traction and massage. In D. X. Cifu (Ed.), *Braddom's Physical Medicine and Rehabilitation* (5th Ed). Philadelphia, PA: Elsevier, pp. 347–367(p. e3).

Won, A. S., Bailenson, J., Lee, J., & Lanier, J. (2015). Homuncular flexibility in virtual reality. *Journal of Computer-Mediated Communication, 20*(3), 241–259.

Yaghoubinia, F., Navidian, A., Sheikh, S., Safarzai, E., & Tabatabaei, S. M. N. A. D. (2016). Effect of music therapy and reflexology on pain in unconscious patients: A randomized clinical trial. *International Journal of Medical Research & Health Sciences, 5*(9), 288–295.

Yuan, S. L. K., Matsutani, L. A., & Marques, A. P. (2015). Effectiveness of different styles of massage therapy in fibromyalgia: a systematic review and meta-analysis. *Manual Therapy, 20*(2), 257–264.

Zarchi, A. R., Hosseini, M. A., Khankeh, H. R., Roghani, R. S., & Biglarian, A. (2016). Evaluation of the effect of reflexology massage on pain severity after abdominal surgery. *Medical-Surgical Nursing Journal, 5*(3), 12–17.

Zegarra-Parodi, R., & Cerritelli, F. (2016). The enigmatic case of cranial osteopathy: Evidence versus clinical practice. *International Journal of Osteopathic Medicine, 21*, 1–4.

Zou, G., Wang, G., Li, J., Wu, G., Huang, J., & Huang, S. (2017). Danger of injudicious use of tui-na therapy in ankylosing spondylitis. *European Spine Journal, 26*(1), 178–180.

Chapter 25 Spirituality as a Component of Multimodal Pain Management

Susan O'Conner-Von, Ann Quinlan-Colwell

CHAPTER OUTLINE

Spirituality, pg. 673

Prayer, pg. 674

  Evidence for Pain Management, pg. 674

  Cautions, pg. 674

Meditation, pg. 675

  Centering Prayer (Spiritual Meditation), pg. 678

  Kabbalah (Qabalah), pg. 679

  Loving Kindness Meditation, pg. 679

  Mindfulness Meditation, pg. 680

  Reflective Walking, Labyrinth Walking, and Movement Meditation, pg. 680

  Ridhwan School Diamond Approach, pg. 680

  Self-Realization Fellowship, pg. 681

  Tibetan Buddhist Meditation, pg. 681

  Transcendental Meditation, pg. 681

  Zen Buddhism/Ch'an, pg. 682

General Cautions and Precautions Regarding Meditation, pg. 682

Key Points, pg. 683

Case Scenario, pg. 683

References, pg. 684

Spirituality

Many definitions of spirituality exist in the literature. Consistent among these definitions is the concept that spirituality is deeply personal and complex. Broader than the concept of religion, spirituality crosses the boundaries of culture. Furthermore, culture influences all aspects of a patient's life, especially the patient's beliefs about health and well-being. Although the terms *spirituality* and *religion* are frequently used interchangeably, religion is often defined as a formalized system of doctrine, beliefs, and practices (Timmins & Neill, 2013). Spirituality, on the other hand, has a more broad and inclusive nature (Koenig, 2004) involving what gives meaning to the life of the individual (Fogerite & Goldberg, 2008). Religion can be thought of as the structure through which a person expresses spirituality; however, religion is not essential to spirituality.

Given the need to advance research in this area, a commonly accepted definition of spirituality was developed at a 2009 national interprofessional consensus conference on the importance of spirituality in quality palliative care (Puchalski et al, 2009). That definition states: "Spirituality is the aspect of humanity that refers to the way individuals seek and express meaning and purpose and the way they experience their connectedness to the moment, to self, to nature, and to the significant or sacred" (Puchalski et al., 2009, p. 887).

Patients with chronic pain often turn to religion or spirituality to cope with their condition (Dedeli & Kaptan, 2013). Although a significant proportion of patients living with chronic pain or with a life-threatening illness express a desire to discuss their spirituality and spiritual needs, these patients often find this important aspect of their being is not assessed or explored by health professionals (Balboni et al., 2013; Pearce, Coan, Herndon, Koenig, & Abernethy, 2012). Nurses play a critical role in the assessment of spiritual, religious, and cultural needs for patients in pain. "Spiritual views can have a substantial impact on patients' understanding of pain and decisions about pain management" (Unruh, 2007, p. 67). As described in provision 1 of the American Nurses Association *Code of Ethics for Nurses* (2015), nurses are to consider such factors as culture, value systems, and religious or spiritual beliefs when planning patient- and family-centered care. This is important because patients can use "spirituality as a positive and constructive coping strategy, with religious rituals, meditation, prayer and mindfulness among the spiritual resources to help them cope with the intensity of their pain and suffering" (HealthCare Chaplaincy Network and Spiritual Care Association, 2017, p, 7).

Prayer

Prayer is the most common spiritual ritual practiced by religious and nonreligious patients. Common in every culture, at a minimum prayer is used during times of stress, uncertainty, and end of life (Young & Koopsen, 2011). There are a number of forms of prayer: intercessory prayer is praying on behalf of another, ritual prayer involves using readings or formal prayers, and petitionary prayer asks *the Sacred* for a specific request (Young & Koopsen, 2011). Centering prayer is considered a spiritual or religious form of meditation. The goal is to open a space for *the Sacred* or that which holds ultimate meaning or purpose (Keating, 2002; Steinhauser et al., 2017).

Evidence for Pain Management

There is a growing body of research examining the connection among mind, body, and spirit. One of the first national government surveys to examine the use of complementary and alternative medicine (CAM) was conducted in 2002 by the National Institutes of Health (NIH) and the Centers for Disease Control and Prevention's (CDC's) National Center for Health Statistics (National Center for Complementary and Integrative Health [NCCIH], 2017). The results of that survey consisted of responses from 31,044 adults aged 18 years and older. The results revealed that 36% of the respondents used some form of CAM. When *prayer for health reasons* was added to the definition of CAM in the survey, the percent of adults using CAM in the United States rose to 62%. The most frequently reported conditions of those seeking CAM therapies were back pain, neck pain, cancer, chronic pain, human immunodeficiency virus (HIV), anxiety, depression, headaches, arthritis, and fatigue (NCCIH, 2017).

Since that initial NIH and CDC survey, numerous studies have explored the benefits of prayer for health reasons, including to control pain. In a cross-sectional study, Ezenwa et al. (2017) examined the coping strategies of 52 adults with sickle cell pain. The mean age of the sample was 34 years, and the majority were African American (92%) and women (79%). Of particular importance was investigating the potential association between health care injustice and what strategies these patients used to cope with their sickle cell pain, given that the population consisted mostly of patients of African descent who have historically experienced health care inequalities (Ezenwa et al., 2017). Results revealed that patients who reported health care justice, that is, in their view they were treated fairly by physicians and nurses, more often reported the use of praying and hoping, heat or cold, massage, diverting attention, or using calming self-statements to cope with their pain (Ezenwa et al., 2017). Patients who reported health care injustice, that is, in their view they were not treated fairly by physicians and nurses, were more likely to use isolation, catastrophizing, and self-statements of fear or anger to cope with their pain (Ezenwa et al., 2017). These investigators stressed the importance of assessing and understanding a patient's coping style and belief system to develop patient-centered interventions to help them cope more effectively with sickle cell pain.

Clinicians can learn about how a patient copes by asking, "Would you please tell me how you deal with the challenges/difficulties/problems in your life?" An example of how a clinician can learn about the belief system of the patient is to ask an open-ended, nonjudgmental question, such as, "Would you please tell me what spirituality means to you?" Or by asking, "What gives meaning to your life?" Another question may be, "Do you participate in any formal religious practices?" In the clinical setting, a more formal assessment can be accomplished with one of the most widely used spiritual assessment tools, entitled the *FICA Tool* (*Faith, Importance and Influence, Community and Address*), which was developed by Christina Puchalski, MD (Borneman, Ferrell, & Puchalski, 2010) (Fig. 25.1).

There is little evidence that proves prayer is effective as a pain management intervention; however, there are studies that lend credence to that concept. The effect on patients of the Muslim meditation prayer practice of *salat* was seen with electroencephalogram (EEG) tracings, which showed significantly increased activity in the occipital and parietal areas of the brain during *salat* (Doufesh, Ibrahim, Ismail, & Wan Ahmad, 2014). Those findings indicated an increase in parasympathetic activity with a reduction in sympathetic activity. The authors of that work suggest that with sustained daily practice the person performing *salat* will have less anxiety and greater ability to relax, which can be beneficial in controlling pain. (See Chapter 21 for discussion of relaxation and pain control.) A case series study evaluated the effect of intense Islamic prayer practices on cerebral blood flow (Newberg et al., 2015). The authors of that study found participants who prayed intensely had reduced cerebral blood flow in the prefrontal cortex, frontal lobe structures, and parietal lobe. This is early research, and the implications regarding how the experience of pain is affected in such situations is not clear. Since the findings were different from those obtained when focused meditation is practiced (see Newberg later in centering prayer), the authors theorized the findings with the intense Islamic prayer may be related to an Islamic prayer goal of surrendering and being connected with God.

Cautions

No evidence was found that directly examined the alleviation of pain with solely the use of spiritual or religious interventions. However, a Cochrane Review conducted by Roberts, Ahmed, and Davison (2014) examined the use of intercessory prayer for the alleviation of illness and recovery from surgery. The sample consisted of 10 randomized trials of patients (N = 7646) with heart disease, rheumatic disease, leukemia, alcohol abuse, or psychological conditions. The review revealed no significant differences in recovery from illness or surgery in those patients for whom others prayed and those for whom others did not pray. However, it was concluded that intercessory prayer was not harmful for patients

FICA Tool	
F–Faith, Belief, Meaning	**Religious/Religiosity**–Pertains to one's beliefs, behaviors, values, rules for conduct, and rituals associated with a specific religious tradition or denomination (O'Brien, 1999). **Spirituality**–Generally, an "individual's attitude and beliefs related to transcendence (God) or to the nonmaterial forces of life and of nature...the dimension of a person that is concerned with ultimate ends and values" and meaning (O'Brien, 1982, p. 88: Taylor, 2006)
• Do you consider yourself spiritual or religious?	
• Do you have spiritual beliefs that help you cope with stress?	
• What gives your life meaning?	
I–Importance and Influence	
• What importance does your faith or belief have in your life?	
• On a scale of 0 (not important) to 5 (very important), how would you rate the importance of faith/belief in your life?	
• Have your beliefs influenced you in how you handle stress?	
• What role do your beliefs play in your health care decision making?	
C–Community	
• Are you a part of a spiritual or religious community?	
• Is this of support to you and how?	
• Is there a group of people you really love or who are important to you?	
A–Address in Care	**We have talked a lot about your spirtuality and/or religious beliefs and how they may or may not be of help to you during your illness. How can your health care providers best support your spirituality?**
• How would you like your health care provider to use this information about your spirtuality as they care for you?	

Fig. 25.1 | **FICA Tool.** (Borneman, T., Ferrell, B., & Puchalski, C. M. (2010). Evaluation of the FICA tool for spiritual assessment. *Journal of Pain and Symptom Management, 40*[2], 163–173.)

who are ill or undergoing surgery, because no negative effects were reported in the sample (Roberts et al., 2014). Additional research is needed to explore the effect of different spiritual practices within the brain and body, particularly with the role of prayer as part of a multimodal plan for managing pain.

Meditation

The word *meditation* comes from the Latin *meditari,* which means to engage in reflection or contemplation (Jantos, 2012). From an Eastern spiritual perspective, meditation is a tool used to enhance spiritual growth, peace, and positive emotions along with reducing stress and negative emotions (Fingelkurts, Fingelkurts, & Kallio-Tamminen, 2015). Although meditation has a long history in the Hebrew bible,

since the 1950s in Western countries, Eastern meditation has become a complementary therapy and a spiritual practice. The authors of a secondary analysis of the 2012 National Health Institute Survey reported that approximately 9.3 million adults in the United States used meditation in the previous year, with 12% of them using it to manage back pain (Cramer, et al., 2016). Often the goal of meditation as practiced in Western countries is to examine the connection between the body and mind, in conjunction with how the person's mental and spiritual dimensions affect well-being (Jantos, 2012). Although the actual practice may be different among religious beliefs (e.g., *davening* among those of the Jewish faith, *centering prayers* among Christians, *praying the rosary* among Roman Catholics), the general concept of joining with the greater whole is similar across traditions (Schwartz, 2011) (Table 25.1). Ultimately, meditation

Table 25.1 | Systems of Meditation

	Centering Prayer/ Contemplation	Kabbalah (Qabalah)	Mindfulness Meditation	Ridhwan School Diamond Approach	Self-Realization Fellowship (SRF)	Transcendental Meditation	Tibetan Buddhism	Zen Buddhism/ Ch'an
Traditional background	Catholic/Christian	Jewish mystical	Vipassana/insight; mindfulness-based stress reduction medical	Sufi Islam, mystical psychology	Hindu Kriya yoga	Vedic Hindu	Various Tibetan lineages	Numerous Chinese and Japanese lineages
Teachers	Thomas Keating; Thomas Merton; Cynthia Bourgeault; M. Basil Pennington; William Meninger	Yehuda Ashlag; David Cooper; Michael Laitman	Jon Kabat-Zinn; Bhante Gunaratana; Sharon Salzberg; Jack Kornfield; Thich Nhat Hanh	A.H. Almaas (Hameed Ali)	Paramahansa Yogananda; Sri Daya Mata	Maharishi Mahesh Yogi (Various)	Fourteenth Dalai Lama; Panchen Lama; Chogyam Trungpa; Seventeenth Karmapa	Bodhidharma; Eisai; Dogan; Huang Po; Charlotte Joko Beck; Claude A. Thomas
Technique	Sacred word; prayer; lectio divina	Kabbalah	Breath/body awareness	Inquiry	Kriya yoga; Hong-Sau; Aum	Personalized mantra	Mantra; visualization; chanting	Zazen
Body/Activity Focus	Contemplative walking	Self-directed	Mindful walking; Hatha yoga; body scan	Breathing exercises	Energization exercises	Self-directed	Rlung-sgom walking; mudras	Martial arts (Kungfu); Zen arts (ceramics, archery, calligraphy)
Readings/ Books	*New Seeds of Contemplation* (Merton); *Open Mind Open Heart* (Keating)	*A Beginner's Guide to Kabbalah* (CD); *A Heart of Stillness* (Cooper)	*Mindfulness in Plain English* (Gunaratana); *Full Catastrophe Living* (Kabat-Zinn); *A Path with Heart* (Kornfield)	*Essence; The Diamond Heart Series I–IV; Inner Journey Home* (by Almaas)	*Autobiography of a Yogi; SRF Lessons* (Yogananda)	*Science of Being and Art of Living; Transcendental Meditation* (Maharishi)	*The World of Tibetan Buddhism; Path to Bliss* (Gyatso); *Start Where You Are* (Chodron)	*Zen Mind Beginner's Mind* (Suzuki); *The Three Pillars of Zen* (Kapleau); *Everyday Zen* (Beck)
Coursework	Retreats; contemplative outreach	Tree of Life; Ten Sefirot; Devekut; teacher-directed	Mindfulness-based stress reduction/ cognitive therapy	Diamond approach lessons; retreats	Mailed lessons; retreats; guru relationship; interviews with monks	Seven-step coursework; interviews; personal mantra; retreats	Teacher-student; lineage-directed	Teacher-student

Main Sites/Headquarters	Abbey of Gethsemani, Trappist, KY; Snowmass, CO; multiple/regional	Multiple	Insight Meditation Society, MA; University of Massachusetts (for mindfulness-based stress reduction); Spirit Rock, CA; Plum Village, France; multiple	Berkeley, CA; Boulder, CO; multiple	Los Angeles; Multiple (see also Yogoda Satsanga Society of India, sister organization to SRF)	Fairfield, IA; multiple; (Transcendental Meditation Independent UK)	Lhasa, Tibet; Dharamsala, India; multiple	Shaolin Temple, China (birthplace); multiple centers
Websites/Contact Information	http://www.centeringprayer.com (also see Christian Meditation: http://www.wccm.org)	http://www.kabbalah.info; http://www.kabbalah.com; 1-800-kabbalah	http://www.dharma.org; http://www.umassmed.edu/cfm/mbsr; http://www.eomega.org; http://www.spiritrock.org; http://www.plumvillage.org	http://www.ahalmaas.com; http://www.ridhwan.org	http://www.srf-yogananda.org	http://www.tm.org; 1-888-learnTM; (http://www.tm-meditation.co.uk, independent, less expensive)	http://www.tibet.com; http://www.deerparkcenter.org; http://www.dawnmountain.org	http://www.dharmanet.org; http://www.tricycle.com
Comments	Contemplation dates back to St. Anthony and the Desert Fathers; revived after Vatican II; in the tradition of Christian saints and mystics	Ancient oral tradition of wisdom and mystery; tells of Light of Creation; Jewish renewal movement	Popularized in the 1980s; from an 8-wk course in a medical/research setting; many vipassana/insight sanghas or groups	Founded in the 1970s; called the Work, draws from psychology and integrates a spiritual approach to self-liberation	Founded in 1920; popularized yoga-meditation in the United States; teaches a direct path to self-realization through ancient Kriya yoga	Popularized in the 1960s; expanded meditation in the United States; large corpus of health research at Maharishi Vedic University	Model of nonviolence, loving compassion for sentient beings; ongoing dialogue with neuroscience researchers	Chinese/Japanese tradition arrived in the United States after World War II; most Zen meditation research is in Japanese

From Fortney, L. (2017). Recommending meditation. In D. Rakel (Ed.), *Integrative medicine* (4th ed., pp. 945–953.e2). Philadelphia, PA: Elsevier.

is considered to be a relaxation response, and there is no doubt there are therapeutic effects of relaxation for patients with chronic pain who practice meditation (Jantos, 2012). Patients can use meditation to assist with pain symptoms and during painful treatments as a positive coping method through distraction, easing of muscle tension, and a general sense of calm. In addition, once mastered, meditation has the benefit of being cost free, requiring no special attire or equipment, and totally portable (Ricard, Lutz, & Davidson, 2014).

There is some evidence that the concentration aspects of meditation affect the theta band of the brain during meditation, which results in greater ability of the person to focus attention and to relax (Tanaka, et al, 2014). This may be important for patients who are coping with pain to enable them to ease tension and achieve a sense of greater calm. The investigators of a large (N = 2409) survey reported meditators endorsed less depression and emotional distress with greater resilience and compassion than those who did not meditate (O'Connor et al., 2015). Another study compared magnetic resonance imaging (MRI) evaluation of novice meditators with experienced meditators and found greater integration of the alpha band functional network topography in the meditators who were more experienced in meditating (van Lutterveld et al., 2017). Although the role and implications of alpha and theta wave activity in the brain regarding pain is not clear, there are preliminary data that indicate EEGs of people with neuropathic pain demonstrate increased activity of these waves (dos Santos Pinheiro et al., 2016). This is another area in which research is needed to clarify the physiologic benefits of meditation and how it can best be used in a multimodal approach to help people better manage pain.

Centering Prayer (Spiritual Meditation)

Centering prayer is a contemplative form of prayer in the Christian tradition, which dates at least to the third century. In recent years, it was rejuvenated by Roman Catholic Abbot Thomas Keating and priests William Meninger and M. Basil Pennington (Keating, 2006; Minichiello, 2018; Pennington, 2010). Centering prayer is considered a general Christian meditation based in Catholic mysticism (Knabb, 2012). With centering prayer, there is a major focus of meditation in the concept of Christian Devotion Meditation that incorporates a variety of techniques that "foster awareness and attention on God" (Frederick & White, 2015, p. 850). Although it is taught by different people with some variation, the essence of centering prayer is to sit quietly, connect with God, focus on a word consistent with love, return to that word whenever distracted, and conclude with a prayer or prayer word (Pennington, 2010). The similarity of centering prayer with mindfulness meditation and mindfulness based cognitive therapy was discussed by Knabb (2012) who identified centering prayer as a potential therapy for Christians who are in remission from depression.

Evidence for Pain Management

Little research exists regarding the effects of centering prayer on those who practice it and even less with the effect on painful conditions. Although not specific about pain, an older study with students (N = 36) reported students who practiced devotional meditation, of which centering prayer is a form, reported less anger and anxiety compared to those who practiced muscle relaxation or who were wait listed (Carlson, Bacaseta, & Simanton, 1988). An interesting older study was done with Franciscan nuns in which cerebral blood flow was monitored before and after 40 minutes of centering prayer in which they internally repeated a spiritual phrase (Newberg, Pourdehnad, Alavi, & d'Aquili, 2003). In that study, the blood flow to the brains of the nuns was monitored and was seen to increase in the prefrontal cortex and the inferior parietal and inferior frontal lobes with an inverse correlation with change in blood flow in the ipsilateral superior parietal lobe (P < .01). Although these are considered positive physiologic responses, and the role of the prefrontal cortex has been studied with regard to pain, the significance of these results in relation to pain is unclear. Centering prayer is also associated with diminishing activity in the amygdala area of the brain (Bingaman, 2013). Again, any specific implication for pain is not clear. A more recent but very small study with centering prayer (N = 9) reported reduced anxiety and stress in participants after 6 weeks of participating in centering prayers (Fox, Gutierrez, Haas, & Durnford, 2016). Because reducing anxiety and depression are correlated with pain management (see Chapters 8 and 22), this is interesting as well as potentially beneficial for pain management. Additional research is needed to clarify the role of centering prayer as part of a multimodal analgesia (MMA) plan of care.

Two studies specifically assessed pain among people using what was described as spiritual meditation compared with what was described as secular meditation (Wachholtz & Pargament, 2005, 2008). In the first study (N = 68), after meditating for 20 minutes for 14 days, the participants who used spiritual meditation (n = 25) reported greater reductions in anxiety and were able to tolerate cold pressor pain for nearly twice as long as those in either the secular meditation group (n = 21) or the relaxation group (n = 22) (Wachholtz & Pargament, 2005). This ability to tolerate the cold pressor pain was an important finding because it was consistent with the earlier work of Keefe et al. (2001) in spiritual coping with pain. In that work, *spiritual coping*, the use of spiritual beliefs or practices to control or manage pain, was correlated with less pain.

The second study was done using spiritual meditation with people living with migraine headaches (n = 92) who were randomized to one of four groups (Wachholtz & Pargament, 2008). The results of that study showed that after 1 month of practice, the participants in the spiritual meditation group (n = 25) had less pain and anxiety and marked increases in pain tolerance compared to the participants in the two nonspiritual meditation groups (n = 22, n = 23) and the relaxation group (n = 22). Although these results are promising, additional research is needed to identify the potential benefit of centering prayer from a holistic health perspective (physiologically, psychologically, and spiritually) (Bingaman, 2013; Fox, Gutierrez, Haas, & Dumford, 2016) and with painful conditions in particular.

Kabbalah (Qabalah)

Kabbalah meditation originated in the Jewish mystical tradition (Fortney, 2018). The term Kabbalah also signifies Jewish mysticism as a general concept in which it is believed human beings need to partner with God to restore creation or for the world to be whole (LaGrone, 2018). The term also is used to designate the indescribable experience of transcendence, which is understood as a sense of increased awareness, unadulterated consciousness or a sense of being one with the universe (Wahbeh, Sagher, Back, Pundhir, & Travis, 2018). Kabbalah has recently garnered increased interest and has been considered one of the postmodern spiritualities (Huss, 2007). The mystical, mysterious, nonmaterial aspects of Kabbalah are consistent with the concepts of postmodern spirituality (Lee, 2016).

Evidence for Pain Management

Although no research studies were found in which Kabbalah meditation was evaluated for pain management, Kabbalah teaches that it is possible to end suffering (Berg, 2001). As with most of the spiritually based meditations, research with regard to controlling pain and how it can be used with multimodal pain management is warranted.

Loving Kindness Meditation

Loving kindness meditation (LKM) is a type of meditation derived from the Buddhist tradition that intends to elicit and convey warm, kind, compassionate, and loving responses for self and other people (Fredrickson, Cohn, Coffey, Pek, & Finkel, 2008; Keng & Tan, 2018; Lumma, Kok, & Singer, 2015). LKM begins with expressing love for those people for whom the person meditating usually feels love, then for self. Next the meditating person expands the feelings of love toward others including those people who are less likeable and even to those who have been harmful to the person (Fredrickson et al., 2008; Lippelt, Hommel, & Colzato, 2014) (Box 25.1).

Evidence for Pain Management

Very little research has been done using LKM and even less using it with patients experiencing pain. In early research (N = 139), participants who practiced LKM for 7 weeks on a regular basis, experienced more positive emotions, greater intrapersonal resources, fewer

---

| **Box 25.1** | Stages of Loving Kindness Meditation |

1. Focus on self
2. Focus on a loved one who is alive and for whom there is no sexual desire
3. Focus on a person who does not elicit positive or negative feelings
4. Focus on a person who is associated with negative feelings
5. Focus on self, loved one, neutral person, and challenging person
6. Focus on the entire universe

From Hofmann, S. G., Grossman, P., & Hinton, D. E. (2011). Loving-kindness and compassion meditation: Potential for psychological interventions. *Clinical Psychology Review, 31*(7), 1126–1132.

---

symptoms of illness, fewer depressive symptoms, and increased satisfaction with life (Fredrickson et al., 2008). In that study, no attention was paid to any pain that may have been experienced by the participants. The authors of a systematic review of kindness-based meditation studies (N = 22) concluded that although the quality of evidence was low to moderate, there is evidence of health benefits (Galante, Galante, Bekkers, & Gallacher, 2014). However, Carson et al. (2005) conducted a small but important research study using LKM with patients with chronic back pain (N = 18). In that study, not only were pain and anger significantly reduced with the practice of LKM but the longer people participated in LKM, the greater was the reduction in pain ($P < .01$) and anger ($P < .09$) during the day in which LKM was practiced. In another study, audio-recorded guided LKM was compared with audio-recorded relaxing music and standard of care among women undergoing breast biopsies (N = 138) (Soo et al., 2016). Although both the LKM (n = 46) and music groups (n = 46) had significantly less anxiety ($P = .05$) compared to the standard of care group (n = 46), only those in the LKM group had significantly less pain ($P = .03$)

The effect of LKM, or compassion meditation as it is sometimes called, does not seem to be limited to spiritual, emotional, or cognitive effects. When MRI testing was done on the brains of people who practiced these meditations for long durations, the results demonstrated structural changes (Engen, Bernhardt, Skottnik, Ricard, & Singer, 2017). From a pain perspective the results of that study were particularly interesting because some of the areas of the brain where there were changes were areas in which opioid receptors are plentiful. In a recent study assessing the perception of imagined pain for self and others, it was found that people who used loving kindness language perceived their own imagined pain as less intense and perceived the imagined pain of others as more intense when compared to that of controls (Williams, Poljacik, Decety, & Nusbaum, 2017). In that study, those using loving kindness language did not demonstrate a significant difference between their rating of pain intensity of themselves and others, whereas those in the control group rated their own pain significantly higher than they rated the pain of others. This along with other research indicates LKM is not only a positive intervention for patients living with chronic pain to use to manage pain but it is also an intervention clinicians can use to increase compassion and better help patients control pain (Williams & Nusbaum, 2016). (See Chapter 27 for discussion of compassion as a component of multimodal pain management.) Based on results of a study in which LKM meditators made significantly fewer errors on continuous performance tasks, clinicians can also use LKM to enhance safe pain management as well (Britton, Lindahl, Cahn, Davis, & Goldman, 2014).

Additional rigorous research is needed to further assess the benefit of LKM for pain management within MMA plans of care. Further research is needed to identify the potential benefits for patients when clinicians practice LKM and gain greater compassion for the pain and suffering of patients (Williams et al., 2017; Wright & Pendry, 2016). Research also would be valuable to assess the effect on patients living with chronic pain and the compassion felt by their significant others if the significant others practiced LKM (Ruchelli et al., 2014).

Mindfulness Meditation

Mindfulness meditation arose from the Buddhist tradition; however, mindfulness meditation is commonly known today as a secular, cognitive type of meditation and for that reason in Chapter 22, it is discussed from an MMA perspective as a valuable component of cognitive-behavioral therapies when working with people living with painful conditions such as fibromyalgia (Grossman, Tiefenthaler-Gilmer, Raysz, & Kesper, 2007).

Reflective Walking, Labyrinth Walking, and Movement Meditation

Although meditation is generally associated with sitting quietly, meditation also can be effectively combined with movement and activity (e.g., yoga movements, walking, biking, dance) (Fortney, 2018). Reflective walking provides a unique opportunity to combine exercise with cognitive and spiritual processing. When the person is attentive to the sensations occurring in the body, there can be a grounding or anchoring component that supports the person being present in the current time (Fortney, 2018).

One form of reflective walking is *labyrinth walking,* which involves following the solitary continuous path

within a particular pattern, which is often designed to symbolize the individual spiritual journey (Sandor, 2005; Zucker, Choi, Cook, & Croft, 2016). Although labyrinth walking has ancient roots in spirituality, during the last few decades it has been considered an important component for reducing stress and promoting health (Heard, Scott, & Yeo, 2015; Sandor, 2005, 2008). Labyrinths are used in a variety of settings, including schools, medical centers, behavioral health centers, correctional facilities, parks, and churches (Heard et al., 2015; Maruca & Shelton, 2016; Sandor, 2005; Zucker et al., 2016). As with other types of reflective walking, a unique quality of labyrinth walking is that it incorporates the physical (walking) with the cognitive (focus) with the spiritual aspects of the walker (Sandor, 2008).

Evidence for Pain Management

Although no research was found regarding reflective walking or labyrinth walking as an intervention for pain management, researchers have evaluated labyrinth walking in a variety of settings, including medical centers (Sandor, 2005; Sandor & Froman, 2006), behavioral health centers (Heard et al., 2015), correctional facilities (Zucker & Sharma, 2012), and academia (Cook & Croft, 2015; Zucker et al., 2016). When labyrinth walking was evaluated in a pilot study (N = 20), at the end of the 2-month study the women who walked the labyrinth demonstrated less anxiety, perceived stress, and verbal aggression compared to the control group in which participants walked a track (Sandor, 2008). In that study, both groups had significant reductions in cortisol levels with no significant differences between the two groups. When the effects of labyrinth walking were evaluated in a study with community-dwelling adults (N = 25); however, results were not strong enough to support or refute any health benefit (Sandor & Forman, 2006).

Research is needed to identify potential benefit of labyrinth walking as part of a multimodal plan for pain management, how it can be used in such a plan, and education needed for clinicians regarding this mind-body-spirit modality.

Research is also needed to explore how reflective walking, meditative movement, and labyrinth walking may be used to support clinicians in managing stress, including compassion fatigue, and for supporting reflective practice (Dalley-Hewer, Opie & Knowles, 2015; Sandor, 2005). It is conceivable labyrinth walking, which incorporates gentle exercise (slow walking) with meditation, is beneficial as a component of a multimodal approach for pain management. Exploring that idea is an opportunity for clinical research.

Ridhwan School Diamond Approach

The Ridhwan School Diamond Approach of spirituality was originated by A. H. Almaas with a background in mystical psychology and Sufi Islam (Fortney, 2018; Woelm,

2006). From this perspective the person is encouraged to uncover and integrate his or her essence and uniqueness with absolutely no judgment (Woelm, 2006). Meditation involves breathing exercises, inquiry, and a spiritual method toward self-liberation (Fortney, 2018).

Evidence for Pain Management

No information was found in which Ridhwan School Diamond Approach meditation was studied as an intervention for pain management. However, the nonjudgmental acceptance and integration of self would be interesting to research with regard to controlling pain and how it can be used to better control pain using a multimodal approach.

Self-Realization Fellowship

Within the self-realization fellowship (SRF) belief system, there is a strong emphasis on thought, with positive thinking as well as aligning what is said outwardly with what is thought inwardly. An example of this is the inconsistency that occurs when a person says out loud to others "I am going to control my pain," but inwardly thinks "I will never be without pain." In this situation, the person needs to reconcile the difference between what is thought inwardly with what is being said verbally. With SRF, there is the belief that through learning to know oneself, the person becomes one with God. There is also the belief that thoughts are powerful and can be manifested into reality (Self-Realization Fellowship, 1982, 1984; Thompson, 2017; Yogananda, 2000, 2006, 2016).

Evidence for Pain Management

No information was found in which SRF was studied as an intervention for pain management. However, the belief system of aligning internal thought with what is said and behavior would be an interesting concept to research regarding controlling pain. It is consistent with cognitive-behavioral therapy concepts discussed in Chapter 22 and could be used as part of a multimodal approach as a spiritual component in conjunction with them.

Tibetan Buddhist Meditation

Tibetan Buddhist meditation dates to the 14th century Dalai Lama (Fortney, 2018). It is characterized by the concept of *non-duality awareness*; thus there is no inside versus outside or good versus evil, and rather the totality of experience is appreciated (Josipovic, Dinstein, Weber, & Heeger, 2012). Typically, in Tibetan Buddhism, people bring their attention and focus on a particular word, phrase, or image in their mind and absorb themselves in the image (Roggenkamp, Waldman, & Newberg, 2009). The goal of the development stage in the Tibetan Buddhist meditation practice is to modify the perception of what is taken in through the senses and to modify the sense of perception as an entity (Dahl, Lutz, & Davidson, 2015).

Evidence for Pain Management

No evidence specific to pain management was identified; however, research that demonstrates the effect of meditation on portions of the human brain can be used to formulate hypotheses for future research. People meditating in a Tibetan Buddhist tradition were assessed with cerebral blood flow monitoring and were found to have increased activity in the prefrontal cortex and cingulate gyrus (Roggenkamp et al., 2009). This is interesting from a pain perspective because some instances of chronic pain have been correlated with the prefrontal cortex (Seminowicz & Moayedi, 2017). During EEG studies, experienced Tibetan Buddhist meditators had greater gamma power both at baseline and during meditation (Britton et al., 2014). Recent research has shown a relationship between muscle pain and the gamma band activity of the brain (Li et al., 2016). This is another area in which research is needed to gain evidence to support meditation as part of an MMA plan of care.

Transcendental Meditation

Transcendental meditation (TM) is a type of meditation in which, without effort, the mind experiences thought processes that are increasingly higher until thought is transcended and more pure consciousness is experienced (Schneider & Carr, 2014). TM, also known as *automatic self-transcending*, originated in Indian and Chinese meditative methods and involves deep physical relaxation and suspension of mental activity, and alertness is increased (Simkin & Black, 2014). In this type of meditation there is no effort to control or monitor what is occurring because that type of mental activity is thought to interfere with the transcending process (Schneider & Carr, 2014; Simkin & Black, 2014). A single word or *mantra* is silently repeated to block interrupting thoughts. TM is designed to be used after education and training with someone who is certified in educating and leading the TM process (Simkin & Black, 2014).

Evidence for Pain Management

There is no evidence of TM being used to help manage pain; however, the research in other areas, such as with loving kindness meditation and mindfulness meditation (see Chapter 22), indicates it may be beneficial. When the transcendental state is reached, it is compared to a *wakeful hypometabolic state* or a *fourth state of consciousness* in which there is relaxation with the added benefits of reduced respirations, cortisol, plasma lactate, catecholamines, and increased galvanic skin tone (Schneider & Carr, 2014). TM has been used in clinical situations and studied with regard to health from a relaxation perspective, particularly with cardiovascular disorders (Leong, 2014; Shi et al., 2017). TM also has been used effectively with people diagnosed with substance use disorder and alcoholism (Shankar, Rosenberg, Dhawan, & Vedamurthachar, 2014).

Zen Buddhism/Ch'an

Zen meditation continues in the Buddhist tradition (Marchand, 2012) in which it originated, incorporating Chinese Taoism and becoming Ch'an, but is best known today as Zen (De Benedittis, 2015). The actual seated Zen meditation posture is referred to as *Zazen*, which translates to "sitting in the position of Buddha" (Hauswald, Übelacker, Leske, & Weisz, 2015, p. 266). Rather than trying to control thoughts with thoughts, from a Zen perspective, thoughts and cognition are controlled by regulating Zazen, breathing, and concentration; this philosophy of "enter(ing) the mind through the body" is in stark contrast to the belief that only the mind can control the mind (Kushner, 2012, p. 243).

Evidence for Pain Management

Zen has a long history of being assessed from a physiologic perspective dating back to a study in 1966 in which EEG monitoring of Zen monks showed alpha tracing within a minute after they began meditating, which initially increased in amplitude but then decreased in frequency (Hauswald et al., 2015). One thought is that the changes in alpha power in coordination with theta activity in the brain support the focus of attention that occurs during meditation (Cahn, Delomore, & Polich, 2013). Also impressive in the monk study was that the effects lasted after the monks stopped meditating (De Benedittis, 2015). In that study, as seen in subsequent research, the longer durations of meditation were correlated with greater thickness of the anterior cingulate. From an analgesia perspective that is interesting because the anterior cingulate is involved in both acute and chronic pain (Bliss, Collingridge, Kaang, & Zhuo, 2016). EEG monitoring of people using Zen meditation revealed activation of both the anterior and prefrontal cortex, which were correlated with greater serum serotonin levels as well (Yu et al., 2011). More recently, in a small study, EEG tracings (N = 11) showed effects in cerebral areas affecting awareness and attention with structural changes in activity and connectivity (Hauswald et al., 2015).

Although recent research using Zen with pain management (Box 25.2) is scarce, it does appear that Zen can be an effective component of an MMA plan of care (Marchand, 2012) to modify sensory and affective facets of pain (Grant, Courtemanche, Duerden, Duncan, & Rainville, 2010). In one small study, people (N = 13) who were well trained in Zen meditation had less sensitivity to pain and experienced analgesia while using Zen meditation (Leong, 2014). In another study (N = 35), compared with controls (n = 18), people who practiced Zen meditation (n = 17) had less pain sensitivity (Grant et al., 2010). In that study, structural MRI scanning showed that the Zen meditators also had denser cortex in the pain-related regions of the brain (dorsal anterior cingulate and somatosensory). Those findings were supported and expanded upon with a subsequent small study (N = 13), in which functional MRI evaluation was used to assess the effect of Zen meditation on ther-

mal pain (Grant, Courtemanche, & Rainville, 2011). The researchers of that subsequent study reported that MRI results showed Zen meditators had less activity in the prefrontal cortex, the amygdala, and hippocampus, and they reported less pain sensitivity, which was strongly predicted by less purposeful interaction between the pain-related and executive cortices. These studies (Table 25.2) are supportive of a potential analgesic benefit of Zen meditation and a cost-effective component of multimodal analgesia.

General Cautions and Precautions Regarding Meditation

Meditation is a generally safe activity; however, as with all activities, considering some cautions and precautions can improve the experience and lead to greater success. Meditation is an intervention that develops over time and thus potential benefit is greater with practice. For some people the time involved in becoming proficient with meditation may be an obstacle (Day, Thorn, & Rubin, 2014). It is important to remember there are a variety of types of meditation (see Table 25.1), and no one meditation technique is right for everyone. Selecting the meditation that is consistent with the spiritual values and beliefs of the individual person is important and likely to be more beneficial. Assuming the most comfortable position and avoiding positions that might cause discomfort despite such positions

---

Box 25.2 | Clinical Application

The nurses noticed that immediately after receiving any opioid pain medicine Martin closed his eyes and was very still with a slight smile on his face. The nurses wondered if Martin did not really need the medicine for pain but just wanted the opioids to "get high." They consulted the Pain Management Advanced Practice Nurse (PM-APN) who reviewed Martin's medical record and found that he had an acute episode of pancreatitis. When the PM-APN interviewed Martin, he reported almost always having severe pain that never was less than 7 on a scale of 0 to 10. The PM-APN asked Martin about his behavior when he received opioid medications. He explained that he has been a Zen Buddhist meditator for many years and found that when he meditates after receiving the medication, he relaxes, and the medication seems to be more effective for his pain. The PM-APN encouraged him to continue this practice, relayed what he explained to the nurses, and explained to them what is known about Zen Buddhist meditation and pain management. The nurses were impressed with this information. They included the meditation as part of his analgesic plan of care and supported Martin in his meditation.

Table 25.2	**Key Web Resources**	
A nonprofit online resource that includes definitions/descriptions of a variety of relaxation techniques, scripts for practicing these techniques, and links to free audio files for meditation, guided imagery, and others. Developed by Jeanne Segal, PhD.	http://www.helpguide.org/articles/stress/relaxation-techniques-for-stress-relief.htm
A website developed by the University of Texas, Austin, to promote student wellness. Includes free access to audio files of relaxation techniques, including deep breathing, progressive muscle relaxation, guided imagery, and other meditations.	http://cmhc.utexas.edu/mindbodylab.html
A collection of free audio files and video lectures discussing the keys of mindfulness practice. Multiple guided meditations of varying lengths developed by the University of Wisconsin-Madison Integrative Medicine and Mindfulness Center faculty.	http://www.fammed.wisc.edu/mindfulness
"Headspace" Mobile Application A mobile application that introduces the listener to mindfulness meditation in a step-by-step fashion. A good resource for people with no previous background in contemplative practices. The first 10 recordings are free.	http://www.headspace.com
"Buddhify 2" mobile application designed for the busy mind and constantly on-the-go person, this application has a large selection of guided meditations that help to promote mindfulness in a variety of common daily activities. Costs $2.99.	http://buddhify.com/

From Minichiello, V. J. (2018). Relaxation techniques. In D. Rakel (Ed.), *Integrative medicine.* (4th ed., pp. 909–913.e1). Philadelphia, PA: Elsevier.

seeming to be congruent with information about successful meditation are important precautions. Patients need to be aware that meditation may bring to conscious attention stressors or experiences that may trigger emotional or psychological responses that can be distressing. Knowing how to contact a therapist if this occurs is important. Processing insights gained from meditation will result in a more fulfilling experience. This can be done through art, music, journaling, or discussions with a meditation teacher or therapist or a trusted person (Fortney, 2018).

Key Points

- Patients use spirituality as a positive and constructive coping strategy, with religious rituals, meditation, prayer, and mindfulness among the spiritual resources to help them cope with the intensity of their pain and suffering.
- Spirituality and religion are not the same.
- Religion often provides a structure through which a person expresses spirituality.
- Although there is not a great deal of research regarding the relationship between spirituality and pain management, what is known indicates that benefits of fostering the relationship are possible.
- Spirituality can be expressed in many different ways. There is no one *right way.*
- Patients' spiritual needs are not assessed by most health care professionals and therefore are not being met as fully as possible.

Case Scenario

Mary is a nurse on the renal unit where patients frequently return and remain for long hospitalizations. She is interested in gaining a better understanding of the relationship between spirituality and pain management. Last year Mary did a process improvement project on her unit in which she surveyed nurses about the spiritual needs of patients. The results strongly indicated most nurses do not feel comfortable talking about religion and spirituality with patients, many nurses do not know about any religion other than the one they practice, and many nurses have heard about meditation but do not understand it as a spiritual practice. This year Mary is developing an education module for the nurses who work on the renal unit about spirituality and how spirituality can be helpful as part of a multimodal approach for pain management.

1. What information should Mary include about spirituality?
2. How should Mary explain the relationship between spirituality and meditation?
3. What information can Mary include to support spirituality as a component of multimodal pain management?
4. What resources can Mary include for the nurses to help patients use spirituality to manage pain?
5. What opportunities can Mary share with clinicians who would like to research the role of spirituality and multimodal pain management?

References

American Nurses Association. (2015). *Code of ethics for nurses with interpretive statements*. Silver Spring, MD: Nursingbooks.org.

Balboni, M., Sullivan, A., Amobi, A., Phelps, A., Gorman, D., Zollfrank, A., & Balboni, T. (2013). Why is spiritual care infrequent at the end of life? Spiritual care perceptions among patients, nurses, and physicians and the role of training. *Journal of Clinical Oncology*, 31(4), 461–467.

Berg, M. (2001). *The Way: Using the Wisdom of Kabbalah for Spiritual Transformation and Fulfillment*. New York, NY: John Wiley & Sons, Inc.

Bingaman, K. A. (2013). The promise of neuroplasticity for pastoral care and counseling. *Pastoral Psychology*, 62(5), 549–560.

Bliss, T. V., Collingridge, G. L., Kaang, B. K., & Zhuo, M. (2016). Synaptic plasticity in the anterior cingulate cortex in acute and chronic pain. *Nature Reviews Neuroscience*, 17(8), 485.

Borneman, T., Ferrell, B., & Puchalski, C. M. (2010). Evaluation of the FICA tool for spiritual assessment. *Journal of Pain and Symptom Management*, 40(2), 163–173.

Britton, W. B., Lindahl, J. R., Cahn, B. R., Davis, J. H., & Goldman, R. E. (2014). Awakening is not a metaphor: the effects of Buddhist meditation practices on basic wakefulness. *Annals of the New York Academy of Sciences*, 1307(1), 64–81.

Cahn, B. R., Delorme, A., & Polich, J. (2013). Event-related delta, theta, alpha and gamma correlates to auditory oddball processing during Vipassana meditation. *Social Cognitive and Affective Neuroscience*, 8(1), 100–111.

Carlson, C. R., Bacaseta, P. E., & Simanton, D. A. (1988). 9.1 A controlled evaluation of devotional meditation and progressive relaxation. *Psychological Perspectives on Prayer: A Reader*, 285.

Carson, J. W., Keefe, F. J., Lynch, T. R., Carson, K. M., Goli, V., Fras, A. M., & Thorp, S. R. (2005). Loving-kindness meditation for chronic low back pain results from a pilot trial. *Journal of Holistic Nursing*, 23, 287–304. https://doi.org/10.1177/0898010105277651.

Cook, M., & Croft, J. B. (2015). Interactive mindfulness technology: A walking labyrinth in an academic library. *College & Research Libraries News*, 76(6), 318–322.

Cramer, H., Hall, H., Leach, M., Frawley, J., Zhang, Y., Leung, B., ... Lauche, R. (2016). Prevalence, patterns, and predictors of meditation use among US adults: A nationally representative survey. *Scientific Reports*, 6, 36760.

Dahl, C. J., Lutz, A., & Davidson, R. J. (2015). Reconstructing and deconstructing the self: cognitive mechanisms in meditation practice. *Trends in Cognitive Sciences*, 19(9), 515–523.

Dalley-Hewer, J., Opie, J., & Knowles, N. (2015). A creative alternative to reflective writing: promoting skills of reflection through walking a labyrinth. *Physiotherapy*, 101(Supp 1), e766–e777.

Day, M. A., Thorn, B. E., & Rubin, N. J. (2014). Mindfulness-based cognitive therapy for the treatment of headache pain: A mixed-methods analysis comparing treatment responders and treatment non-responders. *Complementary Therapies in Medicine*, 22(2), 278–285.

De Benedittis, G. (2015). Neural mechanisms of hypnosis and meditation. *Journal of Physiology-Paris*, 109(4), 152–164.

Dedeli, O., & Kaptan, G. (2013). Spirituality and religion in pain and pain management. *Health Psychology Research*, 1, 154–159.

dos Santos Pinheiro, E. S., de Queirós, F. C., Montoya, P., Santos, C. L., do Nascimento, M. A., Ito, C. H., ... Sá, K. N. (2016). Electroencephalographic patterns in chronic pain: a systematic review of the literature. *PLoS One*, 11(2), e0149085.

Doufesh, H., Ibrahim, F., Ismail, N. A., & Wan Ahmad, W. A. (2014). Effect of Muslim prayer (Salat) on α electroencephalography and its relationship with autonomic nervous system activity. *The Journal of Alternative and Complementary Medicine*, 20(7), 558–562.

Engen, H. G., Bernhardt, B. C., Skottnik, L., Ricard, M., & Singer, T. (2017). Structural changes in socio-affective networks: Multi-modal MRI findings in long-term meditation practitioners. *Neuropsychologia.*, 116(Pt. A), 26–33.

Ezenwa, M., Yao, Y., Molokie, R., Wang, Z., Mandernach, M., Suarez, M., & Wilkie, D. (2017). Coping with pain in the face of healthcare injustice in patients with sickle cell disease. *Journal of Immigrant Minority Health*, 19, 1449–1456.

Fingelkurts, A. A., Fingelkurts, A. A., & Kallio-Tamminen, T. (2015). EEG-guided meditation: a personalized approach. *Journal of Physiology-Paris*, 109(4), 180–190.

Fogerite, S. G., & Goldberg, G. L. (2008). Overview of mind-body therapies. In: Complementary therapies for Physical Therapy: A Clinical Decision-Making Approach. In J. Deutsch, & E. Z. Anderson (Eds.) (pp. 84–120). St. Louis, MO: Elsevier.

Fortney, L. (2018). Recommending Meditation. In D. Rakel (Ed.), *Integrative Medicine* (4th ed., pp. 945–953.e2). Philadelphia, PA: Elsevier.

Fox, J., Gutierrez, D., Haas, J., & Durnford, S. (2016). Centering prayer's effects on psycho-spiritual outcomes: a pilot outcome study. *Mental Health, Religion & Culture*, 19(4), 379–392.

Frederick, T., & White, K. M. (2015). Mindfulness, Christian devotion meditation, surrender, and worry. *Mental Health, Religion & Culture*, 18(10), 850–858.

Fredrickson, B. L., Cohn, M. A., Coffey, K. A., Pek, J., & Finkel, S. M. (2008). Open hearts build lives: positive emotions, induced through loving-kindness meditation, build consequential personal resources. *Journal of Personality and Social Psychology*, 95(5), 1045–1062.

Galante, J., Galante, I., Bekkers, M. J., & Gallacher, J. (2014). Effect of kindness-based meditation on health and well-being: a systematic review and meta-analysis. *Journal of Consulting and Clinical Psychology*, 82(6), 1101.

Grant, J. A., Courtemanche, J., & Rainville, P. (2011). A non-elaborative mental stance and decoupling of executive and pain-related cortices predicts low pain sensitivity in Zen meditators. *PAIN®*, 152(1), 150–156.

Grant, J. A., Courtemanche, J., Duerden, E. G., Duncan, G. H., & Rainville, P. (2010). Cortical thickness and pain sensitivity in Zen meditators. *Emotion*, 10(1), 43.

Grossman, P., Tiefenthaler-Gilmer, U., Raysz, A., & Kesper, U. (2007). Mindfulness training as an intervention for fibromyalgia: evidence of postintervention and 3-year follow-up benefits in well-being. *Psychotherapy and Psychosomatics*, 76(4), 226.

Hauswald, A., Übelacker, T., Leske, S., & Weisz, N. (2015). What it means to be Zen: Marked modulations of local and interareal synchronization during open monitoring meditation. *NeuroImage*, 108, 265–273.

HealthCare Chaplaincy Network and Spiritual Care Association. (2017). *Spiritual care and nursing: A nurse's contribution and practice.* New York, NY: Author.

Heard, C. P., Scott, J., & Yeo, R. D. S. (2015). Walking the Labyrinth: Considering Mental Health Consumer Experience, Meaning Making, and the Illumination of the Sacred in a Forensic Mental Health Setting. *Journal of Pastoral Care & Counseling, 69*(4), 240–250.

Hofmann, S. G., Grossman, P., & Hinton, D. E. (2011). Loving-kindness and compassion meditation: Potential for psychological interventions. *Clinical Psychology Review, 31*(7), 1126–1132.

Huss, B. (2007). The new age of Kabbalah: Contemporary Kabbalah, the new age and postmodern spirituality. *Journal of Modern Jewish Studies, 6*(2), 107–125.

Jantos, M. (2012). Prayer and meditation. In M. Cobb, C. Puchalski, & B. Rumbold (Eds.), *Oxford Textbook of Spirituality in Healthcare* (pp. 359–365). New York, NY: Oxford University Press.

Josipovic, Z., Dinstein, I., Weber, J., & Heeger, D. J. (2012). Influence of meditation on anti-correlated networks in the brain. *Frontiers in Human Neuroscience, 5*, 183. https://doi.org/10.3389/fnhum.2011.00183.

Keating, T. (2002). *Foundations for centering prayer and the Christian contemplative tradition.* New York, NY: Continuum International.

Keating, T. (2006). *Open Mind, Open Heart: 20th Anniversary Edition.* New York, NY: Continuum International.

Keefe, F. J., Affleck, G., Lefebvre, J., Underwood, L., Caldwell, D. S., Drew, J., … Pargament, K. (2001). Living with rheumatoid arthritis: The role of daily spirituality and daily religious and spiritual coping. *The Journal of Pain, 2*(2), 101–110.

Keng, S. L., & Tan, H. H. (2018). Effects of brief mindfulness and loving-kindness meditation inductions on emotional and behavioral responses to social rejection among individuals with high borderline personality traits. *Behaviour Research and Therapy, 100*, 44–53.

Knabb, J. J. (2012). Centering prayer as an alternative to mindfulness-based cognitive therapy for depression relapse prevention. *Journal of Religion and Health, 51*(3), 908–924.

Koenig, H. (2004). Religion, spirituality, and medicine: Research findings and implications for clinical practice. *Southern Medical Journal, 97*(12), 1194–1200.

Kushner, K. (2012). You cannot wash off blood with blood: Entering the mind through the body. *EXPLORE, 8*(4), 243–248.

LaGrone, M. (2018). Judaism and the Anthropocene. In D. A. DellaSala, & M. I. Goldstein (Eds.), *Encyclopedia of the Anthropocene* (pp. 169–174). Waltham, MA: Elsevier.

Lee, D. (2016). The Buddha and the numen: postmodern spirituality and the problem of transcendence in Buddhism. *International Journal of Dharma Studies, 4*(1), 14.

Leong, F. C. (2014). Complementary and alternative medications for chronic pelvic pain. *Obstetrics and Gynecology Clinics, 41*(3), 503–510.

Li, L., Liu, X., Cai, C., Yang, Y., Li, D., Xiao, L., … Qiu, Y. (2016). Changes of gamma-band oscillatory activity to tonic muscle pain. *Neuroscience Letters, 627*, 126–131.

Lippelt, D. P., Hommel, B., & Colzato, L. S. (2014). Focused attention, open monitoring and loving kindness meditation: effects on attention, conflict monitoring, and creativity–A review. *Frontiers in Psychology.* https://doi.org/10.3389/fpsyg.2014.01083. Article 1083.

Lumma, A. L., Kok, B. E., & Singer, T. (2015). Is meditation always relaxing? Investigating heart rate, heart rate variability, experienced effort and likeability during training of three types of meditation. *International Journal of Psychophysiology, 97*(1), 38–45.

Marchand, W. R. (2012). Mindfulness-based stress reduction, mindfulness-based cognitive therapy, and Zen meditation for depression, anxiety, pain, and psychological distress. *Journal of Psychiatric Practice®, 18*(4), 233–252.

Maruca, A. T., & Shelton, D. (2016). Correctional nursing interventions for incarcerated persons with mental disorders: an integrative review. *Issues in Mental Health Nursing, 37*(5), 285–292.

Minichiello, V. J. (2018). Relaxation techniques. In D. Rakel (Ed.), *Integrative Medicine* (4th Ed., pp. 909–913.e1). Philadelphia, PA: Elsevier.

National Center for Complementary and Integrative Health. (2017). *More than one-third of U.S. adults use complementary and alternative medicine.* Retrieved April 23, 2020 from https://nccih.nih.gov/news/2004/052704.htm.

Newberg, A., Pourdehnad, M., Alavi, A., & d'Aquili, E. G. (2003). Cerebral blood flow during meditative prayer: preliminary findings and methodological issues. *Perceptual and Motor Skills, 97*(2), 625–630.

Newberg, A. B., Wintering, N. A., Yaden, D. B., Waldman, M. R., Reddin, J., & Alavi, A. (2015). A case series study of the neurophysiological effects of altered states of mind during intense Islamic prayer. *Journal of Physiology-Paris, 109*(4), 214–220.

O'Connor, L. E., Rangan, R. K., Berry, J. W., Stiver, D. J., Rick, H., Ark, W., & Li, T. (2015). Empathy, compassionate altruism and psychological well-being in contemplative practitioners across five traditions. *Psychology, 6*(08), 989.

Pearce, M., Coan, A., Herndon, J., Koenig, H., & Abernethy, A. (2012). Unmet spiritual care needs impact emotional and spiritual wellbeing in advanced cancer patients. *Supportive Care in Cancer, 20*(10), 2269–2276.

Pennington, B. (2010). *Centering prayer: Renewing an ancient Christian prayer form.* New York, NY: Image.

Puchalski, C., Ferrell, B., Virani, R., Otis-Green, S., Baird, P., Bull, J., & Sulmasy, D. (2009). Improving the quality of spiritual care as a dimension of palliative care: The report of the consensus conference. *Journal of Palliative Medicine, 12*(10), 885–904.

Ricard, M., Lutz, A., & Davidson, R. J. (2014). Mind of the meditator. *Scientific American, 311*(5), 39–45.

Roberts, L., Ahmed, I., & Davison, A. (2014). Intercessory prayer for the alleviation of ill health. *Cochrane Database of Systematic Reviews,* (6). https://doi.org/10.1002/14651858.CD000368.pub3.

Roggenkamp, H., Waldman, M. R., & Newberg, A. B. (2009). Religious experience: Psychology and neurology. In *Encyclopedia of Consciousness* (pp. 273–287).

Ruchelli, G., Chapin, H., Darnall, E., Seppala, E., Doty, J., & Mackey, S. (2014). Compassion meditation training for people living with chronic pain and their significant others: a pilot study and mixed-methods analysis. *The Journal of Pain, 15*(4), s117. Supp.

Sandor, M. K. (2005). The labyrinth: A walking meditation for healing and self-care. *Explore: The Journal of Science and Healing, 1*(6), 480–483.

Sandor, M. K. (2008). Biobehhavioral and spiritual responses of women in a labyrinth walking program. *Brain, Behavior, and Immunity*, 22(4), 34. Supp.

Sandor, M. K., & Froman, R. D. (2006). Exploring the effects of walking the labyrinth. *Journal of Holistic Nursing*, 24(2), 103–110.

Schneider, R. H., & Carr, T. (2014). Transcendental Meditation in the prevention and treatment of cardiovascular disease and pathophysiological mechanisms: An evidence-based review. *Advances in Integrative Medicine*, 1(3), 107–112.

Schwartz, S. A. (2011). Meditation—The controlled psychophysical self-regulation process that works. *Explore: The Journal of Science and Healing*, 7(6), 348–353.

Self-Realization Fellowship. (1982). *Undreamed-of possibilities*. Los Angeles, CA: Author.

Self-Realization Fellowship. (1984). *Self-realization fellowship worldwide prayer circle*. Los Angeles, CA: Author.

Seminowicz, D. A., & Moayedi, M. (2017). The dorsolateral prefrontal cortex in acute and chronic pain. *The Journal of Pain*, 18(9), 1027–1035.

Shankar, S. S. R., Rosenberg, K. P., Dhawan, A., & Vedamurthachar, A. (2014). Meditation and Spirituality-Based Approaches for Addiction. In *Behavioral Addictions* (pp. 343–360). San Diego, CA: Elsevier.

Shi, L., Zhang, D., Wang, L., Zhuang, J., Cook, R., & Chen, L. (2017). Meditation and blood pressure: a meta-analysis of randomized clinical trials. *Journal of Hypertension*, 35(4), 696–706.

Simkin, D. R., & Black, N. B. (2014). Meditation and mindfulness in clinical practice. *Child and Adolescent Psychiatric Clinics*, 23(3), 487–534.

Soo, M. S., Jarosz, J. A., Wren, A. A., Soo, A. E., Mowery, Y. M., Johnson, K. S., ... Shelby, R. A. (2016). Imaging-guided core-needle breast biopsy: impact of meditation and music interventions on patient anxiety, pain, and fatigue. *Journal of the American College of Radiology*, 13(5), 526–534.

Steinhauser, K. E., Fitchett, G., Handzo, G. F., Johnson, K. S., Koenig, H. G., Pargament, K. I., ... Balboni, T. A. (2017). State of the science of spirituality and palliative care research part I: Definitions, measurement, and outcomes. *Journal of Pain and Symptom Management*, 54(3), 428–440.

Tanaka, G. K., Peressutti, C., Teixeira, S., Cagy, M., Piedade, R., Nardi, A. E., ... Velasques, B. (2014). Lower trait frontal theta activity in mindfulness meditators. *Arquivos de Neuropsiquiatria*, 72(9), 687–693.

Thompson, V. D. (2017). The Power of Prayer. *SIT Digital Collections- Capstone Collection.*, 2976.

Timmins, F., & Neill, F. (2013). Teaching nursing students about spiritual care. A review of the literature. *Nurse Education in Practice*, 13(6), 499–505.

Unruh, A. (2007). Spirituality, religion and pain. *Canadian Journal of Nursing Research*, 39(2), 66–86.

van Lutterveld, R., van Dellen, E., Pal, P., Yang, H., Stam, C. J., & Brewer, J. (2017). Meditation is associated with increased brain network integration. *NeuroImage*, 158(1), 18–25.

Wachholtz, A. B., & Pargament, K. I. (2005). Is spirituality a critical ingredient of meditation? Comparing the effects of spiritual meditation, secular meditation, and relaxation on spiritual, psychological, cardiac, and pain outcomes. *Journal of Behavioral Medicine*, 28(4), 369–384.

Wachholtz, A. B., & Pargament, K. I. (2008). Migraines and meditation: does spirituality matter? *Journal of Behavioral Medicine*, 31(4), 351–366.

Wahbeh, H., Sagher, A., Back, W., Pundhir, P., & Travis, F. (2018). A systematic review of transcendent states across meditation and contemplative traditions. *Explore: The Journal of Science and Healing*, 14(1), 19–35.

Williams, P. B., & Nusbaum, H. C. (2016). Toward a neuroscience of wisdom. In J. Absher, & J. Cloutier (Eds.), *Neuroimaging Personality, Social Cognition, and Character* (pp. 383–395). Elseveier Academic Press.

Williams, P. B., Poljacik, G., Decety, J., & Nusbaum, H. C. (2018). Loving-kindness language exposure leads to changes in sensitivity to imagined pain. *The Journal of Positive Psychology*, 13(4), 429–433.

Woelm, E. (2006). Ridwan School/Diamond Approach (Almaas) pp 37. In E. Woelm. *Hypnotherapy and the Inner Judge: Relevance, Methods and Spiritual Aspects*. Verlag-Haus Monsenstein und Vannerdat.

Wright, V., & Pendry, B. (2016). Compassion and its role in the clinical encounter–An argument for compassion training. *Journal of Herbal Medicine*, 6(4), 198–203.

Yogananda, P. (2000). *Journey to self-realization: Collected talks and essays on realizing god in daily life. Volume III*. Los Angeles, CA: Self-Realization Fellowship Publishers.

Yogananda, P. (2006). *Autobiography of a yogi*. Los Angeles, CA: Self-Realization Fellowship Publishers.

Yogananda, P. (2016). *Scientific healing affirmations*. Los Angeles, CA: Stellar Editions.

Young, C., & Koopsen, C. (2011). *Spirituality, Health and Healing: An Integrative Approach*. Sudbury, MA: Jones and Bartlett Publishers.

Yu, X., Fumoto, M., Nakatani, Y., Sekiyama, T., Kikuchi, H., Seki, Y., ... Arita, H. (2011). Activation of the anterior prefrontal cortex and serotonergic system is associated with improvements in mood and EEG changes induced by Zen meditation practice in novices. *International Journal of Psychophysiology*, 80(2), 103–111.

Zucker, D. M., & Sharma, A. (2012). Labyrinth walking in corrections. *Journal of Addictions Nursing*, 23(1), 47–54.

Zucker, D. M., Choi, J., Cook, M. N., & Croft, J. B. (2016). The Effects of Labyrinth Walking in an Academic Library. *Journal of Library Administration*, 56(8), 957–973.

Chapter 26 Natural Products: Supplements, Botanicals, Vitamins, and Minerals as a Component of Multimodal Pain Management

Ann Quinlan-Colwell

CHAPTER OUTLINE

Dietary Supplements, pg. 688

Botanicals and Herbs, pg. 688

Cannabis (*Cannabis sativa, Cannabis indica,* and *Cannabis Indica*), pg. 688

Cat's Claw (*Uncaria tomentosa*), pg. 692

Cayenne (*Capsicum frutescens*), pg. 693

Devil's Claw (*Harpagophytum procumbens, Harpagophytum zeyheri*), pg. 693

Feverfew (*Tanacetum parthenium* L.), pg. 694

Frankincense or Olibanum (*Boswellia serrata*), pg. 694

Ginger (*Zingiber officinale Roscoe*), pg. 696

Turmeric (*Curcuma longa* or *Curcuma domestica*), pg. 698

Willow Bark (*Salicis Cortex*) and White Willow Bark (*Salix alba*), pg. 700

Other Herbs and Botanicals Used for Pain Management, pg. 701

Pharmaconutrients: Nutritional Modulators of Pain, pg. 702

Avocado and Soybean Unsaponifiables (*Persea gratissma* and *Glycine max*) (Piascledine), pg. 702

Bromelain (*Ananas comosus*) (Pineapple Plant), pg. 704

Flavocoxid, pg. 705

Green Tea (*Camellia sinensis*), pg. 705

Honey, pg. 706

Supplements, pg. 707

Acetyl-L-Carnitine, pg. 707

Coenzyme Q_{10} (Ubiquinone-10), pg. 708

Glucosamine Hydrochloride or Sulfate and Chondroitin Sulfate, pg. 709

Hyaluronic Acid, pg. 710

Lactic Acid–Producing Bacteria (*Lactobacillus acidophilus, casei, fermentum, gasseri, johnsonii, paracasei, plantarum, reuteri, rhamnosus,* and *salivarius; Bacillus coagulans*), pg. 711

Magnesium, pg. 712

Methylsulfonylmethane, pg. 713

Omega-3 Polyunsaturated Fatty Acids (Eicosapentaenoic Acid and Docosahexaenoic Acid), pg. 714

Vitamins, pg. 716

B Vitamins, pg. 716

Vitamin D, pg. 719

Vitamin E, pg. 721

Key Points, pg. 723

Case Scenario, pg. 723

References, pg. 723

Dietary Supplements

Dietary supplements are described in the United States by *The Dietary Supplement Health and Education Act of 1994* (DSHEA), which includes vitamins, minerals, herbs, other botanicals, amino acids, or other dietary substances and any metabolites or extracts, either alone or in combination, that are used for human consumption to enhance dietary intake (U.S. Department of Health and Human Services [DHHS], 1994). These substances, excluding vitamins and minerals, continue to be the most common integrative health care intervention used in the United States (Clarke, Black, Stussman, Barnes, & Nahin, 2015). It is important to educate patients to tell clinicians about all botanicals, herbs, vitamins, and supplements they are taking (NCCIH, 2020). Sharing the information enables clinicians to educate and advise patients about potential interactions with medications, contraindications with comorbidities, and any potential adverse effects. From those perspectives it is important for clinicians to have knowledge about the products.

In this chapter, botanicals/herbs, vitamins, and minerals that can be used as part of a multimodal pain management program are discussed. For each product, the indications, available evidence for pain management, cautions, contradictions, and interactions with medications will be described. Unless otherwise specified, discussion is of the products used by the oral route.

Botanicals and Herbs

Evolving from Neanderthal times, plant products are the oldest element of health care, with use as traditional healing preparations and continuing as a component of modern pharmaceuticals (Chugh, Bali, & Koul, 2018; Faqi & Yan, 2017). The World Health Organization (WHO) estimates that 80% of the international population use herbs medicinally (Biniaz, 2013). The U.S. Food and Drug Administration (FDA) defines botanicals as "products that include plant materials, algae, macroscopic fungi, and combinations thereof," excluding animal products unless they are a component of a traditional botanical preparation (FDA, 2016, p. 2). An important consideration regarding the use of all botanicals is that because of geographic variations, time of harvesting, cultivation, quality control, processing methodology, formulation as fresh or dried, and other factors, there is wide variability in the products, quality, strength, potency, and impurities of each plant (Arablou & Aryaeian, 2017; Faqi & Yan, 2017).

There is also wide variation in how botanicals are regulated in different countries, yet many countries are working to improve safety (Alostad, Steinke, & Schafheutle, 2018) (Table 26.1). For instance, in Australia, botanicals are covered by the *good manufacturing practice* or *GMP* code and if they are considered to be a medicinal plant, they are regulated by the *Therapeutics Goods Act of 1989* (Liu & Wang, 2008). The WHO (2003) and the FDA (2007, 2016, 2018, 2020) have issued guidelines and guidance to improve quality control of botanicals.

Although it is important to know and to remind patients that in the United States herbal preparations are generally not regulated for quality (Sengar et al., 2017), the majority of botanicals available in the United States are generally considered safe, with few adverse events reported (Gardniner, Filipelli, & Low Dog, 2018). That, at least in part, is related to the 1994 DHSEA, which holds manufacturers responsible to prove safety and evidence regarding dietary supplements (FDA, 2007, 2018). In 2007, through the DHSEA, the FDA was assigned "by delegation, the express authority to issue regulations establishing current good manufacturing practice (CGMP) requirements for dietary supplements" (FDA, 2007). That action was intended to promote accuracy of labeling and safety in manufacturing of dietary supplements addressing the purity, potency, and strength with the goal of promoting confidence among consumers. Despite these efforts, additional rigorous research and manufacturing regulations are necessary for natural products to clearly be known as safe products (Chugh et al., 2018). These needs are important because the botanical products are promising as important components of a multimodal approach to pain management (Table 26.2).

It is beyond the scope of this chapter to discuss all herbs, botanicals, and supplements used to relieve pain; thus the most commonly used and more frequently studied ones used for analgesia are discussed in some detail in this chapter. Herbs used to a lesser extent and with less research to support use for analgesia are briefly mentioned. Numerous books are available with in-depth discussions of herbs and plants used for health purposes; the reader is referred to such texts for more information. Table 26.3 lists reputable evidence-based resources.

Cannabis (*Cannabis sativa, Cannabis indica, and Cannabis indica*)

For centuries, *C. sativa*, which is the most common variety of the flowering cannabis herb, containing many cannabinoids and flavonoids, has been used for medicinal purposes (Farag & Kayser, 2017). During the late 19th and early 20th centuries, it was marketed for medicinal use in the United States, but despite the opposition of the American Medical Association cannabis was removed from the U.S. Pharmacopeia by the Cannabis Tax Act of 1937 (Savage et al., 2016). Although it continues to be a Schedule I controlled substance, it remains the most extensively used recreational substance (Abalo & Martín-Fontelles, 2017). Yet, the National Academies of Sciences, Engineering, and Medicine (NASEM, 2017) reported that considerable evidence is available to support using cannabis for chronic pain among adult patients. In an effort to reduce the use of prescription opioids, there is growing interest in using medical cannabis as part of multimodal pain management (Vyas, LeBaron, & Gilson, 2018).

Table 26.1 Summary Comparison of Herbal Medicine (HM) Main Registration Requirements in the Drug Regulatory Authority Systems of the United Kingdom, Germany, United States, United Arab Emirates (UAE), and Kingdom of Bahrain

Main Registration Requirements	Regulatory Authority				
	UK	Germany	USA	UAE	Kingdom of Bahrain
Evidence of quality	GMP standards and QC tests for THR and MA	GMP standards and QC tests for THR and MA	Not required for dietary supplements GMP standards and QC tests for botanical drugs	GMP standards and QC tests for traditional HMs and HMs Declaration of pork-free contents Declaration of alcohol content	GMP standards and QC tests for health products and medicines with a vegetable substance Declaration of pork-free contents Declaration of alcohol content
Evidence of safety	Bibliographic data for THR Toxicologic tests for MA	Bibliographic data for THR Toxicologic tests for MA	Not required for dietary supplements unless it is an NDI Toxicologic tests for botanical drugs	Bibliographic data for traditional HMs Toxicologic studies for HMs	Bibliographic data for health products Toxicologic studies for medicines with a vegetable substance
Evidence of efficacy	Long tradition of use for at least 30 y (including 15 y in the EU) for THR Clinical studies for MA	Long tradition of use for at least 30 y (including 15 y in the EU) for THR Clinical studies for MA	Not required for dietary supplements Clinical studies for botanical drugs	Copies of at least two traditional HMs for each herbal ingredient for traditional HMs Clinical studies for HMs	Copies of published scientific literature or international monographs for health products Clinical studies for medicines with a vegetable substance
Label requirement	For THR: Must include a statement that the product is exclusively based on long-standing use Must include a certification mark (THR)	For THR: Must include the words "traditional medicines" and "traditionally used"	For dietary supplements: Must include a disclaimer: "This statement has not been evaluated by the FDA. This product is not intended to diagnose, treat, cure, or prevent any disease" Must state on the label that it is a dietary supplement	No requirements	No requirements

EU, European Union; FDA, U.S. Food and Drug Administration; GMP, Good Manufacturing Practice; MA, marketing authorization; NDI, new dietary ingredients; QC, quality control; THR, traditional herbal registration.

From Alostad, A. H., Steinke, D. T., & Schafheutle, E. I. (2018). International comparison of five herbal medicine registration systems to inform regulation development: United Kingdom, Germany, United States of America, United Arab Emirates and Kingdom of Bahrain. *Pharmaceutical Medicine, 32*(1), 39–49.

Table 26.2	Information on Testing Dietary Supplement and Herbal Products		
Organization		**What to Look for on the Label**	**Web Address**
NSF is a nonprofit public health organization. NSF's certification service includes product testing, Good Manufacturing Practices (GMPs) inspections, ongoing monitoring, and use of the NSF Mark.		NSF	http://www.nsfconsumer.org/food/dietary_supplements.asp
The United States Pharmacopeia (USP)—testing for contamination, adulteration, and good manufacturing processes. USP also examines products for pharmacologic properties.		USP	http://www.usp.org/usp-verification-services/usp-verified-dietary-supplements
Consumer Labs evaluates commercially available dietary supplement products for composition, potency, purity, bioavailability, and consistency of products.		ConsumerLab.com	http://www.consumerlab.com/
U.S. government—GRAS. "GRAS" is an acronym for the phrase Generally Recognized As Safe. Under sections 201(s) and 409 of the Federal Food, Drug, and Cosmetic Act (the Act), any substance that is intentionally added to food is a food additive, that is subject to premarket review and approval by the FDA, unless the substance is generally recognized, among qualified experts, as having been adequately shown to be safe under the conditions of its intended use, or unless the use of the substance is otherwise excluded from the definition of a food additive.		GRAS	http://www.fda.gov/food/ingredientspackaginglabeling/gras/default.htm
Health Canada—In Canada, dietary supplements are regulated by the government in a natural health products category ensuring safety and efficacy of these products. This link includes all dietary supplements that are licensed for sale in Canada.			http://www.hc-sc.gc.ca/

From Gardiner, P., Filipelli, A. C., & Low Dog, T. (2018). Prescribing botanicals. In D. Rakel (Ed.), *Integrative medicine* (4th ed., pp. 979–985e1). St. Louis: Elsevier.

Evidence for Pain Management

Support of cannabis for analgesic purposes is based on understanding the analgesic action of the endogenous cannabinoids that are naturally produced in the human body (Savage et al., 2016). Reports range between 45% and 80% of people using medicinal cannabis are using it specifically to relieve pain (Nugent et al., 2017). The authors of a large systematic review and meta-analysis (N = 79 trials; n = 6462 subjects) reported evidence supporting use of cannabis to relieve chronic pain and spasticity is of moderate quality (Whiting et al., 2015). The National Academies of Sciences (2017) concluded that there is some evidence to conclude people with chronic pain are likely to significantly reduce pain symptoms by using cannabis. In one large Australian study (N = 1514) the 16% of the participants with noncancer pain who had

used cannabis for analgesia reported on the average 70% pain relief when using cannabis, compared to 50% pain relief when not using cannabis, but they also reported greater pain severity and pain interference than those participants who did not use cannabis (Degenhardt et al., 2015). The authors of a 2015 updated systematic review (N = 11 studies) reported cannabinoids that are currently available are at least moderately effective as a component of a multimodal analgesia (MMA) plan of care for chronic noncancer pain (Lynch & Ware, 2015). The authors of that review noted their two systematic reviews (2011 and 2015) included 29 randomized controlled trials (RCTs) and in the three reviews, safe and modest analgesic benefit with cannabinoids was seen in 22 of 25. Based on systemic review, the Guideline Development Subcommittee of the American Academy of Neurology reported oral

Table 26.3 | Evidence-Based Resources for Dietary Supplements

Subscription Services

Dynamed: Reference tool powered by Ebscohost with summaries for more than 3200 topics. There is a mobile application available as well ($395/year for physician subscription).	http://www.dynamed.com/home/
Natural Medicines: You can search by supplement or commercial product name. Also includes information about pregnancy and lactation, as well as adverse events (inquire for pricing).	https://naturalmedicines.therapeuticresearch.com/
HerbMed: HerbMed is an herbal database that provides scientific data underlying the use of herbs for health. HerbMedPro, an enhanced version of HerbMed, is available for subscription, licensing, and data streaming. The public site has 20 herbs; HerbMedPro has an additional 233 herbs and continuous updating (individual subscriber $45.00/year).	http://www.herbmed.org

Nonsubscription Services

The National Center for Complementary and Alternative Medicine (NCCAM): NCCAM is the federal government's lead agency for scientific research on CAM. *Herbs at a Glance*, a series of 42 patient information sheets, are listed at http://nccam.nih.gov/health/herbsataglance.htm	http://nccam.nih.gov/
NIH Office of Dietary Supplements: Provides overview of vitamins, minerals, and dietary supplements with two levels of information—Health Professional and QuickFacts.	http://ods.od.nih.gov/
Dietary Supplement Labels Database: Dietary supplement labels database offers information about label ingredients, enabling users to compare label ingredients in different brands. Each dietary supplement has additional links to other government-created HDS resources such as Medline, ClinicalTrials.gov, and NCCAM.	https://ods.od.nih.gov/Research/Dietary_Supplement_Label_Database.aspx
MedlinePlus—Dietary Supplements—For Free: This consumer health database from the National Library of Medicine offers extensive information on dietary supplements. http://www.nlm.nih.gov/medlineplus/druginformation.html	http://medlineplus.gov
American Botanical Council: This nonprofit organization has helpful information and continuing medical education resources.	http://www.herbalgram.org
Health Canada: The Canadian government regulates natural health products in Canada licensing products with proof of safety and efficacy. This is a very helpful site—it lists products licensed in Canada and has helpful monographs.	http://www.hc-sc.gc.ca

From Gardiner, P., Filipelli, A. C., & Low Dog, T. (2018). Prescribing botanicals. In D. Rakel (Ed.), *Integrative medicine* (4th ed., pp. 979–985e1.). St. Louis: Elsevier.

cannabis extract is effective in reducing central pain and painful spasms in people living with multiple sclerosis (Koppel et al., 2014). (See Chapter 2 for discussion of central pain.)

Strongest evidence for medicinal use of cannabis is for neuropathic pain. The authors of a meta-analysis (N = 5 studies) using a hierarchal Bayesian methodology to assess the benefit of inhaled cannabis for chronic neuropathic pain reported at least short-term benefit among at least 20% of the participants, but inadequate data for assessment of benefit over time (Andreae et al., 2015). In a double-blind, placebo-controlled, crossover study (N = 39), the researchers found central and peripheral neuropathic pain were reduced with both low and moderate doses of vaporized cannabis, with a 30% reduction in pain intensity (Wilsey et al., 2013). The results of a subsequent RCT cross-over pilot with people with chemotherapy-induced neuropathic pain (N = 18), trended toward significance with average decrease in pain intensity scores of 2.6 on the 0 to 10 numeric analogue scale (NAS) with treatment of

an oral mucosal cannabinoid extract spray (Lynch, Cesar-Rittenberg, & Hohmann, 2014).

An innovative use of cannabis was topically in the treatment of painful wounds (Maida & Corban, 2017). In three cases in which topical cannabis was used to treat the pain associated with wounds resulting from pyoderma gangrenosum, pain was significantly less, and the use of opioids were meaningfully reduced with each person. Rigorous research is needed to identify the benefit of cannabis as an analgesic agent for treatment of nociceptive and neuropathic pain as well as cultivation for medical use (Savage et al., 2016). Research is also needed to assess the benefit of different routes of delivery (oral, inhalation, topical) and long-term benefits versus risks (Andreae et al., 2015). Studies are also needed to identify therapeutic doses and ranges (Zengion & Yarnell, 2011). Finally, screening tools for risk of use disorder need to be evaluated to identify validity and reliability when cannabis is used for medicinal pain control (Sznitman & Room, 2018).

Cautions and Contraindications

The most common physical adverse effects are mild, including dry mouth, nausea, fatigue, dizziness, loss of balance of mild to moderate intensity (Lynch & Ware, 2015; Whiting et al., 2015). Some evidence indicates that hyperalgesia can develop with higher doses (Zengion & Yarnell, 2011). There is concern that cannabis may increase the action of warfarin (Krishna & Purushothaman, 2015), and in people with hepatitis C it may intensify hepatic fibrosis (Zengion & Yarnell, 2011).

Cognitive adverse effects of cannabis use include difficulty in concentrating, anxiety, disorientation, confusion, hallucination, and problems with memory, learning, and psychomotor abilities (Andreae et al., 2015; Whiting et al., 2015). The authors of a Canadian literature review caution smoked cannabis is contraindicated with personal or family histories of substance use disorder, psychosis, cardiovascular or respiratory disorders, and during pregnancy (Kahan, Srivastava, Spithoff, & Bromley, 2014). In addition, those authors advised against driving a motor vehicle within 4 hours of smoking and within 6 hours of ingesting cannabis orally.

Contraindications

Cannabis is considered by some to be contraindicated in anyone who is at risk for mental illness, particularly teenagers (Zengion & Yarnell, 2011).

Potential Interactions With Medications

Risk for potentially substantial negative outcomes related to opioid misuse and alcohol abuse are related to using medicinal cannabis alone (Davis, Walton, Bohnert, Bourque, & Ilgen, 2018; Shah, Craner & Cunningham, 2017), and in conjunction with chronic opioid therapy (Nugent et al., 2017). However, in another study, with people using cannabis from a medical cannabis clinic, there was no relationship seen between those who used prescription pain medication and those who did not with development of abuse of alcohol or other substances (Perron, Bohnert, Perone, Bonn-Miller, & Ilgen, 2015). In people receiving medication-assisted therapy for substance use disorder (see Chapter 14), concomitant use of cannabis with opioids is also associated with greater connections between pain with anxiety and depression, which may be related to less self-efficacy (Wilson et al., 2018). There is need for additional research regarding the risks versus benefits of concomitant use of opioids with cannabis.

Cat's Claw (Uncaria tomentosa)

Cat's claw (*Uncaria tomentosa* or *Uncaria guianensis*) is a woody vine plant with thorns similar to the claws of a cat that grows naturally in the Amazon rainforest and tropical regions of Central and South America (de Paula et al., 2015; National Center for Complementary and Integrative Health [NCCIH], 2020a). Since the time of the

Inca civilization cat's claw has been used by Ashaninka priests of the Amazon region in the treatment of people to diminish inflammation, arthritis, gastritis, colitis, viral infections, and cancer and to stimulate the immune system (Chauhan, Singh, Bajaj, & Chauhan, 2015; Hardin, 2007; NCCIH, 2020a). Today the root and bark of *U. tomentosa*, which is the most commercially prepared species, are used for a variety of conditions, including arthritis, colitis, diverticulitis, and gastritis (Hardin, 2007; NCCIH, 2020a). In the United States it is sold as a phytomedicine (plant used for medicinal purposes) (Hardin, 2007).

Evidence for Pain Management

It is thought that the analgesic effect of cat's claw occurs through inhibition of nitrate formation and activation of tumor necrosis factor (TNF–α), an antioxidant with antiinflammatory properties with quinovic acid glycosides, sterols, and oxindole alkaloids being the active ingredients (Akhtar & Haqqi, 2011; Hardin, 2007). However, it is suggested that the antiinflammatory effects do not depend on the alkaloid content (Akhtar & Haqqi, 2011). When studied in Jurkat T (leukemic) cells, cat's claw (*U. tomentosa*) inhibited both COX-1 and COX-2 by impeding activation of TNF–α (Akhtar & Haqqi, 2011). In a small study (N = 51) with adult patients with cancer, aside from any antiinflammatory action, cat's claw was found to have some benefit to reduce fatigue and improve general quality of life (de Paula et al., 2015).

The data regarding cat's claw in treating pain with osteoarthritis (OA) is mixed. In one older study, pain during activity was reported to be significantly reduced but pain at night was not lessened (Akhtar & Haqqi, 2011). There is no definitive evidence to support using cat's claw as an analgesic; therefore additional rigorous research is needed to clarify the benefit of cat's claw as part of MMA treatment (Akhtar & Haqqi, 2011; NCCIH, 2020a). Research is also needed to control for variability of harvesting while controlling for temperature and method of extraction of the therapeutic ingredients (Froeling & Stebbing, 2014).

Cautions

Scant adverse effects have been reported when small doses of cat's claw are used (NCCIH, 2020a). Although current information indicates that cat's claw is nontoxic in vitro, additional research is needed with animals regarding the safety profile (Akhtar & Haqqi, 2011).

Contraindications

It should be avoided in pregnant women or women wanting to become pregnant because it has a history of use for contraception and aborting pregnancies (NCCIH, 2020a).

Potential Interactions With Medications

An interesting potential interaction is that cat's claw may have a gastrointestinal (GI) protective effective when used in conjunction with nonsteroidal antiinflammatory drugs (NSAIDs) (Sandoval et al., 2002). A concern for using cat's claw is the inhibition in laboratory studies of CYP3A4, which is involved in the breakdown of numerous compounds that could increase serum levels of medications taken concomitantly with cat's claw (Froeling & Stebbing, 2014). There is a potential that it may increase the serum level of human immunodeficiency virus (HIV) protease inhibitors; however, it is considered a very low risk (Bone & Mills, 2013a). That action is most likely related to the immune stimulating effects and should be avoided with immunosuppressive medications (Chauhan et al., 2015). Cat's claw may increase the effect of cyclo-SPORINE (Boullata, 2005). It has been associated with increased action of diazepam (Quílez, Saenz, & García, 2012). It also has been associated with blood thinning and should be used with caution by people prescribed antihypertensive medications, and it should not be used when antacids are being used (Chauhan et al., 2015).

Cayenne *(Capsicum frutescens)*

Capsicum is a substance found in several types of hot peppers and has been used as a traditional antiinflammatory agent for centuries, with particular benefit for neuropathic pain (Zampieron & Kamhi, 2015). Because capsicum is now used frequently for analgesia as a prescription medication, it is discussed fully in Chapter 16 from that perspective.

Devil's Claw *(Harpagophytum procumbens, Harpagophytum zeyheri)*

Devil's claw refers collectively to *H. procumbens* and *H. zeyheri,* which are taxonomically close and used equivalently (Mncwangi, Vermaak, & Viljoen, 2014). They are found primarily in the Kalahari Desert of South Africa (Singh et al., 2017). Devil's claw has a centuries long history of use as an analgesic in African countries and since the middle of the last century has been used in various formulations to treat rheumatoid illness in Europe (Akhtar & Haqqi, 2011). During the last decade, Devil's claw was recommended for OA and low back pain as well as dyspepsia and anorexia by the European Scientific Cooperative on Phytotherapy (Fiebich, Muñoz, Rose, Weiss, & McGregor, 2012). The European Pharmacopoeia states that the iridoid glycoside ingredient *harpagoside* should constitute at least 1.2% of devil's claw products (Georgiev, Ivanovska, Alipieva, Dimitrova, & Verpoorte, 2013).

Evidence for Pain Management

The analgesic action of devil's claw is thought to be through inhibition of cyclooxygenase 2 (COX-2) and nitric oxide synthase with particular action on interleukin-6 (IL-6) and IL-1β, thromboxane B2, prostaglandin E_2, and TNF but not with the arachidonic acid pathway (Akhtar & Haqqi, 2011; Fiebich et al., 2012; Smithson, Kellick, & Mergenhagen, 2017). In mouse studies, harpagoside was found to have strong inhibition of COX-1 and portions of the plant were

effective in inhibition of COX-2 and proinflammatory mediators, including nitric oxide and prostaglandin E_2 (Dimitrova, Georgiev, Khan, & Ivanovska, 2013).

Analysis of 15 different studies led to a recommendation that at least 50 mg of the active ingredient harpagoside in Devil's claw is an effective treatment of arthritis, including OA of the knees (Georgiev et al., 2013). A 2006 Cochrane review reported that 50 to 100 mg of harpagoside may be more effective than placebo and was comparable to the COX selective medication rofecoxib (Vioxx) (Gagnier, Van Tulder, Berman, & Bombardier, 2006), which was available at that time but is no longer available in the United States. In a more recent Cochrane review, findings were similar (Oltean et al., 2014). The authors of an analysis of five systematic reviews reported strong evidence for using devil's claw with low back and OA pains of hips and knees, with it not being inferior to the effect of NSAIDs (Lemmon & Roseen, 2018). In addition to devil's claw being reported to reduce back and OA pain, it has been associated with a reduction in the use of NSAID when used by people also taking NSAIDs for those conditions (Smithson et al., 2017).

An interesting application of devil's claw was evaluating the effect on neuropathic pain in rodent studies, in which there was a positive analgesic benefit not only for chronic neuropathic pain but also for postoperative pain (Lim, Kim, Han, & Kim, 2014). Further research is needed to explore the potential role of devil's claw with neuropathic pain. Additional research is needed to determine the possible benefit for rheumatoid arthritis (RA) (Smithson et al., 2017). Studies are needed to identify the biosynthesis, optimal doses, and preferred routes of administration (Georgiev et al., 2013).

Cautions

Other than minor GI side effects (Akhtar & Haqqi, 2011), devil's claw is considered safe in recommended doses even during chronic use (Al-Harbi, Al-Ashban, & Shah, 2013). One caution is that it can increase the effects of warfarin (Zengion & Yarnell, 2011).

Although *H. procumbens* and *H. zeyheri* are used interchangeably, they are not identical, with *H. zeyheri* containing less *Harpagophytum,* which can be identified by infrared hyperspectral imaging (Mncwangi et al., 2014).

Contraindications

Use of devil's claw is contraindicated in people with diarrhea, acute peptic ulcers, and hyperchlorhydria (high levels of stomach acid) (Zengion & Yarnell, 2011).

Potential Interactions With Medications

There are no known interactions with other medicinal products according to the European Medicines Agency (EMA, 2016); however, caution is needed in the presence of anticoagulant medications (Lemmon & Roseen, 2018). There is particular concern with warfarin because the effect may be increased (Krishna & Purushothaman, 2015).

Feverfew (*Tanacetum parthenium* L.)

Feverfew or *T. parthenium* L. is a perennial herb in the Asteraceae family that is native to Asia Minor and the Balkan Peninsula and has been used as an antiinflammatory agent to treat arthritis, headaches, and dysmenorrhea since ancient Roman and Greek times (Mannelli et al., 2015; Pareek, Suthar, Rathore, & Bansal, 2011; Wider, Pittler, & Ernst, 2015). It is now grown worldwide and is most frequently used as an intervention to both prevent and alleviate migraine headaches (Wider et al., 2015). Feverfew is increasingly being studied with growing support for a variety of health care purposes, including pain, gastric disturbances, skin disorders, gynecologic issues, and vertigo, among many others (Pareek et al., 2011).

Evidence for Pain Management

Although the precise mechanism of action is not known, analgesic effects are thought to be primarily the result of the presence of sesquiterpene lactones and polar flavonoids, especially the lipophilic parthenolide, which noncompetitively inhibits serotonin (5-HT) (Mannelli et al., 2015; Pareek et al., 2011; Wider et al., 2015). Prostaglandin synthesis is interrupted and prevented by *tanetin,* which is a lipophilic flavonoid from the leaves, flowers, and seeds of the plant (Pareek et al., 2011). Finally, parthenolides most likely act in the blood vessels to interrupt the contracting and relaxing mechanisms in those vessels (Wider et al., 2015). The researchers of a mouse study proposed that feverfew is effective for migraine headaches as a result of the action of parthenolide as a partial agonist at transient receptor potential, including ankyrin 1 (TRPA1), which then inhibits calcitonin gene-related peptide (CGRP), which is known to trigger the onset of migraine headaches (Materazzi et al., 2013).

Feverfew has been most extensively studied as a treatment for headaches, particularly migraine headaches (Mannelli et al., 2015), for which it is often used prophylactically (Materazzi et al., 2013). However, study results have been inconsistent, which may be at least in part caused by variability in the strength of the plant used and stability of the preparation (Wider et al., 2015). Despite this, feverfew can be an effective treatment in a multimodal approach for migraine and has been suggested as a potentially effective option by the American Academy of Neurology and the American Headache Society (Holland et al., 2012). The benefit of feverfew with migraine is likely related to inhibiting prostaglandin synthesis and reducing spasms of vascular smooth muscle and interrupting the secretion of platelet granule and release of serotonin from them (Bega, 2017; Pareek et al., 2011). In a large study (N = 180) the feverfew extract (MIG-99) in a carbon dioxide base at a dose of 6.25 mg three times per day was effective ($p = 0.0456$) in preventing migraine headaches (Diener, Pfaffenrath, Schnitker, Friede, & Henneicke-von Zepelin, 2005). In a more recent study of 60 participants reporting 151 headaches, sublingual feverfew in combination with ginger was effective in treating migraine with 63% of the participants reporting pain relief within 2 hours of taking sublingual combination (Cady et al., 2011). The authors of a 2015 Cochrane Library review concluded there was low-quality evidence to support feverfew as effective in migraine prevention and noted many of the studies in the review were small with diverse methodology (Wider et al., 2015). Those authors also noted a more recent study with more participants; there was a (0.6) difference in effect in the frequency of migraines with feverfew compared to placebo. They added that feverfew seems to be well tolerated with no significant safety concerns. It is clear that additional research with larger samples and rigorous methodology is needed.

Feverfew does have potential for use with other painful conditions, including RA (Pourianezhad, Tahmasebi, Nikfar, & Mirhoseini, 2016). When used in mice with a variety of pain models, including OA and chemotherapy-induced neuropathic pain, feverfew was an effective analgesic (Mannelli et al., 2015). Relief of diabetic neuropathy was reported from rat studies (Galeotti, Maidecchi, Mattoli, Burico, & Ghelardini, 2014). Additional research is needed to explore the role of feverfew with neuropathic pain in animals and then in humans.

Cautions

Feverfew is considered safe with only relatively minor and reversible side effects, including oral ulcers, loss of taste, skin rashes, nausea and bloating, and muscle and joint discomfort (NCCIH, 2019a; Wider et al., 2015). Chewing leaves or seeds may result in oral swelling and ulcers of the mouth (Mariotti, 2016). Because it is in the family with ragweed and chamomile, it should be avoided by people with allergies to those plants (Pizzorno, Murray & Joiner-Bey, 2016). People who stop taking feverfew after prolonged use may experience sleeping difficulties, headaches, nervousness, and joint stiffness or pain (Mariotti, 2016; NCCIH, 2019a).

Contraindications

Because of the uterine stimulating effect and the folk history of it being used as an abortifacient, feverfew should be avoided during pregnancy (Pareek et al., 2011; Zengion & Yarnell, 2011).

Potential Interactions With Medications

Feverfew can inhibit platelet activity; therefore, it may cause increased bleeding when anticoagulants are taken at the same time (Pareek et al., 2011).

Frankincense or Olibanum (*Boswellia serrata*)

B. serrata is an herb from the resin extracted from the genus *Boswellia,* also known as frankincense or olibanum, and derived from the deciduous *Boswellia* trees that have grown in the Arabian Peninsula and Northern Africa for centuries, with frankincense oils being available in a variety of the *Boswellia* species (Hussain, Al-Harrasi, & Green, 2016). In addition, *B. serrata* grows in India, where it has been used since prehistoric times and in Ayurvedic medicine to treat various health conditions, including chronic inflammatory conditions such as asthma, chronic colitis, ulcerative colitis, Crohn's disease, skin irritations, and RA; chronic pain; diabetes; memory loss; and some cancers (Hamidpour, Hamidpour, Hamidpour, & Shahlari, 2013; Iram, Khan, & Husain, 2017). The benefits of *Boswellia* are due to the antiinflammatory, analgesic, and antiarthritic properties (Bone & Mills, 2013b; Smithson et al., 2017).

Evidence for Pain Management

In some literature, *B. serrata* is considered to be one of the botanical agents with the strongest evidence for use as an analgesic agent (Chiramonte, D'Adamo, & Morrison, 2014); however, in other literature it is considered to be promising but needing more research (Perlman, Rosenberger, & Ali, 2018). The four boswellic acids that are the active compounds of frankincense, inhibit proinflammatory enzymes (Merolla & Cerciello, 2017). Of the four, acetyl-11-keto-β-boswellic acid (AKBA) is the most effective because AKBA is what inhibits the enzyme 5-lipoxygenase (LOX) by binding to it as a noncompetitive inhibitor (Hamidpour et al., 2013; Merolla & Cerciello, 2017) (Fig. 26.1). It is also believed that *Boswellia* inhibits leukotriene biosynthesis and thus reduces the white blood cell count, which is why it is so beneficial with RA (Smithson et al., 2017). Antiinflammatory effects were seen in both human peripheral mononuclear blood cells and mouse macrophages when tested with AKBA from unadulterated *B. serrata* (Merolla & Cerciello, 2017). In addition, AKBA is thought to have a synergistic effect on NSAIDS (Bishnoi, Patil, Kumar, & Kulkarni, 2006). Additional research is needed to explore that relationship

because using the two together could lead to a reduction in standard doses of NSAIDs, thus reducing adverse effects of the NSAIDS (Merolla & Cerciello, 2017) (Box 26.1).

Between 2003 and 2011, the researchers of five RCTs reported pain was reduced statistically and clinically (Chiramonte et al., 2014). One of those studies compared *B. serrata* with valdecoxib (a COX selective medication that is no longer available in the United States) and found *B. serrata* to be statistically significant in reducing pain after 2 months of therapy, with results lasting for 1 month after *B. serrata* was no longer taken (Sontakke et al., 2007). The authors of a virtual Nursing Alliance Leadership Academy Cochrane review reported that *B. serrata* demonstrated potential benefit for OA and needed additional research (Cameron & Chrubasik, 2014). That review was followed by a 2016 Cochrane review that reported that *B. serrata* combined with the soybean and avocado in the herbal supplement *Piascledine* in a 300 mg/day dose demonstrated short-term effects for symptoms associated with OA (Rodriguez-Merchan, 2016).

B. serrata was used successfully in small older studies with patients with inflammatory bowel disorders. In two studies with people living with ulcerative colitis, *B. serrata* was effective in reducing symptoms (Parian, Mullin, Langhorst, & Brown, 2018). In one of those studies with patients with ulcerative colitis and Crohn's disease, *Boswellia* was as effective as sulfasalazine in relieving symptoms. In the second study with patients living with Crohn's disease, *B. serrata* was considered noninferior to mesalamine.

An innovative study used *B. serrata* or frankincense in combination with myrrh to evaluate the effect of the combined herbs in a water formulation on neuropathic pain in mice (Hu et al., 2017). In that study, the researchers reported a nociceptive response plus alleviation of thermal hypersensitivity and mechanical allodynia. Because neuropathic pain is the source of much suffering and

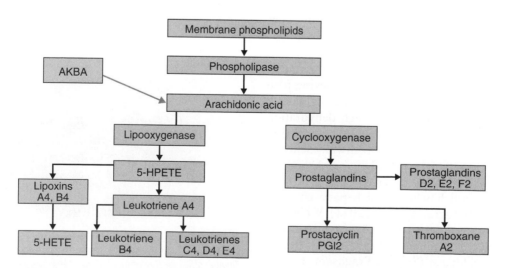

Fig. 26.1 | *AKBA*, Acetyl-11-keto-β-boswellic acid. (From Merolla, G., & Cerciello, S. [2017]. Conservative and postoperative coanalgesic therapy for upper limb tendinopathy using dietary supplements. In R. R. Watson, & S. Zibadi [Eds.]. *Nutritional modulators of pain in the aging population* [pp. 235–243]. London: Elsevier.)

treatment of it can be challenging, additional research is definitely warranted. In another pioneering study in India, an emulsion form of *B. serrata* and another herbal agent (*Withania somnifera*) was developed for topical use with greater permeability (Goyal, Ramchandani, Shrivastava, & Dubey, 2011). That work is important because *B. serrata* has a short elimination half-life and does not have good oral bioavailability, but the high lipophilicity has impeded topical absorption. This new emulsion formulation is promising for topical analgesic use.

Cautions

B. serrata is considered safe, well tolerated, and to have no major side effects (Hamidpour et al., 2013). Rare GI (diarrhea) and skin side effects (urticaria and contact dermatitis) have been reported (Chiramonte et al., 2014; Zengion & Yarnell, 2011).

Contraindications

No contraindications were found.

Potential Interactions With Medications

Information from the Italian Surveillance System of Natural Health Products reported that when *B. serrata* was taken concomitantly with warfarin, at least five patients had increased international normalized ratio (INR) levels, but INR returned to previous levels when the *B. serrata* was discontinued (Paoletti et al., 2011) (Box 26.1).

Ginger (*Zingiber officinale Roscoe*)

Ginger is the rhizome, or root, of the perennial flowering *Zingiber officinale Roscoe* plant, which is one of the hot spices used medicinally for more than 4000 years in Asian countries, where it is native (Arablou & Aryaeian, 2017; Biniaz, 2013; Inserra & Brooks, 2017; Mbaveng & Kuete, 2017; Srinivasan, 2017). It is traditionally and commonly used as a seasoning, supplement, and aromatherapy agent (see Chapter 27), health supplement, and medicinal therapeutic (Inserra & Brooks, 2017) (Fig. 26.2).

The therapeutic effect of ginger in reducing inflammation, preventing or alleviating nausea, and relieving pain are linked with the phytochemical gingerol components, which are transformed to shogaols through dehydration of the gingerols, which are unstable with temperature changes (Inserra & Brooks, 2017; Semwal, Semwal, Combrinck, & Viljoen, 2015; Soltani, Jangjoo, Aghaei, & Dalili, 2017). Ginger is reported to have hepatoprotective benefit in lowering total bilirubin and hepatic enzymes (Alqasoumi, Yusufoglu, Farraj, & Alam, 2011). When ginger was administered in doses of 30 mg/kg in mice, it was reported to be protective against acetaminophen hepatotoxicity similar to silymarin (Sabina, Pragasam, Kumar, & Rasool, 2011). It is also reported to have immunomodulatory, antimicrobial, antiobesity, antiallergic, antiangiogenic, antiatherosclerotic, and antiplatelet aggregation

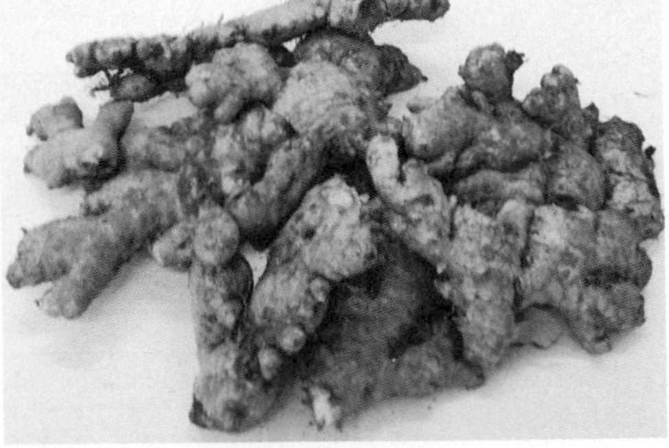

Box 26.1 | Clinical Example

Having dealt with chronic migraine and cervicogenic headaches for over 20 years, I thought I had tried everything. Too many drugs to mention, acupuncture, massage, physical therapy, ice, heat, orthopedic pillows, multiple nutritional supplements, and dietary changes didn't make much of a difference. Botox works well for about 8 weeks. Unfortunately, one can only receive it every 3 months.

I then visited a headache specialist who is a neurologist and psychiatrist. Besides the intervention medical combinations he prescribed, he also suggested that I try a product that was shown in studies to be effective on indomethacin-responsive headaches. I had tried and been very responsive to indomethacin in the past but had to stop taking it because of GI side effects, so I gave the supplement a try. The name brand of the product was Gilacin, but it can be bought in many vitamin or supplement shops, as it is actually *Boswellia serrata* (Indian frankincense). I currently take 300 mg three times daily and it has decreased the frequency of my headaches by at least 50%! It is meant to be used as a preventive, not an abortive, medication. The side effects have been minimal, and most noted has been indigestion. The trick is to drink plenty of water to wash the capsules down. If the powder is released in the esophagus it can burn and does not taste very good. Also noted for me was some hair loss, but no more than I had on another medication (topiramate [Topamax]) and certainly not so much that I wanted to stop the supplement. It seems to work well for me, and it is one more tool in the toolbox that is not an expensive prescription that causes miserable intolerable side effects.
Cindy Kerwick, RN, ACM, CCM
Wilmington, NC

Fig. 26.2 | Ginger is the rhizome or root of the perennial flowering *Zingiber officinale Roscoe* plant. (From Mbaveng, A. T., & Kuete, V. [2017]. *Zingiber officinale*. In V. Kuete [Ed.], *Medicinal spices and vegetables from Africa: Therapeutic potential against metabolic, inflammatory, infections and systematic diseases* [pp. 627–639]. London: Academic Press.)

properties (Semwal et al., 2015). Relevant to those properties, ginger is traditionally used to prevent and treat many conditions, including common upper respiratory tract infections, diabetes, GI symptoms, and pain, and for cardiovascular protective and cancer preventive purposes (Mbaveng & Kuete, 2017; Srinivasan, 2017). Ginger is cleared quickly from the blood of rats and metabolized in the liver, with glucuronide conjugates being excreted through bile with scant amounts of polar metabolites excreted in urine (Arablou & Aryaeian, 2017).

Evidence for Pain Management

Even though ginger is widely used in cooking and complementary health care, little evidence exists concerning the bioavailability of its compounds in humans (Arablou & Aryaeian, 2017). It has long been used in traditional Eastern medicine as an intervention to relieve and prevent nausea with the thought that the effect is due to the inhibitory effect of the gingerol and shogaol components of ginger at M3 and 5-HT3 receptors (Semwal et al., 2015). When compared to ondansetron, when both were administered 1 hour before patients (n = 100) undergoing laparoscopic cholecystectomy, those who received 500 mg oral ginger reported significantly less severity of nausea (Soltani et al., 2017).

Ginger is thought to have antiinflammatory properties related to inhibiting COX, LOX, leukotriene, and prostaglandin synthesis (Rahnama, Montazeri, Huseini, Kianbakht, & Naseri, 2012; Shirvani, Motahari-Tabari, & Alipour, 2017). In animals those properties of ginger were reported to have greater potency than aspirin (Inserra & Brooks, 2017). These antiinflammatory effects of ginger are reported to be beneficial in a variety of painful conditions, including dysmenorrhea, musculoskeletal disorders, RA, and potentially with neuropathic pain situations (Biniaz, 2013; Ha et al., 2012).

Ginger has long been used as a treatment for dysmenorrhea because of what is thought to be inhibition of prostaglandin synthesis and COX (Rahnama et al, 2012). Compared to placebo in students with dysmenorrhea (N = 102), ginger was statistically significant (P = .015) for reducing pain intensity and in pain duration (P = .017) (Rahnama et al., 2012). A second study comparing ginger (n = 35) to placebo (n = 34), ginger was significantly (P < .001) more effective in relieving pain of dysmenorrhea (Jenabi, 2013). In a placebo-controlled randomized study (N = 137) individually comparing zinc (n = 56) with ginger (n = 48) with placebo (n = 46), both zinc and ginger were reported as statistically significant (P < .01) in reducing pain associated with dysmenorrhea (Kashefi, Khajehei, Tabatabaeichehr, Alavinia, & Asili, 2014). However, when ginger (n = 61) was compared to stretching exercises (n = 61) to manage dysmenorrhea pain, ginger was reported as statistically effective in reducing pain intensity (P < .001) but was less effective than exercise and significantly less effective over time and with the duration of time pain was experienced compared with exercise (Shirvani et al., 2017).

The antiinflammatory and analgesic properties of ginger are basic to its benefit with musculoskeletal conditions (Mbaveng & Kuete, 2017) including RA (Biniaz, 2013). The authors of a systematic review of seven studies in which ginger was used for muscle fatigue and pain concluded that when approximately 2 g/day of ginger is taken for at least 5 days, it may help reduce muscle pain after resistance exercise and extended periods of running (Wilson, 2015). In a number of older studies with humans, 400 to 600 mg/day of ginger in divided doses was effective in reducing pain in patients with arthritic knees (Srinivasan, 2017). Ginger was also found to be effective in reducing nitric oxide and C-reactive protein in patients with OA of the knees (N = 120) and those effects continued over 3 months (Naderi, Mozaffari-Khosravi, Dehghan, Nadjarzadeh, & Huseini, 2016). When in a very small study ginger (n = 21) was compared to the NSAID diclofenac (n = 22), ginger was reported to be equally as effective without the distressing GI symptoms (Drozdov, Kim, Tkachenko, & Varvanina, 2012). The authors of a meta-analysis of five randomized placebo-controlled trials evaluating the effect of ginger in patients with OA concluded that ginger had modest benefit with modest quality of evidence; however, the studies were not large enough to perform adequate intent to treat analyses (Bartels et al., 2015). When 1000 mg of ginger in capsule form was taken daily, in patients with pain related to OA of the knees (N = 77), those who received the ginger (n = 37) reported significantly less pain (p = 0.001) and satisfaction with pain control was significantly greater (P = .012) than those who did not receive ginger (n = 40) (Alipour et al., 2017).

Although current information is supportive of ginger having antiinflammatory properties and analgesic benefit, rigorous research is needed to determine the efficacy of ginger as an antiinflammatory and analgesic agent (Hillinger, Wolever, McKernan, & Elam, 2017; Terry, Posadzki, Watson, & Ernst, 2011). Research is also needed regarding parameters of oxidative stress if 1 g of ginger is taken daily (Naderi et al., 2016). The 6-shogaol component of ginger was evaluated in in vivo laboratory studies, which showed neuroprotective effects (Ha et al., 2012). Considering that neuropathic pain can cause significant distress and is difficult to treat, this is an area that needs additional research.

Cautions

Ginger is generally considered to be a safe product and adverse effects are rare (Arablou & Aryaeian, 2017; Bartels et al., 2015; Soltani et al., 2017). Ginger has been reported as safe for the treatment of pregnancy-related nausea and vomiting (Viljoen, Visser, Koen, & Musekiwa, 2014). However, more recently it is recommended that women who are pregnant should avoid using ginger and at a minimum need to confer with clinicians before use (Kim & Choi, 2017), as should all people taking medications. The few side effects that have been reported include mild GI distress (mild heartburn, flatus, belching), diarrhea (Arablou & Aryaeian, 2017; Bartels et al., 2015; Kashefi et al., 2014) and oral irritation if taken in large doses. The GI effects can be minimized by taking it with meals or in a capsule form.

Contraindications

Contraindications are discussed in the section on potential interactions with medications.

Potential Interactions With Medications

Ginger is contraindicated with bleeding disorders and when using anticoagulant medications and is contraindicated when NIFEdipine is being used (Bone & Mills, 2013a; Krishna & Purushothaman, 2015). It may reduce the effectiveness of antacids (Bone & Mills, 2013a). Because ginger is associated with reduction of serum lipid levels it should be used with caution by people taking medications to treat diabetes and cardiac conditions, including hypertension (Arablou & Aryaeian, 2017).

Turmeric (*Curcuma longa* or *Curcuma domestica*)

Turmeric, or *Curcuma longa* or *C. longa* or *C. domestica*, is a perennial herb of several varieties grown in tropical Asia, with the constituent curcumin isolated from the rhizome (Miyazaki et al., 2014) (Fig. 26.3). Curcumin is a polyphenol and active biomolecule in the Indian spice turmeric (Peddada, Peddada, Shukla, Mishra, & Verma, 2015). It has been used for centuries as a traditional Eastern medicine with the belief that it is strong in promoting an antioxidant response (Belcaro et al., 2014) and antiinflammatory properties

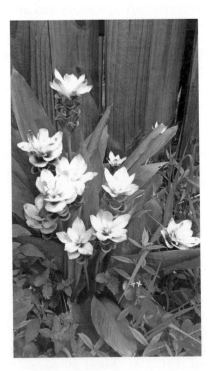

Fig. 26.3 | Curcumin plant flowering.

(Srivastava, Saksena, Khattri, Kumar, & Dagur, 2016). Daily doses of 2 to 10g were considered safe for most people in research studies (Lopez, 2012). The recommended daily dose of turmeric is approximately 1200mg (Smithson, 2017).

Evidence for Pain Management

Curcumin decreases inflammation by suppressing the expression of inflammatory cytokines that curcumin decreases inflammation (Arablou & Kolahdouz-Mohammadi, 2017). The antioxidant and antiinflammatory properties are why curcumin has been a source of interest for treatment of painful conditions that have inflammatory components such as arthritis. For many years, laboratory evidence has supported curcumin, in nontoxic doses demonstrating direct selective COX-2 inhibitor properties when used to treat human colon cancer cells (Goel, Boland, & Chauhan, 2001). Two promising benefits of curcumin are based on reports showing that in vivo it has nephroprotective properties related to mitochondrial fission and autophagy (Molina-Jijón et al., 2016) and promotes hepatic detoxification in part through antioxidant properties (Nabavi, Daglia, Moghaddam, Habtemariam, & Nabavi, 2014). This is particularly encouraging from an analgesic perspective because many medications are contraindicated with kidney and liver disorders.

Numerous research studies have evaluated the antiinflammatory and antinociceptive properties of curcumin in rodents. In addition to antiinflammatory properties it is likely curcumin has additional analgesic properties, including benefit with neuropathic pain. Curcumin was studied with neuropathic sciatic pain in rats with the rats demonstrating fewer pain behaviors and reduced COX-2 serum levels after receiving curcumin (Zanjani, Ameli, Labibi, Sedaghat, & Sabetkasaei, 2014). In another study evaluating the benefit of curcumin with neuropathic pain in rats, the rats who received curcumin had reductions of brain-derived neurotrophic factor and COX-2 in the spinal cord that were dose dependent (Zhu et al., 2014). When curcumin was repeatedly injected intrathecally in another rat model study there was glial cell activation and production of several inflammatory mediators in the spinal cord (Chen et al., 2015). In addition, the results of a study using curcumin in mice with hind paw surgery are promising for using curcumin postoperatively (Sahbaie, Sun, Liang, Shi, & Clark, 2014). In that study, the mice demonstrated less spontaneous pain and abnormal gait and less inflammation at the incisions and nociceptive sensitization (Box 26.2). Finally, when *C. longa* was combined with *Morus alba*, a root bark to treat edema in the paws of rats, the combination inhibited both COX and LOX enzyme functions and had bradykinin receptor antagonist properties as well (Yimam et al., 2016).

The authors of a literature review reported curcumin is potentially beneficial in treatment of a variety of musculoskeletal conditions in humans, including OA, sarcoma, musculocartilaginous disorders, and osteoporosis

The fact that the mice exhibited less abnormal gait is interesting to this author because of a recent patient report. An 85-year-old man started taking curcumin for chronic back, hip, and knee pain. After 2 weeks of taking curcumin on a daily basis, he reported that not only did his back, hip, and knee pain dramatically lessen, but also the neuropathic pain in his feet improved, and he was able to walk without shoes for the first time in years. He asked if the curcumin could also affect his balance and steadiness walking. Coincidentally, he and his wife both noticed that since taking curcumin, he was markedly more steady when walking, with only rare instances of unsteadiness. She was very happy about the improvement in his gait since she was very concerned about him falling. He was very pleased with the improvements in steadiness and pain, especially the reduction in neuropathic pain in his feet.

(Peddada et al., 2015). When used in a large study with people living with chronic pain due to OA of the knees (N = 331), those who received extracts from *C. domestica* (n = 171) had no statistical difference in reports of pain or function compared to those who were treated with ibuprofen (n = 160) (Kuptniratsaikul et al., 2014). In that study the reported side effects were comparable, but GI side effects were less among the *C. domestica* group. More recently, from a 4-month randomized double-blind, placebo-controlled study with people living with OA of the knees (N = 160), it was reported that curcumin suppressed inflammation with reduced biomarkers, decreased oxidative stress, and was associated with greater physical function (Srivastava et al., 2016).

Curcumin also has been evaluated as a treatment for pain other than musculoskeletal pain in humans. In a human experimental heat pain threshold study, curcumin did not affect the pain thresholds but did significantly reduce spontaneous pain intensity and the unpleasantness associated with them (Domenico, Linsehbardt, Haney, & Meagher, 2015). It is reportedly effective as an anti-inflammatory and analgesic agent with wound healing in preclinical studies as well as with burns (Cheppudira et al., 2013). Through a literature review (N = 8 studies) curcumin was reported to be effective for treating endometriosis not only by reducing inflammation but also by inhibiting the invasion, attachment, and angiogenesis of endometrial lesions and by inhibiting proliferation of cells (Arablou & Kolahdouz-Mohammadi, 2017). Early studies investigating the effect of curcumin as a protective treatment for inflammatory bowel disease are encouraging; however, additional research is needed (Loganes et al., 2017).

The major limitation in the use of curcumin is that it has poor bioavailability through the GI tract (Gopi et al., 2017). Recent research in Europe and Asia resulted in the development of products to compensate for that limitation. One product with an improved delivery formulation of *C. longa* (Meriva) is manufactured in Italy (Belcaro et al., 2014) and uses a lecithin (fat) delivery complex with phosphatidylcholine (Hillinger et al., 2017; Dell'Agli et al., 2016). In one laboratory rat study, curcumin by the improved formulation was found in the frontal lobe of the brains of rats at 30 minutes, with peaks at 1 hour, which was more efficient than with simple curcumin administration (Dell'Agli et al., 2016). In Italy the lecithin formulation of curcumin (n = 63) combined with glucosamine was compared with chondroitin and glucosamine (n = 61) among people living with knee OA (Belcaro et al., 2014). In that study, after 4 months the subjects who received the curcumin formulation with glucosamine had significantly greater function with less stiffness, pain, hospitalizations, GI side effects, and use of analgesic medications. Preventive actions were noted in another study using the lecithin delivery system when muscle pain was induced and subjects who received the curcumin in the lecithin delivery system (200 mg bid) not only reported lower pain intensity but also significantly less muscle trauma was found on magnetic resonance imaging (MRI) (Drobnic et al., 2014).

A different curcumin formulation available in Europe is made in Brussels (Flexofytol) and uses a very thin dispersion of curcumin in a galenic form that is designed to enable dispersion through the intestines (Appelboom, Maes, & Albert, 2014). In a large study using that formulation with people with OA (N = 820), the findings were supportive of the formulation in reducing pain and improving function, quality of life, and patient satisfaction. Another product with curcumin in a matrix of natural products is reported to have greater bioavailability than other products developed to improve absorption and transportation of curcumin (Gopi et al., 2017); however, additional research is needed. A curcumin product was developed in China with a soft lipid formation to increase both solubility and bioavailability of curcumin through intestinal absorption (Ji et al., 2016).

These improved delivery systems offer an opportunity for studies in which the amount and delivery of curcumin is more consistent. Research is needed to identify the most efficacious method of delivering curcumin to optimize the bioavailability (Cheppudira et al., 2013). Because in rat studies the lecithin formulation of curcumin seemed to have a more efficient delivery of curcumin to the brain (Dell'Agli et al., 2016) and there is considerable variability in curcumin formulations, it is quite possible that some of the variation seen in research studies is related to variation in the products used. Additional research is needed to clarify the quality of the various hybrids of *C. longa* (Dell'Agli et al., 2016; Hayakawa et al., 2011; Miyazaki et al., 2014). Additional research is also needed to determine efficacy over longer periods (Domenico et al., 2015; Ha & Nesteby, 2017) and to assess side effects over time.

Cautions

Curcumin is listed by the FDA as one of the *generally recognized as safe* (GRAS) products when used in amounts of 60 mg per serving (FDA, 2019). However, it is important to know there are large variations in the genetics, quality, and quantity of curcumin with *C. longa* or *C. domestica*, which is the gold standard of curcumin, but data are insufficient to know the differences and quality of hybrids (Hayakawa et al., 2011; Miyazaki et al., 2014). It is important to remember that research generally uses pure compounds and what is available commercially may have a variety of additives that may be problematic for some people, especially those with inflammatory gastric conditions (Holt, 2016).

There are a few specific cautions with curcumin, but as with all botanicals, using curcumin should be discussed with all clinicians providing care. Curcumin may not be advised in the presence of gallstones; it may slow clotting of blood and interfere with absorption of iron so likely will need to be stopped before surgery; and because it may stimulate contractions of the uterus, it is not advised during pregnancy (Yadav & Tarun, 2017). To avoid exacerbating kidney stones, it is advised to ingest the product turmeric with high-calcium or high-fiber food products; however, this is not a concern with natural curcumin (Zengion & Yarnell, 2011).

Contraindications

Curcumin in dosage larger than 15 g/day is contraindicated when a person is taking anticoagulants and among those who have biliary obstruction (Zengion & Yarnell, 2011).

Potential Interactions With Medications

In addition to hypoglycemic properties, curcumin has anticoagulant properties and should not be used in conjunction with anticoagulant medications (Yadav & Tarun, 2017). The actions of vancomycin, tetracycline, cefixime, and cephotoxime have reportedly increased, whereas there is an opposite effect seen with nalidixic acid when curcumin is used with them (Padmanaban & Nagaraj, 2018). It may affect the action of omeprazole, famotidine, esomeprazole, cimetidine, and lansopraxole (Sahoo, Dandapat, Dash, & Kanhar, 2018).

Willow Bark (*Salicis cortex*) and White Willow Bark (*Salix alba*)

Willow bark has a long history of being used as an antiinflammatory and analgesic agent (Smithson et al., 2017). It is frequently dated by reports of Greeks using it during the time of Hippocrates having patients chewing on white willow bark to ease pain (Srivali, Cheungpasitporn, Chongnarungsin, & Edmonds, 2013).

However, earlier reports of willow bark date back to the 17th century BCE as described in the *Surgical Papyrus* (Schweim, 2017). Willow bark was first isolated and produced as acetylsalicylic acid (aspirin) in 1899 (Grodetsky, 2014). Although aspirin was derived from white willow bark, the herb is noted to take longer to become therapeutic but then has a longer duration of action (Malone & Gloyer, 2013).

Evidence for Pain Management

The antiinflammatory and analgesic effect is generally thought to be the result of the prodrug *salicin*, which after ingestion is readily absorbed (~80%) and metabolized to *saligenin* and other salicylate derivatives by the flora of the intestines (Smithson et al., 2017) and liver into salicylic acid, which is the active medication (Uehleke, Müller, Stange, Kelber, & Melzer, 2013). It is thought through the combined effect of salicin with flavonoids and polyphenols there is an antiinflammatory and analgesic effect through inhibition of both COX-1 and COX-2 (Lemmon & Roseen, 2018; Vlachojannis, Magora, & Chrubasik, 2011; Uehleke et al., 2013). Although similar to aspirin, it does not irritate the GI tract or affect coagulation as does aspirin and has a broader spectrum of action (Lemmon & Roseen, 2018; Vlachojannis et al., 2011). Acting as a nonselective inhibitor of both COX-1 and COX-2, it is thought to block inflammatory prostaglandins (Smithson et al., 2017). It was recently suggested that two other ingredients, salicylates and polyphenols, also may have nociceptive action (Shara & Stohs, 2015).

The most common uses for willow bark are musculoskeletal conditions. White willow bark relieves musculoskeletal pain from OA and back disorders, but the efficacy is very inconsistent (Lemmon & Roseen, 2018; Smithson et al., 2017). The authors of a 2015 systematic review reported white willow bark, when standardized to daily dosages of 120 and 240 mg of the ingredient salicin, was effective for treatment of low back pain (Berberian, Obimba, Glickman-Simon, & Sethi, 2015). The dose of 240 mg of salicin is approximately equivalent to 87 mg of aspirin (Kuphal, 2018). In a 2016 Cochrane review the authors concluded it was more effective than placebo in patients with low back pain with moderate quality of evidence (Gagnier et al., 2016). In a large observational study (N = 436) an over-the-counter German product (Proaktiv) that contains white willow bark was effective as a first-line treatment for musculoskeletal conditions and could safely be used with NSAIDs if needed (Uehleke, 2013). The most common uses for willow bark are musculoskeletal conditions. When it is used for dysmenorrhea, it is most effective when started the day before anticipated symptoms (Kuphal, 2018). More research, with rigorous methodology, is needed to assess the benefit of willow bark alone and in combination with other agents in large samples with additional painful situations (Smithson et al., 2017).

Cautions

Adverse effects of, or reactions to, white willow bark are not common; however, one serious situation occurred when a woman had a severe reaction resulting in acute respiratory distress syndrome that responded well to corticosteroids, antihistamines, and respiratory support (Srivali, et al., 2013). White willow bark minimally affects platelet thrombosis (Gagnier et al., 2016). Considering the relationship between white willow bark with aspirin, it is prudent to avoid willow bark in children with viral infections to minimize the chance of Reye's syndrome, as well as in patients who are allergic to aspirin and those with kidney disorders (Kuphal, 2018).

Contraindications

Willow bark is contraindicated in anyone who has an allergy to salicylate (Zengion & Yarnell, 2011). It should be avoided in any in situations in which aspirin is contraindicated (Patidar, Birla, Patel, Chaturvedi, & Manocha, 2014).

Potential Interactions With Medications

The most significant concern for a potential interaction is between willow bark and warfarin because it may potentiate the effects (Bone & Mills, 2013a). In light of the concern with warfarin, it is also prudent to be cautious with other anticoagulant products as well. Considering the potential for interference with clotting, the American Society of Anesthesiologists suggests for willow bark to be discontinued 2 weeks before any planned surgery (Gayle, Kaye, Kaye, & Shah, 2010).

Other Herbs and Botanicals Used for Pain Management

Many herbs and botanicals have effects related to pain management. The following are lesser used, but potentially important herbal products with varying degrees of efficacy as part of an MMA plan. Although they are not discussed in detail, they deserve at least brief mention as having possible analgesic benefit. As with all the botanicals, additional research with larger samples and greater rigor is needed

Brazilian arnica (Solidago chilensis)

Although some beneficial effect was reported, the 2016 Cochrane review reported very low quality of evidence for Brazilian arnica compared to placebo to reduce the perception of pain in the one very small study (N = 20) in which an ointment formulation was reviewed (Gagnier et al., 2016).

Butterbur (Petasites hybridus)

Butterbur is a traditional phytomedicinal reported to have an antispasmodic and vasodilatory effect on vasculature as well as antiinflammatory effects by inhibiting leukotriene synthesis and activity of lipoxygenase with positive effects on migraine and alleviating dysmenorrhea (Bega, 2017; Pizzorno et al., 2016). Butterbur is effective as a first-line therapy comparable with naproxen for chronic daily headaches (Clark, Padilla, & Dionne, 2016). The American Academy of Neurology and the American Headache Society noted that butterbur may be effective for migraine headaches and is appropriate to use both prophylactically and as treatment (Holland et al., 2012). It is recommended to be used daily for up to 6 months prophylactically to reduce migraine headaches and is reported to reduce the frequency of migraines by up to 60% (Pizzorno et al., 2016). Typical treatment of migraines is twice daily doses of 50 to 75 mg (Bega, 2017). It currently is not endorsed by any U.S. professional medical organizations for migraine prophylaxis (Falzon & Balabanova, 2017).

Butterbur should be avoided during pregnancy and lactation and by people allergic to plants in the Asteraceae family (marigolds, ragweed, chrysanthemums, daises) (Pizzorno et al., 2016). It should be avoided when anticholinergic medications are prescribed because it may intensify the side effects of medications in that category (Falzon & Balabanova, 2017). Raw unprocessed butterbur should be avoided because it may contain hepatotoxic and carcinogenic alkaloids (Bega, 2017), including the pyrrolizidine alkaloid, and products should be certified as pyrrolizidine alkaloid free (Falzon & Balabanova, 2017).

Comfrey (Symphytum officinale L.)

Comfrey continues to be a common product in the United Kingdom, where it has been used at least since the middle ages (Frost, O'Meara, & MacPherson, 2014). Topically, it is used to treat muscle, tendon, and ligament pain and sprains, fractures, and wounds (Frost, O'Meara, & MacPherson, 2014). Although some benefit was reported, in a 2016 Cochrane review, the one study (N = 120) in which an ointment formulation comparing comfrey to placebo to reduce the perception of pain was reported as low quality of evidence (Gagnier et al., 2016).

A caution is that pyrrolizidine alkaloid components are hepatotoxic (Kotsiou & Christine, 2017). Because of increasing evidence of the hepatotoxic effects of comfrey, in 2014, the FDA advised all manufacturers of botanical products to eliminate comfrey from production (Hudson et al., 2018). Topical extracts that contain unsaturated pyrrolizidine alkaloids (uPAs) do have minor risk for being carcinogenic and hepatotoxic, but the extracts that do not contain uPA do not pose a risk when used topically on skin that is intact (Zengion & Yarnell, 2011).

Ginseng (Panax ginseng)

Although ginseng is more commonly known for having a positive effect on cognition, memory, and cancer-related fatigue, it also is thought to have antiinflammatory properties (Falzon & Balabanova, 2017). Ginseng can cause bleeding so should be avoided with warfarin and other anticoagulants (Paik & Lee, 2015). No serious adverse effects are known (Falzon & Balabanova, 2017); however, misuse and abuse of ginseng can result in a cardiac, renal, hepatic, and gynecologic toxicity (Paik & Lee, 2015). Ginseng is known to potentially counteract the action of warfarin (Krishna & Purushothaman, 2015).

Myrrh (Commiphora molmol)

Myrrh is a gum resin from the *Commiphora molmol* tree that grows in the Arabian Peninsula and Africa (Aronson, 2016a). When studied with rodents in Egypt, myrrh was reported to have significant antiinflammatory and analgesic effects, which is consistent with the historical use of myrrh (Shalaby & Hammouda, 2014). In another rodent study, when myrrh was combined with frankincense, it was found to have an analgesic effect and relieved mechanical allodynia (Hu et al., 2017). A tincture of myrrh is used to treat recurrent benign apotheosis (i.e., canker sores) (Schmidt-Westhausen, 2017) and was associated with greater pain reduction when compared to aloe (Mansour, Ouda, Shaker, & Abdallah, 2014). In the United States, myrrh is available as a food and beverage flavor enhancer and in cosmetics (Shalaby & Hammouda, 2014).

Adverse effects tend to be mild, including fatigue, drowsiness, and giddiness (Aronson, 2016a). Because it is possible that myrrh acts as a uterine stimulant, it should be avoided during pregnancy (Al-Jaroudi, Kaddour, & Al-Amin, 2016).

St. John's Wort (Hypericum perforatum)

St. John's wort is more commonly known as an agent to treat depression rather than pain; however, it has antinociceptive properties (hypericin and pseudohypercin) that are exerted at the spinal and central levels of the opioid receptor system and the inhibition of serotonin, dopamine, and noradrenalin reuptake because of the action of hyperforin (Singh et al., 2017; Galeotti et al., 2014). St. John's wort and feverfew demonstrated analgesic effects on rats with diabetic neuropathy (Galeotti et al., 2014). This is interesting because several antidepressant medications are used in the treatment of neuropathic pain. The potential benefit of St. John's wort is that in animal studies it was found to markedly improve the analgesic effect of morphine but did not change the blood levels of morphine (Zengion & Yarnell, 2011).

There are numerous cautions regarding use of St. John's wort in conjunction with other medications. It may increase the adverse effects of several medications and could result in serotonin syndrome, so St. John's wort should not be taken with antidepressant medications (selective serotonin reuptake inhibitors, tricyclic antidepressants, monamine oxidase inhibitors, and nefazodone), triptans, and dextromethorphan (Bone & Mills, 2013a). St. John's wort may reduce the effectiveness of antihistamines, warfarin, digoxin, theophylline, and immune suppressant medications and increase the sedating effect of sedative medications and alcohol. It can reduce the blood levels of some medication that are metabolized in the GI tract and may interfere with the effectiveness of contraceptive agents (Zengion & Yarnell, 2011). It also interacts with protease inhibitors, nonnucleoside reverse transcriptase inhibitors, reserpine, birth control pills, antifungal medications, statins, and calcium channel blockers (Bone & Mills, 2013a). St. John's wort also has been associated with impairment of the action of warfarin (Krishna & Purushothaman, 2015). It is recommended for patients to consult with a clinician to review potential interactions before beginning use of St. John's wort.

Pharmaconutrients: Nutritional Modulators of Pain

Increasingly it is recognized that a multimodal approach to pain management includes nutritional interventions (Table 26.4). Important benefits are that they tend to be safe, with few adverse effects, yet improve analgesia and other symptoms, and in some instances slow disease progression (Lopez, 2012).

Avocado and Soybean Unsaponifiables (Persea gratissma and Glycine max) (Piascledine)

Avocado and soybean unsaponifiables (ASUs) is a hydrolyzed lipid fraction that is sterol rich, consisting of one-third avocado and two-thirds soy unsaponifiables, available as a proprietary product with the trade name Piascledine (Piaxledine 1300, ASU-E; Laboratoires Expanscience, Paris, France) (Cameron & Chrubasik, 2014; Maheu et al., 2014; Perlman et al., 2018). Research using that formulation showed inhibition of inflammatory cytokines and stimulation of collagen formation by ASU (Lopez, 2012). Because the published research has been done with this product with a patented formulation, it is possible that the effects reported are to at least some degree attributable to the particular formulation (Henrotin, Lambert, Couchourel, Ripoll, & Chiotelli, 2011; Perlman et al., 2018). Generic ASU combination products are available in the United States but have not been the source of formal research studies. Recommended dosing is 300 mg/day (Lopez, 2012).

Evidence for Pain Management

ASU was used in a small experimental blinded randomized controlled block study with horses that received either ASU and molasses or placebo molasses and began treadmill exercises, which continued for 8 weeks along with the ASU and molasses (Frisbie, Kawcak, & McIlwraith, 2008). The horses that received ASU had significant improvement in synovial membrane condition and in retarding cartilage erosion; however, other outcomes were not significant. Additional research is

Table 26.4 | Summary of Nutritional Modulators of Pain

Name	Proposed Mechanism	Dosage	Types of Pain
Green tea	• Antiinflammatory properties	• 300–400 mg/day	
Omega-3 polyunsaturated fatty acids	• Reduce cytokine secretion • Competitively inhibit cyclooxygenase and lipoxygenase	• 2.7 g of EPA and DHA daily	• Rheumatoid arthritis • Inflammatory bowel disease • Dysmenorrhea
Magnesium	• Mediates neurogenic inflammation • Smooth muscle relaxant	• 300–600 mg daily • Maintain serum levels of 1.7–2.4 mg/dL	• Fibromyalgia • Menstrual pain • Neuropathic pain
Vitamin D	• Calcium and phosphorous homeostasis • Found in most tissue and muscle cells	• Maintains serum levels above 20 ng/mL	• Polymyalgia rheumatica • Fibromyalgia • Osteoarthritis • Elderly • Nonspecific pain • Statin myopathies
Willow bark	• Nonselective inhibitor of cyclooxygenase	• Salicin 120–240 mg/day	• Joint/knee pain • Acute back pain • Osteoarthritis • Headache • Menstrual cramps • Tendinitis • Generalized pain
Lactobacillus	• Secretes cytokines that affect visceral pain	• 1–10 billion organisms/day	• Abdominal pain
Turmeric (curcumin)	• Nonselective inhibitor of cyclooxygenase	• 1200 mg/day	• Osteoarthritis • Joint pain
Glucosamine and chondroitin	• Glucosamine: Component of cartilage proteoglycans • Chondroitin: Joint matrix substrate	• Glucosamine 500 mg tid • Chondroitin 400 mg tid	• Osteoarthritis • Joint pain
Boswellia	• Inhibits leukotriene biosynthesis	• 300–500 mg bid to tid	• Rheumatoid arthritis • Osteoarthritis
Devil's claw	• COX-2 inhibition	• 600 mg qid	• Osteoarthritis • Rheumatoid arthritis • Back pain
MSM	• Inhibits oxidative damage	• 3–6 g/day	• Osteoarthritis
Green tea	• Inhibits IL-1	• 300–400 mg/day	• Osteoarthritis

COX, Cyclooxygenase; *DHA*, docosahexaenoic acid; *EPA*, eicosapentaenoic acid; *IL*, interleukin; *MSM*, methylsulfonylmethane.

From Smithson, J., Kellick, K. A., & Mergenhagen, K. (2017). Nutritional modulators of pain in the aging population. In R. R. Watson & S. Zibadi (Eds.), *Nutritional modulators of pain in the aging population* (pp. 1919–1998). London: Academic Press.

warranted with larger samples and more diverse samples, including humans.

A Cochrane review reported moderate quality of evidence that ASU probably, but only slightly, improved both pain control and function; however, joint space may not be preserved (Cameron & Chrubasik, 2014). A multicenter (N = 122 sites) study in France that lasted 3 years was impressive in that 233 of 345 participants with OA

of the hip continued for the full duration of the study (Maheu et al., 2014). At the closure of that study, the researchers concluded that ASU decreased the percentage of joint space widening, which indicated a reduction in disease progression and possible modification in the hip OA, but there was no statistical difference in pain intensity between the ASU group (n = 132) and those who received placebo (n = 147). When ASU was used for 4 months in a very small study with women living with arthralgia and OA of the temporomandibular joint (TMJ) (N = 19), the women taking ASU (n = 9) reported reductions in pain, less need to use rescue medicine, and improved quality of life, compared to those who received placebo (n = 10) (Catunda, Vasconcelos, Andrade, & Costa, 2016). Additional rigorous research is needed with larger samples, including the investigation of potential benefit with conditions such as TMJ (Catunda et al., 2016). Research with formulations other than the proprietary product and with different manufacturers is also warranted (Henrotin et al., 2011; Perlman et al., 2018).

Cautions

Data is limited (NCCIH, 2014) but ASU is considered safe and in one study was at least as safe as placebo (Maheu et al., 2014).

Contraindications

The only contraindications found were that anyone with allergy to avocado, soybean, or latex needs to avoid this product.

Potential Interactions With Medications

Soy that is fermented is high in vitamin K and thus can reduce the action of anticoagulants including warfarin (Krishna & Purushothaman, 2015).

Bromelain (Ananas comosus) (Pineapple Plant)

Bromelain is a monocotyledon enzymatic (proteinases, peroxidase, and acid phosphatase) (Wijeratnam, 2016) and nonenzymatic mixture, which is a basic extract of the pineapple plant used for many years by a variety of people living on islands of the Pacific Ocean (Abdul Muhammad & Ahmad, 2017). It is considered as the active ingredient in the *Ananas comosus*, or pineapple, plant and is available only in the natural fresh fruit because bromelain is destroyed during the process of canning pineapple (Mallory, 2018). The analgesic benefit of bromelain is direct through effect on bradykinin and indirectly related to the antiinflammatory effects with digestion of fibrin, thus facilitating elimination of edema (Maluegha, Widodo, Pardjianto, & Widjajanto, 2015). The most effective dosing is considered to be 500 to 1000 mg/day in two to four divided doses (Hameed, 2018; Sarmento, Moura, Lopes, & Silva, 2010; Singh, More, Fatima, Karpe, Aleem, & Prameela, 2016; Spar, 2018).

Evidence for Pain Management

The antiinflammatory effect of bromelain is thought to be from reducing prostaglandin E_2 and impeding the generation of bradykinin at the site of inflammation and possibly reducing concentration of substance P while inhibiting the expression of COX-2 (Sarmento et al., 2010). It is used to relieve pain associated with joint injuries and OA (Wijeratnam, 2016). Yet, results of research with bromelain as an oral analgesic with musculoskeletal pain have been variable, with many of the studies involving bromelain in combination with other agents (Sarmento et al., 2010). It is hypothetically recommended for treatment of gout pain (Hameed, 2018).

Traditionally, bromelain has been used to reduce inflammation and promote healing related to blunt trauma and surgery (Abdul Muhammad & Ahmad, 2017; Maluegha et al., 2015; Wijeratnam, 2016; Sarmento et al., 2010). In two older studies, when it was used preoperatively bromelain was reported to be effective in reducing postoperative inflammation and pain while enhancing healing (Sarmento et al., 2010).

Bromelain is reportedly effective in postoperative dental pain after impacted molars (Majid & Al-Mashhadani, 2014; Ordesi, et al, 2014). Bromelain 250 mg qid was compared with diclofenac 25 mg qid and placebo in patients after extraction of impacted molars (Majid & Al-Mashhadani, 2014). The results of that study (N = 45) showed significant improvement of both bromelain (n = 15) and diclofenac (n = 15) compared to placebo (n = 15) in reducing pain with no significant difference between the two. In that study there was significantly greater reduction in swelling among the diclofenac group compared to the bromelain and placebo groups. In a larger study, bromelain was compared with standard of care as-needed analgesia in people (N = 80) undergoing extraction of impacted molars (Ordesi et al., 2014). In that study the subjects who received bromelain reported significantly less edema and pain with less analgesic medication needed.

Bromelain as a treatment used for chronic prostatitis/chronic pelvic pain syndrome in combination with the bioflavonoid *quercetin,* and papain was effective in reducing perineal and anal tenderness/pain (Spar, 2018). It is also reported to lessen pain associated with blunt trauma, childbirth, episiotomy (Abdul Muhammad & Ahmad, 2017), and angina pectoris (Wijeratnam, 2016). In rodent models it was effective in treating colitis and in two case reports of ulcerative colitis in humans (Parian et al., 2018). Additional rigorous research is needed to clarify the antiinflammatory and analgesic benefits of bromelain alone and in combination with other agents.

Cautions

Bromelain supplementation is considered safe with minimal side effects but should be used with caution in people with hypertension, because tachycardia was reported among people with hypertension who consumed bromelain in high doses (Sarmento et al., 2010). Because it impairs fibrinogen synthesis and exacerbates fibrinolysis, bleeding risk may be increased (Zengion & Yarnell, 2011).

There are no known risks during pregnancy, and caution is not supported by research; however, bromelain is broadly suggested in folk medicine to induce uterine contractions (Mallory, 2018). For that reason, bromelain may need to be used with caution during pregnancy.

Contraindications

No contraindications were found other than the potential contraindication during pregnancy.

Potential Interactions With Medications

Bromelain is reported to increase serum levels of at least some antibiotics and may potentially enhance the effect of anticoagulants as a result of inhibition of platelet aggregation (Sarmento et al., 2010; Wijeratnam, 2016).

Flavocoxid

Flavocoxid is a botanical medical food product that is a proprietary blend of the flavonoids *baicalin* from *Scutellaria baicalensis* and *catechins* from *Acacia catechu*, which both have known antiinflammatory properties (Bitto et al., 2014; Chalasani et al., 2012; Laev & Salakhutdinov, 2015). These flavonoids inhibit both COX-1 and COX-2 and significantly inhibit 5-lipoxygenase (5-LOX) (Bitto et al., 2014).

Evidence for Pain Management

Baicalin and the by-product *baicalein* both have antiinflammatory properties that reduce COX-2, prostaglandin, cytokine, and leukotriene activity (Laev & Salakhutdinov, 2015; Levy, Saikovsky, Shmidt, Khokhlov, & Burnett, 2009). Catechins reduce COX-2 proinflammatory gene expression and in vivo impede the degradation of human cartilage (Bitto et al., 2014; Levy et al., 2009). Both in vitro and in vivo research has demonstrated potent antioxidant qualities of catechin, which is most likely the source of the antiinflammatory, analgesic, and tissue-protecting actions (Stohs & Bagchi, 2015).

An early study (N = 104) compared flavocoxid with naproxen among people with painful OA of the knee. Flavocoxid was statistically effective in reducing pain ($P \leq .001$), and there was no statistical difference between flavocoxid and naproxen, with no serious adverse effects with either product (Levy et al., 2009). A subsequent study (N = 79) compared flavocoxid (500 mg/day) and naproxen (440 mg/day) in middle-aged and older adults with OA (Arjmandi et al., 2014). In that study, the people who received the flavocoxid had significant reductions in pain ($P = .009$) and stiffness ($P = .002$) and increases in range of motion ($P = .04$), with no significant differences from those who received naproxen.

Research was conducted exploring the potential benefit of flavocoxid with other disorders. One study that used flavocoxid with rodents with acutely induced pancreatitis found COX-2 and 5-LOX were inhibited as expected, and in addition serum lipase and amylase levels were reduced, as was pancreatic edema (Polito et al., 2010). It was also investigated with Duchenne muscular dystrophy (DMD) in both rodent models and people living with DMD (N = 20) (Messina et al., 2014). There was positive benefit in both studies and in the one with people living with DMD, flavocoxid was determined to be safe with children.

Additional research is needed to further demonstrate benefit and adverse effect profile (Stohs & Bagchi, 2015). Research was planned to explore the role of flavocoxid as an antiviral medication in treatment of hepatitis B virus (Pollicino et al., 2013), with pancreatitis and other inflammatory disorders (Bitto et al., 2014). Further research is also needed to identify safe 5-LOX inhibitors (Steinhilber & Hofmann, 2014) and explore the potential benefit of other medical foods (Davey, Davey, & Singh, 2016).

Cautions

Flavocoxid was reported to have few if any side effects and is well tolerated in the GI tract (Bitto et al., 2014; Levy et al., 2009; Stohs & Bagchi, 2015). In an original safety study (N = 59), flavocoxid (250 mg bid) it was determined to be as safe as placebo (Morgan, Baggott, Moreland, Desmond, & Kendrach, 2009). More recently, it was reported to have been associated with causing acute liver injury in at least four people (Chalasani et al., 2012), which was reversed when treatment with flavocoxid was discontinued (Davey et al., 2016; Steinhilber & Hofmann, 2014). However, in December 2017 the FDA issued a caution not to use this product because of concern for drug-induced injury to the liver, possible pulmonary complications, and other potential harm (FDA, 2017a). *As of this writing, flavocoid manufactured as Limbrel has been recalled and is no longer available in the United States.* In January of 2018 the manufacturer Primus recalled all unexpired products (FDA, 2018).

Contraindications

It is contraindicated in people with allergies to any ingredient or foods rich in flavonoids (dark chocolate, tea, green tea, Brazil nuts, red wine, and colored fruits and vegetables) (Primus Pharmaceuticals, 2017). There is no evidence about use with pregnant or lactating women or children so should be avoided by those groups (Primus Pharmaceuticals, 2017).

Potential Interactions With Medications

There are no reported problematic interactions with medications, and flavocoxid reportedly does not affect enzymes that metabolize medications or inhibit the hepatic metabolizing enzymes (Primus Pharmaceuticals, 2017). As with other botanical preparations, where it is still available, it is prudent for patients to consult with clinicians before use.

Green Tea (Camellia sinensis)

Although currently green tea is a commonly consumed beverage with approximately 3 billion kg produced annually (Shen et al., 2014), the medicinal qualities have been appreciated in Eastern countries since ancient times (Coppock & Dziwenka, 2016) (Fig. 26.4). The chemistry and processes involved with green tea extracts are vast and complex, with more than 2000 chemical substances

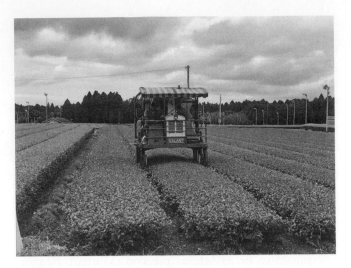

Fig. 26.4 | Green tea being harvested in Kagoshima, Japan. Photo courtesy of Brian Quinlan.

involved and intellectual property issues dating back through history (Coppock & Dziwenka, 2016). Among the substances in green tea are catechins (polyphenols), which are involved with modulating inflammation and musculoskeletal repair in people with OA (Hashempur, Sadrneshin, Mosavat, & Ashraf, 2018). The antiinflammatory dosing of green tea extract is 300 to 400 mg/day (Smithson et al., 2017).

Evidence for Pain Management

The analgesic mechanism of action of green tea is thought to be through the antiinflammatory effects of the catechins and inhibiting collagen degradation through activity of epigallocatechin-3-galate (Smithson et al., 2017). Laboratory studies with rodents (Katiyar & Raman, 2011) and human tissue (Akhtar & Haqqi, 2011) suggest beneficial effect among people living with OA. A small, randomized open-label study compared green tea extract with diclofenac (n = 20) with diclofenac alone (n = 20) in people with OA of the knee. In that study, the people who received the green tea extracts reported significantly less pain intensity (P = .038) and improved function (P = .004), but the pain and function scores of those who received the diclofenac alone did not show significant improvement (Hashempur et al., 2018). In an experimental mouse study, green tea reportedly was effective in providing analgesia and enhancing the analgesic effects of morphine (Lee et al., 2018).

It seems there also may be a preventive effect of green tea with musculoskeletal conditions with positive relationships reported between green tea drinking and bone density and health (Shen et al., 2014). The preventive concept is consistent with the findings of green tea polyphenols being protective of bone health in an earlier study with rodents (Shen, Wang, Guerrieri, Yeh, & Wang, 2008). Additional research with rigorous methodology with animals and humans is needed to clarify the role and potential benefit of green tea as part of a multimodal approach in treating OA and other painful conditions (Shen et al., 2014).

Cautions

Generally green tea extracts are safe; however, in high doses, abdominal pain, muscle pain, GI distress, bloating, and stimulation of the CNS have been reported (Coppock & Dziwenka, 2016; Smithson et al., 2017). Hepatotoxicity associated with green tea is a concern and seems to be a greater risk when other ingredients are combined with the tea (e.g., chromium, usnic acid, goji berries, aloe vera, garcinia cambogia) (Mazzanti, Di Sotto, & Vitalone, 2015). Transfer of pesticides from the tea to people is also a potential concern (Coppock & Dziwenka, 2016).

Contraindications

No specific contraindications to using green tea were found other than the concern for concomitant use with anticoagulants noted in the following section.

Potential Interactions With Medications

Caution is recommended in using green tea extracts when also using a number of medications, including analgesics, antiepileptics, antilipemics, antivirals, β-adrenoceptor blockers, CYP450-metabolized medications, hepatoxic products, hormonal medications, and sedatives (Coppock & Dziwenka, 2016, p. 639). Green tea is advised not to be used with anticoagulant and antiplatelet medications (Krishna & Purushothaman, 2015). As with all products, patients need to review the product in consideration of comorbidities and other medications with a clinician before using (Mazzanti et al., 2015).

Honey

Honey is the natural sweetener product of honey bees *(Apis mellifera)* and has been considered medicinal at least since 2100 to 2000 BCE, when it was written about on a Sumerian tablet (Lazim & Baharudin, 2017). Honey varies greatly by region, whether it is from one type of flora or multiple flora and whether it is pure or adulterated (Jandrić, Frew, Fernandez-Cedi, & Cannavan, 2017; Jandrić et al., 2015). It is more commonly known for the antibacterial and wound healing that result from reducing prostaglandin levels and increasing nitric oxide levels, which also help reduce inflammation and thus pain and pain perception (Al-Waili, Salom, & Al-Ghamdi, 2011; Lazim & Baharudin, 2017; Meo, Al-Asiri, Mahesar, & Ansari, 2016).

Evidence for Pain Management

Although honey has been researched fairly extensively as an antibacterial agent, there has been little research investigating the antinociceptive effect or mechanism of action of honey (Lazim & Baharudin, 2017). It is reported that honey lowers the concentration of plasma prostaglandins with that effect increasing over time, and it is suggested that the locale of action may be COX-1 or COX-2 or even both (Al-Waili et al., 2011). The presence of cytokines, histamine, nitrous oxide, and TNF-alpha (TNF-α) biomarkers are supportive that honey has antinociceptive potential (Lazim & Baharudin, 2017). Phenolic and flavonoids in some forms of honey (i.e., Tualang) possibly have analgesic benefit as well (Aziz, Ismail, Hussin, & Mohamad, 2014) by inhibiting COX-2 and antagonizing the N-methyl-D-aspartate (NMDA) receptor of the central nervous system (CNS) (Lazim & Baharudin, 2017). In animal studies the investigators found honey possibly decreased perception of pain with results suggestive through action of autonomic receptors (Owoyele, Oladejo, Ajomale, Ahmed, & Mustapha, 2014).

Honey has been studied several times with patients who have undergone tonsillectomy with mixed but promising study results (Lazim & Baharudin, 2017). In one study, honey was evaluated in a study with people 8 years of age or older (N = 104) who underwent tonsillectomy, the patients who received acetaminophen plus honey (n = 52) reported significantly lower pain intensity scores and used significantly less analgesic medications compared to those in the placebo group (n = 52) (Boroumand et al., 2013). In another study (N = 63) comparing antibiotics alone (n = 28) with antibiotics with honey (n = 35) intraoperatively during tonsillectomy and for 5 days postoperatively, those who received the honey reported slightly lower pain intensity scores during the early postoperative period, but the difference was not statistically significant (Abdullah, Lazim, & Salim, 2015), results that were similar to the results in another study using honey with patients postoperatively after a tonsillectomy (Amani, Kheiri, & Ahmadi, 2015). Yet, a meta-analysis of four studies using honey after tonsillectomy reported honey having positive benefit for wound healing and pain control, with the need for further research to replicate the studies (Hwang, Song, Jeong, Lee, & Kang, 2016).

When honey was studied with people receiving it as a topical treatment for burns and other wounds primarily as an antibiotic agent and to promote healing (Al-Waili et al., 2011) it was noted to have analgesic benefit as well (Al-Waili et al., 2011; Yaghoobi, Kazerouni, & Kazerouni, 2013). The antiinflammatory effects of honey are associated with greater healing and less pain of skin grafts (Maghsoudi & Moradi, 2015; Meo et al., 2016).

The investigators of a promising study (N = 69) used honey to treat pain in patients with painful radiation-induced mucositis and reported statistically significant reduction in pain intensity ($P < .001$) as well as fewer interruptions in treatment among the 36 participants who received honey compared to the control group (n=33) (Samdariya, Lewis, Kauser, Ahmed, & Kumar, 2015). Although pain was not specifically reported in another study using honey with children with chemotherapy oral mucositis, the severity of the mucositis in the children who received medicinal honey was significantly less and they recovered more quickly (Bulut & Tüfekci, 2016). Thyme honey was used with patients with head and neck cancer (N = 62); those patients who received the thyme honey (n = 32) had significant reductions in pain

intensity ($P < .001$) compared to those who did not (n = 32) (Charalambous et al., 2017). Initial research is promising for analgesic benefit from honey, and the proposed mechanisms of action make sense, but additional research with rigorous methodology and larger samples is needed (Yaghoobi et al., 2013).

Cautions

Although no serious adverse events are reported with using honey as a medicinal agent, stinging pain and atopic reactions have been reported (Yaghoobi et al., 2013). In addition, not all honey is safe for consumption if it contains toxins or hazardous elements, including bacterial spores and traces of metal (Lazim & Baharudin, 2017). Some honey contains *grayanatoxin*, which can cause *mad honey intoxication* and result in a variety of adverse effects, with hypotension, bradycardia, syncope, dizziness, vomiting, and visual disturbances being the most common (Silici & Atayoglu, 2015). Mad honey intoxication is most associated with Turkey and importation of products from Turkey (Jansen et al., 2012).

Contraindications

Anyone with a known allergy to honey should avoid it medicinally and nutritionally.

Potential Interactions With Medications

No interactions were found between honey with medications.

Supplements

Acetyl-L-Carnitine

Acetyl-L-carnitine, which is a carnitine acetyl ester derived from an amino acid, is a molecule involved in the oxidation of fatty acid metabolism and mitochondrial function as well as tubulin acetylation (Alexa-Stratulat, Luca, Bădescu, Bohotin, & Alexa, 2017). It also is essential for acetyl-coenzyme A (CoA) availability to ensure the elimination of toxic by-products of metabolism (Hershman et al., 2013).

Evidence for Pain Management

The analgesic effect of acetyl-L-carnitine is believed to occur through the modulating role it plays in the glutamatergic and cholinergic pathways (Alexa-Stratulat et al., 2017). It is considered potentially helpful in controlling peripheral neuropathic pain (PNP) (Li et al., 2015), most likely related to a role in regeneration of peripheral nerves (Alexa-Stratulat et al., 2017). Although the pathophysiology of PNP is not fully understood, it is thought to be due to a reduction of available acetyl groups that are essential for choline synthesis, and acetyl-L-carnitine deficiency is identified as causing myelin sheath damage, so it is reasonable that acetyl-L-carnitine and L-carnitine are possibly involved in alleviating PNP (Veronese et al.,

2017). A systematic review and meta-analysis of three studies was done using acetyl-L-carnitine via oral and intramuscular routes as treatment for PNP in patients with diabetes and without diabetes (Li et al., 2015). The authors of that review reported acetyl-L-carnitine was statistically effective in relieving pain intensity ($p = .006$) by both routes and was more effective in patients with diabetes ($p < .00001$) compared to those without diabetes ($p = .05$). Another systematic review and meta-analysis of five studies also concluded that acetyl-L-carnitine is effective in reducing PNP of diabetes (Veronese et al., 2017).

In a study with women with fibromyalgia syndrome (FMS) (N = 51), acetyl-L-carnitine (1500 mg/day) (n = 22) was compared to DULoxetine (60 mg/day) (n = 29); no significant improvement was seen in pain intensity and subsequently patients with chemotherapy-induced peripheral neuropathy were advised not to use acetyl-L-carnitine (Leombruni et al., 2015). There were several studies investigating acetyl-L-carnitine with chemotherapy-induced peripherial neuropathy, and earlier studies reported positive results (Alexa-Stratulat et al., 2017). However, a large prospective study (N = 409) with women undergoing taxane-based treatment for breast cancer reported that compared to placebo (n = 201), there was no statistical improvement at 12 weeks among the women who received acetyl-L-carnitine (N = 208) (Hershman et al., 2013). But after 24 weeks, among those who received oral acetyl-L-carnitine there was increased neuropathy and decreased function.

Cautions

GI side effects can occur with doses of approximately 3 g/day, with rare instances of muscle weakness (patients with uremia) and seizures (patients with seizure disorders) and possible increased risk for developing cardiovascular disease (National Institutes of Health [NIH], 2017).

Contraindications

No clear contraindications were found.

Potential Interactions With Medications

There is potential interaction with valproic acid for developing hepatotoxicity, but interestingly acetyl-L-carnitine also may be used as an antidote for valproic acid toxicity (NIH, 2017).

Coenzyme Q$_{10}$ (Ubiquinone-10)

Coenzyme Q$_{10}$, or ubiquinone-10, is a lipid, mitochondrial enzyme, associated with the oxidative phosphorylation pathway and integral to cellular metabolism with the production of adenosine triphosphate (ATP) (Lee et al., 2013). It is also a powerful antioxidant (Alcocer-Gómez, Cano-García, & Cordero, 2013) and is beneficial to good muscle function (Bonakdar, 2018). Regardless of the deficiency, oral coenzyme Q$_{10}$ supplements are effective in reversing the deficit for which it is intended (Alcocer-Gómez et al.,

2013). Recommended dose ranges between 100 and 300 mg/day (Bonakdar, 2018; Coeytaux & Mann, 2018).

Evidence for Pain Management

The antioxidant properties of coenzyme Q$_{10}$ are thought to be helpful with central pain syndrome (see Chapter 3), which is thought to generate significant oxidative stress (Bonakdar, 2018). It is thought oxidative stress is also involved in diabetic neuropathic pain (DNP). Coenzyme Q$_{10}$ was effective in a study with rodents (N = 56) with DNP, supporting the theory that damage resulting from neuronal oxidation as the result of hyperglycemia may be a causative factor of DNP (Zhang et al., 2013). Another benefit of coenzyme Q$_{10}$ with DNP is that it is thought to have a small effect on reducing fasting blood sugar (Moradi, Haghighatdoost, Feizi, & Azadbakht, 2016).

Coenzyme Q$_{10}$ is reported to be effective in reducing frequency of migraine headaches (Sirianni, Ibrahim, & Patwardhan, 2015). The relationship is due to patients with chronic headaches often having reduced phosphorylation potentials (Coeytaux & Mann, 2018). Coenzyme Q$_{10}$ supplementation is also helpful in some children with migraine headaches who have coenzyme Q$_{10}$ deficiency (Mathew, Kim, & Zempsky, 2016).

Deficiency of coenzyme Q$_{10}$ is associated with myofascial pain syndrome (Bonakdar, 2018) and in people with myopathy (Alcocer-Gómez et al., 2013). Low levels of coenzyme Q$_{10}$ are also associated with painful muscular symptoms while on statin therapy (Zagorodnikova, 2015). Although it is recommended by some clinicians (5%–10%) for the muscle symptoms while on statin therapy, there is little evidence supporting any benefit (Jacobson, Khan, Maki, Brinton, & Cohen, 2018). The lack of benefit was supported in a fairly large randomized trial (N = 120) in which no benefit was found in statin-related muscle pain when coenzyme Q$_{10}$ was supplemented (Taylor, Lorson, White, & Thompson, 2015).

Coenzyme Q$_{10}$ was reported to have antiinflammatory effect in people with coronary artery disease by decreasing inflammatory marker IL-6 (Gupta & Prakash, 2015). That antiinflammatory effect may be helpful in pain situations as well. The studies using coenzyme Q$_{10}$ with people with FMS are generally small. One small study (N = 20) generated information implicating involvement of the inflammasome complex in FMS that was mediated by coenzyme Q$_{10}$ (Cordero et al., 2014). A report of four women diagnosed with FMS, who were treated with oral coenzyme Q$_{10}$ supplements noted that each of the four women reported clinical improvement, including reductions in pain intensity with 4- to 5-point decreases on a scale of 0 to 10 and 2- to 5-point decreases on the Widespread Pain Index (Alcocer-Gómez et al., 2013).

Cautions

The rare side effects that occur with coenzyme Q$_{10}$ supplementation are GI, and it may cause hypoglycemia. There is some information indicating coenzyme Q$_{10}$

may interfere with the activity of warfarin, so it should be avoided or only used with increased monitoring of INR levels (Krishna & Purushothaman, 2015). It also may increase the action of antihypertensive medications (Zengion & Yarnell, 2011). It is generally considered safe during pregnancy; however, research is needed to confirm this. Another consideration is that it can be expensive to purchase (Coeytaux & Mann, 2018).

Contraindications

No frank contraindications were found.

Potential Interactions with Medications

Coenzyme Q_{10} should be used only when approved by a clinician when patients are taking chemotherapy medications, antihypertensive medications, anticoagulants, and insulin (Garrido-Maraver et al., 2014).

Glucosamine Hydrochloride or Sulfate and Chondroitin Sulfate

Glucosamine and chondroitin are nutraceutical supplements involved in sustaining synovial fluid viscosity and supporting cartilage (Loveless & Fry, 2016). Glucosamine, which is available in both sulfate and hydrochloride forms, is a constituent of cartilage proteoglycans derived from marine animal exoskeletons, which triggers synovial tissue chondrocyte metabolism and cartilage (Loveless & Fry, 2016; Smithson et al., 2017). Because it is thought to retard degradation of articular cartilage, it is considered beneficial for people with OA (Kwoh et al., 2014). Chondroitin sulfate is a substrate for the development of joint matrix that is derived from the cartilage of sharks and cows (Smithson et al., 2017). Recommended daily doses are 500 mg of glucosamine and 400 mg chondroitin three times per day (Smithson et al., 2017).

Evidence for Pain Management

The results of research investigating the effectiveness of glucosamine and chondroitin as a treatment for OA-related pain are inconsistent (Erickson & Messer, 2013; Hillinger et al., 2017; Malone & Gloyer, 2013; Nahin, Boineau, Khalsa, Stussman, & Weber, 2016; Rodriguez-Merchan, 2016; NCCIH, 2016). The authors of a 2013 literature review concluded there was no evidence to support clinical benefit with glucosamine and chondroitin in treatment of knee OA (Júnior & Inácio, 2013). Later in 2015 the authors of a large systematic review (N = 13 studies) concluded glucosamine and chondroitin sulfate may be protective of cartilage and retard progression of OA in the knee, and in three of the studies there was significant reduction in the loss of cartilage (Gallagher et al., 2015). In a recent very small study (N = 15) comparing the effect of a commercial product containing glucosamine, chondroitin, and hyaluronic acid with placebo in working dogs with OA of the hip, no significant benefit was found over placebo (Alves, Santos, & Jorge, 2017). One older

Cochrane review reported no benefit over placebo with glucosamine (Towheed et al., 2005) and another reported low-quality evidence that chondroitin had benefit greater than placebo when it was used alone or in combination with glucosamine (Singh, Noorbaloochi, MacDonald, & Maxwell, 2015). In an RCT with 2-year follow-up, glucosamine was compared with chondroitin and with the combination and with placebo (Fransen et al., 2015). In that study, no significant difference in pain intensity was reported, but there was significantly less ($P = 0.046$) joint space narrowing over 2 years in those subjects who received the combination of glucosamine and chondroitin. In a large multicenter trial (N = 606), a combination of glucosamine and chondroitin was found to be as effective as celecoxib in relieving pain and swelling (Hochberg et al., 2015).

Although most of the research with the combination of glucosamine and chondroitin has been done with OA, two large studies evaluated using it with chronic low back pain. In the first study (N = 8598), pain at rest and with activity were significantly reduced ($P < .0001$, $P < .0001$) with reductions of pain by approximately 3.5 at rest and 4.5 with movement after 3 months (Singh et al., 2014). In the second study (N = 4588), pain reduced significantly (Singh et al., 2016). In that study both pain at rest and pain on movement were statistically improved ($P < .0001, P < .0001$) with more than 5-point reductions on the 11-point numerical scale for both types of pain.

It is possible the variation in research findings is related to using different formulations of glucosamine, chondroitin, and the combination of the two and difference in doses (Ericksen, 2014; Smithson et al., 2017; Taylor, 2017). This concept was supported in a systematic review that concluded that despite variation in study results, one formulation (Rottapharm/Madaus) of glucosamine had greater beneficial effect than other brands (Ericksen, 2014). This concept was supported by the endorsement of the European Society for Clinical and Economic Aspects of Osteoporosis and Osteoarthritis (ESCO) for the same prescription formulation (Rottapharm/Madaus) of 1500 mg/day dosage as a first-line therapy for OA of the knee (Bruyère et al., 2016). Another factor involved in variability of results is the possibility that different people have physiologically different responses to the products, and this difference may be determined by testing biomarkers (Kraus, Martinez, Herrero, & Verges, 2016). Additional research with rigorous methodology is needed with a variety of OA conditions and comparison of products (Ericksen, 2014; Erickson & Messer, 2013) as well as the accuracy of biomarker predictability (Kraus et al., 2016).

Cautions

The safety profile of glucosamine and chondroitin is reported to be comparable to placebo with only mild GI (i.e., nausea, diarrhea, dyspepsia) side effects (Erickson & Messer, 2013; Nahin et al., 2016; Rodriguez-Merchan, 2016). Glucosamine is known to increase blood glucose

(Smithson et al., 2017). Even though there are no reported reactions, because glucosamine is often extracted from shellfish, people with shellfish allergies need to be cautious (Loveless & Frye, 2016; Malone & Gloyer, 2013).

Contraindications

Glucosamine is contraindicated for anyone who is allergic to shellfish or iodine (Zengion & Yarnell, 2011). When shellfish allergy is a concern, patients can be made aware of a glucosamine formulation made from corn with no shellfish (Malone & Gloyer, 2013). Chondroitin may be contraindicated during pregnancy because of the similarity to the medication heparin (Zengion & Yarnell, 2011).

Potential Interactions With Medications

Concern needs to be given for potential interaction with warfarin and medications used to treat diabetes (Loveless & Frye, 2016).

Hyaluronic Acid

Hyaluronic acid (HA) is a polysaccharide mucoid-like material that forms the gelatinous extracellular matrix in bodily tissues and is resistant to water (Box 26.3) (Bone & Mills, 2013b; Owen, Kuo, & Prestwich, 2017). HA is a natural constituent of synovial fluid and knee cartilage (Altman et al., 2016; Loveless & Fry, 2016) and it is highly viscous (Dym, Bowler, & Zeidan, 2016). Supplemental injection is considered an appropriate treatment for OA of the knee when conservative treatment has not been successful (Hatoum, Fierlinger, Lin, & Altman, 2014). The basis of treatment is the belief that HA increases lubrication of the joint and may cause greater production of hyaluronate within the joint (Loveless & Fry, 2016).

The European Society for Clinical and Economic Aspects of Osteoporosis, Osteoarthritis and Musculoskeletal Diseases (ESCEO) determined that when hyaluronic acid is administered intraarticularly as a viscosupplemention, it is an effective intervention for OA of the knee (Bruyère et al., 2016; Maheu, Rannou, & Reginster, 2016). The American College of Rheumatology (ACR) guidelines recommend intraarticular hyaluronic acid injections (IHAI) for patients for whom conventional therapy has not been successful (Hatoum et al., 2014). There has been much research evaluating HA injections to relieve localized pain in various joints but is approved (at this time) by the FDA only for injections in the knee and is available under several product names (Loveless & Fry, 2016; Owen et al., 2017).

Although it does not have a rapid action, the analgesic benefit for function has a potential duration of action lasting for as long as 6 months after administration (Bruyère et al., 2016). The actual mechanism of action is not clear. Some scientists theorize that exogenous HA is locally effective by restoring homeostasis of the joint, whereas others theorize the action is systemic, suggesting that intravenous administration is as effective as intraarticular administration (Owen et al., 2017).

Evidence for Pain Management

Viscosupplementation through IHAI has long been used as a second-line treatment for OA of the knee with generally positive research findings (Altman et al., 2016; Richette, 2017). One exception to this is from the authors of a large systematic review of chondroprotection and prevention of OA (N = 13 studies), who concluded there was inconsistent effectiveness demonstrated for using IHAI to decrease cartilage loss in knees (Gallagher et al., 2015). The authors of an even larger systematic review and meta-analysis (N = 29 studies) reported IHAI as effective to manage pain and improve function with large treatment effects from 1 and 6 months after injection with statistically significant results (Miller & Block, 2013). The results of a subsequent and larger-yet meta-analysis (N = 129 trials; n = 32,129 subjects) showed that when compared to acetaminophen, NSAIDs (celecoxib, diclofenac, ibuprofen, naproxen), intraarticular corticosteroid injections and placebo, IHAI was the most efficacious treatment for OA of the knee with an effect size of 0.63 (Bannuru et al., 2015). In a recent meta-analysis, when IHAI was compared to intraarticular corticosteroids injections, the corticosteroid injections were more effective sooner during the first month, but the IHAI was more effective over time with effects lasting as long as 6 months (He et al., 2017).

IHAI is reported to maintain optimal function and delay surgical intervention among patients with OA of the knee. In two retrospective studies, the length of time between diagnosis of OA of the knee and total knee replacement (TKR) surgery was extrapolated for patients who received IHAI compared with those who did not. In the first study (N = 182,022), people who underwent TKR surgery after receiving IHAI (27.7%) had a mean time interval from diagnosis to TKR surgery of 1.4 years after one course of IHAI and 3.6 years after five or more courses compared

---

Box 26.3 | Clinical Example

After presenting with multiple bone spurs (osteophytes) on the head of my humerus that caused significant joint pain, I had a course of hyaluronic acid injections. I had two injections per week for six weeks in my left shoulder at an orthopedic clinic in Japan.

Unlike cortisone injections, I noticed no side effects. I was able to resume intense physical training immediately after the shots were administered.

After three weeks, in combination with a range of daily dumbbell and cable (resistance) exercises, I had no pain, and I have not had any pain in the 18 months since I had the injections.

Brian Quinlan, Kagoshima, Japan

with those who did not have IHAI with a mean time interval of 0.7 years from diagnosis to surgery (Altman, Lim, Steen, & Dasa, 2015). In the subsequent study (N = 22,555), the people who received IHAI had a median time from diagnosis to surgery of 908 days compared to 582 days for those who did not have IHAI which represented 1.6 years longer duration between diagnosis and surgery (Altman et al., 2016). In addition, bioengineered IHAI is considered cost-effective with greater benefit when compared to conventional care (Hatoum et al., 2014).

IHAI has been used with painful situations other than OA. It was shown to be effective in reducing pain and increasing the interincisal opening ability (Ouanounou, Goldberg, & Haas, 2017). When compared to other antiinflammatory injections (including corticosteroid), IHAI was most effective in relieving pain of people (N = 100) with TMJ disorder (Gencer, Özkiriş, Okur, Korkmaz, & Saydam, 2014). The authors of a systematic review of IHAI used as treatment for TMJ disorders concluded IHAI can be effective in reducing pain; however, more research is needed (Goiato, da Silva, de Medeiros, Túrcio, & Dos Santos, 2016). IHAI was significantly effectively used as a treatment for pain and wound healing among people (N = 50) who had undergone tonsillectomy (Hancı & Altun, 2015).

Additional research is needed, including comparison of the effectiveness and safety of various product formulations and the possible placebo effect of a substance being injected intraarticularly (Hatoum, Fierlinger, Lin, & Altman, 2014; Maheu et al., 2016). Research is also needed to explore the role of IHAI as treatment with other painful conditions such as TMJ disorder (Dym et al., 2016) and to gain evidence to support clinical guidelines for IHAI initiation and treatment (Altman, Schemitsch, & Bedi, 2015).

Cautions

HA is considered to be as safe as placebo control (Miller & Block, 2013). Since it is a biodegradable polymer it is generally safe; however, the source of the HA can affect safety with inconsistency among different products (Owen et al., 2017). Adverse effects include topical or local reactions, including swelling and stiffness of the joint (He et al., 2017) and pain at the site of injection (Loveless & Fry, 2016). Although still low, with high molecular weight cross-linked formulations of HA, local reactions and postinjection nonseptic arthritis is reported with greater incidence (Maheu et al., 2016).

Contraindications

No specific contraindications were found; however, see the interactions with medications discussed in the following section.

Potential Interactions With Medications

When used for injection, HA is not to be mixed with local anesthetic products (Loveless & Fry, 2016). Although interactions generally are not serious, it is recommended to avoid HA when taking benzodiazepines, phenytoin, furosemide, DOPamine, and alpha-adrenergic agonist products (King, 2016). The effect of HA may be impaired by antiinflammatory medications, antihistamines, flavonoids, antioxidant medications, mast cell stabilizers, and vitamin C, which can be antagonists to HA (King, 2016).

Lactic Acid–Producing Bacteria (*Lactobacillus acidophilus, casei, fermentum, gasseri, johnsonii, paracasei, plantarum, reuteri, rhamnosus,* and *salivarius; Bacillus coagulans*)

L. acidophilus is a probiotic that is often used to restore or enhance healthy microflora (microbiota) in the intestinal tract (Smithson et al., 2017). There are a number of different subspecies that belong to the phylogenetically homogeneous species *Lactobacillus* (McFarland, 2016). The International Scientific Association for Probiotics and Prebiotics identified probiotics as "live microorganisms that, when administered in adequate amounts, confer a health benefit on the host" (Hill et al., 2014).

Although the exact mechanism of action is not known, it is suggested *L. acidophilus* induces expression of opioid and cannabinoid receptors, which have an analgesic action on the cytokines secreted in the GI tract, potentially reducing visceral pain (Smithson et al., 2017). *L. casei* may be used to reduce inflammation and pain in OA with the action thought to be through action on cytokines and cartilage degradation biomarkers (Lopez, 2012). The recommended daily dosing for GI purposes is between 1 and 10 billion organisms daily (Smithson et al., 2017). The antiinflammatory and immunomodulating effects of *B. coagulans* are of interest as treatment for pain and symptoms of arthritis (Mandel, Eichas, & Holmes, 2010).

Evidence for Pain Management

It is suggested that probiotics have an effective role in treatment of patients with irritable bowel syndrome (IBS) and the actions are probably specific to the species or subspecies (Ortiz-Lucas, Tobias, Saz, & Sebastián, 2013); however, their role remains unclear (Alvarez-Sánchez & Rey, 2013) within an MMA plan of care. *L. acidophilus* was found to effectively modulate the expression and activity of mu opioid receptors among a small sample of women (N = 20) with mild to moderate functional abdominal pain (Ringel-Kulka et al., 2014). When *L. reuteri* was used for 30 days with infants who had colic, they had significantly less crying time (P = .001) (Savino, Garro, Montanari, Galliano, & Bergallo, 2018). *L. plantarum* was reported as effective in relieving pain among patients (N = 40) with IBS (Darby & Jones, 2017); however, in a larger study (N = 81), no analgesic benefit was found (Stevenson, Blaauw, Fredericks, Visser, & Roux, 2014). The authors of a meta-analysis of 10 studies in which a probiotic was used to treat IBS concluded pain related to IBS was relieved by probiotics containing

Bifidobacterium breve, Bifidobacterium longum, and *L. acidophilus* (Ortiz-Lucas et al., 2013).

Data on the use of *L. acidophilus* with musculoskeletal pain are only recently emerging, but the data are promising (Lopez, 2012) as a component of a multimodal approach to pain management for arthritic conditions. In laboratory research, with an arthritic model induced by collagen, *Lactobacillus* treatment alleviated the inflammatory responses (Amdekar et al., 2017). *L. acidophilus* was statistically effective ($P < .0001$) in reducing arthritic symptoms in rodents (Amdekar & Singh, 2016). When *B. coagulans* was studied with people with RA (N = 45) the results were promising for analgesia with significant pain intensity ($P = .046$) (Mandel et al., 2010).

Although probiotics seem to have promise as part of an MMA plan of care for people with abdominal and arthritic pain, there is a need for greater research with rigorous methodology. Research is also needed to differentiate the effectiveness of the various subspecies, their effect on different pain situations, and the interaction with patient-specific profiles (Ortiz-Lucas et al., 2013).

Cautions

Lactobacillus has a good safety record (Lopez, 2012), with some GI symptoms when taken in high doses. However, caution is advised for people being treated with chemotherapeutic medications and those with central venous catheters because infections are rare but do occur (Williams, 2010). It is also wise for people who have had cardiac valve replacements to avoid lactobacillus. Because *acidophilus* has been reported in at least some studies to lower fasting blood glucose levels (Nikbakht et al., 2018), people with diabetes should discuss any potential concerns or cautions with a clinician before beginning use.

Contraindications

No frank contraindications were found, but for certain patients with immune system compromise the previously mentioned cautions may be considered contraindications. This needs to be a decision by the clinician caring for the person.

Potential Interactions With Medications

The only identified potential interaction with a medication is that *L. acidophilus* is reported to speed up the metabolism of sulfasalazine, which can be beneficial in patients with painful ulcerative colitis (Li et al., 2016; Paroschi, Breganó, Simão, Dichi, & Miglioranza, 2015).

Magnesium

Magnesium is a mineral abundant in the human body involved in protein synthesis, energy production, bone structure, muscle function, nervous system function, and active intracellular transport of calcium and potassium ions. It is present in green leafy vegetables, whole grains, legumes, nuts, and seeds; is added to some prepared foods;

and is available in some laxatives (NIH, 2020b). From an MMA perspective, magnesium supplementation is of interest not only for analgesic properties but also because of the opioid-sparing effects and the benefit that has been studied between magnesium with depression (Rajizadeh, Mozaffari-Khosravi, Yassini-Ardakani, & Dehghani, 2017; Yary, et al, 2016). The adult recommended daily dosage ranges from 200 to 420 mg/day to maintain serum level between 1.7 and 2.4 mg/dL (Bonakdar, 2018; NIH, 2020b; Smithson et al., 2017).

Evidence for Pain Management

The mechanism of action is thought to be through mediation of the neurogenic inflammation and relaxation of smooth muscle (Smithson et al., 2017). It is also believed to inhibit prostaglandins (Zengion & Yarnell, 2011). Magnesium blocks the NMDA receptor in the CNS with several physiologic activities (Pickering et al., 2011; Venturini et al., 2015) (Box 26.4).

Magnesium has been used in several pain situations. When added to standard of care postoperative tonsillectomy pain management in adults (N = 54), the patients who received the magnesium reported significantly lower pain scores ($P = .001$) with no difference in side effects (Tugrul et al., 2015). Moderate improvement in migraine headaches was reported in three of four studies using a total of 600 mg/day of magnesium (NIH, 2020b); however, the authors of a review of 10 studies concluded the

---

Box 26.4	Analgesic Influences of Magnesium With Inflammation and Neuropathic Pain

Substance P, & glutamate, & calcitonin gene related peptide in spinal cord release & activity

MAGNESIUM POTENTIATES:

Morphine activity in dorsal horn presynaptic areas

MAGNESIUM REDUCES:

N-Methyl-D-aspartate receptor action
Substance P synthesis
Pre- & postsynaptic calcium channel activity
Thromboxane A2, proinflammatory eicosanoids, & cytokines outside the CNS

MAGNESIUM BLOCKS:

Receptor-coupled calcium channel

Data from Venturini, M. A., Zappa, S., Minelli, C., Bonardelli, S., Lamberti, L., Bisighini, L., . . . & Latronico, N. (2015). Magnesium-oral supplementation to reduce pain in patients with severe peripheral arterial occlusive disease: The MAG-PAPER randomised clinical trial protocol. *BMJ Open, 5*(12), e009137, p. 1).

evidence remains limited and there may be greater benefit to obtaining magnesium through dietary means rather than supplementation (Teigen & Boes, 2015). In a small but innovative study, transdermal magnesium was pilot tested on patients (N = 24) with FMS, with significant improvement in all subscales of the Revised Fibromyalgia Impact Questionnaire, including pain intensities and function (Engen et al., 2015). The results in all these areas are encouraging and warrant additional research.

Data regarding the benefit of magnesium with neuropathic pain demonstrates mixed results (Venturini et al., 2015). In a month-long trial (N = 45) with patients with neuropathic pain, no difference was seen between those treated with magnesium (n = 23) compared with those treated with placebo (n = 22) (Pickering et al., 2011). In other studies, magnesium was effective with neuropathic pain when administered at least initially by the intravenous route (Venturini et al., 2015). In one such study (N = 80) in patients with chronic low back pain with neuropathic symptoms, 50% of the participants received 2 weeks of intravenous magnesium infusion, then received oral magnesium for an additional 4 weeks while the other half of the participants received placebo (Yousef & Al-deeb, 2013). In that study, all participants continued with their standard of care multimodal treatment of anticonvulsants, antidepressants, and analgesics. The participants who received the magnesium interventions had significant reduction in reported pain intensity (P = 0.034) and in flexion, extension, and lateral extension ability (P = 0.018), (P = 0.039), and (P = 0.035), respectively. Magnesium sulfate (MgSO4) was compared with ketamine with older patients with intractable postherpetic neuralgia pain (N = 30) with significant benefit from both agents and no statistical difference in reported pain intensity between the two groups (Kim, Lee, & Oh, 2015). Additional research is needed with the different populations.

MgSO4 is reported to enhance opioid-induced analgesia and thus reduces the quantity of opioids needed for adequate pain control (Bujalska-Zadrożny, Tatarkiewicz, Kulik, Filip, & Naruszewicz, 2016). When MgSO4 was added to morphine in studies with rodents, the analgesic benefit of morphine was significantly increased (Bujalska-Zadrożny & Duda, 2014; Bujalska-Zadrożny et al., 2016). A large meta-analysis, with 25 trials, was done in which magnesium by bolus and continuous infusion was compared with placebo among perioperative patients receiving opioids (Albrecht, Kirkham, Liu, & Brull, 2013). The authors of that analysis reported that regardless of mode of administration, during the first 24 hours postoperatively, magnesium perioperatively reduced consumption of intravenous opioid (morphine) by 24.4% and pain intensity reports were significantly less at both rest (P < .0001) and with activity (P < .009). Those results are important not only for the role of magnesium in an MMA plan but also from the perspective of opioid sparing and safety during the first 24 hours postoperatively when patients are at increased risk for opioid-induced respiratory depression. (See Chapter 13 for detailed discussion of opioid induced respiratory depression.)

Cautions

Magnesium is generally considered very safe (Venturini et al., 2015). However, at high doses magnesium can cause untoward effects of the cardiovascular, metabolic, endocrine, renal, respiratory, ophthalmologic, and peripheral nervous systems and the CNS (Bujalska-Zadrożny et al., 2016). Magnesium can also cause diarrhea (NIH, 2020b; Zengion & Yarnell, 2011).

Contraindications

No frank contraindications were found.

Potential Interactions With Medications

Consultation is advised with a clinician, about the advisability of taking and how to take supplemental magnesium with bisphosphonates, antibiotics, diuretics, and proton pump inhibitors (NIH, 2020b).

Methylsulfonylmethane

Methylsulfonylmethane (MSM), is an organosulfur compound that occurs naturally and is found in a variety of green plants, algae, vegetables, fruits, grains, fish, and milk but can be destroyed with overcooking and processing (Ahn et al., 2015; Butawan, Benjamin, & Bloomer, 2017; Sengar et al., 2017; Smithson et al., 2017; Tennent, Hylden, Kocher, Aden, & Johnson, 2017). MSM results from ingested dimethyl sulfoxide (DMSO), through which it supplies sulfur for formation of amino acids (Smithson et al., 2017). It is commonly available and also known as dimethyl sulfone, methyl sulfone, sulfonylbismethane, organic sulfur, and crystalline dimenthyl sulfoxide (Butawan et al., 2017). Daily dosage recommendation ranges from 1000 to 3000 mg/day (Perlman et al., 2018) and reportedly is well tolerated in doses as high as 3000 to 6000 mg/day (Smithson et al., 2017). It is available in oral (tablets, capsules, and powders) and topical (creams) preparations (Rajasekaran, 2017).

Evidence for Pain Management

The mechanism of action is through the inhibition of oxidative damage (Smithson et al., 2017) and degeneration when augmented with this organic sulfur nutrient (Lopez, 2012), because sulfur is essential for connective tissue development (Perlman et al., 2018). The results of laboratory studies indicate MSM reduces COX-2, cytokines, and inducible nitric oxide expression, and in animal studies, cytokine expression was reduced with MSM (Butawan et al., 2017). In animal research, MSM seemed to reduce inflammation of joint disease (Perlman et al., 2018). Although evidence to support analgesia with MSM is limited, what is available is promising, with trends toward improved function with less pain (Perlman et al., 2018).

The benefit of MMS for arthritis-related pain as reported is inconsistent. It has antiinflammatory assets when used orally and topically and in one study was effective in managing pain and swelling but not stiffness related to OA (Rajasekaran, 2017; Smithson et al., 2017) and RA (Ahn et al., 2015). In an RCT study, those who received 6 g/day of MSM reported small but significant improvement in pain intensity and function (Nahin et al., 2016). However, when 3 g of MSM was evaluated as a preventive measure among military trainees (N = 180), no improvement was seen after 8 weeks of use (Tennent et al., 2017). Despite benefit for arthritis reported from some studies, meta-analyses did not find support for clinical effectiveness of analgesia (Raditic & Bartges, 2014).

When MSM was compared to placebo in women (N = 22) who had run a half marathon, the 50% of participants who received the MSM reported less pain in both muscles and joints (Withee et al., 2017). These findings were consistent with those of an earlier study that found that 10-day supplementation with MSM appeared to reduce muscle damage (Barmaki, Bohlooli, Khoshkhahesh, & Nakhostin-Roohi, 2012). Additional research is needed with rigorous methodology with larger human studies and comparison of MSM products and evaluation of adverse events.

Cautions

In research studies, MSM safety was comparable to placebo (Lopez, 2012). It is a GRAS product with few adverse effects, which tend to be mild (Butawan et al., 2017) and may include nausea, diarrhea, and headache (Perlman et al., 2018).

Contraindications

No contraindications were found.

Potential Interactions With Medications

No information on real or potential interaction with medications was found in the available literature.

Omega-3 Polyunsaturated Fatty Acids (Eicosapentaenoic Acid and Docosahexaenoic Acid)

Omega-3 polyunsaturated fatty acids (omega-3 PUFAs) contain antiinflammatory properties and are necessary for human health (Souza & Norling, 2015). Two omega-3 PUFAs most commonly used for pain control are eicosapentaenoic acid (EPA) and docosahexaenoic acid (DHA) (Gioxari, Kaliora, Marantidou, & Panagiotakos, 2018; Souza & Norling, 2015), which are only contained in oily fish and fish oil supplements (Abdulrazaq, Innes, & Calder, 2017). The omega-3 PUFAs function as substrates for development of resolvins, maresins, and pro-

tectins (neuroprotectins when initiated in neural tissues), which are mediators for resolving inflammation (Uranga, López-Miranda, Lombo, & Abalo, 2016). Their mechanism of action is thought to be reduction of inflammation through reduction of cytokine secretion and competitive inhibition of COX and LOX in part by displacing arachidonic acid, making it less available for prostaglandin synthesis (Abdulrazaq et al., 2017; Smithson et al., 2017) (Table 26.5). Recommended daily dosing ranging from 2.7 to 3.6 g/day was effective (Abdulrazaq et al., 2017; Smithson, Kellick, & Mergenhagen, 2017).

Evidence for Pain Management

Much of the research regarding the analgesic role of omega-3 PUFAs has been among people living with RA. The authors of a 2012 systematic review reported modest benefit in relieving RA symptoms, with reports of less pain, joint swelling, morning stiffness, and need for NSAID use (Miles & Calder, 2012). Despite research of omega-3 PUFAs as an intervention with RA for more than 25 years, the evidence supporting it remains inconsistent, with one meta-analysis reporting omega-3 PUFA only reduced leukotriene B4 (Gioxari et al., 2018). In that review (N = 18 studies; n = 1143 subjects), patients or clinicians reported less pain in patients taking the omega-3 PUFAs, although there was no significant reduction in pain in the remaining 8 studies. In a recent study (N = 591) with people living with RA who were treated with methotrexate, the authors reported omega-3 PUFA was inversely related to refractory but not inflammatory pain (Lourdudoss et al., 2018).

The possible benefit of omega-3 PUFAs as a treatment for irritable bowel disorders (IBDs) such as Crohn's disease or ulcerative colitis, was initially sparked by observation that Eskimos, who eat large amounts of oily fish and thus omega-3 PUFAs, rarely have IBD (Uranga et al., 2016). The results of clinical trials, however, have been inconsistent, with no strong evidence of benefit (Calder, 2013). In experimental models and mice studies, marine omega-3 PUFAs were effective in reducing the colonic damage, and resolvins, in particular, were seen to be protective in colitis situations that were chemically induced (Calder, 2013; Uranga et al., 2016). Clinical studies with fish oil as a treatment for IBD were inconsistent (Calder, 2015).

Less frequent research has been done evaluating omega-3 PUFAs with other painful conditions. They were evaluated with a prophylactic diet high in omega-3 PUFAs among people with spinal cord injury; it was noted that the biomarkers for inflammatory substances were significantly less among people eating the diet high in omega-3 PUFAs (Figueroa et al., 2013). The authors of that study concluded there was prophylactic benefit of omega-3 PUFAs with chronic pain from spinal cord injury. Other researchers with omega-3 PUFAs and spinal cord injury agree that there is promising potential benefit for them as part of a multimodal treatment plan, but more research is needed (Michael-Titus & Priestley, 2014). When used

Table 26.5 | Summary of the Antiinflammatory Actions of Marine n − 3 Fatty Acids and the Likely Mechanisms Involved

Antiinflammatory Effect	Likely Mechanism Involved
Decreased leukocyte chemotaxis	Decreased production of some chemoattractants (e.g., LTB_4); Downregulated expression of receptors for chemoattractants
Decreased adhesion molecule expression and decreased leukocyte-endothelium interaction	Downregulated expression of adhesion molecule genes (via NF-κB, PPAR-γ, GPR120, etc.)
Decreased production of eicosanoids from arachidonic acid	Lowered membrane content of arachidonic acid; Inhibition of cyclooxygenase; Downregulated expression of cyclooxygenase-2 gene (by NF-κB, PPAR-γ, GPR120, etc.)
Decreased production of arachidonic acid containing endocannabinoids	Lowered membrane content of arachidonic acid
Increased production of "weak" eicosanoids from EPA	Increased membrane content of EPA
Increased production of antiinflammatory EPA and DHA containing endocannabinoids	Increased membrane content of EPA and DHA
Increased production of proresolution resolvins, protectins, and maresins	Increased membrane content of EPA and DHA; Presence of aspirin
Decreased production of inflammatory cytokines	Downregulated expression of inflammatory cytokine genes (by NF-κB, PPAR-γ, GPR120, etc.)
Modified T cell reactivity	Disruption of membrane rafts and intracellular signaling (by increased content of EPA and DHA in specific membrane regions)

DHA, Docosahexaenoic acid; *EPA*, eicosapentaenoic acid; *GPR120*, G protein–coupled receptor 120; *LTB4*, leukotriene B4; *NF-κB*, nuclear factor-kappa B; *PPAR-γ*, peroxisome proliferator-activated receptor-gamma.

From Table 3 "A summary of the anti-inflammatory actions of marine n − 3 fatty acids and the likely mechanisms involved. Modified from [1]." on page 478 of Calder, P. C. (2015). Marine omega-3 fatty acids and inflammatory processes: Effects, mechanisms and clinical relevance. *Biochimica et Biophysica Acta (BBA) Molecular and Cell Biology of Lipids, 1851*(4), 469–484.

with teens with migraine headaches, those treated with omega-3 PUFAs had fewer headaches but there was not significant difference from placebo (Nahin et al., 2016). However, in another study of people with chronic headaches (N = 56), compared to those who reduced omega-3 and increased n-6 fatty acids in their diets, those who increased omega-3 PUFAs and reduced n-6 fatty acids in their diets had significantly greater improvement in headache symptoms ($P < .001$) and headache frequency ($P = .02$) (Ramsden et al., 2013).

The authors of one large systematic review and meta-analysis assessing studies of omega-3 PUFAs with chronic pain conditions reported the largest positive effect was found with people with dysmenorrhea (Prego-Domínguez, Hadrya, & Takkouche, 2016). This is reasonable because proinflammatory prostaglandins are increased when arachidonic acid is released from endometrial cell membranes, and higher intake of omega-3 PUFAs results in less menstrual pain and less NSAID need (Kuphal, 2018). In one study (N = 95), women with primary dysmenorrhea who received omega-3 PUFAs, after 3 months reported significantly less pain ($P < .05$) and fewer ibuprofen rescue doses ($P = .001$) (Rahbar, Asgharzadeh, & Ghorbani, 2012).

Further research is needed with strong methodology, larger samples, and subjects with a variety of painful conditions and to clarify effectiveness, side effects, and potential risks. Research is also warranted to identify if there is a difference in the effect of high levels of omega-3 PUFAs in diet consumption compared to supplementation.

Cautions

Generally, omega-3 PUFAs are considered safe with a few minor and predominantly GI side effects (indigestion, diarrhea, gas), but it is not clear if there is cross allergy with shellfish and if they contribute to increased risk for developing prostate cancer (NCCIH, 2015). They have been associated with bruising and clotting inhibition (Zengion & Yarnell, 2011).

Contraindications

PUFAs may be considered contraindicated before surgery because of their anticoagulant properties (Zengion & Yarnell, 2011).

Potential Interactions With Medications

As with all supplements, patients are advised to discuss using omega-3 PUFAs with a clinician before starting supplementation. People being treated with anticoagulants, such as coumadin, need to be aware of the possible interactions with anticoagulant or blood thinning medications with which the effects may be increased by omega-3 PUFAs (NIH, 2019c; Walz, Barry, & Koshman, 2016).

Vitamins

B Vitamins

All eight of the B vitamins are water soluble (not stored by the body) and assist in the conversion of carbohydrates to glucose and in the metabolism of amino acids, proteins, and fats (Khalil, Chambers, Khalil, & Ang, 2016). They are important in nervous system function (Alexa-Stratulat et al., 2017) and to a lesser degree with liver function and with type 2 diabetes (Nix et al., 2015). Deficiency of the B vitamins is characterized by cognitive difficulties, impaired motor coordination, and peripheral neuropathy (Khalil et al., 2016), yet these dysfunctions are potentially reversible with vitamin supplementation and/or dietary modifications (Saulino, 2014). When the analgesic effects of high-dose B vitamins (B1, B6, and B12) on neuropathic pain among rodents was evaluated, it was reported they caused inhibition of thermal hyperalgesia that is immediate but dose dependent (Song, 2017). Even though there is no identified mechanism of action for pain control, with increasing frequency, B vitamins are investigated and used to improve neurologic conditions, including diabetic neuropathy and neuralgia, and inflammatory conditions (Mikkelsen, Stojanovska, Prakash, & Apostolopoulos, 2017; Tan, 2014).

Vitamin B$_1$ (Thiamine)

Vitamin B$_1$ is essential for production of ATP, myelin, and neurotransmitter synthesis in the nervous system (Alexa-Stratulat et al., 2017; Fattal-Valevski, 2011). Thiamine deficiency is also correlated with depression (Mikkelsen et al., 2017), which can be an important complicating factor with chronic pain (see Chapters 8 and 22). Thiamine is found in red meat, legumes, whole grain cereals, nuts, wheat germ, rice (except polished rice), fish, seafood, and poultry (DiNicolantonio, Liu, & O'Keefe, 2018; Fattal-Valevski, 2011; NIH, 2018c). Lack of vitamin B$_1$ is seen in neuropathic disorders such as nutritional polyneuropathy and Wernicke-Korsakoff syndrome (Alexa-Stratulat et al., 2017). Thiamine deficiency is also correlated with anxiety and depression (Mikkelsen et al., 2017). Animal research indicates deficiency of thiamine may be correlated with Alzheimer's disease (NIH, 2019d). Recommendations for adult daily intake are 1.2 to 1.5 mg/day for men and 1.0 to 1.1 for women, with increases to 1.5 during pregnancy and 1.6 when breastfeeding (Fattal-Valevski, 2011).

Evidence for Pain Management Even though it seems logical that thiamine has an important role with neuropathic activity and potentially neuropathic pain, the evidence for thiamine and pain management is scarce. When the relationship between B$_1$ and DPN was studied in male rodents (N = 40), there was a reversal of the pathologic effects of DPN (uneven thickness of myelin of the sciatic nerve and lamellar separation) in the rodents who received B$_1$ (Song, Chen, & Zhao, 2017). This is a promising study that requires additional research. The researchers of another rodent study compared the antiinflammatory benefit of thiamine with that of indomethacin and reported that indomethacin was more effective during the acute phase but that thiamine was more effective over time with chronicity (Zaringhalam et al., 2016).

When vitamin B$_1$ (100 mg/day) and vitamin E (400 units/day) were used for dysmenorrhea (N = 90), both vitamins were statistically significant in reducing pain intensity ($P < .001$), ($P < .002$) and pain duration ($P < .001$), ($P < .001$) (Nayeban, Jafarnejad, Nayeban, & Sefidgaran, 2014). This is consistent with other studies that reported thiamine improved mental and physical symptoms of premenstrual syndrome (PMS) (Abdollahifard, Koshkaki, & Moazamiyanfar, 2014) and that dietary thiamine and riboflavin were associated with risk for developing PMS (Chocano-Bedoya et al., 2011).

In an innovative Italian study, postoperative pain control was compared using interscalene blocks with levobupivacaine alone compared with levobupivacaine with thiamine (Alemanno et al., 2016). In that study the patients in both groups had similar analgesia but those who received the levobupivacaine with thiamine had significantly ($P < .001$) longer periods of analgesia. These results indicate a multimodal approach for perineural analgesia to provide longer duration of postoperative analgesia.

Cautions Vitamin B$_1$ is generally safe with few mostly mild side effects, including pruritus, cyanosis, feeling warm, and symptoms of anaphylaxis (e.g., angioedema, diaphoresis, urticaria). Caution is advised during pregnancy, breastfeeding, and renal compromise (Martel & Franklin, 2017). As with all vitamins and supplements, consultation with a clinician is advised before use.

Contraindications No frank contraindications were found.

Potential Interactions With Medications Vitamin B$_1$ can potentially decrease absorption of some antibiotics, increase metabolism of phenytoin, and increase renal elimination of some antihypertensives and digoxin (Karadima, Kraniotou, Bellos, & Tsangaris, 2016).

Vitamin B$_2$ (Riboflavin)

Like the other B vitamins, riboflavin is involved in production of energy and is necessary to convert vitamins B$_6$ and B$_9$ into usable forms in the body (Khalil et al., 2016). Riboflavin also has strong association with the neurologic system, with deficiencies related to cognition,

CNS changes, and depression, particularly in older adults (Mikkelsen et al., 2017). Riboflavin is found in beef, almonds, fortified cereal grains, dairy products (yogurt, milk, cheese), seafood, chicken, eggs, and fish (NIH, 2020d). Recommended adult daily dosing is 1.1 to 1.3 mg/day.

Evidence for Pain Management Vitamin B_2 was found to have moderate evidence for preventing migraine headaches by the American Academy of Neurology, with vitamin B_6 and combinations of B_6 with B_{12} and folic acid having potential benefits (Wells, Baute, & Wahbeh, 2017). It is suggested that the benefit of riboflavin is related to the possibility of a mitochondrial flaw in brain metabolism causing migraine headaches, and riboflavin as an important cofactor in the oxidative metabolism may correct the flaw (Colombo, Saraceno, & Comi, 2014).

Cautions Vitamin B_2 is considered generally safe with few side effects. The side effects reported include diarrhea and polyuria (Wells et al., 2017).

Contraindications No frank contraindications were found.

Potential Interactions With Medications Although no clinically relevant interactions are listed by the National Institutes of Health (NIH, 2020d), there are potential interactions listed in the literature. The two potential interactions identified were between B_2 and antibiotics and psychotherapeutic medications (Karadima et al., 2016). Before taking vitamin B_2 use should be discussed with a clinician.

Vitamin B_6 (Pyridoxine, Pyridoxal, and Pyridoxamine)

Vitamin B_6 is available in three forms, pyridoxine, pyridoxal, and pyridoxamine, that occur naturally (Combs & McClung, 2017b). Vitamin B_6 is readily available in food sources, particularly fish, organ meats, legumes, nuts, avocados, noncitrus fruits, whole grains, vegetables, and egg yolks (Stover & Field, 2015). Vitamin B_6 is needed for absorption of vitamin B_{12}; it is necessary for development of a number of neurotransmitters that transmit signals between nerve cells and dopamine, serotonin, norepinephrine, and γ-aminobutyrate (GABA), which are instrumental in nociception (Combs & McClung, 2017b; Stover & Field, 2015). B_6 is also needed for metabolism of amino acids and is essential for the formation of myelin (Khalil et al., 2016). Low levels of plasma pyridoxal 5′-phosphate of vitamin B_6 is associated with a number of inflammatory disorders (Ueland, McCann, Midttun, & Ulvik, 2017). B_6 deficiency is seen with myofascial pain syndrome (Bonakdar, 2018), migraine headaches, and depression (Mikkelsen et al., 2017). Usual recommended adult doses of vitamin B_6 is between 1.3 and 1.7 mg in adult men and between 1.3 and 1.5 mg in adult women, with increase to 1.9 mg during pregnancy and 2 mg when lactating, and should not exceed 100 mg unless approved by a clinician (NIH, 2020e).

Evidence for Pain Management Vitamin B_6 has been studied with a variety of pain conditions with a neurologic component or basis; however, there is no strong support that it is beneficial in any of them. People living with painful autoimmune conditions, such as RA, ulcerative colitis, Crohn's disease, and IBD may need greater amounts of vitamin B_6 because that vitamin may be reduced with the chronic inflammation (NIH, 2020e); however, this is an area needing research. According to the American Academy of Neurology, vitamin B_6 has potential benefit in preventing migraine headaches (Wells et al., 2017).

Pyridoxine has been studied in women with PMS symptoms and is listed as likely to be beneficial by the International Association for the Study of Pain (IASP) (Berkley, 2013). Because primary dysmenorrhea is the result of a cascade of prostaglandins and leukotrienes in the wall of the uterus, substances with antiinflammatory properties are effective (Tridenti & Vezzani, 2018). When vitamin B_6 was compared to auriculotherapy (see Chapter 27), both were statistically significant with no statistical difference between the two interventions (Koleini & Valiani, 2017). There is a need for further research with more rigorous design to evaluate the benefit of vitamin B_6 with dysmenorrhea (NIH, 2020e), which affects up to 85% of women (Tridenti & Vezzani, 2018).

Cautions Vitamin B_6 in high doses has side effects that include skin reactions, photosensitivity, nausea, vomiting, epigastric pain, and painful skin lesions; with increased dosing, neurologic symptoms such as ataxia, lower limb paresthesia, and imbalance issues may occur (Kumar, Kaur, & Singh, 2017; NIH, 2020e). Isolated single instances of congenital defects when pyridoxine was taken in early pregnancy have been reported, but no current research has supported that relationship (NIH, 2020e).

An interesting investigation of vitamin B_6 was with idiopathic burning mouth syndrome (iBMS), which is characterized by painful burning sensations of the mouth; it occurs primarily in perimenopausal women and the cause is unknown (Dieb & Boucher, 2017). When vitamin B_6 levels were assessed in women with iBMS (N = 42), elevated serum levels that correlated to greater pain were found in 17% of the women and when the levels were decreased in two of the women their pain also decreased (Dieb, Moreau, Rochefort, & Boucher, 2017). These findings may be related to what is called the *vitamin B_6 paradox*, which is that although vitamin B_6 is implicated with relieving neuropathic pain, high doses of supplementation of vitamin B_6 are implicated with neuropathic pain (Vrolijk et al., 2017).

Contraindications No frank contraindications were found except the cautions given in the following section regarding concomitant therapy with certain medications.

Potential Interactions With Medications Supplemental vitamin B_6 should not be taken without clinician approval if the following medications are taken: cycloSPORINE, theophylline, and antiseizure medications (e.g., phenytoin, carBAMazepine, valproic acid) (NIH, 2020e).

Vitamin B$_9$ (Folate or Folic Acid)

Vitamin B$_9$ or folic acid is another water-soluble vitamin considered essential for metabolism and is found in many plants, especially those with a foliar origin and green leafy vegetables (Combs & McClung, 2017a). It is available in the diet by eating green leafy vegetables, legumes (i.e., lentils and chickpeas), almonds, chestnuts, eggs, and liver (Sharma, Gaikwad, & Kulkarni, 2017). Low levels of folate are linked to low response to antidepressant medications with some improvement in response to those medications when folate is added (Mikkelsen et al., 2017). Absorption of folate is necessary for maintaining healthy bones and development of the CNS and neurologic function (Combs & McClung, 2017a). Recommended daily allotments for adults is 400 mcg for adults, with 600 mg recommended during pregnancy and 500 mg recommended when lactating (NIH, 2020f).

Evidence for Pain Management Neurologic symptoms are increasingly seen after bariatric surgery and may be due to nutritional deficiencies, including vitamins B$_1$, B$_9$, and B$_{12}$ (Landais, 2014).

Cautions Higher than recommended levels of folic acid are concerning for interacting with vitamin B$_{12}$; for possibly masking neurologic damage of megaloblastic anemia; and possibly related to accelerating the activity of preneoplastic lesions in colorectal cancer (NIH, 2020f).

Contraindications No frank contraindications were found, except the cautions in the following section regarding concomitant therapy with certain medications.

Potential Interactions With Medications Folic acid should be avoided when taking methotrexate, sulfaSALAzine, and antiepileptic medications (e.g., phenytoin, carBAMazepine, and valproate (NIH, 2020f). Because folic acid can have undesirable interactions with other medications as well, it is recommended that anyone who is regularly prescribed medications consult a clinician before supplementing with this vitamin (NIH, 2020f).

B$_{12}$ (Cyanocobalamin or Cobalamin)

Vitamin B$_{12}$ is not found in vegetables or plants, but rather in animal tissues, and deficiency is generally found only among people who adhere to a strict vegan diet with no animal products and those with congenital disorders interfering with absorption or transportation of B$_{12}$ (Combs & McClung, 2017c; NIH, 2020c). Absorption of vitamin B$_{12}$ from food requires an adequate amount of stomach acid, and the ability to absorb declines with increasing age (Tick, 2015). B$_{12}$ deficiency is seen with neurologic changes and anemia (Combs & McClung, 2017c), myofascial

pain syndrome (Bonakdar, 2018), depression, agitation (Mikkelsen et al., 2017), and other chronic pain disorders (Tick, 2015). It is also associated with neuronal dysfunction in people with spinal cord injuries (Saulino, 2014) and was recently reported among the Chinese population with diabetic neuropathy (Wang, Zhai, & Liu, 2017). Recommended daily allowance from the NIH (2020c) for adults is 2.4 mcg, with 2.6 mcg during pregnancy and 2.8 mcg while lactating.

Evidence for Pain Management There is less research available for B$_{12}$ than the other B vitamins and the studies have been with a variety of painful conditions. Inadequate levels of vitamin B$_{12}$ is associated with atrophic glossitis (atrophy of the dorsal surface of the tongue) with burning, stinging, and eventually lesions and paresthesia if not corrected with supplementation (Pedersen, Forssell, & Grinde, 2016). Vitamin B$_{12}$ was used successfully in several studies to treat painful aphthous ulcers or canker sores, which are an inflammation of the inside of the mouth that may be related to a vitamin B$_{12}$ deficiency (Liu, 2017).

Injections of vitamin B$_{12}$ were administered to people with chronic pain who did not have vitamin B$_{12}$ deficiency, yet the patients receiving the injections reported less pain and less analgesic medication use (Tick, 2015). An interesting treatment combination was vitamin B$_{12}$ combined with ketorolac (N = 60) which was statistically ($P \leq .001$) effective in reducing edema and pain compared to placebo with either B$_{12}$ or ketorolac alone in rodents (Rahman, 2017). Laboratory research is needed to investigate the role of vitamin D in musculoskeletal conditions including myofascial pain syndrome (Bonakdar, 2018) and diabetic neuropathy (Wang et al., 2017).

Cautions Vitamin B$_{12}$ is considered safe, with little toxicity reported (NIH, 2020c). The Institute of Medicine reported that no adverse effects were noted concerning vitamin B$_{12}$ in people who are healthy, even with excessive amounts from food or supplementation (Institute of Medicine [IOM], 1998; NIH, 2016a). However, on rare occasions, with high doses, acne has been reported (Aronson, 2016b).

Contraindications No frank contraindications were found.

Potential Interactions With Medications Vitamin B$_{12}$ can interact with chloramphenicol, proton pump inhibitors, histamine (H$_2$) receptor agonists, and metFORMIN (NIH, 2020c). It is advisable for patients to consult with a clinician before beginning supplementation when taking those medications.

Vitamin B Complex and Combinations

Evidence for Pain Management A vitamin B complex (vitamins B$_1$, B$_6$, and B$_{12}$) was used for 7 to 14 days to treat rodents in which a temporary ischemic neuropathic pain condition was created (Yu et al., 2014). In that study, there was a significant reduction in thermal hyperalgesia with a series of cellular changes indicating a neuroprotection and analgesic benefit of the vitamin B complex. Of particular interest in that study was the B complex and a reduction in an enzyme (GAD65) necessary for synthesis of the GABA inhibitory neurotransmitter (Tan, 2014; Yu et al., 2014). Additional research is needed, but these results are hopeful for a relatively benign intervention for neuropathic pain, which is so disabling for so many people.

When vitamin B complex (vitamins B_1, B_6, and B_{12}) was used in people living with chronic temporomandibular joint (TMJ) disorder (N = 26), pain intensity was significantly reduced in the 50% who received vitamin B complex compared to placebo ($P > .05$) (Rajaran & Choi, 2016). Combinations of B_6 with B_{12} and folic acid having potential benefits for preventing migraine headaches were reported by the American Academy of Neurology (Wells et al., 2017). Vitamin B_{12} also has been used for more than 20 years in combination with vitamins B_1 and B_6 to reduce inflammation and nociceptive and neuropathic pain, but was not effective when used alone in animal studies (Imtiaz et al., 2016). In a preventive type of study that also combined vitamin B_{12} combined with B_1 and vitamin B_6, in intramuscular injections, the asymptomatic people treated with the B vitamins had better myelinated peripheral nerve conductivity than did controls (Brito et al., 2016).

Cautions Adverse effects are reported with high doses, including skin irritations and rare allergic reactions (Aronson, 2016b); however, the reader is referred to potential interactions with the individual B vitamins.

Contraindications No frank contraindications were found.

Potential Interactions With Medications No potential interactions with medications are noted (Aronson, 2016b); however, the reader is referred to potential interactions with the individual B vitamins.

Vitamin D

Vitamin D is one of the fat-soluble vitamins that interacts with calcium homeostasis, with bone metabolism, and in supporting the musculoskeletal system (Gendelman, Itzhaki, Makarov, Bennun, & Amital, 2015; NIH, 2020g). Rather than being an actual vitamin, the group of molecules known as vitamin D are essential substances obtained solely from food intake (Girgis, Clifton-Bligh, Hamrick, Holick, & Gunton, 2013). Recent studies indicate that vitamin D functions like a hormone necessary to all systems and cell types (Tick, 2015) (Fig. 26.5). In addition to the more common role it plays in bone health, it is involved with immune system regulation (Sedighi, 2017) (Fig. 26.3).

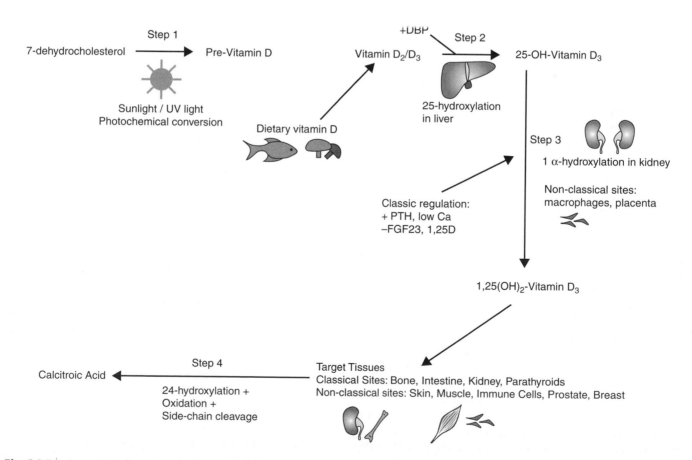

Fig. 26.5 | **The metabolic pathway of vitamin D.** (From Girgis, C. M., Clifton-Bligh, R. J., Hamrick, M. W., Holick, M. F., & Gunton, J. E. [2013]. The roles of vitamin D in skeletal muscle: form, function, and metabolism. *Endocrine Reviews, 34*[1], 33–83.)

Increasing evidence also is supporting the role of vitamin D in maintaining strength in skeletal muscles (Gendelman et al., 2015; Girgis et al., 2013), thus providing additional support to the musculoskeletal system and improving strength (Tick, 2015). Other effects of vitamin D include antiinflammatory, antifibrotic, and antiapoptotic activities (Antony & Ding, 2017). Vitamin D is also considered a neuroprotective neurosteroid with detoxifying activities and is thought to potentially temper the inflammatory cascade, including nitric oxide, substance P, and glutamate, that occurs when vertebral discs are herniated (Sedighi, 2017). Considering the relationship between vitamin D and the substances of the inflammatory cascade, it is not surprising that significant deficiencies of this vitamin are associated with chronic pain (Tick, 2015).

Evidence for Pain Management

The role of vitamin D with chronic pain is not clear (Lemmon & Roseen, 2018). People who are obese, who live in the northern hemisphere, who have more skin pigmentation, and older adults are at higher risk for vitamin D deficiency (Tick, 2015). Epidemiologic studies have reported an association between deficiencies of vitamin D and chronic musculoskeletal pain and the association occurring in as many as 90% of the people in one study (Lemmon & Roseen, 2018). Low levels of vitamin D are correlated with increased inflammation (Tick, 2015) and musculoskeletal pain. Vitamin D deficiency also has been associated with myofascial pain syndrome and increasing sensitivity to pain with that condition (Bonakdar, 2018) and, as with vitamin B_{12}, vitamin D is associated with neuronal dysfunction in people with spinal cord injuries (Saulino, 2014). Low levels of vitamin D were found in 21% of patients with chronic pain (N = 174) and those with lower levels had significantly greater severity of pain intensity, which led the researchers to speculate that low levels of vitamin D may contribute to increased pain sensitivity (von Känel, Müller-Hartmannsgruber, Kokinogenis, & Egloff, 2014).

Research considering the potential role of vitamin D as an analgesic has evolved from the identification of low vitamin D levels in people with musculoskeletal pain (Gendelman et al., 2015). In a longitudinal study in Canada, low vitamin D levels were predictive of knee pain (P = .002) and hip pain (P = .083) (Laslett et al., 2014). The relationship may be related to osteomalacia, which is caused by vitamin D deficiency and can cause localized or diffuse dull, achy pains (Lemmon & Roseen, 2018). One proposal is that inadequate vitamin D activates cytokines and inflammatory stimuli, which result in inflammatory pain, and these low levels are also correlated with pain sensitization (Antony & Ding, 2017) (Fig. 26.6). From this perspective, supplemental vitamin D at least in part can potentially modify musculoskeletal pain by correcting the deficiency that contributed to the pain. Theoretically, vitamin D has potential benefit in an MMA plan of care.

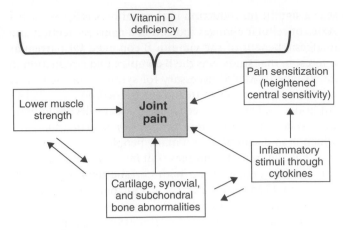

Fig. 26.6 | (From Antony, B., & Ding, C. [2017]. Vitamin D deficiency in joint pain: Effects of vitamin D supplementation. In R. R. Watson, & S. Zibadi (Eds.). *Nutritional modulators of pain in the aging population* [pp. 183–189]. London: Academic Press.)

Research regarding the benefit of supplemental vitamin D for chronic musculoskeletal pain is inconsistent; however, there is no strong evidence to support vitamin D as being helpful with preexisting musculoskeletal pain. Two Cochrane reviews reported insufficient evidence to support vitamin D as being superior to placebo for any chronic pain condition (Straube, Derry, Moore, & McQuay, 2010; Straube, Derry, Straube, & Moore, 2015). One more recent meta-analysis reviewing the effect of vitamin D on OA of the knee concluded vitamin D may have no clinically significant benefit for pain control or disease progression with OA (Diao, Yang, & Yu, 2017). A second recent meta-analysis (N = 4 studies) with the use of vitamin D in the same population concluded that vitamin D was helpful in pain and function but not in preventing cartilage loss (Gao, Chen, & Deng, 2017); however, the veracity of those results was challenged (Hussain, Singh, Akhtar, & Najmi, 2017). The authors of both recent meta-analyses think additional research is needed.

The authors of an analysis of three studies in which vitamin D supplementation was used with people living with chronic nonspecific musculoskeletal pain, reported no benefit from vitamin D (Gaikwad, Vanlint, Mittinity, Moseley, & Stocks, 2017). The investigators of a 2-year randomized placebo-controlled, double-blind clinical trial (N = 146) reported that compared with controls (n = 73) raising vitamin D levels (n = 73) did not reduce pain intensity or improve cartilage volume in patients with OA of the knees (McAlindon et al., 2013). Similar results were reported from a 2-year multicenter, double-blind, placebo-controlled clinical trial in Australia (n = 413) with no improvement in tibial cartilage volume or reduction in pain scores (Jin et al., 2016).

Considering the role of vitamin D with knee OA from a preventive perspective may be more viable and important. In an Australian study (N = 413) older adults with knee OA and varying degrees of vitamin D insufficiency were followed for 24 months (Zheng et al., 2017). In that study, the researchers concluded there are advantageous benefits for maintaining adequate levels of vitamin D for delaying or preventing loss of cartilage and effusion-synovitis and maintaining function among older adults with OA of the knee.

However, in another study (N = 74) with various musculoskeletal pains, the group who received 4000 IU of vitamin D (n = 36) in addition to their usual analgesic regimen reported significantly less pain intensity at 6 weeks ($P < .001$) and 12 weeks ($P < .001$) compared to those who did not receive the vitamin D supplement (n = 38) (Gendelman et al., 2015). Similarly, in a study using vitamin D supplementation among veterans (N = 28) with chronic pain and vitamin D deficiency, after vitamin D supplementation the participants who received it had significant improvements in pain ($P < .001$) as well as with improvements in sleep, general health, and quality of life (Huang, Shah, Long, Crankshaw, & Tangpricha, 2013).

Vitamin D is potentially important as an intervention to prevent pain; several studies have identified the ingestion of vitamin D supplements with improving muscle performance and lowering the instance of falls among older adults taking 800 to 1000 IUs daily (Dawson-Hughes, 2017). The mechanisms through which vitamin D is protective is not clear (Dhaliwal & Aloia, 2017). In related studies, an association of increased risk for falling was associated with low levels of vitamin D (serum levels of 25(OH)D) among older adults (Dhaliwal & Aloia, 2017). Interestingly, although it is not particularly surprising that doses lower than the recommended allowance were not effective in reducing falls, higher doses seemed to increase the fall risk (Dawson-Hughes, 2017). Study results are inconsistent, ranging from no improvement to 43% improvement (Dhaliwal & Aloia, 2017). Additional research is needed to clarify the mechanism of action by which vitamin D is protective of falling and with large, diverse samples and strong methodology.

Another interesting relationship was seen between vitamin D and people with carpal tunnel syndrome, with levels of vitamin D being significantly lower ($P = .003$) in patients with mild carpal tunnel syndrome (n = 36) compared to those with no such symptoms (n = 40) (Demiryurek & Gundogdu, 2017). Additional research is needed to explore the possible relationship between vitamin D deficiency with carpal tunnel syndrome and to determine if it may be therapeutic either from a preventive or treatment perspective in an MMA plan of care.

Laboratory research is needed to investigate the role of vitamin D in musculoskeletal conditions, including myofascial pain syndrome (Bonakdar, 2018). Further studies are needed to guide recommendations for dosages of vitamin D in people with painful musculoskeletal conditions, and additional research is needed with larger samples for longer durations (Girgis et al., 2013; Huang et al., 2013; Laslett, 2014; Lemmon & Roseen, 2018). Although it seems sensible to check the vitamin D level in patients who have chronic musculoskeletal pain and start a trial with vitamin D supplements if the level is low and vitamin D is not contraindicated, vitamin D is not innocuous (Laslett, 2014; Lemmon & Roseen, 2018).

Cautions

The adverse effect level from vitamin D supplementation is considered to be greater than 4000 IU per day (Tick, 2015). The NIH recommends daily doses as a dietary supplement are 600 IU for adults but 800 IU for those over 70 years of age with 600 IU during pregnancy and when lactating (NIH, 2020g). Other sources recommend 800 to 1000 IU daily particularly for older adults (Bonakdar, 2018; Dawson-Hughes, 2017).

There are few adverse effects with vitamin D (Straube et al., 2015). When taken in excess the following have been reported: poor appetite (anorexia), weight loss, cardiac arrhythmias, polyuria, vascular/tissue calcification, renal calculi, and cardiac and renal complications (NIH, 2018f). Vitamin D is recommended to be used with caution in the presence of calcium oxalate nephrolithiasis (Zengion & Yarnell, 2011). More is not better; fall risk increases in older adults when taking more than 1000 IU daily (Dawson-Hughes, 2017). As with other supplements, patients are advised to discuss possible supplementation with a clinician before starting.

Contraindications

Vitamin D is contraindicated in the presence of hypercalcemia, hyperphosphatemia, sarcoidosis, and toxicity of vitamin D (Zengion & Yarnell, 2011).

Potential Interactions With Medications Corticosteroids, orlistat, PHENobarbital, phenytoin, and cholesterol-lowering agents are some of the medications that are concerning when taken with vitamin D (NIH, 2018f). It is prudent for all patients who regularly take medications to consult with a clinician before beginning supplementation with vitamin D.

Vitamin E

Vitamin E is the common general name for the fat-soluble antioxidant tocopherols (four) and tocotrienol (four) derivatives (Combs & McClung, 2017d; Jiang, 2014). It is available in the oils of wheat germ, safflower, sunflower, and grains and seeds (Combs & McClung, 2017d), dark leafy green vegetables, nuts (e.g., almond, hazelnuts), peanuts, soybean oil, kiwis, and mangos (Jiang, 2014; NIH, 2020c). Recommended dietary intake is between 3 and 15 mg/day (Galli et al., 2017).

Evidence for Pain Management

It is reasonable that vitamin E is involved in controlling pain because it is essential for function of the neurologic systems and is neuroprotective and deficiency is seen with neuromuscular and neurologic pathology

(Alexa-Stratulat et al., 2017; Galli et al, 2017). Vitamin E deficiency has been associated with neurologic conditions such as Alzheimer's and Parkinson's diseases (Combs & McClung, 2017d). It also has a role in bone health guarding against disease (Peh, Tan, Liao, & Wong, 2016). In one study the tocotrienol component of vitamin E was effective in relieving pain of diabetic neuropathy in rodents (Kuhad, Bishnoi, Tiwari, & Chopra, 2009). In another study with people living with pain from diabetic neuropathy, 88% (N = 70) of those who received vitamin E and oil of evening primrose had mild to moderate benefit after 2 weeks of treatment (Ogbera, Ezeobi, Unachukwu, & Oshinaike, 2014). The authors of a third study using oral vitamin E to treat painful diabetic neuropathy (N = 92) reported that people who received vitamin E (n = 46) reported significantly less pain (P < .01) compared to the standard of care group (n = 46), who were treated with pregabalin (Rajanandh, Kosey, & Prathiksha, 2014). When it was studied in patients with chemotherapy-induced peripheral neuropathy with positive benefit seen in small studies, but the benefit was not supported in a larger study (Pachman, Loprinzi, Grothey, & Ta, 2014). However, the researchers of a more recent small study with rodents (N = 8) who had partial sciatic nerve ligation and were treated with pregabalin, vitamin E, or a combination of the two, concluded that both had antinociceptive and neuroprotective effects alone and in combination (Meymandi et al., 2017).

Vitamin E gamma-tocotrienol was demonstrated to suppress cytokine-triggered activation of the nuclear factor NK-κB (Wang, Park, Jang, Ma, & Jiang, 2015), which is thought to be a proinflammatory signaling pathway (Lawrence, 2009), and upstream regulation. Forms of vitamin E also have been seen to inhibit COX-1, COX-2, prostaglandins, leukotrienes, and other components of the inflammatory cascade (Jiang, 2014). In animal models antiinflammatory effects were noted on pancreatic gene expression when vitamin E supplementation was administered (Bhardwaj, Yadav, & Garg, 2017). Considering the intensity of pain associated with pancreatitis, additional research is needed in humans. Although the antiinflammatory benefit of vitamin E seems to be clear (Alexa-Stratulat et al., 2017; Jiang, 2014), clinical trials have not supported the use of vitamin E supplementation to reduce risk for developing inflammatory disorders such as RA (Combs & McClung, 2017d).

However, reports from older RCTs were that in high doses (100–600 IU per day) it was effective in reducing inflammation and pain in people with RA and rhabdomyolysis in horses (Combs & McClung, 2017d). Vitamin E showed slow onset of antiinflammatory and analgesic effects in a rodent model that were promising (Rossato et al., 2015). There have been a few recent studies investigating the benefit of vitamin E with dysmenorrhea with positive results (Kashanian, Lakeh, Ghasemi, & Noori, 2013). In a recent study, vitamin E was effective in statistically improving function and reducing pain intensity reported by people living with OA of the knees (N = 72) (Tantavisut et al., 2017).

Vitamin E has been used as an intervention in several interesting studies. When compared with vitamin B$_6$, to reduce pain related to mastalgia (painful breast tissue), vitamin E was equally effective in reducing pain during subsequent menstrual cycles (N = 80) (Shobeiri, Oshvandi, & Nazari, 2015). Results of studies using vitamin E to treat the symptoms of tardive dyskinesia (repetitive involuntary movements of the face) also have been mixed and limited by poor methodology (Bergman, Walker, Nikolakopoulou, Soares-Weiser, & Adams, 2017). The researchers of a laboratory study showed that a tocotrienol substance from vitamin E was effective in improving bone structure with testosterone-deficient rodents (Chin & Ima-Nirwana, 2014). In another study (N = 30), when compared to standard of care, patients who were treated with dressings with a tocotrienol substance from vitamin E reported significantly less pain while undergoing painful skin graft donor site dressing changes (Stanizzi, Bottoni, Tartaglione, Bolletta, & Benedetto, 2017). Studies have shown that on some inflammatory biomarkers of pancreatic gene expression in rodents, supplementation of vitamin E has antiinflammatory benefit (Monteiro, Silva, Ambrosio, Zucoloto, & Vannucchi, 2012). Research is needed to further explore the role of vitamin E in the nociceptive process and adverse events that may occur with supplementation (Galli et al., 2017) and with muscle activity, bone health, skin grafts, pancreatitis, and mastalgia.

Cautions

Vitamin E is considered to be one of the safest of vitamins, but in high doses it can interfere with the action of other fat-soluble vitamins (Combs & McClung, 2017d). Adverse side effects include diarrhea, GI distress, pulmonary emboli, thromboemboli, thrombophlebitis, hypertension, fatigue, gynecomastia, and breast tumor, but there are few data about how often these occur (Aronson, 2016c).

Contraindications

No frank contraindications were found other than the potential contraindications with concomitant medications discussed in the following section.

Potential Interactions With Medications

Bleeding risk increases with acetylsalicylic acid (e.g., aspirin) and anticoagulants (e.g., warfarin, clopidogrel) and it interferes with vitamin K (Aronson, 2016c; Krishna & Purushothaman, 2015) so should be avoided by people with risk for bleeding or taking medications in those categories. People who are prescribed niacin, simvastatin, anticoagulant/antiplatelet, chemotherapeutic medications, and radiotherapy should consult with a clinician before taking vitamin E (NIH, 2018f).

Key Points

- Botanicals, herbs, supplements, and vitamins offer promising benefit as components of a multimodal analgesic plan of care.
- Early research is promising for many of the botanicals, herbs, supplements, and vitamins, but additional research is needed.
- Patients need to be educated that just because something is natural does not mean that it is without harm, and they need to consult with clinicians before and while using botanicals, herbs, supplements, and vitamins.

Case Scenario

Rodney is a 46-year-old man who works in construction and lives with chronic arthritis of both knees and his left ankle. He has been on opioids (oxyCODONE 5–15 mg every 4–6 hours as needed for pain) but wants to reduce the amount he is taking because of severe constipation. He tells you his girlfriend has been reading about botanicals and supplements and asks if you think any of them could help him. He is concerned about taking more medication because he takes NSAIDs and medication for controlling diabetes (glipiZIDE) as well as an anticoagulant. He also tells you that his girlfriend is interested because she has severe dysmenorrhea.

1. What information will you give him about botanicals, herbs, supplements, and vitamins that may be helpful for his arthritic pain?
2. What can you tell him about his girlfriend using them for dysmenorrhea?
3. What cautions does Rodney need to know about side effects?
4. What cautions does Rodney need to know about interactions with the medications he is already taking?
5. What limitations does he need to know about using the botanicals, herbs, supplements, and vitamins?

References

Abalo, R., & Martín-Fontelles, I. (2017). Cannabis, cannabinoids, and visceral pain. In A. Farr (Ed.), *Handbook of Cannabis and Related Pathologies: Biology, Pharmacology, Diagnosis, and Treatment* (pp. 439–449). London: Academic Press.

Abdollahifard, S., Koshkaki, A. R., & Moazamiyanfar, R. (2014). The effects of vitamin B1 on ameliorating the premenstrual syndrome symptoms. *Global Journal of Health Science, 6*(6), 144–153.

Abdul Muhammad, Z., & Ahmad, T. (2017). Therapeutic uses of pineapple-extracted bromelain in surgical care-A review. *JPMA: Journal of the Pakistan Medical Association, 67*(1), 121–125.

Abdullah, B., Lazim, N. M., & Salim, R. (2015). The effectiveness of Tualang honey in reducing post-tonsillectomy pain. *Kulak Burun Bogaz Ihtis Derg, 25*(3), 137–143.

Abdulrazaq, M., Innes, J. K., & Calder, P. C. (2017). Effect of ω-3 polyunsaturated fatty acids on arthritic pain: A systematic review. *Nutrition, 39*, 57–66.

Ahn, H., Kim, J., Lee, M. J., Kim, Y. J., Cho, Y. W., & Lee, G. S. (2015). Methylsulfonylmethane inhibits NLRP3 inflammasome activation. *Cytokine, 71*(2), 223–231.

Akhtar, N., & Haqqi, T. M. (2011). Epigallocatechin-3-gallate suppresses the global interleukin-1beta-induced inflammatory response in human chondrocytes. *Arthritis Research & Therapy, 13*(3), R93.

Al-Harbi, N. O., Al-Ashban, R. M., & Shah, A. H. (2013). Toxicity studies on *Harpagophytum procumbens* (Devils claw) capsules in mice. *Journal of Medicinal Plants Research, 7*(42), 3089–3097.

Al-Jaroudi, D., Kaddour, O., & Al-Amin, N. (2016). Risks of myrrh usage in pregnancy. *JBRA Assisted Reproduction, 20*(4), 257–258.

Al-Waili, N., Salom, K., & Al-Ghamdi, A. A. (2011). Honey for wound healing, ulcers, and burns; data supporting its use in clinical practice. *The Scientific World Journal, 11*, 766–787.

Albrecht, E., Kirkham, K. R., Liu, S. S., & Brull, R. (2013). Perioperative intravenous administration of magnesium sulphate and postoperative pain: a meta-analysis. *Anaesthesia, 68*(1), 79–90.

Alcocer-Gómez, E., Cano-García, F. J., & Cordero, M. D. (2013). Effect of coenzyme Q 10 evaluated by 1990 and 2010 ACR Diagnostic Criteria for Fibromyalgia and SCL-90-R: Four case reports and literature review. *Nutrition, 29*(11), 1422–1425.

Alemanno, F., Ghisi, D., Westermann, B., Bettoni, A., Fanelli, A., La Colla, L., … Cesana, B. M. (2016). The use of vitamin B1 as a perineural adjuvant to middle interscalene block for postoperative analgesia after shoulder surgery. *Acta Bio Medica Atenei Parmensis, 87*(1), 22–27.

Alexa-Stratulat, T., Luca, A., Bădescu, M., Bohotin, C. R., & Alexa, I. D. (2017). Nutritional Modulators in Chemotherapy-Induced Neuropathic Pain. In R. R. Watson, & S. Zibadi (Eds.), *Nutritional Modulators of Pain in the Aging Population* (pp. 9–33). London: Academic Press.

Alipour, Z., Asadizaker, M., Fayazi, S., Yegane, N., Kochak, M., & Zadeh, M. H. H. (2017). The Effect of Ginger on Pain and Satisfaction of Patients with Knee Osteoarthritis. *Jundishapur Journal of Chronic Disease Care, 6*(1). https://doi.org/10.17795/jjcdc-34798.

Alostad, A. H., Steinke, D. T., & Schafheutle, E. I. (2018). International Comparison of Five Herbal Medicine Registration Systems to Inform Regulation Development: United Kingdom, Germany, United States of America, United Arab Emirates and Kingdom of Bahrain. *Pharmaceutical Medicine, 32*(1), 39–49.

Alqasoumi, S., Yusufoglu, H., Farraj, A., & Alam, A. (2011). Effect of 6-shogaol and 6-gingerol on diclofenac sodium induced liver injury. *International Journal of Pharmacology, 7*(8), 868–873.

Altman, R., Lim, S., Steen, R. G., & Dasa, V. (2015). Hyaluronic acid injections are associated with delay of total knee replacement surgery in patients with knee osteoarthritis: evidence from a large US health claims database. *PLoS One, 10*(12), e0145776.

Altman, R., Fredericson, M., Bhattacharyya, S. K., Bisson, B., Abbott, T., Yadalam, S., & Kim, M. (2016). Association between hyaluronic acid injections and time-to-total knee replacement surgery. *The Journal of Knee Surgery, 29*(07), 564–570.

Altman, R. D., Schemitsch, E., & Bedi, A. (2015, October). Assessment of clinical practice guideline methodology for the treatment of knee osteoarthritis with intra-articular hyaluronic acid. *Seminars in Arthritis and Rheumatism*, 45(2), 132–139.

Alvarez-Sánchez, A., & Rey, E. (2013). Probiotics for irritable bowel syndrome: should we give them full names? *Revista Espanola de Enfermedades Digestivas: Organo Oficial de la Sociedad Espanola de Patologia Digestiva*, 105(1), 1–2.

Alves, J. C., Santos, A. M., & Jorge, P. I. (2017). Effect of an oral joint supplement when compared to carprofen in the management of hip osteoarthritis in working dogs. *Topics in Companion Animal Medicine*, 32, 126–129.

Amani, S., Kheiri, S., & Ahmadi, A. (2015). Honey versus diphenhydramine for post-tonsillectomy pain relief in pediatric cases: a randomized clinical trial. *Journal of clinical and diagnostic research: Journal of Clinical and Diagnostic Research*, 9(3), SC01–SC04.

Amdekar, S., & Singh, V. (2016). *Lactobacillus acidophilus* maintained oxidative stress from reproductive organs in collagen-induced arthritic rats. *Journal of Human Reproductive Sciences*, 9(1), 41–46.

Amdekar, S., Kumar, A., & Singh, V. (2017). Transcriptional activity of cytokines induced by oral administration of *Lactobacillus casei* and *Lactobacillus acidophilus* in experimental model of arthritis. *AIMS Molecular Science*, 4(2), 164–174.

Andreae, M. H., Carter, G. M., Shaparin, N., Suslov, K., Ellis, R. J., Ware, M. A., ... Johnson, M. (2015). Inhaled cannabis for chronic neuropathic pain: a meta-analysis of individual patient data. *The Journal of Pain*, 16(12), 1221–1232.

Antony, B., & Ding, C. (2017). Vitamin D deficiency in joint pain: Effects of vitamin D supplementation. In R. R. Watson, & S. Zibadi (Eds.), *Nutritional Modulators of Pain in the Aging Population* (pp. 183–189). London: Academic Press.

Appelboom, T., Maes, N., & Albert, A. (2014). A new curcuma extract (Flexofytol®) in osteoarthritis: results from a Belgian real-life experience. *The Open Rheumatology Journal*, 8, 77–81.

Arablou, T., & Aryaeian, N. (2017). The effect of ginger *(Zingiber officinale)* as an ancient medicinal plant on improving blood lipids. *Journal of Herbal Medicine.*, 12, 11–15.

Arablou, T., & Kolahdouz-Mohammadi, R. (2017). Curcumin and endometriosis: Review on potential roles and molecular mechanisms. *Biomedicine & Pharmacotherapy*, 97, 91–97.

Arjmandi, B. H., Ormsbee, L. T., Elam, M. L., Campbell, S. C., Rahnama, N., Payton, M. E., ... Daggy, B. P. (2014). A combination of *Scutellaria baicalensis* and *Acacia catechu* extracts for short-term symptomatic relief of joint discomfort associated with osteoarthritis of the knee. *Journal of Medicinal Food*, 17(6), 707–713.

Aronson, J. K. (Ed.) (2016a). Myrrh. In: J. K. Aronson (Editor in Chief). *Meyler's Side Effects of Drugs: The International Encyclopedia of Adverse Drug Reactions and Interactions* (16th Ed, p. 1158)). New York: Elsevier.

Aronson, J. K. (Ed.) (2016b). Vitamin B$_{12}$ (cobalamins). In: J. K. Aronson (Editor in Chief). *Meyler's Side Effects of Drugs: The International Encyclopedia of Adverse Drug Reactions and Interactions* (16th Ed). New York, NY: Elsevier. (p. 475–477).

Aronson, J. K. (Ed.) (2016c). Vitamin E (cobalamins). In: J. K. Aronson (Editor in Chief). *Meyler's Side Effects of Drugs: The International Encyclopedia of Adverse Drug Reactions and Interactions* (16th Ed). New York, NY: Elsevier. (p. 488–493).

Aziz, C. B. A., Ismail, C. A. N., Hussin, C. M. C., & Mohamed, M. (2014). The antinociceptive effects of Tualang honey in male Sprague-Dawley rats: a preliminary study. *Journal of Traditional and Complementary Medicine*, 4(4), 298–302.

Bannuru, R. R., Schmid, C. H., Kent, D. M., Vaysbrot, E. E., Wong, J. B., & McAlindon, T. E. (2015). Comparative Effectiveness of Pharmacologic Interventions for Knee Osteoarthritis: A Systematic Review and Network Meta-analysis Pharmacologic Interventions for Knee OA. *Annals of Internal Medicine*, 162(1), 46–54.

Barmaki, S., Bohlooli, S., Khoshkhahesh, F., & Nakhostin-Roohi, B. (2012). Effect of methylsulfonylmethane supplementation on exercise: Induced muscle damage and total antioxidant capacity. *Journal of Sports Medicine and Physical Fitness*, 52(2), 170–174.

Bartels, E. M., Folmer, V. N., Bliddal, H., Altman, R. D., Juhl, C., Tarp, S., ... Christensen, R. (2015). Efficacy and safety of ginger in osteoarthritis patients: a meta-analysis of randomized placebo-controlled trials. *Osteoarthritis and Cartilage*, 23(1), 13–21.

Bega, D. (2017). Complementary and Integrative Interventions for Chronic Neurologic Conditions Encountered in the Primary Care Office. *Primary Care: Clinics in Office Practice*, 44(2), 305–322.

Belcaro, G., Dugall, M., Luzzi, R., Ledda, A., Pellegrini, L., Cesarone, M. R., ... Errichi, M. (2014). Meriva (R) + Glucosamine versus Chondroitin + Glucosamine in patients with knee osteoarthritis: an observational study. *European Review of Medical Pharmacology and Science*, 18(24), 3959–3963.

Berberian, P., Obimba, C., Glickman-Simon, R., & Sethi, T. (2015). Herbs for low-back pain, acupuncture for psychological distress, osteopathic manipulative therapy for chronic migraine, honey dressings for burns, vegetarian diet and risk of colorectal cancer. *Explore (New York, NY)*, 11(5), 410–414.

Bergman, H., Walker, D. M., Nikolakopoulou, A., Soares-Weiser, K., & Adams, C. E. (2017). Systematic review of interventions for treating or preventing antipsychotic-induced tardive dyskinesia. *Health Technology Assessment*, 21(43), 1–248.

Berkley, K. J. (2013). Primary dysmenorrhea: an urgent mandate. *International Association for the Study of Pain*, 21(3), 1–8.

Bhardwaj, P., Yadav, R. K., & Garg, P. K. (2017). Pain relief in chronic pancreatitis: role of nutritional antioxidants. In R. R. Watson, & S. Zibadi (Eds.), *Nutritional Modulators of Pain in the Aging Population* (pp. 265–273). London: Academic Press.

Biniaz, V. (2013). A review of the world-wide researches on the therapeutic effects of ginger during the past two years. *Jentashapir Journal of Health Research*, 4(4), 333–337.

Bishnoi, M., Patil, C. S., Kumar, A., & Kulkarni, S. K. (2006). Potentiation of antinociceptive effect of NSAIDs by a specific lipooxygenase inhibitor, acetyl 11-keto-beta boswellic acid. *Indian Journal of Experimental Biology*, 44(2), 128–132.

Bitto, A., Squadrito, F., Irrera, N., Pizzino, G., Pallio, G., Mecchio, A., ... Altavilla, D. (2014). Flavocoxid, a nutraceutical approach to blunt inflammatory conditions. *Mediators of Inflammation, 2014*. https://doi.org/10.1155/2014/790851.

Bonakdar, R. A. (2018). Myofascial pain syndrome. In D. Rakel (Ed.), *Integrative Medicine* (4th Ed, pp. 651-661.e2). Philadelphia, PA: Elsevier.

Bone, K., & Mills, S. (2013a). Appendix C: Potential herb-drug interactions for commonly used herbs. In K. Bone, & S. Mills (Eds.), *Principles and Practice of Phytotherapy* (2nd Ed., pp. 970–996). London: Elsevier.

Bone, K., & Mills, S. (2013b). Herbal approaches to system dysfunction. In K. Bone, & S. Mills (Eds.), *Principles and Practice of Phytotherapy* (2nd Ed., pp. 183–350). London: Elsevier.

Boroumand, P., Zamani, M. M., Saeedi, M., Rouhbakhshfar, O., Motlagh, S. R. H., & Moghaddam, F. A. (2013). Post tonsillectomy pain: can honey reduce the analgesic requirements? *Anesthesiology and Pain Medicine*, 3(1), 198–202.

Boullata, J. (2005). Natural health product interactions with medication. *Nutrition in Clinical Practice*, 20(1), 33–51.

Brito, A., Verdugo, R., Hertrampf, E., Miller, J. W., Green, R., Fedosov, S. N., … Matamala, J. M. (2016). Vitamin B-12 treatment of asymptomatic, deficient, elderly Chileans improves conductivity in myelinated peripheral nerves, but high serum folate impairs vitamin B-12 status response assessed by the combined indicator of vitamin B-12 status. *The American Journal of Clinical Nutrition*, 103(1), 250–257.

Bruyère, O., Cooper, C., Pelletier, J. P., Maheu, E., Rannou, F., Branco, J., … Martel-Pelletier, J. (2016). A consensus statement on the European Society for Clinical and Economic Aspects of Osteoporosis and Osteoarthritis (ESCEO) algorithm for the management of knee osteoarthritis: from evidence-based medicine to the real-life setting. *Seminars in Arthritis and Rheumatism*, 45(4), S3–S11.

Bujalska-Zadrożny, M., & Duda, K. (2014). Additive effect of combined application of magnesium and MK-801 on analgesic action of morphine. *Pharmacology*, 93(3-4), 113–119.

Bujalska-Zadrożny, M., Tatarkiewicz, J., Kulik, K., Filip, M., & Naruszewicz, M. (2016). Magnesium enhances opioid-induced analgesia: What we have learnt in the past decades? *European Journal of Pharmaceutical Sciences*, 99(1), 113–127.

Bulut, H. K., & Tüfekci, F. G. (2016). Honey prevents oral mucositis in children undergoing chemotherapy: A quasi-experimental study with a control group. *Complementary Therapies in Medicine*, 29, 132–140.

Butawan, M., Benjamin, R. L., & Bloomer, R. J. (2017). Methylsulfonylmethane: Applications and Safety of a Novel Dietary Supplement. *Nutrients*, 9(3), 290–311.

Cady, R. K., Goldstein, J., Nett, R., Mitchell, R., Beach, M. E., & Browning, R. (2011). A Double-Blind Placebo-Controlled Pilot Study of Sublingual Feverfew and Ginger (LipiGesicTMM) in the Treatment of Migraine. *Headache: The Journal of Head and Face Pain*, 51(7), 1078–1086.

Calder, P. C. (2013). Omega-3 polyunsaturated fatty acids and inflammatory processes: nutrition or pharmacology? *British Journal of Clinical Pharmacology*, 75(3), 645–662.

Calder, P. C. (2015). Marine omega-3 fatty acids and inflammatory processes: effects, mechanisms and clinical relevance. *Biochimica et Biophysica Acta (BBA)-Molecular and Cell Biology of Lipids*, 1851(4), 469–484.

Cameron, M., & Chrubasik, S. (2014). Oral herbal therapies for treating osteoarthritis. *The Cochrane Library*. https://doi.org/10.1002/14651858.CD002947.pub2.

Catunda, I. S., Vasconcelos, B. D. E., Andrade, E. D. S., & Costa, D. F. N. (2016). Clinical effects of an avocado–soybean unsaponifiable extract on arthralgia and osteoarthritis of the temporomandibular joint: preliminary study. *International Journal of Oral and Maxillofacial Surgery*, 45(8), 1015–1022.

Chalasani, N., Vuppalanchi, R., Navarro, V., Fontana, R., Bonkovsky, H., Barnhart, H., & Hoofnagle, J. H. (2012). Acute liver injury due to flavocoxid (Limbrel), a medical food for osteoarthritis: a case series. *Annals of Internal Medicine*, 156(12), 857–860.

Charalambous, A., Lambrinou, E., Katodritis, N., Vomvas, D., Raftopoulos, V., Georgiou, M., … Charalambous, M. (2017). The effectiveness of thyme honey for the management of treatment-induced xerostomia in head and neck cancer patients: A feasibility randomized control trial. *European Journal of Oncology Nursing*, 27, 1–8.

Chauhan, R., Singh, V., Bajaj, H., & Chauhan, S. B. (2015). Cat's Claw: A miracle herb from the rain forest of Peru. *Indian Journal of Drugs*, 3(4), 96–101.

Chen, J. J., Dai, L., Zhao, L. X., Zhu, X., Cao, S., & Gao, Y. J. (2015). Intrathecal curcumin attenuates pain hypersensitivity and decreases spinal neuroinflammation in rat model of monoarthritis. *Scientific Reports*, 5, 10278. https://doi.org/10.1038/srep10278.

Cheppudira, B., Fowler, M., McGhee, L., Greer, A., Mares, A., Petz, L., … Clifford, J. L. (2013). Curcumin: a novel therapeutic for burn pain and wound healing. *Expert Opinion on Investigational Drugs*, 22(10), 1295–1303.

Chinn, K. Y., & Ima-Nirwana, S. (2014). Effects of annatto-derived tocotrienol supplementation on osteoporosis induced by testosterone deficiency in rats. *Clinical Interventions in Aging*, 9, 1247–1259.

Chiramonte, D., D'Adamo, C., & Morrison, B. (2014). Integrative approaches to pain management. In B. Benny, M. Grabois, & K.-T. Chan (Eds.), *Practical Management of Pain* (5th Ed., pp. 658–668.e3). Philadelphia, PA: Mosby.

Chocano-Bedoya, P. O., Manson, J. E., Hankinson, S. E., Willett, W. C., Johnson, S. R., Chasan-Taber, L., … Bertone-Johnson, E. R. (2011). Dietary B vitamin intake and incident premenstrual syndrome. *The American Journal of Clinical Nutrition*, 93(5), 1080–1086.

Chugh, N. A., Bali, S., & Koul, A. (2018). Integration of Botanicals in Contemporary Medicine: Road Blocks, Checkpoints and Go-ahead Signals. *Integrative Medicine Research.*, 7(2), 109–125.

Clark, G. T., Padilla, M., & Dionne, R. (2016). Medication treatment efficacy and chronic orofacial pain. *Oral and Maxillofacial Surgery Clinics*, 28(3), 409–421.

Clarke, T. C., Black, L. I., Stussman, B. J., Barnes, P. M., & Nahin, R. L. (2015). Trends in the use of complementary health approaches among adults: United States, 2002–2012. *National Health Statistics Reports*, 79, 1–55.

Coeytaux, R. R., & Mann, J. D. (2018). Headache. In D. Rakel (Ed.), *Integrative Medicine* (4th Ed, pp. 108–119.e3). Philadelphia, PA: Elsevier.

Colombo, B., Saraceno, L., & Comi, G. (2014). Riboflavin and migraine: the bridge over troubled mitochondria. *Neurological Sciences*, 35(1), 141–144.

Combs, G. F., & McClung, J. P. (2017a). Folate. In *The Vitamins* (5th Ed., pp. 419–429). London: Academic Press.

Combs, G. F., & McClung, J. P. (2017b). Vitamin B6. pp. 351–370 In *The Vitamins (5th Ed.) The Vitamins* (5th Ed., pp. 419–429). London: Academic Press.

Combs, G. F., & McClung, J. P. (2017c). Vitamin B12. In *The Vitamins* (5th Ed., pp. 431–452). London: Academic Press.

Combs, G. F., & McClung, J. P. (2017d). Vitamin E. In *The Vitamins* (5th Ed., pp. 207–242). London: Academic Press.

Coppock, R., & Dziwenka, M. (2016). Green tea extract. In R. C. Gupta (Ed.), *Nutraceuticals: Efficacy Safety and Toxicity* (pp. 633–652). London: Academic Press.

Cordero, M. D., Alcocer-Gómez, E., Culic, O., Carrión, A. M., de Miguel, M., Díaz-Parrado, E., ... & Sánchez-Alcazar, J. A. (2014). NLRP3 inflammasome is activated in fibromyalgia: the effect of coenzyme Q10. *Antioxidants & Redox Signaling*, 20(8), 1169–1180.

Darby, T. M., & Jones, R. M. (2017). Beneficial influences of *Lactobacillus plantarum* on human health and disease. In *The Microbiota in Gastrointestinal Pathophysiology* (pp. 109–117) Academic Press.

Davey, S., Davey, A., & Singh, J. V. (2016). Untapped potential of "medical foods" in developed and developing nations: A mixed method study by a systematic review with scientometric analysis. *Journal of Scientometric Research*, 5(1), 420–430.

Davis, A. K., Walton, M. A., Bohnert, K. M., Bourque, C., & Ilgen, M. A. (2018). Factors associated with alcohol consumption among medical cannabis patients with chronic pain. *Addictive Behaviors*, 77, 166–171.

Dawson-Hughes, B. (2017). Vitamin D and muscle function. *The Journal of Steroid Biochemistry and Molecular Biology*, 137(4), 313–316.

Degenhardt, L., Lintzeris, N., Campbell, G., Bruno, R., Cohen, M., Farrell, M., & Hall, W. D. (2015). Experience of adjunctive cannabis use for chronic non-cancer pain: findings from the Pain and Opioids IN Treatment (POINT) study. *Drug and Alcohol Dependence*, 147, 144–150.

Dell'Agli, M., Sangiovanni, E., Risè, P., Rossetti, A. C., Morazzoni, P., Riva, A., ... Molteni, R. (2016). Bioavailability of curcumin in the rat frontal lobe and hippocampus after repeated administration of MERIVA®. *Planta Medica*, 81(S 01), P895.

Demiryurek, B. E., & Gundogdu, A. A. (2017). The Effect of Vitamin D Levels on Pain in Carpal Tunnel Syndrome. *Orthopaedics & Traumatology: Surgery & Research*, 103(6), 919–922.

de Paula, L. C. L., Fonseca, F., Perazzo, F., Cruz, F. M., Cubero, D., Trufelli, D. C., ... del Giglio, A. (2015). Uncaria tomentosa (cat's claw) improves quality of life in patients with advanced solid tumors. *The Journal of Alternative and Complementary Medicine*, 21(1), 22–30.

Dhaliwal, R., & Aloia, J. F. (2017). Effect of vitamin D on falls and physical performance. *Endocrinology and Metabolism Clinics*, 46(4), 919–933.

Diao, N., Yang, B., & Yu, F. (2017). Effect of vitamin D supplementation on knee osteoarthritis: A systematic review and meta-analysis of randomized clinical trials. *Clinical Biochemistry*, 50(10), 1312–1316.

Dieb, W., & Boucher, Y. (2017). Burning Mouth Syndrome and Vitamin B6. *Pain Medicine*, 18(8), 1593–1594.

Dieb, W., Moreau, N., Rochefort, J., & Boucher, Y. (2017). Role of vitamin B6 in idiopathic burning mouth syndrome: some clinical observations. *Médecine Buccale Chirurgie Buccale*, 23(2), 77–83.

Diener, H., Pfaffenrath, V., Schnitker, J., Friede, M., & Henneicke-von Zepelin, H. H. (2005). Efficacy and safety of 6.25 mg tid feverfew CO2-extract (MIG-99) in migraine prevention: a randomized, double-blind, multicentre, placebo-controlled study. *Cephalalgia*, 25(11), 1031–1041.

Dimitrova, P., Georgiev, M., Khan, M., & Ivanovska, N. (2013). Evaluation of *Verbascum* species and harpagoside in models of acute and chronic inflammation. *Open Life Sciences*, 8(2), 186–194.

DiNicolantonio, J. J., Liu, J., & O'Keefe, J. H. (2018). Thiamine and Cardiovascular Disease: A Literature Review. *Progress in Cardiovascular Diseases.*, 61(10), 27–32.

Domenico, C., Linsenbardt, H., Haney, R., & Meagher, M. (2015). (544) Evaluating the anti-hyperalgesic and anti-inflammatory potential of curcumin in a human model of experimental pain. *The Journal of Pain*, 16(4), S112.

Drobnic, F., Riera, J., Appendino, G., Togni, S., Franceschi, F., Valle, X., ... Tur, J. (2014). Reduction of delayed onset muscle soreness by a novel curcumin delivery system (Meriva®): a randomised, placebo-controlled trial. *Journal of the International Society of Sports Nutrition*, 11(1), 31.

Drozdov, V. N., Kim, V. A., Tkachenko, E. V., & Varvanina, G. G. (2012). Influence of a specific ginger combination on gastropathy conditions in patients with osteoarthritis of the knee or hip. *The Journal of Alternative and Complementary Medicine*, 18(6), 583–588.

Dym, H., Bowler, D., & Zeidan, J. (2016). Pharmacologic treatment for temporomandibular disorders. *Dental Clinics of North America*, 60(2), 367–379.

Engen, D. J., McAllister, S. J., Whipple, M. O., Cha, S. S., Dion, L. J., Vincent, A., ... Wahner-Roedler, D. L. (2015). Effects of transdermal magnesium chloride on quality of life for patients with fibromyalgia: a feasibility study. *Journal of Integrative Medicine*, 13(5), 306–313.

Eriksen, P. R. (2014). Risk of bias and brand explain the observed inconsistency in trials on glucosamine for osteoarthritis: a meta-analysis of placebo-controlled trials. *Osteoarthritis and Cartilage*, 22, S26–S27.

Erickson, J. M., & Messer, T. M. (2013). Glucosamine and chondroitin sulfate treatment of hand osteoarthritis. *Journal of Hand Surgery*, 38(8), 1638–1640.

European Medicines Agency (EMA). (2016). European Union herbal monograph on *Harpagophytum procumbens DC.* and/or *Harpagophytum zeyheri Decne.*, radix EMA/HMPC/627057/2015 http://www.ema.europa.eu/docs/en_GB/document_library/Herbal_-_Herbal_monograph/2016/11/WC500216102.pdf Retrieved 11/14/2017.

Falzon, C. C., & Balabanova, A. (2017). Phytotherapy: An introduction to herbal medicine. *Primary Care: Clinics in Office Practice*, 44(2), 217–227.

Faqi, A. S., & Yan, J. S. (2017). Nonclinical safety assessment of botanical products. In A. S. Faqi (Ed.), *A Comprehensive Guide to Toxicology in Nonclinical Drug Development* (2nd Ed, pp. 813–823). London: Academic Press.

Farag, S., & Kayser, O. (2017). The cannabis plant: Botanical aspects. In A. Farr (Ed.), *Handbook of Cannabis and Related Pathologies: Biology, Pharmacology, Diagnosis, and Treatment* (pp. 3–12). London: Academic Press.

Fattal-Valevski, A. (2011). Thiamine (vitamin B1). *Journal of Evidence-Based Complementary & Alternative Medicine*, 16(1), 12–20.

Fiebich, B. L., Muñoz, E., Rose, T., Weiss, G., & McGregor, G. P. (2012). Molecular Targets of the Antiinflammatory Harpagophytum procumbens (devil's claw): Inhibition of TNFα and COX-2 Gene Expression by Preventing Activation of AP-1. *Phytotherapy Research*, 26(6), 806–811.

Figueroa, J. D., Cordero, K., Serrano-Illan, M., Almeyda, A., Baldeosingh, K., Almaguel, F. G., & De Leon, M. (2013). Metabolomics uncovers dietary omega-3 fatty acid-derived metabolites implicated in anti-nociceptive responses after experimental spinal cord injury. *Neuroscience*, 255(26), 1–18.

Fransen, M., Agaliotis, M., Nairn, L., Votrubec, M., Bridgett, L., Su, S., ... Woodward, M. (2015). Glucosamine and chondroitin for knee osteoarthritis: a double-blind randomised placebo-controlled clinical trial evaluating single and combination regimens. *Annals of the Rheumatic Diseases*, 74(5), 851–858.

Frisbie, D. D., Kawcak, C. E., & McIlwraith, C. W. (2008). 518 Evaluation of oral avocado/soybean unsaponifiables using an experimental model of equine osteoarthritis. *Osteoarthritis and Cartilage*, 16, S222–S223.

Froeling, F. E., & Stebbing, J. (2014). Uncaria tomentosa, the cat's whiskers or claws? *The Lancet Oncology*, 15(12), 1299–1300.

Frost, R., O'Meara, S., & MacPherson, H. (2014). The external use of comfrey: A practitioner survey. *Complementary Therapies in Clinical Practice*, 20(4), 347–355.

Gagnier, J. J., Van Tulder, M., Berman, B., & Bombardier, C. (2006). Herbal medicine for low back pain. *Cochrane Database Systematic Review*, 2, CD004504.

Gagnier, J. J., Oltean, H., van Tulder, M. W., Berman, B. M., Bombardier, C., & Robbins, C. B. (2016). Herbal medicine for low back pain: A Cochrane review. *Spine*, 41(2), 116–133.

Gaikwad, M., Vanlint, S., Mittinity, M., Moseley, G. L., & Stocks, N. (2017). Does vitamin D supplementation alleviate chronic nonspecific musculoskeletal pain? A systematic review and meta-analysis. *Clinical Rheumatology*, 36(5), 1201–1208.

Galeotti, N., Maidecchi, A., Mattoli, L., Burico, M., & Ghelardini, C. (2014). St. John's wort seed and feverfew flower extracts relieve painful diabetic neuropathy in a rat model of diabetes. *Fitoterapia*, 92, 23–33.

Gallagher, B., Tjoumakaris, F. P., Harwood, M. I., Good, R. P., Ciccotti, M. G., & Freedman, K. B. (2015). Chondroprotection and the prevention of osteoarthritis progression of the knee: a systematic review of treatment agents. *The American Journal of Sports Medicine*, 43(3), 734–744.

Galli, F., Azzi, A., Birringer, M., Cook-Mills, J. M., Eggersdorfer, M., Frank, J., ... Özer, N. K. (2017). Vitamin E: Emerging aspects and new directions. *Free Radical Biology and Medicine*, 102, 16–36.

Gao, X. R., Chen, Y. S., & Deng, W. (2017). The effect of vitamin D supplementation knee osteoarthritis: a meta-analysis of randomized controlled trials. *International Journal of Surgery*, 46(1), 14–20.

Gardiner, P., Filipelli, A. C., & Low Dog, T. (2018). Prescribing botanicals. In D. Rakel (Ed.), *Integrative Medicine* (4th Ed., pp. 979–985.e1). St. Louis: Elsevier.

Garrido-Maraver, J., Cordero, M. D., Oropesa-Avila, M., Vega, A. F., de la Mata, M., Pavon, A. D., ... de Lavera, I. (2014). Clinical applications of coenzyme Q10. *Frontiers in Bioscience (Landmark Ed)*, 19, 619–633.

Gayle, J. A., Kaye, A. D., Kaye, A. M., & Shah, R. (2010). Anticoagulants: newer ones, mechanisms, and perioperative updates. *Anesthesiology Clinics*, 28(4), 667–679.

Gencer, Z. K., Özkiriş, M., Okur, A., Korkmaz, M., & Saydam, L. (2014). A comparative study on the impact of intra-articular injections of hyaluronic acid, tenoxicam and betametazon on the relief of temporomandibular joint disorder complaints. *Journal of Cranio-Maxillofacial Surgery*, 42(7), 1117–1121.

Gendelman, O., Itzhaki, D., Makarov, S., Bennun, M., & Amital, H. (2015). A randomized double-blind placebo-controlled study adding high dose vitamin D to analgesic regimens in patients with musculoskeletal pain. *Lupus*, 24(4-5), 483–489.

Georgiev, M. I., Ivanovska, N., Alipieva, K., Dimitrova, P., & Verpoorte, R. (2013). Harpagoside: from Kalahari Desert to pharmacy shelf. *Phytochemistry*, 92, 8–15.

Gioxari, A., Kaliora, A. C., Marantidou, F., & Panagiotakos, D. P. (2018). Intake of ω-3 polyunsaturated fatty acids in patients with rheumatoid arthritis: A systematic review and meta-analysis. *Nutrition*, 45, 114–124.

Girgis, C. M., Clifton-Bligh, R. L., Hamrick, M. W., Holick, M. F., & Gunton, J. E. (2013). The roles of vitamin D in skeletal muscle: Form, function, and metabolism. *Endocrine Reviews*, 34(1), 33–83.

Goel, A., Boland, C. R., & Chauhan, D. P. (2001). Specific inhibition of cyclooxygenase-2 (COX-2) expression by dietary curcumin in HT-29 human colon cancer cells. *Cancer Letters*, 172(2), 111–118.

Goiato, M. C., da Silva, E. V. F., de Medeiros, R. A., Túrcio, K. H. L., & Dos Santos, D. M. (2016). Are intra-articular injections of hyaluronic acid effective for the treatment of temporomandibular disorders? A systematic review. *International Journal of Oral and Maxillofacial Surgery*, 45(12), 1531–1537.

Gopi, S., Jacob, J., Varma, K., Jude, S., Amalraj, A., Arundhathy, C. A., ... Stohs, S. J. (2017). Comparative Oral Absorption of Curcumin in a Natural Turmeric Matrix with Two Other Curcumin Formulations: An Open-label Parallel-arm Study. *Phytotherapy Research*, 31(12), 1883–1891.

Goyal, S., Sharma, P., Ramchandani, U., Shrivastava, S. K., & Dubey, P. K. (2011). Novel anti-inflammatory topical herbal gels containing with aniasomnifera and *Boswellia serrata*. *International Journal of Pharmaceutical & Biological Archive*, 2(4), 1087–1094.

Grodetsky. (2014). Acetylsalicylic acid. In *Encyclopedia of Toxicology Reference Module in Biomedical Sciences* (3rd Ed., pp. 54–55). New York: Elsevier.

Gupta, C., & Prakash, D. (2015). Nutraceuticals for geriatrics. *Journal of Traditional and Complementary Medicine*, 5(1), 5–14.

Ha, L. H., & Nesteby, A. (2017). The effects of curcumin in decreasing pain in patients with osteoarthritis. *School of Physician Assistant Studies*, 606. https://commons.pacificu.edu/pa/606.

Ha, S. K., Moon, E., Ju, M. S., Kim, D. H., Ryu, J. H., Oh, M. S., & Kim, S. Y. (2012). 6-Shogaol, a ginger product, modulates neuroinflammation: A new approach to neuroprotection. *Neuropharmacology*, 63(2), 211–223.

Hameed, F. A. (2018). Gout. In D. Rakel (Ed.), *Integrative Medicine* (4th Ed., pp. 689–696.e2). Philadelphia, PA: Elsevier.

Hamidpour, R., Hamidpour, S., Hamidpour, M., & Shahlari, M. (2013). Frankincense (乳香 Rǔ Xiāng; *Boswellia* Species): From the selection of traditional applications to the novel phytotherapy for the prevention and treatment of serious diseases. *Journal of Traditional and Complementary Medicine*, 3(4), 221–226.

Hancı, D., & Altun, H. (2015). Effectiveness of hyaluronic acid in post-tonsillectomy pain relief and wound healing: a prospective, double-blind, controlled clinical study. *International Journal of Pediatric Otorhinolaryngology*, 79(9), 1388–1392.

Hardin, S. R. (2007). Cat's claw: an Amazonian vine decreases inflammation in osteoarthritis. *Complementary Therapies in Clinical Practice*, 13(1), 25–28.

Hashempur, M. H., Sadrneshin, S., Mosavat, S. H., & Ashraf, A. (2018). Green tea *(Camellia sinensis)* for patients with knee osteoarthritis: A randomized open-label active-controlled clinical trial. *Clinical Nutrition, 37*(1), 85–90.

Hatoum, H. T., Fierlinger, A. L., Lin, S. J., & Altman, R. D. (2014). Cost-effectiveness analysis of intra-articular injections of a high molecular weight bioengineered hyaluronic acid for the treatment of osteoarthritis knee pain. *Journal of Medical Economics, 17*(5), 326–337.

Hayakawa, H., Minaniya, Y., Ito, K., Yamamoto, Y., & Fukuda, T. (2011). Difference of curcumin content in *Curcuma longa* L. (Zingiberaceae) caused by hybridization with other *Curcuma* species. *American Journal of Plant Sciences, 2*(2), 111–119.

He, W. W., Kuang, M. J., Zhao, J., Sun, L., Lu, B., Wang, Y., … Ma, X. L. (2017). Efficacy and safety of intraarticular hyaluronic acid and corticosteroid for knee osteoarthritis: A meta-analysis. *International Journal of Surgery, 39*(1), 95–103.

Henrotin, Y., Lambert, C., Couchourel, D., Ripoll, C., & Chiotelli, E. (2011). Nutraceuticals: do they represent a new era in the management of osteoarthritis? a narrative review from the lessons taken with five products. *Osteoarthritis and Cartilage, 19*(1), 1–21.

Hershman, D. L., Unger, J. M., Crew, K. D., Minasian, L. M., Awad, D., Moinpour, C. M., … Wade, J. L., III. (2013). Randomized double-blind placebo-controlled trial of acetyl-L-carnitine for the prevention of taxane-induced neuropathy in women undergoing adjuvant breast cancer therapy. *Journal of Clinical Oncology, 31*(20), 2627–2633.

Hill, C., Guarner, F., Reid, G., Gibson, G. R., Merenstein, D. J., Pot, B., … Calder, P. C. (2014). Expert consensus document: The International Scientific Association for Probiotics and Prebiotics consensus statement on the scope and appropriate use of the term probiotic. *Nature Reviews Gastroenterology & Hepatology, 11*(8), 506–514.

Hillinger, M. G., Wolever, R. Q., McKernan, L. C., & Elam, R. (2017). Integrative Medicine for the Treatment of Persistent Pain. *Primary Care: Clinics in Office Practice, 44*(2), 247–264.

Hochberg, M. C., Martel-Pelletier, J., Monfort, J., Möller, I., Castillo, J. R., Arden, N., … & Henrotin, Y. (2015). Combined chondroitin sulfate and glucosamine for painful knee osteoarthritis: a multicentre, randomised, double-blind, non-inferiority trial versus celecoxib. *Annals of the Rheumatic Diseases,* annrheumdis-2014. 206792. https://doi.org/10.1136.

Holland, S., Silberstein, S. D., Freitag, F., Dodick, D. W., Argoff, C., & Ashman, E. (2012). Evidence-based guideline update: NSAIDs and other complementary treatments for episodic migraine prevention in adults: report of the Quality Standards Subcommittee of the American Academy of Neurology and the American Headache Society. *Neurology, 78*(17), 1346–1353.

Holt, P. R. (2016). Curcumin for inflammatory bowel disease: a caution. *Clinical Gastroenterology and Hepatology, 14*(1), 168.

Hu, D., Wang, C., Li, F., Su, S., Yang, N., Yang, Y., … Gu, L. (2017). A Combined Water Extract of Frankincense and Myrrh Alleviates Neuropathic Pain in Mice via Modulation of TRPV1. *Neural Plasticity, 2017,* 3710821.

Huang, W., Shah, S., Long, Q., Crankshaw, A. K., & Tangpricha, V. (2013). Improvement of pain, sleep, and quality of life in chronic pain patients with vitamin D supplementation. *The Clinical Journal of Pain, 29*(4), 341–347.

Hudson, A., Lopez, E., Almalki, A. J., Roe, A. L., & Calderón, A. I. (2018). A review of the toxicity of compounds found in herbal dietary supplements. *Planta Medica, 84*(09/10), 613–626.

Hussain, H., Al-Harrasi, A., & Green, I. R. (2016). Frankincense *(Boswellia)* oils. In V. Preedy (Ed.), *Essential Oils in Food Preservation, Flavor and Safety* (pp. 431–440). Amsterdam: Elsevier.

Hussain, S., Singh, A., Akhtar, M., & Najmi, A. K. (2017). Letter to the editor on the article. The effect of vitamin D supplementation on knee osteoarthritis: A meta-analysis of randomized controlled trials. *International Journal of Surgery, 48*(12), 309–310.

Hwang, S. H., Song, J. N., Jeong, Y. M., Lee, Y. J., & Kang, J. M. (2016). The efficacy of honey for ameliorating pain after tonsillectomy: a meta-analysis. *European Archives of Oto-Rhino-Laryngology, 273*(4), 811–818.

Imtiaz, M., Begum, N., Ali, T., Gomes, R. R., Saha, S., Tasfi, R. F., … Kamal, N. (2016). Pain & Inflammation: Effects of short-term daily administration of Vitamin B12 & Folic acid in long Evans rats. *Bangladesh Critical Care Journal, 4*(1), 33–37.

Inserra, P., & Brooks, A. (2017). Getting the root of chronic inflammation: Ginger's antiinflammatory properties. In R. R. Watson, & S. Zibadi (Eds.), *Nutritional Modulators of Pain in the Aging Population* (pp. 67–73). London: Academic Press.

Institute of Medicine. (IOM). (1998). *Food and Nutrition Board. Dietary Reference Intakes: Thiamin, Riboflavin, Niacin, Vitamin B6, Folate, Vitamin B12, Pantothenic Acid, Biotin, and Choline* (p. 1998). Washington, DC: National Academies Press.

Iram, F., Khan, S. A., & Husain, A. (2017). Phytochemistry and potential therapeutic actions of Boswellic acids: A mini-review. *Asian Pacific Journal of Tropical Biomedicine, 7*(6), 513–523.

Jacobson, T. A., Khan, A., Maki, K. C., Brinton, E. A., & Cohen, J. D. (2018). Provider recommendations for patient-reported muscle symptoms on statin therapy: Insights from the Understanding Statin Use in America and Gaps in Education survey. *Journal of Clinical Lipidology., 12*(1), P78–P88.

Jandrić, Z., Frew, R. D., Fernandez-Cedi, L. N., & Cannavan, A. (2017). An investigative study on discrimination of honey of various floral and geographical origins using UPLC-QToF MS and multivariate data analysis. *Food Control, 72*(2), 189–197. Part B.

Jandrić, Z., Haughey, S. A., Frew, R. D., McComb, K., Galvin-King, P., Elliott, C. T., & Cannavan, A. (2015). Discrimination of honey of different floral origins by a combination of various chemical parameters. *Food Chemistry, 189*(1), 52–59.

Jansen, S. A., Kleerekooper, I., Hofman, Z. L., Kappen, I. F., Stary-Weinzinger, A., & van der Heyden, M. A. (2012). Grayanotoxin poisoning: 'mad honey disease' and beyond. *Cardiovascular Toxicology, 12*(3), 208–215.

Jenabi, E. (2013). The effect of ginger for relieving of primary dysmenorrhea. *Journal of the Pakistan Medical Association, 63*(1), 8–10.

Ji, H., Tang, J., Li, M., Ren, J., Zheng, N., & Wu, L. (2016). Curcumin-loaded solid lipid nanoparticles with Brij78 and TPGS improved in vivo oral bioavailability and in situ intestinal absorption of curcumin. *Drug Delivery, 23*(2), 459–470.

Jiang, Q. (2014). Natural forms of vitamin E: metabolism, antioxidant, and anti-inflammatory activities and their role in disease prevention and therapy. *Free Radical Biology and Medicine, 72,* 76–90.

Jin, X., Jones, G., Cicuttini, F., Wluka, A., Zhu, Z., Han, W., … Ding, C. (2016). Effect of vitamin D supplementation on tibial cartilage volume and knee pain among patients with symptomatic knee osteoarthritis: a randomized clinical trial. *JAMA, 315*(10), 1005–1013.

Júnior, O. V. L., & Inácio, A. M. (2013). Use of glucosamine and chondroitin to treat osteoarthritis: a review of the literature. *Revista Brasileira de Ortopedia, 48*(4), 300–306.

Kahan, M., Srivastava, A., Spithoff, S., & Bromley, L. (2014). Prescribing smoked cannabis for chronic noncancer pain. *Canadian Family Physician, 60*(12), 1083–1090.

Karadima, V., Kraniotou, C., Bellos, G., & Tsangaris, G. T. (2016). Drug-micronutrient interactions: food for thought and thought for action. *EPMA Journal, 7*(1), 10. https://doi.org/10.1186/s13167-016-0059-1.

Kashanian, M., Lakeh, M. M., Ghasemi, A., & Noori, S. (2013). Evaluation of the effect of vitamin E on pelvic pain reduction in women suffering from primary dysmenorrhea. *The Journal of Reproductive Medicine, 58*(1-2), 34–38.

Kashefi, F., Khajehei, M., Tabatabaeichehr, M., Alavinia, M., & Asili, J. (2014). Comparison of the effect of ginger and zinc sulfate on primary dysmenorrhea: a placebo-controlled randomized trial. *Pain Management Nursing, 15*(4), 826–833.

Katiyar, S. K., & Raman, C. (2011). Green tea: a new option for the prevention or control of osteoarthritis. *Arthritis Research & Therapy, 13*(4), 121–122.

Khalil, H., Chambers, H., Khalil, V., & Ang, C. D. (2016). Vitamin B for treating diabetic peripheral neuropathy: Intervention protocol. *The Cochrane Library., 6,* CD012237.

Kim, J. Y., & Choi, J. S. (2017). Single-dose oral toxicity and acute dermal irritation of steamed and dried ginger extract in rat and white rabbit. *The Journal of Animal & Plant Sciences, 27*(6), 1822–1828.

Kim, Y. H., Lee, P. B., & Oh, T. K. (2015). Is magnesium sulfate effective for pain in chronic postherpetic neuralgia patients comparing with ketamine infusion therapy? *Journal of Clinical Anesthesia, 27*(4), 296–300.

King, M. (2016). The use of hyaluronidase in aesthetic practice. *Aesthetic Complications Expert Group, The Use of Hyaluronidase in Aesthetic Practice,* 1–9. https://www.visage-aesthetics.com/wp-content/uploads/2016/02/ACEGUIDESHYALASE.pdf. Retrieved 12/23/2017.

Koleini, S., & Valiani, M. (2017). Comparing the effect of auriculotherapy and vitamin B6 on the symptoms of premenstrual syndrome among the students who lived in the dorm of Isfahan University of Medical Sciences. *Iranian Journal of Nursing and Midwifery Research, 22*(5), 354–358.

Koppel, B. S., Brust, J. C., Fife, T., Bronstein, J., Youssof, S., Gronseth, G., & Gloss, D. (2014). Systematic review: Efficacy and safety of medical marijuana in selected neurologic disorders Report of the Guideline Development Subcommittee of the American Academy of Neurology. *Neurology, 82*(17), 1556–1563.

Kotsiou, A., & Christine, T. (2017). Hepatotoxicity of herbal medicinal products. *Journal of Medicinal Plants, 5*(3), 80–88.

Kraus, V. B., Martinez, H., Herrero, M., & Verges, J. (2016). A proteomic panel predicts drug response to the combination of glucosamine and chondroitin sulfate. *Osteoarthritis and Cartilage, 24,* S89.

Krishna, S., & Purushothaman, A. (2015). Warfarin interactions with complementary medicines, herbs and dietary supplements. *Journal of Chemical and Pharmaceutical Research, 7*(6), 71–75.

Kuhad, A., Bishnoi, M., Tiwari, V., & Chopra, K. (2009). Suppression of NF-κβ signaling pathway by tocotrienol can prevent diabetes associated cognitive deficits. *Pharmacologic Biochemical Behavior, 92*(2), 251–289.

Kumar, A., Kaur, H., & Singh, A. (2017). Neuropathic Pain models caused by damage to central or peripheral nervous system. *Pharmacological Reports., 70*(2).

Kuphal, G. J. (2018). Dysmenorrhea. In D. Rakel (Ed.), *Integrative Medicine* (4th Ed., pp. 569–577.e2). Philadelphia, PA: Elsevier.

Kuptniratsaikul, V., Dajpratham, P., Taechaarpornkul, W., Buntragulpoontawee, M., Lukkanapichonchut, P., Chootip, C., … Laongpech, S. (2014). Efficacy and safety of *Curcuma domestica* extracts compared with ibuprofen in patients with knee osteoarthritis: a multicenter study. *Clinical Interventions in Aging, 9,* 451–459.

Kwoh, C. K., Roemer, F. W., Hannon, M. J., Moore, C. E., Jakicic, J. M., Guermazi, A., … Boudreau, R. (2014). Effect of oral glucosamine on joint structure in individuals with chronic knee pain: a randomized, placebo-controlled clinical trial. *Arthritis & Rheumatology, 66*(4), 930–939.

Laev, S. S., & Salakhutdinov, N. F. (2015). Anti-arthritic agents: progress and potential. *Bioorganic & Medicinal Chemistry, 23*(13), 3059–3080.

Landais, A. (2014). Neurological complications of bariatric surgery. *Obesity Surgery, 24*(10), 1800–1807.

Laslett, L. L., Quinn, S., Burgess, J. R., Parameswaran, V., Winzenberg, T. M., Jones, G., & Ding, C. (2014). Moderate vitamin D deficiency is associated with changes in knee and hip pain in older adults: a 5-year longitudinal study. *Annals of the Rheumatic Diseases, 73*(4), 697–703.

Lawrence, T. (2009). The nuclear factor NF-κB pathway in inflammation. *Cold Spring Harb Perpect Biol, 1*(a001651), 1–10.

Lazim, N. M., & Baharudin, A. (2017). Chapter 10 Honey: A Natural remedy for pain relief. In R. R. Watson, & S. Zibadi (Eds.), *Nutritional Modulators of Pain in the Aging Population* (pp. 123–134). London: Academic Press.

Lee, J., Hong, Y. S., Jeong, J. H., Yang, E. J., Jhun, J. Y., Park, M. K., … Cho, M. L. (2013). Coenzyme Q10 ameliorates pain and cartilage degradation in a rat model of osteoarthritis by regulating nitric oxide and inflammatory cytokines. *PLoS One, 8*(7), e69362.

Lee, Y. H., Huang, Y. F., Chou, H. H., Lin, W. T., Yang, H. W., & Lin-Shiau, S. Y. (2018). Studies on a novel regimen for management of orofacial pain and morphine tolerance. *Journal of Dental Sciences., 13*(2), 131–137.

Lemmon, R., & Roseen, E. J. (2018). Chronic low back pain. In D. Rakel (Ed.), *Integrative Medicine* (4th Ed., pp. 662–675.e3). Philadelphia, PA: Elsevier.

Leombruni, P., Miniotti, M., Colonna, F., Sica, C., Castelli, L., Bruzzone, M., … Torta, R. G. (2015). A randomised controlled trial comparing duloxetine and acetyl L-carnitine in fibromyalgic patients: preliminary data. *Clinical and Experimental Rheumatology, 33*(Suppl. 88), S82–S85.

Levy, R. M., Saikovsky, R., Shmidt, E., Khokhlov, A., & Burnett, B. P. (2009). Flavocoxid is as effective as naproxen for managing the signs and symptoms of osteoarthritis of the knee in humans: a short-term randomized, double-blind pilot study. *Nutrition Research, 29*(5), 298–304.

Li, S., Li, Q., Li, Y., Li, L., Tian, H., & Sun, X. (2015). Acetyl-L-carnitine in the treatment of peripheral neuropathic pain: a systematic review and meta-analysis of randomized controlled trials. *PLoS One, 10*(3), e0119479.

Li, Z. M., Li, X. J., Tan, Z. H., Xie, L. M., & Deng, X. Z. (2016). Effect of bifidobacteria combined with sulfasalazine on serum inflammatory factors and immune functions in patients with ulcerative colitis. *Journal of Hainan Medical University, 22*(21), 40–43.

Lim, D. W., Kim, J. G., Han, D., & Kim, Y. T. (2014). Analgesic effect of *Harpagophytum procumbens* on postoperative and neuropathic pain in rats. *Molecules, 19*(1), 1060–1068.

Liu, H.-L. (2017). Vitamin B$_{12}$ for relieving pain in aphthous ulcers. In R. R. Watson, & S. Zibadi (Eds.), *Nutritional Modulators of Pain in the Aging Population* (pp. 217–223). London: Elsevier.

Liu, Y., & Wang, M. W. (2008). Botanical drugs: challenges and opportunities: contribution to Linnaeus Memorial Symposium 2007. *Life Sciences, 82*(9-10), 445–449.

Loganes, C., Lega, S., Bramuzzo, M., Vecchi Brumatti, L., Piscianz, E., Valencic, E., ... Marcuzzi, A. (2017). Curcumin Anti-Apoptotic Action in a Model of Intestinal Epithelial Inflammatory Damage. *Nutrients, 9*(6), 578.

Lopez, H. L. (2012). Nutritional interventions to prevent and treat osteoarthritis. Part II: Focus on micronutrients and supportive nutraceuticals. *Physical Medicine & Rehabilitation, 4*(5S), S156–S168. https://doi.org/10.1016/j.pmrj.2012.02.023.

Lourdudoss, C., Di Giuseppe, D., Wolk, A., Westerlind, H., Klareskog, L., Alfredsson, L., ... Lampa, J. (2018). Dietary Intake of Polyunsaturated Fatty Acids and Pain in spite of Inflammatory Control among Methotrexate Treated Early Rheumatoid Arthritis Patients. *Arthritis Care & Research., 70*(2), 2015–2212.

Loveless, M. S., & Fry, A. L. (2016). Pharmacologic therapies in musculoskeletal conditions. *Medical Clinics of North America, 100*(4), 869–890.

Lynch, M. E., Cesar-Rittenberg, P., & Hohmann, A. G. (2014). A double-blind, placebo-controlled, crossover pilot trial with extension using an oral mucosal cannabinoid extract for treatment of chemotherapy-induced neuropathic pain. *Journal of Pain and Symptom Management, 47*(1), 166–173.

Lynch, M. E., & Ware, M. A. (2015). Cannabinoids for the treatment of chronic non-cancer pain: an updated systematic review of randomized controlled trials. *Journal of Neuroimmune Pharmacology, 10*(2), 293–301.

Maghsoudi, H., & Moradi, S. (2015). Honey: a skin graft fixator convenient for both patient and surgeon. *Indian Journal of Surgery, 77*(3), 863–867.

Maheu, E., Rannou, F., & Reginster, J. Y. (2016). Efficacy and safety of hyaluronic acid in the management of osteoarthritis: evidence from real-life setting trials and surveys. *Seminars in Arthritis and Rheumatism, 45*(4), S28–S33.

Maheu, E., Cadet, C., Marty, M., Moyse, D., Kerloch, I., Coste, P., ... Grouin, J. M. (2014). Randomised, controlled trial of avocado–soybean unsaponifiable (Piascledine) effect on structure modification in hip osteoarthritis: the ERADIAS study. *Annals of the Rheumatic Diseases, 73*(2), 376–384.

Maida, V., & Corban, J. (2017). Topical Medical Cannabis: A New Treatment for Wound Pain: Three Cases of Pyoderma Gangrenosum. *Journal of Pain and Symptom Management, 54*(5), 732–736.

Majid, O. W., & Al-Mashhadani, B. A. (2014). Perioperative bromelain reduces pain and swelling and improves quality of life measures after mandibular third molar surgery: a randomized, double-blind, placebo-controlled clinical trial. *Journal of Oral and Maxillofacial Surgery, 72*(6), 1043–1048.

Mallory, D. J. (2018). Postdates pregnancy. In D. Rakel (Ed.), *Integrative Medicine* (4th Ed., pp. 535–541.e1). Philadelphia, PA: Elsevier.

Malone, M. A., & Gloyer, K. (2013). Complementary and alternative treatments in sports medicine. *Primary Care Clinical Office Practice, 40*(4), 945–968.

Maluegha, D. P., Widodo, M. A., Pardjianto, B., & Widjajanto, E. (2015). The effects of bromelain on angiogenesis, nitric oxide, and matrix metalloproteinase-3 and-9 in rats exposed to electrical burn injury. *Wound Medicine, 9*, 5–9.

Mandel, D. R., Eichas, K., & Holmes, J. (2010). *Bacillus coagulans*: a viable adjunct therapy for relieving symptoms of rheumatoid arthritis according to a randomized, controlled trial. *BMC Complementary and Alternative Medicine, 10*(1), 1.

Mannelli, L. D. C., Tenci, B., Zanardelli, M., Maidecchi, A., Lugli, A., Mattoli, L., & Ghelardini, C. (2015). Widespread pain reliever profile of a flower extract of *Tanacetum parthenium*. *Phytomedicine, 22*(7), 752–758.

Mansour, G., Ouda, S., Shaker, A., & Abdallah, H. M. (2014). Clinical efficacy of new aloe vera-and myrrh-based oral mucoadhesive gels in the management of minor recurrent aphthous stomatitis: a randomized, double-blind, vehicle-controlled study. *Journal of Oral Pathology & Medicine, 43*(6), 405–409.

Mariotti, A. J. (2016). Appendix. In F. J. Dowd, B. Johnson, & A. Mariotti (Eds.), *Pharmacology and Therapeutics for Dentistry* (7th Ed., pp. 642–647). St. Louis, MO: Elsevier.

Martel, J. L., & Franklin, D. S. (2017). Vitamin, B1 (Thiamine). *StatPearls Publishing, LLC* PMID: 29493982. https://www.ncbi.nlm.nih.gov/books/NBK482360/ Accessed 05/06/2018.

Materazzi, S., Benemei, S., Fusi, C., Gualdani, R., De Siena, G., Vastani, N., ... Dussor, G. (2013). Parthenolide inhibits nociception and neurogenic vasodilatation in the trigeminovascular system by targeting the TRPA1 channel. *PAIN®, 154*(12), 2750–2758.

Mathew, E., Kim, E., & Zempsky, W. (2016). Pharmacologic treatment of pain. (pp. 209-219). In *Seminars in pediatric neurology* (Vol. 23, No. 3) Philadelphia: WB Saunders.

Mazzanti, G., Di Sotto, A., & Vitalone, A. (2015). Hepatotoxicity of green tea: an update. *Archives of Toxicology, 89*(8), 1175–1191.

Mbaveng, A. T., & Kuete, V. (2017). Zingiber Officinale. In V. Kuete (Ed.), *Medicinal Spices and Vegetables from Africa: Therapeutic potential against metabolic, inflammatory, infections and systematic diseases* (pp. 627–639). London: Academic Press.

McAlindon, T., LaValley, M., Schneider, E., Nuite, M., Lee, J. Y., Price, L. L., ... Dawson-Hughes, B. (2013). Effect of vitamin D supplementation on progression of knee pain and cartilage volume loss in patients with symptomatic osteoarthritis: a randomized controlled trial. *JAMA, 309*(2), 155–162.

McFarland, L. V. (2016). An observation on inappropriate probiotic subgroup classifications in the meta-analysis by Lau and Chamberlain. *International Journal of General Medicine, 9*, 333–334.

Meo, S. A., Al-Asiri, S. A., Mahesar, A. L., & Ansari, M. J. (2016). Role of honey in modern medicine. *Saudi Journal of Biological Sciences, 24*(5), 975–978.

Merolla, G., & Cerciello, S. (2017). Conservative and postoperative coanalgesic therapy for upper limb tendinopathy using dietary supplements. In R. R. Watson, & S. Zibadi (Eds.), *Nutritional Modulators of Pain in the Aging Population* (pp. 235–243). London: Elsevier.

Messina, S., Vita, G. L., Licata, N., Sframeli, M., Bitto, A., Distefano, M. G., & Barcellona, C. ... Vita, G. (2014). G. P. 100 Pilot study of flavocoxid in ambulant DMD patients. *Neuromuscular Disorders*, 24(2014), 825. no. 9.

Meymandi, M. S., Sepehri, G., Abdolsamadi, M., Shaabani, M., Heravi, G., Yazdanpanah, O., & Abhati, M. M. (2017). The effects of co-administration of pregabalin and vitamin E on neuropathic pain induced by partial sciatic nerve ligation in male rats. *Inflammopharmacology*, 25(2), 237–246.

Michael-Titus, A. T., & Priestley, J. V. (2014). Omega-3 fatty acids and traumatic neurological injury: from neuroprotection to neuroplasticity? *Trends in Neurosciences*, 37(1), 30–38.

Mikkelsen, K., Stojanovska, L., Prakash, M., & Apostolopoulos, V. (2017). The effects of vitamin B on the immune/cytokine network and their involvement in depression. *Maturitas*, 96, 58–71.

Miles, E. A., & Calder, P. C. (2012). Influence of marine n-3 polyunsaturated fatty acids on immune function and a systematic review of their effects on clinical outcomes in rheumatoid arthritis. *British Journal of Nutrition*, 107(S2), S171–S184.

Miller, L. E., & Block, J. E. (2013). US-approved intra-articular hyaluronic acid injections are safe and effective in patients with knee osteoarthritis: systematic review and meta-analysis of randomized, saline-controlled trials. *Clinical Medicine Insights. Arthritis and Musculoskeletal Disorders*, 6(1), 57–63.

Miyazaki, A., Hayakawa, H., Kobayashi, T., Aoki, Y., Kurita, S., Kashiwagi, T., & Yamamoto, Y. (2014). Effects of Rhizome Yield and Curcumin Content on Curcumin Yield from Curcuma. *Tropical Agriculture and Development*, 58(4), 163–168.

Mncwangi, N., Vermaak, I., & Viljoen, A. M. (2014). Mid-infrared spectroscopy and short wave infrared hyperspectral imaging: A novel approach in the qualitative assessment of *Harpagophytum procumbens* and *H. zeyheri* (devil's claw). *Phytochemistry Letters*, 7, 143–149.

Molina-Jijón, E., Aparicio-Trejo, O. E., Rodríguez-Muñoz, R., León-Contreras, J. C., del Carmen Cárdenas-Aguayo, M., Medina-Campos, O. N., ... Arreola-Mendoza, L. (2016). The nephroprotection exerted by curcumin in maleate-induced renal damage is associated with decreased mitochondrial fission and autophagy. *BioFactors*, 42(6), 686–702.

Monteiro, T. H., Silva, C. S., Ambrosio, L. M. C. S., Zucoloto, S., & Vannucchi, H. (2012). Vitamin E alters inflammatory gene expression in alcoholic chronic pancreatitis. *Journal of Nutrigenetics and Nutrigenomics*, 5(2), 94–105.

Moradi, M., Haghighatdoost, F., Feizi, A., & Azadbakht, L. (2016). Effect of coenzyme Q10 supplementation on diabetes biomarkers: a systematic review and meta-analysis of randomized controlled clinical trials. *Archives of Iranian Medicine*, 19(8), 588.

Morgan, S. L., Baggott, J. E., Moreland, L., Desmond, R., & Kendratch, A. C. (2009). The safety of flavocoxid, a medical food, in the dietary management of knee osteoarthritis. *Journal of Medicinal Food*, 12(5), 1143-1148.

Nabavi, S. F., Daglia, M., Moghaddam, A. H., Habtemariam, S., & Nabavi, S. M. (2014). Curcumin and liver disease: from chemistry to medicine. *Comprehensive Reviews in Food Science and Food Safety*, 13(1), 62–77.

Naderi, Z., Mozaffari-Khosravi, H., Dehghan, A., Nadjarzadeh, A., & Huseini, H. F. (2016). Effect of ginger powder supplementation on nitric oxide and C-reactive protein in elderly knee osteoarthritis patients: A 12-week double-blind randomized placebo-controlled clinical trial. *Journal of Traditional and Complementary Medicine*, 6(3), 199–203.

Nahin, R. L., Boineau, R., Khalsa, P. S., Stussman, B. J., & Weber, W. J. (2016). Evidence-based evaluation of complementary health approaches for pain management in the United States. *Mayo Clinic Proceedings*, 91(9), 1292–1306.

National Academies of Sciences (NAS). (2017). *The Health Effects of Cannabis: Chapter Highlights*. Washington, D. C.: National Academies Press. https://www8.nationalacademies.org/onpinews/newsitem.aspx?RecordID=24625&mod=article_inline. Accessed 8/21/2020.

National Academies of Sciences, Engineering and Medicine (NASEM). (2017). *The Health Effects of Cannabis and Cannabinoids*. Washington, D.C.: National Academies Press.

National Center for Complementary and Integrative Health (NCCIH). (2016). *Osteoarthritis in depth*. https://www.nccih.nih.gov/health/osteoarthritis-in-depth. Accessed 8/16/2020.

National Center for Complementary and Integrative Health (NCCIH). (2018). *Omega-3 Supplements: In Depth*. NCCIH Publication No.: D482. https://nccih.nih.gov/health/omega3/introduction.htm. Accessed 8/21/2020.

National Center for Complementary and Integrative Health (NCCIH). (2020a). *Cat's claw*. NCCIH Publication No.: D334. https://nccih.nih.gov/health/catclaw#hed1. Accessed 8/16/2020.

National Center for Complementary and Integrative Health (NCCIH). (2019a). *Feverfew*. NCCIH Publication No.: D342. https://nccih.nih.gov/health/feverfew. Accessed 8/16/2020.

National Institutes of Health Office of Dietary Supplements (NIH). (2017). *Carnitine: what is it?*. https://ods.od.nih.gov/factsheets/Carnitine-HealthProfessional. Accessed 11/28/2017.

National Institutes of Health Office of Dietary Supplements (NIH). (2019b). *Omega-3 Fatty Acids fact sheet for health professionals*. https://ods.od.nih.gov/factsheets/Omega3FattyAcids-HealthProfessional/. Accessed 8/17/2020.

National Institutes of Health Office of Dietary Supplements (NIH). (2019c). *Omega-3 Fatty Acids fact sheet for health professionals*. https://ods.od.nih.gov/factsheets/Omega3FattyAcids-HealthProfessional/. Accessed 8/21/2020.

National Institutes of Health Office of Dietary Supplements (NIH). (2019d). *Thiamine fact sheet for health professionals*. https://ods.od.nih.gov/factsheets/Thiamin-HealthProfessional/. Accessed 8/17/2020.

National Institutes of Health Office of Dietary Supplements (NIH). (2020b). *Magnesium dietary supplement fact sheet*. https://ods.od.nih.gov/factsheets/Magnesium-HealthProfessional. Accessed 8/21/2020.

National Institutes of Health Office of Dietary Supplements (NIH). (2020c). *Vitamin B12 dietary supplement fact sheet*. https://ods.od.nih.gov/factsheets/VitaminB12-HealthProfessional/#h9. Accessed 8/17/2020.

National Institutes of Health Office of Dietary Supplements (NIH). (2020d). *Riboflavin fact sheet for health professionals*. https://ods.od.nih.gov/factsheets/Riboflavin-HealthProfessional/. Accessed 8/21/2020.

National Institutes of Health Office of Dietary Supplements (NIH). (2020e). *Vitamin B6 fact sheet for health professionals*. https://ods.od.nih.gov/factsheets/VitaminB6-HealthProfessional/#h2. Accessed 8/17/2020.

National Institutes of Health Office of Dietary Supplements (NIH). (2020f). *Folate fact sheet for health professionals*. https://ods.od.nih.gov/factsheets/Folate-HealthProfessional/. Accessed 8/17/2020.

National Institutes of Health Office of Dietary Supplements (NIH). (2020g). *Vitamin D fact sheet for health professionals*. https://ods.od.nih.gov/factsheets/VitaminD-HealthProfessional/. Accessed 8/17/2020.

Nayeban, S., Jafarnejad, F., Nayeban, S., & Sefidgaran, A. (2014). A Comparison of the Effects of Vitamin E and Vitamin B1 on the Severity and Duration of Pain in Primary Dysmenorrhea. *Journal of Midwifery and Reproductive Health*, 2(2), 143–146.

Nikbakht, E., Khalesi, S., Singh, I., Williams, L. T., West, N. P., & Colson, N. (2018). Effect of probiotics and synbiotics on blood glucose: a systematic review and meta-analysis of controlled trials. *European Journal of Nutrition*, 57(1), 95–106. https://doi.org/10.1007/s00394-016-1300-3.

Nix, W. A., Zirwes, R., Bangert, V., Kaiser, R. P., Schilling, M., Hostalek, U., & Obeid, R. (2015). Vitamin B status in patients with type 2 diabetes mellitus with and without incipient nephropathy. *Diabetes Research and Clinical Practice*, 107(1), 157–165.

Nugent, S. M., Yarborough, B. J., Smith, N. X., Dobscha, S. K., Deyo, R. A., Green, C. A., & Morasco, B. J. (2017). Patterns and correlates of medical cannabis use for pain among patients prescribed long-term opioid therapy. *General Hospital Psychiatry*, 50(1), 104–110.

Ogbera, A. O., Ezeobi, E., Unachukwu, C., & Oshinaike, O. (2014). Treatment of diabetes mellitus-associated neuropathy with vitamin E and Eve primrose. *Indian Journal of Endocrinology and Metabolism*, 18(6), 846–849.

Oltean, H., Robbins, C., van Tulder, M. W., Berman, B. M., Bombardier, C., & Gagnier, J. J. (2014). Herbal medicine for low-back pain. *Cochrane Database of Systematic Reviews*, 12, 1–68.

Ordesi, P., Pisoni, L., Nannei, P., Macchi, M., Borloni, R., & Siervo, S. (2014). Therapeutic efficacy of bromelain in impacted third molar surgery: a randomized controlled clinical study. *Quintessence International*, 45(8), 679–684.

Ortiz-Lucas, M., Tobias, A., Saz, P., & Sebastián, J. J. (2013). Effect of probiotic species on irritable bowel syndrome symptoms: A bring up to date meta-analysis. *Revista Espanola De Enfermedades Digestivas*, 105(1), 19–36.

Ouanounou, A., Goldberg, M., & Haas, D. A. (2017). Pharmacotherapy in Temporomandibular Disorders: A Review. *Journal of the Canadian Dental Association*, 83(h7), 1488–2159.

Owen, S. C., Kuo, J.-W., & Prestwich, G. D. (2017). 2.214 – Hyaluronic acid. In *Reference Module in Materials Science and Materials Engineering: Comprehensive Biomaterials II* (pp. 239–259). New York: Elsevier.

Owoyele, B. V., Oladejo, R. O., Ajomale, K., Ahmed, R. O., & Mustapha, A. (2014). Analgesic and anti-inflammatory effects of honey: the involvement of autonomic receptors. *Metabolic Brain Disease*, 29(1), 167–173.

Pachman, D. R., Loprinzi, C. L., Grothey, A., & Ta, L. E. (2014). The search for treatments to reduce chemotherapy-induced peripheral neuropathy. *The Journal of Clinical Investigation*, 124(1), 72–74.

Padmanaban, G., & Nagaraj, V. A. (2018). Curcumin From Turmeric as an Adjunct Drug? *Studies in Natural Products Chemistry*, 57, 179–202.

Paik, D. J., & Lee, C. H. (2015). Review of cases of patient risk associated with ginseng abuse and misuse. *Journal of Ginseng Research*, 39(2), 89–93.

Paoletti, A., Gallo, E., Benemei, S., Vietri, M., Lapi, F., Volpi, R., … Vannacci, A. (2011). Interactions between natural health products and oral anticoagulants: spontaneous reports in the Italian Surveillance System of Natural Health Products. *Evidence-based Complementary and Alternative Medicine*, 2011. https://doi.org/10.1155/2011/612150. Article ID 612150.

Pareek, A., Suthar, M., Rathore, G. S., & Bansal, V. (2011). Feverfew (*Tanacetum parthenium* L.): A systematic review. *Pharmacognosy Reviews*, 5(9), 103–110.

Parian, A. M., Mullin, G. E., Langhorst, J., & Brown, A. (2018). Inflammatory bowels disease. In D. Rakel (Ed.), *Integrative Medicine* (4th Ed., pp. 501–516.e8). Philadelphia, PA: Elsevier.

Paroschi, T. P., Breganó, J. W., Simão, A. N. C., Dichi, I., & Miglioranza, L. H. S. (2015). Effects of Sulfasalazine, *Lactobacillus Plantarum* (Lp-115) and Fish Oil in Experimental Colitis. *SM Journal of Food Nutritional Disorders*, 1(1), 1005.

Patidar, A., Birla, D., Patel, V., Chaturvedi, M., & Manocha, N. (2014). A Review on advantages of Natural Analgesics over Conventional Synthetic Analgesics. *International Journal of Pharmacy & Life Sciences*, 5(5), 3534–3549.

Peddada, K. V., Peddada, K. V., Shukla, S. K., Mishra, A., & Verma, V. (2015). Role of curcumin in common musculoskeletal disorders: a review of current laboratory, translational, and clinical data. *Orthopaedic Surgery*, 7(3), 222–231.

Pedersen, A. M. L., Forssell, H., & Grinde, B. (2016). Orofacial pain conditions: Pain and oral mucosa. *Den Norske Tannlegeforen TIDENDE*, 126(2), 96–102.

Peh, H. Y., Tan, W. D., Liao, W., & Wong, W. F. (2016). Vitamin E therapy beyond cancer: Tocopherol versus tocotrienol. *Pharmacology & Therapeutics*, 162, 152–169.

Perlman, A. I., Rosenberger, L., & Ali, A. (2018). Osteoarthritis. In D. Rakel (Ed.), *Integrative Medicine* (4th Ed., pp. 639–650. e3). Philadelphia, PA: Elsevier.

Perron, B. E., Bohnert, K., Perone, A. K., Bonn-Miller, M. O., & Ilgen, M. (2015). Use of prescription pain medications among medical cannabis patients: Comparisons of pain levels, functioning, and patterns of alcohol and other drug use. *Journal of Studies on Alcohol and Drugs*, 76(3), 406–413.

Pickering, G., Morel, V., Simen, E., Cardot, J. M., Moustafa, F., Delage, N., … Dubray, C. (2011). Oral magnesium treatment in patients with neuropathic pain: a randomized clinical trial. *Magnesium Research*, 24(2), 28–35.

Pizzorno, J. E., Murray, M. T., & Joiner-Bey, H. (2016). Migraine headache. In J. E. Pizzorno, M. T. Murray, & H. Joiner-Bey (Eds.), *The Clinician's Handbook of Natural Medicine* (3rd Ed., pp. 658–677). St. Louis, MO: Elsevier.

Polito, F., Bitto, A., Irrera, N., Sqiadrotp, F., Fazzari, C., Minutoli, L., & Altavilla, D. (2010). Flavocoxid, a dual inhibitor of cyclooxygenase-2 and 5-lipoxygenase, reduces pancreatic damage in an experimental model of acute pancreatitis. *British Journal of Pharmacology*, 161, 1002–1011.

Pollicino, T., Musolino, C., Bitto, A., Raimondo, G., Squadrito, F., & Altavilla, D. (2013). Antiviral Activity of Flavocoxid against Hepatitis B Virus. *Hepatology*, *58*, 717A.

Pourianezhad, F., Tahmasebi, S., Nikfar, S., & Mirhoseini, M. (2016). Review on feverfew, a valuable medicinal plant. *Journal of HerbMed Pharmacology*, *5*(2), 45–49.

Prego-Domínguez, J., Hadrya, F., & Takkouche, B. (2016). Polyunsaturated Fatty Acids and Chronic Pain: A Systematic Review and Meta-analysis. *Pain Physician*, *19*(8), 521–535.

Primus Pharmaceuticals, Inc. (2017). *Limbrel® Product Insert*. http://www.limbrel.com/downloads/limbrel_pi.pdf. Accessed 11/26/2017.

Quílez, A., Saenz, M. T., & García, M. D. (2012). *Uncaria tomentosa* (Willd. ex. Roem. & Schult.) DC. and *Eucalyptus globulus Labill*: interactions when administered with diazepam. *Phytotherapy Research*, *26*(3), 458–461.

Raditic, D. M., & Bartges, J. W. (2014). The role of chondroprotectants, nutraceuticals, and nutrition in rehabilitation. In D. Mills, & D. Levine (Eds.), *Canine Rehabilitation and Physical Therapy* (2nd Ed., pp. 254–276). St. Louis, MO: Elsevier.

Rahbar, N., Asgharzadeh, N., & Ghorbani, R. (2012). Effect of omega-3 fatty acids on intensity of primary dysmenorrhea. *International Journal of Gynecology & Obstetrics*, *117*(1), 45–47.

Rahman, M. (2017). (107) Vitamin B12 and Ketorolac on pain and inflammation in Long Evans rats. *The Journal of Pain*, *18*(4), S3–S4.

Rahnama, P., Montazeri, A., Huseini, H. F., Kianbakht, S., & Naseri, M. (2012). Effect of *Zingiber officinale* R. rhizomes (ginger) on pain relief in primary dysmenorrhea: a placebo randomized trial. *BMC Complementary and Alternative Medicine*, *12*(1), 92.

Rajanandh, M. G., Kosey, S., & Prathiksha, G. (2014). Assessment of antioxidant supplementation on the neuropathic pain score and quality of life in diabetic neuropathy patients: A randomized controlled study. *Pharmacological Reports*, *66*(1), 44–48.

Rajaran, J. R., & Choi, W. S. (2016). Effectiveness of vitamin b complex in reducing chronic temporomandibular joint disorder pain: double blind randomised clinical trial. *International Journal of Oral and Maxillofacial Surgery*, *46*(Supp 1), 235.

Rajasekaran, A. (2017). Nutraceuticals. In J. Reedijk (Ed.), *Reference Module in Chemistry, Molecular Sciences and Chemical Engineering: Comprehensive Medicinal Chemistry III* (pp. 107–134). London: Elsevier.

Rajizadeh, A., Mozaffari-Khosravi, H., Yassini-Ardakani, M., & Dehghani, A. (2017). Effect of magnesium supplementation on depression status in depressed patients with magnesium deficiency: A randomized, double-blind, placebo-controlled trial. *Nutrition*, *35*, 56–60.

Ramsden, C. E., Faurot, K. R., Zamora, D., Suchindran, C. M., MacIntosh, B. A., Gaylord, S., … Mann, D. (2013). Targeted alteration of dietary n-3 and n-6 fatty acids for the treatment of chronic headaches: a randomized trial. *PAIN®*, *154*(11), 2441–2451.

Richette, P. (2017). Hyaluronic acid: Still useful in knee osteoarthritis? *Joint Bone Spine*, *84*(6), 655–656.

Ringel-Kulka, T., Goldsmith, J. R., Carroll, I. M., Barros, S. P., Palsson, O., Jobin, C., & Ringel, Y. (2014). *Lactobacillus acidophilus* NCFM affects colonic mucosal opioid receptor expression in patients with functional abdominal pain-a randomised clinical study. *Alimentary Pharmacology & Therapeutics*, *40*(2), 200–207.

Rodriguez-Merchan, E. C. (2016). Conservative treatment of acute knee osteoarthritis: A review of the Cochrane Library. *Journal of Acute Disease*, *5*(3), 190–193.

Rossato, M. F., Hoffmeister, C., Tonello, R., de Oliveira Ferreira, A. P., & Ferreira, J. (2015). Anti-inflammatory effects of vitamin E on adjuvant-induced arthritis in rats. *Inflammation*, *38*(2), 606–615.

Sabina, E. P., Pragasam, S. J., Kumar, S., & Rasool, M. (2011). 6-Gingerol, an active ingredient of ginger, protects acetaminophen-induced hepatotoxicity in mice. *Zhong Xi Yi Jie He Xue Bao, (Journal of Chinese Integrative Medicine)*, *9*(11), 1264–1269.

Sahbaie, P., Sun, Y., Liang, D. Y., Shi, X. Y., & Clark, J. D. (2014). Curcumin treatment attenuates pain and enhances functional recovery after incision. *Anesthesia & Analgesia*, *118*(6), 1336–1344.

Sahoo, A. K., Dandapat, J., Dash, U. C., & Kanhar, S. (2018). Features and outcomes of drugs for combination therapy as multi-targets strategy to combat Alzheimer's disease. *Journal of Ethnopharmacology*, *215*(1), 42–73.

Samdariya, S., Lewis, S., Kauser, H., Ahmed, I., & Kumar, D. (2015). A randomized controlled trial evaluating the role of honey in reducing pain due to radiation induced mucositis in head and neck cancer patients. *Indian Journal of Palliative Care*, *21*(3), 268–273.

Sandoval, M., Okuhama, N. N., Zhang, X. J., Condezo, L. A., Lao, J., Angeles, F. M., … Miller, M. J. S. (2002). Anti-inflammatory and antioxidant activities of cat's claw (*Uncaria tomentosa* and *Uncaria guianensis*) are independent of their alkaloid content. *Phytomedicine*, *9*(4), 325–337.

Sarmento, D. M., Moura, D. P., Lopes, S. L., & Silva, S. C. (2010). Bromelain monograph. *Alternative Medicine Review*, *15*(4), 361–368.

Saulino, M. (2014). Spinal cord injury pain. *Physical Medicine and Rehabilitation Clinics*, *25*(2), 397–410.

Savage, S. R., Romero-Sandoval, A., Schatman, M., Wallace, M., Fanciullo, G., McCarberg, B., & Ware, M. (2016). Cannabis in pain treatment: clinical and research considerations. *The Journal of Pain*, *17*(6), 654–668.

Savino, F., Garro, M., Montanari, P., Galliano, I., & Bergallo, M. (2018). Crying Time and RORγ/FOXP3 Expression in *Lactobacillus reuteri* DSM17938-Treated Infants with Colic: A Randomized Trial. *The Journal of Pediatrics*, *192*. 171-177.e1.

Schmidt-Westhausen, A. M. (2017). Medical management of oral mucosal lesions. In P. A. Brennan, H. Schliephake, G. E. Ghali, & L. Cascarini (Eds.), *Maxillofacial Surgery* (3rd Ed., pp. 1544–1555). St. Louis, MO: Elsevier.

Schweim, H. G. (2017). Synergistic effects—Is it possible to make 'the devil an angel'? *Synergy*, *4*, 8.

Sedighi, M. (2017). Vitamin D and disc herniation associated pain. In: R. R. Watson, & S. Zibadi. *Nutritional Modulators of Pain in the Aging Population*. (pp. 275-280). London: Elsevier.

Semwal, R. B., Semwal, D. K., Combrinck, S., & Viljoen, A. M. (2015). Gingerols and shogaols: Important nutraceutical principles from ginger. *Phytochemistry*, *117*, 554–568.

Sengar, G. S., Deb, R., Chakraborty, S., Mondal, K., Venkatasan, B., & Singh, U. (2017). Overview of pain in livestock: Mechanism to nutritional control. In R. R. Watson, & S.

Zibadi (Eds.), *Nutritional Modulators of Pain in the Aging Population* (pp. 3–8). London: Elsevier.

Shah, A., Craner, J., & Cunningham, J. L. (2017). Medical cannabis use among patients with chronic pain in an interdisciplinary pain rehabilitation program: Characterization and treatment outcomes. *Journal of Substance Abuse Treatment*, 77, 95–100.

Shalaby, M. A., & Hammouda, A. A. E. (2014). Analgesic, anti-inflammatory and anti-hyperlipidemic activities of *Commiphora molmol* extract (Myrrh). *Journal of Intercultural Ethnopharmacology*, 3(2), 56.

Shara, M., & Stohs, S. J. (2015). Efficacy and safety of white willow bark *(Salix alba)* extracts. *Phytotherapy Research*, 29(8), 1112–1116.

Sharma, N., Gaikwad, A. B., & Kulkarni, Y. A. (2017). Folic acid in pain: An epigenetic link. In R. R. Watson, & S. Zibadi (Eds.), *Nutritional Modulators of Pain in the Aging Population* (pp. 245–251). London: Academic Press.

Shen, C. L., Wang, P., Guerrieri, J., Yeh, J. K., & Wang, J. S. (2008). Protective effect of green tea polyphenols on bone loss in middle-aged female rats. *Osteoporosis International*, 19(7), 979–990.

Shen, C. L., Mo, H., Smith, B. J., Chen, C. H., Chen, L., Chyu, M. C., & Kwun, I. S. (2014). Green Tea and other Fruit Polyphenols Attenuate Deterioration of Bone Microarchitecture. In R. R. Watson, V. R. Preedy, & S. Zibadi (Eds.), *Polyphenols in Human Health and Disease* (pp. 681–693). London: Elsevier Academic Press.

Shirvani, M. A., Motahari-Tabari, N., & Alipour, A. (2017). Use of ginger versus stretching exercises for the treatment of primary dysmenorrhea: a randomized controlled trial. *Journal of Integrative Medicine*, 15(4), 295–301.

Shobeiri, F., Oshvandi, K., & Nazari, M. (2015). Clinical effectiveness of vitamin E and vitamin B6 for improving pain severity in cyclic mastalgia. *Iranian Journal of Nursing and Midwifery Research*, 20(6), 723–727.

Silici, S., & Atayoglu, A. T. (2015). Mad honey intoxication: A systematic review on the 1199 cases. *Food and Chemical Toxicology*, 86(12), 282–290.

Singh, G., Alekseeva, L., Alekseev, V., Barinov, A., Goriachev, D., & Nasonov, E. (2014). THU0341 Combination Treatment with Glucosamine–Chondroitin Sulfate Reduces Pain, Disability and NSAID Consumption in Patients with Chronic Low Back Pain: Final Results from A Large, Community-Based, Pilot, Open Prospective Interventional Study. *Annals of the Rheumatic Diseases*, 73(Suppl 2), 300.

Singh, G., Alekseeva, L., Alekseev, V., Goriachev, D., Barinov, A., Nasonov, E., … Pyanykh, S. (2016). SAT0505 Severely-Disabling Chronic Low Back Pain: Combination Treatment with Glucosamine–Chondroitin Sulfate Reduces Disability, Pain and NSAID Consumption: Results from A Large, Community-Based, Pilot, Open Prospective Interventional Study. *Annals of the Rheumatic Diseases*, 75(Suppl 2), 652–853.

Singh, H., Bhushan, S., Arora, R., Buttar, H. S., Arora, S., & Singh, B. (2017). Alternative treatment strategies for neuropathic pain: Role of Indian medicinal plants and compounds of plant origin—A review. *Biomedicine & Pharmacotherapy*, 92(8), 634–650.

Singh, J. A., Noorbaloochi, S., MacDonald, R., & Maxwell, L. J. (2015). Chondroitin for osteoarthritis. *Cochrane Database of Systematic Reviews*, 2015(1). https://doi.org/10.1002/14651858.CD005614.pub2.

Singh, T., More, V., Fatima, U., Karpe, T., Aleem, M. A., & Prameela, J. (2016). Effect of proteolytic enzyme bromelain on pain and swelling after removal of third molars. *Journal of International Society of Preventive & Community Dentistry*, 6(Suppl 3), S197.

Sirianni, J., Ibrahim, M., & Patwardhan, A. (2015). Chronic pain syndromes, mechanisms, and current treatments. In *Progress in Molecular Biology and Translational Science, Vol 131* (pp. 565–611). San Diego, CA: Academic Press.

Smithson, J., Kellick, K. A., & Mergenhagen, K. (2017). Nutritional modulators of pain in the aging population. In R. R. Watson, & S. Zibadi (Eds.), *Nutritional Modulators of Pain in the Aging Population* (pp. 191–198). London: Academic Press.

Soltani, E., Jangjoo, A., Aghaei, M. A., & Dalili, A. (2017). Effects of preoperative administration of ginger (*Zingiber officinale* Roscoe) on postoperative nausea and vomiting after laparoscopic cholecystectomy. *Journal of Traditional and Complementary Medicine.*, 8(3), 387–390.

Song, R., Chen, X., & Zhao, Z. (2017). Protective effect of vitamin B1 on diabetic peripheral neuropathy (DPN) and its mechanism. *Biomedical Research*, 28(14), 6210–6215.

Song, X.-J. (2017). B Vitamins & analgesia & neuroprotective. In R. R. Watson, & S. Zibadi (Eds.), *Nutritional Modulators of Pain in the Aging Population* (pp. 255–264). London: Academic Press.

Sontakke, S., Thawani, V., Pimpalkhute, S., Kabra, P., Babhulkar, S., & Hingorani, L. (2007). Open, randomized, controlled clinical trial of Boswellia serrata extract as compared to valdecoxib in osteoarthritis of knee. *Indian Journal of Pharmacology*, 39(1), 27.

Souza, P. R., & Norling, L. V. (2016). Implications for eicosapentaenoic acid-and docosahexaenoic acid-derived resolvins as therapeutics for arthritis. *European Journal of Pharmacology*, 785, 165–173.

Spar, M. (2018). Chronic prostatitis/chronic pelvic pain syndrome. In D. Rakel (Ed.), *Integrative Medicine* (4th Ed., pp. 616–622.e1). Philadelphia, PA: Elsevier.

Srinivasan, K. (2017). Ginger rhizomes *(Zingiber officinale)*: A spice with multiple health beneficial potentials. *PharmaNutrition*, 5(1), 18–28.

Srivali, N., Cheungpasitporn, W., Chongnarungsin, D., & Edmonds, L. C. (2013). White willow bark induced acute respiratory distress syndrome. *North American Journal of Medical Sciences*, 5(5), 330.

Srivastava, S., Saksena, A. K., Khattri, S., Kumar, S., & Dagur, R. S. (2016). *Curcuma longa* extract reduces inflammatory and oxidative stress biomarkers in osteoarthritis of knee: a four-month, double-blind, randomized, placebo-controlled trial. *Inflammopharmacology*, 24(6), 377–388.

Stanizzi, A., Bottoni, M., Tartaglione, C., Bolletta, E., & Benedetto, G. D. (2017). Associated use of silicone–vitamin E gauzes and α-tocopherol acetate oil in healing of skin graft donor sites. *International Wound Journal*, 14(5), 813–817.

Steinhilber, D., & Hofmann, B. (2014). Recent Advances in the Search for Novel 5-Lipoxygenase Inhibitors. *Basic & Clinical Pharmacology & Toxicology*, 114(1), 70–77.

Stevenson, C., Blaauw, R., Fredericks, E., Visser, J., & Roux, S. (2014). Randomized clinical trial: effect of Lactobacillus plantarum 299 v on symptoms of irritable bowel syndrome. *Nutrition*, 30(10), 1151–1157.

Stohs, S. J., & Bagchi, D. (2015). Antioxidant, anti-inflammatory, and chemoprotective properties of *Acacia catechu* heartwood extracts. *Phytotherapy Research, 29*(6), 818–824.

Stover, P. J., & Field, M. S. (2015). Vitamin B-6. *Advances in Nutrition: An International Review Journal, 6*(1), 132–133.

Straube, S., Derry, S., Moore, R. A., & McQuay, H. J. (2010). Vitamin D for the treatment of chronic painful conditions in adults. *Cochrane Database Syst Rev, 1*, CD007771.

Straube, S., Derry, S., Straube, C., & Moore, R. A. (2015). Vitamin D for the treatment of chronic painful conditions in adults. *The Cochrane Library., 5*, CD007771.

Sznitman, S. R., & Room, R. (2018). Rethinking indicators of problematic cannabis use in the era of medical cannabis legalization. *Addictive Behaviors, 77*(1), 100–101.

Tan, A. (2014). B vitamins for pain following spinal cord trauma. *European Journal of Pain, 18*(1), 1–2.

Tantavisut, S., Tanavalee, A., Honsawek, S., Suantawee, T., Ngarmukos, S., Adisakwatana, S., & Callaghan, J. J. (2017). Effect of vitamin E on oxidative stress level in blood, synovial fluid, and synovial tissue in severe knee osteoarthritis: a randomized controlled study. *BMC Musculoskeletal Disorders, 18*(1), 281–290.

Taylor, B. A., Lorson, L., White, C. M., & Thompson, P. D. (2015). A randomized trial of coenzyme Q10 in patients with confirmed statin myopathy. *Atherosclerosis, 238*(2), 329–335.

Taylor, N. (2017). Nonsurgical management of osteoarthritis knee pain in the older adult. *Clinics in Geriatric Medicine, 33*(1), 41–51.

Teigen, L., & Boes, C. J. (2015). An evidence-based review of oral magnesium supplementation in the preventive treatment of migraine. *Cephalalgia, 35*(10), 912–922.

Tennent, D. J., Hylden, C. M., Kocher, B. K., Aden, J. K., & Johnson, A. E. (2017). A randomized controlled trial evaluating methylsulfonylmethane versus placebo to prevent knee pain in military initial entry trainees. *US Army Medical Department Journal*, (3-17), 21–25.

Terry, R., Posadzki, P., Watson, L. K., & Ernst, E. (2011). The use of ginger *(Zingiber officinale)* for the treatment of pain: a systematic review of clinical trials. *Pain Medicine, 12*(12), 1808–1818.

Tick, H. (2015). Nutrition and pain. *Physical Medicine and Rehabilitation Clinics of North America, 26*(2), 309–320.

Towheed, T., Maxwell, L., Anastassiades, T. P., Shea, B., Houpt, J. B., Welch, V., … Wells, G. A. (2005). Glucosamine therapy for treating osteoarthritis. *The Cochrane Library, 2*(2), CD002946.

Tridenti, G., & Vezzani, C. (2018). Dysmenorrhea. In *Good Practice in Pediatric and Adolescent Gynecology* (pp. 77–97). Cham, Switzerland: Springer.

Tugrul, S., Degirmenci, N., Eren, S. B., Dogan, R., Veyseller, B., & Ozturan, O. (2015). Analgesic effect of magnesium in post-tonsillectomy patients: a prospective randomised clinical trial. *European Archives of Oto-Rhino-Laryngology, 272*(9), 2483–2487.

Uehleke, B., Müller, J., Stange, R., Kelber, O., & Melzer, J. (2013). Willow bark extract STW 33-I in the long-term treatment of outpatients with rheumatic pain mainly osteoarthritis or back pain. *Phytomedicine, 20*(11), 980–984.

Ueland, P. M., McCann, A., Midttun, Ø., & Ulvik, A. (2017). Inflammation, vitamin B6 and related pathways. *Molecular Aspects of Medicine, 53*, 10–27.

Uranga, J. A., López-Miranda, V., Lombo, F., & Abalo, R. (2016). Food, nutrients and nutraceuticals affecting the course of inflammatory bowel disease. *Pharmacological Reports, 68*(4), 816–826.

U. S. Department of Health and Human Services-Federal Drug Administration (FDA). (2016). Botanical drug development guidance for industry. (Revision 1). Silver Springs, MD: *Center for Drug Evaluation and Research, Food and Drug Administration.* Retrieved November 13, 2017 from https://www.fda.gov/media/93113/download.

U.S. Department of Health and Human Services (DHSS). (1994). *The Dietary Supplement Health and Education Act of 1994 Public Law 103-417.* 103ʳᵈ Congress (Approved October 25, 1994). USA.gov. https://ods.od.nih.gov/About/DSHEA_Wording.aspx#sec3. Retrieved 11/11/2017.

U.S. Food and Drug Administration (FDA). (2004). *Botanical Drug Product Guidance.* U. S. Department of Health and Human Services. https://ods.od.nih.gov/About/DSHEA_Wording.aspx. Accessed 8/16/2020.

U.S. Food and Drug Administration (FDA). (2007). Backgrounder on the final rule for current good manufacturing practices (CGMPs) for dietary supplements. In *U.S. Food & Drug Administration: Current Good Manufacturing Practices (CGMPs).* https://www.fda.gov/food/guidanceregulation/cgmp/ucm110863.htm. Accessed May 5, 2018.

U.S. Food and Drug Administration (FDA). (2014). Dietary supplement current manufacturing practices (CGMPs) and interim final rule (IFR) facts. In *U.S. Food & Drug Administration: Current Good Manufacturing Practices (CGMPs).* https://www.fda.gov/food/guidanceregulation/cgmp/ucm110858.htm. Accessed May 5, 2018.

U.S. Food and Drug Administration (FDA). (2016). *Botanical Drug Development Guidance for Industry.* U. S. Department of Health and Human Services. https://www.fda.gov/downloads/drugs/guidancecomplianceregulatoryinformation/guidances/ucm458484.pdf. Retrieved 11/11/2017.

U.S. Food and Drug Administration (FDA). (2017). *FDA Alerts Consumers About Potentially Life-threatening Health Problems Linked to Limbrel.* U. S. Department of Health and Human Services. https://www.fda.gov/Food/RecallsOutbreaksEmergencies/SafetyAlertsAdvisories/ucm585992.htm. Retrieved 5/5/2018.

U.S. Food and Drug Administration (FDA). (2018). *Dietary Supplements Guidance Documents & Regulartory Information.* Retrieved August 21, 2020 from https://www.fda.gov/food/guidance-documents-regulatory-information-topic-food-and-dietary-supplements/dietary-supplements-guidance-documents-regulatory-information.

U.S. Food and Drug Administration (FDA). GRAS *Notices: GRAS No. 66 Curcumin from turmeric (Curcuma longa L.).* U. S. Department of Health and Human Services. https://www.accessdata.fda.gov/scripts/fdcc/?set=GRASNotices&id=686 Retrieved 11/11/2017.

U.S. Food and Drug Administration (FDA). (2018). *Limbrel Capsules by Primus Pharmaceuticals: FDA Advisory Linked to Potentially Life-Threatening Health Problems.* Retrieved August 21, 2020 from https://www.fda.gov/safety/recalls-market-withdrawals-safety-alerts/primus-announces-voluntary-nationwide-recall-all-lots-within-expiry-prescription-medical-food.

U.S. Food and Drug Adminiatration (FDA). (2019). *GRAS Notices: GRAS No. 000822 Synthetic Curcumin from turmeric*

(Curcuma longa L.). U. S. Department of Health and Human Services. Retrieved August 22, 2020 from https://www.fda.gov/media/130730/download.

Venturini, M. A., Zappa, S., Minelli, C., Bonardelli, S., Lamberti, L., Bisighini, L., ... Latronico, N. (2015). Magnesium-oral supplementation to reduce Pain in patients with severe Peripheral arterial occlusive disease: the MAG-PAPER randomised clinical trial protocol. *BMJ Open, 5*(12), e009137.

Veronese, N., Sergi, G., Stubbs, B., Bourdel-Marchasson, I., Tessier, D., Sieber, C., ... Maggi, S. (2017). Effect of acetyl-l-carnitine in the treatment of diabetic peripheral neuropathy: A systematic review and meta-analysis. *European Geriatric Medicine, 8*(2), 117–122.

Viljoen, E., Visser, J., Koen, N., & Musekiwa, A. (2014). A systematic review and meta-analysis of the effect and safety of ginger in the treatment of pregnancy-associated nausea and vomiting. *Nutrition Journal, 13*(1), 20.

Vlachojannis, J., Magora, F., & Chrubasik, S. (2011). Willow species and aspirin: different mechanism of actions. *Phytotherapy Research, 25*(7), 1102–1104.

von Känel, R., Müller-Hartmannsgruber, V., Kokinogenis, G., & Egloff, N. (2014). Vitamin D and central hypersensitivity in patients with chronic pain. *Pain Medicine, 15*(9), 1609–1618.

Vrolijk, M. F., Opperhuizen, A., Jansen, E. H., Hageman, G. J., Bast, A., & Haenen, G. R. (2017). The vitamin B6 paradox: supplementation with high concentrations of pyridoxine leads to decreased vitamin B6 function. *Toxicology In Vitro, 44,* 206–212.

Vyas, M. B., LeBaron, V. T., & Gilson, A. M. (2018). The use of cannabis in response to the opioid crisis: A review of the literature. *Nursing Outlook, 66*(1), 56–65.

Walz, C. P., Barry, A. R., & Koshman, S. L. (2016). Omega-3 polyunsaturated fatty acid supplementation in the prevention of cardiovascular disease. *Canadian Pharmacists Journal/ Revue de Pharmaciens du Canada, 149*(3), 166–173.

Wang, D., Zhai, J. X., & Liu, D. W. (2017). Serum folate, vitamin B12 levels and diabetic peripheral neuropathy in type 2 diabetes: a meta-analysis. *Molecular and Cellular Endocrinology, 443,* 72–79.

Wang, Y., Park, N. Y., Jang, Y., Ma, A., & Jiang, Q. (2015). Vitamin E γ-tocotrienol inhibits cytokine-stimulated NF-κB activation by induction of anti-inflammatory A20 via stress adaptive response due to modulation of sphingolipids. *The Journal of Immunology, 195*(1), 126–133.

Wells, R. E., Baute, V., & Wahbeh, H. (2017). Complementary and Integrative Medicine for Neurologic Conditions. *The Medical Clinics of North America, 101*(5), 881–893.

Whiting, P. F., Wolff, R. F., Deshpande, S., Di Nisio, M., Duffy, S., Hernandez, A. V., ... Schmidlkofer, S. (2015). Cannabinoids for medical use: a systematic review and meta-analysis. *JAMA, 313*(24), 2456–2473.

Wider, B., Pittler, M. H., & Ernst, E. (2015). Feverfew for preventing migraine. *The Cochrane Library,* CD002286.

Wijeratnam, S. W. (2016). Pineapple. In *Reference Module in Food Science: Encyclopedia of Food and Health* (pp. 380–384). St. Louis, MO: Elsevier.

Williams, N. T. (2010). Probiotics. *American Journal of Health-System Pharmacy, 67*(6), 449–458.

Wilsey, B., Marcotte, T., Deutsch, R., Gouaux, B., Sakai, S., & Donaghe, H. (2013). Low-dose vaporized cannabis sig-

nificantly improves neuropathic pain. *The Journal of Pain, 14*(2), 136–148.

Wilson, M., Gogulski, H. Y., Cuttler, C., Bigand, T. L., Oluwoye, O., Barbosa-Leiker, C., & Roberts, M. A. (2018). Cannabis use moderates the relationship between pain and negative affect in adults with opioid use disorder. *Addictive Behaviors, 77,* 225–231.

Wilson, P. B. (2015). Ginger *(Zingiber officinale)* as an analgesic and ergogenic aid in sport: a systemic review. *The Journal of Strength & Conditioning Research, 29*(10), 2980–2995.

Withee, E. D., Tippens, K. M., Dehen, R., Tibbitts, D., Hanes, D., & Zwickey, H. (2017). Effects of Methylsulfonylmethane (MSM) on exercise-induced oxidative stress, muscle damage, and pain following a half-marathon: a double-blind, randomized, placebo-controlled trial. *Journal of the International Society of Sports Nutrition, 14*(1), 24.

World Health Organization (WHO). (2003). *WHO guidelines on good agricultural and collection practices (GACP) for medicinal plants* (pp. 1–72). Geneva: World Health Organization.

Yadav, R. P., & Tarun, G. (2017). Versatility of turmeric: A review the golden spice of life. *Journal of Pharmacognosy and Phytochemistry, 6*(1), 41–46.

Yaghoobi, R., Kazerouni, A., & Kazerouni, O. (2013). Evidence for clinical use of honey in wound healing as an anti-bacterial, anti-inflammatory anti-oxidant and anti-viral agent: A review. *Jundishapur Journal of Natural Pharmaceutical Products, 8*(3), 100–1004.

Yary, T., Lehto, S. M., Tolmunen, T., Tuomainen, T. P., Kauhanen, J., Voutilainen, S., & Ruusunen, A. (2016). Dietary magnesium intake and the incidence of depression: A 20-year follow-up study. *Journal of Affective Disorders, 193,* 94–98.

Yimam, M., Lee, Y. C., Moore, B., Jiao, P., Hong, M., Nam, J. B., ... Jia, Q. (2016). Analgesic and anti-inflammatory effects of UP1304, a botanical composite containing standardized extracts of *Curcuma longa* and *Morus alba. Journal of Integrative Medicine, 14*(1), 60–68.

Yousef, A. A., & Al-deeb, A. E. (2013). A double-blinded randomised controlled study of the value of sequential intravenous and oral magnesium therapy in patients with chronic low back pain with a neuropathic component. *Anaesthesia, 68*(3), 260–266.

Yu, C. Z., Liu, Y. P., Liu, S., Yan, M., Hu, S. J., & Song, X. J. (2014). Systematic administration of B vitamins attenuates neuropathic hyperalgesia and reduces spinal neuron injury following temporary spinal cord ischaemia in rats. *European Journal of Pain, 18*(1), 76–85.

Zagorodnikova, K. (2015). Coenzyme Q10 levels in Patients on low dose statins in relation to their therapeutic and adverse effects. *Clinical Therapeutics, 37*(8), e82.

Zampieron, E., & Kamhi, E. (2015). Topical and Oral Herbal Pain Remedies. *International Journal of Complementary & Alternative Medicine, 1*(4), 00021.

Zanjani, M. T., Ameli, H., Labibi, F., Sedaghat, K., & Sabetkasaei, M. (2014). The attenuation of pain behavior and serum COX-2 concentration by curcumin in a rat model of neuropathic pain. *The Korean Journal of Pain, 27*(3), 246–252.

Zaringhalam, J., Akbari, A., Zali, A., Manaheji, H., Nazemian, V., Shadnoush, M., & Ezzatpanah, S. (2016). Long-term treatment by vitamin B1 and reduction of serum proinflammatory cytokines, hyperalgesia, and paw edema in adjuvant-induced arthritis. *Basic and Clinical Neuroscience, 7*(4), 331–340.

Zengion, A. H., & Yarnell, E. (2011). Herbal and nutritional supplements for painful conditions. In T. A. Lennard, S. Walkowski, A. K. Singla, & D. G. Vivian (Eds.), *Pain Procedures in Clinical Practice* (3rd Ed., pp. 187–204). St. Louis, MO: Saunders.

Zhang, Y. P., Eber, A., Yuan, Y., Yang, Z., Rodriguez, Y., Levitt, R. C., ... Candiotti, K. A. (2013). Prophylactic and antinociceptive effects of coenzyme Q10 on diabetic neuropathic pain in a mouse model of type 1 diabetes. *Anesthesiology: The Journal of the American Society of Anesthesiologists, 118*(4), 945–954.

Zheng, S., Jin, X., Cicuttini, F., Wang, X., Zhu, Z., Wluka, A., ... Blizzard, L. (2017). Maintaining vitamin D sufficiency is associated with improved structural and symptomatic outcomes in knee osteoarthritis. *The American Journal of Medicine, 130*(10), 1211–1218.

Zhu, X., Li, Q., Chang, R., Yang, D., Song, Z., Guo, Q., & Huang, C. (2014). Curcumin alleviates neuropathic pain by inhibiting p300/CBP histone acetyltransferase activity-regulated expression of BDNF and cox-2 in a rat model. *PLoS One, 9*(3), e91303.

Chapter 27 Additional Nonpharmacologic Interventions as Components of Multimodal Pain Management

Ann Quinlan-Colwell

CHAPTER OUTLINE

Aromatherapy, pg. 739

Evidence for Pain Management, pg. 739

Cautions, pg. 740

Caring, Empathy, and Compassion by Caregivers, pg. 742

Evidence for Pain Management, pg. 743

Cautions, pg. 743

Crossing Hands and/or Arms Over the Midline, pg. 743

Evidence for Pain Management, pg. 744

Cautions, pg. 745

Dietary Choices, pg. 745

Antiinflammatory Diet, pg. 745

Ketogenic Diet, pg. 747

Environmental Modifications, pg. 747

Lighting, pg. 748

Sound, pg. 748

Temperature, pg. 748

Position, pg. 749

Evidence for Pain Management, pg. 749

Caution, pg. 749

Hypnosis, pg. 749

Evidence for Pain Management, pg. 750

Caution, pg. 751

Mirror Therapy or Mirror Visual Feedback Therapy, pg. 751

Evidence for Pain Management, pg. 752

Mirror Visual Feedback Therapy and Other Chronic Pain Conditions, pg. 753

Virtual Reality Mirror Visual Feedback Therapy, pg. 753

Mirror Visual Feedback Therapy in Home Settings, pg. 753

Mirror Visual Feedback Therapy and Referred Sensations, pg. 753

Cautions for Using Mirror Visual Feedback Therapy, pg. 754

Obesity and Weight Management, pg. 754

Evidence for Pain Management, pg. 755

Cautions, pg. 756

Static Magnet Therapy, pg. 756

Evidence for Pain Management, pg. 756

Cautions, pg. 756

Temperature Modalities, pg. 756

Therapeutic Superficial Heat, pg. 756

Therapeutic Cold, Ice, Cryotherapy, pg. 758

Alternating or Contrasting Temperature Therapy, pg. 759

Evidence for Pain Management, pg. 760

Cautions, pg. 760

Valsalva Maneuver, pg. 760

Evidence for Pain Management, pg. 760

Cautions, pg. 761

Contraindications, pg. 761

Key Points, pg. 761

Case Scenario, pg. 761

References, pg. 762

SOME nonpharmacologic interventions do not easily fit into one of the major categories discussed in other chapters. They include aromatherapy, empathy and caring of clinicians, crossing arms and hands, diet and food choices, environment, heat and cold application, hypnosis, magnets, mirror therapy, Valsalva maneuver, and weight loss. Each of them will be discussed in this chapter, including an explanation of the intervention, how it can be used, the evidence for use as a pain management strategy, and any cautions or contraindications. Although each method will be reviewed individually, many of them can be used together, as can other nonpharmacologic interventions and pharmacologic preparations as part of a multimodal approach to pain management.

Aromatherapy

Aromatherapy involves using concentrated essential oils. These oils are aromatic, complex, volatile, and semivolatile concentrated compounds, which for medicinal purposes are extracted from portions of a plant, including the flowers, fruits, leaves, and barks (Ali et al., 2015; Dimitriou, Mavridou, Manataki, & Damigos, 2017; Manion & Widder, 2017; Moghaddam & Mehdizadeh, 2017). It is thought that signals arising from the aromatherapy oils transmit through the olfactory bulb to reach the limbic and hypothalamus areas of the brain, then subsequently cause a release of endorphins and enhance serotonin in the plasma circulation (Ali et al., 2015; Sut & Kahyaoglu-Sut, 2017). (See Chapter 3 for discussion of the physiology of nociception, including endorphins and serotonin.)

The essential oil is transmitted through either inhalation or topical absorption through massage or bathing (Ali et al., 2015; Metin & Ozdemir, 2016; National Cancer Institute [NCI], 2018). Inhalation may be done directly with a small amount of the oil or indirectly, for example, using a nebulizer with ultrasonic diffusion to flow throughout a room (NCI, 2018). Aromatherapy is reported as an effective intervention for a wide range of conditions, including pain, myalgia, headache, sleeping disturbances, and depression (Ali et al., 2015). During the last few decades, use of aromatherapy has grown exponentially and it is important that clinicians are familiar with this therapy and how it may interface with other components of a multimodal pain management plan (Manion & Widder, 2017).

Evidence for Pain Management

Internationally, there are many reports of research using aromatherapy through both massage and inhalation in a wide variety of patient groups. In one report, aromatherapy was considered effective ($P = .001$) in helping manage labor pain in pregnant women (n = 120) (Yazdkhasti & Pirak, 2016). Nurses in Minnesota and

Wisconsin conducted a multisite study (n = 10,262) assessing the use of several essential aromatherapy oils, including lavender, ginger, sweet marjoram, mandarin, and a combination of oils (Johnson et al., 2016). In that study the majority of aromatherapy was by inhalation and the most frequently used essential oil was lavender. The authors reported that ginger had the strongest effect on nausea, lavender and sweet marjoram were equally effective in reducing anxiety, and sweet marjoram had that greatest effect in controlling pain. In another study, lavender aromatherapy was effective in reducing pain ($P = .01$) and anxiety ($P < .001$) compared to standard of care in a trial using lavender during the common but painful procedure of venous cannulation that can negatively affect the satisfaction of the patient (Karaman et al., 2016). Similar results were reported with the effect of lavender aromatherapy among patients (n = 92) receiving insertion of a needle into a fistula for hemodialysis (Bagheri-Nesami, Espahbodi, Nikkhah, Shorofi, & Charati, 2014). In that study, the patients who received lavender oil aromatherapy reported significantly less ($P = .009$) pain after three sessions compared to controls, who only received aromatherapy but no lavender. In another study, patients on hemodialysis reported inhaling aromatherapy with lavender and sweet orange essential oils was effective in decreasing fatigue and improving sleep (Muz & Taşcı, 2017), which conceivably can have a positive effect on pain control as well. (See Chapter 8 for discussion of the relationship between pain and sleep.)

The authors of a systematic review of nine randomized controlled trials (RCTs) (n = 644 subjects) reported there is insufficient evidence to conclude aromatherapy is effective in reducing the intensity of postoperative pain (Dimitriou et al., 2017). That was reported prior to five studies in the review in which aromatherapy was seen as helpful in reducing pain intensity and four in which no significant difference was found. Another review with seven RCTs involving aromatherapy among patients with dementia revealed no efficacy in that population; however, a positive effect on reducing stress among nurses and others working in critical care environments was noted (Anderson, Deng, Anthony, Atalla, & Monroe, 2017). In a subsequent study, nurses and patient care technicians working in trauma units and intensive care units reported statistically fewer incidences of feeling stressed when essential oil of lavender was constantly diffused over 30 days into a specific nursing work area (Johnson et al., 2017).

Among people living with rheumatoid arthritis (RA), aromatherapy massage using a combination of *Lavandula angustifolia, Juniperus officinalis, Cananga odorata,* and *Rosmarinus officinalis* (n = 17) was compared with reflexology (n = 17) (Metin & Ozdemir, 2016). (See Chapter 24 for discussion of reflexology.) In that study, pain and fatigue were significantly less ($P < .05$) in both groups compared to a control group (n = 17), but those in the reflexology group experienced pain control in 1 week compared to 2 weeks for the aromatherapy massage group ($P < .05$). When aromatherapy massage (n = 30) was compared with aromatherapy inhalation (n = 30) among patients with burns, the reduction in anxiety and pain were statistically greater in both groups compared to the control group (n = 30) (Seyyed-Rasooli et al., 2016). Interestingly, although both interventions in that study were significant compared to controls, inhalation aromatherapy ($P = .002$) was more effective than massage aromatherapy ($P = .007$) in reducing anxiety and aromatherapy massage ($P < 0.001$) was more effective than aromatherapy inhalation in reducing pain ($P = .001$). Differences in the two interventions were that more essential lavender oil was used in the inhalation group, who also received *Rosa damascene* and the massage group received almond oil with the lavender. The authors of a meta-analysis (n = 6 studies; n = 362 subjects) reported abdominal aromatherapy massage was used effectively to control pain in women with dysmenorrhea compared to massage with placebo oils (Sut & Kahyaoglu-Sut, 2017). In that analysis, the most commonly used essential oil was lavender, either alone or in combination with other essential oils.

Rigorous research is needed to determine the efficacy of aromatherapy (Dimitriou et al., 2017; Karaman, 2016) in different populations and efficacy with different strengths and combinations of the various essential oils (Bagheri-Nesami et al., 2014; Seyyed-Rasooli et al., 2016; Sut & Kahyaoglu-Sut, 2017). The difference between essential oils used in aromatherapy inhalation versus aromatherapy massage (Seyyed-Rasooli et al., 2016), including the possibly confounding effect of massage, needs to be studied as well. Research is also needed to determine safety, identify adverse events, and address ethical considerations and implementation of aromatherapy within facilities.

Finally, clinicians must bear in mind that the effectiveness of the essential oil can be affected by a variety of factors specific to the plant, the environment, and the extraction process (Manion & Widder, 2017; Moghaddam & Mehdizadeh, 2017). Continuing critical review of current literature and research is important (Manion & Widder, 2017). Courses and programs are available, and certification in aromatherapy is advised. Certification can be obtained through several reputable sources, including the National Association for Holistic Aromatherapy (http://www.naha.org) and the Canadian Federation of Aromatherapists (http://www.cfacanada.com) (NCI, 2018).

Cautions

When used as intended, aromatherapy with pure essential oils is generally recognized as safe, yet it is important to remember that there can be toxicity and contraindications with these natural products (Buckle, 2015b; Manion & Widder, 2017; NCI, 2018). An important caution is to use only pure essential oils of good quality. Although essential oils are readily available in many areas, there

---

Box 27.1 | Characteristics of Reputable Essential Oils

- Product will be labeled clearly as: "Pure 100% essential oil."
- Bottle is colored glass with an integral stopper.
- It is produced by a reputable supplier who can provide information regarding origin of the oil, expiration date, material safety data sheets, and gas-chromatography/mass spectrometry data.
- The label will have cautions and precautions clearly stated.
- A list of reputable suppliers of essential oils is available at http://www.rjbuckle.com

Collated from Buckle, J. (2015a). Basic plant taxonomy, basic essential oil chemistry, extraction, biosynthesis, and analysis. In J. Buckle. *Clinical aromatherapy: Essential oils in healthcare* (3rd ed., pp. 37–72). St. Louis, MO: Elsevier.

---

can be significant differences in the quality of the oil and many are diluted with alcohol or other oils (Buckle, 2015a). Box 27.1 presents points to consider when purchasing essential oils. It is important to remember that essential oils are flammable and may have a flash point between 50° and 60° C (122° and 140° F) (Tisserand & Young, 2013). Box 27.2 provides advice on storage and controlling quality of essential oils. Finally, essential oils are not intended for ingestion in the United States or the United Kingdom (NCI, 2018).

Reported adverse reactions include varying degrees of allergic reactions, skin irritations, vomiting, hepatotoxicity, nephrotoxicity, mental status changes, neuromuscular issues, and respiratory issues (Buckle, 2015b; NCI, 2018).

Box 27.2 | Advice for Storing and Controlling Quality of Essential Oils

- Store in cool area (ideally under refrigeration).
- After opening, replace the cap immediately after use.
- Store out of the reach of children.
- Adhere to expiration dates and if none is on the bottle use within 12 months of purchase or first use.
- Dispose of essential oils that are prone to oxidation within 6 months of purchase or first use.
- Keep out of direct sunlight and away from heat, flames, vaporizers, and candles.

Tisserand, R., & Young, R. (2013). *Essential oil safety-E-book: A guide for health care professionals.* London: Churchill Livingstone.

Both dermatologic and respiratory allergic reactions are reported (Aronson, 2016).

Caution is advised if using essential oils topically and with covering the skin where essential oil has been applied before going out of doors because there may be sensitivity to the sun (U.S. Department of Health and Human Services [DHHS], 2014; NCI, 2018). One patient with a history of migraine headaches reported headache after exposure to lavender by an oxygen mask (Dimitriou et al., 2017). The essential oils of both tea tree and lavender are reported to have properties similar to those of estrogen and can reduce the effect of androgens (NCI, 2018). Table 27.1 presents cases in which there were overdoses of common essential oils.

Table 27.1 | Reported Cases of Overdose With Common Essential Oils

Essential Oil	Amount (mL or Drops)	Symptoms	Author
Cinnamon *Cinnamomum verum*	60 mL	Dizziness, double vision, nausea, vomiting, collapse.	Pilapil, 1989
Citronella *Cymbopogon nardus*	15 mL	12-month-old girl: Vomiting, shock, frothing at the mouth, deep rapid respiration, cyanosis, convulsions, brain hemorrhage. Died.	Mant, 1961
	25 mL	16-month-old boy: Gastric lavage. Survived.	Temple et al., 1991
Clove *Syzygium aromaticum*	5 mL	7-month-old child: Severe acidosis, central nervous system depression, ketones in urine; gastric lavage. Survived.	Lane, et al 1991
	5–10 mL	2-year-old boy: Clove plus paracetamol; acidosis, deteriorating liver function, extremely low blood glucose, generalized seizure, deep coma; given heparin; conscious after 6 days. Survived.	Hartnoll et al., 1993
	10 mL	15-month-old boy: Liver failure; given intravenous injection of N-acetylcysteine; liver function returned within 4 days. Survived.	Janes et al., 2005
	8 mL	32-year-old woman: Self-injected intravenously; acute respiratory distress, noncardiogenic pulmonary edema; abnormal chest radiograph; medical intervention for 7 days. Survived.	Kirsch et al., 1990
	less than 8 mL	3-month-old girl: Fulminant hepatic failure; gastric lavage; intravenous injection of *N*-acetylcysteine. Survived.	Eisen et al., 2004
Eucalyptus (cineole-rich species)	5 mL	Vertigo, loss of coordination, abnormal respiration, epigastric pain, cold sweats.	Craig, 1953
		Lesser amounts = excess respiratory tract mucus; greater amounts = decreased respiratory tract mucus, pinpoint pupils, rapid drowsiness, unconsciousness.	Patel & Wiggins, 1980
		109 children (mean age 23 months) over 10 years; gastric lavage, nasogastric charcoal and medical intervention. All survived.	Tibballs, 1995
Hyssop *Hyssopus officinalis*	10–20 drops 30 drops 10 drops	6-year-old boy: Convulsions, hospitalized. Survived. 18-year-old girl: Unconscious, seizure. Survived. 26-year-old girl: Seizure. Survived.	O'Mullane et al., 1982 O'Mullane et al., 1982 Millet et al., 1981
Pennyroyal *Mentha pulegium*	10 mL	4 case studies including 1 death. Review of 18 cases in adult women with moderate to severe toxicity. 1 death.	Anderson et al., 1996
Pine *Pinus sylvestris*	400–500 mL	Suicide attempt; hospitalization; hemoperfusion with activated charcoal plus Amberlite and hemodialysis. Survived.	Koppel et al., 1982

Continued

Table 27.1 | Reported Cases of Overdose With Common Essential Oils—cont'd

Essential Oil	Amount (mL or Drops)	Symptoms	Author
Dalmatian sage *Salvia officinalis*	7 mL	44-year-old woman took sage for asthma: Convulsions, dyspnea, cardiac failure, death.	Whitling, 1908
	Unspecified	33-day-old baby boy: Accidentally given sage oil for colic; seizures, nystagmus, hyperreflexia, and irritability; hospitalization; IV diazepam and midazolam. Survived.	Halicioglu et al., 2011
	5 mL	5-year-old girl: Given sage oil for colic; seizures; hospitalized; gastric lavage and active charcoal treatment. Survived.	Halicioglu et al., 2011
Tea tree *Melaleuca alternifolia*	15 mL	17-month-old boy: Ataxia, drowsiness; recovered within 8 hours.	Del Beccaro, 1995
	10 mL	23-month-old boy.	Jacobs & Hornfeldt, 1994
	"Small amount"	4-year-old boy: Ataxic, nonresponsive, intubated. Survived.	Morris et al., 2003
Wintergreen *Gaultheria fragrantissima*	1 oz	5 mL of wintergreen is equivalent to 22 adult aspirin tablets. Wintergreen is 98% methyl salicylate. 44-year-old man: Seizure; hospitalized. Died 18 hours later.	Botma et al., 2001 Davis, 2007 Cauthen & Hester, 1989

From Buckle, J. (2015b). Essential oil toxicity and contraindications. In J. Buckle. *Clinical aromatherapy: Essential oils in healthcare* (3rd ed., pp. 73–94). St. Louis, MO: Elsevier.

Caring, Empathy, and Compassion by Caregivers

Historically, relationships between clinicians and patients were considered to have a therapeutic affect beyond the treatments and medications that were administered (Decety & Fotopoulou, 2015). Caring for patients in pain involves the clinician synchronizing their brain with their hands and heart to effectively assist the patient who is not able to adequately achieve pain relief or pain control alone. This caring can be profound. When patients experience a sense of caring, they feel safe (Dempsey, 2018) and experience greater satisfaction with pain control even when specific pain intensity goals may not be met (Decety & Fotopoulou, 2015; Quinlan-Colwell, 2009). For many years, it has been known that patients are more satisfied with their care, feel less anxious, and have better outcomes when they feel empathy and compassion from clinicians (Vogus & McClelland, 2016). Compassion is a discrete innate ability that enables one to affectively understand and respond to the suffering of others and to have empathy for them; it is distinctly different from other emotions, such as distress, love, or sadness (Kagan, 2014; Wright & Pendry, 2016). With compassion there is a communication of caring. Compassionate care is a vehicle through which a meaningful link or bond occurs between clinicians and patients and helps the clinician understand the individual experience of pain (Burnell, 2009). It is based on the caring and empathy of the clinician being in harmony with the emotions of another person (Wright & Pendry, 2016).

Kagan (2015) suggested that it is necessary to convey empathy and compassion for patients to feel they have dignity, which is an essential component of being a person. An important component of sharing empathy and caring is verbally and nonverbally conveying empathic messages. An example of this is a clinician telling a patient, "I can't feel your pain, but I believe you have pain and that it is hard for you to control. I am going to work with you to better control it." Although pain is a subjective, private, and personal experience, it can be shared through verbal and nonverbal expression, and then it is no longer a private experience (Bouchard, 2013). Research supports the concept that caregiver interactions meaningfully affect the pain experiences of people and their ability to control their own pain (Vervoort & Trost, 2017). Interactions between patients and clinicians occur frequently, and it is easy for clinicians to think of them as being routine. The literature tells us that for patients the communications are often very impactful with profound effects (Darlow et al., 2013; Dempsey, 2018). Many clinicians have experienced a patient reminding the clinician of something they said to the patient during an earlier encounter which the clinician had long forgotten, but continued to impact the patient. Improving communication can help improve interactions between patients with pain and the clinicians working with them (Bouchard, 2013). It is hypothesized that a compassionate clinician can enhance the nociceptive benefit of interventions provided to patients with chronic pain (Smith, Fortin, Dwamena, & Frankel, 2013).

Evidence for Pain Management

Research indicates that pain perception can be lessened and pain tolerance can be increased with experiences perceived as supportive and safe which are influenced by positive supportive interpersonal interactions (Decety & Fotopoulou, 2015). The results of a large systematic review (n = 51 studies) indicated there is at least a small effect of reduced pain perception when communication of positive messages are conveyed by clinicians (Howick et al., 2017). The results of a survey of patients who were veterans (n = 1075) revealed patient perception of pain and even pain intensity was found to be correlated with clinician communication (Ruben, Meterko, & Bokhour, 2018). Box 27.3 lists characteristics of positive communication between clinicians and patients with pain.

Collaborative work among psychologists, developmental scientists, and neuroscientists theorize that through evolution, the brains of mammals have developed and honed empathy as an ability to connect with others for survival (Decety & Fotopoulou, 2015). Neuroimaging studies indicate that when pain relief is expected, pain intensity can be lessened when the prefrontal cortex and mesolimbic reward circuits are activated and neurotransmitters are released (Jensen et al., 2014). The anterior insular part of the brain of patients who were treated in a particularly empathic manner by clinicians showed less pain response on functional magnetic resonance imaging (fMRI) compared to controls (Sarinopoulos, et al, 2013). In a study that evaluated the effect of physician interaction on patients, fMRI results showed that when physicians felt compassionate toward patients in pain, there was selective activation of the ventral striatum and ventrolateral and dorsolateral prefrontal cortices of

their brains, which are involved with senses of value and reward (Jensen et al., 2014).

Investigators evaluated patient satisfaction surveys of people who frequently used emergency department (ED) care for pain (n = 305) and found that, among other factors, patient satisfaction was most significantly influenced by the perception that the physician cared (empathically) for the patient (P < .001), perception nurses cared (empathically) for the patient (P < .001), compassion conveyed by nurses (P < .001), and degree of pain control (P < .001) (Newcomb et al., 2017). In another study, when the clinician-patient relationship was explored with patients receiving opioid treatment for chronic pain, it was clear that compassionate patient-centered partnerships in which the clinicians communicated well with patients were most effective (Esquibel & Borkan, 2014). In that study it was reported opioid prescriptions could be avoided when the care was considered compassionate.

Compassion can be developed, replenished, and refined through numerous techniques such as introspection, mindfulness practice, and loving kindness meditation. Clinicians are well advised to remember that compassion for others begins with self-compassion and self-care (Beaumont & Martin, 2016). Box 27.4 presents specific examples and ideas for developing, honing, or re-creating compassion.

Research with strong methodology using a variety of multimodal interventions conveyed with compassion, empathy, and caring needs to be conducted among patients with both acute and chronic pain conditions (Frankel, 2017). Additional rigorous studies to investigate the effect of communication on the patient-clinician relationship and on the perception of pain are warranted (Howick et al., 2017). Research is also needed to explore the role of compassion in selecting health care as a career and how compassion may change over time while working in health care, particularly with caring for patients who live with pain.

Cautions

The primary caution needed in conveying compassion and a sense of caring is to maintain healthy boundaries to avoid compassion fatigue (Cross, 2019; Seppala, Hutcherson, Nguyen, Doty, & Gross, 2014; Wright & Pendry, 2016). One precautionary activity to prevent compassion fatigue and burn out is the practice of loving kindness meditation (see Chapter 25).

Crossing Hands and/or Arms Over the Midline

When the hands of the person experiencing pain are crossed over the midline of the body, it is thought to interfere with the ability for the person to understand where tactile stimuli occur, and early research indicates this is likely true for pain stimuli as well (Gallace, Torta, Moseley,

---

Box 27.3	Clinician-Patient Communication

- Increase awareness of where there may be potential areas of miscommunication, including pronunciation, semantics, grammar, and lexicon.
- Listen to what patients think about their condition and pain management needs and therapies.
- Be attentive to nonverbal communication and where it may be inconsistent with what is being said.
- When there seems to be a disconnect between verbal and nonverbal communication, acknowledge it and ask the patient to explain it.
- Ask the source of what patients' believe about pain (other clinicians, family, literature, internet, etc.).
- Develop an awareness of personal experiences, feelings, and biases regarding pain, patients experiencing pain, their behaviors, and the variety of multimodal options for pain control.

Box 27.4   Key Attributes of Compassion, Skills of Compassion, and Interventions Designed to Increase Levels of Compassion

Gilbert's (2009) First Psychology of Compassion (Compassionate Attributes)

- *Care for well-being:* Caring for oneself and other people with a desire and a caring motivation to notice and turn toward suffering with a wish to alleviate distress and stimulate well-being.
- *Sensitivity to distress:* Developing self-awareness and being attentive to one's own suffering (through physical and emotional clues) and other people's distress.
- *Sympathy:* Acknowledging and feeling emotionally moved by past and present experiences of suffering and distress.
- *Distress tolerance:* Turning toward suffering and learning to tolerate difficult emotions with an open-hearted acceptance and kindness.
- *Empathy:* A desire to learn, understand, and discover the reasons we and other people behave, think, and feel in situations and environments (e.g., thinking about why we are self-critical and when we first noticed self-criticism).
- *Nonjudgement:* Individuals are taught techniques that aim to help them learn to notice and let go of self-attacking and self-criticism without judgement.

Gilbert's (2009) Second Psychology of Compassion (Compassionate Skills)

- *Attention:* Linked to mindfulness, focusing on the present moment without judgment or criticism.
- *Reasoning:* Training the mind to think and reason in helpful ways (focusing on a balanced perspective, for example, asking oneself "how can I think in a way that will help me in this situation").
- *Behavior:* Behaving in ways that help individuals move through suffering, toward their life goals. This can be difficult and requires courage because it may involve facing fears or refraining from using unhelpful safety behaviors.
- *Sensory:* Learning to stimulate the affect regulation system by using breathing practices, vocal tones, and body postures.

- *Feeling:* Noticing and responding to emotions using compassion.
- *Imagery:* Using imagery exercises that aim to stimulate the soothing affiliative system.

Gilbert's (2009) Compassionate Mind Training (Interventions Include)

- *Mindfulness and focused attention:* Learning to notice that our attention can be directed by us.
- *Soothing rhythm breathing (SRB):* Exploration of breathing methods that have been found to be connected with heart rate variability, positive health outcomes, and cerebral activity (Gilbert, 2014). SRB can help regulate the threat system.
- *Creating a safe place:* Creating a place in the mind that provides affiliative feelings.
- *Compassion focused imagery:* Using imagery exercises to stimulate the soothing systems and manage distress. When anxious or worried, individuals may imagine negative, critical, or scary images that tend to add to distress.
- *Compassion as a flow:* Exercises designed to increase levels of compassion for self and others would be introduced.
- *Developing the compassionate self:* Using acting skills and imagery techniques to create and develop a compassionate ideal self that may be used to cultivate compassion for others and self.
- *Developing our ideal compassionate other:* Using imagery techniques to create an image of an ideal compassionate other (an image that offers compassion).
- *Our different parts:* Exploration of the different emotional parts (e.g., angry, anxious, and critical). Using a compassionate mind to relate to our different parts.
- *Engaging with self-criticism using the compassion self:* The compassionate self will direct compassionate behavior, thoughts, and feelings to the critical self.

Data from Beaumont, E., & Martin, C. J. H. (2016). A proposal to support student therapists to develop compassion for self and others through Compassionate Mind Training. *The Arts in Psychotherapy, 50*, 111–118.

& Iannetti, 2011; Sambo et al., 2013; Torta, et al, 2013). Although this is an area with little and novel research, it has potential for a safe, effective method of modulating pain by interrupting painful messages (Gallace et al., 2011).

Evidence for Pain Management

In a very small study (n = 7), although not statistically significant, the participants had greater difficulty identifying the location of painful stimuli when their arms were crossed (Sambo et al., 2013). Another small, yet interesting study compared the effect of interference of painful stimuli when hands were crossed over the chest in patients who had a stroke, both those with *spatial neglect* (i.e., lack of awareness of things or people on the side of the body opposite to the location of the stroke, more commonly with strokes affecting the right brain) (n = 11), and those without *spatial* neglect (n = 16) (Vizzari et al., 2017).

The researchers of that study found that although patients with spatial neglect did not experience analgesia when arms were crossed, 81% of the patients without spatial neglect did achieve analgesia. This seems to support the theory that crossing the arms or hands interferes with an awareness of the body and thus the location of where painful stimuli are occurring.

The underlying concepts of how crossing the arms over the midline supports pain control are based in research in neurobiology. That research has broadened the knowledge base of nociception to include an understanding that cortical processes of nociception are encoded within a representation of the *peripersonal space* (i.e., the multifaceted body and space around it) of the person (Jones, 2014). The relationship of what is occurring in the peripersonal space with pain awareness is rooted in awareness of and defense by the body of potential threats exemplified by painful stimuli (Filbrich, Alamia, Blandiaux, Burns, & Legrain, 2017). This corresponds to the concepts of somatosensory mapping, which enables the person to identify where tactile and nociceptive stimuli are located (Sambo et al., 2013). Analgesia can conceivably occur through interruption of the integration of nociceptive signaling that can attenuate pain perception (Jones, 2014). When researchers used fMRI to investigate these concepts (n = 17), they found that analgesia produced by crossing hands involved a number of areas of the brain, including the cingulate, insular, frontal cortices of the pain neuromatrix and the posterior parietal area, which are involved with proprioception (Torta et al., 2013). (See Chapter 3 for discussion of nociception and the neuromatrix.) Because crossing the arms costs nothing and is generally innocuous yet feasible for most people, this is an area in which additional research is needed (De Paepe, Crombez, & Legrain, 2015). This is a pain intervention that is very amenable to nursing research.

Cautions

No concerns or cautions were identified or reported; however, research is very early and additional work is needed on this topic.

Dietary Choices

Internationally there is recent heightened interest in the relationship between diet and activation of nociception, pain perception, and analgesia (Bjørklund, et al., 2019). Vegetarian, vegan, and gluten-free diets have been associated with pain relief in people with RA (Perlman, Rosenberger, & Ali, 2018). Because two diet programs are presented in the literature as specific interventions for potentially helping to manage pain, they are discussed here. These are the antiinflammatory diet and the ketogenic diet.

Antiinflammatory Diet

In general, an antiinflammatory diet is similar to the Mediterranean diet in that rather than omega-6 fatty acids, consumption of omega-3 fatty acids, which are in deep water fish, is encouraged, along with fruits, vegetable, beans, nuts, and whole grains, with possible addition of fish oil supplements (Kohatsu & Karpowicz, 2018; Viveky, Dahl, & Whiting, 2013). The antiinflammatory diet also may include full-fat dairy products and some lean protein such as chicken, with a limitation of refined food products (Viveky et al., 2013). Antiinflammatory diets are also high in fiber and low in unhealthy oils, sugar, and starchy carbohydrates (Tick, 2015). Other dietary products that are considered antiinflammatory include turmeric (curcumin) (see Chapter 26), wine, cocoa (particularly dark chocolate), ginger, chili pepper, basil, rosemary, thyme, and oregano (Kohatsu & Karpowicz, 2018). Compared with the proinflammatory diets that are high in processed foods and sugar, which increase inflammation, antiinflammatory diets are effective in reducing the inflammation of painful conditions and inflammatory diseases (Arranz, 2017; Tick, 2015). Fig. 27.1 presents a patient handout of the antiinflammatory diet.

Evidence for Pain Management

The premise underlying the antiinflammatory diet is the role of inflammation in chronic pain and in some of the conditions from which pain arises, such as OA, RA (Arranz, 2017), and myofascial pain syndrome (Bonakdar, 2018). When inflammation becomes chronic there is a recurrent stimulation to synthesize cytokines, which are proinflammatory and contribute to several chronic conditions (Viveky et al., 2013). The antiinflammatory diet is of particular interest considering it is designed to help prevent chronic inflammation from developing and subsequently the risk factors associated with the nonsteroidal antiinflammatory drugs (NSAIDs) (Kohatsu & Karpowicz, 2018). (See Chapter 10 for a detailed discussion of NSAIDS.)

Omega-3 fatty acids are polyunsaturated fatty acids (PUFAs) that support antiinflammatory mechanisms (Tick, 2015) and are involved in the production of the antiinflammatory eicosanoids (Arranz, 2017). PUFAs are known to have antinociceptive properties (Ramsden et al., 2013) and have been associated with reducing pain and joint stiffness in people living with RA (Norling & Perretti, 2013). A meta-analysis of RCTs (n = 10 studies) in which omega-3 PUFAs were administered in dosages of at least 2.7 g/d to people with RA showed there was reduced NSAID use, with no statistical difference in joint swelling or morning stiffness between those who used NSAIDs and those who consumed omega-3 PUFAs (Lee, Bae, & Song, 2012). In a study supported by the National Institutes of Health (NIH) (n = 67), a reduction of proinflammatory fatty acids and an increase in omega-3 PUFAs was correlated with a reduction in Headache Impact Test scores ($P < .001$), hours per

Patient Handout: The Antiinflammatory Diet

Inflammation in the body is known to contribute to chronic disease such as diabetes, heart disease, asthma, inflammatory gut disorders, arthritis, obesity, cancer, and dementia. Eating an antiinflammatory diet may reduce inflammation and decrease chronic disease. Food as medicine is powerful! Here are some simple guidelines:

Antiinflammatory diet guidelines:

1) Choose healthy fats.
   • Substitute extra-virgin olive oil for other vegetable oils, trans-fats, or butter in your cooking for health benefits.
   • Eat two servings (4 ounces each) of fatty fish per week.
   • Reduce use of omega-6 fats (hydrogenated vegetable oils) to keep ratio of omega-6: omega-3 in range of 2:1–4:1.

2) Increase vegetable and fruit intake (especially vegetables)
   • Eat at least 5 servings of vegetables and fruit per day, with more than half as vegetables.
   • Color your diet! - deeply-colored fruits and vegetables contain higher amounts of protective phytochemicals.
   • Use the plate method - the biggest portion (half the plate) is where the vegetables go (excluding potatoes).

3) Choose whole grain carbohydrates and limit the portion sizes.
   • Choose carbs that are whole grain (requires chewing!), and aim for at least 25 grams of fiber per day.
   • Rx: double your vegetable intake, and halve your intake of refined carbohydrates (anything with flour and/or added sugar)!

4) Get your protein from plant sources such as legumes, nuts, and seeds, and/or choose lean, natural animal sources of protein in moderate amounts.

5) Spice it up! Include antiinflammatory herbs and spices such as garlic, turmeric, rosemary, ginger, oregano, cumin, and cayenne in your diet.

6) Eat mindfully
   • Be mindful of your food portions. Quality AND quantity matter. Regardless of how healthy your food choices are, excess calories from any source can increase inflammation and obesity.
   • Chew slowly and savor your food.

7) Adopt the Okinawan philosophy of *"hara hachi bu"*–stopping when nearly 8/10 full and paying attention to your hunger and satiety signals. Remember to focus on the whole diet pattern, not just components. Choose food that is closest to its natural form (i.e., less processed).

8) Best dietary advice in 7 words: "Eat food. Not too much. Mostly plants."

9) Adopt an antiinflammatory LIFESTYLE
   • Incorporate regular exercise that you enjoy into your life.
   • Keep weight under control. It is important to prevent and reduce obesity, especially abdominal obesity, as obesity itself sets up chronic inflammation in the body. Maintain body mass index (BMI) between 18.5–24.9.
   • Be aware of, and find healthy ways to reduce stress.

10) Enjoy 1-2 ounces of dark chocolate (at least 70%) as an occasional treat!

Eat more:	Eat less:
Foods high in omega-3 fats • Cold mater fish (Salmon, Spanish Mackerel, Anchovies, Sardines, Herring) • Flax seeds, flax oil, chia, or hemp seeds • Walnuts Vegetables • Yellow. orange, and red veggies (peppers, carrots, beets) • Dark leafy greens (spinach, kale, arugula, broccoli) Deeply-colored fruit • Berries, melons, citrus fruit Whole grains • Steel-cut or whole rolled cats • Sprouted-grain breads Antiinflammatory spices • Turmeric • Ginger • Rosemary • Oregano • Cayenne	Foods high in trans- and saturated fats • Processed and red meats • Dairy products • Partially hydrogenated oils Foods high in omega-6 fats (in order to get a better omega 6:3 ratio) • Corn, cottonseed, grapeseed, peanut, soy oils Refined carbohydrates (with a high glycemic load) • White breads or bagels • English muffins • Instant or white rice • Rice and corn cereals • Crackers, cookies, cakes Sodas and juices • Including "diet" drinks

Fig. 27.1 | **Patient Handout: Antiinflammatory Diet.** (From Kohatsu, W., & Karpowicz, S. [2018]. Antiinflammatory diet. In D. Rakel [Ed.], *Integrative medicine* [4th ed.]. St. Louis, MO: Elsevier.

day of headache pain ($P < .001$), and number of days per month headaches were experienced ($P < .02$) (Ramsden et al., 2013). From that study, it also was reported that there were significant increases in the antinociceptive n-3 pathway markers ($P < .001$). (See Chapter 26 for greater discussion of the role of PUFAs as a component of a multimodal analgesia [MMA] plan of care.)

Although it is clear there is potential benefit in following an antiinflammatory diet, there also is a need for additional research to more clearly identify the benefits for people living with chronic pain and the mechanisms by which the diet affects pain (De Von, Piano, Rosenfeld, & Hoppensteadt, 2014).

Cautions

Even though the antiinflammatory diet seems to be balanced and a reasonable dietary choice, it is important to remember that additional research is needed with regard to patients with chronic pain. One caution is that people living with chronic illnesses such as RA may already have poor nutrition, and new dietary restrictions could be harmful, particularly if adherence is selective or poor (Smedslund, Byfuglien, Olsen, & Hagen, 2010). It is prudent for anyone considering using the antiinflammatory diet as part of an MMA approach to pain management to discuss it with a clinician.

Ketogenic Diet

The ketogenic diet was originated by Dr. Russel Wilder in 1921 as a high-fat and low-carbohydrate diet by which ketone bodies were produced as a treatment for epilepsy in children (Wilder, 1921). It was based on the concept that fasting and minimal sugar intake best controlled epilepsy and that the ketogenic diet could accomplish a long-term starvation-like state with adequate nutrition through a formula with a ratio of 4 fats to 1 protein/carbohydrate combination (Messer & Kossoff, 2015).

Evidence for Pain Management

Reports of benefits of a ketogenic diet for painful conditions are variable (Totsch, Waite, & Sorge, 2015). When a ketogenic diet was fed to rats, they displayed less sensitivity to thermal pain (Ruskin, Suter, Ross, & Masino, 2013). Two months after a ketogenic diet was fed to mice with diabetic neuropathy, the neuropathy was considered reversed through gene expression and histology testing (Poplawski et al., 2011). When tested among people with neuropathic (sciatic nerve) pain, no analgesic effect was found (Masino & Ruskin, 2013).

Since the ketogenic diet was originally developed as a treatment for epilepsy, it is interesting that more positive results are seen in humans with headache. A ketogenic diet was effective in a very small group of patients (n = 5) with cluster headaches who reported no headaches after 1 month on

the ketogenic diet (Di Lorenzo, Coppola, Sirianni, Rossi, & Pierelli, 2015). The ketogenic diet was also effective with people experiencing migraine headaches (n = 16), with a reported reduction in the frequency of headaches from an average of 4.1 to 1.4 per month ($P < .001$) (Bracaglia, Coppola, Di Lorenzo, Di Lenola, & Pierelli, 2015). When used with adolescents who had migraine headaches (n = 16), there was marked attrition because of noncompliance (n = 5) with the treatment regimen and negative gastrointestinal effects (n = 2) (Farkas, Mak, Richter, & Farkas, 2014). In that study, there was variable benefit with the remaining (n = 9) participants because some reported a benefit (n = 3) and some reported marked benefit (n = 3), but no one was headache free during the 3-month study. It is not known why there was such disparity in the two studies using a ketogenic diet in people with migraines, but in the second study, it may at least in part be related to the metabolism of adolescent subjects. Clearly, additional research is needed to explore the potential benefit of the ketogenic diet for treatment of headache (Barbanti, Fofi, Aurilia, Egeo, & Caprio, 2017) and other painful conditions.

Cautions

Adverse effects, which can occur in up to half of people adhering to the ketogenic diet, include abdominal pain, nausea, vomiting, and constipation (Martin, Jackson, Levy, & Cooper, 2016; Messer & Kossoff, 2015). Additional adverse effects of the ketogenic diet reported in children include hypoglycemia, lethargy, and reluctance to eat (Lin, Turner, Doerrer, Stanfield, & Kossoff, 2017). Clearly, it is important for any person considering using the ketogenic diet as part of a multimodal pain management plan to review it with a clinician who is aware of any comorbidities the person may have. If it is used, it is also important for clinicians to guide patients to follow the ketogenic diet, which has evidence for pain management rather than any modifications that have been popularized for general weight loss.

Environmental Modifications

The hospital setting is the environment in which clinicians spend a large part of their lives, so it is easy to understand how clinicians can be unaware of the stress the hospital environment can cause patients. Yet, hospitals are environments with a multitude of noises, lights, odors, and temperatures that may be uncomfortable, unpleasant, or stressful to the patient and the patient's family (Roque & Carraro, 2015). It is difficult for people to control pain when they are physically uncomfortable, including when the environment around them is not conducive to their comfort.

Consideration of environmental factors when caring for patients dates to Florence Nightingale who wrote in *Notes on Nursing*: "the role of the nurse is to put the patient in the best possible condition for nature to act so healing can occur" (Nightingale, 1860). Her theory, principles, and methodology continue as central elements of nursing today (McDonald, 2014). Fundamental in Nightingale's metaparadigm theory is the interconnection of person, health, nursing, and environment, with one of her basic assumptions being that nursing care is accomplished through alteration of the environment (Rahim, 2013). As Helen Erickson (2015) described, when creating a nurturing space where healing and analgesia can occur, it is important to minimize sounds, odors, and lights that the patient finds uncomfortable or distracting.

What constitutes environmental comfort is specific for each person; thus there may be particular challenges in promoting comfort through modification of environmental factors when the hospital or facility room is shared with another person. When the differences in environmental preferences are significant and it is feasible to do so, changing the allocation of rooms to facilitate sharing of rooms by people with similar preferences can be very helpful.

Lighting

Illuminance is the degree of the perceived power of natural and artificial light per room or other area (Taneli & Kovach, 2015). Illuminance is individually appreciated, with some people wanting brighter lighting and others preferring softer or dimmer lighting (Quinlan-Colwell, 2012). Nonglare lights can improve comfort, particularly for older adults (Pappas, 2015). In hospital settings, lights may be bright, and frequently the control of lighting is not within the reach of the patient. Asking patients about their preference and respecting the preference as much as possible is important, as is turning bright lights off after using them for assessment or treatment. Creating quiet times when lights are dimmed is an intervention that can promote rest for patients, particularly in critical care areas where lights and noises can be excessive (Halm, 2016). In addition, blinds or shades can be adjusted to facilitate less brightness (De Giuli, Zecchin, Salmaso, Corain, & De Carli, 2013).

Being attentive to the location of equipment can be helpful for patients at night. Many pieces of equipment have bright indicator lights that can be disturbing to patients trying to sleep. Trying to arrange all equipment with indicator lights on one side of the room and turning lights off after an intervention may enable the patient to fall back to sleep and rest easier. It also may be difficult for patients to return to sleep after a nighttime intervention, if the lights are not turned off when the clinician leaves. For people who are sensitive to light, leaving the bathroom light on after emptying a catheter or urinal can interfere with being able to return to sleep. Recently a patient in one hospital had a large sign posted to the door of his room that read "Please turn the overhead light off before you leave."

Sound

Acoustic comfort is how contented from a sound perspective a person is within their environment (Taneli & Kovach, 2015). That comfort is significantly influenced by the intensity of sound. Conversely, *noise* is sound that is not wanted and is considered disagreeable (Memoli, Dawson, Barham & Grounds, 2012). As with light, sound appreciation and tolerance are individual and depend on quality of hearing ability and personal preference (Quinlan-Colwell, 2012). Acoustic comfort or discomfort can affect how comfortable the person feels (Pappas, 2015). Noise-induced stress can occur as a result of the sounds from various machines and equipment, closing doors, ice machines, and staff discussions (Halm, 2016; Memoli et al., 2012). Noise often interferes with sleeping and has been associated with poor patient satisfaction and impaired recovery (McGough et al., 2018; Memoli et al., 2012). When sounds cannot be identified, they can cause anxiety or even fear, as with a patient who is unfamiliar with a hospital tubing system and may perceive the clamor to be a gunshot or another frightening sound. Some patients are comforted by having a radio or television playing, whereas others find it annoying. For some patients, white noise, ambient sound, or relaxing sound machines may be helpful to increase acoustic comfort and help with pain control (Karakoç & Türker, 2014). Scheduling quiet times has been shown to improve patient satisfaction (McGough et al., 2018).

Temperature

The environmental temperature is an important factor in achieving patient comfort (Kolcaba, 2015). In an environment that is *thermally comfortable* there is no stress from feeling too warm or too cold (Wagner, Byrne, & Kolcaba, 2006). From an anecdotal perspective, it is not possible to be comfortable when the environment feels too warm or too cold. Environmental temperature preference is also highly individual, with some people preferring warmer temperatures and others preferring cooler ones (Khodakarami & Nasrollahi, 2012). Older adults, who often have less subcutaneous fat beneath thinning skin, are generally more sensitive to cooler temperatures and are less able to adjust their response to heat (Quinlan-Colwell, 2012). When there is significant reduction in heat, the person may feel anxious and have difficulty getting comfortable (O'Brien, Greenfield, Anderson, Smith, & Morris, 2010). Warmed blankets are an intervention that is welcomed by many patients, particularly in the perioperative area, as are *warming gowns, some with forced air* (Leeth, Mamaril, Oman, & Krumbach, 2010). When warmed blankets were compared preoperatively with patient-controlled warming gowns, both were effective for improved thermal comfort, but the patient-controlled warming gowns were also correlated with less anxiety before surgery

(Wagner, et al., 2006). Research is needed to better define the relationship between uncomfortable and comfortable environmental temperatures and pain control.

Position

Assisting patients into positions of comfort is a basic health care intervention. When patients have a certain position they prefer, helping them to achieve that position can increase their ability to better manage pain (Czarnecki et al., 2011; Drew et al., 2014; Quinlan-Colwell, 2012). Using pillows, towels, blankets, and assistive devices can be helpful in assisting patients to achieve and maintain a comfortable position (Quinlan-Colwell, 2012). Pillows can be placed to support the back of a side-lying patient, and patients can be taught to hold a pillow to support the surgical site.

Although positioning for comfort seems to be something that patients may intuitively know, there are instances when patients need education regarding how to position themselves to optimize pain control. An example of this is lying in a left lateral position after a colonoscopy to facilitate passing flatus, thus relieving bloating and pain (Devitt, Shellman, Gardner, & Wemett, 2011). Another example is seen in patients with headaches of an orthostatic origin. The patient may experience increased pain intensity when in an upright position but pain being eased when in a recumbent position (Ali, Singh, Hassan, & Naqash, 2017). Educating laboring women about position is important because certain maternal positions during different stages of labor are correlated with reduced length of labor and better pain control (Mertz & Earl, 2018).

Evidence for Pain Management

The importance of coordinating an environment that is pleasant and comfortable for the patient and thus conducive to controlling pain seems reasonable and is supported by anecdotal information; however, no specific evidence or research on this topic could be found. Clearly, research is needed to provide evidence-based support of the importance of improving patient comfort through environmental efforts to promote pain reduction (Krinsky, Murillo, & Johnson, 2014). Research is also needed to explore the potential analgesic benefit of chairs and beds that are designed to prevent skin breakdown by being programmed to trigger the person to move and change position (Smith & Cooper, 2006). This is another area that is most appropriate for nursing research.

Caution

The only caution in modifying the environment to be most comfortable for the patient is rather than assuming what the patient prefers, ask the patient what he or she prefers for light, sound, temperature, and position. Adjustments then can be made congruent with the preferences of the patient whenever possible. Thus, rather than following the golden rule: *do unto others as you would have them do unto you,* the patient will be more comfortable and better able to control pain when following the *platinum rule* which advises: *do unto others what they would have you do unto them* (Geller, 2015). With the platinum rule applied, the patient will be able to be more comfortable congruent with his or her preferences and hopefully better able to control pain.

Hypnosis

Hypnosis has a long, intricate history dating back to the ancient Roman temples of Aesculapius and then progressing through the 18th-century influence of Mesmer into the 19th century with Charcot and Freud, to the 20th-century work of Hilgard and Milton Erickson (Kihlstrom, 2016; Norelli, 2009; Peter, 2015). The Hypnosis Definition Committee of the Division 30 of the American Psychological Association most recently officially defined hypnosis as "a state of consciousness involving focused attention and reduced peripheral awareness characterized by an enhanced capacity for response to suggestion" (American Psychological Association, 2019, p. 5). It is more simply defined as "the art of creating an alternative reality by imagination, which ideally should be experienced like a hallucination or illusion" (Peter, 2015, p. 458). Hypnosis incorporates a number of components, such as relaxation, focused attention, imagery or visualization, interpersonal processing, and suggestion. There continue to be differences in expert opinion regarding which of these elements represents the core component(s) of hypnosis, making it difficult to determine if a specific treatment should be classified as hypnosis or not.

Hypnosis is also described as a social interactive process during which the hypnotist offers suggestions of imaginative experiences to the subject (the person undergoing hypnosis), who responds to them (Kihlstrom, 2016). Those suggestions involve modifications of perception, memory, and the voluntary control of the person over actions. The hypnotist guides the person being hypnotized to respond to suggestions for modification in what is being experienced by changing how it is sensed and perceived and how the person feels, thinks, or responds to the experience (Brugnoli, 2014). Although the hypnotist leads the process, the effectiveness of hypnosis is less related to the technique or skill of the hypnotist than to the ability and capacity of the person experiencing hypnosis to be absorbed in the experience, and in that very important sense "all hypnosis is self-hypnosis" (Kihlstrom, 2016, p. 362). The person experiencing hypnosis must allow it to occur and for the experience to be fully experienced (Peter, 2015). In that sense, the person must relinquish conscious control of his or her physical reality, and dissociate from it, to allow the hypnotic trance state to become real. The quality of the hypnotic trance response depends on several qualities (Peter, 2015) (Box 27.5).

Hypnosis is used in clinical settings to help manage pain related to a variety of acute pain situations, including burns, childbirth, and procedures (e.g., bone marrow aspiration, dental work) (Kihlstrom, 2016) with little to moderate documented effectiveness (Tefikow et al., 2013). Hypnosis is also used in management of chronic pain, cancer-related pain, disability, and palliative care (Brugnoli, 2014). It is thought that two critical factors influencing the ability to successfully use hypnosis to control pain are the suggestibility of the person being hypnotized or their hypnotizability and the particular characteristics of the pain involved (Peter, 2015). *Hypnotizability* describes the ease with which a person can be hypnotized or their capacity to enter into a hypnotic trance (Brugnoli, 2014) (see Box 27.5).

Evidence for Pain Management

Although hypnosis has been used for centuries across cultures to treat all types of painful conditions (Pintar & Lynn, 2009), evidence supporting the use of hypnosis in pain management has become more robust over the last 20 years. This is seen with the application of hypnosis to chronic pain with the reduction of sensory pain and suffering through the process of hypnotic suggestion known as *hypnotic analgesia* (Kihlstrom, 2016). Recent advances in understanding arose from studies examining brain functions associated with hypnosis and hypnotic

analgesia (Barabasz & Barabasz, 2008; Oakley, 2008; Oakley & Halligan, 2010). As the 21st century began, it was proposed that the physiology of hypnotic analgesia was similar to that of distraction of attention; however, that hypothesis was not supported by laser electrocortical testing (Friederich et al., 2001). In a more recent study evaluating laser-evoked potentials in the brains of people with chronic pain, the amplitude changes during hypnosis were again different from those during relaxation and distraction (Matinella et al., 2017). This supports using hypnosis in conjunction with relaxation and distraction as part of an MMA plan of care.

The authors of a meta-analysis of functional neuroimaging studies of human brains during hypnotic analgesic suggestions (HASs) (n = 8 studies; n = 75 subjects) noted during painful stimulation that HASs were associated with significant activation of cortical and subcortical cerebral activity and inhibition of the thalamus (Del Casale et al., 2015). These areas of the brain are also involved in the nociceptive process; therefore it is reasonable that there can be an analgesic effect. The authors of that study concluded the neuroimaging is confirmatory of the use of hypnosis as an analgesic intervention. (See Chapter 3 for discussion of the nociception process.) In a more recent study (n = 57) using fMRI, during hypnosis reduced activity was noted in the dorsal anterior cingulate cortex (ACC), with increased connectivity recorded between the dorsolateral prefrontal cortex and the insula, which is consistent with the observable characteristics of a person in a hypnotic trance (Jiang, White, Greicius, Waelde, & Spiegel, 2017). The decreased activity in the ACC is important from an analgesic perspective. The researchers of a small study with men with irritable bowel syndrome (n = 15) conducted dopamine receptor imaging during hypnotic analgesia (Fukudo et al., 2014). Those researchers reported that their data suggested dopamine release in the brain was induced by hypnosis in the presence of visceral sensory inputs.

People living with a variety of chronic pain conditions have been helped with hypnosis. In a meta-analysis of research studies using hypnosis to treat chronic pain situations (n = 12 studies), the authors concluded hypnosis had good efficacy compared to wait-list control as an intervention to treat chronic pain (Adachi, Fujino, Nakae, Mashimo, & Sasaki1, 2014). Those authors also concluded there were larger effect sizes with hypnosis compared with other psychological treatments for chronic pain that is not headache related. They also noted that hypnosis and other psychological treatments can coexist within a multimodal approach for managing chronic pain. Recently hypnosis was used to treat the persistent pain involved with burns. After 4 sessions, hypnosis was found to be effective in reducing the pain intensity of daily chronic pain and pain-related anxiety (Jafarizadeh, Lotfi, Ajoudani, Kiani, & Alinejad, 2018). A small (n = 20) but important study done in France evaluated the use of hypnosis before physical therapy in people with complex

---

| **Box 27.5** | Variables Influencing Quality of the Hypnotic Response |

- The degree to which the person being hypnotized possesses hypnotic suggestibility or hypnotizability
- Presence and depth of the trance state
- Type of hypnotic phenomenon that is intended to occur
- The wording and way suggestions intended to achieve the phenomenon are presented
- Factors related to the setting in which suggestions are offered
- Motivation and expectations of the person experiencing hypnosis
- Quality and type of relationship between the hypnotherapist and the person being hypnotized
- The skills and rapport of the hypnotherapist

From Peter, B. (2015). *Hypnosis: International encyclopedia of the social & behavioral sciences* (2nd ed., Vol. 11.). Oxford, U.K.: Elsevier. Retrieved May 12, 2018 from https://doi.org/10.1016/B978-0-08-097086-8.21069-6; *International encyclopedia of the social & behavioral sciences* (2nd ed., Vol. 11). Oxford, U.K. https://doi.org/10.1016/B978-0-08-097086-8.21069-6.

regional pain syndrome (CRPS) of the hands and wrists (Lebon, Rongières, Apredoaei, Delclaux, & Mansat, 2017). After an average of 5.4 sessions, the results of that work were impressive, with improvement noted in functional pain scores, physical function, and patient satisfaction. In addition, 80% of the participants of that study returned to work while pain intensity and analgesic requirements decreased. In a three-arm study with people living with chronic pain (n = 415), psychoeducation plus physiotherapy (n = 169) was compared with self-hypnosis plus self-care education (n = 157) and controls who had no intervention (n = 89) (Vanhaudenhuyse et al., 2018). In that study, people in both intervention groups had improvements in pain; however, those in the self-hypnosis group also had less disability and reported an awareness of being able to use hypnosis to manage pain rather than relying on analgesic medications.

Hypnosis is also used effectively with acute pain. A meta-analysis was done of RCTs using hypnosis among people having surgery or medical procedures (n = 34 RCTs; n = 2597 subjects) (Tefikow et al., 2013). Although in that analysis positive effects were reported for pain, emotional distress, medication consumption, procedure time, and recovery when hypnosis was used, the internal validity of the individual RCTs was considered limited because of methodologic flaws. Although it has rarely been used in the ED, a novel acute care use of hypnosis is in the ED, where many procedures are performed (Iserson, 2014) (Box 27.6).

Hypnosis is considered a common intervention to help manage pain involved with the care of burn wounds (Meyer et al., 2017). Barber's Rapid Induction Analgesia (RIA) technique for quickly eliciting relaxation and analgesia is commonly used with people undergoing burn wound care (Barber, 1977; Scheffler, Koranyi, Meissner, Straub, & Rosendahl, 2018). An alternative method is for hypnosis to be done before the wound care, with nurses giving posthypnotic suggestions during the procedure (Meyer et al., 2017). The results of a meta-analysis of nonpharmacologic interventions for people to manage pain during wound care of burns (n = 21 studies), showed hypnosis and distraction, particularly virtual reality distraction (see Chapter 21) had the largest effect sizes in controlling pain during the painful wound care (Scheffler et al., 2018).

Hypnosis has been used in combination with virtual reality (see Chapter 21). One advantage to this combination intervention is that a hypnotist does not need to be present. A second advantage may be that because images are supplied and presented, the person undergoing hypnosis does not need to conceptualize the alternative state (Meyer et al., 2017). Research is needed to identify if there is a difference in effect or results of traditional hypnosis, in which an important component is the person imagining the cues, compared with the virtual hypnosis, in which the cues are presented similar to a distraction. The use of virtual reality hypnosis also needs to be studied with a variety of acute, procedural, and chronic pain situations.

Research has begun to study the neuroscience involved with hypnosis and the effect on the brain, but more work is needed, including on the relationships among hypnosis, nociception, pain sensation, and analgesia (De Benedittis, 2015; Del Casale et al., 2015). Research with strong methodology is needed to explore the role of hypnosis with both chronic pain conditions (Kihlstrom, 2016), including pain related to cancer (Wortzel & Spiegel, 2017), and acute pain situations (e.g., surgery, procedures) (Tefikow et al., 2013). Considering the number of procedures for which hypnosis has been effective that are routinely done in the ED, use of hypnosis in that setting is promising and warrants research (Iserson, 2014).

Caution

Hypnosis is considered safe with rare negative effects, that include thoughts, feelings, or behaviors the person does not want to experience and occasional nausea, dizziness, or headaches (Norelli, 2009).

Mirror Therapy or Mirror Visual Feedback Therapy

Mirror visual feedback therapy (MVFT) or mirror therapy was presented by Ramachandran and Rogers-Ramachandran (1992) as an intervention to treat patients with limbs affected by chronic central pain and hemiparesis resulting from a stroke. Mirror therapy is a simple and noninvasive therapeutic technique in which a mirror or mirror box is used to reflect movement or stimulation of an unaffected limb corresponding to a painful or paralyzed limb (Ramachandran & Altschuler, 2009; Ramachandran, & Rogers-Ramachandran, 2000) (Fig. 27.2). Today, in addition to the original indications,

---

Box 27.6	Potential Benefits of Using Hypnosis in the Emergency Department

- It is safe with no serious risks.
- Time for onset of use is short.
- It can be readily available (particularly with virtual reality hypnosis).
- It is cost effective.
- Minimal clinicians are needed.
- No equipment is needed unless virtual reality system is used.
- Patients in any age group are appropriate.
- There is a potential for reduced cost of patient care.

From Iserson, K. V. (2014). An hypnotic suggestion: Review of hypnosis for clinical emergency care. *The Journal of Emergency Medicine*, 46(4), 588–596.

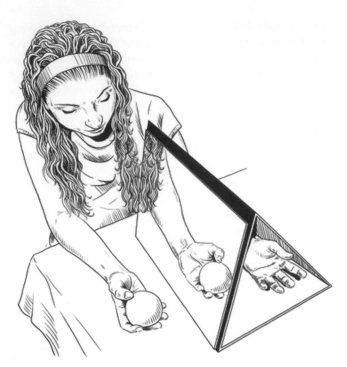

Fig. 27.2 | **Mirror Box Therapy.** (From Liebenson, C. [2012]. Musculoskeletal myths. *Journal of Bodywork & Movement Therapies*, 16[2], 165–182.)

mirror therapy is increasingly used with people living with phantom limb pain (PLP) and CRPS (Al Sayegh et al, 2013; Barbin, Seetha, Casillas, Paysant, & Perennou, 2016; Ramachandran & Altschuler, 2009).

Mirror therapy uses a large mirror placed in a sagittal position in the middle of a box from which the top and one side have been removed (see Fig. 27.2). With the painful or phantom limb placed behind the mirror, the person sees a reflection of the unaffected limb in the mirror that is in the location of the painful or phantom limb, generating an illusion of the painful or phantom limb being healthy and intact. As the unaffected limb moves, the person perceives the painful or phantom limb also moving with the impression that it is functioning in response to commands to move (Ramachandran & Altschuler, 2009).

Evidence for Pain Management

The authors of a systematic review (n = 20 studies) of mirror therapy used with patients with phantom limbs after amputation concluded there is insufficient evidence to recommend mirror therapy as a treatment for PLP (Barbin et al., 2016). One of the challenges evaluating the benefit of mirror therapy with people with PLP is that the studies are generally small. Nevertheless, the results are often compelling. Two small studies were done with soldiers at the Walter Reed and Brooke Army Medical Centers (WRBAC) who had amputations. In the first study, participants with lower extremity amputations (n = 29) received mirror therapy each day for 4 weeks (Griffin,

Curran, Pasquina, & Tsao, 2015). The soldiers in that study who reported baseline visual analogue score (VAS) pain less than 60 (n = 19) reported dramatic reductions in pain after 1 week of mirror therapy and those with baseline VAS scores greater than 60 (n = 10) reported significant reduction ($P < .003$) in pain after 2 or more weeks of mirror therapy. That indicates that although more sessions with mirror therapy are needed when pain intensity is greater, it can still be effective to reduce pain and improve function. This time factor may be an important consideration both when educating about mirror therapy and when conducting research with it. In the second small study at WRBAC, the soldiers volunteered to participate in mirror therapy (n = 9) for 15 minutes, or 5 days per week for 4 weeks, or be in a control group (n = 6) (Finn et al., 2017). In that study the men who underwent mirror therapy reported significant decreases in pain intensity ($P < .002$) and frequency of pain ($P < .003$). Compared to transcutaneous electrical nerve stimulation (TENS) (n = 13) (see Chapter 20), mirror therapy (n = 13) was equally effective over 4 days for people with PLP, with significantly less pain in both groups after the interventions (Tilak et al., 2016). When fMRI analysis was used with people who had PLP using mirror therapy over 4 weeks, the fMRI data showed in the primary somatosensory cortex a reversal of dysfunctional cortical organization and less activity in the inferior parietal cortex after mirror therapy (Foell, Bekrater-Bodmann, Diers, & Flor, 2014). Since these are areas of the brain involved with pain perception (Wang et al., 2019), additional investigation is needed with mirror therapy.

The authors of a review of the literature (n = 9 studies) concluded that mirror therapy is an intervention with positive benefits for pain reduction and motor function improvement among people living with CRPS (Al Sayegh et al., 2013). Most of the research using mirror therapy with people who live with CRPS was done in those who have CRPS type 1, in which there is no evidence of nerve injury; very few were done in those who have CRPS type 2, in which the pain syndrome occurs after injury of a major nerve (Al Sayegh et al., 2013; Breivik, Allen, & Stubhaug, 2013). In a fairly early study using mirror therapy with people with CRPS type 1 (n = 48), those who received mirror therapy had significant reductions in pain intensity and allodynia ($P < .001$) and there were statistically significant differences in those areas when compared to controls at 6-month follow-up ($P < .001$) (Cacchio, De Blasis, De Blasis, Santilli, & Spacca, 2009). When mirror therapy was used with people who had a stroke and also had CRPS type 1 (n = 30), the patients who received standard rehabilitation therapy mirror therapy for 2 to 4 hours on 5 days per week plus mirror therapy for 4 weeks reported significantly less pain ($P < .03$) and greater mobility ($P < .001$) compared to patients who received standard rehabilitation therapy without mirror therapy (Vural, Yuzer, Ozcan, Ozbudak, & Ozgirgin, 2016).

Mirror Visual Feedback Therapy and Other Chronic Pain Conditions

MVFT is being used with chronic pain conditions other than PLP and CRPS. When used with patients (n = 69) who had chronic pain with limited range of motion, patients experienced significant reduction in pain intensity ($P = .014$), less pain catastrophizing ($P < .001$), and kinesiophobia ($P = .012$), with significant improvement in flexion on active range of motion ($P < .001$) (Louw et al., 2017). MVFT was used with patients who had chronic post-stroke pain (n = 40) with some benefit in function and some nonsignificant pain reduction with repeated interventions (Michielsen et al., 2011).

Virtual Reality Mirror Visual Feedback Therapy

A contemporary and future use of mirror therapy is in coordination with electronics and telehealth. *Virtual reality mirror visual feedback therapy* (VRMVFT) is a very exciting advancement in mirror therapy in which movements can be specifically addressed and the patient can be more fully immersed in the experience (Sato et al, 2010) (Fig. 27.3). When used in a very small study in Japan with patients with CRPS, four of the five participants reported more than 50% less pain intensity, with two of them stopping treatment after the five beneficial interventions and not completing the course of eight sessions (Sato et al., 2010). VRMVFT was used in a pilot study with three

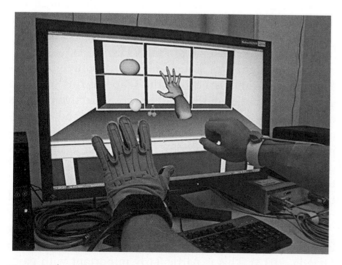

Fig. 27.3 | A personal computer–based desktop virtual reality system for mirror visual feedback therapy. The arm on the affected side *(right)* and the targets appear in the virtual environment. Finger motion is simulated by the CyberGlove on the nonaffected side *(left)* and arm motion is simulated by FASTRAK on the affected side. (From Sato, K., Fukumori, S., Matsusaki, T., Maruo, T., Ishikawa, S., Nishie, H., & Matsumi, M. [2010]. Nonimmersive virtual reality mirror visual feedback therapy and its application for the treatment of complex regional pain syndrome: An open-label pilot study. *Pain Medicine, 11*[4], 622–629.)

patients diagnosed with RA of the wrists who reported improvement in function with some analgesic benefit as well (Choi, Heo, Hwang, & Koo, 2016). Although use of MVFT and VRMVFT is reported most often in people with chronic pain, an innovative study in Korea used VRMVFT with patients (n = 22) after total knee arthroplasty (Koo, et al, 2015). In that study there were impressive reductions in pain intensity and improvements in movement (Koo et al., 2015). In one feasibility study, use of VRMVFT in conjunction with participating in a virtual reality game was evaluated (Ortiz-Catalan, Sander, Kristoffersen, Håkansson, & Brånemark, 2014). In that study VRMVFT was effective in relieving pain and restoring active movement of a residual upper limb of a person who had not been able to move the limb for nearly 50 years. With VRMVFT he had a telescopic effect of perceiving his hand in an anatomically correct position (Ortiz-Catalan et al., 2014).

Research with VRMVFT is young, with interesting and exciting findings being reported. One aspect that calls for more research is that the distance between the corporal limb and the virtual limb seems to affect the degree of analgesic effect (Nierula, Martini, Matamala-Gomez, Slater, & Sanchez-Vives, 2017). Another area of potential interest is in VRMVFT being used with PLP that is particularly promising for people who have bilateral amputations. In traditional MT, it is necessary for the person to have an intact contralateral limb, but that is not necessary with VRMVFT (Gackenbach, Wijeyaratnam, & Flockhart, 2017).

Mirror Visual Feedback Therapy in Home Settings

The feasibility of using VRMVFT was tested in the home setting (n = 7) using a head-mounted display set (Trojan et al., 2014). The participants between the ages of 22 and 53 reported no technical difficulties and demonstrated improvements in hand movement. Two patients with PLP successfully used mirror therapy at home after they electronically received detailed instructions from the clinician (Gover-Chamlou & Tsao, 2016). Both patients had complete resolution of pain within 8 weeks. The Patient Centered Telerehabilitation (PACT) study is a multicenter RCT conducted in Germany and the Netherlands to assess the effect of mirror therapy on PLP in the context of telerehabilitation (McAuley, 2015). It is expected the results of the PACT study will increase the evidence on mirror therapy using mirror therapy in the context of telehealth.

Mirror Visual Feedback Therapy and Referred Sensations

Referred sensation is an unusual phenomenon that occurs when a person with a phantom limb experiences the sense of being touched on the phantom limb when a different part of the body receives sensory stimulation, which can occur regardless of whether the person generally experiences phantom sensations (Collins et al., 2017). In a very small study using virtual reality technology (n = 9) participants with PLP repeatedly touched an object with a virtual limb representing the phantom limb while the corresponding facial cheek was touched (Ichinose et al., 2017). When compared to controls, the participants who participated in the intervention had significantly greater reduction in pain (P < .05). Additional study of virtual mirror therapy among people with referred sensations is needed. To improve the quantity and quality of evidence, additional research with good methodology and larger sample sizes is needed to determine the benefit of MT with PLP and phantom limb mobility (Barbin et al., 2016). The variations between studies warrants further research, as do potential adverse effects of mirror therapy (Hagenberg & Carpenter, 2014).

Cautions for Using Mirror Visual Feedback Therapy

All jewelry needs to be removed and tattoos or scars on the unaffected limb need to be covered to not cause confusion in the mirror image (Rothgangel, Braun, Witte, Beurskens, & Smeets, 2016). Such covering could be done by applying an opaque stocking or glove over the scars or tattoos.

Untoward or adverse effects reported after mirror therapy tend to be mild and tend to resolve after a few sessions (Rothgangel et al., 2016). The adverse effects include increase in physical pain, sensory alterations, freezing temperature sensation in the phantom limb, boredom, emotional responses, depression, grief reactions, dizziness, diaphoresis, and nausea and vomiting, with some type of emotional response being most common followed by an increase in pain (Hagenberg & Carpenter, 2014; Rothgangel et al., 2016). To address or minimize the chance of these occurring, it is important to advise patients of the possibility of adverse events occurring and be prepared for the possibility of them doing so. It is advisable to have blankets available to minimize any sensation of freezing of the phantom limb (Hagenberg & Carpenter, 2014). It is recommended that patients be assessed before participating in mirror therapy to ensure that they have adequate strength to control the trunk of their body, do not have pain in the intact limb, and are psychologically appropriate for mirror therapy (Rothgangel et al., 2016). In addition, it is important to remember that this therapy is not necessarily helpful for all patients with pain. As noted, MVFT has been reported to increase pain for at least some people living with fibromyalgia syndrome (McCabe, Cohen, & Blake, 2007) and in at least some people who had whiplash-associated disorder (Daenen, et al, 2012).

Obesity and Weight Management

When caloric intake is greater than caloric expenditure, the consequence is an increase in fat storage and body weight or obesity (Arranz, 2017; Rodgers, 2017), which is a disproportionate accumulation of fat in adipose tissue (Okifuji & Hare, 2015). Obesity negatively affects quality of life, including sleep, activity, pain intensity, and pain relief (Thomazeau et al., 2014).

Based on available evidence it is clear that reduction in weight is a crucial and fundamental intervention for any patient with chronic musculoskeletal pain who is overweight or obese (Aaboe, Bliddal, Messier, Alkjaer, & Henriksen, 2011).

With data from the most recent state of U.S. health (1990-2010), it was estimated that poor dietary choices and practices were the leading risk factor contributing to marked disability with more than 70,000 associated deaths (Murray, 2013). More recent data from Centers for Disease Control and Prevention (CDC) identified at least 72 million people in the United States as obese with the cost for health care for each of those individuals being $1429.00 more per year compared to individuals who are not obese (CDC, 2019).

It is estimated that the cost of health conditions related to obesity annually consumes more than 200 billion health care dollars for adult Americans (Okifuji & Hare, 2015). The range of a normal BMI is between 18.5 and 25.0 and there are a number of grades of obesity for BMI greater than 25.0 (National Center for Health Statistics [NCHS], 2017). Data from 2016 shows that more than 71% of women and more than 76% of men between 65 and 74 years of age are overweight or obese, with more than 35% of each group having a BMI greater than 30.0 (NCHS, 2017).

The exploration of potentially effective weight management programs is beyond the scope of this book. In addition, the program that will be most effective depends on patient-specific characteristics, abilities, and willingness to change. Some patients may need behavior modification programs in addition to education in nutritious diet and exercise (Okifuji & Hare, 2015). Clinicians need to discuss the importance of reducing weight and maintaining a healthy body mass index (BMI) to help control pain and numerous other health-related conditions.

Maintaining a recommended BMI is an important component to effective pain control (Kieser, et al., 2019; Lozada, 2013). This is particularly important with painful musculoskeletal conditions, including low back pain (LBP) (NIH, 2014) and OA of the knees when obesity causes varus or valgus malalignments (Lozada, 2013). With advancing age, OA becomes more frequently diagnosed, with approximately 50% of older adults living with the condition (Glover et al., 2015). Weight loss can help prevent musculoskeletal disorders such as OA and can reduce pain and disability (Lozada, 2013; Perlman et al., 2018). Even a 10% reduction in weight can help to

Box 27.7	Clinical Application: A Weight Loss Experience

I have been overweight since I was 5 years old. My mother can remember me saying to my grandmother, "Me-maw I'm bored; can I have a sandwich?"

I don't remember physical pain when I was younger, but there was definitely a lot of emotional pain from bullying and not fitting in with others or in a Brownie uniform and unable to perform activities in gym like rope climbing.

Physical pain came much later. The first time I remember having physical pain from being overweight was when I worked 12-hour shifts in an ICU after nursing school. I had reached my all-time high weight of 420 pounds and developed plantar fasciitis and a bone spur in my heel. I was also unable to groom myself properly at that point.

I had gastric bypass surgery, and the first thing I noticed after losing weight aside from increased energy was the absence of pain, and it was exhilarating!! I had decreased pain in my feet and knees mainly, but also my back. I had no idea how the presence of daily pain affected my life until it was no longer present!

Denise Kuhn, MSN, RN, CPHQ

reduce the load on lower knee joints and improve walking (Messier et al., 2011). Box 27.7 presents a clinical application of the effect of obesity and weight reduction with chronic pain.

Evidence for Pain Management

A number of factors have been linked to the pain and obesity relationship (Arranz, 2017; Okifuji & Hare, 2015). Both chronic pain and obesity can limit function and activity, which can lead to increased obesity and pain in a circular pattern (Arranz, 2017). Socioeconomic and lifestyle factors are associated with obesity. Characteristics of patients at nine integrative medicine centers (n = 2015) revealed that when compared to patients of normal weight or underweight (n = 1135), and even to those who were overweight (n = 580), patients who were obese (n = 300) were more likely to be nonwhite, single, and uninsured, with lower income, at least one chronic comorbidity, and greater pain intensity (Yang et al., 2017). From a preventive perspective, lifestyle changes, including healthy diet choices, maintaining a low BMI, and adequate physical activity of at least 30 minutes per day can be employed to improve health (Tick, 2015). From a public health perspective, the provision of education and avenues through which people who are at high risk for obesity and chronic pain can learn and be supported in achieving a healthy weight are warranted. Prevention and treatment of obe-

sity are important health care imperatives that can literally prevent a lifetime of pain. A longitudinal British study (n = 1866) assessed weight and back pain at 20, 30, 40, and 50 years of age and found that obesity and increased abdominal girth were correlated with radiating LBP (Frilander et al., 2015).

The relationship between obesity and chronic pain may be grounded in physiology and body chemistry. Recent research indicates that nociceptive sensitivity may be different in the presence of obesity (Rodgers, 2017). It is known there is an association and similar pathologic processes between obesity and increased inflammation (De Von et al., 2014; Seaman, 2013). Obese rats that were stimulated with noxious stimuli displayed increased sensitivity to pain and an increased inflammatory response, which may indicate obesity is a type of low-grade inflammatory disorder, and, as a result, responses to other inflammatory situations are increased (Iannitti, Graham, & Dolan, 2012). Glover et al. (2015) noted that obese individuals with pain from OA of the knee had lower than normal levels of vitamin D; however, the underlying mechanism of this is not known. It is possible excess weight limits exercise and time spent out of doors and sun exposure, which could result in lower levels of vitamin D (Glover et al., 2015). The degree of obesity also seems to be a factor in pain, with obese older adults being twice as likely as their lean counterparts to have chronic pain, and those who were severely obese with a BMI greater than 40 kg/m^2 being more than four-fold more likely to have chronic pain (Rodgers, 2017). However, the relationship between pain and obesity is not limited to older adults with arthritis. The relationship is also seen in young adults, teens, and children as young as 3 years old (Deere et al., 2012; Okifuji & Hare, 2015; Smith, Sumar, & Dixon, 2014).

Reducing weight is shown to have positive benefit among people living with chronic pain. The investigators of a 2011 Danish study reported that during a 4-month weight loss program participants (n = 157) reduced their weight by an average of 13.7 kg (~30 lb), which corresponded to an average 13.5% loss of baseline weight (Aaboe et al., 2011). In that study, the participants also experienced a 7% reduction in knee joint loading, with 13% reduction in axial impulse and 12% less abductor movement of the internal knees with statistically significant ($P < .0001$) less pain intensity reported.

Research is needed to better understand the factors involved in the relationship between obesity and pain (Glover et al., 2015; Okifuji & Hare, 2015) and the relationships among obesity, pain, inflammation, and cytokines (De Von et al., 2014). How dietary modification and nutrition can be used to best help patients who are obese and experience pain needs to be better understood (Rodgers, 2017). There is a definite need to research which weight reduction methods are most effective for people living with chronic pain and how best to motivate them to comply with weight reduction methods (Yang et al., 2017).

Cautions

No specific cautions were found for reducing weight among people who are overweight. However, it seems reasonable to ensure that the method of weight loss is medically sound with adequate nutrition and consideration of any comorbidity dietary requirements.

Static Magnet Therapy

Static magnet therapy in the form of rings, bracelets, and necklaces to treat arthritis has a long history dating back to the Greeks during the first century CE to treat arthritis and continued through the Middle Ages (Basford, 2001). Today magnets are also available in insoles for shoes, as bandages, and in mattress pads. Contrasted with electromagnets, static magnets have magnetic fields that do not change within a therapeutic range of 300 to 5000 gauss (G) (the unit by which magnetic fields are measured). No possible mechanism of action for how magnets might be effective to control pain has been identified. The most plausible theory is that in some way they cause an increase in blood flow by action on charged ions; however, physiologically this does not seem likely and there is no evidence to support it (Malone & Gloyer, 2013; Millis & Levine, 2014; NIH, 2013).

Evidence for Pain Management

It is theorized that magnets are effective in controlling pain through reducing conduction of nerves and depolarization; however, physiologically it is thought this would require a far stronger magnetic field (24 T) than is used therapeutically (Millis & Levine, 2014). Although the efficacy of magnets has been studied in a variety of models since the 1600s in both humans and animals, high-quality evidence and research are limited (Millis & Levine, 2014; Wells, Baute, & Wahbeh, 2017). Research results are also inconsistent. An older research study with people with post-polio syndrome pain (n = 50) reported significant differences ($P < .0001$) in pain relief among those who received magnet therapy (Vallbona, Hazlewood & Jurida, 1997). However, since that study, there has been little benefit reported. The authors of a systematic review (n = 9 studies) concluded static magnet therapy is not supported by evidence as an effective pain treatment (Pittler, Brown, & Ernst, 2007). In a 12-week study (n = 194), people with OA of the knee or hip who wore magnetic bracelets (170 to 200 mT strength) reported changes in pain intensity. However, another study using magnetic bracelets for OA symptoms, including pain, showed no benefit (Malone & Gloyer, 2013). Positive effects were reported when magnet therapy was combined with walking in people with OA (Lozada, 2013). When magnetic knee sleeves were compared to nonmagnetic sleeves in people with OA of the knee (n = 29), pain relief was noted at four hours, but there were no significant differences in pain relief at 6 weeks (Malone & Gloyer, 2013; Lozada, 2013). Yet, small studies have shown that magnet therapy reduced pain in patients with carpal tunnel syndrome (Wells et al., 2017). Static magnet therapy was used when dental pain was induced in mice that were placed within a static magnet field; the researchers concluded that it could be effective to control dental pain in mice (Zhu et al., 2017). Much more research with rigorous methodology is needed to establish dosing, duration, and benefit for pain management with magnet therapy (Millis & Levine, 2014; Wells et al., 2017).

Cautions

There are no known major negative or adverse effects associated with magnet therapy; however, magnets should not be used by people with pacemakers, insulin pumps, or other electronic devices (Malone & Gloyer, 2013; Millis & Levine, 2014; NIH, 2013). It is important to also not use static magnets as a replacement or to delay assessment and treatment of pain (NIH, 2013). The National Center for Complementary and Integrative Health noted that although static magnets are frequently sold for pain control, there is no scientific evidence that they are effective to relieve pain (NIH, 2013).

Temperature Modalities

Temperature therapy, either superficial heat or cold, is generally most effective when used with joints close to the skin, such as wrists, ankles, elbows, knees, and shoulders (Lozada, 2013). Temperature changes will also occur more quickly in people with less subcutaneous tissue (Galloway, 2017). It is thought that by exciting the thermoreceptors transmitting messages to the dorsal horn by either heat or cold change in temperature may impede transmission of pain stimuli (Galloway, 2017).

Therapeutic Superficial Heat

Therapeutic heat is another analgesic modality with ancient origins (Petrofsky et al., 2013). It can be implemented through warm soaks, heating pads, hot water bags, hot packs, hot gel packs (hydrocollator packs), heat wraps, paraffin baths, heat mittens, fluid therapy, heat lamps and whirlpool baths, heated swimming pools, showers in temperatures no greater than 45° C (113° F) for 30 minutes or less to increase circulation, relieve pain, ease muscle spasms, decrease stiffness of joints, and help with preventing contractures (Ahmad-Shirvani & Ganji, 2016; Alvarado-García & Salazar-Maya, 2017; Benny, Grabois, & Chan, 2014; Corti, 2014; Galloway, 2017; Lozada, 2013; Perlman et al., 2018). Warm baths are a frequent self care intervention for people living with sickle cell disease. Homemade hot packs are made with rice or beans placed in a cloth such as a sock then slightly heated in the microwave (Corti, 2014). It is important to avoid extreme temperatures, including prolonged microwave heating. As with all sources of heat, a towel should be placed between the hot pack and the skin.

Superficial heat is effective through increasing vasodilatation, facilitating an increase in oxygen, nutrients, metabolites, and enzyme activities, and improving extensibility and pliability of tissue (Corti, 2014; Galloway, 2017). Superficial heat can also facilitate increased range of motion (Szekeres, MacDermid, Grewal, & Birmingham, 2017). Recent research suggests that tissue repair may be accelerated through enhancement of angiogenic (stimulation of or formation of blood vessels) and myogenic (smooth muscle activity) expression (Kim et al., 2017).

The analgesic effect of heat is thought to be the result of mediation by calcium channels, which are heat sensitive and cause an increase in intracellular calcium (Petrofsky et al., 2013). It is thought that heat can affect structures distant from the skin through conduction heating (Arankalle, Wardle, & Nair, 2016; Galloway, 2017). Superficial heat is a commonly used self-care treatment that may be an effective addition to MMA when people are hospitalized (McDonald, Soutar, Chan, & Afriyie, 2015). Finally, Jones, Moseley, and Carus (2013) suggested that heat contributes to antinociception by introducing a new sensory input and creating a feeling of safety.

Evidence for Pain Management

Superficial heat is a conventional nonpharmacologic treatment for musculoskeletal pain. Heat therapy is a common self-care tool for managing pain that is used by patients of all ages; it is a preferred treatment of older adults (Alvarado-García & Salazar-Maya, 2017) but also popular with younger people living with chronic pain conditions, such as Ehlers-Danlos syndrome (Arthur, Caldwell, Forehand, & Davis, 2016) and temporomandibular joint pain (Rashid, Matthews, & Cowgill, 2013). Although superficial heat is a frequently used self-care treatment (Dommerholt, Finnegan, Grieve, & Hooks, 2016) and is often recommended for relief of acute LBP (Lichentenstein & Miles, 2018; Shaheed et al., 2016), clinicians rarely include it in a multimodal approach to managing pain in the hospital setting.

The authors of a Cochrane systematic review reported that there is low evidence for long-term benefit of heat for chronic LBP (Kamper et al., 2015). Members of a Canadian and U.S. task force on neck pain and associated disorders (OPTIMa Collaboration) reported that heat as a passive therapy is not effective for neck pain and should not be used (Wong et al., 2016). Although there is little research evidence that heat is effective for musculoskeletal injury (Malanga, Yan, & Stark, 2015), heat application is a primary recommendation, with moderate quality evidence, as treatment of acute, subacute, and chronic LBP by the American College of Physicians (Qaseem, Wilt, McLean,

& Forciea, 2017). Moist heat was used effectively in conjunction with mindfulness meditation (see Chapter 22) in a multimodal protocol to manage pain and increase function of people with chronic orofacial pain (Merrill & Goodman, 2016). The investigators of a study (n = 150) with older women with knee pain in Japan randomized the women into four groups: exercise (n = 37), health education (n = 37), heat with steam-generating sheets (HSGS) (n = 38), and exercise with HSGS (n = 38). The researchers in that study reported the women who received heat application in conjunction with exercise had significant improvement in movement and function with less pain compared to the women who received education and either treatment exercise or heat alone (Kim et al., 2013).

In the guidelines for postoperative pain management, the task force members noted that they could neither recommend nor dissuade the use of several physical modalities, including heat, in the management of postoperative pain (Chou et al., 2016). Although heat is not recommended in treatment of acute injuries (Lin, Lin, Jan, Lin, & Cheng, 2014), it is used in some acute situations. Several studies, including the ones that are discussed here, have investigated the effect of heat on exercise-induced muscle damage and reported positive results. When dry heat was compared with moist heat among people doing squat exercises (n = 100) there was similar but somewhat enhanced benefit with the moist heat (Petrofsky et al., 2013). In a small study (n = 11), subjects who received heat generated via a circulating sleeve garment immediately after exercise reported less pain than the controls (Kim et al., 2017). Warm showers have been used effectively with women. In one study (n = 80), during labor women used warm showers to significantly reduce pain intensity. This intervention is also reported to help the mother feel comforted and facilitate a fuller sense of participation by the mother in the birth process (Lee, Liu, Lu, & Gau, 2013). Heat therapy was provided to Iranian women in the form of hot packs made with hot towels that were applied to the sacrum-perineum of women in labor (Taavoni, Abdolahian, & Haghani, 2013). Interestingly, when compared with controls, as labor progressed, the women with the heat therapy had greater statistically significant differences in pain control at 30 minutes ($P = .056$), 60 minutes ($P = .008$), and 90 minutes ($P = .007$).

Despite the long history of use and acceptance by many people, there remains a need for research with rigorous methodology to establish the efficacy of superficial moist and dry heat as part of a multimodal approach to pain management (Chou et al., 2016; Kamper et al., 2015; Malanga et al., 2015). Research is also needed to more fully explore the role of heat with acute pain situations.

Cautions

Temperatures greater than 45° C can cause damage to tissues and need to be avoided (Galloway, 2017). Caution is needed when using heat with wounds and superficial metal implants (Perlman et al., 2018).

Box 27.8 Contraindications to Therapeutic Heat

- Insensate skin
- Atrophic skin
- Inability to communicate or respond to pain
- Acute inflammation
- Malignancy
- Ischemia
- Growth plates
- Peripheral vascular disease
- Demyelinating disease

From Benny, B., Grabois, M., & Chan, K. T. (2014). Physical medicine techniques in pain management. In H. T. Benzon, J. P. Rathmell, C. L. Wu, C. E. Argoff, & D. C. Turk. *Practical management of pain* (5th ed., pp. 629–641.e2). St. Louis, MO: Elsevier.

Important precautions are to protect the skin, follow manufacturer recommendations for preparation for use, prescribe treatments for specific time frames and intervals (Benny et al., 2014), and educate patients in the importance of adhering to the specified time frames. Commercial hot packs need to be limited to 15 to 30 minutes with adjustments for the individual (Perlman et al., 2018). Hot packs should be placed on top of the affected area rather than beneath to avoid impairment of circulation and dispersion of heat (Benny et al., 2014). These same precautions are important to advise when homemade hot water bottles or hot packs made with grains or beans are used.

Contraindications

Heat should be avoided near the testicles; with neuropathy, poor vascular circulation, and severe cardiac insufficiency; and in the presence of cancer (Lozada, 2013). Box 27.8 discusses contraindications to therapeutic heat.

Therapeutic Cold, Ice, Cryotherapy

Ice, therapeutic cold, and cryotherapy all involve reducing the temperature of the involved area of the body with the intention of relieving pain and reducing edema and possibly muscle spasm (Benny et al., 2014; Galloway, 2017; Guillot et al., 2017; Lozada, 2013). By lowering the temperature of the injured area, cold therapy or cryotherapy can be effective with acute injuries because lower tissue temperature results in a slower metabolic rate and less need for oxygen limiting the degree of damage and lessening the excitability of muscle spindles (Galloway, 2017). There is also a reduction in edema and pain by reducing cellular metabolism and lessening leukocyte-mediated tissue destruction (Sferopoulos, 2017). Although cold therapy is most often thought of

with acute injury or surgery, beneficial effects also have been reported with chronic conditions (Lozada, 2013). In fact, cryotherapy has been used since Hippocrates for a variety of conditions, including rheumatic conditions (Guillot et al., 2017).

Today, in addition to the traditional crushed ice, there are a variety of methods through which cryotherapy can be delivered, including gel packs, a cuff device (Cryocuff) with cold water, continuously flowing cold water (Galloway, 2017), computer-controlled cryotherapy (Rashkovska, Trobec, Avbelj, & Veselko, 2018), cryotherapy with compression (Kraeutler, Reynolds, Long, & McCarty, 2015), gaseous cryotherapy in which there is a projection of carbon dioxide microcrystals (Galloway, 2017), ice slushes, rubs, and whirlpools (Benny et al., 2014).

Evidence for Pain Management

Surprisingly, when ice pack application was compared to no cold application among young adults undergoing impacted mandibular molar surgeries, there was no difference in pain, edema, or patient satisfaction; however, for 2 days both groups received ibuprofen 400 mg tid, which may have been a confounding factor (Zandi, Amini, & Keshavarz, 2016). When cold gel packs were used with a group of patients (n = 34) who underwent median sternotomies, the patients in the half of the sample who had the gel packs reported minimal pain increase with breathing exercises compared with the half of the sample who did not have the gel packs, who reported significant increase in pain (Zencir & Eser, 2016). In a study using ice packs with patients (n = 55) who had midline abdominal incisions, those who received the ice packs (n = 28) reported significantly lower pain intensity scores ($P < .005$) and used significantly less opioids than those who did not use ice packs (n = 27) ($P < .008$) (Watkins et al., 2014).

An appropriate use of cryotherapy is with women who breastfeed their infants, because it is an inexpensive, nonpharmacologic, effective analgesic that does not interfere with breastfeeding (Paiva et al., 2016). In one study (n = 50) of women with episiotomy-related pain after vaginal birth, the women who received crushed ice to the perineum (n = 24) had greater pain relief after 20 minutes compared with those who did not receive crushed ice to the perineum (n = 26) (Beleza, Ferreira, Driusso, dos Santos, & Nakano, 2017). Furthermore, pain relief in the treatment group continued for 1 hour with the lower pain intensity correlated to lower perineal region temperature. Similar results with the same durations of action were reported in another study of postpartum women using ice packs (n = 50) (Paiva et al., 2016).

When cold therapy (cryo/cuff) was used at 2 hours and 6 hours postoperatively in patients who underwent knee arthroplasty (n = 60), those who received the cold therapy (n = 27) had markedly reduced pain on postoperative days 1 through 5 compared with those who did not receive cold therapy (n = 33) (Kuyucu, Bülbül, Kara, Koçyiğit, & Erdil,

2015). Using cold therapy after anterior cruciate ligament reconstruction is common; however, one study compared cooling with the use of traditional gel packs compared to computer-controlled cryotherapy (temperature of the affected area is measured by the computer device, which then promotes optimal cooling) with pads designed for the knee after anterior cruciate ligament reconstruction (Rashkovska et al., 2018). In that study, the researchers found that the patients who received computer-controlled cryotherapy had more effective cooling that was better controlled. In a review of studies (n = 8 studies; n = 187 subjects) in which cold was used after total knee arthroplasties, it was found that pain was relieved more effectively in the studies in which a device circulated a continuous cold flow compared to those in which a cold pack was used (Chughtai et al., 2017). However, when compressive cryotherapy was compared to a common ice elastic wrap after rotator cuff repair, no difference was found in pain intensity or opioid use (Kraeutler et al., 2015). These studies support cryotherapy as an important component of MMA with the added benefit of reducing the quantity of analgesia required in some postoperative patients as well as for acute trauma situations.

Cold therapy also has been used effectively with some chronic pain conditions. For example, it can reduce pain and ease muscle spasms (Galloway, 2017). It has been studied in people with arthritis, hemophilia, and cancer, among other conditions. When ice (n = 15) was compared with cold carbon dioxide (n = 15), the therapies were equally effective in reducing pain among people with OA of the knee (Guillot et al., 2017). Although there is no evidence supporting the use of ice for back pain, it may assist in reducing inflammation and promoting analgesia (National Institute of Neurological Disorders and Stroke [NINDS, 2017]). Ice is effective for articular bleeds and painful joint swelling in hemophilia (Rodriguez-Merchan, 2018). A review of the use of cryotherapy for adverse symptoms of chemotherapy among patients with cancer reported positive effects for painful oral mucositis both in intensity and duration and for onycholysis (a loosening or detaching of the nail) (Kadakia, Rozell, Butala, & Loprinzi, 2014).

A more involved use of cold is *cryoablation,* which causes disruption of the myelinated fibers but does not disrupt the endoneurium, so subsequent regeneration can occur. Cryoablation has been used effectively in a small number of situations (after thoracotomy pain and intercostal neuralgia) under direct visualization with ultrasonography (Connelly, Malik, Madabushi, & Gibson, 2013). It also has been used in the treatment of Barrett's esophagus (Chen & Pasricha, 2011).

Cautions

Adverse effects of therapeutic cold can range from minor skin irritation and burns to frostbite and nerve injuries when certain cold applications or topical anesthetic skin refrigerants are used (Galloway, 2017; Sferopoulos,

| Box 27.9 | Contraindications to Therapeutic Cold |

- Insensate skin
- Ischemia
- Peripheral vascular diseases
- Raynaud's phenomenon
- Cold insensitivity
- Cold urticaria
- Cryoglobulinemia
- Paroxysmal cold hemoglobinuria

From Benny, B., Grabois, M., & Chan, K. T. (2014). Physical medicine techniques in pain management. In H. T. Benzon, J. P. Rathmell, C. L. Wu, C. E. Argoff, & D. C. Turk. *Practical management of pain* (5th ed., pp. 629–641.e2). St. Louis, MO: Elsevier.

2017). Headaches were reported when cold was used with oral mucositis or as treatment on the head (Kadakia et al., 2014). Caution is needed when using cold therapy with people with diabetes for two reasons. First, people who have non–insulin-dependent diabetes are reported to have a prolonged recovery time after any exposure to cold. Second, if the person has peripheral neuropathy, there may be an impairment in sensation to coldness (Galloway, 2017).

To avoid injury, there should be a material or cloth between the coolant and skin, appropriate/recommended length of time should not be exceeded, and appropriate evaluation to rule out fracture or other serious injury needs to occur in a timely manner (Corti, 2014; Sferopoulos, 2017). Fifteen minutes is the time for maximum cooling of muscles to take place, and the muscle then can remain cool for approximately 50 minutes (Galloway, 2017). From that perspective, reasonable duration of cold application may be 15 minutes, no more often than every hour, but greater caution is needed for patients with diabetes and other neuropathies.

Contraindications

Ice should not be used on burned tissue; rather, cool running water is indicated for minor thermal burns (Warner, Coffee, & Yowler, 2014). Box 27.9 details additional contraindications to using therapeutic cold.

Alternating or Contrasting Temperature Therapy

Although they are generally considered two separate therapies, therapeutic heat and cold also can be combined in a *contrast bath.* As the name indicates the affected portion of the body is alternately placed in warm (e.g., 38° to 43° C) and cold baths (e.g., 13° to 18° C) several times for short periods (e.g., 6 minutes warm, then 4 minutes cold) (Benny et al., 2014; Galloway, 2017). A variation is using *alternating compresses* of heat and cold with the same concept; however, the compresses are applied to the affected area rather than immersing the affected area (Arankalle et al., 2016). Another variation alternates warm water bags and ice (Ahmad-Shirvani & Ganji, 2016).

Evidence for Pain Management

Contrast baths have been used for the treatment of CRPS, after carpal tunnel release, and with other pain conditions that are sympathetically mediated (Benny et al., 2014; Galloway, 2017). Alternating compresses, as described, were used for different lengths of time, with the warm compress in place for 15 to 20 minutes followed by the cold compress for 0.5 to 1 minute, and was reported effective for reducing heel pain (Arankalle et al., 2016). One study (n =96) used warm water bags and ice bags both alone and intermittently to manage labor pain and found that there was no statistical difference in pain relief or condition of the neonates among the three groups, but greater satisfaction was reported by those who received heat and intermittent heat and cold compared to those who only received cold therapy (Ahmad-Shirvani & Ganji, 2016).

Cautions

Cautions for contrasting temperature treatments are the same for heat and cold individually (see Boxes 27.8 and Box 27.9).

Valsalva Maneuver

In a person who is awake, the Valsalva maneuver occurs subsequent to a forceful expiration against a glottis that is closed for at least 16 seconds, resulting in increased intrathoracic pressure with a reduction in venous return (Verghese et al., 2002; Kumar et al., 2016). This can be accomplished by bending forward, coughing, or sneezing (Kirby & Purdy, 2014). The antinociceptive effect is thought to occur as a result of the increased intrathoracic pressure activating either the sinoaortic baroceptor reflex arc or the cardiopulmonary baroreceptor (Kumar et al., 2016; Vijay, Meenakshi, Sukhpal, & Ashish, 2013; Zaidi, 2015). It also has been suggested that an analgesic effect is derived directly from stimulation of the vagus nerve (Basaranoglu et al., 2006).

Evidence for Pain Management

Early use of the Valsalva maneuver for pain involved using it to control the pain of angina pectoris and atypical chest pain (Levine, McIntyre, & Glovsky, 1966). Today it is most commonly used to control pain associated with venipuncture or venous cannulation, which not only is done often but also is painful and distressing to patients.

The Valsalva maneuver is reported to reduce physical pain and psychological distress during venipuncture or venous cannulation (Agarwal, Sinha, Tandon, Dhiraaj, & Singh, 2005; Vijay et al., 2013). Having the patient use this technique is a simple, noninvasive, cost-effective, practical approach that takes minimal time to implement for managing the pain and stress involved with the venipuncture procedures (Akdas et al., 2014; Vijay et al., 2013).

Researchers have evaluated this antinociceptive effect in a number of locations eliciting the Valsalva maneuver by stimulating the vagus nerve with a variety of methods. One simple way in which patients can be encouraged to do this is by closing the mouth, pinching the nose, and attempting to exhale (Zaidi, 2015). In an early study (n = 75), investigators taught participants to elicit the Valsalva maneuver by raising a column of mercury to 30 mm Hg and then holding for at least 30 seconds (Agarwal et al., 2005). After venipuncture, the reports of pain by patients in that group were compared with reports of pain by participants in a distraction group who pressed a rubber ball and by a control group (n = 25). The researchers in that study reported there was significantly less pain reported among the Valsalva group ($P < .001$) compared to either of the other two groups. In another study (n = 100), the Valsalva maneuver was elicited by having participants raise the needle of an aneroid blood pressure apparatus by 20 points by forcefully blowing into a rubber tube connected to the device (Vijay et al., 2013). The researchers of that study reported that the mean pain intensity scores of the participants who used the Valsalva maneuver were also significantly less ($P < .01$) compared to the control group. In a more recent larger study (n = 200) participants were divided into four groups of 50 each (Shivashankar, Nalini, & Rath, 2018). When compared to the other two intervention groups, distraction pressing a rubber ball) (36% pain) and being photographed with a bright light (44%), the incidence of pain among the participants using the Valsalva maneuver was greater (46% pain) but was markedly less than in the control group (100% pain) (Shivashankar et al., 2018).

Valsalva maneuver was compared with eutectic mixture of local anesthetic (EMLA) in one group and petroleum jelly in another group with each applied 30 minutes before venipuncture (Suren et al., 2013). In that study (n = 182), those who used the Valsalva maneuver had pain intensity scores comparable to those who received EMLA but significantly lower than the controls. An additional interesting finding in that study was that successful venipuncture was significantly greater ($P < .001$) in the Valsalva group compared to either of the other two groups. In a smaller study with children (n = 60), the Valsalva maneuver was compared with EMLA applied 60 minutes before venipuncture and a control group (Akdas et al., 2014). Although the children in the Valsalva maneuver group had statistically more pain than those in the EMLA group ($P < .05$), they had less pain than the control group.

The Valsalva maneuver is also used to distend the neck veins in children who are intubated to facilitate placement of central lines (Farrelly & Stitelman, 2016). In 2002, researchers reported simulated Valsalva maneuver maximized the cross-sectional area of the internal jugular vein in infants more than either liver compression or Trendelenburg position alone, but the three maneuvers combined were most effective in both infants and children (Verghese et al., 2002). Those researchers reported the simulation was accomplished by applying sustained increase in airway pressure through inflation of the anesthesia machine bag for 10 seconds. Although this use of the Valsalva maneuver does not directly involve pain control, it may contribute to preventing or minimizing pain by facilitating easier access, less trauma, and fewer complications.

The Valsalva maneuver was recently explored with other procedures akin to venipuncture. In patients undergoing a spinal needle puncture, the Valsalva maneuver was compared with distraction and control (n = 82), with the investigators reporting significant reductions in pain among the patients who used the Valsalva maneuver by blowing into sphygmomanometer tube and raising the mercury to 30 mm Hg for a minimum of 20 seconds (Kumar et al., 2016). The Valsalva maneuver was also evaluated among people undergoing needle insertion to arteriovenous fistulas for hemodialysis. In one study with people undergoing that procedure (n = 70) the Valsalva maneuver was compared to ice placed on an acupressure point; even though both interventions reduced pain, the Valsalva maneuver was more effective (Davtalab, Naji, & Shahidi, 2016). When it was subsequently evaluated with people undergoing hemodialysis with fistula insertion (n = 35) the patients reported significantly less pain ($P < .001$) after they used the Valsalva maneuver (Davtalab & Naji, 2017). Additional research is needed to explore use of the Valsalva maneuver with other types of pain, how it can best be used, and to clarify contraindications and cautions.

Cautions

Successful use of the Valsalva maneuver depends on the patient fully understanding the technique and adequately activating the maneuver (Zaidi, 2015). Although simple and easy to use, there are several cautions for using the Valsalva maneuver. It can cause increase in intracranial pressure (Brooks, 2015) so should be avoided in patients who are recovering from neurosurgical procedures. Because it may cause epistasis, the maneuver should be avoided after rhinoplasty, at least during the first week postoperatively (Cuzalina, 2018). The Valsalva maneuver may also aggravate back pain (Dewitte et al., 2016). Increased venous pressure through the Valsalva maneuver may cause a subconjunctival hemorrhage (Tarff & Behrens, 2017). If a patient develops a headache as a result of the Valsalva maneuver, this is considered a red flag indicating the need for a neurologic evaluation of the headache (Kirby & Purdy, 2014).

Contraindications

This intervention is not appropriate to use in any situation in which the Valsalva maneuver needs to be avoided or is contraindicated.

Key Points

- An important component of pain management is caring and compassionate clinicians.
- The mechanism of how many nonpharmacologic interventions provide analgesia is understood, but additional research is needed to define which therapy works best for which type of pain and painful condition.
- It is important to remember that products and modalities that are natural may have side effects and can produce adverse reactions.
- Caution in the use of natural products, as with any therapy, is warranted.
- Clinicians need to be well informed of nonpharmacologic interventions so they can implement them properly and educate and advise patients on their use.
- Too much of a good thing may be too much, especially with aromatherapies, heat, and cold.
- There are a variety of nonpharmacologic interventions that are promising for pain management and need additional research.

Case Scenario

Donald is a 43-year-old man who is admitted to the hospital today reporting worsening low back pain and pain in his lower leg that has been diagnosed as complex regional pain syndrome. His current weight is 182 kg. He is divorced, lost his job as a construction worker, and does not participate in any exercise program. He is diaphoretic and squinting. He was recently assessed, and the large overhead light is still on. He is drinking a sugary soft drink while he tells you that he needs more or different medication for these pains in his back and leg. Donald tells you that he thinks everyone thinks he is "drug seeking."

1. What additional information do you want to know about Donald and his environment?
2. What education would you provide to Donald?
3. What nonpharmacologic interventions may be beneficial for him?
4. Because he is not working, what interventions could be included in a multimodal analgesic plan for him at discharge?
5. What cautions would you advise him?
6. How would you address his perception that he is being labeled as "drug seeking"?

References

Aaboe, J., Bliddal, H., Messier, S. P., Alkjaer, T., & Henriksen, M. (2011). Effects of an intensive weight loss program on knee joint loading in obese adults with knee osteoarthritis. *Osteoarthritis and Cartilage*, 19(7), 822–828.

Adachi, T., Fujino, H., Nakae, A., Mashimo, T., & Sasaki1, J. (2014). A meta-analysis of hypnosis for chronic pain problems: A comparison between hypnosis, standard care, and other psychological interventions. *International Journal of Clinical and Experimental Hypnosis*, 62(1), 1–28.

Agarwal, A., Sinha, P. K., Tandon, M., Dhiraaj, S., & Singh, U. (2005). Evaluating the efficacy of the Valsalva maneuver on venous cannulation pain: a prospective, randomized study. *Anesthesia & Analgesia*, 101(4), 1230–1232.

Ahmad-Shirvani, M., & Ganji, J. (2016). Comparison of separate and intermittent heat and cold therapy in labour pain management. *Nursing Practice Today*, 3(4), 179–186.

Akdas, O., Basaranoglu, G., Ozdemir, H., Comlekci, M., Erkalp, K., & Saidoglu, L. (2014). The effects of Valsalva maneuver on venipuncture pain in children: comparison to EMLA® (lidocaine–prilocaine cream). *Irish Journal of Medical Science (1971-)*, 183(4), 517–520.

Al Sayegh, S., Filén, T., Johansson, M., Sandström, S., Stiewe, G., & Butler, S. (2013). Mirror therapy for Complex Regional Pain Syndrome (CRPS) A literature review and an illustrative case report. *Scandinavian Journal of Pain*, 4(4), 200–207.

Ali, B., Al-Wabel, N. A., Shams, S., Ahamad, A., Khan, S. A., & Anwar, F. (2015). Essential oils used in aromatherapy: A systemic review. *Asian Pacific Journal of Tropical Biomedicine*, 5(8), 601–611.

Ali, Z., Singh, S., Hassan, N., & Naqash, I. (2017). Pain management. In H. Prabhakar (Ed.), *Essentials of Neuroanesthesia* (pp. 835–851). London: Academic Press.

Alvarado-García, A. M., & Salazar-Maya, Á. M. (2017). Everything is valid in chronic pain: Interventions by older adults for pain relief. *Enfermería Clínica (English Edition)*, 27(1), 11–20.

Anderson, A. R., Deng, J., Anthony, R. S., Atalla, S. A., & Monroe, T. B. (2017). Using Complementary and Alternative Medicine to Treat Pain and Agitation in Dementia. *Critical Care Nursing Clinics*, 29(4), 519–537.

American Psychological Association (APA). (2019). *Policy & procedures manual of APA Division 30 The Society of Psychological Hypnosis*. Retrieved August 8, 2020 from https://www.apadivisions.org/division-30/search?query=manual.

Arankalle, D., Wardle, J., & Nair, P. M. (2016). Alternate hot and cold application in the management of heel pain: A pilot study. *The Foot*, 29, 25–28.

Aronson, J. K. (2016). Complementary and alternative medicine. In *Meyler's Side Effects of Drugs* (pp. 560–578). St. Louis: MO: Elsevier.

Arranz, L. I. (2017). Effects of obesity on function and quality of life in chronic pain. In R. R. Watson, & S. Zibadi (Eds.), *Nutritional Modulators of Pain in the Aging Population* (pp. 151–170). London: Elsevier.

Arthur, K., Caldwell, K., Forehand, S., & Davis, K. (2016). Pain control methods in use and perceived effectiveness by patients with Ehlers–Danlos syndrome: a descriptive study. *Disability and Rehabilitation*, 38(11), 1063–1074.

Bagheri-Nesami, M., Espahbodi, F., Nikkhah, A., Shorofi, S. A., & Charati, J. Y. (2014). The effects of lavender aromatherapy on pain following needle insertion into a fistula in hemodialysis patients. *Complementary Therapies in Clinical Practice*, 20(1), 1–4.

Barabasz, A. F., & Barabasz, M. (2008). Hypnosis and the brain. In M. R. Nash, & A. Barnier (Eds.), *The Oxford handbook of hypnosis: Theory, research, and practice* (pp. 337–364). Oxford, England: Oxford University Press.

Barbanti, P., Fofi, L., Aurilia, C., Egeo, G., & Caprio, M. (2017). Ketogenic diet in migraine: rationale, findings and perspectives. *Neurological Sciences*, 38(1), 111–115.

Barber, J. (1977). Rapid induction analgesia: A clinical report. *American Journal of Clinical Hypnosis*, 19(3), 138–147.

Barbin, J., Seetha, V., Casillas, J. M., Paysant, J., & Perennou, D. (2016). The effects of mirror therapy on pain and motor control of phantom limb in amputees: A systematic review. *Annals of Physical and Rehabilitation Medicine*, 59(4), 270–275.

Basaranoglu, G., Basaranoglu, M., Erden, V., Delatioglu, H., Pekel, A. F., & Saitoglu, L. (2006). The effects of Valsalva manoeuvres on venepuncture pain. *European Journal of Anaesthesiology*, 23(7), 591–593.

Basford, J. R. (2001). A historical perspective of the popular use of electric and magnetic therapy. *Archives of Physical Medicine and Rehabilitation*, 82(9), 1261–1269.

Beaumont, E., & Martin, C. J. H. (2016). A proposal to support student therapists to develop compassion for self and others through Compassionate Mind Training. *The Arts in Psychotherapy*, 50, 111–118.

Beleza, A. C. S., Ferreira, C. H. J., Driusso, P., dos Santos, C. B., & Nakano, A. M. S. (2017). Effect of cryotherapy on relief of perineal pain after vaginal childbirth with episiotomy: a randomized and controlled clinical trial. *Physiotherapy*, 103(4), 453–458.

Benny, B., Grabois, M. & Chan, K. T. (2014). Physical medicine techniques in pain management. In: H. T. Benzon, J. P. Rathmell, C. L. Wu, C. E. Argoff & D. C. Turk. *Practical Management of Pain* (5th Ed.) St. Louis, MO: Elsevier. pp 629-641.e2.

Bjørklund, G., Aaseth, J., Doşa, M. D., Pivina, L., Dadar, M., Pen, J. J., & Chirumbolo, S. (2019). Does diet play a role in reducing nociception related to inflammation and chronic pain? *Nutrition*, 66, 153–165.

Bonakdar, R. A. (2018). Myofascial pain syndrome. In D. Rakel (Ed.), *Integrative Medicine* (4th Ed., pp. 651–661.e2.). Philadelphia, PA: Elsevier.

Bouchard, L. (2013). Using a linguistic approach in pain medicine: advances in doctor-patient communication. *The Journal of Pain*, 14(4), S7.

Bracaglia, M., Coppola, G., Di Lorenzo, C., Di Lenola, D., & Pierelli, F. (2015). O017. Cortical functional correlates of responsiveness to short-lasting preventive intervention with ketogenic diet (KD) in migraine: a multimodal evoked potentials study. *The Journal of Headache and Pain*, 16(S1), A58.

Breivik, H., Allen, S. M., & Stubhaug, A. (2013). Mirror-therapy: An important tool in the management of Complex Regional Pain Syndrome (CRPS). *Scandinavian Journal of Pain*, 4(4), 198–199.

Brooks, C. (2015). Critical care nursing in acute postoperative neurosurgical patients. *Critical Care Nursing Clinics*, 27(1), 33–45.

Buckle, J., & Buckle, J. (2015a). Basic plant taxonomy, basic essential oil chemistry, extraction, biosynthesis, and analysis. In *Clinical Aromatherapy: Essential Oils in Healthcare* (3rd Ed, pp. 37–72). St. Louis, MO: Elsevier.

Buckle, J. (2015b). Essential oil toxicity and contraindications. In J. Buckle (Ed.), *Clinical Aromatherapy: Essential Oils in Healthcare* (3rd Ed., pp. 73–94). St. Louis, MO: Elsevier.

Brugnoli, M. P. (2014). Clinical Hypnosis and Relaxation in Surgery Room. Critical Care and Emergency, for Pain and Anxiety Relief. *Journal of Anesthesia & Critical Care: Open Access, 1*(3), 00018.

Burnell, L. (2009). Compassionate care: A concept analysis. *Home Health Care Management & Practice, 21*(5), 319–324.

Cacchio, A., De Blasis, E., De Blasis, V., Santilli, V., & Spacca, G. (2009). Mirror therapy in complex regional pain syndrome type 1 of the upper limb in stroke patients. *Neurorehabilitation and Neural Repair, 23*(8), 792–799.

Centers for Disease Control and Prevention (CDC). (2019). Disability and Obesity. *Disability and Health Promotion*, Retrieved August 8, 2020 from https://www.cdc.gov/ncbddd/disabilityandhealth/obesity.html.

Chen, A. M., & Pasricha, P. J. (2011). Cryotherapy for Barrett's esophagus: Who, how, and why? *Gastrointestinal Endoscopy Clinics of North America, 21*(1), 111–118.

Choi, S. W., Heo, S., Hwang, C. H., & Koo, K. I. (2016). Mirror Therapy Using Virtual Reality on the Wrist of Rheumatoid Arthritis; Pilot Trial. *Brain & Neurorehabilitation, 9*(1), 48–55.

Chou, R., Gordon, D. B., de Leon-Casasola, O. A., Rosenberg, J. M., Bickler, S., Brennan, T., ... Griffith, S. (2016). Management of Postoperative Pain: a clinical practice guideline from the American Pain Society, the American Society of Regional Anesthesia and Pain Medicine, and the American Society of Anesthesiologists' committee on regional anesthesia, executive committee, and administrative council. *The Journal of Pain, 17*(2), 131–157.

Chughtai, M., Sodhi, N., Jawad, M., Newman, J. M., Khlopas, A., Bhave, A., & Mont, M. A. (2017). Cryotherapy Treatment after Unicompartmental and Total Knee Arthroplasty: A Review. *The Journal of Arthroplasty, 32*(12), 3822–3832.

Collins, K. L., McKean, D. L., Huff, K., Tommerdahl, M., Favorov, O. V., Waters, R. S., & Tsao, J. W. (2017). Hand-to-Face remapping But no Differences in Temporal Discrimination Observed on the intact hand Following Unilateral Upper limb amputation. *Frontiers in Neurology, 8*.

Connelly, N. R., Malik, A., Madabushi, L., & Gibson, C. (2013). Use of ultrasound-guided cryotherapy for the management of chronic pain states. *Journal of Clinical Anesthesia, 25*(8), 634–636.

Corti, L. (2014). Nonpharmaceutical approaches to pain management. *Topics in Companion Animal Medicine, 29*(1), 24–28.

Cross, L. A. (2019). Compassion fatigue in palliative care nursing: A concept analysis. *Journal of Hospice and Palliative Nursing, 21*(1), 21–28.

Cuzalina, A., & Niamtu, J. (2018). Rhinoplasty. In *Cosmetic Facial Surgery* (2nd Ed, pp. 323–392). St. Louis, MO: Elsevier.

Czarnecki, M. L., Turner, H. N., Collins, P. M., Doellman, D., Wrona, S., & Reynolds, J. (2011). Procedural pain management: A position statement with clinical practice recommendations. *Pain Management Nursing, 12*(2), 95–111.

Daenen, L., Nijs, J., Roussel, N., Wouters, K., Van Loo, M., & Cras, P. (2012). Sensorimotor incongruence exacerbates symptoms in patients with chronic whiplash associated disorders: an experimental study. *Rheumatology, 51*(8), 1492–1499.

Darlow, B., Dowell, A., Baxter, G. D., Mathieson, F., Perry, M., & Dean, S. (2013). The enduring impact of what clinicians say to people with low back pain. *The Annals of Family Medicine, 11*(6), 527–534.

Davtalab, E., & Naji, S. (2017). The evaluation of Valsalva maneuver on pain intensity within the needle insertion to the arteriovenous fistula for patients undergoing hemodialysis in the selected hospitals in Isfahan in 2015. *Annals of Tropical Medicine and Public Health, 10*(5), 1322–1327.

Davtalab, E., Naji, S., & Shahidi, S. (2016). Comparing the effects of Valsalva maneuver and ice massage at Hoku point methods on pain intensity within the needle insertion to the arteriovenous fistula (AVF) for patients undergoing hemodialysis in the selected hospitals in Isfahan in 2015. *International Journal of Medical Research & Health Sciences, 5*(5), 101–107.

De Benedittis, G. (2015). Neural mechanisms of hypnosis and meditation. *Journal of Physiology – Paris, 109*(4-6), 152–164.

De Giuli, V., Zecchin, R., Salmaso, L., Corain, L., & De Carli, M. (2013). Measured and perceived indoor environmental quality: Padua Hospital case study. *Building and Environment, 59*, 211–226.

De Paepe, A. L., Crombez, G., & Legrain, V. (2015). From a somatotopic to a spatiotopic frame of reference for the localization of nociceptive stimuli. *PloS One, 10*(8), e0137120.

De Von, H. A., Piano, M. R., Rosenfeld, A. G., & Hoppensteadt, D. A. (2014). The association of pain with protein inflammatory biomarkers: a review of the literature. *Nursing Research, 63*(1), 51–62.

Decety, J., & Fotopoulou, A. (2015). Why empathy has a beneficial impact on others in medicine: unifying theories. *Frontiers in Behavioral Neuroscience, 8*, 457.

Deere, K. C., Clinch, J., Holliday, K., McBeth, J., Crawley, E. M., Sayers, A., ... Tobias, J. H. (2012). Obesity is a risk factor for musculoskeletal pain in adolescents: findings from a population-based cohort. *PAIN®, 153*(9), 1932–1938.

Del Casale, A., Ferracuti, S., Rapinesi, C., De Rossi, P., Angeletti, G., Sani, G., ... Girardi, P. (2015). Hypnosis and pain perception: An Activation Likelihood Estimation (ALE) meta-analysis of functional neuroimaging studies. *Journal of Physiology-Paris, 109*(4), 165–172.

Dempsey, C. (2018). *The Antidote to Suffering: How Compassionate and Connected Care Can Improve Safety, Quality, and Experience*. NY: NY: McGraw Hill.

Devitt, J., Shellman, L., Gardner, K., & Nichols, L. W. (2011). Using positioning after a colonoscopy for patient comfort management. *Gastroenterology Nursing, 34*(2), 93–100.

Dewitte, V., Peersman, W., Danneels, L., Bouche, K., Roets, A., & Cagnie, B. (2016). Subjective and clinical assessment criteria suggestive for five clinical patterns discernible in nonspecific neck pain patients. A Delphi-survey of clinical experts. *Manual Therapy, 26*(1), 87–96.

Di Lorenzo, C., Coppola, G., Sirianni, G., Rossi, P., & Pierelli, F. (2015). O045. Cluster headache improvement during Ketogenic Diet. *The Journal of Headache and Pain, 16*(S1), A99.

Dimitriou, V., Mavridou, P., Manataki, A., & Damigos, D. (2017). The Use of Aromatherapy for Postoperative Pain Management: A Systematic Review of Randomized Controlled Trials. *Journal of PeriAnesthesia Nursing, 32*(6), 530–541.

Dommerholt, J., Finnegan, M., Grieve, R., & Hooks, T. (2016). A critical overview of the current myofascial pain literature—January 2016. *Journal of Bodywork and Movement Therapies*, 20(1), 156–167.

Drew, D., Gordon, D., Renner, L., Morgan, B., Swensen, H., & Manworren, R. (2014). The Use of "As-Needed" Range Orders for Opioid Analgesics in the Management of Pain. *Pain Management Nursing*, 15(2), 551–554.

Erickson, H. (2015). Helen Erickson, Evelyn Tomlin, and Mary Ann Swain's theory of Modeling and Role Modeling. In M. C. Smith, & M. E. Parker (Eds.), *Nursing Theories and Nursing Practice* (4th Ed, pp. 185–206). Philadelphia, PA: F. A. Davis Company.

Esquibel, A. Y., & Borkan, J. (2014). Doctors and patients in pain: Conflict and collaboration in opioid prescription in primary care. *PAIN®*, 155(12), 2575–2582.

Farkas, M. K., Mak, E., Richter, E., & Farkas, V. (2014, December). EHMTI-0336. Metabolic diet therapy in the prophylactic treatment of migraine headache in adolescents by using ketogenic diet. In *The Journal of Headache and Pain (Vol. 15, No. S1, p. G9)*: Springer Milan.

Farrelly, J. S., & Stitelman, D. H. (2016, December). Complications in pediatric enteral and vascular access. *Seminars in Pediatric Surgery*, 25(6), 371–379.

Filbrich, L., Alamia, A., Blandiaux, S., Burns, S., & Legrain, V. (2017). Shaping visual space perception through bodily sensations: Testing the impact of nociceptive stimuli on visual perception in peripersonal space with temporal order judgments. *PloS One*, 12(8), e0182634.

Finn, S. B., Perry, B. N., Clasing, J. E., Walters, L. S., Jarzombek, S. L., Curran, S., ... Pasquina, P. F. (2017). A randomized, controlled trial of mirror therapy for upper extremity phantom limb pain in male amputees. *Frontiers in Neurology*, 8, 267.

Foell, J., Bekrater-Bodmann, R., Diers, M., & Flor, H. (2014). Mirror therapy for phantom limb pain: brain changes and the role of body representation. *European Journal of Pain*, 18(5), 729–739.

Frankel, R. M. (2017). The Evolution of Empathy Research: Models, Muddles, and Mechanisms. *Patient Education and Counseling*, 100(11), 2128–2130.

Friederich, M., Trippe, R. H., Özcan, M., Weiss, T., Hecht, H., & Miltner, W. H. (2001). Laser-evoked potentials to noxious stimulation during hypnotic analgesia and distraction of attention suggest different brain mechanisms of pain control. *Psychophysiology*, 38(5), 768–776.

Frilander, H., Solovieva, S., Mutanen, P., Pihlajamäki, H., Heliövaara, M., & Viikari-Juntura, E. (2015). Role of overweight and obesity in low back disorders among men: a longitudinal study with a life course approach. *BMJ Open*, 5(8), e007805.

Fukudo, S., Morishita, J., Watanabe, S., Kawabata, K., Ishizu, N., Tanaka, Y., ... Yanai, K. (2014). 241 Evidence of Dopamine Release During Hypnotic Analgesia Under Visceral Stimulation in Humans. *Gastroenterology*, 146(5), S–57.

Gackenbach, J., Wijeyaratnam, D., & Flockhart, C. (2017). The video gaming frontier. In J. Gackenbach, & J. Brown (Eds.), *Boundaries of Self and Reality Online - Implications of Digitally Constructed Realities* (pp. 161–185). London: Elsevier.

Gallace, A., Torta, D. M. E., Moseley, G. L., & Iannetti, G. D. (2011). The analgesic effect of crossing the arms. *Pain*, 152(6), 1418–1423.

Galloway, K. (2017). Cryotherapy and moist heat. In J. D. Placzek, & D. A. Boyce (Eds.), *Orthopaedic Physical Therapy Secrets* (3rd Ed, pp. 54–59). St. Louis, MO: Elsevier.

Geller, E. S. (2015). Seven life lessons from humanistic behaviorism: how to bring the best out of yourself and others. *Journal of Organizational Behavior Management*, 35(1-2), 151–170.

Gilbert, P. (2009). Introducing compassion-focused therapy. *Advances in Psychiatric Treatment*, 15(3), 199–208.

Gilbert, P. (2014). The origins and nature of compassion focused therapy. *British Journal of Clinical Psychology*, 53(1), 6–41.

Glover, T. L., Goodin, B. R., King, C. D., Sibille, K. T., Herbert, M. S., Sotolongo, A. S., ... Redden, D. T. (2015). A Cross-sectional Examination of Vitamin D, Obesity, and Measures of Pain and Function in Middle-aged and Older Adults With Knee Osteoarthritis. *The Clinical Journal of Pain*, 31(12), 1060–1067.

Gover-Chamlou, A., & Tsao, J. W. (2016). Telepain management of phantom limb pain using mirror therapy. *Telemedicine and e-Health*, 22(2), 176–179.

Griffin, S. C., Curran, S. E. A. N., Pasquina, P. F., & Tsao, J. W. (2015). Time course of therapeutic response to mirror therapy for phantom limb pain. *Journal of the Neurological Sciences*, 357, e94.

Guillot, X., Tordi, N., Prati, C., Verhoeven, F., Pazart, L., & Wendling, D. (2017). Cryotherapy decreases synovial Doppler activity and pain in knee arthritis: A randomized-controlled trial. *Joint Bone Spine*, 84(4), 477–483.

Hagenberg, A., & Carpenter, C. (2014). Mirror visual feedback for phantom pain: international experience on modalities and adverse effects discussed by an expert panel: a Delphi study. *PM&R*, 6(8), 708–715.

Halm, M. (2016). Making Time for Quiet. *American Journal of Critical Care*, 25(6), 552–555.

Howick, J., Lewith, G., Mebius, A., Fanshawe, T. R., Bishop, F., van Osch, M., ... Mistiaen, P. (2017). Positive messages may reduce patient pain: A meta-analysis. *European Journal of Integrative Medicine*, 11, 31–38.

Iannitti, T., Graham, A., & Dolan, S. (2012). Increased central and peripheral inflammation and inflammatory hyperalgesia in Zucker rat model of leptin receptor deficiency and genetic obesity. *Experimental Physiology*, 97(11), 1236–1245.

Ichinose, A., Sano, Y., Osumi, M., Sumitani, M., Kumagaya, S. I., & Kuniyoshi, Y. (2017). Somatosensory Feedback to the Cheek During Virtual Visual Feedback Therapy Enhances Pain Alleviation for Phantom Arms. *Neurorehabilitation and Neural Repair*, 31(8), 717–725.

Iserson, K. V. (2014). An hypnotic suggestion: review of hypnosis for clinical emergency care. *The Journal of Emergency Medicine*, 46(4), 588–596.

Jafarizadeh, H., Lotfi, M., Ajoudani, F., Kiani, A., & Alinejad, V. (2018). Hypnosis for reduction of background pain and pain anxiety in men with burns: A blinded, randomised, placebo-controlled study. *Burns*, 44(1), 108–117.

Jensen, K. B., Petrovic, P., Kerr, C. E., Kirsch, I., Raicek, J., Cheetham, A., ... Kaptchuk, T. J. (2014). Sharing pain and relief: neural correlates of physicians during treatment of patients. *Molecular Psychiatry*, 19(3), 392–398.

Jiang, H., White, M. P., Greicius, M. D., Waelde, L. C., & Spiegel, D. (2017). Brain activity and functional connectivity associated with hypnosis. *Cerebral Cortex*, 27(8), 4083–4093.

Johnson, J. R., Rivard, R. L., Griffin, K. H., Kolste, A. K., Joswiak, D., Kinney, M. E., & Dusek, J. A. (2016). The effectiveness of nurse-delivered aromatherapy in an acute care setting. *Complementary Therapies in Medicine, 25*, 164–169.

Johnson, K., West, T., Diana, S., Todd, J., Haynes, B., Bernhardt, J., & Johnson, R. (2017). Use of aromatherapy to promote a therapeutic nurse environment. *Intensive and Critical Care Nursing, 40*(1), 18–25.

Jones, G. (2014). Where in Space is My Pain? The Role of the Defensive Peripersonal Space & its Influence on Pain Perception. *Pain and Rehabilitation-the Journal of Physiotherapy Pain Association, 2014*(37), 4–12.

Jones, L., Moseley, G. L., & Carus, C. (2013). Pain. In S. B. Porter (Ed.), *Tidy's Physiotherapy* (15th Ed., pp. 381–401). Edinburgh: Elsevier.

Kadakia, K. C., Rozell, S. A., Butala, A. A., & Loprinzi, C. L. (2014). Supportive cryotherapy: A review from head to toe. *Journal of Pain and Symptom Management, 47*(6), 1100–1115.

Kagan, S. H. (2014). Compassion. *Geriatric Nursing, 35*(1), 69–70.

Kagan, S. H. (2015). Dignity, evidence, and empathy. *Geriatric Nursing, 36*(5), 394–396.

Kamper, S. J., Apeldoorn, A. T., Chiarotto, A., Smeets, R. J. E. M., Ostelo, R. W. J. G., Guzman, J., & van Tulder, M. W. (2015). Multidisciplinary biopsychosocial rehabilitation for chronic low back pain: Cochrane systematic review and meta-analysis. *BMJ, 350*, h444.

Karakoç, A., & Türker, F. (2014). Effects of white noise and holding on pain perception in newborns. *Pain Management Nursing, 15*(4), 864–870.

Karaman, T., Karaman, S., Dogru, S., Tapar, H., Sahin, A., Suren, M., … Kaya, Z. (2016). Evaluating the efficacy of lavender aromatherapy on peripheral venous cannulation pain and anxiety: A prospective, randomized study. *Complementary Therapies in Clinical Practice, 23*, 64–68.

Khodakarami, J., & Nasrollahi, N. (2012). Thermal comfort in hospitals: A literature review. *Renewable and Sustainable Energy Reviews, 16*(6), 4071–4077.

Kieser, D. C., Wyatt, M. C., Boissiere, L., Hayashi, K., Cawley, D. T., Yilgor, C., … Kleinstueck, F. (2019). The effect of increasing body mass index on the pain and function of patients with adult spinal deformity. *Journal of Spine Surgery, 5*(4), 535.

Kihlstrom, J. F. (2016). Hypnosis. In *Reference Module in Neuroscience and Biobehavioral Psychology: Encyclopedia of Mental Health* (2nd Ed., pp. 361–365): Elsevier. ISBN: 978-0-12-809324-5.

Kim, H., Suzuki, T., Saito, K., Kim, M., Kojima, N., Ishizaki, T., … Yoshida, H. (2013). Effectiveness of exercise with or without thermal therapy for community-dwelling elderly Japanese women with non-specific knee pain: A randomized controlled trial. *Archives of Gerontology and Geriatrics, 57*(3), 352–359.

Kim, K., Nie, Y., Boersma, D., Song, Q., Kuang, S., Gavin, T. P., & Roseguini, B. T. (2017). Heat therapy alters the expression of myogenic and angiogenic factors and accelerates functional recovery following exercise-induced muscle damage in humans. *The FASEB Journal, 31*(1 Supplement), 1086–1094.

Kirby, S., & Purdy, R. A. (2014). Headaches and brain tumors. *Neurologic Clinics, 32*(2), 423–432.

Kohatsu, W., & Karpowicz, S. (2018). Antiinflammatory diet. In D. Rakel (Ed.), *Integrative Medicine* (4th Ed.). St. Louis, MO: Elsevier.

Kolcaba, K. (2015). Katharine Kolcaba's Comfort Theory. In M. C. Smith, & M. E. Parker (Eds.), *Nursing Theories and Nursing Practice* (4th Ed, pp. 381–391). Philadelphia, PA: F. A. Davis Company.

Koo, K. I., Cho, S. D., Chee, Y. J., Heo, S. C., Park, D. K., & Hwang, C. H. (2015). The post-operative analgesia of the virtual reality using a mirror therapy after total knee arthroplasty. *Journal of the Neurological Sciences, 357*, e83.

Kraeutler, M. J., Reynolds, K. A., Long, C., & McCarty, E. C. (2015). Compressive cryotherapy versus ice: a prospective, randomized study on postoperative pain in patients undergoing arthroscopic rotator cuff repair or subacromial decompression. *Journal of Shoulder and Elbow Surgery, 24*(6), 854–859.

Krinsky, R., Murillo, I., & Johnson, J. (2014). A practical application of Katharine Kolcaba's comfort theory to cardiac patients. *Applied Nursing Research, 27*(2), 147–150.

Kumar, S., Gautam, S. K. S., Gupta, D., Agarwal, A., Dhirraj, S., & Khuba, S. (2016). The effect of Valsalva maneuver in attenuating skin puncture pain during spinal anesthesia: a randomized controlled trial. *Korean Journal of Anesthesiology, 69*(1), 27–31.

Kuyucu, E., Bülbül, M., Kara, A., Koçyiğit, F., & Erdil, M. (2015). Is cold therapy really efficient after knee arthroplasty? *Annals of Medicine and Surgery, 4*(4), 475–478.

Lebon, J., Rongières, M., Apredoaei, C., Delclaux, S., & Mansat, P. (2017). Physical therapy under hypnosis for the treatment of patients with type 1 complex regional pain syndrome of the hand and wrist: Retrospective study of 20 cases. *Hand Surgery and Rehabilitation, 36*(3), 215–221.

Lee, S. L., Liu, C. Y., Lu, Y. Y., & Gau, M. L. (2013). Efficacy of warm showers on labor pain and birth experiences during the first labor stage. *Journal of Obstetric, Gynecologic, & Neonatal Nursing, 42*(1), 19–28.

Lee, Y. H., Bae, S. C., & Song, G. G. (2012). Omega-3 polyunsaturated fatty acids and the treatment of rheumatoid arthritis: a meta-analysis. *Archives of Medical Research, 43*(5), 356–362.

Leeth, D., Mamaril, M., Oman, K. S., & Krumbach, B. (2010). Normothermia and patient comfort: A comparative study in an outpatient surgery setting. *Journal of PeriAnesthesia Nursing, 25*(3), 146–151.

Levine, H. J., McIntyre, K. M., & Glovsky, M. M. (1966). Relief of angina pectoris by Valsalva maneuver. *New England Journal of Medicine, 275*(9), 487–489.

Lichentenstein, S., & Miles, C. (2018). Acute low back pain. In R. Olympia, R. O'Neill, & M. Silvis (Eds.), *Urgent Care Medicine Secrets* (pp. 187–190). Philadelphia, PA: Elsevier.

Lin, A., Turner, Z., Doerrer, S. C., Stanfield, A., & Kossoff, E. H. (2017). Complications during ketogenic diet initiation: prevalence, treatment, and influence on seizure outcomes. *Pediatric Neurology, 68*, 35–39.

Lin, Y. F., Lin, D. H., Jan, M. H., Lin, C. H. J., & Cheng, C. K. (2014). Orthopedic physical therapy. In: *Reference Module in Biomedical Sciences: Comprehensive Biomedical Physics* (Vol 10, pp. 379–400). St. Louis, MO: Elsevier. https://doi.org/10.1016/B978-0-444-53632-7.01024-8.

Louw, A., Puentedura, E. J., Reese, D., Parker, P., Miller, T., & Mintken, P. (2017). Immediate effects of mirror therapy in patients with shoulder pain and decreased range of motion. *Archives of Physical Medicine and Rehabilitation, 98*(10), 1941–1947.

Lozada, C. J. (2013). Treatment of osteoarthritis. In G. S. Firestein, R. C. Budd, S. E. Gabriel, I. B. McInness, & J. R. O'Dell (Eds.), *Vol 2. Kelley's Textbook of Rheumatology* (9th Ed., pp 1646–1659.e4.). Elsevier.

Malanga, G. A., Yan, N., & Stark, J. (2015). Mechanisms and efficacy of heat and cold therapies for musculoskeletal injury. *Postgraduate Medicine, 127*(1), 57–65.

Malone, M. A., & Gloyer, K. (2013). Complementary and alternative treatments in sports medicine. *Primary Care: Clinics in Office Practice, 40*(4), 945–968.

Manion, C. R., & Widder, R. M. (2017). Essentials of essential oils. *AM J Health-Syst Pharm, 74*(9), 153–162. doi:https://doi.org/10.2146/ajhp151043.

Martin, K., Jackson, C. F., Levy, R. G., & Cooper, P. N. (2016). Ketogenic diet and other dietary treatments for epilepsy. *The Cochrane Library., 2*, CD001903.

Masino, S. A., & Ruskin, D. N. (2013). Ketogenic diets and pain. *Journal of Child Neurology, 28*(8), 993–1001.

Matinella, A., Brugnoli, M. P., Pasin, E., Segatti, A., Concon, E., & Squintani, G. (2017). 70. Laser-evoked potentials (LEPs) in chronic pain conditions during hypnotic analgesia. *Clinical Neurophysiology, 128*(12), e432.

McAuley, J. (2015). Commentary to: The PACT trial: PAtient Centered Telerehabilitation Effectiveness of software-supported and traditional mirror therapy in patients with phantom limb pain following lower limb amputation: protocol of a multicentre randomised controlled trial. *Journal of Physiotherapy, 61*(1), 42.

McCabe, C. S., Cohen, H., & Blake, D. R. (2007). Somaesthetic disturbances in fibromyalgia are exaggerated by sensory–motor conflict: implications for chronicity of the disease? *Rheumatology, 46*(10), 1587–1592.

McDonald, D. D., Soutar, C., Chan, M. A., & Afriyie, A. (2015). A closer look: alternative pain management practices by heart failure patients with chronic pain. *Heart & Lung: The Journal of Acute and Critical Care, 44*(5), 395–399.

McDonald, L. (2014). Florence Nightingale and Irish nursing. *Journal of Clinical Nursing, 23*(17-18), 2424–2433.

McGough, N. N., Keane, T., Uppal, A., Dumlao, M., Rutherford, W., Kellogg, K., … Fields, W. (2018). Noise reduction in progressive care units. *Journal of Nursing Care Quality, 33*(2), 166–172.

Memoli, G., Dawson, D., Barham, R., & Grounds, M. (2012, April). Distributed noise monitoring in intensive care units. *Acoustics* 2012, Apr 2012, Nantes, France. ffhal-00811377f.

Merrill, R. L., & Goodman, D. (2016). Chronic orofacial pain and behavioral medicine. *Oral and Maxillofacial Surgery Clinics of North America, 28*(3), 247–260.

Mertz, M. J., & Earl, C. J. (2018). Labor pain management. In D. Rakel (Ed.), *Integrative Medicine* (4th Ed., pp. 526–534.e3.). Philadelphia, PA: Elsevier.

Messer, R. D., & Kossoff, E. H. (2015). Ketogenic diets for the treatment of epilepsy. In R. R. Watson, & V. R. Preedy (Eds.), *Bioactive Nutraceuticals and Dietary Supplements in Neurological and Brain Disease* (pp. 441–448). St. Louis, MO: Elsevier.

Messier, S. P., Legault, C., Loeser, R. F., Van Arsdale, S. J., Davis, C., Ettinger, W. H., & DeVita, P. (2011). Does high weight loss in older adults with knee osteoarthritis affect bone-on-bone joint loads and muscle forces during walking? *Osteoarthritis and Cartilage, 19*(3), 272–280.

Metin, Z. G., & Ozdemir, L. (2016). The effects of aromatherapy massage and reflexology on pain and fatigue in patients with rheumatoid arthritis: a randomized controlled trial. *Pain Management Nursing, 17*(2), 140–149.

Meyer, W. J., Jeevendra Martyn, J. A., Wiechman, S., Thomas, C. R., & Woodson, L. (2017). Management of pain and other discomforts in burned patients. In D. Herndon (Ed.), *Total Burn Care* (5th Ed.) (pp. 679-699 e.6): Elsevier Inc.

Michielsen, M. E., Selles, R. W., van der Geest, J. N., Eckhardt, M., Yavuzer, G., Stam, H. J., … Bussmann, J. B. (2011). Motor recovery and cortical reorganization after mirror therapy in chronic stroke patients: a phase II randomized controlled trial. *Neurorehabilitation and Neural Repair, 25*(3), 223–233.

Millis, D., & Levine, D. (2014). Other modalities in veterinary rehabilitation. In *Canine Rehabilitation and Physical Medicine* (2nd Ed, pp. 393–400). St. Louis, MO: Elsevier.

Moghaddam, M., & Mehdizadeh, L. (2017). Chemistry of essential oils and factors influencing their constituents. In A. M. Grumezescu, & A. M. Holban (Eds.), *Soft Chemistry and Food Fermentation: Handbook of Food Bioengineering, Volume 3* (pp. 379–419). London, UK: Academic Press.

Murray, C. J., Abraham, J., Ali, M. K., Alvarado, M., Atkinson, C., Baddour, L. M., … Bolliger, I. (2013). The state of US health, 1990-2010: burden of diseases, injuries, and risk factors. *JAMA, 310*(6), 591–606.

Muz, G., & Taşcı, S. (2017). Effect of aromatherapy via inhalation on the sleep quality and fatigue level in people undergoing hemodialysis. *Applied Nursing Research, 37*, 28–35.

National Cancer Institute. (2018). Aromatherapy and essential oils (PDQ®) – Professional Version. *Cancer Treatment.* https://www.cancer.gov/about-cancer/treatment/cam/hp/aromatherapy-pdq Accessed 05/12/2018.

National Center for Health Statistics. (NCHS). (2017). *Health, United States, 2016: With Chartbook on Long-term Trends in Health.* Hyattsville, MD: The Center.

National Institutes of Health (NIH). (2013). *Magnets.* https://nccih.nih.gov/health/magnet/magnetsforpain.htm. Retrieved 10/21/2017.

National Institutes of Health (NIH). (2020). *Low Back Pain Fact Sheet.* Retrieved August 8, 2020 from https://search.usa.gov/search?utf8=%E2%9C%93&affiliate=ninds&query=low+back+pain+fact+sheet.

National Institute of Neurological Disorders and Stroke (NINDS). (2017). *Low back pain fact sheet.* https://www.ninds.nih.gov/Disorders/Patient-Caregiver-Education/Fact-Sheets/Low-Back-Pain-Fact-Sheet. Accessed 05/12/2018.

Newcomb, P., Wilson, M., Baine, R., McCarthy, T., Penny, N., Nixon, C., & Orren, J. (2017). Influences on Patient Satisfaction Among Patients Who Use Emergency Departments Frequently for Pain-Related Complaints. *Journal of Emergency Nursing, 43*(6), 553-559. doi.org/https://doi.org/10.1016/j.jen.2017.03.022.

Nierula, B., Martini, M., Matamala-Gomez, M., Slater, M., & Sanchez-Vives, M. V. (2017). Seeing an embodied virtual hand is analgesic contingent on colocation. *The Journal of Pain, 18*(6), 645–655.

Nightingale, F. (1860). *Notes on Nursing: What It Is, and What It Is Not.* New York, NY: Appleton.

Norelli, L. J. (2009). Hypnotic analgesia. In H. S. Smith (Ed.), *Current Therapy in Pain* (pp. 518–520). Philadelphia, PA: Saunders.

Norling, L. V., & Perretti, M. (2013). The role of omega-3 derived resolvins in arthritis. *Current Opinion in Pharmacology*, 13(3), 476–481.

Oakley, D. A. (2008). Hypnosis, trance and suggestion: Evidence from neuroimaging. In M. R. Nash, & A. Barnier (Eds.), *The Oxford handbook of hypnosis: Theory, research, and practice* (pp. 365–392). Oxford, England: Oxford University Press.

Oakley, D. A., & Halligan, P. W. (2010). Psychophysiological foundations of hypnosis and suggestion. In S. J. Lynn, J. W. Rhue, & I. Kirsch (Eds.), *Handbook of clinical hypnosis* (2nd ed., pp. 79–117). Washington, DC: American Psychological Association.

O'Brien, D., Greenfield, M. L. V., Anderson, J. E., Smith, B. A., & Morris, M. (2010). Comfort, satisfaction, and anxiolysis in surgical patients using a patient-adjustable comfort warming system: a prospective randomized clinical trial. *Journal of PeriAnesthesia Nursing*, 25(2), 88–93.

Okifuji, A., & Hare, B. D. (2015). The association between chronic pain and obesity. *The Journal of Pain Research*, 8, 399–408.

Ortiz-Catalan, M., Sander, N., Kristoffersen, M. B., Håkansson, B., & Brånemark, R. (2014). Treatment of phantom limb pain (PLP) based on augmented reality and gaming controlled by myoelectric pattern recognition: a case study of a chronic PLP patient. *Frontiers in Neuroscience*, 8, 24. https://doi.org/10.3389/fnins.2014.00024.

Paiva, C. D. S. B., de Oliveira, S. M. J. V., Francisco, A. A., da Silva, R. L., Mendes, E. D. P. B., & Steen, M. (2016). Length of perineal pain relief after ice pack application: A quasi-experimental study. *Women and Birth*, 29(2), 117–122.

Pappas, C. (2015). *Is There a Difference in Pain Management of Patients with Upper Extremity Injuries in Relation to Age? Masters' Thesis. Rhode Island College. Via Digital commons @ RIC.* https://digitalcommons.ric.edu/cgi/viewcontent.cgi?referer=https://scholar.google.com/scholar?hl=en&as_sdt=0%2C34&q=Pappas%2C+C.+%282015%29.+Is+There+a+Difference+in+Pain+Management+of+Patients+with+Upper+Extremity+Injuries+in+Relation+to+Age%3F&btnG=&httpsredir=1&article=1123&context=etd. Accessed 05/12/2018.

Perlman, A. I., Rosenberg, L., & Ali, A. (2018). Osteoarthritis. In D. Rakel (Ed.), *Integrative Medicine* (4th Ed., pp 639–650e.). Philadelphia, PA: Elsevier.

Petrofsky, J., Berk, L., Bains, G., Khowailed, I. A., Hui, T., Granado, M., ... Lee, H. (2013). Moist heat or dry heat for delayed onset muscle soreness. *Journal of Clinical Medicine Research*, 5(6), 416–425.

Peter, B. (2015). *Hypnosis: International encyclopedia of the social & behavioral sciences.* (2nd ed., Vol. 11). Oxford, U.K.: Elsevier. Retrieved August 29, 2017 from https://doi.org/10.1016/B978-0-08-097086-8.21069-6.

Pintar, J., & Lynn, S. J. (2009). *Hypnosis: A brief history.* John Wiley & Sons.

Pittler, M. H., Brown, E. M., & Ernst, E. (2007). Static magnets for reducing pain: systematic review and meta-analysis of randomized trials. *Canadian Medical Association Journal*, 177(7), 736–742.

Poplawski, M. M., Mastaitis, J. W., Isoda, F., Grosjean, F., Zheng, F., & Mobbs, C. V. (2011). Reversal of diabetic nephropathy by a ketogenic diet. *PLoS One*, 6(4), e18604.

Qaseem, A., Wilt, T. J., McLean, R. M., & Forciea, M. A. (2017). Noninvasive Treatments for Acute, Subacute, and Chronic Low Back Pain: A Clinical Practice Guideline From the American College of Physicians Noninvasive Treatments for Acute, Subacute, and Chronic Low Back Pain. *Annals of Internal Medicine*, 166(7), 514–530.

Quinlan-Colwell, A. (2012). *Pain Management for Older Adults: A Clinical Guide for Nurses.* NY: Springer Publishing Company.

Quinlan-Colwell, A. D. (2009). Understanding the paradox of patient pain and patient satisfaction. *Journal of Holistic Nursing*, 27(3), 177–182.

Rahim, S. (2013). Clinical Application of Nightingale's Environmental Theory. *i-Manager's Journal on Nursing*, 3(1), 43.

Ramachandran, V. S., & Altschuler, E. L. (2009). The use of visual feedback, in particular mirror visual feedback, in restoring brain function. *Brain*, 132(7), 1693–1710.

Ramachandran, V. S., & Rogers-Ramachandran, D. (2000). Phantom limbs and neural plasticity. *Archives of Neurology*, 57(3), 317–320.

Ramachandran, V. S., Stewart, M., & Rogers-Ramachandran, D. C. (1992). Perceptual correlates of massive cortical reorganization. *Neuroreport*, 3(7), 583–586.

Ramsden, C. E., Faurot, K. R., Zamora, D., Suchindran, C. M., MacIntosh, B. A., Gaylord, S., ... Barden, A. (2013). Targeted alteration of dietary n-3 and n-6 fatty acids for the treatment of chronic headaches: a randomized trial. *PAIN®*, 154(11), 2441–2451.

Rashid, A., Matthews, N. S., & Cowgill, H. (2013). Physiotherapy in the management of disorders of the temporomandibular joint—perceived effectiveness and access to services: a national United Kingdom survey. *British Journal of Oral and Maxillofacial Surgery*, 51(1), 52–57.

Rashkovska, A., Trobec, R., Avbelj, A., & Veselko, M. (2018). 52 – Efficacy of cryotherapy for pain control after anterior ligament reconstruction. In C. Prodromos (Ed.), *The Anterior Cruciate Ligament* (2nd Ed). Philadelphia, PA: Elsevier.

Rodgers, H. M. (2017). The interrelationship of obesity, pain, and diet/nutrition. In R. R. Watson, & S. Zibadi (Eds.), *Nutritional Modulators of Pain in the Aging Population* (pp. 143–149). London: Elsevier. ISBN: 978-0-12-805186-3.

Rodriguez-Merchan, E. C. (2018). Treatment of musculoskeletal pain in haemophilia. *Blood Reviews*, 32(2), 116–121.

Roque, A. T. F., & Carraro, T. E. (2015). Perceptions about the hospital environment from the perspective of high-risk puerperal women based on Florence Nightingale's theory. *Revista Gaucha de Enfermagem*, 36(4), 63–69.

Rothgangel, A., Braun, S., Witte, L., Beurskens, A., & Smeets, R. (2016). Development of a Clinical Framework for Mirror Therapy in Patients with Phantom Limb Pain: An Evidence-based Practice Approach. *Pain Practice*, 16(4), 422–434.

Ruben, M. A., Meterko, M., & Bokhour, B. G. (2018). Do patient perceptions of provider communication relate to experiences of physical pain? *Patient Education and Counseling*, 101(2), 209–213.

Ruskin, D. N., Suter, T. A., Ross, J. L., & Masino, S. A. (2013). Ketogenic diets and thermal pain: dissociation of hypoalgesia, elevated ketones, and lowered glucose in rats. *The Journal of Pain*, 14(5), 467–474.

Sambo, C. F., Torta, D. M., Gallace, A., Liang, M., Moseley, G. L., & Iannetti, G. D. (2013). The temporal order judgement of tactile and nociceptive stimuli is impaired by crossing the hands over the body midline. *Pain, 154*(2), 242–247.

Sarinopoulos, I., Hesson, A. M., Gordon, C., Lee, S. A., Wang, L., Dwamena, F., & Smith, R. C. (2013). Patient-centered interviewing is associated with decreased responses to painful stimuli: An initial fMRI study. *Patient Education and Counseling, 90*(2), 220–225.

Sato, K., Fukumori, S., Matsusaki, T., Maruo, T., Ishikawa, S., Nishie, H., … Matsumi, M. (2010). Nonimmersive virtual reality mirror visual feedback therapy and its application for the treatment of complex regional pain syndrome: an open-label pilot study. *Pain Medicine, 11*(4), 622–629.

Scheffler, M., Koranyi, S., Meissner, W., Straub, B., & Rosendahl, J. (2018). Efficacy of non-pharmacological interventions for procedural pain relief in adults undergoing burn wound care: A systematic review and meta-analysis of randomized controlled trials. *Burns, 44*(7), 1709–1720.

Seaman, D. R. (2013). Body mass index and musculoskeletal pain: is there a connection? *Chiropractic Manual Therapies, 21*(1), 15.

Seppala, E. M., Hutcherson, C. A., Nguyen, D. T., Doty, J. R., & Gross, J. J. (2014). Loving-kindness meditation: a tool to improve healthcare provider compassion, resilience, and patient care. *Journal of Compassionate Health Care, 1*(1), 5.

Seyyed-Rasooli, A., Salehi, F., Mohammadpoorasl, A., Goljaryan, S., Seyyedi, Z., & Thomson, B. (2016). Comparing the effects of aromatherapy massage and inhalation aromatherapy on anxiety and pain in burn patients: A single-blind randomized clinical trial. *Burns, 42*(8), 1774–1780.

Sferopoulos, N. K. (2017). Skin burns following cryotherapy in misdiagnosed pediatric injuries. *Journal of Bodywork and Movement Therapies., 22*(3), 556–559. doi.org/10.1016/j.jbmt.2017.09.006.

Shaheed, C. A., McFarlane, B., Maher, C. G., Williams, K. A., Bergin, J., Matthews, A., & McLachlan, A. J. (2016). Investigating the primary care management of low back pain: a simulated patient study. *The Journal of Pain, 17*(1), 27–35.

Shivashankar, A., Nalini, K. B., & Rath, P. (2018). The role of nonpharmacological methods in attenuation of pain due to peripheral venous cannulation: A randomized controlled study. *Anesthesia Essays and Researches, 12*(1), 7–10.

Smith, R. C., Fortin, A. H., Dwamena, F., & Frankel, R. M. (2013). An evidence-based patient-centered method makes the biopsychosocial model scientific. *Patient Education and Counseling, 91*(3), 265–270.

Smedslund, G., Byfuglien, M. G., Olsen, S. U., & Hagen, K. B. (2010). Effectiveness and safety of dietary interventions for rheumatoid arthritis: a systematic review of randomized controlled trials. *Journal of the American Dietetic Association, 110*(5), 727–735.

Smith, S. M., Sumar, B., & Dixon, K. A. (2014). Musculoskeletal pain in overweight and obese children. *International Journal of Obesity, 38*(1), 11–15.

Smith, T. E., & Cooper, C. L. (2006). *Apparatus and method for reducing the risk of decubitus ulcers. US7030764B2 U. S. Grant.* Washington. D.C.: United States Patent and Trademark Office.

Suren, M., Kaya, Z., Ozkan, F., Erkorkmaz, U., Arıcı, S., & Karaman, S. (2013). Comparison of the use of the Valsalva maneuver and the eutectic mixture of local anesthetics (EMLA®) to relieve venipuncture pain: a randomized controlled trial. *Journal of Anesthesia, 27*(3), 407–411.

Sut, N., & Kahyaoglu-Sut, H. (2017). Effect of aromatherapy massage on pain in primary dysmenorrhea: A meta-analysis. *Complementary Therapies in Clinical Practice, 27*, 5–10.

Szekeres, M., MacDermid, J. C., Grewal, R., & Birmingham, T. (2017). The short-term effects of hot packs vs therapeutic whirlpool on active wrist range of motion for patients with distal radius fracture: A randomized controlled trial. *Journal of Hand Therapy., 31*(3), 276–281.

Taavoni, S., Abdolahian, S., & Haghani, H. (2013). Effect of sacrum-perineum heat therapy on active phase labor pain and client satisfaction: a randomized, controlled trial study. *Pain Medicine, 14*(9), 1301–1306.

Taneli, Y., & Kovach, C. R. (2015). Advancing Theory and Practice Through Collaborative Research in Environmental Gerontology. *Research in Gerontological Nursing, 8*(2), 58–60.

Tarff, A., & Behrens, A. (2017). Ocular Emergencies. *Medical Clinics, 101*(3), 615–639.

Tefikow, S., Barth, J., Maichrowitz, S., Beelmann, A., Strauss, B., & Rosendahl, J. (2013). Efficacy of hypnosis in adults undergoing surgery or medical procedures: A meta-analysis of randomized controlled trials. *Clinical Psychology Review, 33*(5), 623–636.

Thomazeau, J., Perin, J., Nizard, R., Bouhassira, D., Collin, E., Nguyen, E., … Lloret-Linares, C. (2014). Pain management and pain characteristics in obese and normal weight patients before joint replacement. *Journal of Evaluation in Clinical Practice, 20*(5), 611–616.

Tick, H. (2015). Nutrition and pain. *Physical Medicine and Rehabilitation Clinics, 26*(2), 309–320.

Tilak, M., Isaac, S. A., Fletcher, J., Vasanthan, L. T., Subbaiah, R. S., Babu, A., … Tharion, G. (2016). Mirror therapy and transcutaneous electrical nerve stimulation for management of phantom limb pain in amputees—a single blinded randomized controlled trial. *Physiotherapy Research International, 21*(2), 109–115.

Tisserand, R., & Young, R. (2013). General safety guidelines. In *Essential Oil Safety-E-Book: A Guide for Health Care Professionals.* London: Churchill Livingstone.

Torta, D. M., Diano, M., Costa, T., Gallace, A., Duca, S., Geminiani, G. C., & Cauda, F. (2013). Crossing the line of pain: fMRI correlates of crossed-hands analgesia. *The Journal of Pain, 14*(9), 957–965.

Totsch, S. K., Waite, M. E., & Sorge, R. E. (2015). Dietary influence on pain via the immune system. *In Progress in molecular biology and translational science* (Vol. 131, pp. 435–469). Academic Press.

Trojan, J., Diers, M., Fuchs, X., Bach, F., Bekrater-Bodmann, R., Foell, J., … Flor, H. (2014). An augmented reality home-training system based on the mirror training and imagery approach. *Behavior Research Methods, 46*(3), 634–640.

U.S. Department of Health and Human Services (US DHHS). (2014). Aromatherapy. In *Federal Drug Administration.* https://www.fda.gov/cosmetics/productsingredients/products/ucm127054.htm. Accessed 05/12/2018.

Vallbona, C., Hazlewood, C. F., & Jurida, G. (1997). Response of pain to static magnetic fields in postpolio patients: a double-blind pilot study. *Archives of Physical Medicine and Rehabilitation, 78*(11), 1200–1203.

Vanhaudenhuyse, A., Gillet, A., Malaise, N., Salamun, I., Grosdent, S., Maquet, D., ... Faymonville, M. E. (2018). Psychological interventions influence patients' attitudes and beliefs about their chronic pain. *Journal of Traditional and Complementary Medicine, 8*(2), 296–302.

Verghese, S. T., Nath, A., Zenger, D., Patel, R. I., Kaplan, R. F., & Patel, K. M. (2002). The effects of the simulated Valsalva maneuver, liver compression, and/or Trendelenburg position on the cross-sectional area of the internal jugular vein in infants and young children. *Anesthesia & Analgesia, 94*(2), 250–254.

Vervoort, T., & Trost, Z. (2017). Examining Affective-Motivational Dynamics and Behavioral Implications Within The Interpersonal Context of Pain. *The Journal of Pain.*.

Vijay, V., Meenakshi, A., Sukhpal, K., & Ashish, B. (2013). Effect of Valsalva maneuver prior to peripheral intravenous cannulation on intensity of pain. *Nursing and Midwifery Research Journal, 9*(4), 143–151.

Viveky, N., Dahl, W. J., & Whiting, S. J. (2013). Should an anti-inflammatory diet be used in long-term care homes? *Healthy Aging Research, 2*, 1–9.

Vizzari, V., Barba, S., Gindri, P., Duca, S., Giobbe, D., Cerrato, P., ... Torta, D. M. (2017). Mechanical pinprick pain in patients with unilateral spatial neglect: The influence of space representation on the perception of nociceptive stimuli. *European Journal of Pain, 21*(4), 738–749.

Vogus, T. J., & McClelland, L. E. (2016). When the customer is the patient: Lessons from healthcare research on patient satisfaction and service quality ratings. *Human Resource Management Review, 26*(1), 37–49.

Vural, S. P., Yuzer, G. F. N., Ozcan, D. S., Ozbudak, S. D., & Ozgirgin, N. (2016). Effects of mirror therapy in stroke patients with complex regional pain syndrome type 1: a randomized controlled study. *Archives of Physical Medicine and Rehabilitation, 97*(4), 575–581.

Wagner, D., Byrne, M., & Kolcaba, K. (2006). Effects of comfort warming on preoperative patients. *AORN Journal, 84*(3), 427–448.

Wang, W. E., Roy, A., Misra, G., Ho, R. L., Ribeiro-Dasilva, M. C., Fillingim, R. B., & Coombes, S. A. (2019). Altered neural oscillations within and between sensorimotor cortex and parietal cortex in chronic jaw pain. *NeuroImage: Clinical, 24*, 101964.

Warner, P. M., Coffee, T. L., & Yowler, C. J. (2014). Outpatient burn management. *Surgical Clinics of North America, 94*(4), 879–892.

Watkins, A. A., Johnson, T. V., Shrewsberry, A. B., Nourparvar, P., Madni, T., Watkins, C. J., ... Master, V. A. (2014). Ice packs reduce postoperative midline incision pain and narcotic use: a randomized controlled trial. *Journal of the American College of Surgeons, 219*(3), 511–517.

Wells, R. E., Baute, V., & Wahbeh, H. (2017). Complementary and Integrative Medicine for Neurologic Conditions. *The Medical Clinics of North America, 101*(5), 881–893.

Wilder, R. M. (1921). The effects of ketonemia on the course of epilepsy. In *Vol. 2. Mayo Clin Proc* (pp. 307–308).

Wong, J. J., Shearer, H. M., Mior, S., Jacobs, C., Côté, P., Randhawa, K., ... van der Velde, G. (2016). Are manual therapies, passive physical modalities, or acupuncture effective for the management of patients with whiplash-associated disorders or neck pain and associated disorders? An update of the Bone and Joint Decade Task Force on Neck Pain and Its Associated Disorders by the OPTIMa collaboration. *The Spine Journal, 16*(12), 1598–1630.

Wortzel, J., & Spiegel, D. (2017). Hypnosis in Cancer Care. *American Journal of Clinical Hypnosis, 60*(1), 4–17.

Wright, V., & Pendry, B. (2016). Compassion and its role in the clinical encounter: An argument for compassion training. *Journal of Herbal Medicine, 6*(4), 198–203.

Yang, N. Y., Wolever, R. Q., Roberts, R., Perlman, A., Dolor, R. J., Abrams, D. I., ... & Simmons, L. A. (2017). Integrative health care services utilization as a function of body mass index: A BraveNet practice-based research network study. *Advances in Integrative Medicine, 4*(1), 14–21.

Yazdkhasti, M., & Pirak, A. (2016). The effect of aromatherapy with lavender essence on severity of labor pain and duration of labor in primiparous women. *Complementary Therapies in Clinical Practice, 25*, 81–86.

Zaidi, N. (2015). Attenuation of Peripheral Venous Cannulation Pain: A Review of Various Strategies in Practice. *Journal of Anesthesia Clinical Care, 2*(010).

Zandi, M., Amini, P., & Keshavarz, A. (2016). Effectiveness of cold therapy in reducing pain, trismus, and oedema after impacted mandibular third molar surgery: a randomized, self-controlled, observer-blind, split-mouth clinical trial. *International Journal of Oral and Maxillofacial Surgery, 45*(1), 118–123.

Zencir, G., & Eser, I. (2016). Effects of Cold Therapy on Pain and Breathing Exercises Among Median Sternotomy Patients. *Pain Management Nursing, 17*(6), 401–410.

Zhu, Y., Wang, S., Long, H., Zhu, J., Jian, F., Ye, N., & Lai, W. (2017). Effect of static magnetic field on pain level and expression of P2X3 receptors in the trigeminal ganglion in mice following experimental tooth movement. *Bioelectromagnetics, 38*(1), 22–30.

Chapter 28 Improving Institutional Commitment for Effective Multimodal Pain Management

Ann Quinlan-Colwell, Sue Ballato, Greg Scott Firestone, Eva Pittman

CHAPTER OUTLINE

Organizational Commitment to Quality and Pain Management, pg. 770

    Customer Satisfaction, pg. 771

    Patient Safety, pg. 772

    Clinical Care, pg. 772

Organizational Initiatives to Support Quality of Safe and Effective Multimodal Pain Management, pg. 772

    Interdisciplinary Pain Oversight Committee, pg. 772

    Medication Safety Committee, pg. 778

    Opioid Risk Initiatives and Safety Interventions, pg. 778

Quality Improvement, pg. 781

    Plan-Do-Study-Act, pg. 781

    Lean Methodology, pg. 782

    A3 Methodology, pg. 783

    Clinical Research Programs, pg. 786

Clinical Nursing Efforts to Support Organizational Initiatives, pg. 787

    Nursing Shared Governance, pg. 787

    Pain Resource Nurse Program, pg. 788

Education of Clinicians, pg. 789

Future Opportunities for Improvement, pg. 790

    Innovation, pg. 790

    Resources for Guiding Improvements in Institutional Commitment to Safe and Effective Pain Management, pg. 790

Key Points, pg. 790

Case Scenario, pg. 792

References, pg. 792

Organizational Commitment to Quality and Pain Management

High-quality and safe care are at the heart of excellence in health care organizations and should be the underpinning of every patient interaction (Groves, 2014). It is essential that the strategic plan of every health care organization has a focus on quality to improve outcomes and patient satisfaction (Weiner, Balijepally, & Tanniru, 2015). In addition to a fiduciary responsibility, hospital boards are responsible for developing an organizational strategy and a culture to support the delivery of high-quality, safe care for the community they serve (Millar, Freeman, & Mannion, 2015). Further, since the passage of the United States 2010 Patient Protection and Affordable Care Act (ACA), hospital boards have been required to proactively govern with sufficient attention being paid to quality and patient safety (Belmont et al., 2011).

The new framework for the delivery of health care in the United States was created by the ACA, which provided health care organizations a comprehensive strategy for quality improvement (QI) (Wherry & Miller, 2016). The foundation for this QI included clinical integration, reduction of waste, increased transparency, and a systematic approach to care (Belmont et al., 2011). The goal is coordinated patient care across the continuum to achieve optimal results. Coordinated care is accomplished by eliminating waste and reducing costs, increasing patient safety and care quality, and improving efficiency throughout the system (Tsai et al., 2015). The ACA expanded many programs and developed several programs under the umbrella of a value-based purchasing program, as illustrated in Fig. 28.1.

In an era in which quality and cost effectiveness are increasingly essential characteristics of differentiation, prudent organizations are aligning their organizational initiatives to best position themselves in the market

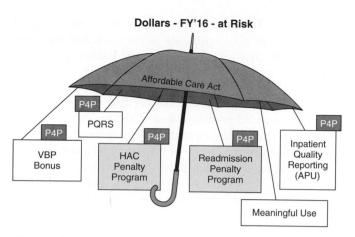

Dollars - FY'16 - at Risk

Fig. 28.1 | **Value Based Purchasing Umbrella.** *APU*, Annual payment update; *FY*, fiscal year; *HAC*, hospital-acquired condition; *P4P*, pay for performance; *PQRS*, Physician Quality Reporting System; *VBP*, value-based purchasing. (Copyrighted Sue Ballato©. Used with permission.)

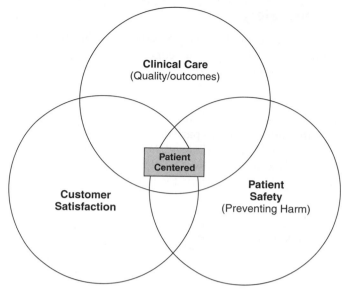

Fig. 28.2 | **Domains of Quality.** (Copyrighted Sue Ballato©. Used with permission.)

(Weiner et al., 2015). Greater transparency has become a priority because the Centers for Medicare and Medicaid Services (CMS) and the Joint Commission (TJC) have accelerated efforts to promote better outcomes, patient safety, and effective care. An important component of achieving those efforts is requiring hospitals to collect data on the core measures (national standards of care and processes to reduce complications) and other quality metrics (Chilgren, 2008). This transparency continued to advance, as evidenced by the CMS recently publishing patient satisfaction, mortality rates, and readmission rates (Belmont et al., 2011). All results are published online for public access, including availability at the http://www.quality-check.org and https://www.medicare.gov/hospitalcompare/search.html websites. These publicly available data have increased accountability of hospitals and health care providers across the country (Burwell, 2015). To maintain current levels of reimbursement, increase volumes, and compete in the marketplace, hospitals must differentiate their services based on quality (French, Homer, Gumus, & Hickling, 2016). This increased high profile for quality and patient safety has provided the impetus for hospital leadership to provide additional resources to achieve a successful result (Jones, Lankshear, & Kelly, 2016).

Quality has been defined in many ways, including by the Institute of Medicine (IOM; now the National Academy of Medicine). The IOM's (2001) definition of health care quality is, "Quality of care is the degree to which health services for individuals and populations increase the likelihood of desired health outcomes and are consistent with current professional knowledge." This definition provides clear and consistent language that can be used as a conceptual framework to compare other definitions of health care quality. This conceptual framework can be organized into three domains: (1) clinical care domain, (2) patient safety domain, and (3) customer service domain with the overlap depicted in Fig. 28.2 as patient centered.

In a health care setting, quality can be defined in eight ways. According to these definitions, quality is classified as (1) customer satisfaction, (2) meeting requirements, (3) continuous process improvement, (4) teamwork and empowerment, (5) outstanding service, (6) cost control and resource utilization, (7) doing the right things right the first time, and (8) how business is done.

Continuous quality improvement (CQI) is not any one thing; it cannot be easily reduced to a slogan, a method of problem-solving, or even a process of cultural change (Laverentz & Kumm, 2017). CQI creates an enormous impact on all aspects of a culture of a hospital, from the way in which patients are treated, to how departments interact, to the language used to describe improvement activities (Laverentz & Kumm, 2017). Whether they are admitting patients, preparing meals, performing heart transplants, or negotiating the budget, staff members are asked to reexamine how their work is planned, executed, and evaluated. CQI can help them do this, but only if it is defined in terms they can understand and use (McFadden, Stock, & Gowen III, 2015).

Customer Satisfaction

Unlike in other parts of the world where health care is supply driven, in the United States, health care is consumer or customer driven (Chilgren, 2008). In today's health care environment, customer satisfaction rises to the top of the list for many health care organizations. A customer can be described in a variety of ways, including as a patient, employee, physician, care provider, or family member. Satisfying the health care consumer can be a daunting task, especially when there are variations in the definition of quality by each individual. It is important to determine who the customer is, what the customer needs, and how the particular service can be delivered in a manner that provides value to the individual.

Patient Safety

In health care quality, patient safety can imply what is based on the Hippocratic conception of "first do no harm" (Donabedian, 2003). (See Chapter 2 for discussion of ethics and pain management.) A care provider should not intentionally harm a patient or create an environment in which harm could occur (IOM, 2001). Doing no harm is simply not enough as patients seek care or a cure when pursuing medical care (Parand, Dopson, Renz, & Vincent, 2014). Quality initiatives designed around improving quality and patient safety by both staff and managers have indicated a support for a culture of clinical excellence from senior leaders and the hospital board of directors (Chilgren, 2008). Parand et al. (2014) performed a systematic review on the role of managers in quality and patient safety. The results of that study indicated senior management involvement in quality and patient safety work was directly related to improved performance in those areas.

Clinical Care

The concerns discussed in this chapter are not unique to health care in the United States. A multinational study was conducted to explore if there was an association between hospital leadership and quality (Tsai et al., 2015). The specific focus of the study was to determine if there was a relationship between quality of care provided with hospital board involvement and the management of care by front-line managers (Tsai et al., 2015). Data were collected from hospitals across the United States and United Kingdom (Tsai et al., 2015). Those data indicated a positive correlation between hospitals with effective management practices such as higher attention to quality, effective use of metrics to drive improvement, and the delivery of higher quality care. Additionally, hospitals that had highly engaged boards had excellent performance by management and staff (Tsai et al., 2015). With the increasing financial pressure by the CMS hospital value-based purchasing programs to link quality payment to quality performance, it is imperative for hospitals to look at processes and structure to improve clinical outcomes (French et al., 2016).

Organizational Initiatives to Support Quality of Safe and Effective Multimodal Pain Management

With a quality focus, health care organizations have responsibility to pursue and support strategies within a culture dedicated to ensuring all patients receive safe and effective pain management (ECRI, 2017). A critical component of achieving that is supporting an interdisciplinary multimodal approach to pain management for people with acute and/or chronic pain (IOM, 2011; Kress

et al., 2015). To date no one strategy has been identified as effective for all institutions to improve and optimize safe and effective pain management. Rather, guidelines have been presented through several diverse resources (Box 28.1). It is incumbent upon each organization to assess the population served, the needs of the population, the education and proficiency of clinicians caring for the population, and barriers within the system that prevent patients from having optimal pain management. To best address the needs of each patient, the organization leadership needs to evaluate information, pursue QI, and implement necessary measures (e.g., guidance, education, technology) to create a culture in which clinicians use an integrative multimodal approach to best care for patients with pain. An underlying organizational responsibility is to use appropriate evidence to support standards of care that both ensure consistently effective care and enable that care to be individualized to address the painful experience of each patient (ECRI, 2017; IOM, 2011). This approach is consistent with patient-centered care.

Much of the literature discussing QI efforts and research focuses on improvement activities within an acute care hospital setting. To ensure continuity of safe and effective pain management, it is imperative these efforts are used by clinicians working in ambulatory care, long-term care, rehabilitation, public health, home health, palliative care, hospice, and any other settings in which health care is provided. QI, research, and publication of such efforts in these settings are sorely needed.

Interdisciplinary Pain Oversight Committee

Pain oversight committees are often developed to guide overall pain management within an organization, or they can be developed with a more particular focus such as education or changing prescription practices (Schell, Abramcyzk, Fominaya, Friedman, & Castle, 2017). Generally, the members of the oversight committee assesses the current state of pain management in the organization, conducts gap and needs analyses, leads improvement activities, and then oversees ongoing pain-related processes (ECRI, 2017) (Fig. 28.3). As a team, the committee members need to have the authority to implement change based on QI activities (Kaplan, Provost, Froehle, & Margolis, 2012). From a continuous improvement perspective, the committee needs to plan for and then conduct regular reassessments of activities and improvements (Australian Commission on Safety and Quality in Health Care [ACSQHC], 2012).

Developing an interdisciplinary committee to guide and improve how pain is assessed and managed within the organization is vital (ECRI, 2017). The Australian Commission on Safety and Quality in Health Care (2012) advised it is important for the oversight team to be collaborative and accountable and include representative frontline staff who can identify real or potential barriers to safe care. Although each organization is unique and no

Box 28.1 Recommendations for Organizational Strategies to Achieve Safe and Effective Multimodal Pain Management

- Develop an interdisciplinary team and identify support from leadership and frontline staff who are dedicated to improve safe and effective multimodal pain management as a moral and professional responsibility.
- Create gap analyses related to safe and effective pain management that includes policies, practices, tools, and resources and identifying where disparities exist.
- Examine data (e.g., adverse events, naloxone use), outcomes, processes, and systems to identify opportunities to improve safe and effective multimodal pain management.
- Reduce or remove barriers that impede optimal pain management, compromise safety, and create disparities, and improve safe multimodal pain management for all patients.
- Identify current and potential resources to support safe and effective multimodal pain management, including people and technology.
- Review and evaluate policies, procedures, protocols, and education to ensure standardization of evidence-supported processes that are done in conjunction with clinical assessment, thinking, and judgment.
- Develop facility standard of care with clinical strategies that balance standardized work processes and pathways with provision for clinical assessment, thinking, and judgement.
- Provide clinicians and staff with available evidence-supported education to enable them to provide safe and effective multimodal pain management consistent with policies and procedures of the organization.
- Increase awareness of the importance of minimizing and preventing pain when possible and effectively treating acute pain to minimize the development of chronic pain.
- Educate all clinicians regarding the importance of appropriately assessing, then safely and effectively managing pain with a multimodal approach to prevent

undertreated pain, adverse effects, negative outcomes, and impaired quality of life.
- Ensure all patients are appropriately assessed and reassessed for pain and side effects, including function, psychosocial impact, sedation, and respiratory sedation.
- Educate and empower clinicians to intervene appropriately without delays based on assessment findings.
- Encourage and support multimodal and multidisciplinary pain management of the person with acute and/or chronic pain throughout the continuum of care.
- Encourage collaboration of clinicians from all disciplines across the continuum of health care.
- Provide and encourage the use of positive feedback and constructive criticism within a supportive framework to encourage improvement through shared goals that encourage challenging existing processes with innovative options.
- Educate patients and families to dispel myths and misinformation as well as about multimodal resources available to support multimodal pain management.
- Encourage and support the use of continuous quality improvement and interdisciplinary clinical research at both academic and nonacademic organizations.

Based on and expanded from the ECRI Institute. (1011). Action Recommendations: Organizational Strategies in the 2017 *ECRI Institute PSO deep dive opioid use in acute care* (p. 9). Washington, D.C.: Institute of Medicine. Kress, H. G., Aldington, D., Alon, E., Coaccioli, S., Collett, B., Coluzzi, F., . . . & Mangas, A. C. (2015). A holistic approach to chronic pain management that involves all stakeholders: Change is needed. *Current Medical Research and Opinion, 31*(9), 1743–1754; Mackey, S. (2016). Future directions for pain management: Lessons from the Institute of Medicine pain report and the national pain strategy. *Hand Clinics, 32*(1), 91–98; and Manss, G. (2017). Implementation of daily senior leader rounds using a transformational leadership approach. *Nurse Leader, 15*(1), 65–69.

recommendations were found in the literature to guide the structure or composition of an interdisciplinary pain oversight committee, there are some key players who need to participate. From a generic perspective, members are needed from organization leadership, medicine (e.g., hospitalist, anesthesia, surgery, behavioral health, addictionology), nursing, pharmacy, physical therapy, complementary modalities, clinical education, and pain management specialists.

Regardless of the composition or agenda of the committee, success depends on the support of both leadership and clinicians (ECRI, 2017). The importance of leadership

involvement is seen in the latest TJC standards (TJC, 2017a). Those standards require all hospitals accredited by TJC to have members of the medical staff with leadership responsibilities to be involved with pain, QI, and safety improvement activities. Aspects of effective pain management influenced by leadership include creating a pain-sensitive culture, commitment to continual improvement, supporting open team communication (e.g., truth over harmony), valuing cohesive collaborative team functioning, and empowering clinicians (Kaplan et al., 2012).

There are some examples of successful pain-focused teamwork in the literature. St. Joseph's Hospital in

Text continued on page 778

**PAIN MANAGEMENT PRACTICES
INSTITUTIONAL ASSESSMENT CHECKLIST**

Name of institution: _____

Person completing checklist/date: _____

ASSESSMENT QUESTIONS	YES	NO	COMMENTS
Does the hospital have a multidisciplinary pain committee? What disciplines and how often do they meet? If no formal pain committee, do any other councils or committees focus on pain?			
Does the hospital have a pain service/team? If so, who coordinates it and who are team members? If no formal pain service or team, is there an individual(s) who evaluates patients' pain other than the primary nurses?			
Does the hospital have a pain resource nurse (PRN) program? Describe the requirements to be a PRN and how they are utilized.			
Does the hospital have a quality improvement process in place for pain management? What aspects and outcomes are monitored?			
Does the hospital have a multidisciplinary high-risk medication safety oversight committee? What disciplines and how often do they meet? If no high-risk medication committee, how does the hospital identify and monitor risk/safety issues related to high-risk medications?			
Does the hospital have an opioid safety committee? If not, how is opioid adverse event risk and prevention identified and addressed?			

Fig. 28.3 | **Pain Management Practices Institutional Assessment Checklist.** (Courtesy Chris Pasero.)

continued

ASSESSMENT QUESTIONS	YES	NO	COMMENTS
Is there multidisciplinary support to improve/change pain management practices? Give examples.			
Does the hospital administration support pain management practice improvements/changes? Give examples.			
Are there major obstacles to improving pain management? Give examples.			
Are decision-making tools such as pain management decision trees, algorithms, or scripting used?			
Is pain management education provided regularly for all disciplines? What is taught, who teaches it, and how often? Is it mandatory?			
Are patients taught about pain assessment management techniques? What is taught, who teaches it, and when?			
Are patients taught about opioid side effects and how these can be minimized and treated? What is taught, who teaches it, and when?			
Are patients given the option of not taking an opioid to avoid opioid side effects?			
Is the concept of multimodal analgesia understood by most nurses, physicians, and pharmacists? If not, what are the barriers to increasing understanding?			

Fig. 28.3, Cont'd

continued

ASSESSMENT QUESTIONS	YES	NO	COMMENTS
Do multimodal practices/order sets exist? If not, what are the barriers to implementing them?			
Does the hospital formulary allow orders for a variety of nonopioid options, such as acetaminophen, NSAIDs, local anesthetics, ketamine, clonidine, muscle relaxants?			
Are non-opioids (see above examples) given before opioids are given, i.e., are they used as a foundation of pain management therapy?			
Are nonpharmacologic methods, such as ice, heat, massage, music, TV comfort channel, used routinely? Which methods are used and who provides them most often?			
Are all patients screened for risk for opioid-induced respiratory depression on admission?			
Are all patients screened for risk for opioid-induced respiratory depression during opioid therapy, such as with changes in patient condition, introduction of iatrogenic risk?			
Is documentation of risk screening and ongoing opioid risk assessment for opioid-induced respiratory depression audited? What tool is used? How is the staff informed of audit findings?			

Fig. 28.3, Cont'd

continued

ASSESSMENT QUESTIONS	YES	NO	COMMENTS
Is unwanted sedation assessed during opioid administration in the postanesthesia care unit (PACU)? If yes, what scale is used?			
Is unwanted sedation assessed during opioid administration on the clinical units? Is a scale used for sedation assessment? If yes, what scale is used?			
Is pulse oximetry (oxygen saturation monitoring) used? Is it used in continuous or intermittent mode? Is it limited to certain clinical units or patients?			
Is capnography (end-tidal CO_2 monitoring) used? Is it limited to certain clinical units or patients?			
Is documentation of risk screening and ongoing opioid risk assessment for opioid-induced respiratory depression audited? What tool is used? How is the staff informed of audit findings?			
Is unwanted sedation assessed during opioid administration in the postanesthesia care unit (PACU)? If yes, what scale is used?			
Is unwanted sedation assessed during opioid administration on the clinical units? Is a scale used for sedation assessment? If yes, what scale is used?			

Fig. 28.3, Cont'd

continued

ASSESSMENT QUESTIONS	YES	NO	COMMENTS
Is pulse oximetry (oxygen saturation monitoring) used? Is it used in continuous or intermittent mode? Is it limited to certain clinical units or patients?			
Is capnography (end-tidal CO$_2$ monitoring) used? Is it limited to certain clinical units or patients?			
Are centralized capnography and pulse oximetry utilized whereby all monitoring of these parameters can be seen from the nurse's station? If yes, on which units?			
Does the hospital own an adequate number of pulse oximetry and capnography monitors or have plans to purchase an adequate number?			

Fig. 28.3, Cont'd

Marshfield, Michigan, formed an interdisciplinary steering committee with oversight to implement an initiative to improve pain management and foster patient-centered care across the continuum (Lutz, 2017). That committee uses evidence-based best practices to standardize care and continually reevaluates where there are opportunities to further improve. There is an interdisciplinary pain management oversight committee at the Veterans Administration Medical Center in Charleston, South Carolina (Isaacks, 2015). That committee consists of representatives from pain management, primary care, pharmacy, behavioral health, and the quality department who work to establish appropriate protocols and standards for safe pain management throughout the continuum of care.

There is a need for research to better identify what constitutes successful oversight committees, what are the characteristics of those committees, what was involved with their successful efforts, and what the members learned from efforts that were not effective. Subsequent publication of that research is also important to disseminate the information and assist other organizations with their efforts to improve pain management.

Medication Safety Committee

Medication safety committees are generally multidisciplinary teams that follow and assess trends in the use of medications, adverse events, and medication errors and then initiate education for both clinicians and patients (Dinescu et al., 2012; Khalil, Shahid, & Roughead, 2017). Within the California Hospital Association, members of the medication safety committees are the designated experts in medication safety. The association has a "Medication Safety Toolkit" that can be used to assess and then improve medication safety in an organization. Among other areas addressed are ways to enhance safety with opioids, reducing adverse drug events and reducing diversion of controlled substances (CHA, 2020). Researchers who evaluated the effectiveness of another medication safety program reported success depended on collecting baseline data, analyzing the data, explaining it to clinicians, identifying what errors occurred, and transforming the organizational culture to one of safety (Khalil & Lee, 2018). The ISMP Medication Safety Self-Assessment Tool for High-Alert Medications is an excellent organizational tool for assessing the safety and practices regarding opioids and other high-risk medications within an organization (ISMP, 2018).

Opioid Risk Initiatives and Safety Interventions

Opioids have been a mainstay in acute, chronic, and palliative pain management for many years. Concerns and cautions have progressively increased regarding adverse events such as respiratory depression and the prevalence of opioid use disorder, which in 2017 was estimated to involve 2 million Americans (St. Marie, Arnstein, & Zimmer, 2018). These topics are discussed in detail in other chapters. (See Chapter 11 for discussion of opioids, Chapter 12 for discussion of opioid side effects, Chapter 13 for discussion of advancing sedation and opioid-induced respiratory depression, and Chapter 14 for a detailed discussion of substance use disorder.) In this chapter the discussion is from the perspective of how institutions can improve their commitment to safe and effective multimodal pain management by addressing opioid risk initiatives and safety interventions.

Health care leaders are challenged to scrutinize opioid prescribing in the facility by conducting a self-assessment of the organization (ECRI, 2017). This scrutiny needs to include investigating any risks to patient safety, inadequate education of clinicians, barriers to safe opioid prescribing (e.g., cumbersome system for clinicians to check the state monitoring database), barriers to safe opioid administration, barriers to appropriate use of multimodal analgesia including nonpharmacologic interventions, and inadequate education of patients in preparation for discharge. There is a requirement for leadership oversight of opioid prescribing in the most recent TJC standards (TJC, 2017a; TJC, 2017b). The American Society for Pain Management Nurses (ASPMN, 2018) has developed a tool kit to assist organizational leadership with meeting the TJC standards. The ASPMN toolkit can be accessed at: https://customer.aspmn.org/aspmnwcm/Store/Shared_Content/Store_Home_Custom.aspx.

From a national perspective, the President's Commission on Combating Drug Addiction and the Opioid Crisis (PCCDOC) drafted an interim report that called for several actions (PCCDOC, 2017). Improvements in education of clinicians regarding safe opioid prescribing and assessing patient risk are important and basic needs. The PCCDOC also identified the need to enhance prescription drug monitoring programs, including access across states, and recognized the need for naloxone to be available to patients and first responders in the community. The Commission also called for increased resources for behavioral health services, substance use disorder facilities, and medication-assisted therapy.

Organizational efforts have been undertaken in diverse areas of the United States to address concerns regarding appropriate and safe opioid prescription and administration while improving safe and effective multimodal pain management. In 2014 the Hospital and Healthsystem Association of Pennsylvania–Hospital Improvement Innovation Network (HAP HIIN) advised each participating hospital to create an interdisciplinary team with representatives, similar to those previously described, as appropriate members for a pain oversight committee but with greater leadership representation and risk management representation (HAP HIIN, 2014). The HAP HIIN developed a self-assessment tool to identify areas of specific risk and opportunities for improvement. They share this tool, which can be completed as a group activity by hospital interdisciplinary teams.

The U.S. Veterans Health Administration (VHA) was a pioneer in addressing these concerns. One VHA effort was the Stratification Tool for Opioid Risk Mitigation (STORM), which evolved from the VHA's integrative Opioid Safety Initiative and Overdose Education and Naloxone Distribution program (Oliva et al., 2017). STORM uses electronic medical record (EMR) data to predict the likelihood of each individual patient being at high risk for an opioid-related adverse event and overdose.

New Hanover Regional Medical Center in North Carolina took a different approach by partnering with representatives of behavioral health facilities, substance use treatment centers, schools (public school system, colleges, universities), local churches, government agencies (state public health, local public health, Medicaid, legislature, court system), first responders, law enforcement, transportation, recovery support groups, families, and others. This interdisciplinary group, with many subcommittees, was working in an ongoing fashion at the time of publication to address multimodal pain management, opioid use, opioid misuse, and abuse from a supportive community perspective (Herndon, Pino, Quinlan-Colwell, 2017).

Regardless of the scope of the initiative (facility based, system wide, community, state, or federal), a commonality among these efforts is the active participation of leaders, interdisciplinary clinicians, and front-line staff, as well as patients and families, when appropriate or possible. It is also important to include representatives of disciplines and support services who can sustain efforts for continued success. In a hospital setting, this likely will include representatives from informatics, respiratory therapy, physical therapy, social work, and behavioral health, among others. In the community, it is important to include representatives from government agencies, treatment centers, behavioral health, public health, police, first responders, schools, churches, housing, and transportation, among others (Herndon et al., 2017).

Naloxone Availability

In recent years, overdoses from opioids and other pharmaceutical products surpassed motor vehicle accidents as the number one cause of death because of injury (Centers for Disease Control and Prevention [CDC], 2012). Naloxone is an opioid antagonist that can reverse respiratory depression and sequelae of opioid overdose and save lives (Rudd-Barnard, Pangarkar, Moaleji, & Glassman, 2016). Education about the importance of using naloxone appropriately is imperative. Naloxone education needs to be focused on several groups, including bedside clinicians, first responders (emergency medical service [EMS], law enforcement), patients, and families. Clinicians need to be educated and competent in administering naloxone to any patient who has received an opioid and is nonresponsive with slowed respirations. Many organizations include as-needed (prn) orders for naloxone on order sets with opioid prescriptions, with some linking naloxone use to sedation assessment score on a tool such as the Pasero

Opioid Sedation Scale (POSS). (See Chapters 11 and 13 for more information on naloxone and Chapter 13 for more information on the POSS.)

In an effort to monitor opioid adverse events, medication safety teams frequently collect organization-specific naloxone data; however, this can be an imprecise gauge because naloxone can be used for reasons other than respiratory depression (ECRI, 2017; Gordon & Pellino, 2005). For example, a small dose of naloxone in a slow intravenous infusion is used as an effective treatment for pruritus, nausea, and vomiting (Gan et al., 1997). Naloxone has been used to successfully reverse valproic acid intoxication (Thanacoody, 2007). Naloxone also can be used in an effort to reverse sedation when the cause of sedation may be related to comorbidities, that is, cause other than opioids (Gordon & Pellino, 2005). However, naloxone data collection does provide the opportunity for the committee to review the event and identify additional information to follow up appropriately (Rudd-Barnard, Pangarkar, Moaleji, & Glassman, 2016) and monitor trends.

EMS and other first responders often are the first people who identify the overdose situation. The importance of educating EMS was highlighted in the report of a recent study in Rhode Island (Sumner et al., 2016). In that study, it was found that naloxone was administered by EMS to only 66% of patients who overdosed with opioids. The authors also reported females and people who did not have signs of opioid abuse were three-fold less likely to receive naloxone. Similarly, older adults were less likely to receive it. The authors of a 4-year-long retrospective review (2009–2013) of EMS-administered naloxone reported patients who were more frequently transported to the emergency department (ED) were also more likely to receive naloxone than those who were less often transported to the ED (Lindstrom et al., 2015). Using national data from the U.S. National Medical Services Information System, the use of multiple administrations of naloxone by EMS providers to the same person during one event increased between 2012 and 2015, which may be related to the potency or dose of the opioids causing the overdose (Faul et al., 2017). One hindrance of naloxone being used by emergency medical technicians (EMTs) is that in some states, EMTs in some categories are not allowed to administer it (Faul et al., 2015). Unfortunately, this limited ability is more frequently true in rural areas where other resources are also limited.

Firefighters and police officers who are not paramedics are also often the first to respond to an overdose situation and are increasingly being trained in appropriate naloxone use. To date, at least 43 states have some use of naloxone by law enforcement officers (North Carolina Harm Reduction Coalition [NCHRC], 2018). In Massachusetts, several communities have provided naloxone education and accorded the ability to administer naloxone to nonparamedic first responders (Davis, Ruiz, Glynn, Picariello, & Walley, 2014). In Ohio the use of intranasal naloxone by police officers was associated with a reduction in deaths as a result of overdose (Rando,

Broering, Olson, Marco, & Evans, 2015). As of February 2018, there were 1084 instances of successful naloxone rescues by law enforcement officers reported in North Carolina alone (NCHRC, 2018). This was a dramatic increase from the 185 rescues in the summer of 2016.

The third group of people who need education about naloxone are patients and their family members and friends. Current research studies indicate bystanders and those who are personally at risk for overdose are willing to learn how to administer naloxone (Clark, Wilder, & Winstanley, 2014; Mueller, Walley, Calcaterra, Glanz, & Binswanger, 2015). The effort of making naloxone available to those individuals (bystanders and those at risk) has increased during the past 20 years with more than 50,000 people in the United States having received community *overdose education and naloxone (OEN)* rescue kits between 1996 and 2010 (CDC, 2012). Concern over arrest traditionally dissuaded people in the community from using naloxone. To counteract that concern and encourage use when needed, at the time of this writing, at least 40 states and the District of Columbia enacted immunity laws (i.e., *Good Samaritan* laws) (PCCDOC, 2017). In some states, only first responders and family members are allowed to possess naloxone (e.g., West Virginia), whereas in other states, naloxone is legalized and sold over the counter (e.g., Massachusetts) and available to anyone (Beheshti et al., 2015).

A survey conducted with people who participated in OEN training in the northeast United States (n = 126) showed the responders were predominantly white (95%), female (78%), and parents of an opioid user (85%) and wanted to have a naloxone kit in their residence (72%) (Bagley et al., 2015). Of those responding, 16 were parents who had witnessed an overdose in their son or daughter. Five of the training attendees had successfully administered naloxone to someone after an overdose.

One of the recommendations in *The CDC Guideline for Prescribing Opioids for Chronic Pain* is that providers need to discuss and consider coprescribing naloxone when prescribing opioids (Dowell, Haegerich, & Chou, 2016). Most recently it was recommended in the 2017 President's Commission on Combating Drug Addiction and the Opioid Crisis draft report that naloxone needs to be prescribed whenever *high-risk opioids* are prescribed (PCCDOC, 2017). This is not a novel idea. Scotland was the pioneer in establishing a nationally funded program to provide *take-home naloxone* as a health policy (Bird, Parmar, & Strang, 2015). In that program, naloxone is provided to all individuals who are determined to be at risk for overdose of an opioid (Bird, McAuley, Perry, & Hunter, 2016). Further, many hospitals in the United States now require automatic prescription of naloxone whenever opioids are prescribed in the inpatient setting. To further these efforts, in April of 2018, the Office of the Surgeon General issued a public health advisory stressing the need to educate people (e.g., clinicians, opioid users, family, first responders, community members) about naloxone while making it available and encouraging the use of it to save lives (Adams, 2018). That public health advisory supports the importance of institutional and community collaboration and efforts to address this serious health situation.

There are many benefits for naloxone to be available to reverse opioid-induced respiratory depression in a non–health care environment. Despite successful efforts with OEN, there continues to be disagreement as to whether naloxone should be readily available to those in the community (Beheshti et al., 2015). The topic of community-available naloxone needs to be researched to assess safety, benefits versus potential undesirable effects or risk, pitfalls, and inappropriate use (Zuckerman, Weisberg, & Boyer, 2014). The influence of layperson administration and more accurate identification of an opioid overdose during a 911 call also need to be explored (Faul et al., 2017). Another area in need of research is the effect of intranasal naloxone on overdoses involving opioids other than heroin, such as higher potency fentaNYL (Wermeling, 2015). Finally, the long-term effect of the increased availability of naloxone on substance misuse/abuse and seeking help with substance use disorder recovery needs to be researched (Moore, Lloyd, Oretti, Russell, & Snooks, 2015).

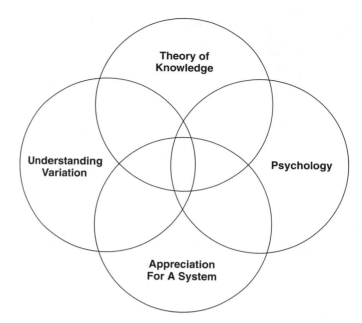

Fig. 28.4 | Deming's Four Elements of the System of Profound Knowledge. (From Koyle, M. A., Koyle, L. C. C., & Baker, G. R. (2018). Quality improvement and patient safety: Reality and responsibility from Codman to today. *Journal of Pediatric Urology, 14*, 16–18.)

Quality Improvement

QI can be considered a process in which existing information, data, or knowledge are used in active efforts to improve the system or process (Koyle, Koyle, & Baker, 2018). In that sense, QI efforts are designed to assess data to determine the level of performance of a unit or agency when compared to professional standards and to identify barriers to care or improvement. After identification of a problem, the next step in QI is to plan how to improve to enable meeting or surpassing the standard (Baker et al., 2014; IOM, 2011). Using collected data, analyzing it, and then making appropriate changes are not only necessary steps for improving health care, but it is essential that the changes to be made through a continuous improvement process (Curcin, Woodcock, Poots, Majeed, & Bell, 2014). Following implementation, it is necessary to monitor activities, maintain efforts, and facilitate continuing progress (Baker et al., 2014; IOM, 2011).

Current QI processes largely grew from the *System of Profound Knowledge* by William Edwards Deming, who identified four elements in that system. Those elements are (1) having a theory of knowledge, (2) understanding psychology and human behavior, (3) appreciating the system, and (4) understanding variation in the system and the need to eliminate it (Koyle et al., 2018) (Fig. 28.4).

Plan-Do-Study-Act

One QI method commonly used in health care is *Plan-Do-Study-Act (PDSA)*, which is a rapid cycle process designed to provide structure for making and testing change to

improve quality within health care systems (Koyle et al., 2018; Taylor et al., 2014). The PDSA process originated in 1950 when Deming introduced to Japanese engineers the scientific methodology of Walter Shewhart. This became known as the Deming wheel, Deming circle, or Deming cycle. The wheel focused on a rotation of four steps: *design, production, sales,* and *research.* This was altered and adopted by the Japanese engineers as the PDCA cycle of *plan* (design), *do* (production), *check* (sales), and *act* (research). Subsequently, Deming revised the circle into the Shewhart Cycle for Learning and Improvement with the four components of *plan, do, study,* and *act* (Moen & Norman, 2010).

As envisioned today, the four steps of the PDSA process are consistent with the last revision by Deming (Fig. 28.5). The *plan* step of the cycle involves identifying the goal or objective, asking questions, and developing a plan to reach the goals. The *do* step includes implementing the plan and collecting and analyzing data. *Study* comprises completing data analysis, assessing progress, summarizing findings, and reflecting on what has been learned. *Act* involves identifying what needs to be done next, including any necessary refinements to the plan and ensuring all advances are realized (Donnelly & Kirk, 2015; Moen & Norman, 2010; Wainwright, Immins, & Middleton, 2016) (Fig. 28.5). The continuous improvement perspective of PDSA is an important aspect through which each cycle involves adjustments for further enhancement (Koyle et al., 2018). This occurs when the fourth step, *act,* leads to another PDSA cycle, with each cycle resulting in small changes. These small incremental changes are thought to result in the greatest chance for sustaining improvements (Donnelly & Kirk, 2015).

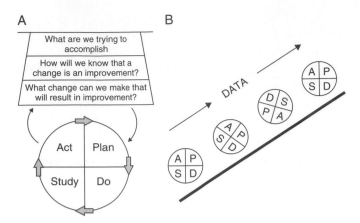

Fig. 28.5 | The concept of promoting change in a system using Plan-Do-Study-Act (PDSA) (A). PDSA cycles are repeatedly employed in a "ramping up" or escalating fashion so that a hunch ultimately leads to sustainable changes that result in improvement (B). (From Koyle, M. A., Koyle, L. C. C., & Baker, G. R. (2018). Quality improvement and patient safety: Reality and responsibility from Codman to today. *Journal of Pediatric Urology, 14,* 16–18.)

The PDSA method is easily used to support continuous improvement in health care. It was used to improve clinical care of patients with hip osteoarthritis in the United Kingdom (Wainwright et al., 2016). In that QI initiative, *plan,* or the objective, was to identify a nonsurgical alternative to surgical hip replacements. *Do* was implementing a cycling program designed to improve mobility and lessen pain. That was done with three consecutive groups for whom data were collected. *Study* involved analyzing the data, including patient responses to open-ended questions about the experiences. Those components of data were then compared with the current literature. In that QI effort, *act* involved continuing the activity and acknowledging the need for research to further explore the benefit to a larger population.

The PDSA methodology was used by nurses in a pain resource nurse (PRN) program in Wisconsin (Greeneway & Corsten, 2016). Their *plan* step was to improve pain management, patient satisfaction scores, and compliance with organization and TJC standards. Their *do* step was to implement nonpharmacologic interventions (i.e., music therapy, guided imagery, comfort menu, individual education) and provide information about the effort to nurses by huddles and a newsletter. Their *act* step was to assess the results, which showed improvements. They recycled with the PDSA and the following year implemented additional strategies, including education regarding the pain scale, a newly developed pain-specific staff newsletter, and nursing pain competency tool. They are continuing to monitor results and work to improve care and scores.

Lean Methodology

Lean is a QI philosophy, methodology, management system, and tool set that enables individuals and organizations to improve quality, safety, and efficiency through the elimination of waste and redundancy (Collar et al., 2012; Simons et al., 2015). Many people credit Toyota Motor Corporation with the genesis of Lean methodology, because in 1945 they developed the Toyota Production System model for process improvement and refined it over several decades (Graban, 2012; Spear & Bowen, 1999). This is not completely accurate because Toyota was inspired by others, including Henry Ford and Edwards Deming, who visited the Toyota plant (Graban, 2012). As with PDSA, Lean theory is deep-rooted in the scientific method concepts developed by Deming's friend and mentor Walter A. Shewhart (Simon & Canacari, 2012).

Although Lean started in the manufacturing industry, it can be applied in any environment. Over the past two decades, leaders in health care have gradually adopted Lean methodology to continually improve patient safety and quality of care and reduce waste while improving efficiency (D'Andreamatteo, Ianni, Lega, & Sargiacomo, 2015). Lean is a superb strategy for achieving operational excellence, continuous improvement, and continuous learning. Similar to PDSA, an important aspect of Lean is the focus on continuous small incremental improvements that increase over time (Olesen, Powell, Hvolby, & Fraser, 2015). Therefore organizations are encouraged to move away from viewing issues and failures negatively. Instead they are encouraged to carefully examine failures and view them as learning opportunities to guide improvements.

Lean provides a road map to view problems objectively, guiding the problem solver by providing a standardized, structured way of assessing process issues and difficulties (Knechtges & Decker, 2014). In that sense, Lean is a format for problem solving that is simple to use, is logical, and follows the design of the PDSA model (Simon & Canacari, 2012), which is an important component within the Lean process (Knechtges & Decker, 2014). By applying rules of observation with gathering relevant facts and details about how the process functions, the user can identify the true root cause of the dysfunction. Rather than blaming individuals (i.e., the *root who*), Lean is a process designed to identify malfunctions within the system and rectify the breakdowns to enable people using the system to succeed (Ashok Sarkar, Ranjan Mukhopadhyay, & Ghosh, 2013; Furman & Kuczyńska-Chałada, 2016; Yushak, Hashimb, Chulc, & Bakard, 2016). Thus searching for and identifying the root cause of the problem are critical.

From a Lean perspective, functions and activities are categorized based on their value as either *value added,* or *non–value added* or *muda,* which is the Japanese word for activity that is wasteful (Collar et al., 2012; Graban, 2012). Value-added components or activities are those tangible or intangible elements in a process that contribute directly to the service being delivered (Graban, 2012). Direct patient interactions with clinicians, including pain assessment and developing an analgesic plan of care, are elements contributing direct value to what is experienced by the patient. Non–value-added items are things or activities that waste time and delay or block the delivery of care or service (Collar et al., 2012; Graban, 2012). An example of non–value added in patient care is when a patient must wait for a clinician to locate the medical record, assessment tools, supplies, or medication. Ineffective communication, confusion regarding clinician orders, searching for essential equipment and medications, or any work that contains duplication or waste, requires rework, or is redundant are all non–value-added functions.

A true Lean transformation will be accomplished only if employees feel safe in their positions and environment. It is important to set the stage and change the culture of the organization to approach issues in a way that cultivates respect and safety (Simons et al., 2015). When Lean permeates the culture of an organization, there is *respect for people* (Gabow & Goodman, 2015). Using Lean methodology moves the organization toward a focus of fixing any dysfunctional aspects of the process. Using Lean moves the organization away from a culture of blaming (i.e., *root who did it wrong*), which leads to fear and typically a reluctance to report issues, which can lead to more serious situations and compromise safety (Barnas & Adams, 2014; Mullaney, 2010). When using Lean methods, blame is replaced with accountability and staff having necessary resources to succeed and time and support to most effectively problem solve issues. People who function from a Lean perspective seek to understand failures. They also want to understand processes impeding performance and obstructing the natural productive flow within a given system, which can lead to dissatisfied patients and clinicians (customers) (Liker & Trachilis, 2014). With Lean methodology, when things do not go as planned, the entire process is analyzed to identify the root causes of obstructions or failures, to prevent continuing harm to patients and clinicians (Collar et al., 2012).

A3 Methodology

A3 problem solving is a systematic, consistent, concise, objective, logical, consensus building component of Lean methodology (Kimsey, 2010). The A3 format is so named for the size of paper used to diagram the process (Estrada, 2018). By using a standardized template, participants are encouraged to consistently and more fully understand the problem as it occurs across the system in the active current state (Rotter et al., 2017; Sobek & Smalley, 2008). The A3 template is a visual process improvement tool that encourages synthesis and distillation of information, including a statement of the problem, depiction of the issues of the current work environment, critical examination of the root causes, identifying the targeted state, and then developing a plan (Brateanu, Thomascik, Koncilja, Spencer, & Colbert, 2017; Estrada, 2018; Mullaney, 2010). This process also facilitates time management skills.

Initially it is important to assemble a team of stakeholders, making sure the people who are doing the work and the people being affected by possible decisions to change the process are represented. Identify a team leader to maintain team focus on the A3 in progress. It is important to have the voice of the people doing the work present and active throughout the process and gain their input. Problem solving should be performed in real time, not saved to be performed at another meeting (Kimsey, 2010). Table 28.1 presents the specific steps in the A3 process.

Use of the A3 methodology is undertaken by a process owner together with a team of appropriate stakeholders, including frontline staff. The team members gather information and then analyze the information to gain a consensus understanding of how best to repair the process to improve process alignment. The team directly observes the process by going to where the work is performed. This is also known as *Gemba walk* or going to *Gemba*, which is the Japanese word to identify the place where the work happens (Rotter et al., 2017). This type of information gathering may involve interviewing workers, performing direct observations of the process, and timing different components of the process. Going to the *Gemba* is an effective way to learn about the process and identify where waste occurs in the process (Mullaney, 2010). In this way, the Lean A3 method minimizes the influence of bias or prejudicial theorizing and posing premature solutions (Shook, 2008). In addition to facilitating coherence of problem solving and accelerating process improvement, the A3 approach can improve communication because within an A3 gathering truth is more important than harmony in a confidential setting.

As the information is depicted on the A3 template, participants see the workflow process visually in a clear, concise, distilled display of the generalized flow of problem solving, resulting from the diligence of the team. Box 28.2 presents an example of a completed A3 template. Using this methodology, stakeholders collectively endeavor to construct an accurate, reliable, consistent and nonarbitrary representation of the problem (Toussaint, Billi, & Graban, 2017). The A3 documentation progresses as information is collected; processing of information occurs, and problem solving generates countermeasures to correct the problem (Brateanu et al., 2017). This is illustrated in the Clinical Application in Box 28.2. Elements of the A3 document may be used for future coaching of frontline staff, to explain the reasons why the countermeasures were chosen to make necessary improvements in the desired state. This shared learning style allows participants to anticipate what information would be helpful to resolve the issue.

A3: Pitfalls

It is important to remember that when performing any type of process improvement, issues will arise, such as *scope creep,* which involves taking on an issue that is too big for an A3 (Smith, Wood, & Beauvais, 2011).

Table 28.1	**The A3 Process Using Plan-Do-Study-Act (PDSA) Cycles**
Plan: Formulate the issue statement.	This is a one- or two-sentence objective statement of the actual problem, rather than just the symptoms that exist because of the problem.
Plan: Identify key background information and baseline measurements.	This is a brief description of why the current situation is a problem with data or information supporting the reasons, severity, and impact on the customer and/or organization. It is essential to have data or metrics illustrating the extent of the problem. This is a key step in the process to measure improvement from baseline.
Plan: Identify the current state using value stream mapping (VSM).	This is a description of the process as it currently exists. The team goes to the Gemba. They observe and interview the staff doing the work using humble inquiry (creating a relationship based on interest and inquisitiveness rather than interrogation). Based on Gemba observations, the team creates a visual representation on the A3 template of all aspects of the process. This template guides problem solving and prioritizing efforts.
Plan: Conduct the analysis of the problem.	The process begins by reviewing the areas of concern in the bursts in the VSM of the A3. As possible concerns are consolidated into similar factors and prioritized. Next the team asks the question *why* and continues to ask why to each response until the root cause is identified. This is a drill down process to identify the root cause and effect of each individual issue. Visualizing the value stream mapping assists in this analysis.
Plan: Identify the target condition or future state	In this step the team identifies an appropriate, yet challenging goal that is identified as the target condition or future state. This answers the questions of *what do you want to achieve* and *when do you want to achieve it?* It is important to identify measurable indicators for the future state.
Plan: Create the countermeasures.	After the future state has been identified, the team needs to take actions to reduce or eliminate the root causes or problems by implementing countermeasures. These are the changes that need to happen to counteract the root cause/s to enable the team to move closer to the target condition.
Do: Implement the plan.	All countermeasures should be tested on a small scale before fully implementing them. An implementation plan is established with details of how to ensure the countermeasures will be activated, who will be responsible for what action, and when will the expected outcome for each action be operational. Such a plan is important to ensure progress and accountability of all members.
Study: Evaluate the results of the trial.	The next step is to review and evaluate the impact of the countermeasures on the new target condition by conducting a cost/benefit analysis during a trial period. Assess if progress was made in reaching the target condition. If no progress was made, what barriers were encountered? Assess the costs versus benefits (e.g., financial, time, quality, safety) of implementation. Results will determine if the countermeasures and new process need to be implemented. These results will be evaluated in coordination with the value stream to determine if the countermeasures and new process need to be fully implemented or modified and retested. If the plan is to be implemented, it needs to be communicated to stakeholders and staff. Often, standard work for the new process or better way of doing the work is developed. When that is done stakeholders and staff must be educated about the standard work.
Act: Monitor	Once countermeasures are fully implemented, ongoing monitoring of *leading* and *lagging indicators* is done using leading and lagging indicators to support sustainment and ensure the target is achieved. *Leading indicators* are human behaviors that are performed daily and are monitored on a regular basis to assess compliance with the new standard work of the target condition. To achieve the target condition, it is important that staff have accountability with the new standard work process. *Lagging indicators* are assessments of the overall results at 30-, 60-, 90-day intervals.

Modified from Barnas, K., & Adams, E. (2014). Beyond heroes: A lean management system for healthcare. Appleton, WI: ThedaCare Center for Healthcare Value; Graban, M. (2012). Lean hospitals: Improving quality, patient safety, and employee engagement (2nd ed.). Boca Raton, FL: CRC Press; Liker, J. K., & Trachilis, G. (2014) Developing Lean leaders at all levels: A practical guide. Winnipeg, Manitoba, Canada: Lean Leadership Institute Publications; Rotter, T., Plishka, C. T., Adegboyega, L., Fiander, M., Harrison, E. L., Flynn, R., . . . & Kinsman, L. (2017). Lean management in health care: Effects on patient outcomes, professional practice, and healthcare systems. The Cochrane Library, CD012831; Schein, E. H. (2014). Humble inquiry: The gentle art of asking instead of telling. San Francisco, CA: Berrett-Koehler, Inc.

Box 28.2 | Clinical Application: A3 Example: Increasing Pain Management Scores on Hospital Consumer Assessment of Healthcare Providers and Systems (HCAHPS)/Press Ganey Survey

A multidisciplinary team comprising frontline staff and representation from the administration was convened with a Lean Coach to use the A3 process to explore factors contributing to the low HCAPS/Press Ganey scores on one particular unit. The team reviewed the survey comments, observed the pain management process on the unit, interviewed patients, spoke with staff, and mapped pain-related processes. The top issues identified are highlighted in red and visually displayed on the current state map as Kaizen bursts shown in the following figure. After the current state analysis was complete, the team used the *5 Whys* to drill down to the root cause, which was subsequently identified as no defined plan or process for staff to communicate with patients about pain control.

Once this true, *root cause* was identified, it was time to move to the right side of the A3 paper to develop the *future state or target condition*. A clear *target condition* was "to meet/exceed the organizational target of reaching the 76th percentile or greater on the survey rankings." Two *countermeasures* were developed to counteract the root cause. Thus standard work for creating and communicating an individualized pain management plan was developed, trialed on a small scale using the PDSA process, and then rolled out to the entire unit.

Staff were educated and held accountable to follow the new standard format of communicating the plan for pain management with patients. Leadership monitored the process daily until sustainment was evident before moving onto weekly monitoring. When the new process became part of the unit culture, assessment was done with monthly checks. In this case the percentile ranking on the HCAPS/Press Ganey survey went from the 12th to the 99th percentile, exceeding the organizational target days of implementation.

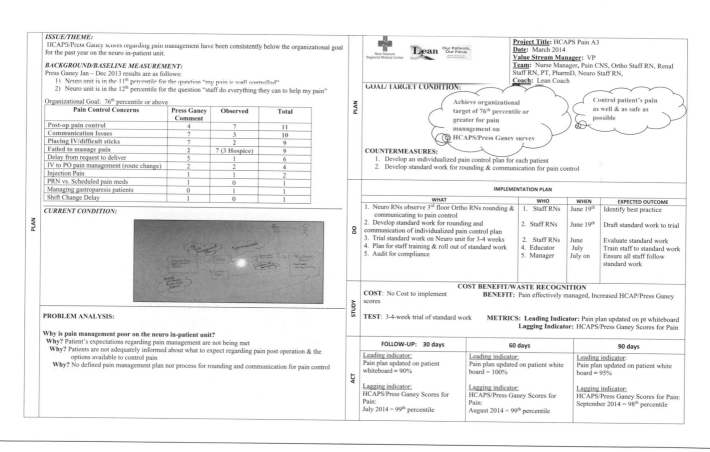

Two indicators of scope creep are issues that involve more than one department or issues that occur outside the sphere of influence of the Lean group. One way to make sure that important issues outside of the scope of the A3 are addressed is to have a *parking lot* document on which all of these issues to be addressed in the future are recorded. Other pitfalls that can lead to poor results are initially failing to identify a true root cause, not testing the new processes before rolling out to full implementation, and not following up for sustainment. These can all eventually lead to process breakdown and failure.

Clinical Research Programs

Nurses have conducted important pain-related research in the clinical setting with patients of all ages from a variety of perspectives. A few examples of this diverse research are reported here. Hunt et al. (2015) explored a number of variables regarding pain in older community-dwelling adults with dementia (Hunt et al., 2015). Quinlan-Colwell, Thear, Miller-Baldwin, and Smith (2017) explored the effective use of the POSS in pediatric patients (Box 28.3). Another group of nurses evaluated the impact of preoperative education on postoperative pain-related outcomes in patients undergoing coronary artery bypass graft surgery (Watt-Watson, Stevens, Costello, Katz, & Reid, 2016). A feasibility study evaluating the effect of using a guided internet-based psychoeducational intervention employing cognitive-behavioral therapy and self-management was done among people living with chronic pain (Perry, VanDenKerkhof, Wilson, & Tripp, 2017). Pizzi, Chelly, and Marlin (2014) studied the time involved in administering oral prn pain management and found that nurses spend approximately 11 minutes to administer each prn oral analgesic medication. A group of nurses in Canada conducted a pilot study to assess the benefit of using distraction kits to help children manage their pain when undergoing painful procedures in the ED (Ballard et al., 2017). A recent study explored the experiences of pain among urban African Americans who were living with cancer (Maly, Singh, & Vallerand, 2018). The influence of pain management nursing research on health policy was explored by Schreier (2017). She advised some areas in which nursing research is needed include opioid/substance use disorder, the role of opioids in pain management, and the various aspects of integrative multimodal therapies for pain management.

Several researchers have investigated the challenges that limit nursing engagement in research in the clinical setting, including inadequate time, knowledge, authority, and organizational support (Scala, Price, & Day, 2016). When the Barriers to Nurses' Participation in Research Questionnaire (BNPRQ) was used at one academic center, lack of time, inadequate resources for conducting research, and lack of *personal relevance* were identified as substantial barriers (Hagan & Walden, 2017). To counteract the knowledge deficit, inadequate research resources, and apprehension about participating in research, nurses who aspire to conduct clinical research can collaborate or partner with nurse researchers in an academic institution. Such a partnership brings nurses with research expertise to work jointly with nurses with clinical questions who desire to improve practice (Balakas, Bryant, & Jamerson, 2011). Another professional collaboration that can be very positive is between shared governance, including unit-based practice councils and QI councils with nursing research committees. Box 28.3 provides an example of how collaboration can be beneficial for patients and nurses.

Box 28.3	Clinical Application: Moving From Why Can't We? in Wilmington, North Carolina, to an International Presentation in Madrid, Spain

In 2015 a pediatric staff nurse at New Hanover Regional Medical Center (NHRMC) asked why the pediatric nurses could not use the Pasero Opioid Sedation Scale (POSS) to assess sedation in pediatric patients who were being treated with opioids to manage pain. She brought the question to the Pediatric Unit Based Practice Committee. The nurses were advised they could not use the POSS with pediatric patients because there was no evidence to support it being used within that population. The nurses contacted the nurse educator for the pediatric unit, who they knew is also a member of the NHRMC Nursing Research Committee. The nurse educator brought the question to the Nursing Research Committee, where it was decided that she, the chair of that committee, and two of the pediatric nurses would undertake a research study to explore whether the POSS could be used safely and effectively with pediatric patients who were receiving opioid medications for pain management. After completing the research, they published the study and their findings that it could be used safely and effectively with pediatric patients. After the publication, the researchers were invited to present at numerous national and international conferences. NHRMC supported them to present at a conference in Madrid, Spain, in December 2017. To date the POSS has been safely and effectively used with pediatric patients. An interesting addendum is that since beginning use of the POSS documentation of assessment/reassessment of both pain and sedation has markedly increased and the increase has been sustained over more than 2 years.

All nurses work with patients who experience pain at one time or another. As a result, they have the opportunity and population to facilitate being involved in pain-related research in the clinical setting. There are many topics regarding pain in clinical settings in which research is needed. These include, but are not limited to, pain assessment, patient perceptions of pain, clinician perception of patients' pain, effectiveness of the various nonpharmacologic interventions (see Chapters 20 to 27), and effectiveness of patient education regarding pain. A specific area in which clinical research is needed is to explore the risks and safety needs of patients receiving opioids who are transported from one area or facility to another (ECRI, 2017).

Clinical Nursing Efforts to Support Organizational Initiatives

Safe and effective multimodal pain management can be achieved for all patients when the relationship between clinicians and leadership is collaborative in support of organizational initiatives. There are a variety of ways in which clinicians can be supportive. For example, members of nursing shared governance committees and nurses who belong to PRN programs may be excellent sources for support and collaboration.

Nursing Shared Governance

Hess defined shared governance as an "organizational innovation that legitimatizes health care professionals' decision-making control over their practice, while extending their influence on administrative areas previously controlled by managers" (Hess, 2011, p. 235). Although the origin of nursing shared governance is often attributed to Tim Porter-O'Grady and Sharon Finnegan (1984), the University of Iowa initiated shared governance in 1975 (Cullen, Wagner, Matthews, & Farrington, 2017). Nursing shared governance provides a framework for all nurses working within an organization to not only participate in decision making and policy development but also have ownership, authority, and accountability to influence decisions affecting nursing that are made within the organization (Bieber & Joachim, 2016; Dearmon, Riley, Mestas, & Buckner, 2015; Porter-O'Grady, 1989; Porter-O'Grady, 1991; Meyers & Costanzo, 2015; Slatyer, Coventry, Twigg, & Davis, 2016). The word *shared* is crucial because shared governance is designed to be a process in which nursing leadership empowers frontline nurses with authority while the frontline nurses commit to being competent, autonomous, accountable, and responsible; each group communicates with one another to make the most advantageous shared decisions (Meyers & Costanzo, 2015).

The specific structure through which shared governance is implemented can vary by organization, but generally it consists of committees or councils. The key committees or councils include those involved with evidence-based practice (QI and research); clinical education or professional development; policy review and updates; quality, safety, and nursing practice; informatics; and documentation (Cullen et al., 2017).

Often, unit-based practice committees (UBPCs) are part of a shared governance model (Joseph & Bogue, 2016). These are committees of nurses who work on a particular clinical unit and affect practice decisions on that unit. The UBPC may be a component of an organizational nursing shared governance program or independent but aligned with such a program. Joseph and Bogue (2016) identified nine effective competencies that are characteristic of nursing practice councils. These competencies are delineated in Fig. 28.6.

Although no specific correlation was found in the literature for the effect of nursing shared governance on pain management, nursing shared governance is correlated with high-quality and safe patient care (Kutney-Lee et al., 2016). Those correlations are consistent with safe and effective pain management. Three nursing shared governance councils that are particularly appropriate for being involved with improving pain management across the organization are the outcomes and improvements or QI council, the practice council, and the professional development council overseeing clinical ladder projects. Box 28.3 presents a clinical application of a nursing shared governance council improving pain management. The relationship between nursing shared governance and pain management is also an area much in need of nursing research.

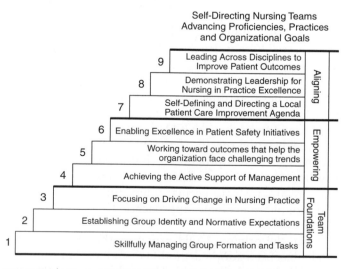

Fig. 28.6 | The Staged Competencies of Effective Nursing Practice Councils. (From Joseph, M. L., & Bogue, R. J. (2016). A theory-based approach to nursing shared governance. *Nursing Outlook, 64*(4), 339–351.)

Leadership can assess effectiveness of shared governance using the 86-question Index of Professional Nursing Governance (IPNG) tool that provides information regarding personnel issues, organizational data, areas of influence, organizational involvement, professional practice, decision making, and goal setting with conflict resolution process (Meyers & Costanzo, 2015). The IPNG is a valid and reliable tool that measures the nurses' perceptions of their organization's shared governance program (Lamoureux, Judkins-Cohn, Butao, McCue, & Garcia, 2014; Wilson, 2014). The information gained from the IPNG enables administrative assessment and guides intervention for support and improvement (Hess, 2016). It allows for comparison of the individual hospital with other hospitals with nursing shared governance (Wilson, 2014).

Pain Resource Nurse Program

Another organization-wide initiative that has been used in a variety of health care settings, including ambulatory care, is known as the *Pain Resource Nurse (PRN)* program. Although some facilities have modified the title (e.g. *Pain Star, Pain Champion, Link Nurses*), *PRN* program is the most common name to describe a team of nurses who are identified as having a particular interest, knowledge, or expertise with helping manage pain, receive pain-specific education, and are supported to coordinate process improvement efforts to improve pain management within their area of work (Paice, Barnard, Creamer, & Omerod, 2006). Consistent with this, the term *PRN* often is used to refer to a nurse who is a member of that program or group.

The PRN program concept originated in 1993 at the City of Hope (COH) National Medical Center. In that program, staff nurses received 40 hours of structured education in various aspects of pain, ongoing support designed to empower the nurses to be active in pain management processes, and working with colleagues to improve pain management among the patients for whom they provide care (Ferrell, Grant, Ritchey, Ropchan, & Rivera, 1993). The original program began as a quality-assurance project to survey nurses at COH to evaluate their knowledge and attitudes regarding pain. A carefully designed educational program was developed based on the data from the survey, and from that the PRN program evolved. In addition to education specific to the PRN role, the curriculum for the COH PRN program included physiology, ethical psychosocial aspects, myths about pain, assessment of pain, pharmacologic agents, interventional approaches, and nonpharmacologic approaches to managing pain (Table 28.2).

Since the original COH program, the PRN Program model has been adopted, modified, and used in countless hospitals around the world. The authors of a systematic review (n = 11 studies) of the effect of PRN programs on pain management imprent reported significant variability among programs in relation to design (Crawford, Boller,

Table 28.2	Curriculum of the Pain Resource Nurse Training Program
Day 1	Welcome and introduction, 1/2 hr
	Pre knowledge and attitudes survey, 1/4 hr
	Definition of pain, 1-1/2 hr
	Nurses' role in pain management
	Anatomy and physiology
	Assessment of pain, 2 hr
	Myths and misconceptions related to pain
	Behaviors of the patient in pain
	Pain assessment, 1-1/2 hr
	Clinical on inpatient units
	Discussion of clinical experience, 1 hr
Day 2	Pharmacologic management of pain, 2-1/4 hr
	Opioids
	NSAIDs
	Adjuvants
	Potentiators and inhibitors
	Agonists and antagonists
	Equianalgesia, 1-1/2 hr
	Pharmacology lab practice session, 3-1/4 hr
	Case studies/small groups
	CADD pump demonstration
Day 3	Surgical approaches to pain management, 1-1/2 hr
	Side effects of opioid analgesia, 1-1/4 hr
	Constipation
	Nausea and vomiting
	Sedation
	The role of pharmacy in pain management, 1/2 hr
	Side effects, 1/2 hr
	Group work
	The use of radiation therapy in pain
	Management, 2-1/2 hr
	The process of case analysis: the nurses' role, 1/2 hr
	Epidural analgesia, 1 hr
	Clinical validation
	Case studies, 1 hr
	Clinical on inpatient units
Day 4	Discussion of clinical experience and homework from day 3, 1 hr
	Introduction to nondrug comfort measures, 1/2 hr
	Acupuncture, 3/4 hr
	Application of heat, 1 hr
	Demonstration and lab
	Application of cold, 1 hr
	Demonstration and lab
	Massage, 1-1/2 hr
	Demonstration and lab
	Relaxation and distraction, 3/4 hr
	Demonstration and lab
	Imagery, 1/2 hr

Table 28.2 | Curriculum of the Pain Resource Nurse Training Program—cont'd

Day 5	Ethical issues of pain management, 1/2 hr
	Spiritual aspects of pain and suffering, 1/2 hr
	Cultural aspects, 1/2 hr
	Resources for patient education, 1/2 hr
	Open discussion: problem solving and goal setting, 1-3/4 hr
	Psychosocial aspects, 1 hr
	Implementing the role of the pain resource nurse, 1/2 hr
	Course evaluation, 1/2 hr
	Post-knowledge and attitudes survey
	Graduation and reception, 1 hr

NSAIDs, Non-steroidal anti-inflammatory drugs.
From Ferrell, B. R., Grant, M., Ritchey, K. J., Ropchan, R., & Rivera, L. M. (1993). The pain resource nurse training program: A unique approach to pain management. *Journal of Pain and Symptom Management, 8*(8), 549–556.

Jadalla, & Cuenca, 2016). In that review, the authors concluded there was low to moderate support for their effectiveness. The authors also concluded that the following four characteristics are essential for PRN programs to be successful:

1. Commitment, support, and active involvement of management in establishing effective pain management are priorities throughout the facility.
2. Challenges are addressed regarding barriers to effective pain management within the organization and among staff.
3. Several strategies are combined to counter the barriers.
4. There is a culture of cooperative interdisciplinary communication and collaboration.

Internationally, the critical factor in the success of a PRN program is identified as the ongoing support of nursing leadership and management (Crawford et al., 2016; Ladak et al., 2013; Paice et al., 2006; Vickers, Wright & Staines, 2014; Williams et al., 2012). Without support from nursing leadership, it is difficult to sustain a PRN program and almost impossible for it to be successful. If nursing leadership does not consider the PRN effort to be a priority, nursing management will not support the individual PRN nurses with time to participate in education, QI activities, and PRN meetings or retreats. Their active and consistent participation in those activities are essential to success.

Education of Clinicians

Ensuring continuing pain-related education for clinicians is essential to ensure that the high quality of the organization is maintained and continues to improve

(Tulchinsky & Varavikova, 2014). A critical component of all institutional QI efforts is closing the circle by teaching and periodically reeducating all clinicians with targeted evidence-based information regarding policies, guidelines, and best practices adapted by the organization to provide the safest and most effective pain management for all patients. Members of ECRI (created as the Emergency Care Research Institute) highlighted the need for clinician education in their Deep Dive document, when they reported knowledge deficit was the third most frequent factor that contributed to adverse events involving opioids (ECRI, 2017). It is also identified in TJC prepublication requirements for the revised standards regarding assessment and management of pain (TJC, 2017a; TJC, 2017b). TJC lists an element of performance for hospitals to provide educational resources and programs with resources designed to support staff, including licensed independent practitioners, "to improve pain assessment, pain management and the safe use of opioid medications based on the identified needs of its patient population" (TJC, 2017a; TJC, 2017b). Appropriate clinician instruction provides information and tools that enable clinicians to appropriately assess pain, prescribe multimodal analgesia, safely administer analgesic medications, advocate for and implement appropriate nonpharmacologic interventions, and provide meaningful evidence-based information to other clinicians, patients, and their families.

Education provided by the organization may be either proactive or reactive. *Proactive education* is done when it is anticipated that some aspect within the system could be problematic before an actual occurrence or real difficulties or errors occur. These are frequently identified through QI activities (e.g., Lean or Six Sigma). An example of proactive education can be seen when there are no adverse events, but the results of a knowledge and attitude survey about pain indicate that nurses in a certain area have inadequate knowledge about pain medications; proactive education is then undertaken to prevent errors related to pain medications from occurring (Box 28.4). *Reactive education* is provided in response to an untoward event or malfunction in the system (ECRI, 2017). An example of reactive education is when education aimed at improving sedation assessment and earlier intervention is conducted after a medication safety committee reports an increase in the amount of naloxone used to reverse opioid-induced respiratory depression.

No one component of an institutional effort will be the solution for all problems or challenges; however, education is essential for all efforts. Education is essential for helping ensure clinicians will adhere to policies, procedures, guidelines, safety needs, and standards of care. There are many opportunities, avenues, and methods to provide education to clinicians. For example, the Michigan Health & Hospital Association Keystone Center provides monthly webinars and coaching calls with clinicians (ECRI, 2017). Box 28.4 presents opportunities to improve delivery of current information about pain to clinicians.

Box 28.4	Opportunities for Providing Education to Clinicians

- Specific mandatory in-person classes
- Webinars and online education
- Informational posters (e.g., stairway posters; potty pages)
- Staff huddles and huddle boards
- Education and discussions during staff meetings
- Morbidity and mortality conferences
- One-on-one education and coaching
- Prompt follow-up education of all *near misses* (errors for which there is intervention and patient safety is not affected)
- Showcasing successful use of multimodal analgesia
- Peer support and education (e.g., pain champion nurses)
- Unit or professional specialty targeted education
- Organizational newsletters
- Electronic education modules
- Grand rounds
- Interactive media
- Simulation
- Regional professional-specific continuing education events

It is important for education to include current data, evidence-based principles, organization-specific information, policies, and procedures. TJC advised education of clinicians be based on analysis of clinician observations, adverse events, and near misses (TJC, 2012). A near miss is an error or malfunction that occurs but is interrupted or corrected before reaching the patient (Crane et al., 2015). An example is when an incorrect dose of an opioid is stored in the medication administration device, but the nurse finds the error and does not administer it to the patient. In that example, an error occurred but it was interrupted before reaching the patient. The *Safe Use of Opioid Medications in Acute Care* is available through the ECRI and can be modified to include organization-specific practice information as an educational strategy (ECRI, 2017). It is imperative for organization leadership to understand that education alone is not sufficient to make change. There needs to be follow-up evaluation of care, processes, effectiveness of the education, implementation of the education, and continuing practice. The CMS has partnered with the CDC and the Agency for Healthcare Research and Quality (AHRQ) to share guidance and promote educational tools and information that are evidence-based and population-needs specific (CMS, 2017).

Future Opportunities for Improvement

Research is needed to assess the effectiveness of various QI tools and processes to determine how often they are used, how consistently they are used as intended, and to what degree they are effective (Taylor et al., 2014). Research is also needed to identify the most effective ways to use data stored within EMRs to support continuing improvement efforts (Curcin et al., 2014). Original research is needed for those aspects of pain management and institutional support for pain management in categories in which currently there is no evidence or insufficient evidence to ascertain an appropriate standard for practice (Baker et al., 2014).

Innovation

It is imperative for organizations to be open to new and innovative ways to safely help patients who have pain to more effectively manage their pain. An example of such innovation is at a Veterans Administration Hospital in Wisconsin that offers a telephone-based clinic with a pharmacist-staffed consultation service for people with neuropathic pain (Collins, Ebert, Hentzen, Johnson, & Stevenson, 2013). It is anticipated that other innovative telehealth processes will evolve as the result of the COVID-19 pandemic.

Resources for Guiding Improvements in Institutional Commitment to Safe and Effective Pain Management

There are many resources available to organizations to guide and assist with improving an institutional commitment to safe and effective pain management. A sampling of these resources is presented in Box 28.5.

Key Points

- All patients are ethically entitled to effective pain management.
- It is imperative for organization leaders to be actively involved in initiatives that promote and ensure safe and effective multimodal pain management.
- Health care organization leaders need to be aware of the variety of resources and best practice efforts supporting multimodal analgesia.
- Lean is an incremental continuous improvement methodology used to improve processes.
- Lean is supported by a coach working with facility leadership and employees who do the work of improving processes within the facility.
- Leadership coaching and accountability to standard work drives sustainment of improvement efforts.

Box 28.5 | Resources for Guiding Improvements in Institutional Commitment

GENERAL RESOURCES

- American Academy of Pain Medicine: http://www.painmed.org/
- American Society for Pain Management Nursing: http://www.aspmn.org/documents
- American Society for Pain Management Nursing Joint Commission Tool Kit: http://www.aspmn.org/pages/newsandannouncements.aspx#ASPMN®'sJointCommissionToolKit
- American Society of Anesthesiologists: http://www.asahq.org
- American Society of Health-System Pharmacists (ASHP): https://www.ncbi.nlm.nih.gov/pubmed/20208056
- Anesthesia Patient Safety Foundation: https://www.apsf.org/
- Centers for Disease Control and Prevention: https://www.cdc.gov
- Centers for Medicare and Medicaid: https://www.cms.gov
- Centers for Medicare and Medicaid Transforming Clinical Practice Initiative: https://innovation.cms.gov/initiatives/Transforming-Clinical-Practices/
- Clinical Tools, Inc.: https://www.opioidrisk.com
- ECRI Institute and Patient Safety Organization: https://www.ecri.org
- Institute for Clinical Systems Improvement: https://www.icsi.org/
- Institute for Safe Medication Practice: http://ismp.org
- National Center for Complementary and Integrative Health (NIH): https://nccih.nih.gov
- National Institute on Drug Abuse (NIH): https://www.drugabuse.gov/
- National Quality Forum: https://www.qualityforum.org/
- National Quality Measures Clearinghouse (Agency for Health care Research and Quality): https://www.qualitymeasures.ahrq.gov/
- Society of Hospital Medicine Toolkit: Reducing adverse drug events related to opioids (RADEO): implementation guide, 2015: http://tools.hospitalmedicine.org/resource_rooms/imp_guides/radeo/radeo_implementation_guide.pdf
- The Hospital and Healthsystem Association of Pennsylvania–Hospital Improvement Innovation Network (HAP HIIN): https://partnershipforpatients.cms.gov/about-the-partnership/hospital-engagement-networks/thehospitalengagementnetworks.html
- The Joint Commission (TJC). (2017b). Requirement, rationale, reference. *R3 Report* (11), 1-7: https://www.jointcommission.org/-/media/tjc/documents/standards/r3-reports/r3_report_issue_11_2_11_19_rev.pdf
- United States Drug Enforcement Administration (USDEA). https://www.dea.gov/diversion-control-division
- United States Food and Drug Administration: https://www.fda.gov
- United States Veterans Administration/Department of Defense: https://www.healthquality.va.gov

LEAN RESOURCES

- Cheaper Better Faster: Toyota help feed Hurricane Sandy (2013, September 7): https://www.youtube.com/watch?v=wz28yMcDvVM NUMIT video
Contributor, S. (2017, April 30). Job Instruction Training: http://www.shmula.com/job-instruction-training/23003/
- Countermeasures in Lean. (2016, September 27): http://www.velaction.com/countermeasures/
- Creating A Value Stream Map. (2018): http://leanmanufacturingtools.org/551/creating-a-value-stream-map/
- Lean Toolbox: Current State, Ideal State, and Future State (2016, August 3): https://medcom.uiowa.edu/theloop/announcements/lean-toolbox-current-state-ideal-state-and-future-state
- Simon, K. (n.d.). Pareto principle (80/20 Rule): https://www.isixsigma.com/tools-templates/pareto/pareto-principle-8020-rule/
- Toussaint, J., Billi, J., & Graban, M. (2017, January). Lean for Doctors [Editorial]. Catalysis. http://www.createvalue.org

CLINICAL NURSING RESEARCH RESOURCES

- National Institute of Nursing Research: http://www.ninr.nih.gov
- Nursing Research from the American Nurses Association: http://www.nursingworld.org/
- EspeciallyForYou/Nurse-Researchers EBSCO Nursing Resources that Support Nursing Research: https://www.ebscohost.com/nursing

NALOXONE RESOURCES

- North Carolina Harm Reduction Coalition: http://www.nchrc.org/law-enforcement/us-law-enforcement-who-carry-naloxone/

- True improvement is based on identifying the root cause of the problem and implementing countermeasures.
- Health care organization leaders need to ensure all clinicians are educated in appropriate pain assessment and safe multimodal pain management.
- Health care organization leadership needs to support clinicians in quality improvement activities and research.
- Health care organization leaders need to support clinicians who are involved in clinical improvement efforts such as shared governance and pain resource nurses.

Case Scenario

Medical Center XYZ is a 650-bed level 1 trauma center located in the middle of a busy inner-city neighborhood. The population served consists of many older adults with chronic, painful medical conditions and a large percentage of young and middle-aged people with substance use disorder and victims of a variety of trauma situations (e.g., motor vehicle accidents, gunshot wounds, assaults, domestic violence, falls). Many patients of all ages who have overdosed are admitted to the emergency department. Sonja was recently hired as the director of quality and patient safety department. In her new role she is responsible for all quality and safety initiatives, including pain management, patient satisfaction, adverse drug events, medication errors, and meeting accreditation standards. She learns there is no oversight of adverse drug events, no one is collecting naloxone data, and there is no nursing shared governance or nursing research at XYZ.

1. With which other medical center departments does Sonja need to collaborate?
2. What baseline data does she need to collect?
3. What medical center committees does she need to make sure are in place and functioning?
4. What other groups could she encourage to be formed be helpful to her in her new position?
5. What outside resources could she access to help in her efforts?
6. What quality improvement efforts does she need to undertake?

References

Adams, J. M. (2018). Increasing Naloxone Awareness and Use: The Role of Health Care Practitioners. *JAMA, 319*(20), 2073–2074.

American Society for Pain Management Nursing (ASPMN). (2018). *ASPMN®'s Joint Commission Tool Kit*. Joint Commission Tool Kit http://www.aspmn.org/pages/newsandannouncements.aspx# (Accessed 02/27/2018).

Ashok Sarkar, S., Ranjan Mukhopadhyay, A., & Ghosh, S. K. (2013). Root cause analysis, Lean Six Sigma and test of hypothesis. *The TQM Journal, 25*(2), 170–185.

Australian Commission on Safety and Quality in Health Care (ACSQHC). (2012). *Safety and Quality Improvement Guide Standard 4 Medication Safety*. Sydney, Australia: Australian Commission on Safety and Quality in Health Care.

Bagley, S. M., Peterson, J., Cheng, D. M., Jose, C., Quinn, E., O'Connor, P. G., & Walley, A. Y. (2015). Overdose education and naloxone rescue kits for family members of individuals who use opioids: characteristics, motivations, and naloxone use. *Substance Abuse, 36*(2), 149–154.

Baker, K. M., Clark, P. R., Henderson, D., Wolf, L. A., Carman, M. J., Manton, A., & Zavotsky, K. E. (2014). Identifying the differences between quality improvement, evidence-based practice, and original research. *Journal of Emergency Nursing, 40*(2), 195–197.

Balakas, K., Bryant, T., & Jamerson, P. (2011). Collaborative research partnerships in support of nursing excellence. *Nursing Clinics, 46*(1), 123–128.

Ballard, A., Le May, S., Khadra, C., Fiola, J. L., Charette, S., Charest, M. C., ... Tsimicalis, A. (2017). Distraction Kits for Pain Management of Children Undergoing Painful Procedures in the Emergency Department: A Pilot Study. *Pain Management Nursing, 18*(6), 418–426.

Barnas, Kim, & Adams, E. (2014). *Beyond Heroes: A Lean Management System for Healthcare*. Appleton, WI: ThedaCare Center for Healthcare Value.

Beheshti, A., Lucas, L., Dunz, T., Haydash, M., Chiodi, H., Edmiston, B., ... Sobota, B. (2015). An evaluation of naloxone use for opioid overdoses in West Virginia: a literature review. *American Medical Journal, 6*(1), 9–13.

Belmont, E., Haltom, C. C., Hastings, D. A., Homchick, R. G., Morris, L., Taitsman, J., ... Peisert, K. (2011). A new quality compass: Hospital boards' increased role under the affordable care act. *Health Affairs, 30*(7), 1282–1289.

Bieber, P., & Joachim, H. (2016). Shared governance: a success story. *Nurse Leader, 14*(1), 62–66.

Bird, S. M., Parmar, M. K., & Strang, J. (2015). Take-home naloxone to prevent fatalities from opiate-overdose: protocol for Scotland's public health policy evaluation, and a new measure to assess impact. *Drugs: Education, Prevention and Policy, 22*(1), 66–76.

Bird, S. M., McAuley, A., Perry, S., & Hunter, C. (2016). Effectiveness of Scotland's National Naloxone Programme for reducing opioid-related deaths: a before (2006–10) versus after (2011–13) comparison. *Addiction, 111*(5), 883–891.

Brateanu, A., Thomascik, J., Koncilja, K., Spencer, A. L., & Colbert, C. Y. (2017). Using Continuous Quality-Improvement Techniques to Evaluate and Enhance an Internal Medicine Residency Program's Assessment System. *The American Journal of Medicine, 130*(6), 750–755.

Burwell, S. M. (2015). Setting value-based payment goals: HHS efforts to improve US health care. *New England Journal of Medicine, 372*(10), 897–899.

California Hospital Association (CHA). (2020). Medication Safety Committee. https://www.calhospital.org/medication-safety-committee. Accessed 8/7/2020.

Centers for Disease Control and Prevention (CDC). (2012). Community-Based Opioid Prevention Programs Providing Naloxone—United States, 2010. MMWR. *Morbidity and Mortality Weekly Report, 61*(6), 101–105.

Centers for Medicare and Medicaid Services (CMS). (2017). *Centers for Medicare and Medicaid Services (CMS) Opioid Misuse Strategy 2016: Executive Summary.* https://www.cms.gov/Outreach-and-Education/Outreach/Partnerships/Downloads/CMS-Opioid-Misuse-Strategy-2016.pdf. Accessed, 2/23/2018.

Chilgren, A. A. (2008). Managers and the new definition of quality. *Journal of Healthcare Management, 53*(4), 221–229.

Clark, A. K., Wilder, C. M., & Winstanley, E. L. (2014). A systematic review of community opioid overdose prevention and naloxone distribution programs. *Journal of Addiction Medicine, 8*(3), 153–163.

Collar, R. M., Shuman, A. G., Feiner, S., McGonegal, A. K., Heidel, N., Duck, M., ... Bradford, C. R. (2012). Lean management in academic surgery. *Journal of the American College of Surgeons, 214*(6), 928–936.

Collins, E., Ebert, J., Hentzen, K., Johnson, D., & Stevenson, K. (2013). Development of a telephone clinic for the management of neuropathic pain. *The Journal of Pain, 14*(4), S39.

Crane, S., Sloane, P. D., Elder, N., Cohen, L., Laughtenschlaeger, N., Walsh, K., & Zimmerman, S. (2015). Reporting and using near-miss events to improve patient safety in diverse primary care practices: a collaborative approach to learning from our mistakes. *The Journal of the American Board of Family Medicine, 28*(4), 452–460.

Crawford, C. L., Boller, J., Jadalla, A., & Cuenca, E. (2016). An integrative review of pain resource nurse programs. *Critical Care Nursing Quarterly, 39*(1), 64–82.

Cullen, L., Wagner, M., Matthews, G., & Farrington, M. (2017). Evidence into practice: integration within an organizational infrastructure. *Journal of PeriAnesthesia Nursing, 32*(3), 247–256.

Curcin, V., Woodcock, T., Poots, A. J., Majeed, A., & Bell, D. (2014). Model-driven approach to data collection and reporting for quality improvement. *Journal of Biomedical Informatics, 52*, 151–162.

D'Andreamatteo, A., Ianni, L., Lega, F., & Sargiacomo, M. (2015). Lean in healthcare: A comprehensive review. *Health Policy, 119*(9), 1197–1209.

Davis, C. S., Ruiz, S., Glynn, P., Picariello, G., & Walley, A. Y. (2014). Expanded access to naloxone among firefighters, police officers, and emergency medical technicians in Massachusetts. *American Journal of Public Health, 104*(8), e7–e9.

Dearmon, V. A., Riley, B. H., Mestas, L. G., & Buckner, E. B. (2015). Bridge to shared governance: developing leadership of frontline nurses. *Nursing Administration Quarterly, 39*(1), 69–77.

Dinescu, L. I., Todorov, D., Biglow, M., Toderika, Y., Cohen, H., & Patel, K. (2012). Medication Safety in Rehabilitation Medicine. *Physical Medicine and Rehabilitation Clinics, 23*(2), 271–303.

Donabedian, A. (2003). *An introduction to quality Assurance in Health Care.* Oxford: England: Oxford University Press Ltd.

Donnelly, P., & Kirk, P. (2015). Use the PDSA model for effective change management. *Education for Primary Care, 26*(4), 279–281.

Dowell, D., Haegerich, T. M., & Chou, R. (2016). CDC guideline for prescribing opioids for chronic pain—United States, 2016. *JAMA, 315*(15), 1624–1645.

ECRI Institute. (2017). *ECRI Institute PSO Deep Dive Opioid Use in Acute Care.* Plymouth Meeting, PA: ECRI Institute.

Estrada, C. R. (2018). Variability in care—What would business people think? *The Journal of Urology, 199*(1), 40–42.

Faul, M., Dailey, M. W., Sugerman, D. E., Sasser, S. M., Levy, B., & Paulozzi, L. J. (2015). Disparity in naloxone administration by emergency medical service providers and the burden of drug overdose in US rural communities. *American Journal of Public Health, 105*(S3), e26–e32.

Faul, M., Lurie, P., Kinsman, J. M., Dailey, M. W., Crabaugh, C., & Sasser, S. M. (2017). Multiple Naloxone administrations among emergency medical service providers is increasing. *Prehospital Emergency Care, 21*(4), 411–419.

Ferrell, B. R., Grant, M., Ritchey, K. J., Ropchan, R., & Rivera, L. M. (1993). The pain resource nurse training program: a unique approach to pain management. *Journal of Pain and Symptom Management, 8*(8), 549–556.

French, M. T., Homer, J., Gumus, G., & Hickling, L. (2016). Key provisions of the Patient Protection and Affordable Care Act (ACA): a systematic review and presentation of early research findings. *Health Services Research, 51*(5), 1735–1771.

Furman, J., & Kuczyńska-Chałada, M. (2016). Change management in lean enterprise. *Ekonomia i Zarzadzanie, 8*(2), 23–30.

Gabow, P. A., & Goodman, P. L. (2015). *The Lean Prescription Powerful Medicine for Our Ailing Healthcare System.* Boca Raton, Fla: CRC Press.

Gan, T. J., Ginsberg, B., Glass, P. S., Fortney, J., Jhaveri, R., & Perno, R. (1997). Opioid-sparing effects of a low-dose infusion of naloxone in patient-administered morphine sulfate. *Anesthesiology: The Journal of the American Society of Anesthesiologists, 87*(5), 1075–1081.

Gordon, D. B., & Pellino, T. A. (2005). Incidence and characteristics of naloxone use in postoperative pain management: a critical examination of naloxone use as a potential quality measure. *Pain Management Nursing, 6*(1), 30–36.

Graban, M. (2012). *Lean Hospitals: Improving Quality, Patient Safety, and Employee Engagement* (2nd Ed). Boca Raton, FL: CRC Press.

Greeneway, M. L., & Corsten, P. (2016). PRN Group Provides Positive Pain Results. *Pain Management Nursing, 17*(2), 104–105.

Groves, P. S. (2014). The relationship between safety culture and patient outcomes: Results from pilot meta-analyses. *Western Journal of Nursing Research, 36*(1), 66–83.

Hagan, J., & Walden, M. (2017). Development and evaluation of the barriers to nurses' participation in research questionnaire at a large academic pediatric hospital. *Clinical Nursing Research, 26*(2), 157–175.

Herndon, O., Pino, J., & Quinlan-Colwell, A. (2017). Answering a call to action for a community with a health care crisis. Presentation at: 27th Society for Pain Management Nursing Annual Conference, Phoenix, AZ, September 13–16, 2017.

Hess, R. G., Jr. (2011). Slicing and dicing shared governance: in and around the numbers. *Nursing Administration Quarterly, 35*(3), 235–241.

Hess, R. G. (2016). Shared governance. *Nursing Outlook, 64*(6), 530.

Hospital and Healthsystem Association of Pennsylvania – Hospital Improvement Innovation Network (HAP HIIN). (2014). *Pennsylvania Hospital Engagement Network: Organizational Assessment of Safe Opioid Practices* (pp. 1–14). Pennsylvania patient Safety Authority. http://patientsafety.pa.gov/pst/Documents/Opioids/organization.pdf. Accessed 02/17/2018.

Hunt, L. J., Covinsky, K. E., Yaffe, K., Stephens, C. E., Miao, Y., Boscardin, W. J., & Smith, A. K. (2015). Pain in community-dwelling older adults with dementia: results from the National Health and Aging Trends Study. *Journal of the American Geriatrics Society, 63*(8), 1503–1511.

Institute of Medicine. (2001). *Crossing the Quality Chasm: A new health system for the 21st century.* Washington, DC: The National Academies Press.

Institute of Medicine (IOM). (2011). *Relieving Pain in America: A Blueprint for Transforming Prevention, Care, Education, and Research.* Washington, DC: The National Academies Press.

Institute for Safe Medication Practice (ISMP). (2018). *ISMP Medication Safety Self-Assessment for High-Alert Medications.* http://ismp.org/selfassessments/SAHAM/Default.aspx. Accessed 02/27/2018.

Isaacks, S. (2015). Ralph H. Johnson VA Medical Center. In *Monthly Report from the Director – March 2015.* https://www.charleston.va.gov/about/directorletter/2015_03.asp. Accessed 02/16/18.

Jones, A., Lankshear, A., & Kelly, D. (2016). Giving voice to quality and safety matters at board level: A qualitative study of the experiences of executive nurses working in England and Wales. *International Journal of Nursing Studies, 59,* 169–176.

Joseph, M. L., & Bogue, R. J. (2016). A theory-based approach to nursing shared governance. *Nursing Outlook, 64*(4), 339–351.

Kaplan, H. C., Provost, L. P., Froehle, C. M., & Margolis, P. A. (2012). The Model for Understanding Success in Quality (MUSIQ): building a theory of context in healthcare quality improvement. *BMJ Quality and Safety, 21*(1), 13–20. https://doi.org/10.1136/bmjqs-2011-000010.

Khalil, H., & Lee, S. (2018). The implementation of a successful medication safety program in a primary care. *Journal of Evaluation in Clinical Practice., 24*(2), 403–407.

Khalil, H., Shahid, M., & Roughead, L. (2017). Medication safety programs in primary care: a scoping review. *JBI Database of Systematic Reviews and Implementation Reports, 15*(10), 2512–2526.

Kimsey, D. B. (2010). Lean methodology in health care. *AORN Journal, 92*(1), 53–60.

Knechtges, P., & Decker, M. C. (2014). Application of Kaizen Methodology to Foster Departmental Engagement in Quality Improvement. *Journal of the American College of Radiology, 11*(12), 1126–1130. https://doi.org/10.1016/j.jacr.2014.08.027.

Koyle, M. A., Koyle, L. C. C., & Baker, G. R. (2018). Quality improvement and patient safety: Reality and responsibility from Codman to today. *Journal of Pediatric Urology., 14,* 16–18. https://doi.org/10.1016/j.jpurol.2017.07.004.

Kress, H. G., Aldington, D., Alon, E., Coaccioli, S., Collett, B., Coluzzi, F., … Mangas, A. C. (2015). A holistic approach to chronic pain management that involves all stakeholders: change is needed. *Current Medical Research and Opinion, 31*(9), 1743–1754.

Kutney-Lee, A., Germack, H., Hatfield, L., Kelly, S., Maguire, P., Dierkes, A., … Aiken, L. H. (2016). Nurse Engagement in Shared Governance and Patient and Nurse Outcomes. *The Journal of Nursing Administration, 46*(11), 605–612.

Ladak, S. S., McPhee, C., Muscat, M., Robinson, S., Kastanias, P., Snaith, K., … Shobbrook, C. (2013). The journey of the pain resource nurse in improving pain management practices:

understanding role implementation. *Pain Management Nursing, 14*(2), 68–73.

Lamoureux, J., Judkins-Cohn, T., Butao, R., McCue, V., & Garcia, F. (2014). Measuring perceptions of shared governance in clinical practice: psychometric testing of the RN-focused Index of Professional Governance (IPNG). *Journal of Research in Nursing, 19*(1), 69–87.

Laverentz, D. M., & Kumm, S. (2017). Concept evaluation using the PDSA cycle for continuous quality improvement. *Nursing Education Perspectives, 38*(5), 288–290. http://www.dx.doi.org.library.capella.edu/10.1097/01.NEP.0000000000000161.

Liker, J. K., & Trachilis, G. (2014). *Developing Lean Leaders at all Levels: A Practical Guide.* Winnipeg, Manitoba, Canada: Lean Leadership Institute Publications.

Lindstrom, H. A., Clemency, B. M., Snyder, R., Consiglio, J. D., May, P. R., & Moscati, R. M. (2015). Prehospital naloxone administration as a public health surveillance tool: a retrospective validation study. *Prehospital and Disaster Medicine, 30*(4), 385–389.

Lutz, P. S. (2017). Evolution of a Cross-Continuum Pain Steering Committee: A Model of Interprofessional Shared Governance. *Pain Management Nursing, 18*(2), 67.

Mackey, S. (2016). Future directions for pain management: Lessons from the Institute of Medicine pain report and the national pain strategy. *Hand Clinics, 32*(1), 91–98.

Maly, A., Singh, N., & Vallerand, A. H. (2018). Experiences of Urban African Americans with Cancer Pain. *Pain Management Nursing, 19*(1), 72–78.

Manss, G. (2017). Implementation of Daily Senior Leader Rounds Using a Transformational Leadership Approach. *Nurse Leader, 15*(1), 65–69.

McFadden, K. L., Stock, G. N., & Gowen, C. R., III. (2015). Leadership, safety climate, and continuous quality improvement: Impact on process quality and patient safety. *Health Care Management Review, 40*(1), 24–34.

Meyers, M. M., & Costanzo, C. (2015). Shared governance in a clinic system. *Nursing Administration Quarterly, 39*(1), 51–57.

Millar, R., Freeman, T., & Mannion, R. (2015). Hospital board oversight of quality and safety: a stakeholder analysis exploring the role of trust and intelligence. *BMC Health Services Research, 15*(1), 196–208.

Moen, R. D., & Norman, C. L. (2010). Circling back. *Quality Progress 43, no., 11*(2010), 22–28.

Moore, C., Lloyd, G., Oretti, R., Russell, I., & Snooks, H. (2015). Paramedic supplied "take home" naloxone: A randomized feasibility study. *Emergency Medical Journal, 32*(5), 421–422.

Mueller, S. R., Walley, A. Y., Calcaterra, S. L., Glanz, J. M., & Binswanger, I. A. (2015). A review of opioid overdose prevention and naloxone prescribing: implications for translating community programming into clinical practice. *Substance Abuse, 36*(2), 240–253.

Mullaney, K. (2010). Improving the Process of Supplying Instruments to the Operating Room Using the Lean Rapid Cycle Improvement Process. *Perioperative Nursing Clinics, 5*(4), 479–487. https://doi.org/10.1016/j.cpen.2010.09.001.

North Carolina Harm Reduction Coalition (NCHRC). (2018). Law enforcement. *NHRMC.* http://www.nchrc.org/law-enforcement/us-law-enforcement-who-carry-naloxone/. Accessed 2/24/2018.

Olesen, P., Powell, D., Hvolby, H. H., & Fraser, K. (2015). Using lean principles to drive operational improvements in intermodal container facilities: A conceptual framework. *Journal of Facilities Management, 13*(3), 266–281.

Oliva, E. M., Bowe, T., Tavakoli, S., Martins, S., Lewis, E. T., Paik, M., … Medhanie, A. (2017). Development and applications of the Veterans Health Administration's Stratification Tool for Opioid Risk Mitigation (STORM) to improve opioid safety and prevent overdose and suicide. *Psychological Services, 14*(1), 34–49.

Paice, J. A., Barnard, C., Creamer, J., & Omerod, K. (2006). Creating organizational change through the pain resource nurse program. *The Joint Commission Journal on Quality and Patient Safety, 32*(1), 24–31.

Parand, A., Dopson, S., Renz, A., & Vincent, C. (2014). The role of hospital managers in quality and patient safety: a systematic review. *BMJ Open, 4*(9), e005055.

Perry, J., VanDenKerkhof, E. G., Wilson, R., & Tripp, D. A. (2017). Guided internet-based psycho-educational intervention using cognitive behavioral therapy and self-management for individuals with chronic pain: A feasibility study. *Pain Management Nursing, 18*(3), 179–189.

Pizzi, L. J., Chelly, J. E., & Marlin, V. (2014). Nursing time study for the administration of a PRN oral analgesic on an orthopedic postoperative unit. *Pain Management Nursing, 15*(3), 603–608.

Porter-O'Grady, T. (1989). Shared governance: Reality or sham? *The American Journal of Nursing, 89*(3), 350–351.

Porter-O'Grady, T. (1991). Shared governance for nursing. *AORN Journal, 53*(2), 458–459.

Porter-O'Grady, T., & Finnigan, S. (1984). *Shared Governance for Nursing: A creative approach to professional accountability.* Rockville, MD: Aspen Systems Corporation.

President's Commission on Combating Drug Addiction and the Opioid Crisis drafted an interim report (PCCDOC). (2017). *Interim Report.* https://www.whitehouse.gov/sites/whitehouse.gov/files/ondcp/commission-interim-report.pdf. Accessed 02/17/2018.

Quinlan-Colwell, A., Thear, G., Miller-Baldwin, E., & Smith, A. (2017). Use of the Pasero Opioid-induced Sedation Scale (POSS) in pediatric patients. *Journal of Pediatric Nursing: Nursing Care of Children and Families, 33*, 83–87.

Rando, J., Broering, D., Olson, J. E., Marco, C., & Evans, S. B. (2015). Intranasal naloxone administration by police first responders is associated with decreased opioid overdose deaths. *The American Journal of Emergency Medicine, 33*(9), 1201–1204.

Rotter, T., Plishka, C. T., Adegboyega, L., Fiander, M., Harrison, E. L., Flynn, R., … Kinsman, L. (2017). Lean management in health care: effects on patient outcomes, professional practice, and healthcare systems. *The Cochrane Library.*, CD012831.

Rudd-Barnard, G., Pangarkar, S., Moaleji, N., & Glassman, P. (2016). (141) Epidemiology of naloxone use for opioid overdose in a tertiary care medical center. *The Journal of Pain, 17*(4), S11.

Scala, E., Price, C., & Day, J. (2016). An integrative review of engaging clinical nurses in nursing research. *Journal of Nursing Scholarship, 48*(4), 423–430.

Schein, E. H. (2014). *Humble Inquiry: The gentle art of asking instead of telling.* San Francisco: Berrett-Koehler, Inc.

Schell, R., Abramcyzk, A., Fominaya, C., Friedman, R., & Castle, S. (2017). Outcomes associated with a multidisciplinary pain oversight committee to facilitate appropriate management of chronic opioid therapy in Veterans. *Pharmacotherapy: The Journal of Human Pharmacology and Drug Therapy, 35*(11), e280–e281.

Schreier, A. M. (2017). Influencing Health policy with pain management nursing research. *Pain Management Nursing, 18*(2), 66.

Shook, J. (2008). *Managing to Learn: Using the A3 management process to solve problems, gain agreement, mentor, and lead.* Cambridge, MA: The Lean Enterprise Institute.

Simon, R. W., & Canacari, E. G. (2012). A Practical Guide to Applying Lean Tools and Management Principles to Health Care Improvement Projects. *AORN Journal, 95*(1), 85–103. https://doi.org/10.1016/j.aorn.2011.05.021.

Simons, P. A., Houben, R., Vlayen, A., Hellings, J., Pijls-Johannesma, M., Marneffe, W., & Vandijck, D. (2015). Does lean management improve patient safety culture? An extensive evaluation of safety culture in a radiotherapy institute. *European Journal of Oncology Nursing, 19*(1), 29–37.

Slatyer, S., Coventry, L. L., Twigg, D., & Davis, S. (2016). Professional practice models for nursing: a review of the literature and synthesis of key components. *Journal of Nursing Management, 24*(2), 139–150.

Smith, C., Wood, S., & Beauvais, B. (2011). Thinking lean: implementing DMAIC methods to improve efficiency within a cystic fibrosis clinic. *Journal for Healthcare Quality, 33*(2), 37–46.

Sobek, D. K., II, & Smalley, A. (2008). *Understanding A3 Thinking: A critical component of Toyota's PDCA management system.* Boca Raton, FL: CRC Press.

Society of Hospital Medicine (SHM). (2015). In T. W. Frederickson, D. B. Gordon, M. De Pinto, et al. (Eds.), *Reducing adverse drug events related to opioids (RADEO): implementation guide.* http://tools.hospitalmedicine.org/resource_rooms/imp_guides/radeo/radeo_implementation_guide.pdf. Accessed 07/31/2020.

Spear, S., & Bowen, K. (1999). Decoding the DNA of the Toyota Production System. *Harvard Business Review (September-October)*, 97–106.

St. Marie, B. S., Arnstein, P., & Zimmer, P. A. (2018). Pain and Opioids: Call for Policy Action. *The Journal for Nurse Practitioners, 14*(1), 40–44.

Sumner, S. A., Mercado-Crespo, M. C., Spelke, M. B., Paulozzi, L., Sugerman, D. E., Hillis, S. D., & Stanley, C. (2016). Use of naloxone by emergency medical services during opioid drug overdose resuscitation efforts. *Prehospital Emergency Care, 20*(2), 220–225.

Taylor, M. J., McNicholas, C., Nicolay, C., Darzi, A., Bell, D., & Reed, J. E. (2014). Systematic review of the application of the plan–do–study–act method to improve quality in healthcare. *BMJ Quality and Safety, 23*, 290–298.

Thanacoody, H. K. R. (2007). Chronic valproic acid intoxication: reversal by naloxone. *Emergency Medicine Journal, 24*(9), 677–678.

The Joint Commission (TJC). (2012). Safe use of opioids in hospitals. *Sentinel Event Alert 2012 Aug 8*, (49), 1–5. https://www.jointcommission.org/sea_issue_49/. Accessed 2/23/2018.

The Joint Commission (TJC). (2017a). *Prepublication requirements: standards revisions related to pain assessment and management.* 2017 Jun 19 [cited 2017 Jul 7] https://www.jointcommission.org/assets/1/18/HAP_Pain_Jan2018_Prepub.pdf. Accessed 2/23/2018.

The Joint Commission (TJC). (2017b). Requirement, rationale, reference. *R3 Report*, (11), 1–7. https://www.jointcommission.org/-/media/tjc/documents/standards/r3-reports/r3_report_issue_11_2_11_19_rev.pdf. Accessed 02/17/2018.

Toussaint, J., & Gerard, R. A. (2012). *On the Mend: Revolutionizing Healthcare to save lives and Transform the Industry*. Cambridge, MA: Lean Enterprise Institute.

Toussaint, J., Billi, J. E., & Graban, M. (2017). *Lean for doctors*. WI: Catalysis: Appleton. https://createvalue.org. Accessed: 7/31/2020.

Tsai, T. C., Jha, A. K., Gawande, A. A., Huckman, R. S., Bloom, N., & Sadun, R. (2015). Hospital board and management practices are strongly related to hospital performance on clinical quality metrics. *Health Affairs*, 34(8), 1304–1311.

Tulchinsky, T. H., & Varavikova, E. A. (2014). Human resources for health. In T. H. Tulchinsky, E. A. Varavikova, & J. D. Bickford (Eds.), *The New Public Health* (3rd Ed., pp. 729–770). San Diego, CA: Academic Press. 3rd Ed.

Vickers, N., Wright, S., & Staines, A. (2014). Surgical nurses in teaching hospitals in Ireland: understanding pain. *British Journal of Nursing*, 23(17), 924–929.

Wainwright, T. W., Immins, T., & Middleton, R. G. (2016). A cycling and education programme for the treatment of hip osteoarthritis: a quality improvement study. *International Journal of Orthopaedic and Trauma Nursing*, 23(1), 14–24.

Watt-Watson, J., Stevens, B., Costello, J., Katz, J., & Reid, G. (2016). Impact of preoperative education on pain management outcomes after coronary artery bypass graft surgery: a pilot. *Canadian Journal of Nursing Research Archive J*, 31(4).

Weiner, J., Balijepally, V., & Tanniru, M. (2015). Integrating strategic and operational decision making using data-driven dashboards: The case of St. Joseph Mercy Oakland Hospital. *Journal of Healthcare Management*, 60(5), 319–330.

Wermeling, D. P. (2015). Review of naloxone safety for opioid overdose: practical considerations for new technology and expanded public access. *Therapeutic Advances in Drug Safety*, 6(1), 20–31.

Wherry, L. R., & Miller, S. (2016). Early coverage, access, utilization, and health effects associated with the Affordable Care Act Medicaid expansions: A quasi-experimental study. *Annals of Internal Medicine*, 16(12), 795–803.

Williams, A. M., Toye, C., Deas, K., Fairclough, D., Curro, K., & Oldham, L. (2012). Evaluating the feasibility and effect of using a hospital-wide coordinated approach to introduce evidence-based changes for pain management. *Pain Management Nursing*, 13(4), 202–214.

Wilson, K. L. (2014). *Nurses Perceptions of Shared Governance Two Years Post Implementation of a Councilor Shared Governance Model*. Dayton, OH: Wright State University.

Yushak, M. S., Hashimb, Y., Chulc, S. W., & Bakard, N. A. (2016). Lean moderates resistance to change: Literature review. In *Proceedings of the 2nd UUM International Qualitative Research Conference. May 24-26, 2016*. Malaysia: Penang.

Zuckerman, M., Weisberg, S. N., & Boyer, E. W. (2014). Pitfalls of intranasal naloxone. *Prehospital Emergency Care*, 18(4), 550–554.

Appendix: Terminology

A

acetaminophen poisoning, /əset'əmin″əfin/, a toxic reaction to the ingestion of excessive doses of acetaminophen. Many over-the-counter and prescription medications contain acetaminophen. Individuals may ingest an overdose accidentally when taking multiple products containing acetaminophen. Dosages exceeding 140 mg/kg can produce liver failure, and larger doses can be fatal. Large amounts of acetaminophen metabolites can overwhelm the glutathione-detoxifying mechanism of the liver, resulting in progressive necrosis of the liver within 5 days. The onset of symptoms may be marked by nausea and vomiting, profuse sweating, pallor, and oliguria. The incidence of nausea and vomiting increases, accompanied by jaundice and pain in the upper abdomen, hypoglycemia, encephalopathy, and kidney failure. Treatment requires acetate ($CH_3 CO_2^-$) 17 acetone–inducing vomiting or performing gastric lavage, depending on the length of time since the ingestion. Acetylcysteine may prevent extensive liver damage if given by nasogastric tube soon after ingestion.

acetylcholine (ACh), /as'ətilkō″lēn, əsē'til-/, a direct-acting cholinergic neurotransmitter agent widely distributed in body tissues, with a primary function of mediating the synaptic activity of the nervous system and skeletal muscles. Its half-life and duration of activity are short because it is rapidly destroyed by acetylcholinesterase. Its activity also can be blocked by atropine at the junctions of nerve fibers with glands and smooth muscle tissue. It is a stimulant of the vagus and autonomic nervous system and functions as a vasodilator and cardiac depressant. It also has an effect at the neuromuscular junction that causes muscle contraction.

acetylsalicylic acid poisoning, /əsē'təlsal'isil″ik, as'itəl-/, the toxic effects of overdosage of the commonly used antipyretic and analgesic drug aspirin. Early symptoms include dizziness, ringing in the ears, changes in body temperature, gastrointestinal discomfort, and hyperventilation. Severe poisoning is marked by respiratory alkalosis, which may lead to metabolic acidosis. Children and the elderly are particularly vulnerable to the potential toxic effects of salicylates. *See also* Reye's syndrome, salicylate poisoning.

adenosine triphosphatase (ATPase), an enzyme in skeletal muscle and other tissues that catalyzes the hydrolysis of adenosine triphosphate to adenosine diphosphate and inorganic phosphate. Among various enzymes in this group, mitochondrial ATPase is involved in obtaining energy for cellular metabolism and myosin ATPase is involved in muscle contraction.

adenosine triphosphate (ATP), a compound consisting of the nucleotide adenosine (A) attached through its ribose group to three phosphoric acid molecules (P). Hydrolysis of ATP to adenosine diphosphate (D) releases energy. By coupling a less favorable reaction in the cell with this hydrolysis, the less favorable reaction may proceed, allowing one to think of ATP as the cellular energy currency, especially in muscle.

advocacy, /ad″vəkas'ē/, 1. A process whereby a health care professional provides a patient with the information to make certain decisions, usually related to some aspect of the patient's health care. 2. A method by which patients, their families, attorneys, health professionals, and citizen groups can work together to develop programs that ensure the availability of high-quality health care for a community. 3. Pleading a cause on behalf of another, such as a nurse advising a colleague on better care of a patient, a physical or occupational therapist lobbying for appropriate professional services, or any health care professional urging others that the patient's desires be honored.

aerobic exercise, any physical exercise that requires additional effort by the heart and lungs to meet the striated muscles' increased demand for oxygen. Aerobic exercise increases the breathing rate and ultimately raises heart and lung efficiency. Prolonged aerobic exercise (at least 20 minutes five times a week) is recommended for the maintenance of a healthy cardiovascular system. Examples of aerobic exercise include running, jogging, swimming, and vigorous dancing or cycling.

afferent pathway, [L, *ad* + *ferre*, to bear; AS, *paeth* + *weg*], the course or route taken, usually by a linkage of neurons, from the periphery of the body toward the central nervous system.

afferent tract, [L, *ad* + *ferre*, to bear, *tractus*], a pathway for nerve impulses traveling inward or toward the brain, the center of an organ, or another body structure. Also called ascending tract.

agonist, /ag″ənist/ [Gk, *agon*, struggle], 1. A contracting muscle whose contraction is opposed by another muscle (an antagonist). Also a muscle that works in support of another muscle, creating the same motion. The brachialis and biceps brachii are agonistic muscles. 2. A drug or other substance having a specific cellular affinity that produces a predictable response.

alpha wave, one of several types of brain waves, characterized by a relatively high voltage or amplitude and a frequency of 8 to 13 Hz. Alpha waves are the "relaxed waves" of the brain and constitute the majority of waves recorded by electroencephalograms registering the activity of the parietal and the occipital lobes and the posterior parts of the temporal lobes when the individual is awake but nonattentive and relaxed, with the eyes closed. Opening and closing the eyes affects the patterns of the alpha waves and the beta waves. Also called alpha rhythm, Berger wave.

amino acid (AA), /əmē″nō/, an organic chemical compound composed of one or more basic amino groups and one or more acidic carboxyl groups. A total of 20 of the more than 100 amino acids that occur in nature are the building blocks of proteins. The 8 essential amino acids are isoleucine, leucine, lysine, methionine, phenylalanine, threonine, tryptophan, and valine. Arginine and histidine are essential in infants. Cysteine and tyrosine are semi-essential because they may be synthesized from methionine and phenylalanine, respectively. The main nonessential amino acids are alanine, asparagine, aspartic acid, glutamine, glutamic acid, glycine, proline, and serine. From their structures, the amino acids can be classified as basic (arginine, histidine, lysine), acidic (aspartic acid, glutamic acid), or neutral (the remainder); each group is transported across cell membranes by different carrier methods. Individual amino acids represent the monomeric units that can be connected via peptide linkages (amide bonds) to produce polymeric structures called proteins.

ankylosing spondylitis, /ang′kilō″sing/, a chronic inflammatory disease associated with human leukocyte antigen B27, first affecting the spine and adjacent structures and commonly progressing to eventual fusion (ankylosis) of the involved joints. In extreme cases a forward flexion of the spine, called a "poker spine" or "bamboo spine," develops. Also called Marie-Strümpell arthritis, Marie-Strümpell disease.

- *Observations:* The disease primarily affects males under 30 years of age and generally follows a course of 20 years. There is a strong hereditary tendency. In addition to the spine, the joints of the hip, shoulder, neck, ribs, and jaw are often involved. When the costovertebral joints are involved, the patient may have difficulty expanding the rib cage while breathing. Ankylosing spondylitis is a systemic disease, often affecting the eyes and

heart. Many patients also have inflammatory bowel disease.

- *Interventions:* The chronic nature of the disease requires a coordinated team approach. The medical aim of treatment is to reduce pain and inflammation in the involved joints, usually with nonsteroidal antiinflammatory drugs and tumor necrosis factor drugs. Physical therapy helps keep the spine as erect as possible to prevent flexion contractures. The occupational therapist examines surroundings (home, school, work environment) to determine the impact of the disease on everyday functions and responsibilities. Nursing care must focus on management of the medication regimen and coping with the chronic nature of the disease. In advanced cases, surgery may be performed to straighten a badly deformed spine.

- *Patient care considerations:* Care is complex, and the patient should be encouraged to take an active role in management. Support groups are an important resource.

antagonist, /antagə″nist/ [Gk, *antagonisma*, struggle], 1. One who contends with or is opposed to another. 2. (in physiology) Any agent, such as a drug or muscle, that exerts an opposite action to that of another or competes for the same receptor sites. Kinds include antimetabolite, associated antagonist, direct antagonist, opioid antagonist. 3. (in dentistry) A tooth in the upper jaw that articulates during mastication or occlusion with a tooth in the lower jaw. — antagonistic, adj

anxiety, /angzī″ətē/ [L, *anxietas*], anticipation of impending danger and dread accompanied by restlessness, tension, tachycardia, and breathing difficulty not necessarily associated with a specific or known stimulus. Kinds include castration anxiety, free-floating anxiety, generalized anxiety disorder, separation anxiety, situational anxiety, panic disorder.

aromatherapy, a form of herbal medicine that uses various oils from plants. The route of administration can be absorption through the skin or through inhalation. The aromatic biochemical structures of certain herbs are thought to act in areas of the brain related to past experiences and emotions (e.g., limbic system).

art therapy, the use of art media to reconcile emotional conflicts, foster self-awareness, and express unspoken and frequently unconscious concerns. Art therapy is often used when traditional forms of verbal psychotherapy have failed or been rejected by an individual and when individuals have difficulty expressing feelings or use verbalization as a defense mechanism.

autohypnosis, [Gk, *autos, hypnos,* sleep], the self-induction of hypnosis by an individual who concentrates on one subject to attain an altered state of consciousness. It also may occur in a person who has become habituated to the process by undergoing hypnosis a number of times.

B

Beck Depression Inventory (BDI), [Aaron T. Beck, American psychiatrist, b. 1921], a system of classifying a total of 18 criteria of depressive illness. It was developed by Aaron T. Beck in the 1960s as a diagnostic and therapeutic tool for the treatment of childhood affective disorders. The BDI is similar to the 21-criteria *Diagnostic and Statistical Manual of Mental Disorders* (DSM) diagnostic system of the 1980s except that the DSM-IV scale includes loss of interest, restlessness, and sulkiness, which are missing from the BDI; the BDI lists somatic complaints and loneliness, which are criteria not included in the DSM-III inventory.

beta wave, one of several types of brain waves, characterized by relatively low voltage and a frequency of more than 13 Hz. Beta waves are the "busy waves" of the brain, recorded by electroencephalograph from the frontal and the central areas of the cerebrum when the patient is awake and alert with eyes open. Also called beta rhythm.

bradykinin, /-kī″nin/ [Gk, *bradys* + *kinein,* to move], a peptide containing nine amino acid residues produced from alpha$_2$-globulin by the enzyme kallikrein. Bradykinin is a potent vasodilator.

bromelain, /brō′məlān/, any of several enzymes that catalyze cleavage of proteins on the carboxyl side of alanine, glycine, lysine, and tyrosine bonds. Differing forms are derived from the fruit (fruit bromelain) and stem (stem bromelain) of the pineapple plant. The enzyme is administered orally as an antiinflammatory agent (especially to relieve swelling in the nasal and paranasal sinuses) and is also used in immunology to render red cells agglutinable by incomplete antibody.

burning mouth syndrome, a burning sensation of the oral mucous membranes and tongue that is often associated with aging in terms of menopause and hormonal changes, although it can also suggest other conditions or infections, such as yeast infections.

C

calcitonin, /kal′sitō″nin/ [L, *calx* + Gk, *tonos,* tone], a hormone produced in parafollicular cells of the thyroid that participates in regulating the blood level of calcium and stimulates bone mineralization. A synthetic preparation of the hormone is used in the treatment of certain bone disorders. Calcitonin acts to reduce the blood level of calcium and to inhibit bone resorption, whereas parathyroid hormone acts to increase blood calcium level and bone resorption. Vitamin D also contributes to the regulation of calcium homeostasis. Also called salmon calcitonin, thyrocalcitonin.

carbon dioxide content (CO$_2$ content) test, a blood test used to measure CO$_2$ content in the blood. It is used to assist in evaluating the patient's pH status and electrolytes. It is usually performed along with other assessments of electrolytes and is used primarily as a rough guide as to the patient's acid-base balance, CO$_2$

inhalation, a carefully controlled procedure in which CO$_2$ gas is administered in the treatment of anxiety or after resuscitation to ameliorate hemorrhagic shock–induced lung injury.

carbon dioxide (CO$_2$) narcosis, a condition of confusion, tremors, convulsions, and possible coma that may occur if blood levels of CO$_2$ increase to 70 mm Hg or higher. Individuals with chronic obstructive pulmonary disease can have CO$_2$ narcosis without these symptoms because they develop a tolerance to elevated CO$_2$. When ventilation is sufficient to maintain a normal oxygen partial pressure in the arteries, the CO$_2$ partial pressure is generally near 40 mm Hg.

caudal anesthesia, the injection of a local anesthetic agent into the caudal (end) portion of the epidural space through the sacral hiatus to anesthetize sacral and lower lumbar nerve roots. Once popular in obstetrics, it is now rarely performed except in pediatric anesthesia. Complications of caudal anesthesia include infection, a high (5% to 10%) rate of failure, frequent neurologic complications, dural puncture, and hypotension. *See also* regional anesthesia.

central nervous system depressant, any drug that decreases the function of the central nervous system, such as alcohol, tranquilizers, barbiturates, and hypnotics. Such drugs can produce tolerance, physical dependence, and compulsive drug use. These substances depress excitable tissue throughout the central nervous system (CNS) by stabilizing neuronal membranes, decreasing the amount of transmitter released by the nerve impulse, and generally depressing postsynaptic responsiveness and ion movement. Larger dosages cause anesthesia and potentially fatal respiratory and cardiovascular depression. CNS depressants elevate the seizure threshold and can produce physical dependence in a relatively short period. After alcohol the most abused depressants are the short-acting barbiturates, especially PENTobarbital, secobarbital, glutethimide, methyprylon, and methaqualone. These substances have popular street names on the illicit market, such as "reds" (secobarbital) and "yellows" (PENTobarbital). Sudden withdrawal of general CNS depressants that have been used in high doses for prolonged periods can be fatal to some individuals.

central nervous system stimulant, a substance that quickens the activity of the central nervous system (CNS), increasing the rate of neuronal discharge or by blocking an inhibitory neurotransmitter. Many natural and synthetic compounds stimulate the CNS, but only a few are used therapeutically. Caffeine, a potent CNS stimulant, is used to help restore mental alertness and overcome respiratory depression, but it may cause nausea, nervousness, tinnitus, tremor, tachycardia, extrasystole, diuresis, and visual disturbances. Amphetamines, sympathomimetic amines with CNS-stimulating activity, are used in treating narcolepsy and obesity, but these drugs have a high potential for abuse and may cause dizziness, restlessness, tachycardia, increased blood pressure, headache, mouth dryness, an unpleasant taste, gastrointestinal symptoms, and urticaria. Various amphetamines, especially deanol acetamidobenzoate, a precursor of acetylcholine, are prescribed for hyperkinetic child syndrome because CNS stimulants may act as depressants in children. Doxapram is used to stimulate the respiratory center and restore consciousness after anesthesia and to treat acute sedative-hypnotic intoxication. Also called analeptic.

central neuronal plasticity, (in chiropractic) the tendency for the neuronal responses to noxious stimuli to spread to other central pathways, producing the symptoms of referred pain.

central sleep apnea, a form of sleep apnea resulting from decreased respiratory center output. It may involve primary brainstem medullary depression resulting from a tumor of the posterior fossa, poliomyelitis, or idiopathic central hypoventilation.

cervical disc syndrome, an abnormal condition characterized by compression or irritation of the cervical nerve roots in or near the intervertebral foramina before the roots divide into the anterior and posterior rami. When it is caused by ruptured intervertebral discs, degenerative cervical disc disease, or cervical injuries, it may produce varying degrees of malalignment, causing nerve root compression. Most cervical disc syndromes are caused by injuries that involve hyperextension. Edema usually occurs in all cases of cervical disc syndrome. Nonsurgical intervention, which is usually a successful treatment, may include immobilization of the cervical vertebrae to decrease irritation and provide rest for the traumatized area. Other treatment may include special exercises, heat therapy, and intermittent traction. Mild analgesics are usually successful in controlling the pain associated with cervical disc syndrome, especially when used with immobilization. Surgery is recommended only when signs and symptoms persist despite nonsurgical treatment. The prognosis for this condition is usually good, but recurrence of symptoms is common. Also called cervical root syndrome.

cervical plexus, the network of nerves formed by the ventral primary divisions of the first four cervical nerves. Each nerve, except the first, divides into the superior branch and the inferior branch, and the branches unite to form three loops. The plexus is located opposite the cranial aspect of the first four cervical vertebrae. It communicates with certain cranial nerves and numerous muscular and cutaneous branches.

cervical plexus block, anesthetic nerve block at any point below the mastoid process from the second cervical vertebra to the sixth cervical vertebra. This method is used for operations on the area between the jaw and clavicle, such as for carotid endarterectomy. Complications may include Horner's syndrome, inadvertent stellate ganglion or brachial plexus block, vertebral artery bleeding or infection, subarachnoid or peridural penetration, phrenic nerve block or palsy manifested by respiratory failure, or laryngeal nerve block, manifested by sudden hoarseness.

cervical radiculopathy, disease of the cervical nerve roots, often manifesting as neck or shoulder pain.

clinical judgment, the application of information based on actual observation of a patient combined with subjective and objective data that lead to a conclusion.

clinical reasoning, higher order thinking in which the health care provider, guided by best evidence or theory, observes and relates concepts and phenomena to develop an understanding of their significance.

cluster headache, a condition characterized by attacks of intense unilateral pain, occurring most often over the eye and forehead. It is accompanied by flushing and watering of the eyes and nose. Cluster headaches are more common in males, occur in cycles, and are exacerbated with alcohol use. The attacks occur in groups, with a duration of several hours.

code of ethics, a statement encompassing the set of rules based on values and the standards of conduct to which practitioners of a profession are expected to conform. Kinds include Code for Nurses, Hippocratic oath.

coenzyme, /kō·en″zīm/ [L, *cum,* together with, *en,* in, *zyme,* ferment], a nonprotein substance that combines with an apoenzyme to form a complete enzyme or holoenzyme. Coenzymes include some of the vitamins, such as B_1 and B_2, and have smaller molecules than enzymes. Coenzymes are dialyzable and heat-stable and usually dissociate readily from the protein portions of the enzymes with which they combine.

coenzyme Q, any of several quinines that function as electron-carrying coenzymes involved in the electron transport chain or in aerobic cellular respiration. Also called ubiquinone, coenzyme Q10.

cognitive-behavioral therapy (CBT), an approach to problem solving that helps persons understand their thoughts and develop strategies to change behaviors. Founded by Dr. Aaron Beck, an American psychiatrist (b. 1921), CBT is effective in the treatment of mood disorders and many other mental health conditions. CBT is accomplished in psychotherapy groups and/or in individual counseling. The goal is to identify how one's own thoughts and beliefs lead to certain behaviors and to make changes in thinking first, become aware of behaviors, and then move toward a positive change in both.

cognitive therapy, any of the various methods of treating mental and emotional disorders that help a person change attitudes, perceptions, and patterns of thinking, from rational to realistic thoughts about self and situations. Kinds include behavior therapy, existential therapy, Gestalt therapy, transactional analysis.

comfort measure, [L, *com,* together, *fortis,* strong], any action taken to promote the soothing of a patient, such as a back rub, a change in position, the prewarming of a stethoscope or bedpan, or administration of selected medications or treatments.

complementary and alternative medicine (CAM), a large and diverse set of systems of diagnosis, treatment, and prevention based on philosophies and techniques other than those used in conventional Western medicine, often derived from traditions of medical practice used in other (non-Western) cultures. Such practices may be described as alternative, that is, existing as a body separate from and as a replacement for conventional Western medicine, or complementary, that is, used in addition to conventional Western practice. CAM is characterized by its focus on the whole person as a unique individual, on the energy of the body and its influence on health and disease, on the healing power of nature and the mobilization of the body's own resources to heal itself, and on the treatment of the underlying causes, rather than symptoms, of disease. Many of the techniques have not been validated by controlled studies.

complex regional pain syndrome, a neuromuscular condition characterized by pain and stiffness in the shoulder and arm, limited joint motion, swelling of the hand, muscle atrophy, and decalcification of the underlying bones. It is thought that a disturbance to the sympathetic nervous system is responsible for this condition. The condition occurs most commonly after myocardial infarction. Also called reflex sympathetic dystrophy syndrome (RSD), causalgia, shoulder-hand syndrome.

compression neuropathy, any of several disorders involving damage to sensory nerve roots or peripheral nerves, caused by mechanical pressure or localized trauma. Compression neuropathy is characterized by paresthesia, weakness, or paralysis. The carpal, peroneal, radial, and ulnar nerves are most commonly involved. *See also* paresthesia.

consultant, /kənsul″tənt/ [L, *consultare,* to deliberate], a person who by training and experience has acquired a special knowledge in a subject area that has been recognized by a peer group and who is invited to guide, teach, or advise others in a professional capacity.

continuous positive airway pressure (CPAP), a method of noninvasive or invasive ventilation assisted by a flow of air delivered at a constant pressure throughout the respiratory cycle. It is performed for patients who can initiate their own respirations but who are not able to maintain adequate arterial oxygen levels without assistance. CPAP may be given through a ventilator and endotracheal tube, through a nasal cannula, or into a hood over the patient's head. Respiratory distress syndrome in the newborn and sleep apnea are often treated with CPAP. Portable CPAP machines are increasingly common in the home to deal with sleep apnea. Also called constant positive airway pressure (CPPB).

continuous quality improvement (CQI), a system that seeks to improve the provision of services with an emphasis on future results. Like total quality management, CQI uses a set of statistical tools to understand subsystems and uncover problems, but its emphasis is on maintaining quality in the future, not just controlling a process. Once a process that needs improvement is identified, a team of knowledgeable individuals is gathered to research and document each step of that process. Once specific expectations and the means to measure them have been established, implementation aims at preventing future failures and involves the setting of goals, education, and the measurement of results. If necessary, the plan may be revised on the basis of the results, so that the improvement is ongoing.

continuous regional anesthesia, [L, *continuare,* to unite], a method for maintaining regional nerve block. A local anesthetic solution is infused at intervals or at a slow rate to infiltrate epidural or spinal spaces, usually by an indwelling catheter.

contrast bath, a bath in which the patient alternately immerses a part of the body, usually the hands or feet, in hot and cold water for a specified period. The procedure is used to increase the blood flow to a particular area. The technique is used most often by physical therapists to reduce inflammation to restore mobility and function.

Controlled Substances Act, a U.S. law enacted in 1970 that regulates the prescribing and dispensing of psychoactive drugs, including stimulants, depressants, and hallucinogens. The act lists five categories of restricted drugs organized by their medical acceptance, abuse potential, and ability to produce dependence. A similar act exists in Canada.

counter-irritant, an agent used to produce an irritation in one part of the body, intended to relieve irritation in some other part.

cramp, [AS, *crammian,* to fill], 1. A spasmodic and often painful contraction of one or more muscles. 2. A pain resembling a muscular cramp. Kinds include heat cramp, writer's cramp. *See also* charley horse, dysmenorrhea, wryneck, torticollis.

cryotherapy, /krī′ōther″əpē/ [Gk, *kryos* + *therapeia*], a treatment using cold as a destructive medium. Cutaneous tags, warts, condyloma acuminatum, and actinic keratosis are some of the common skin disorders responsive to cryotherapy. Solid carbon dioxide or liquid nitrogen is applied briefly with a sterile cotton-tipped applicator or cryospray instrument. Blistering, followed by necrosis, results. The procedure may be repeated.

cultural assimilation, /kul″chərəl/, a process by which members of a minority group lose cultural characteristics that distinguish them from the dominant cultural group or take on the cultural characteristics of another group or cultural event, a unique interaction of values, beliefs, ways, and mannerisms, celebrated and shared.

cultural healer, a member of an ethnic or cultural group who uses traditional methods of healing rather than conventional scientific methods to provide health care for other members of the group or members of another ethnic minority group.

culture, /kul″chər/ [L, *colere,* to cultivate], 1. (in microbiology) A laboratory test involving the cultivation of microorganisms or cells in a special growth medium. 2. (in psychology) A set of learned values, beliefs, customs, and behavior that is shared by a group of interacting individuals. 3. (in the humanities and social sciences) The beliefs of individuals in a group that contribute to their sense of identity, acceptance, and belonging.

culture-bound, (in anthropology) a term that connects the interpretation of an event to the beliefs of a particular culture. In health, examples of culture-bound conditions include diseases that are thought to be related to the "evil eye," illnesses that are attributed to spirits, or beliefs that prayer is necessary for healing.

cupping, a counter-irritant technique from Eastern medicine of applying a suction device to the skin to draw blood to the surface of the body.

cytokine, /sī″təkīn/, one of a large group of low-molecular-weight proteins secreted by various cell types and involved in cell-to-cell communication, coordinating antibody and T-cell immune interactions, and regulating immune reactivity. Kinds include interferon, interleukin, lymphokine.

D

delta wave, 1. The slowest of several types of brain waves, characterized by a frequency of 4 Hz and a relatively high voltage. Delta waves are "deep-sleep waves" associated with a dreamless state from which an individual is not easily aroused. Also called delta rhythm. 2. (in cardiology) A slurring of the QRS portion of an electrocardiogram tracing caused by preexcitation in Wolff-Parkinson-White syndrome.

dendrite, /den″drīt/ [Gk, *dendron,* tree], a slender branching process that extends from the cell body of a neuron and that is capable of being stimulated by a neurotransmitter. Each neuron usually possesses several dendrites, which receive synapses where chemical transmission occurs from axons to dendrites (or an axon, in the case of unipolar neurons). The number of dendrites and thus the number of synapses varies with the functions of a neuron. Also called cytodendrite.

diabetic neuropathy, a noninflammatory disease process associated with diabetes mellitus and characterized by sensory and/or motor disturbances in the peripheral nervous system. Patients commonly experience degeneration of sensory nerves and pathways. Early symptoms, which include pain and loss of reflexes in the legs, may occur in patients with only mild hyperglycemia. Diabetes is associated with a wide range of neuropathies, including mononeuritis multiplex, compression and entrapment mononeuropathies, cranial neuropathies, and autonomic and small fiber neuropathies. Differential diagnosis is difficult because not all sensorimotor neuropathies are caused by diabetes.

diabetic polyneuropathy, a disorder involving a number of nerves, a long-term complication of diabetes mellitus. Central nervous system, autonomic, and peripheral nerves may be affected. Neuropathic ulcers commonly develop on the feet.

diaphragmatic breathing, /dī·əfragmat″ik/ [Gk, *diaphragma,* partition], a pattern of expiration and inspiration in which most of the ventilatory work is done with the diaphragm. Many males normally breathe diaphragmatically, whereas few females do. The technique is taught to patients with chronic obstructive pulmonary disease to facilitate respiration. The patient is trained to strengthen the contractile force of the abdominal wall muscles to elevate the diaphragm and empty the lungs. The patient places a hand on the epigastrium during training to focus attention on that portion of the body. Also called diaphragmatic respiration.

disparities, (for health or related reasons) inequality in health status or in access to health services for a group of individuals based on racial, ethnic, or socioeconomic status.

dissociative anesthesia, /disō″shē·ətiv/, a unique anesthesia characterized by analgesia and amnesia with minimal effect on respiratory function. The patient does not appear to be anesthetized and can swallow and open eyes but does not process information. This form of anesthesia may be used to provide analgesia during brief, superficial operative procedures or diagnostic processes. Ketamine hydrochloride is a phencyclidine derivative that inhibits principally the N-methyl-D-aspartate (NMDA) receptor, used to induce dissociative anesthesia. Ketamine is used in combination with a benzodiazepine or alone for patients with trauma with very unstable, low blood pressure or for elderly patients. Emergence may be accompanied by delirium, excitement, disorientation, and confusion.

disuse phenomena, /disyoos″/ [L, *dis* + *usus,* to make use of; Gk, *phainein,* to show], the physical and psychological changes, usually degenerative, that result from the lack of use of a body part or system. Disuse phenomena are associated with confinement and immobility, especially in orthopedics. Individuals deprived of sufficient interaction with the world around them may lose motivation and acquired abilities because of lack of practice. Pain and therapeutic opioid drugs commonly associated with the treatment of many illnesses and abnormal conditions contribute to disuse phenomena.

drug agonist, a drug that is capable of binding to a neurotransmitter or hormone receptor and causing a response similar to that of the endogenous hormone or neurotransmitter.

drug clearance, the elimination of a drug from the body. Drugs and their metabolites are excreted primarily by the kidneys into the urine, but other routes for elimination include bile, sweat, saliva, breast milk, and expired air. The rate of clearance helps determine the size and frequency of a dosage of a particular medication.

drug concentration, the amount of drug in a given volume of plasma (e.g., number of micrograms per milliliter). Toxic drug levels may be observed when the body's normal mechanisms for metabolizing and excreting drugs are impaired, as commonly occurs in patients with liver or kidney disorders and in infants with immature organs. Dosage adjustments should be made in such individuals to accommodate their impaired metabolism and excretion.

drug distribution, the pattern of distribution of drug molecules by various tissues after the chemical enters the circulatory system. Because of differences in pH, lipid content, cell membrane functions, and other individual tissue factors, most drugs are not distributed equally in all parts of the body. For example, the acidity of aspirin influences a distribution pattern that is different from that of an alkaline product such as amphetamine.

drug-drug interaction, a modification of the effect of a drug when administered with another drug. The effect may be an increase or a decrease in the action of either substance, or it may be an adverse effect that is not normally associated with either drug. The particular interaction may be the result of a chemical-physical incompatibility of the two drugs or a change in the rate of absorption or the quantity absorbed in the body, the binding ability of either drug, or an alteration in the ability of receptor sites and cell membranes to bind either drug. Most adverse drug-drug interactions are either pharmacodynamic or pharmacokinetic in nature.

Drug Enforcement Agency (DEA), an agency of the U.S. Drug Enforcement Administration of the federal government, empowered to enforce regulations that control the import or export of opioid drugs and certain other substances or the traffic of these substances across state lines.

drug-food interaction, the effect produced when some drugs and certain foods or beverages are taken at the same time. For example, grapefruit juice blocks the metabolism of some drugs in the gastrointestinal tract, an action that can cause normal dosages of a drug to reach toxic levels in the plasma.

drug holiday, a period of drug withdrawal to reverse ineffectiveness of a drug resulting from receptor desensitization or adverse effects that may result from chronic treatment. For example, after a 7- to 10-day drug holiday, levodopa responsiveness appears to be enhanced, and lower doses are required to produce a therapeutic effect.

drug metabolism, the transformation of a drug by the body tissues, primarily those of the liver, into a more water-soluble metabolite that can be eliminated. This process inactivates many drugs, but some drugs have metabolites that are also biologically active and others are administered as pro-drugs that must undergo drug metabolism to become biologically active.

drug potency, the amount of drug required to produce a given percentage of its maximal effect, irrespective of the size of maximal effect. A drug can have high potency but poor efficacy, meaning that response is seen at very low doses and remains small even at high doses. Drug potency is seldom an important clinical consideration.

drug sensitivity, an increase in the responsiveness of an individual to a medication because of variations in the way the drug is metabolized. Should not be confused with drug allergy.

drug tolerance, a condition of cellular adaptation to a pharmacologically active substance so that increasingly larger doses are required to produce the same physiologic or psychological effect obtained earlier with smaller doses. Also called metabolic tolerance.

dura mater, /doŏ″rə mā″tər, dyoŏ″rə/ [L, *durus,* hard, *mater,* mother], the outermost and most fibrous of the three membranes surrounding the brain and spinal cord. The dura mater encephali covers the brain, and the dura mater spinalis covers the cord.

dysmenorrhea, /dis′menəre″ə/ [Gk, *dys* + *men,* month, *rhein,* to flow], painful menstruation sufficiently severe that it prevents the performance of normal activities. Primary dysmenorrhea is associated with an excess of prostaglandins, primarily prostaglandin F_2-alpha (PGF$_2$α). Secondary dysmenorrhea may be caused by a clinically identifiable cause, or if not, it is called idiopathic. These causes may be classified as extrauterine (endometriosis, benign and malignant tumors, inflammation, adhesions and, rarely, psychogenic), intramural (adenomyosis, leiomyomata), and intrauterine (leiomyomata, polyps intrauterine contraceptive devices, infection, and cervical stenosis). Treatment depends on identification of the specific cause. Also called menorrhagia. Also spelled dysmenorrhoea.

E

efferent nerve, a nerve that transmits impulses away or outward from a nerve center, such as the brain or spinal cord, usually causing a muscle contraction or release of a glandular secretion.

efferent pathway, [L, *effere,* to carry out; ME, *paeth* + *weg*], 1. The route of nerve fibers carrying impulses away from a nerve center. 2. The system of blood vessels that conveys blood away from a body part.

effleurage, /ef′ləräzh″/ [Fr, skimming the surface], a technique in massage in which long, light, or firm strokes are used, usually over the spine and back. Fingertip effleurage is a light technique performed with the tips of the fingers in a circular pattern over one part of the body or in long strokes over the back or an extremity. Fingertip effleurage of the abdomen is a technique commonly used in the Lamaze method of natural childbirth.

Ehlers-Danlos syndrome, /ā″lərz dan″ləs/ [Edward Ehlers, Danish physician, 1863–1937; Henri A. Danlos, French physician, 1844–1912], a hereditary disorder of connective tissue, marked by hyperplasticity of skin, tissue fragility, and hypermotility of joints. Minor trauma may cause a gaping wound with little bleeding. Sprains, joint dislocations, and synovial effusions are common. Life expectancy is usually normal.

emollient bath, a bath taken in water containing an emollient, such as bran, to relieve irritation and inflammation.

empathic, /empath″ik/ [Gk, *en,* into, *pathos,* feeling], pertaining to or involving the entering of one person into the emotional state of another while remaining objective and distinctly separate.

empathy, /em″pəthē/ [Gk, en, in, pathos, feeling], the ability to recognize and, to some extent, share the emotions and states of mind of another and to understand the meaning and significance of that person's behavior. It is an essential quality for effective psychotherapy.

endogenous, /endoj″ənəs/ [Gk, *endon* + *genein,* to produce], 1. Growing within the body. 2. Originating from within the body or produced from internal causes, such as a disease caused by the structural or functional failure of an organ or system. –endogenic, adj.

endorphin, /endôr″fin/ [Gk, *endon* + *morphe,* shape], one of the three groups of endogenous opioid peptides composed of many amino acids, elaborated by the pituitary gland and other brain areas, and acting on the central and the peripheral nervous systems to reduce pain. There are three known, designated alpha, beta, and gamma. Beta-endorphin has been isolated in the brain and in the gastrointestinal tract and seems to be the most potent of the endorphins. Beta-endorphin is composed of 30 amino acids that are identical to part of the sequence of 91 amino acids of the hormone beta-lipotropin, also produced by the pituitary gland. Behavioral tests indicate that beta-endorphin is a powerful analgesic in humans and animals. Brain-stimulated analgesia in humans releases beta-endorphin into the cerebrospinal fluid.

end-tidal capnography, /end″tīdəl/, the process of continuously recording the level of carbon dioxide in expired air. The percentage of carbon dioxide (CO_2) at the end of expiration can be estimated and gives a close approximation of the alveolar CO_2 concentration. The process, which requires the use of infrared spectroscopy, is used to monitor critically ill patients and in pulmonary function testing. The data are typically recorded automatically on a strip of graph paper on a bedside patient monitor.

end-tidal CO_2, the partial pressure or maximal concentration of carbon dioxide (CO_2) at the end of an exhaled breath, which is expressed as a percentage of CO_2 or millimeters of mercury. The normal values are 5% to 6% CO_2, which is equivalent to 35 to 45 mm Hg.

end-tidal CO_2 determination, the concentration of CO_2 in a patient's end-tidal breath, assumed to reflect arterial CO_2 tension. A significant difference may indicate a change in ventilation/perfusion matching.

enkephalin, /enkef″əlin/ [Gk, *enkepalos,* brain, *in,* within], one of two pain-relieving pentapeptides produced in the body, located in the pituitary gland, brain, and gastrointestinal tract. Axon terminals that release enkephalins are concentrated in the posterior horn of the gray matter of the spinal cord, in the central part of the thalamus, and in the amygdala of the limbic system of the cerebrum. Enkephalins function as neurotransmitters or neuromodulators and inhibit neurotransmitters in the pathway for pain perception, thereby reducing the emotional as well as the physical impact of pain. Methionine-enkephalin and isoleucine-enkephalin are each composed of five amino acids, four of which are identical in both compounds. These two neuropeptides can depress neurons throughout the central nervous system. Although it is not known exactly how these neuropeptides function, the enkephalins are natural pain killers and may be involved, with other neuropeptides, in the development of psychopathologic behavior in some cases. Compare endorphin.

epidural, /ep′idoŏr″əl/ [Gk, *epi* + *dura,* hard], outside or above the dura mater, which surrounds the central nervous system.

epidural blood patch (EBP), a treatment for postdural puncture headache caused by an inadvertent puncture of the dura mater during an epidural anesthetic, in which 15 to 20 mL of a patient's autologous blood is injected into the epidural space at or near the location of a dural puncture. The volume injected displaces cerebrospinal fluid (CSF) from the lumbar CSF space into the area surrounding the brain, often yielding immediate relief. When the blood clots, it seals the dural puncture, prohibiting further leakage of CSF from the subarachnoid space.

epidural hematoma, an accumulation of blood in the epidural space, caused by damage to and leakage of blood from the middle meningeal artery, producing compression of the dura mater and thus of the brain. Unless evacuated, it may result in herniation through the tentorium and death.

equianalgesic dose, /ē′kwē·an′əljē″sik/, a dose of one analgesic that is equivalent in pain-relieving effects to that of another analgesic. This equivalence permits substitution of medications to prevent possible adverse effects of one of the drugs. The term is also applied to equivalent alternative dose sizes and routes of administration of analgesic that is equivalent in pain-relieving effects to that of another analgesic. This equivalence permits substitution of medications to prevent possible adverse effects of one of the drugs.

The term is also applied to equivalent alternative dose sizes and routes of administration.

essential oils, 1. A class of generally aromatic volatile oils. 2. The essences extracted from plants for use in flavoring foods, perfumes, and medicines. Some essential oils have been used therapeutically for thousands of years.

ethical distress, (for health or related reasons) the discomfort a health care provider experiences when he or she is prevented from doing what is thought to be right.

ethics, /eth″iks/ [Gk, *ethikos,* moral duty], the science or study of moral values or principles, including ideals of autonomy, beneficence, and justice. – ethical, adj.

evidence-based practice, the practice of health care in which the practitioner systematically finds, appraises, and uses the most current and valid research findings as the basis for clinical decisions. The term is sometimes used to denote evidence-based medicine specifically but also includes other professions.

excitation, /ek′sitā″shən/ [L, *excitare,* to arouse], nerve or muscle action as a result of impulse propagation; a state of mental or physical excitement.

exercise, /ek″sərsiz/ [L, *exercere,* to exercise], 1. n. The performance of any physical activity for the purpose of conditioning the body, improving health, or maintaining fitness or as a means of therapy for correcting a deformity or restoring the organs and body functions to a state of health. 2. n. Any action, skill, or maneuver that causes muscle exertion and is performed repeatedly to develop or strengthen the body or any of its parts. 3. v. To use a muscle or part of the body in a repetitive way to maintain or develop its strength. Exercise has a beneficial effect on each of the body systems, although in excess it can lead to the breakdown of tissue and cause injury. Kinds include active assisted exercise, active exercise, active resistance exercise, aerobic exercise, anaerobic exercise, isometric exercise, isotonic exercise, muscle-setting exercise, passive exercise, progressive resistance exercise, range-of-motion exercise, therapeutic exercise, underwater exercise.

exercise tolerance, the level of physical exertion an individual may be able to achieve before reaching a state of exhaustion. Exercise tolerance tests are commonly performed on a treadmill under the supervision of a health professional who can stop the test if signs of distress are observed.

exogenous, /igzoj″ənəs/ [Gk, *exo* + *genein,* to produce], 1. Outside the body. 2. Originating outside the body or an organ of the body or produced from external causes, such as a disease caused by a bacterial or viral agent foreign to the body. – exogenic, adj.

F

fibromyalgia, a form of nonarticular rheumatism characterized by musculoskeletal pain, spasms, stiffness, fatigue, and severe sleep disturbance. Common sites of pain or stiffness include the lower back, neck, shoulder region, arms, hands, knees, hips, thighs, legs, and feet. These sites are known as trigger points. Physical therapy, nonsteroidal antiinflammatory drugs, and muscle relaxants provide temporary relief. Also called fibrositis, soft tissue rheumatism.

Food and Drug Administration (FDA), a U.S. federal agency responsible for the enforcement of federal regulations on the manufacture and distribution of food, drugs, medical devices, and cosmetics. The regulations are intended to prevent the sale of impure or dangerous substances.

Fournier's gangrene, /foornyāz″/ [Jean A. Fournier, French syphilographer, 1832–1914], an infective gangrene of the scrotum or vulva caused by an anaerobic hemolytic strain of *Streptococcus.* This form of gangrene is associated with diabetes. It occurs after local trauma, operative procedures, underlying urinary tract disease, or a distant acute inflammatory process. It is relatively rare in the United States. Infective agents are *Bacteroides fragilis* and aerobic *Escherichia coli.* Also called polymicrobial necrotizing fasciitis.

G

gait analysis, evaluation of the manner or style of walking, normally done by observing an individual walking in a straight line. Objective measurement systems that include video recordings, infrared cameras, specialized floor systems, and electromyography may be employed when deviations from normal are present.

general adaptation syndrome (GAS), [L, *genus,* kind; L, *adaptare,* to fit; Gk, *syn,* together, *dromos,* course], the defense response of the body or the psyche to injury or prolonged stress, as described by Hans Selye (1907–1982). It consists of an initial stage of shock or alarm reaction, followed by a phase of increasing resistance or adaptation in which the various defense mechanisms of the body or mind are used, and culminates in a state of adjustment and healing or of exhaustion and disintegration. Also called adaptation syndrome.

glia cells, /glī″ə, glē″ə/ [Gk, *glia,* glue; L, *cella,* storeroom], neural cells that have a connective tissue–supporting function in the central nervous system. Examples include astrocytes and oligodendroglial cells of ectodermal origin and microglial cells of mesodermal origin.

H

habituation, /həbich′oo·ā″shən/ [L, habituare, to become used to], 1. An acquired tolerance gained by repeated exposure to a particular stimulus, such as alcohol. 2. A decline and eventual elimination of a conditioned response by repetition of the conditioned stimulus. 3. Psychological and emotional dependence on a drug, tobacco, or alcohol that results from the repeated use of the substance but without the addictive, physiological need to increase dosage. Also called negative adaptation. Compare addiction. 4. (in occupational therapy) Internal readiness to demonstrate a consistent pattern of behavior guided by habits and roles; this readiness is associated with specific temporal, physical, or social environments.

half-life (T$_{1/2}$), [AS, *haelf* + lif], 1. The time required for a radioactive substance to lose 50% of its activity through decay. Each radionuclide has a unique half-life. Also called radioactive half-life. 2. The amount of time required to reduce a drug level to half of its initial value. Usually the term refers to time necessary to reduce the plasma value to half of its initial value. After five half-lives, 97% of a single drug dose will be eliminated.

hallucinatory neuralgia, /həloo″sənətôr′ē/, a feeling of localized pain that persists after an episode of severe throbbing pain has subsided.

herb, /(h)urb/ [L, *herba,* grass], 1. Any plant that is used for culinary or medicinal purposes. 2. A leafy plant without a wooden stem whose parts growing above the ground die back after the growing season.

herbalist, /hur″bəlist/, 1. A person who specializes in the study of herbs and their health benefits. 2. A practitioner or individual who uses plants or parts of plants for therapeutic benefit. 3. An individual who grows and harvests herbal plants for medicinal purposes.

histamine, /his″təmēn, -min/ [Gk, *histos,* tissue; L, *amine,* ammonia], a compound found in all cells that is produced by the breakdown of histidine. It is released in allergic inflammatory reactions. Cellular receptors of histamine include the H1 receptors, which are responsible for the dilation of blood vessels and the contraction of smooth muscle; the histamine receptors type 2 (H$_2$), which are responsible for the stimulation of heart rate and gastric secretion; and H$_3$ receptors, which are thought to play a role in regulation of the release of histamine and other neurotransmitters from neurons. H$_1$ and H$_2$ receptors also mediate the contraction of vascular smooth muscle.

histamine headache, a headache associated with the release of histamine from the body tissues and marked by symptoms of dilated carotid arteries, fluid accumulation under the eyes, tearing (or lacrimation), and rhinorrhea (runny nose). Symptoms include sudden sharp pain on one side of the head, involving the facial area from the neck to the temple. Treatment includes the use of preparations of antihistamines and ergot that help constrict the arteries. Also called cluster headache, Horton's histamine cephalalgia. *See also* cephalalgia.

holism, /hō″lizəm/ [Gk, *holos,* whole], a philosophical concept in which an entity is seen as more than the sum of its parts. Holism is prominent in current approaches to psychology, biology, medicine, nursing, allied health professions, and other scientific, sociologic, and educational fields of study and practice. Also spelled wholism.

holistic, /hōlis″tik/ [Gk, *holos*], pertaining to the whole; considering all factors, as holistic medicine.

holistic counseling, an alternative form of psychotherapy that focuses on the whole person (mind, body, and spirit) and health. The goal is growth of the whole person.

holistic health, /hōlis″tik/ [AS, *hal,* whole, *haelth*], a concept that concern for health requires a perception of the individual as an integrated system rather than one or more separate parts, including physical, mental, spiritual, and emotional. Also spelled wholistic health.

holistic health care, a system of comprehensive or total patient care that considers the physical, emotional, social, economic, and spiritual needs of the person, his or her response to illness, and the effect of the illness on the ability to meet self-care needs.

holistic nurse, a nurse who focuses on healing the whole person as the goal of care. In practicing holistic nursing, the nurse implements interventions aimed at bio-psycho-social-spiritual-environmental healing.

home assessment, [AS, *ham,* village; L, *assidere,* to sit beside], an examination of the living area of a physically challenged person to make recommendations for the elimination of safety hazards and suggestions for architectural or other modifications that would allow for independent functioning.

homotopic pain, /hō′mōtop″ik/, pain experienced at the point of injury.

Horner's syndrome, [Johann F. Horner, Swiss ophthalmologist, 1831–1886], a neurologic condition characterized by a constricted (miotic) pupil, ptosis, and facial anhidrosis, associated with a lesion in the spinal cord, with damage to a cervical nerve or any ascending part of the sympathetic outflow to the face/head. Signs are ipsilateral (same side) to the injury.

H$_1$ receptor, a type of histamine receptor present in smooth muscles, on vascular endothelial cells, in the heart, and in the central nervous system. Triggering of H$_1$ receptors by histamine mediates vasodilation. *See also* histamine blocking agent.

H$_2$ receptor, a type of histamine receptor on various kinds of cells through which histamine mediates bronchial constriction in asthma and gastrointestinal constriction in diarrhea. *See also* histamine blocking agent.

H$_1$ receptor antagonist, any of a large number of agents that block the action of histamine by competitive binding to the H$_1$ receptor. Such agents also have sedative, anticholinergic, and antiemetic effects, the exact effect varying from drug to drug, and are used for the relief of allergic symptoms and as antiemetics, antivertigo agents, sedatives, and antidyskinetics in parkinsonism. This group is traditionally called the antihistamines.

H$_2$ receptor antagonist, an agent that blocks the action of histamine by competitive binding to the H$_2$ receptor. It is used to inhibit gastric secretion in the treatment of peptic ulcer.

hydrotherapy, /-ther″əpē/ [Gk, *hydor* + *therapeia,* treatment], the use of water in the treatment of various disorders. Hydrotherapy may include continuous tub baths, wet sheet packs, or shower sprays.

hyperalgia, /-al″jə/, extreme sensitivity to pain. Also called hyperalgesia.

hypercapnia, /hī′pərkap″nē·ə/ [Gk, *hyper* + *kapnos,* vapor], greater-than-normal amounts of carbon dioxide in the blood. Also called hypercarbia.

hypercapnic acidosis, /-kap″nik/ [Gk, *hyper* + *kapnos,* vapor; L, *acidus,* sour, *osis,* condition], an excessive acidity in body fluids caused by an increase in carbon dioxide (CO_2) tension in the blood. The condition may be secondary to pulmonary insufficiency. As CO_2 accumulates in the blood, its acidity increases.

hypnosis, /hipnō″sis/ [Gk, *hypnos,* sleep], a passive, trancelike state that resembles normal sleep during which perception and memory are altered, resulting in increased responsiveness to suggestion. The condition is usually induced by the monotonous repetition of words and gestures while the subject is completely relaxed.

hypnotherapy, /hip′nəther″əpē/ [Gk, *hypnos* + *therapeia,* treatment], the induction of a specific altered state (trance) for memory retrieval, relaxation, or suggestion. Hypnotherapy is often used to alter habits (e.g., smoking, obesity), treat biological mechanisms such as hypertension or cardiac arrhythmias, deal with the symptoms of a disease, alter an individual's reaction to disease, and affect an illness and its course through the body.

hypoxia, /hīpok″sē·ə/ [Gk, *hypo* + *oxys,* sharp, *genein,* to produce], inadequate oxygen tension at the cellular level, characterized by tachycardia, hypertension, peripheral vasoconstriction, dizziness, and mental confusion. Mild hypoxia stimulates peripheral chemoreceptors to increase heart and respiration rates. The central mechanisms that regulate breathing fail in severe hypoxia, leading to irregular respiration, Cheyne-Stokes respiration, apnea, and respiratory and cardiac failure. Increased sensitivity to the depressant effect of opiates on the respiratory system is common in chronic hypoxia, causing severe depression of respiration or apnea from relatively small doses. If the availability of oxygen is inadequate for aerobic cellular metabolism, energy is provided by less efficient anaerobic pathways that produce metabolites other than carbon dioxide and water. The tissues most sensitive to hypoxia are the brain, heart, pulmonary vessels, and liver. Treatment may include cardiotonic and respiratory stimulant drugs, oxygen therapy, mechanical ventilation, and frequent analysis of blood gases.

I

iatrogenic, /ī′atrōjen″ik, yat-/ [Gk, *iatros,* physician, *genein,* to produce], caused by treatment or diagnostic procedures. An iatrogenic disorder is a condition that is caused by medical personnel or procedures or that develops through exposure to the environment of a health care facility. *See also* nosocomial. – iatrogeny, iatrogenesis, n.

idiopathic, /-path″ik/ [Gk, *idios* + *pathos,* disease], without a known cause.

indolent, /in″dələnt/ [L, *in* + *dolere,* to suffer pain], 1. Pertaining to an organic disorder that is accompanied by little or no pain. 2. Slow to heal or grow, as in wounds that heal very slowly.

insensible, /insen″sibəl/ [L, *in* + *sentire,* to feel], 1. Pertaining to a person who is unconscious for any reason. 2. Pertaining to a person who is apathetic or deprived of normal sense perceptions.

insomnia, /insom″nē·ə/ [L, *in,* not, *somnus,* sleep], chronic inability to sleep or to remain asleep throughout the night, wakefulness, sleeplessness. Insomnia may be the symptom of a psychiatric disorder. Formerly called agrypnia.

inspiration, /in′spirā″shən/ [L, *inspirare,* to breathe in], the act of drawing air into the lungs. The major muscle of inspiration is the diaphragm, the contraction of which creates a reduced pressure in the chest, causing the lungs to expand and air to flow inward. Accessory inspiratory muscles include the external intercostals, scaleni, scapular elevators, and sternocleidomastoids. Because expiration is usually a passive process, these muscles of inspiration alone produce normal respiration. Lungs at maximal inspiration have an average total capacity of 5.5 to 6 L of air. Also called inhalation.

Instrumental activities of daily living (IADLs), /in′strəmen″təl/, activities that support life within the home and community and that often require more complex interactions than those used in a category called activities of daily living (ADL). IADLs include care of others, care of pets, child rearing, communication management, driving and community mobility, financial management, health management and maintenance, home establishment and management, meal preparation and cleanup, religious and spiritual activities, implementation of safety and emergency precautions, and shopping.

integration, /in′təgrā″shən/ [L, *integrare,* to make whole], 1. The act or process of unifying or bringing together. 2. (in psychology) The organization of all elements of the personality into a coordinated functional whole that is in harmony with the environment, one of the primary goals.

intention, /inten″shən/ [L, *intendere,* to aim], a kind of healing process. Healing by primary intention is the initial union of the edges of a wound, progressing to complete healing without granulation. Healing by secondary intention is wound closure in which the edges are separated, granulation tissue develops to fill the gap, and epithelium grows in over the granulations, producing a scar. Healing by tertiary intention is wound closure in which granulation tissue fills the gap between the edges of the wound, with epithelium growing over the granulation at a slower rate and producing a larger scar than the scar resulting from healing from secondary intention. Suppuration is also usually found.

interleukin, /-loo″kin/, cytokines mainly produced by leukocytes. Interleukins participate in communication among leukocytes and are important in the inflammatory response. Most interleukins direct other cells to divide and differentiate. Each acts on a particular group of cells that have receptors specific to that interleukin.

interoceptive, /in′tərōsep″tiv/ [L, *internus,* inward, *capere,* to take], pertaining to stimuli originating from within the body that are related to the functioning of the internal organs or the receptors they activate.

intervertebral, /in′tərvur″təbrəl/ [L, *inter* + *vertebra,* back joint], pertaining to the space between any two vertebrae, such as the fibrocartilaginous discs.

intraosseous infusion, the injection of blood, medications, or fluids into bone marrow rather than into a vein. The technique may be performed in emergency treatment of a child when intravenous infusion is not feasible.

ischemic pain, unpleasant, often excruciating pain associated with decreased blood flow caused by mechanical obstruction, constricting orthopedic casts, or insufficient blood flow that results from injury or surgical trauma. Ischemic pain caused by occlusive arterial disease is often severe and may not be relieved, even with opioids. The individual with peripheral vascular disease may experience ischemic pain only while exercising because the metabolic demands for oxygen cannot be met as a result of occluded blood flow. The ischemic pain of partial arterial occlusion is not as severe as the abrupt, excruciating pain associated with complete occlusion, such as by an embolus or thrombus.

isometric, /ī′səmet″rik/ [Gk, *isos* + *metron,* measure], maintaining the same length or dimension.

isometric contraction, [Gk, *isos,* equal, *metron,* measure; L, *contractio,* a drawing together], muscular contraction not accompanied by movement of the joint. Resistance applied to the contraction increases muscle tension without producing movement of the joint. Also called muscle-setting exercise.

isometric exercise, a form of active exercise in which muscle tension is increased while pressure is applied against stable resistance. This exercise may be accomplished by pushing or pulling against an immovable object or by simultaneously contracting opposing muscles, such as by pressing the hands together. There is no joint movement, and muscle length remains unchanged, but muscle strength and tone are maintained or improved. *See also* exercise.

-ize, suffix to form verbs from adjectives and nouns. Verbs mean "to make, become, engage in, or use" or "to treat or combine with": oxidize, anesthetize.

J

jogger's heel, [ME, *joggen,* to shake; AS, *hela,* heel], a painful condition characterized by bruising, bursitis, fasciitis, or calcaneal spurs that results from repetitive and forceful striking of the heel on the ground. It is common among joggers and distance runners. Judicious selection of well-fitting running shoes and avoidance of running on hard surfaces are recommended to prevent occurrence or recurrence of the condition.

K

ketogenesis, /-jen″əsis/ [Gk, *keton* + Gk, *genein,* to produce], the formation or production of ketone bodies.

ketogenic amino acid, /-jen″ik/, an amino acid whose carbon skeleton serves as a precursor for ketone bodies.

ketogenic diet, a diet high in fats (often as medium-chain triglycerides) and proteins and low in carbohydrates, primarily used in the treatment of epilepsy.

L

***Lactobacillus* (L),** /lak′tōbəsil″əs/ [L, *lac* + *bacillum,* small rod], any one of a group of nonpathogenic gram-positive rod-shaped bacteria that produce lactic acid from carbohydrates. Many species are normally found in the human intestinal tract and vagina.

Lactobacillus acidophilus, [L, *lac,* milk, *bacillum,* small rod, *acidus,* sour; Gk, *philein,* to love], a bacterium present in the intestinal tract and vagina, as well as in milk and dairy products. The strain is used to manufacture a fermented milk product. Generally considered to be beneficial because it produces vitamin K, lactase, and other antimicrobial substances when ingested.

laminectomy, /lam′inek″təmē/ [L, *lamina* + Gk, *ektomē,* excision], surgical removal of the bony arches of one or more vertebrae. It is performed to treat compression fractures, dislocations, herniated nucleus pulposus, and cord tumors and to stimulate the spinal cord. With the patient under general anesthesia and prone to eliminate lordosis, reduce venous congestion, and keep the abdomen free; the laminae are removed, and the underlying problem is corrected. Spinal fusion with cages, rods, screws, and/or bone graft is used to stabilize the spine if several laminae are removed. If the procedure is a cervical laminectomy, the patient is observed for signs of respiratory distress caused by cord edema. Motor function and sensation in the extremities are evaluated every 2 to 4 hours for 48 hours. The dressing is examined frequently for hemorrhage or leakage of cerebrospinal fluid. The patient is taught to logroll without twisting the spine or hips. – laminectomize, v.

laser, /lā″zər/, a source of intense monochromatic radiation of the visible, ultraviolet, or infrared portions of the spectrum. Lasers are used in surgery to divide or cause adhesions or to destroy or fix tissue in place. Abbreviation for *l*ight *a*mplification by *s*timulated *e*mission of *r*adiation. Also called optic laser, optic maser.

laser pain management, the use of lasers to relieve pain. The laser can be used in place of acupuncture needles at acupuncture points or may be used directly over the source of pain.

level of consciousness (LOC), [OFr, *livel* + L, *conscire*, to be aware of], a degree of cognitive function involving arousal mechanisms of the reticular formation of the brain. The stages of response of the mind to stimuli vary from unconsciousness through vague awareness to full attention. The usual standard levels include coma, in which the patient does not appear to be aware of the environment; stupor, in which the patient is vaguely aware of the environment; drowsiness, in which the patient responds to stimuli but may be slow to react; and alert wakefulness. Impaired LOC may be expressed in obtundation or reduced alertness, stupor, syncope, or unresponsiveness.

liposome, /lip′əsōm/ [Gk, *lipos,* fat, *soma,* body], a small, spherical particle consisting of a bilayer of phospholipid molecules surrounding an aqueous solution.

lumbar plexus, a network of nerves formed by the ventral anterior primary divisions of the first three and the greater part of the fourth lumbar nerves. It is located on the inside of the posterior abdominal wall, either dorsal to the psoas major or among its fibers and ventral to the transverse processes of the lumbar vertebrae. The branches of the lumbar plexus are the iliohypogastric, ilioinguinal, genitofemoral, lateral femoral cutaneous, obturator, accessory obturator, and femoral nerves. The iliohypogastric, ilioinguinal, and genitofemoral nerves supply the caudal part of the abdominal wall. The lateral femoral cutaneous, obturator, accessory obturator, and femoral nerves supply the anterior thigh and the middle of the leg. Only 20% of people have the accessory obturator nerve, which comes from the third and the fourth lumbar nerves.

M

maintenance, 1. Providing a stable state over a long period of time as distinguished from a short-term remedial or prophylactic effect; as in a drug or treatment plan. 2. In anesthesia, the surgical or procedural period of anesthesia delivery, in which a combination of inhaled agents and adjunct medications are administered to allow an appropriate surgical field or procedural conditions.

maintenance dose, /mān″tənəns/ [Fr, *maintenir,* to uphold; Gk, *dosis,* giving], the amount of drug required to keep a desired mean steady-state concentration in the tissues.

malfeasance, /malfē″zəns/ [Fr, *malfaire,* to do evil], performance of an unlawful, wrongful act.

massage, /məsäzh, məsäj″/ [Fr, *masser,* to stroke], the manipulation of the soft tissue of the body through stroking, improve muscle tone, and to relax the patient. The procedure is performed either with the bare hands or through some mechanical means, such as a vibrator. The most common sites for massage are the back, knees, elbows, and heels. Care is taken not to massage inflamed areas, particularly of the extremities, because of the danger of loosening blood clots. Open wounds and areas of rash, tumor, or excessive sensitivity are avoided. Even if the extremities (legs) are not inflamed, they should not be massaged if the client has been immobilized for an extended period. The procedure is performed with the patient prone or on the side, comfortably positioned, with an emollient lotion or cream applied to the area to be massaged. The caregiver's hands are warm, and excessive pressure is avoided to prevent pain or injury. Kinds include cardiac massage, effleurage, flagellation, friction, frôlement, pétrissage, tapotement, vibration.

medical marijuana, cannabis or cannabinoids used in the therapeutic management of a disease or to control symptoms of a disease. It is used to reduce nausea and vomiting and improve appetite and in the management of pain. It is available in many forms, but its use as a medication is not legal in every jurisdiction.

mastalgia, /mastal″jə/ [Gk, *mastos,* breast, *algos,* pain], pain in the breast caused by congestion during lactation, an infection, fibrocystic disease, or advanced cancer. The early stages of breast cancer are rarely accompanied by pain. Hormonal changes also may be a factor. –mastalgic, adj.

medical marijuana, cannabis or cannabinoids used in the therapeutic management of a disease or to control symptoms of a disease. It is used to reduce nausea and vomiting and improve appetite and in the management of pain. It is available in many forms, but its use as a medication is not legal in every jurisdiction.

meditation, /med′itā″shən/ [L, *meditari,* to consider], a state of consciousness in which the individual eliminates environmental stimuli from awareness so that the mind has a single focus, producing a state of relaxation and relief from stress. A wide variety of techniques are used to clear the mind of stressful outside interference.

mental health (MH), a relative state of mind in which a person is able to cope with and adjust to the recurrent stresses of everyday living in an acceptable way.

mEq, abbreviation for milliequivalent.

meta-analysis, a systematic method that takes data from a number of independent studies and integrates them using statistical analysis.

milliequivalent (mEq), /-ikwiv′ələnt/ [L, *mille* + *aequus,* equal, *valere,* to be strong], 1. The number of grams of solute dissolved in 1 mL of a normal (1 N) solution. 2. One-thousandth (10^{-3}) of a gram equivalent.

mind-body medicine, a holistic approach to medicine that takes into account the effect of the mind on physical processes, including the effects of psychosocial stressors and conditioning, particularly as they affect the immune system. Many of the therapeutic techniques used have as their purpose increasing the body's natural resistance to disease by managing the stressors.

mindfulness meditation, a technique of meditation in which distracting thoughts and feelings are not ignored but are rather acknowledged and observed nonjudgmentally as they arise to create a detachment from them and gain insight and awareness.

mineral, /min″ərəl/ [L, *minera,* mine], 1. An inorganic substance occurring naturally in the earth's crust, having a characteristic chemical composition and (usually) crystalline structure. 2. (in nutrition) A compound containing a metal, nonmetal, radical, or phosphate that is needed for proper body function and maintenance of health. The needed substance is usually ingested as a part of such a compound, such as table salt (sodium chloride), instead of as a free element, and the compound is usually referred to by the name of the needed substance.

modality, /mōdal″itē/, 1. The method of application of a therapeutic agent or regimen. 2. A sensory entity, such as the sense of vision or taste.

modulation, /mod′yəlā″shən/, an alteration in the magnitude or any variation in the duration of an electrical current. Modulation, which affects physiologic responses to various waveforms, may be continuous, interrupted, pulsed, or surging.

moist heat, [OFr, *moiste* + AS, *haetu*], the use of hot water, towels soaked in hot water, aquathermia pads, hot water bottles, or hot water vapors to reduce inflammation and pain, stimulate circulation, and/or relieve symptoms as directed by a physician. Hot towels should be wrung out to remove surplus moisture and should not be too hot to be held in the hands of the person applying moist heat.

morbid obesity, [L, *morbidus,* diseased, *obesitas,* fatness], an excess of body fat, or weight of 100 lb over ideal body weight, that increases the risk for developing cardiac and endocrine disturbances, including coronary artery disease, diabetes mellitus, and some kinds of cancer.

Morton's plantar neuralgia, [Thomas G. Morton; L, *planta,* foot sole; Gk, *neuron,* nerve, *algos,* pain], a severe throbbing pain that affects the anastomotic nerve branch between the medial and the lateral plantar nerves.

movement therapy, a movement-based therapeutic technique that aids in release of expressions or feelings and aids in promoting feeling and awareness.

music therapist, a health professional trained to use music within a therapeutic relationship to address a client's needs, such as facilitating movement and physical rehabilitation, motivating the client to cope with treatment, providing emotional support, and providing an outlet for expressing feelings. A baccalaureate or master's degree and clinical internship are required, after which an individual may take an examination to earn the credential music therapist board certified.

music therapy, [Gk, *mousike,* music, *therapeia,* treatment], a form of adjunctive psychotherapy in which music is used as a means of recreation and communication, especially with autistic children, and as a means to elevate the mood of depressed and psychotic patients. It is used to effect positive changes in the psychological, physical, cognitive, or social functioning of individuals with health or educational problems and used for a wide variety of indications, including mental disorders, developmental and learning disabilities, neurologic disabilities, and the management of pain or stress.

myalgia, /mī·al″jə/ [Gk, *mys,* muscle, *algos,* pain], diffuse muscle pain, usually accompanied by malaise. Also called myoneuralgia.

myalgic asthenia, /mī·al″jik/ [Gk, *mys* + *algos,* pain, *a* + *sthenos,* without strength], a condition characterized by a general feeling of fatigue and muscular pain, often resulting from or associated with psychological stress.

myoclonus, /mī′ōklō″nəs/ [Gk, *mys* muscle; + *klonos,* contraction], a spasm of a muscle or a group of muscles. – myoclonic, adj.

myofascial pain, jaw muscle distress associated with chewing or exercise of the masticatory muscles.

myofascial release, a set of massage techniques used to relieve muscle pain resulting from abnormally tight fascia.

myotherapy, /-ther″əpē/, a technique of corrective muscle exercises involving pressure on fingers and joints to relieve pain or spasms.

N

Narcotics Anonymous, an international nonprofit organization with the goal of assisting its members to live drug-free.

National Committee for Quality Assurance (NCQA), a U.S. independent nonprofit accrediting body for managed health care organizations. Its focus is on improving quality of care in the managed care industry by assessing compliance of health plans to NCQA-developed standards for quality improvement, utilization management, credentialing processes, member rights and responsibilities, preventive services, and record management.

National Institute of Mental Health (NIMH), 1. An institute of the U.S. National Institutes of Health whose mission is to provide national leadership in the understanding, treatment, and prevention of mental illnesses through basic research on the brain and behavior, and through clinical, epidemiologic, and services research. 2. A division of the Mental Health Commission of Canada that serves as a catalyst for improving the mental health system and changing the attitudes and behaviors of Canadians surrounding mental health issues. NIMH makes recommendations on how best to improve the systems that are directly related to mental health care.

National Institute of Nursing Research (NINR), an institute of the National Institutes of Health that supports clinical and basic research to establish a scientific basis for the care of individuals across the life span in a variety of ways.

National Institute on Alcohol Abuse and Alcoholism, an institute of the National Institutes of Health that conducts research focused on improving the treatment and prevention of alcoholism and alcohol-related problems.

National Institute on Drug Abuse (NIDA), an institute of the National Institutes of Health that seeks to bring the power of science to bear on drug abuse and addiction through support and conduct of research across a broad range of disciplines, with rapid and effective dissemination of results of the research.

National Institutes of Health (NIH), an agency of the U.S. Department of Health and Human Services made up of several institutions and constituent divisions, including the Bureau of Health Manpower Education, the National Library of Medicine, the National Cancer Institute, and several research institutes and divisions. The NIH is divided into two parts: One part is responsible for the funding of biomedical research outside the NIH, and the other conducts research.

naturopath, /nach″ərōpath′/, a person who practices naturopathy.

naturopathic medicine, a philosophy of medicine that presumes that there is an inherent healing power in nature and in every human being. This major health system includes practices that emphasize diet, nutrition, homeopathy, and various mind-body therapies. Emphasis is placed on self-healing, treatment through changes in lifestyle, and the use of prevention techniques that promote health. Currently, 17 states, the District of Columbia, and the U.S. territories of Puerto Rico and the U.S. Virgin Islands have licensing or regulation laws for naturopathic doctors. In Canada, two sets of provincial licensing board examinations exist.

naturopathy, /nach′ərop″əthē/ [L, *natura* + Gk, *pathos*, disease], a system of therapeutics based on natural foods, light, warmth, massage, fresh air, regular exercise, and the avoidance of medications. Advocates believe that illness can be healed by the natural processes of the body.

nerve accommodation, the ability of nerve tissue to adjust to a constant source and intensity of stimulation so that some change in either intensity or duration of the stimulus is necessary to elicit a response beyond the initial reaction. Accommodation is probably caused by reduced sodium ion permeability, which results in an increased threshold intensity and subsequent stabilization of the resting membrane potential.

nerve compression, a pathologic event that causes harmful pressure on one or more nerves, resulting in nerve damage and muscle weakness, atrophy, or paresthesias over time. Any nerve that passes over a rigid prominence is vulnerable, and the degree of damage depends on the magnitude and duration of the compressive force. Various factors may contribute to susceptibility, such as inherited predisposition, malnutrition, trauma, and disease. Various activities associated with routine occupations may unduly compress especially vulnerable nerves, such as the median nerve, radial nerve, femoral nerve, and plantar nerves. Rest and the cessation or modification of causative activities often heal nerve damage caused by compression. Surgery may be required to correct more severe cases.

nerve endings, the fine branchlike terminations of peripheral neurons. Sensory endings are effectively dendrites lying far from the neuronal cell body, and motor nerve endings are the endings of axons and are called motor endplates. *See also* neuron.

nerve entrapment, an abnormal condition and type of mononeuropathy characterized by nerve damage and muscle weakness or atrophy. The peripheral nerve trunks of the body are especially vulnerable to entrapment in which repeated compression results in significant impairment. Nerves that pass over rigid prominences or through narrow bony and fascial canals are particularly prone to entrapment. The common signs of this disorder are pain and muscular weakness. Nerve damage by entrapment occurs more often when adjacent joints are affected by swelling and inflammation, such as in rheumatoid arthritis, pregnancy, and acromegaly. Signs of nerve entrapment also may develop after repeated bruising of certain nerves by various activities involving repeated motions, such as those associated with knitting and prolonged walking. Kinds include carpal tunnel syndrome.

nerve excitability, [L, *nervus*, nerve, *excitare*, to rouse], the readiness of a nerve cell to respond to a stimulus.

nerve fiber, a slender process, the axon of a neuron. Each fiber is classified as myelinated or unmyelinated. Myelinated fibers are further designated as A or B fibers. C fibers are unmyelinated. The A fibers are somatic. A alpha fibers are large fibers and transport impulses at a velocity of 60 to 100 m/s. A beta fibers are smaller and transmit pressure and temperature impulses at a velocity of 30 to 70 m/s. A gamma fibers transmit touch and pressure impulses. A delta fibers are the smallest and transmit impulses associated with sharp pain sensation. B fibers are more finely myelinated than A fibers. They are both afferent and efferent and are mainly associated with visceral innervation. The unmyelinated C fibers are efferent postganglionic autonomic and afferent fibers that conduct impulses of prolonged, burning pain sensation from the viscera and periphery.

nerve growth factor (NGF), a protein whose hormone-like action affects differentiation, growth, and maintenance of neurons.

nerve plexus, [L, *nervus*, nerve, *plexus*, plaited], an interwoven network of nerves, such as the lumbar plexus formed by the anterior primary branch of the upper four lumbar nerves.

nerve root, the part of a nerve adjacent to the center to which it is connected.

nerve root impingement, the abnormal protrusion of body tissue into the space occupied by a spinal nerve root. Causes may include disc herniation, tissue prolapse, and inflammation.

nerve sheath, [L, *nervus,* nerve; AS, *scaeth*], any of several types of coatings or coverings for nerve fibers and nerve tracts. Kinds include endoneurial nerve sheath, medullary nerve sheath, myelin sheath, neurilemma.

neuralgia, /noǒral″jə/ [Gk, *neuron + algos,* pain], an abnormal condition characterized by severe stabbing pain, caused by a variety of disorders affecting the nervous system. – neuralgic, adj.

neuralgic amyotrophy, /noǒral″jik ā′mīot″rəfē/, a brachial plexus disorder characterized by sudden pain and muscle weakness in the upper limbs and sometimes by muscular wasting or atrophy. The cause is unknown. Also called Parsonage-Turner syndrome.

neuroelectric therapy, the use of a low-amperage electrical current to stimulate nerve endings. The action may stimulate endogenous neurotransmitters, such as endorphins that produce symptomatic relief. Kinds include transcutaneous electrical nerve stimulation (TENS).

neuron, /noǒr″on/ [Gk, *nerve*], the basic nerve cell of the nervous system, containing a nucleus within a cell body and extending one or more processes. Neurons can be classified according to the direction in which they conduct impulses or according to the number of processes they extend. Sensory neurons transmit nerve impulses toward the spinal cord and the brain. Motor neurons transmit nerve impulses from the brain and the spinal cord to the muscles and the glandular tissue. Multipolar neurons, bipolar neurons, and unipolar neurons are classified according to the number of processes they extend to the different kinds of neurons. Multipolar neurons have one axon and several dendrites, as do most of the neurons in the brain and the spinal cord. Bipolar neurons, which are less numerous than the other types, have one axon and only one dendrite. Unipolar neurons have one axon and no dendrites. All primary sensory afferents and some autonomic neurons are unipolar. All neurons have one axon, and most have one or more dendrites and have a slightly gray color when clustered, as in the nuclei of the brain and the spinal cord. As the generators and carriers of nerve impulses, neurons function according to electrochemical processes involving positively charged sodium and potassium ions and the changing electrical potential of the extracellular and the intracellular fluid of the neuron. Also spelled neurone. – neuronal, adj.

neuropathic pain, pain that results from direct stimulation of the myelin or nervous tissue of the peripheral or central nervous system (except for sensitized C fibers), generally felt as burning or tingling and often occurring in an area of sensory loss. It is seen commonly in patients with uncontrolled diabetes.

neuropathic pain syndrome, a condition of autonomic hyperactivity that results in sharp, stinging, or stabbing pain. The disorder is usually noninflammatory but may result in the destruction of peripheral nerve tissue. It also may be accompanied by changes in skin color, temperature, and edema.

neuropathy, /noǒrop″əthē/ [Gk, *neuron + pathos,* disease], inflammation or degeneration of the peripheral nerves, such as that associated with lead poisoning. – neuropathic, adj.

neurotransmitter, /-transmit″ər/ [Gk, *neuron + * L, *transmittere,* to transmit], a chemical that modifies or results in the transmission of nerve impulses between synapses. Neurotransmitters are released from synaptic knobs into synaptic clefts and bridge the gap between presynaptic and postsynaptic neurons. Each vesicle within a synaptic knob stores as many as 10,000 neurotransmitter molecules. When a nerve impulse reaches a synaptic knob, thousands of neurotransmitter molecules squirt into the synaptic cleft and bind to specific receptors. This flow allows an associated diffusion of potassium and sodium ions that causes an action potential. Excitatory neurotransmitters decrease the negativity of postsynaptic membrane potentials; inhibitory neurotransmitters increase such potentials. Kinds include acetylcholine, γ-aminobutyric acid, norepinephrine.

nitrous oxide (N_2O, NOx), /nī′trəs/, a colorless, odorless gas, first used as an anesthetic agent in 1844, is the least potent of currently used inhalation anesthetics. It provides analgesia but not complete amnesia or akinesia and is usually supplemented with other drugs. Because high concentrations of N_2O are required, hypoxia is a risk and supplemental oxygen is needed. N_2O is associated with an increased incidence of nausea and vomiting, environmental pollution, spontaneous abortion in health care workers exposed, and suspected teratogenicity. It has many contraindications to its use. Despite these shortcomings it remains in use in the United States because of its rapid onset and offset, relative lack of cardiac or respiratory depression, and its low cost. It is most often used to supplement other anesthetic agents, especially during an inhalation induction of children. N_2O remains a commonly administered dental anesthetic.

nociceptive, /nō′sēsep″tiv/ [L, *nocere,* to injure, *capere,* to receive], pertaining to a neural receptor for painful stimuli.

nociceptive reflex, [L, *nocere,* to injure, *capere,* to receive, *reflectere,* to bend back], a reflex caused by a painful stimulus.

nociceptive stimulus, [L, *nocere,* to injure, *capere,* to receive, *stimulus,* goad], a painful, sometimes detrimental or injurious, stimulus.

nociceptor, /nō′sēsep″tər/, a somatic and visceral free nerve ending of thinly myelinated and unmyelinated fibers. It usually reacts to tissue injury but also may be excited by endogenous chemical substances.

nonfeasance, /nonfē″zəns/ [L, *non* + *facere,* to do], a failure to perform a task, duty, or undertaking that one has agreed to perform or has a legal duty to perform.

norepinephrine (NE), /nôr′epinef″rin/, an adrenergic hormone (catecholamine) that acts to increase blood pressure by vasoconstriction but does not affect cardiac output. It is synthesized by the adrenal medulla, the peripheral sympathetic nerves, and the central nervous system. It is available as a drug, levarterenol, which is used to maintain the blood pressure in acute hypotension secondary to trauma, heart disease, or vascular collapse.

nutraceuticals, /noo″träsoo′tĭkalz/, 1. Functional foods. 2. Foods thought to have a beneficial effect on human health.

O

obese, /ōbēs″/ [L, *obesus,* swollen], pertaining to an excessive accumulation of body fat. A body mass index of 30.0 or greater indicates obesity.

obesity, /ōbē″sitē/ [L, *obesitas,* fatness], an abnormal increase in the proportion of fat cells, mainly in the viscera and subcutaneous tissues of the body. Obesity may be exogenous or endogenous. Hyperplastic obesity is caused by an increase in the number of fat cells in the increased adipose tissue mass. Hypertrophic obesity results from an increase in the size of the fat cells in the increased adipose tissue mass.

- *Observations:* Obesity is manifested as excess body weight for height. Overweight is determined by a body mass index (BMI) of 25 to 29.9 kg/m^2, and obesity is a BMI = 30 kg/m^2. Body fat distribution can be assessed by waist-to-hip ratios, with a ratio of greater than 1.0 for men and greater than 0.8 for women signaling increased risk for obesity. Morbidity and mortality are increased in the obese. Complications include predisposition to diabetes mellitus, hypertension, hyperlipidemia, coronary artery disease, cerebrovascular disease, osteoarthritis, sleep apnea, and certain cancers.

obstructive sleep apnea (OSA), a form of sleep apnea involving a physical obstruction in the upper airways, most commonly the glottis. Although often described as occurring mainly in obese patients, in fact it is also seen routinely in patients with a normal body mass index (BMI). It is also often associated with patients with secondary pulmonary insufficiency or a constitutional defect. A nonobese person with a congenital abnormality of the upper airways also may experience OSA.

omega-3 fatty acid, a fatty acid with a double bond located at the third carbon atom away from the omega (methyl) end of the molecule. Major sources are cold-water fish and vegetable oils. Omega-3 fatty acids, such as eicosapentaenoic acid and docosahexaenoic acid, appear to have protective functions in preventing the formation of blood clots and reducing the risk for coronary heart disease.

omega-6 fatty acid, an unsaturated fatty acid in which the double bond closest to the omega (methyl) end of the molecule occurs at the sixth carbon from that end. Major sources are vegetable and seed oils.

omega-9 fatty acid, a polyunsaturated fatty acid found in animal and vegetable fats

opiate, /ō″pē·it/ [Gk, *opion,* poppy juice], 1. A drug that contains opium, derivatives of opium, or any of several semisynthetic or synthetic drugs with opium-like activity. 2. *(Informal)* Any soporific or opioid drug. 3. Pertaining to a substance that causes sleep or relief of pain. Morphine and related opiates may produce unwanted side effects such as respiratory depression, nausea, vomiting, dizziness, and constipation. Patients with reduced blood volume are more susceptible to the hypotensive effect of morphine and related drugs. Opiates are used with extreme caution in obese patients and in those with head injuries, emphysema, or other problems associated with decreased respiratory function. Also called opioid.

opiate receptor, [Gk, *opion,* poppy juice; L, *recipere,* to receive], transmembrane proteins that bind to endogenous opioid neuropeptides and exogenous morphine and similar natural or synthetic compounds. The three major classes of these receptors are designated mu, kappa, and delta. Morphine preferentially stimulates mu receptors to produce analgesia, euphoria, respiratory depression, constipation, and pinpoint pupils. Some other drugs (e.g., butorphanol) can selectively block mu receptors while stimulating kappa receptors; this provides moderate to high pain relief with low abuse potential. Stimulation of delta receptors can also contribute to analgesia. The receptors are found in high concentrations in the dorsal horn of the spinal cord and in the brain regions involved with pain modulation or pain transmission (e.g., periaqueductal gray matter). Endogenous agonists at these receptors include endorphins, enkephalins, and dynorphins.

opioid, /ō″pē·oid/ [Gk, *opion,* poppy juice, *eidos,* form], strictly speaking, pertaining to natural and synthetic chemicals that have opium-like effects similar to morphine, though they are not derived from opium. Examples include endorphins or enkephalins produced by body tissues or synthetic methadone. Morphine and related drugs are often included in this category because the term narcotic has lost its original meaning.

opioid antagonist, a drug that blocks mu, kappa, or delta opioid receptors, used primarily in the treatment of opioid-induced mu receptor–mediated respiratory depression. The opioid antagonist naloxone is administered parenterally, whereas naltrexone is administered orally.

opioid receptor, any of a number of types of receptors for opiates and opioids. At least seven different types are postulated at different locations in the body, grouped into three major classes (delta, kappa, and mu) according to the specific substances they bind and to the specific physiologic effect or effects that binding causes or inhibits.

opium, /ō″pē·əm/ [Gk, *opion*, poppy juice], a milky exudate from the unripe capsules of *Papaver somniferum* and *Papaver album* yielding 9.5% or more of anhydrous morphine. It is an opioid analgesic, a hypnotic, and an astringent. Opium contains several alkaloids, including codeine, morphine, and papaverine.

organic headache, a headache caused by any of a wide variety of intracranial disorders, including sinus or ear infections, brain tumors, and subdural hematomas.

osteoarthritis, /os′tē·ō′ärthrī″tis/ [Gk, *osteon* + *arthron*, joint, *itis*, inflammation], a form of arthritis in which one or many joints undergo degenerative changes, including subchondral bony sclerosis, loss of articular cartilage, and proliferation of bone spurs (osteophytes) and cartilage in the joint. Inflammation of the synovial membrane of the joint is common late in the disease. Osteoarthritis is the most common form of arthritis. Its cause is unknown but may include chemical, mechanical, genetic, metabolic, and endocrine factors. Emotional stress often aggravates the condition. The disease usually begins with pain after exercise or use of the joint. Stiffness, tenderness to the touch, crepitus, and enlargement develop. Deformity, incomplete dislocation, and synovial effusion may eventually occur. Involvement of the hip, knee, or spine causes more disability than osteoarthritis of other areas.

outcome measure, a measure of the quality of medical care, the standard against which the end result of the intervention is assessed.

overweight, /-wāt/ [AS, *ofer* + *gewiht*, weight], 1. More than normal in body weight after adjustment for height, body build, and age, or 10% to 20% above the person's "desirable" body weight. 2. A body mass index between 25.0 and 29.9.

oxygen saturation, 1. The fraction of the hemoglobin molecules in a blood sample that are saturated with oxygen at a given partial pressure of oxygen. Normal saturation is 95% to 100%. 2. Percentage of hemoglobin-bound oxygen compared to total capacity of the hemoglobin.

P

pain, [L, *poena*, punishment], an unpleasant sensation caused by noxious stimulation of the sensory nerve endings. It is a subjective feeling and an individual response to the cause. Pain is a cardinal symptom of inflammation and is valuable in the diagnosis of many disorders and conditions. It may be mild or severe, chronic or acute, lancinating, burning, dull or sharp, precisely or poorly localized, or referred. The experience of pain is influenced by physical, mental, biochemical, psychological, physiologic, social, cultural, and emotional factors.

pain and suffering, (in law) an element in a claim for damages that allows recovery for the mental and physical pain, suffering, distress, and trauma that an individual has endured as a result of injury.

pain assessment, an evaluation of the reported pain and the factors that alleviate or exacerbate it, as well as the response to treatment of pain. Responses to pain vary widely among individuals, depending on many different physical and psychological factors, such as specific diseases and injuries and the health, pain threshold, fear, anxiety, and cultural background of the individual involved, as well as the way the person expresses pain experiences.

pain intervention, the attempt to relieve pain by various measures.

pain mechanism, the network that communicates unpleasant sensations and the perceptions of noxious stimuli throughout the body in association with physical disease and trauma involving tissue damage. The gate control theory of pain is an attempt to explain the role of the nervous system in the pain response. It states that pain signals that reach the nervous system excite a group of small neurons that form a "pain pool." When the total activity of these neurons reaches a minimum level, a theoretic gate opens and allows the pain signals to proceed to higher brain centers. The areas in which the gates operate are considered to be in the spinal cord dorsal horn and the brainstem. The pattern theory holds that the intensity of a stimulus evokes a specific pattern, which is interpreted by the brain as pain. This perception is the result of the intensity and frequency of stimulation of a nonspecific end organ. Some authorities think that bradykinin and histamine, two chemical substances produced by the body, cause pain. Recently discovered pain killers produced naturally by the body are the enkephalins and the endorphins. Some studies indicate that the enkephalins are 10 times as potent as morphine in reducing pain. It is known that after histamine and some other naturally occurring chemical substances are released in the body, pain sensations travel along fast-conducting and slow-conducting nerve fibers. These pain-transmitting neuropathways communicate the pain sensation to the dorsal root ganglia of the spinal cord and synapse with certain neurons in the posterior horns of the gray matter. The pain sensation is then transmitted to the reticular formation and the thalamus by neurons that form the anterolateral spinothalamic tract. It is then conveyed to various areas of the brain, such as the cortex and the hypothalamus, by synapses at the thalamus. The immediate reaction to pain is transmitted over the reflex arc by sensory fibers in the dorsal horn of the spinal cord and by synapsing motor neurons in the anterior horn. This anatomic pattern of sensory and motor neurons allows the individual to move quickly at the touch of some harmful stimulus, such as extreme heat or cold. Nerve impulses alerting the individual to move away from such stimuli are simultaneously sent along efferent nerve fibers from the brain. Also called gate theory of pain, pain pathway.

pain receptor, any one of the many free nerve endings throughout the body that warn of potentially harmful changes in the environment, such as excessive pressure or temperature. The free nerve endings constituting most of the pain receptors are located chiefly in the epidermis and in the epithelial covering of certain mucous membranes. They also appear in the stratified squamous epithelium of the cornea, in the root sheaths and the papillae of the hairs, and around the bodies of sudoriferous glands. The terminal ends of pain receptors consist of unmyelinated nerve fibers that often anastomose into small knobs between the epithelial cells. Any kind of stimulus, if it is intense enough, can stimulate the pain receptors in the skin and the mucosa, but only radical changes in pressure and certain chemicals can stimulate the pain receptors in the viscera. Referred pain results only from stimulation of pain receptors located in deep structures, such as the viscera, the joints, and the skeletal muscles and never from pain receptors in the skin.

pain threshold, the point at which a stimulus, usually one associated with pressure or temperature, activates pain receptors and produces a sensation of pain. Individuals with low pain thresholds experience pain much sooner and faster than those with higher thresholds; individuals' reactions to stimulation of pain receptors vary.

palliate, /pal″ē·āt/ [L, *palliare,* to cloak], to soothe or relieve. – palliative, adj., – palliation, n.

palliative treatment, /pal″ē·ətiv′/ [L, *palliare,* to cloak, *tractare,* to handle], therapy designed to relieve or reduce intensity of uncomfortable symptoms but not to produce a cure. Some kinds of palliative treatment are the use of opioids to relieve pain in a patient with advanced cancer, the creation of a colostomy to bypass an inoperable obstructing lesion of the bowel, and the debridement of necrotic tissue in a patient with metastatic malignancy.

paracervical block, a form of regional anesthesia in which a local anesthetic is injected into each side of the uterine cervix to block nerves innervating the uterine cervix. Paracervical block is not the anesthesia of choice for labor and delivery, given the high incidence of fetal bradycardia and its efficacy in only the first stage of labor, but it is an option during abortion and other gynecologic procedures.

parasympathetic, /-sim′pəthet″ik/ [Gk, *para + sympathein,* to feel with], pertaining to the craniosacral division of the autonomic nervous system, consisting of the oculomotor, facial, glossopharyngeal, vagus, and pelvic nerves. The actions of the parasympathetic division are mediated by the release of acetylcholine and primarily involve the protection, conservation, and restoration of body resources. Preganglionic parasympathetic fibers, which emerge from the hypothalamus, other brain areas, and sacral segments of the spinal cord, form synapses in ganglia located near or in the walls of the organs to be innervated. Reactions to parasympathetic stimulation are highly localized and tend to counteract the adrenergic effects of sympathetic nerves. Parasympathetic secretion of lacrimal, salivary, and digestive glands; induce bile and insulin release; dilate peripheral and visceral blood vessels; constrict the pupils, esophagus, and bronchioles; and relax sphincters during micturition and defecation. Postganglionic parasympathetic fibers extend to the uterus, vagina, oviducts, and ovaries in females and to the prostate, seminal vesicles, and external genitalia in males, innervating blood vessels of pelvic organs in both sexes; stimulation of these nerves causes vasodilation in the clitoris and labia minora and erection of the penis.

parasympathetic ganglion, [Gk, *para + sympathein,* to feel with, *ganglion,* knot], a cluster of nerve cell bodies of the parasympathetic division of the autonomic nervous system. The nerves are functionally antagonistic to those of the sympathetic division.

parasympathetic nervous system, *See* autonomic nervous system.

paravertebral block, [Gk, *para + L, vertebra + OFr, bloc*], 1. The blocking of transmission of somatic impulses by the spinal nerves by injection of a local analgesic solution near the point of their emergence. 2. The blocking of the paravertebral sympathetic chain of nerves anterolateral to the vertebral bodies.

patient-controlled analgesia (PCA), a drug-delivery system that dispenses a preset intravascular dose of an opioid analgesic when the patient pushes a switch on an electric cord. The device consists of a computerized pump with a chamber containing the drug. The patient administers a dose of opioid intravenously when the need for pain relief arises. A lockout interval automatically inactivates the system if a patient tries to increase the amount of opioid within a preset period.

perception, /pərsep″shən/ [L, *percipere,* to perceive], 1. The conscious recognition and interpretation of sensory stimuli that serve as a basis for understanding, learning, and knowing or for motivating a particular action or reaction. 2. The result or product of the act of perceiving. Kinds include depth perception, extrasensory perception, facial perception, stereognostic perception. – perceptual, perceptive, adj.

percutaneous absorption, the process of absorption through the skin from topical application.

percutaneous catheter, a catheter inserted through the skin rather than through an orifice, such as a central venous catheter or one used for hemodialysis or peritoneal dialysis

percutaneous catheter placement, a technique in which an intracatheter is introduced through the skin into an artery and placed at a site or structure to be studied by using selective angiography and other diagnostic procedures. The puncture site is infiltrated with a local anesthetic before insertion of the catheter. A special needle is inserted into the artery, and a long, flexible spring guide is passed through the needle for approximately 15 cm. The needle is then removed, the catheter is advanced to the desired position, and the guide is withdrawn. The catheter is withdrawn at the end of the procedure.

pétrissage, /pā′trisäzh″/ [Fr, *petrir,* to knead], a technique in massage in which the skin is gently lifted and squeezed. Pétrissage promotes circulation and relaxes muscles.

phantom limb syndrome, a phenomenon common after amputation of a limb in which sensation or discomfort is experienced in the missing limb. In some people severe pain persists. *See also* pseudesthesia.

pharmacodynamics, /-dīnam′iks/ [Gk, *pharmakon,* drug, *dynamis,* power], the study of how a drug acts on a living organism, including the pharmacologic response and the duration and magnitude of response observed relative to the concentration of the drug at an active site in the organism.

pharmacogenetics, /-jənet″iks/ [Gk, *pharmakon,* drug, *genesis,* origin], the study of the effect of the genetic factors belonging to a group or to an individual on the response of the group or the individual to certain drugs.

pharmacokinetics, /fär′məkōkinet″iks/ [Gk, *pharmakon + kinesis,* motion], the study of the action of drugs within the body, which can, in many respects, be envisioned more accurately as the actions of the body on an administered drug. It includes studies of the mechanisms of drug absorption, distribution, metabolism, and excretion; onset of action; duration of effect; biotransformation; and effects and routes of excretion of the metabolites of the drug.

Pilates method, a gentle but focused exercise-based system that tones, stretches, and strengthens the body in a nonimpact, balanced system of body-mind exercise and mobilizes the body to move with maximum efficiency and minimum effort. Classes include mat work and use of equipment designed to provide resistance against tensioned springs to isolate and develop specific muscle groups. This method can achieve an improvement of body alignment and breathing, increased body awareness, and efficient and graceful movement.

polymyalgia rheumatica, /-mī·al′jə/ [Gk, *polys + mys,* muscle, *algos,* pain, *rheuma,* flux], a chronic, episodic inflammatory disease of the large arteries that usually develops in people over 60 years of age. The disease primarily affects the arteries in muscles. It is characterized by pain and stiffness of the back, shoulder, or neck that is usually more severe on rising in the morning. There also may be a cranial headache, which affects the temporal and occipital arteries, causing a severe throbbing headache. Serious complications of polymyalgia rheumatica include arterial insufficiency, coronary occlusion, stroke, and blindness. Patients with the disease usually have a high erythrocyte sedimentation rate. The disease may follow a self-limited course. However, adrenocorticosteroids have proved highly effective in reducing inflammation and in speeding recovery.

polymyositis, /pol′ēmī′ōsī″tis/ [Gk, *polys + mys,* muscle, *itis*], inflammation of many muscles, usually accompanied by deformity, edema, insomnia, pain, sweating, and tension. Some forms of polymyositis are associated with malignancy.

polyneuralgia, /-noŏral′jə/ [Gk, *polys,* many, *neuron,* nerve, *algos,* pain], a type of neuralgia that affects several nerves at the same time.

polyneuritis, /-noŏrī′tis/ [Gk, *polys,* many, *neuron,* nerve, *itis,* inflammation], an inflammation involving many nerves.

polyneuropathy, /-noŏrop′əthē/ [Gk, *polys,* many, *neuron,* nerve, *pathos,* disease], a condition in which many peripheral nerves are afflicted with a disorder.

polypharmacy, /-fär′məsē/, the use of a number of different drugs, possibly prescribed by different health care providers and filled in different pharmacies, by a patient who may have one or several health problems.

posthypnotic suggestion, /-hipnot″ik/ [L, *post,* after; Gk, *hypnos,* sleep; L, *suggerere,* to suggest], an action suggested to a hypnotized subject during a trance that the subject carries out on awakening from the trance. The action is in response to a cue, and the subject usually does not know why he or she is performing it.

practice guideline, a detailed description of a process of patient care management that will facilitate improvement or maintenance of health status or slow the decline in health status in certain chronic clinical conditions. The purpose of a practice guideline is to assist health care providers to identify preferred treatment by providing links among diagnoses, treatments, and outcomes and by describing alternatives available for each patient. Practice guidelines provide a basis for evaluation of care and allocation of resources.

preganglionic neuron, /-gang′glē·on″·ik/ [L, *prae* + Gk, *gagglion,* knot, *neurom,* nerve], a neuron whose axon terminates in contact with another nerve cell located in a peripheral ganglion.

presence, /prez′əns/, a mode of being available in a situation with the wholeness of one's individual being; a gift of self that can be given freely, invoked, or evoked.

prevertebral ganglia, collections of postganglionic sympathetic neuronal cell bodies in recognizable aggregations along the abdominal prevertebral plexus. They include the celiac, superior mesenteric, aorticorenal, and inferior mesenteric ganglia and play a critical role in innervations of the abdominal viscera.

prn, p.r.n., (in prescriptions) a notation for a Latin phrase meaning "as needed." The administration times are determined by the patient's needs. Abbreviation for pro re nata.

probiotics, microorganisms present in food or supplements that confer health benefits.

progressive assistive exercise, an exercise designed to improve the strength of a muscle group progressively by gradually decreasing assistance required of a therapist for an active motion, thereby increasing the patient's active effort. *See also* progressive resistance exercise.

progressive relaxation, a technique for combating tension and anxiety by systematically tensing and relaxing muscle groups.

progressive resistance exercise (PRE), a method of increasing the strength of a weak or injured muscle by gradually increasing the resistance against which the muscle works, such as by using graduated weights. Also called graduated resistance exercise. *See also* progressive assistive exercise.

proprietary, /-prī′əter′ē/ [L, *proprietas*, property], 1. Pertaining to an institution or other organization that is operated for profit. 2. pertaining to a product, such as a drug or device, that is made for profit.

proprietary medicine, any pharmaceutic preparation or medicinal substance that is protected from commercial competition because its ingredients or method of manufacture is kept secret or is protected by trademark or copyright.

proprioception, /prō′prē·əsep″shən/ [L, *proprius*, one's own, *capere*, to take], sensation pertaining to stimuli originating from within the body related to spatial position and muscular activity or to the sensory receptors that they activate.

prospective study, an analytic study designed to determine the relationship between a condition and a characteristic shared by some members of a group. The population selected is healthy at the beginning of the study. Some of the members of the group share a particular characteristic, such as cigarette smoking. The researcher follows the population group over a period of time, noting the rate at which a condition, such as lung cancer, occurs in the smokers and in the nonsmokers. A prospective study may involve many variables or only two; it may seek to demonstrate a relationship that is an association or one that is causal. Prospective studies produce a direct measure of risk called the relative risk.

pseudesthesia, /soo′desthē″zhə/ [Gk, *pseudes*, false, *aisthesis*, feeling], a sensation experienced without an external stimulus or a sensation that does not correspond to the causative stimulus, such as phantom limb pain occurring after an amputation.

psoas major, /sō″əs/ [Gk, *psoa*, loin], a long muscle originating from the transverse processes of the lumbar vertebrae and the fibrocartilages and sides of the vertebral bodies of the lower thoracic vertebrae and the lumbar vertebrae. It joins the iliacus to form the iliopsoas deep in the pelvis as it passes under the inguinal ligament and inserts in the lesser trochanter. It acts to flex and rotate the thigh and to flex and laterally bend the spine.

psoas minor, a long, slender muscle of the pelvis, ventral to the psoas major. Many individuals do not have this muscle. The psoas minor functions to flex the spine.

psoas part of iliopsoas fascia, the part of the fascia that invests the psoas major muscle.

psoriatic arthritis, /sôr′e·at″ik/, a form of arthritis associated with psoriatic lesions of the skin and nails, particularly at the distal interphalangeal joints of the fingers and toes.

- *Observations:* Stiffness and swelling, as well as joint pain, are the main symptoms of psoriatic arthritis. The health care team should emphasize the importance of joint protection, maintenance of a healthy weight, and appropriate exercise. The control of stress is also an important intervention. .
- *Patient care considerations:* Psoriatic arthritis can occur in people without psoriatic skin lesions. Activity is important, and the medications used to control symptoms can cause fatigue. The patient should be encouraged to remain active.

psychogenic pain, [Gk, *psyche*, mind; L, *poena*, penalty], a functional pain that does not have any known organic cause.

psychotherapist, /-ther″əpist/, one who practices psychotherapy, including psychiatrists, licensed psychologists, psychiatric nurses, psychiatric social workers, and individuals trained in counseling. The specific requirements for education and training differ markedly in content, breadth, and duration, depending on the form of psychotherapy practiced. Licensing procedures and definitions of practice vary from state to state.

psychotherapy, /-ther″əpē/ [Gk, *psyche* + *therapeia*, treatment], any of a large number of related methods of treating mental and emotional disorders by psychological techniques rather than by physical means.

pudendal, /pu-den′dal/, pertaining to or supplying the pudendum, such as pudendal nerves or a pudendal block.

pudendal block, /p(y)ooden″təl/ [L, *pudendus*, shameful; Fr, *bloc*, lump], a form of regional anesthetic block administered to provide anesthesia of the perineum, which is particularly useful during the expulsive second stage of labor. The pudendal nerves are anesthetized by the injection of a local anesthetic near the trunk of each nerve as it passes over the sacrospinous ligament, just below the ischial spine. A 10-mL syringe, a long needle, and a guide are used in the procedure. The injection is most easily performed transvaginally. Pudendal block anesthetizes the perineum, vulva, and perirectal area without affecting the muscular contractions of the uterus. When the block is properly administered, the risk is minimal. Today's obstetric anesthesia is most often epidural analgesia.

purposeful activity, /pur″pəsfoŏl/, activity that depends on consciously planned and directed involvement of the person. It is thought that conscious involvement in body movements enhances the development of sensorimotor control and coordination during therapeutic or rehabilitative exercises.

P value, (in research) the statistical probability of the occurrence of a given finding by chance alone in comparison with the known distribution of possible findings, considering the kinds of data, the technique of analysis, and the number of observations. The *P* value may be noted as a decimal: $P < .01$ means that the likelihood that the phenomena tested occurred by chance alone is less than 1%. The lower the *P* value, the less likely the finding would occur by chance alone.

Q

Qi, /chē/, in traditional Chinese medicine, the vital energy of the human body.

quality, /kwol″itē/ [L, *qualis*], 1. A descriptive specification of the penetrating nature of an x-ray beam. It is influenced by kilovoltage and filtration: a higher kilovoltage produces more penetration, and filtration removes selected wavelengths and "hardens" the beam. 2. (in speech therapy) Refers to the nature of phonation produced by the vocal folds. Disorders of voice quality include hoarseness, harshness, breathiness, and glottal fry.

quality assessment measures, formal systematic organizational evaluation of overall patterns or programs of care, including clinical, consumer, and systems evaluation.

quality assurance, (for health or related reasons) a pledge to the public by those within the various health disciplines that they will work toward the goal of an optimally achievable degree of excellence in the services rendered to every patient. *See also* quality management.

- *Method:* A quality assurance program takes into account the need to define that which is to be measured. Quality assurance implies a clear understanding of what is meant by quality and a valid and reliable method for evaluating the care that is provided. Implementation of a quality assurance program involves the development of criteria based on acceptable standards of care and norms of professional behavior. The norms are established by members of the profession or professions who are expert in the care of a specific patient population. Evaluation is conducted by a review committee and may be retrospective or concurrent.

- *Patient care considerations:* The ultimate goal of both retrospective and concurrent review is improvement of patient care. Individual members of the health care team hold themselves accountable to the public and patient for the caliber of care they provide.

- *Outcome criteria:* Outcome represents a measurable change in the health/illness status of the patient that is the end result of the care the patient received. *Cost/benefit* refers to the expenditure of money, time, and effort in providing health care and the relationship this cost bears to the actual benefits to the recipient of care. It is the promise to evaluate outcomes thoroughly and employ the results of the evaluation for continuous improvement of patient care that is the essence of quality assurance.

quality of life, [L, *qualis,* what kind; AS, *lif*], a measure of the optimum energy or force that endows a person with the power to cope successfully with the full range of challenges encountered in the real world. The term applies to all individuals, regardless of illness or disability, on the job, at home, or in leisure activities. Quality enrichment methods can include activities that reduce boredom and allow a maximum amount of freedom in choosing and performing various tasks. Although assessment tools are available to evaluate physical and social dimensions of quality of life, an individual's general sense of well-being or satisfaction with the attributes of life is often more difficult to evaluate.

quintessence, /kwintes″əns/ [L, *quinta + essentia,* the fifth essence], 1. A highly concentrated extract of any substance. 2. A tincture or extract containing the most essential components of plant materials.

R

radiculitis, /rədik′yəlī″tis/ [L, *radix,* root; Gk, *itis,* inflammation], an inflammation involving a spinal nerve root, resulting in pain and hyperesthesia.

radiculopathy, /rədik′yəlop″əthē/ [L, *radix,* root; Gk, *pathos,* disease], a disease involving a spinal nerve root.

range-of-motion exercise, [OFr, *ranger,* to arrange in a row; L, *motio,* movement], any body action involving the adduction, extension, flexion, pronation, supination, and rotation. Such exercises are usually applied actively or passively in the prevention and treatment of orthopedic deformities, in the assessment of injuries and deformities, and in athletic conditioning. They are important for joint mobility.

rational emotive behavior therapy, (in psychotherapy) a cognitive-behavioral therapy based on the premise that people's beliefs strongly affect their emotional functioning and that the beliefs can be modified to allow individuals to lead happy and productive lives.

referred pain, /rifurd″/ [L, *referre + poena,* punishment], pain felt at a site different from that of an injured or diseased organ or body part. For example, angina, the pain of coronary artery insufficiency, may be felt in the left shoulder, arm, or jaw.

reflexology, /rē′fleksol″əjē/, an alternative medicine technique that uses reflex points on the hands and feet. Pressure is applied at points that correspond to various body parts with the intention of eliminating blockages thought to produce pain or disease. The goal is to bring the body into balance.

reframing, /rēfrā″ming/, changing the conceptual and/or emotional viewpoint in relation to which a situation is experienced and placing it in a different frame that fits the "facts" of a concrete situation equally well, thereby changing its entire meaning.

regional anesthesia, 1. Anesthesia provided by injecting a local anesthetic to block a group of sensory nerve fibers. The tissues are anesthetized layer by layer, as the surgeon approaches the deeper structures of the body. Regional anesthesia has largely replaced local anesthesia for major procedures. Kinds include Bier block, brachial plexus anesthesia, caudal anesthesia, conduction anesthesia, epidural anesthesia/analgesia, paracervical block, pudendal block, spinal anesthesia. *See also* anesthesia. 2. (in dentistry) The loss of sensation to pain, temperature, and pressure of a tooth, teeth, jaw, and soft tissue caused by deposit of a local anesthetic agent in close proximity to a nerve or nerves. Kinds include posterior superior alveolar block, middle superior alveolar block, anterior superior alveolar block.

reiki, /ra'ke/, an Eastern healing tradition whose purpose is to rebalance the complex energy systems that compose the body when they have become out of balance. In this tradition, people are considered to be surrounded by an unlimited universal energy source from which the physical universe is built. The energy systems in the healthy body are in balance, but they can be disrupted by stress, and this unbalancing may have physical manifestations such as pain. The reiki practitioner is trained to channel energy from the universal energy source, which flows through his or her hands to the body of the receiver. The result is the rebalancing of mind and body, the strengthening of body and spirit, the opening of energy blockages, the creation of a sense of well-being, and the healing of illnesses.

reinforcement-extinction, (in psychology) a process of socialization in which one learns to engage in certain behaviors (reinforcement) or to avoid certain behaviors (extinction). The anticipated result is that the reinforced behaviors become habitual and those that undergo extinction disappear.

relative risk, the ratio of the chance of a disease developing among members of a population exposed to a factor compared with a similar population not exposed to the factor. In many cases the relative risk is modified by the duration or intensity of exposure to the causative factors.

relax, /rilaks"/ [L, *relaxare,* to ease], to reduce tension or anxiety.

relaxation, /rē'laksā"shən/ [L, *relaxare,* to ease], 1. A reducing of tension, as when a muscle relaxes between. 2. (in magnetic resonance imaging) The return of excited nuclei to their normal unexcited state by the release of energy.

relaxation response, a protective mechanism against stress that brings about decreased heart rate, lower metabolism, and decreased respiratory rate. It is the physiologic opposite of the "fight or flight," or stress, response.

reliability, /rilī'əbil"itē/ [L, *religare,* to fasten behind], (in research) the extent to which a test measurement or device produces the same results with different investigators, observers, or administration of the test over time. If repeated use of the same measurement

tool on the same sample produces the same consistent results, the measurement is considered reliable.

religiosity, /rilij'ē·os"itē/ [L, *religiosus*], a psychiatric symptom characterized by the demonstration of excessive or affected piety.

REM, /rem, är"ē'em"/, a dream state. Abbreviation for rapid eye movement.

replication, rep'likā"shən/ [L, *replicare,* to fold back], 1. A process of duplicating, reproducing, or copying; literally, a folding back of a part to form a duplicate. 2. (in research) The exact repetition of an experiment, performed to confirm the initial findings. 3. (in genetics) The duplication of the polynucleotide strands of DNA or the synthesis of DNA. The process involves the unwinding of the double helix molecule to form two single strands, each of which acts as a template for the synthesis of a complementary strand. The two resulting molecules of DNA each contain one new and one parental strand, which coil to form the double helix. – replicate, v.

respiratory acidosis, an abnormal condition characterized by a low plasma pH resulting from reduced alveolar ventilation. The hypoventilation inhibits the excretion of carbon dioxide, which consequently combines with water in the body to produce carbonic acid, thus reducing plasma pH. Respiratory acidosis can result from disorders such as airway obstruction, medullary trauma, neuromuscular disease, chest injury, pneumonia, pulmonary edema, emphysema, and cardiopulmonary arrest. It also may be caused by the suppression of respiratory reflexes with opioids, sedatives, hypnotics, or anesthetics. Also called carbon dioxide acidosis.

- *Observations:* Some common signs and symptoms of respiratory acidosis are headache, dyspnea, fine tremors, tachycardia, hypertension, and vasodilation. Confirming diagnosis is usually based on a $PaCO_2$ over the normal 45 mm Hg and an arterial pH below 7.35.

respiratory alkalosis, an abnormal condition characterized by a high plasma pH resulting from increased alveolar ventilation. The consequent acceleration of carbon dioxide excretion lowers the plasma level of carbonic acid, thus raising plasma pH. The hyperventilation may be caused by pulmonary and nonpulmonary problems. Some pulmonary causes are acute asthma, pulmonary vascular disease, and pneumonia. Some nonpulmonary causes are aspirin toxicity, anxiety, fever, metabolic acidosis, inflammation of the central nervous system, gram-negative septicemia, and hepatic failure.

- *Observations:* Deep and rapid breathing at rates as high as 40 breaths/min is a major sign of respiratory alkalosis. Other symptoms are light-headedness, dizziness, peripheral paresthesia, tingling of the hands and feet, muscle weakness, tetany, and cardiac arrhythmia. Confirming diagnosis is often based on a $PaCO_2$ below 35 mm Hg and a pH greater than

7.45. PaO$_2$ may be higher than 100. In the acute stage, blood pH rises in proportion to the fall in PaCO$_2$, but in the chronic stage it remains within the normal range of 7.35 to 7.45. The carbonic acid concentration is normal in the acute stage of this condition but below normal in the chronic stage.

respiratory depression, [L, *respirare,* to breathe, *depremere,* to press down], respiration that has a rate below 12 breaths/min or that fails to provide full ventilation and perfusion of the lungs. Also called respiratory insufficiency.

respiratory failure, the inability of the cardiovascular and pulmonary systems to maintain an adequate exchange of oxygen and carbon dioxide in the lungs. Respiratory failure may be caused by a failure in oxygenation or ventilation. Oxygenation failure is characterized by refractory hypoxemia and occurs in diseases that affect the alveoli or interstitial tissues of the lungs, such as alveolar edema, emphysema, fungal infections, leukemia, lobar pneumonia, lung carcinoma, various pneumoconioses, pulmonary eosinophilia, sarcoidosis, or tuberculosis. Ventilatory failure, characterized by increased arterial tension of carbon dioxide, occurs in acute conditions in which retained pulmonary secretions cause increased airway resistance and decreased lung compliance, as in bronchitis. Ventilation may also be reduced by depression of the respiratory center by barbiturates or opiates, hypoxia, hypercapnia, intracranial diseases, trauma, or lesions of the neuromuscular system or thoracic cage.

respiratory rhythm, a regular, oscillating cycle of inspiration and expiration, controlled by neuronal impulses transmitted between the respiratory centers in the brain and the muscles of inspiration in the chest and diaphragm. The normal breathing pattern may be altered by a variety of conditions.

rheumatoid arthritis (RA), [Gk, *rheuma,* flux, *eidos,* form, *arthron,* joint, *itis,* inflammation], a chronic, inflammatory, destructive, and sometimes deforming collagen disease that has an autoimmune component. It is characterized by symmetric inflammation of synovial membranes and increased synovial exudate, leading to thickening of the membranes and swelling of the joints. Rheumatoid arthritis usually first appears when patients, most often women, are between 36 and 50 years of age. The course of the disease is variable but is most frequently marked by alternating periods of remission and exacerbation.

rhizotomy, /rīzot″əmē/, the surgical resection of the dorsal root of a spinal nerve, performed to relieve pain and sometimes to decrease spasms.

rolling effleurage, a circular rubbing stroke used in massage to promote circulation and muscle relaxation, especially on the shoulder and buttocks. It is performed with the hand flat, the palm and closely held fingers acting as a unit.

S

salicylate, /səlis″əlāt/ [Gk, *salix,* willow, *hyle,* matter], any of several widely prescribed drugs derived from salicylic acid. Salicylates exert analgesic, antipyretic, and antiinflammatory actions. The most important is acetylsalicylic acid, or aspirin. Sodium salicylate also has been used systemically, and it exerts similar effects. Many of the actions of aspirin appear to result from its ability to inhibit cyclooxygenase, a rate-limiting enzyme in prostaglandin biosynthesis. Aspirin is used in a wide variety of conditions, and, in the usual analgesic dosage, it causes only mild adverse effects. Severe occult gastrointestinal (GI) bleeding or gastric ulcers may occur with frequent use. Large doses taken over a long period can cause significant impairment of hemostasis. Occasionally an asthma-like reaction is produced in hypersensitive individuals. Because of the ready availability of aspirin, accidental and intentional overdosage is common. Symptoms of salicylate intoxication include tinnitus, GI disturbances, abnormal respiration, acid-base imbalance, and central nervous system disturbances. Fatalities have resulted from ingestion of as little as 10 grains of aspirin in adults or as little as 4 mL of methyl salicylate (oil of wintergreen) in children. In addition to aspirin and sodium salicylate, which are used systemically, methyl salicylate is used topically as a counter-irritant in ointments and liniments. Methyl salicylate can be absorbed through the skin in amounts capable of causing systemic toxicity. Another salicylate, salicylic acid, is too irritating to be used systemically and is used topically as a keratolytic agent, for example, for removing warts.

Schedule I, a category of drugs not considered legitimate for medical use. Among the substances so classified by the Drug Enforcement Agency are mescaline, lysergic acid diethylamide, heroin, and marijuana. Special licensing procedures must be followed to use these or other Schedule I substances.

Schedule II, a category of drugs considered to have a strong potential for abuse or addiction but that have legitimate medical use. Among the substances so classified by the Drug Enforcement Agency are morphine, cocaine, pentobarbital, oxycodone, alphaprodine, and methadone.

Schedule III, a category of drugs that have less potential for abuse or addiction than Schedule II or I drugs. Among the substances so classified by the Drug Enforcement Agency are glutethimide and various analgesic compounds containing codeine.

Schedule IV, a category of drugs that have less potential for abuse or addiction than those of Schedules I to III. Among the substances so classified by the Drug Enforcement Agency are chloral hydrate, chlordiazepoxide, meprobamate, and oxazepam.

Schedule V, a category of drugs that have a small potential for abuse or addiction. Among the substances so classified by the Drug Enforcement Agency are many commonly prescribed medications that contain small amounts of codeine or diphenoxylate. The specific drugs in Schedule V vary greatly from state to state.

sciatica, /sī·at″ikə/, an inflammation of the sciatic nerve, usually marked by pain and tenderness along the course of the nerve through the thigh and leg. It may result in a wasting of the muscles of the lower leg over time. Also called sciatic neuritis.

sciatic nerve, a long nerve originating in the sacral plexus and extending through the muscles of the thigh, leg, and foot, with numerous branches.

Science of Unitary Human Beings, a conceptual model and theory of nursing proposed by Martha Rogers in 1970. Its four basic concepts focus on the nature and direction of "unitary human development": (1) human and environmental energy fields, (2) complete and continuous openness of the energy fields, (3) human energy fields perceived as single waves that give identity to a field, and (4) "pandimensionality," a nonlinear domain without spatial or temporal attributes.

selective serotonin reuptake inhibitor (SSRI), an antidepressant drug that blocks reuptake of serotonin without blocking reuptake of other biogenic amines such as norepinephrine and dopamine. Advantages over tricyclic antidepressant drugs include fewer anticholinergic side effects (dry mouth, blurred vision, urinary retention) and fewer antihistaminic side effects (sedation, weight gain).

self-advocacy, the process of representing oneself, including making one's own decisions about life, developing a network of support, knowing one's rights and responsibilities, reaching out to others when in need of assistance, mastering self-determination, and learning how to obtain information to gain an understanding about issues of personal interest or importance.

self-anesthesia, self-administered inhalation anesthesia in which whiffs of anesthetic gas are inhaled from a hand-held breathing device controlled by the patient. This form of anesthesia is most common in England.

self-regulation, a plan for patients to eliminate health risk behaviors. It includes self-monitoring, self-evaluation, and self-reinforcement.

self-reinforcing adaptation, (in occupational therapy) a therapeutic technique in which each successful stage of adjustment stimulates the next, more complex step.

sensation, /sensā″shən/ [L, *sentire,* to feel], 1. A feeling, impression, or awareness of a body state or condition that results from the stimulation of a sensory receptor site and transmission of the nerve impulse along an afferent fiber to the brain. Kinds include delayed sensation, epigastric sensation, primary sensation, referred sensation, subjective sensation. 2. A feeling or an awareness of a mental or emotional state, which may or may not result in response to an external stimulus.

sensory integration, the organization of sensory input for use, a perception of the body or environment, an adaptive response, a learning process, or the development of some neural function.

sensory modulation, interpreting and filtering sensory information.

sensory nerve, a nerve consisting of afferent fibers that conduct sensory impulses from the periphery of the body to the brain or spinal cord via the dorsal spinal roots.

sensory neuropathy, neuropathy or polyneuropathy of sensory nerves.

sensory nucleus of trigeminal nerve, a collection of nerve cells in the pons that serves as the main nucleus for reception of tactile fibers of the trigeminal area.

sensory pathway, [L, *sentire,* to feel; AS, *paeth* + *weg*], the route followed by a sensory nerve impulse from an end organ to a reflex center in the brain or spinal cord.

sensory processing, means by which the brain receives, detects, and integrates incoming sensory information for use in producing adaptive responses to one's environment.

sensory receptor, [L, *sentire,* to feel, *recipere,* to receive], a specialized nerve ending that, when stimulated, initiates an afferent or sensory nerve impulse.

serotonin, /ser′ətō″nin, sir′-/ [L, *serum* + Gk, *tonos,* tone], a naturally occurring derivative of tryptophan found in platelets and in cells of the brain and the intestine. Serotonin is released from platelets on damage to the blood vessel walls. It acts as a potent vasoconstrictor. Serotonin in intestinal tissue stimulates the smooth muscle to contract. In the central nervous system, it acts as a neurotransmitter. Lysergic acid diethylamide interferes with the action of serotonin in the brain. The normal concentration of serotonin in the urine is 0.05 to 0.2 µg/mL. Also called 5-hydroxytryptamine.

shared governance, an organizational framework proposed by Tim Porter-O'Grady that provides for the full use of nursing resources. This system is designed to reflect the professional character of the participants in the nursing organization and to promote certain positive behaviors and practices. The purpose of shared governance is the establishment of a system in which staff participate fully in all activities that have an impact on their work and their ultimate goal of meaningful patient care.

Shiatsu, a Japanese form of acupressure involving finger pressure at specific points on the body, mainly for the purpose of balancing energy in the body.

sickle cell crisis, an acute episodic condition that occurs in children with sickle cell anemia. The crisis may be vasoocclusive, resulting from the aggregation of misshapen erythrocytes, or anemic, resulting from bone marrow aplasia, increased hemolysis, folate deficiency, or splenic sequestration of erythrocytes.

- *Observations:* Painful vasoocclusive crisis is the most common of the sickle cell crises. It is usually preceded by an upper respiratory or gastrointestinal infection without an exacerbation of anemia. The clumps of sickled erythrocytes obstruct blood vessels, resulting in occlusion, ischemia, and infarction of adjacent tissue. Characteristics of this kind of crisis are leukocytosis; acute abdominal pain from visceral hypoxia; painful swelling of the soft tissue of the hands and feet (hand-foot syndrome); and migratory, recurrent, or constant joint pain, often so severe that movement of the joint is limited. Persistent headache, dizziness, convulsions, visual or auditory disturbances, facial nerve palsies, coughing, shortness of breath, and tachypnea may occur if the central nervous system or lungs are affected.

side effect, [AS, *side* + L, *effectus*], any reaction to or consequence of a medication or therapy. This can be an effect carried beyond the desired limit, such as hemorrhaging from an anticoagulant, or a reaction unrelated to the primary object of the therapy, such as an anaphylactic reaction to an antibiotic. Usually, although not necessarily, the effect is undesirable and may manifest itself as nausea, dry mouth, dizziness, blood dyscrasias, blurred vision, discolored urine, or tinnitus.

sign, /sīn/ [L, *signum,* mark], an objective finding as perceived by an examiner, such as a fever, a rash, the whisper heard over the chest in pleural effusion, or the light band of hair seen in children after recovery from kwashiorkor. Many signs accompany symptoms. For example, erythema and a maculopapular rash are often seen with pruritus.

significance, signif″ikəns/ [L, *significare,* to signify], 1. In research, the statistical probability that a given finding may have occurred by chance alone. The conventional standard for attributing significance is a finding that occurs fewer than 5 times in 100 by chance alone *(P < .05).* 2. The importance of a study in developing a practice or theory, as in nursing practice.

sleep, [AS, *slaepan,* to sleep], a state marked by reduced consciousness, diminished activity of the skeletal muscles, and depressed metabolism. People normally experience sleep in patterns that follow four observable, progressive stages. A device such as an encephalograph is used to record the recurrent pattern of brain waves during the stages. During stage 1 the brain waves are of the theta type, followed in stage 2 by the appearance of distinctive sleep spindles; during stages 3 and 4 the theta waves are replaced by delta waves. These four stages represent three-fourths of a period of typical sleep and collectively are called nonrapid eye movement sleep. The remaining time is usually occupied with rapid eye movement (REM) sleep, which can be detected with electrodes placed on the skin around the eyes so that tiny electric discharges from contractions of the eye muscles are transmitted to recording equipment. The REM sleep periods, lasting from a few minutes to half an hour, alternate with the NREM periods. Dreaming occurs during REM time. Individual sleep patterns normally change throughout life because daily requirements for sleep gradually diminish from as much as 20 hours a day in infancy to as little as 6 hours a day in old age. Infants tend to begin a sleep period

with REM sleep, whereas REM activity usually follows the four stages of NREM sleep in adults.

sleep apnea, a sleep disorder characterized by periods in which respiration is absent. The person is momentarily unable to contract respiratory muscles or to maintain airflow through the nose and mouth.

somatic pain, generally well-localized pain that results from the activation of peripheral nociceptors without injury to the peripheral nerve or central nervous system.

spasm, /spaz″əm/ [Gk, *spasmos*], 1. An involuntary muscle contraction of sudden onset, such as habit spasms, hiccups, stuttering, or a tic. 2. A convulsion or seizure. 3. A sudden transient constriction of a blood vessel, bronchus, esophagus, pylorus, ureter, or other hollow organ.

spirituality, aspects of human thought and behavior that refer to the way individuals and groups seek and express meaning and purpose, particularly in how they relate to religious deities or to sacred or otherworldly matters.

spiritual healing, the use of spiritual practices, such as prayer, for the purpose of effecting a cure of or an improvement in an illness.

spiritual healing and prayer, the offering of prayers to a higher being or authority for the purpose of reducing stress, promoting healing, or arresting disease. Spiritual healing may be practiced by the individual patient, by groups, or by others with or without the patient's knowledge.

spiritual therapy, [L, *spiritus,* breath; Gk, *therapeia,* treatment], a form of counseling or psychotherapy that involves moral, spiritual, and religious influences on behavior and physical health; the use of spiritual and religious beliefs and values to strengthen the self.

stabilization exercises, exercises to develop proximal control in symptom (pain)-free positions, such as sitting on a gymnastic ball and extending one knee to maintain balance and control without pain.

statistical significance, [L, *status,* condition, *significare,* to signify], an interpretation of statistical data that indicates that an occurrence was probably the result of a causative factor and not simply a chance result. Statistical significance at the 1% level indicates a 1 in 100 probability that a result can be ascribed to chance.

stress, [OFr, *estrecier,* to tighten], any emotional, physical, social, economic, or other factor that requires a response or change. Examples include dehydration, which can cause an increase in body temperature, and a separation from parents, which can cause a young child to cry. Stress can be positive or negative. Ongoing chronic stress can result in physical illness. Stress has been theorized as a major contributing factor in many physical diseases, such as asthma. Stress may also be applied therapeutically to promote change, such as implosive therapy for phobic patients, in which the patient is given support while being exposed to the situation that produces anxiety and is thereby gradually desensitized. The nature and degree of stress observed in a patient are frequently evaluated by the nurse as part of the ongoing holistic nursing assessment.

stress-adaptation theory, a concept that stress depletes the reserve capacity of individuals, thereby increasing their vulnerability to health problems.

stress management, methods of controlling factors that require a response or change within a person by identifying the stressors, eliminating negative stressors, and developing effective coping mechanisms to counteract the response constructively. Kinds include guided imagery, biofeedback, meditation.

stressor, /stres″ər/ [OFr, *estrecier,* to tighten], anything that causes wear and tear on the body's physical or mental resources. *See also* general adaptation syndrome.

stress reaction, an acute maladaptive emotional response to an actual or perceived stressor.

subjective symptoms, [L, *subjectus,* subject; Gk, *symptoma*], symptoms that are observed only by the patient and that cannot be objectively confirmed.

sublingual administration of a medication, the administration of a drug, usually in tablet form, by placing it beneath the tongue until the tablet dissolves. Administering drugs such as nitroglycerin by this route rather than by swallowing avoids the extensive first-pass metabolism of nitroglycerin that occurs in the liver.

substance abuse, the overindulgence in and dependence on a stimulant, depressant, or other chemical substance, leading to effects that are detrimental to the individual's physical or mental health, or the welfare of others.

Substance Abuse and Mental Health Services Administration (SAMHSA), an agency of the U.S. Department of Health and Human Services with the function of disseminating accurate and up-to-date information about and providing leadership in the prevention and treatment of addictive and mental disorders.

substance abuse testing, a screening of the urine or blood, or another kind of test, to identify drug use or drug overdose or poisoning from substances such as lead and carbon monoxide.

substance P, a polypeptide neurotransmitter that stimulates vasodilation and contraction of intestinal and other smooth muscles. It also plays a part in salivary secretion, diuresis, natriuresis, and pain sensation. It has been isolated from certain cells of the gastrointestinal and biliary tracts.

suggestibility, /səjes″tibil″itē/, pertaining to a person's susceptibility to having his or her ideas or actions influenced or altered by others.

suggestion, /səjes″chən/ [L, *suggerere,* to propose], 1. The process by which one thought or idea leads to another, as in the association of ideas. 2. The use of persuasion, exhortation, or another technique to implant an idea, thought, attitude, or belief in the mind of another as a means of influencing or altering behavior or states of mind. *See also* hypnosis. 3. An idea, belief, or attitude implanted in the mind of another.

surrogate, /sur″əgāt/ [L, *surrogare,* to substitute], 1. A substitute; a person or thing that replaces another. 2. A person who represents and acts as a parent, taking the place of the father or mother. 3. (in psychoanalysis) A substitute parental figure, or a symbolic image or representation of another, as may occur in a dream. The identity of the person represented often remains in the unconscious.

Swedish massage, /swē′dish/ [Fr, *masser*], the most commonly used form of classic Western massage, generally performed in the direction of the heart, sometimes with active or passive movement of the joints. It is used especially for relaxation, relief of muscular tension, and improvement of circulation and range of motion.

sympathectomy, /sim′pəthek″təmē/ [Gk, *sympathein,* to feel with, *ektomē,* excision], a surgical interruption of part of the sympathetic nerve pathways to relieve chronic pain or to promote vasodilation in vascular diseases, such as arteriosclerosis, claudication, Buerger's disease, and Raynaud's phenomenon. The sheath around an artery carries the sympathetic nerve fibers that control constriction of the vessel. Removal of the sheath causes the vessel to relax and expand and allows more blood to pass through it. The operation also may be done with a vascular graft to increase the blood flow through the graft area. Preoperatively the physician may assess the effect of surgery by injecting sympathetic ganglia with a local anesthesia to interrupt temporarily the sympathetic nerve impulses. The nerves lie along the spinal column and are approached through the back or the neck, by using local anesthesia. Postoperatively, the adequacy of circulation and peripheral nervous supply in the affected extremity is monitored. An arteriogram shows a widened pathway.

sympathetic, /sim′pəthet″ik/ [Gk, *sympathein,* to feel with], 1. Pertaining to a display of compassion for another's grief. 2. Pertaining to a division of the autonomic nervous system. 3. *See also* sympathy.

sympathy, /sim″pəthē/ [Gk, *sympathein*], 1. An expressed interest or concern regarding the problems, emotions, or states of mind of another. 2. The relation that exists between the mind and body, causing the one to be affected by the other. 3. Mental contagion or the influence exerted by one individual or group on another and the effects produced, such as the spread of panic, uncontrollable laughter, or yawning. 4. The physiologic or pathologic relationship between two organs, systems, or parts of the body.

synapse, /sin″aps, sinaps″/ [Gk, *synaptein,* to join], 1. n. The region surrounding the point of contact between two neurons or between a neuron and an effector organ, across which nerve impulses are transmitted through the action of a neurotransmitter, such as acetylcholine or norepinephrine. When an impulse reaches the terminal point of one neuron, it causes the release of the neurotransmitter. The neurotransmitter diffuses across the gap between the two cells to bind with receptors in the other neuron, muscle, or gland, triggering electric changes that either inhibit or continue the transmission of the impulse. Synapses are polarized so that nerve impulses normally travel in only one direction; they are also subject to fatigue, oxygen deficiency, anesthetics, and other chemical agents. Kinds include axoaxonic synapse, axodendritic synapse, axodendrosomatic synapse, axosomatic synapse, dendrodendritic synapse. 2. v. To form a synapse or connection between neurons. 3. v., (in genetics) To form a synaptic fusion between homologous chromosomes during meiosis. – synaptic, *adj.*

synapsis, /sinap″sis/, the pairing of homologous chromosomes during early meiotic prophase in gametogenesis to form double or bivalent chromosomes.

synaptic junction, the membranes of both the presynaptic neuron and the postsynaptic receptor cell together with the synaptic cleft. *See also* synapse.

synaptic transmission, the passage of a neural impulse across a synapse from one nerve fiber to another by means of a neurotransmitter.

synergy, /sin″ərjē/ [Gk, *syn* + *ergein*, to work], 1. The process in which two organs, substances, or agents work simultaneously to enhance the function and effect of one another. 2. The coordinated action of a set of muscles that work together to produce a specific movement, as in a reflex action. 3. A combined action of different parts of the autonomic nervous system, as in the sympathetic and parasympathetic innervation of secreting cells of the salivary glands, with both systems having a secretory effect. 4. The interaction of two or more drugs to produce a certain effect, as in the exaggerated response to tyramine in a person who is treated with a monoamine oxidase inhibitor. Also called synergism.

systematic reviews, a scientific investigation that asks a specific question and uses explicit, rigorous, prespecified methods to identify, critically appraise, select, and summarize findings of similar but separate studies. Systematic reviews are the cornerstone of evidence-based health care decision making.

T

tai chi, a technique that uses slow, purposeful, motor-physical movements of the body for the purpose of control to increase outer body mass strength and achieve a more balanced physiologic and psychological state. Tai chi has positive effects on the respiratory, cardiovascular, and cerebral functions in both children and older adults, including reducing the incidence of falls in older people.

tallman lettering, a method of writing medications that are commonly confused. Uppercase lettering is used to draw attention to the differences in the medication names. Kinds include acetaZOLAMIDE, acetoHEXAMIDE, chlorproPAMIDE, chlorproMAZINE.

telehealth, the use of telecommunication technologies to provide health care services and access to medical and surgical information for training and educating health care professionals and consumers, to increase awareness and educate the public about health-related issues, and to facilitate medical research across distances.

telemedicine, the use of telecommunication equipment and information technology to provide clinical care to individuals at distant sites and the transmission of medical and surgical information and images needed to provide that care.

temporomandibular joint (TMJ), [L, *tempora* + *mandere*, to chew, *jungere*, to join], one of a pair of joints connecting the mandible of the jaw to the temporal bone of the skull. It is a combined hinge and gliding joint, formed by the anterior parts of the mandibular fossae of the temporal bone, the articular eminences, the condyles of the mandible, and five ligaments. The TMJ is the only joint in the body in which movement of one joint is always synchronous with movement of the other joint.

tension headache, a pain that affects the head as the result of overwork or emotional strain and that involves tension in the muscles of the neck, face, and shoulder.

tetrahydrocannabinol (THC), /-hi′drōkənab′inol/, the active principle, occurring as two psychotomimetic isomers, in the hemp plant *Cannabis sativa*, used in the preparation of marijuana, hashish, bhang, and ganja. THC increases pulse rate and has variable effects on blood pressure. It causes conjunctival reddening and a feeling of euphoria. The drug affects memory, cognition, and the sensorium; decreases motor coordination; and increases appetite. Nonintoxicating doses of THC are used experimentally in the treatment of glaucoma and to relieve nausea and increase the appetite in patients receiving cancer chemotherapy. *See also* cannabis.

thalamic syndrome, [Gk, *thalamos* + *syn*, together, *dromos*, course], a vascular disorder involving the ventral and posterolateral nuclei of the thalamus and related nerve fibers. It causes disturbances of sensation and partial or complete paralysis of one side of the body. A major effect is an increased threshold to all stimuli on the opposite side of the body so that any stimuli may cause an exaggerated response. Also called *Dejerine-Roussy syndrome.*

therapeutic communication, a process in which the nurse consciously influences a client or helps the client to a better understanding through verbal or nonverbal communication. Therapeutic communication involves the use of specific strategies that encourage the patient to express feelings and ideas and that convey acceptance and respect.

therapeutic dose, [Gk, *therapeia*, treatment, *dosis*, giving], the dose that may be required to produce a desired effect.

therapeutic equivalent, a drug that has essentially the same effect in the treatment of a disease or condition as one or more other drugs. A drug that is a therapeutic equivalent may or may not be chemically equivalent, bioequivalent, or generically equivalent.

therapeutic exercise, any exercise planned and performed to attain a specific physical benefit, such as maintenance of the range of motion, strengthening of weakened muscles, increased joint flexibility, or improved cardiovascular and respiratory function.

therapeutic horseback riding, an equestrian experience for those with special needs, promoting the ability to build independence and self-confidence and to help the person reach individualized goals.

Therapeutic Touch (TT), a healing method based on the premise that the body possesses an energy field that can be affected by the focused intention of the healer, using a consciously directed exchange of energy between practitioner and patient. The practitioner uses the hands as a focus to assess the patient's energy field, to release areas where the free flow of energy is blocked, and to balance the patient's energy by transferring energy from a universal life energy force to the patient.

therapeutic use of self, thoughtful and deliberate use of one's personality, opinions, and judgments as a component of the therapeutic process.

thermal, /thur'məl/ [Gk, *therme*, heat], pertaining to the production, application, or maintenance of heat. Also thermic.

thermotherapy, /-ther'əpē/ [Gk, *therme* + *therapeia*, treatment], the treatment of disease by the application of heat. Thermotherapy may be administered as dry heat with heat lamps, diathermy machines, electric pads, or hot water bottles or as moist heat with warm compresses or immersion in warm water. Warm soaks or compresses may be used to treat local infections, relax muscles, and relieve pain in patients with motor problems, and promote circulation in peripheral vascular disorders such as thrombophlebitis. —thermotherapeutic, adj.

theta wave, [Gk, *theta*, eighth letter of Greek alphabet; AS, *wafian*], one of the several types of brain waves, characterized by a relatively low frequency of 4 to 7 Hz and a low amplitude of 10 µV. Theta waves are the "drowsy waves" of the temporal lobes of the brain and appear in electroencephalograms when the individual is awake but relaxed and sleepy. Also called theta rhythm.

threshold, /thresh'ōld/ [AS, *therscold*], the point at which a stimulus is great enough to produce an effect. For example, a pain threshold is the point at which a person becomes aware of pain.

threshold of consciousness, [AS, *therscold* + L, *conscire*, to be aware], the lowest limit of perception of a stimulus.

threshold stimulus, [AS, *therscold* + L, *stimulare*, to incite], a stimulus that is just sufficient to produce a response. Below that level, no action or response is likely without additional intensity of the stimulus. Also called limen, liminal stimulus.

throb, [ME, *throbben*, to beat intensely], a deep, pulsating kind of discomfort or pain. —throbbing, adj., n.

tingling, [ME, *tinklen*, to tinkle], a prickly sensation in the skin or a body part, accompanied by diminished sensitivity to stimulation of the sensory nerves.

tolerance, /tol'ərəns/ [L, *tolerare*, to endure], a phenomenon by which the body becomes increasingly resistant to a drug, substance, or activity through continued exposure. Kinds include work tolerance.

tonus, /tō'nəs/ [Gk, *tonos*, stretching], 1. The normal state of balanced tension in the body tissues, especially the muscles. Partial contraction or alternative contraction and relaxation of neighboring fibers of a group of muscles hold the organ or the part of the body in a neutral functional position without fatigue. Tonus is essential for many normal body functions, such as holding the spine erect, the eyes open, and the jaw closed. Also called muscle tone. 2. The state of the body tissues being strong and fit. Also called tone.

torsades de pointes, /tôrsäd' de pô·aNt', tôr'säd də point'/ [Fr, *torsader*, to twist together, *pointes*, tips], a type of ventricular tachycardia with a spiral-like appearance ("twisting of the points") and complexes that at first look positive and then negative on an electrocardiogram. It is precipitated by a long Q-T interval, which often is induced by drugs (quiNIDine, procainamide, or disopyramide) but may be the result of hypokalemia, hypomagnesemia, or profound bradycardia. The first line of treatment is intravenous magnesium sulfate and defibrillation if the patient is unstable.

total quality management (TQM), an approach to the improvement of the provision of services based on the premise that the overwhelming majority of quality failures are the result of flaws in processes and that quality can be improved by controlling these processes. TQM replaces traditional methods of quality management based on the identification and correction of problems as they occur and requires the participation of all members of an organization in improving processes, products, services, and the culture in which they work. TQM involves creation of an organizational structure for identifying and improving processes, the use of data-based statistical analysis to study processes, and the empowerment of employees to take responsibility for their own tasks in a way that encourages both continuous learning and personal responsibility. In a health care setting, this means a shift from an emphasis on tasks to an emphasis on outcomes of care, which provide the data. *See also* continuous quality improvement.

traction, /trak'shən/ [L, *trahere*, to draw], 1. (in orthopedics) The process of putting a limb, bone, or group of muscles under tension by means of weights and pulleys to align or immobilize the part to reduce muscle spasm or relieve pressure on it. Kinds include Bryant's traction, Buck's traction, Russell's traction, skeletal traction, skin traction, split Russell traction. 2. The process of pulling a part of the body along, through or out of its socket or cavity, such as axis traction with obstetric forceps in delivering an infant.

traction response, the body's reaction to traction applied to the spine. Alterations of certain signs and symptoms of a musculoskeletal disorder may be revealed by traction tests. For example, if traction relieves a symptom, it may indicate impingement of a nerve root. Traction may also be used therapeutically to increase joint range, overcome muscle spasms, shorten soft tissues, or neutralize pressure and relieve pain in various joints.

traditional Chinese medicine (TCM), the diverse body of medical theory and practice that has evolved in China, comprising four branches: acupuncture and moxibustion, herbal medicine, qi gong, and tui na. Although TCM encompasses a variety of theory and practice, all of its forms share certain underlying characteristics. The body and mind are considered together as a dynamic system subject to cycles of change and affected by the environment, and emphasis is on supporting the body's self-healing ability. Fundamental to TCM are the yin-yang principle and the concept of basic substances that pervade the body: qi, jing (essence), and shen (spirit), collectively known as the three treasures, and the blood (a fluid and material manifestation of qi) and body fluids (which moisten and lubricate the body). Disease arises from a disturbance of qi within the body, the particular pathologic process depending on the location of the disturbance; causes are classified into three groups, external (which are environmental), internal (emotions), and miscellaneous (such as diet, fatigue, or trauma). Diagnosis is by visual assessment, listening and smelling, questioning, and palpation; a single biomedical disease may be associated with a large number of TCM diagnoses, and one TCM diagnosis may encompass a number of biomedical diseases. Once a diagnosis is established, therapy aims at restoring the body's homeostasis by treating the root cause of the disease.

Trager approach, service mark for a bodywork technique whose purpose is to train patients to develop awareness of movement patterns that relieve pain and promote relaxation. It consists of two components: tablework, in which the practitioner, in a meditative state, uses touch and gentle passive movement to assist the patient in experiencing new movement patterns, and Mentastics, in which the patient is taught a series of movements designed to relieve tension.

trance, [L, *transire,* to pass across], 1. A sleeplike state characterized by the complete or partial suspension of consciousness and loss or diminution of motor activity, as seen in hypnosis, dissociative disorders, and various cataleptic and ecstatic states. 2. A dazed or bewildered condition; stupor. 3. A state of detachment from one's immediate surroundings, such as in deep concentration or daydreaming. Kinds include alcoholic trance, *death trance,* hypnotic trance, induced trance.

transcendental meditation (TM), a psychophysiologic exercise designed to lower levels of tension and anxiety and increase tolerance of frustration. TM has been described as a state of consciousness that does not require any physical or mental control. During meditation, the person enters a hypometabolic state in which there is reduced activity of the adrenergic component of the autonomic nervous system.

transcutaneous electrical nerve stimulation (TENS), a method of pain control by the application of electric impulses to the nerve endings. This is done through electrodes that are placed on the skin and attached to a stimulator by flexible wires. The electric impulses generated are similar to those of the body but different enough to block transmission of pain signals to the brain. TENS is noninvasive and nonaddictive, with no known side effects. It is contraindicated in patients with a demand-type cardiac pacemaker. Also called transcutaneous nerve stimulation.

transcutaneous oxygen/carbon dioxide (O_2/CO_2) monitoring, a method of measuring the O_2 or CO_2 in the blood by attaching electrodes to the skin. O_2 is commonly measured through an oximeter, which contains heating coils to raise the skin temperature and increase blood flow at the surface. O_2 content is calculated in terms of light absorption at various wavelengths. Transcutaneous CO_2 electrodes are similar to blood gas electrodes, with a Teflon membrane tip that is permeable to gases.

transmission, /-mish″ən/ [L, *transmittere,* to transmit], the transfer or conveyance of a thing or condition, such as a neural impulse, infectious or genetic disease, or a hereditary trait, from one person or place to another. —transmissible, adj.

transversospinales muscles, a group of muscles deep to the erector spinae that consist of the semispinalis, multifidus, and rotatores muscles. When these muscles contract bilaterally, they extend the vertebral column, an action similar to that of the erector spinae group. However, when muscles on only one side contract, they pull the spinous processes toward the transverse processes on that side, causing the trunk to turn or rotate in the opposite direction.

trigeminal neuralgia, a neurologic condition of the trigeminal facial nerve, characterized by paroxysms of flashing, stablike pain radiating along the course of a branch of the nerve from the angle of the jaw. It is caused by degeneration of the nerve or by pressure on it. Any or all of the three branches of the nerve may be affected. Neuralgia of the first branch results in pain around the eyes and over the forehead; of the second branch, in pain in the upper lip, nose, and cheek; of the third branch, in pain on the side of the tongue and the lower lip. The momentary bursts of pain recur in clusters lasting many seconds. Paroxysmal episodes of the pains may last for hours. Also called prosopalgia, tic douloureux.

trigger point, a point on the body that is particularly sensitive to touch and, when stimulated, becomes the site of a painful neuralgia.

trunk balance, the ability to maintain postural control of the trunk, including the shifting and bearing of weight on each side to free an extremity for a particular function such as reaching and grasping. Weight shifting can be anterior, posterior, lateral, or diagonal and involve righting, equilibrium, and protective reactions. Head and neck control allows for dissociation of the shoulder and pelvic girdles from the trunk.

tyramine, /tī″rəmēn/ [Gk, *tyros,* cheese, *amine,* ammonia], an amino acid synthesized in the body from the essential amino acid tyrosine. Tyramine stimulates the release of the catecholamines epinephrine and norepinephrine. People taking monoamine oxidase inhibitors should avoid the ingestion of foods and beverages containing tyramine, particularly aged cheeses and meats, bananas, yeast-containing products, and certain alcoholic beverages, such as red wines. *See also* norepinephrine.

tyrosine (Tyr), /tī″rəsēn/ [Gk, *tyros*], an amino acid synthesized in the body from the essential amino acid phenylalanine. Tyrosine is found in most proteins and is a precursor of melanin and several hormones, including epinephrine and thyroxine.

U

ulcerative colitis, a chronic, episodic, inflammatory disease of the large intestine and rectum. It is characterized by profuse watery diarrhea containing varying amounts of blood, mucus, and pus. Some of the many systemic complications of ulcerative colitis include peripheral arthritis, ankylosing spondylitis, kidney and liver disease, and inflammation of the eyes, skin, and mouth. People with severe disease may develop toxic megacolon, a dangerous complication that may lead to perforation of the bowel, septicemia, and death. Also called inflammatory bowel disease.

underlying assumption, /un″dərlī″ing/, a set of rules one holds about oneself, others, and the world. These rules are regarded by the individual as unquestionably true.

underwater exercise, /un″dərwô′tər/ [AS, *under* + *woeter*], any physical activity performed in a pool or large tub, such as a Hubbard tank, in which the buoyancy of the water facilitates the movement of weak or injured muscles. Also called aquatherapy, aquatic exercise. *See also* exercise.

unitary human conceptual framework, /yoo″niter′ē/, a complex theory in nursing introduced by Martha Rogers that emphasizes the importance of holistic health care and an understanding of the human being in relation to the universal environment.

United States Pharmacopeia (USP), a compendium recognized officially by the U.S. Federal Food, Drug, and Cosmetic Act that contains descriptions, uses, strengths, and standards of purity for selected drugs and for all of their forms of dosage.

USP unit, a dose unit as recommended by the *United States Pharmacopeia.* A unit is used in the United States to measure the potency of a vitamin or drug.

V

vagus nerve, /vā″gəs/ [L, *vagus,* wandering, *nervus,* nerve], either of the longest pair of cranial nerves mainly responsible for parasympathetic control over the heart and many other internal organs, including thoracic and abdominal viscera. The vagus nerves communicate through 13 main branches, connecting to four areas in the brain. Also called nervus vagus, pneumogastric nerve, tenth cranial nerve.

validity, /valid″itē/, (in research) the extent to which a test measurement or other device measures what it is intended to measure. A data collection tool should accurately reflect the concept that it is intended to measure. Kinds include construct validity, content validity, current validity, predictive validity.

Valsalva maneuver, /valsal″və/ [Antonio M. Valsalva, Italian surgeon, 1666–1723; OFr, *maneuvre,* work done by hand], any forced expiratory effort against a closed airway, such as when an individual holds the breath and tightens the muscles in a concerted, strenuous effort to move a heavy object. Most healthy individuals perform Valsalva maneuvers during normal daily activities without any injurious consequences. However, such efforts are dangerous for many patients with cardiovascular disease, especially if they become dehydrated, increasing the viscosity of their blood and the attendant risk of blood clotting. Constipation increases the risk for cardiovascular trauma in such patients, especially if they perform a Valsalva maneuver in trying to move their bowels. On relaxation after each muscular effort with held breath, the blood of such individuals rushes to the heart, often overloading the cardiac system and causing cardiac arrest. Orthopedic patients often use a Valsalva maneuver in changing their position in bed with the aid of an overhead trapeze bar. Patients who may be endangered by performing a Valsalva maneuver are commonly instructed to exhale instead of holding their breath when they move. Exhalation decreases the risk for cardiovascular trauma. Part of the danger is a bradycardia response.

value, /val″yoo/ [L, *valere,* to be strong], a personal belief about the worth of a given idea or behavior.

value system, the accepted mode of conduct and the set of norms, goals, and values binding any social group. Such guidelines for determining what is right or wrong, good or bad, and desirable or undesirable serve as a frame of reference for the individual in reaching decisions and in achieving a meaningful life.

variable, /ver″ē·əbəl/, 1. A factor in an experiment or scientific test that tends to vary, or take on different values, while other elements or conditions remain constant. 2. An attribute of a person that is measurable and that varies (heart rate, age).

visceral afferent fibers, the nerve fibers of the visceral nervous system that receive stimuli, carry impulses toward the central nervous system, and share the sensory ganglia of the cerebrospinal nerves with the somatic sensory fibers. Peripheral distribution of the visceral afferent fibers constitutes the main difference between them and the somatic afferents. The visceral afferent fibers produce sensations different from those of the somatic afferent fibers. The visceral efferent fibers connect with both the somatic and visceral afferent fibers. The number and extent of the visceral afferent fibers is not clearly established. Their peripheral processes reach the ganglia by various routes. Most of the visceral afferent fibers accompany blood vessels for part of their course, and various afferent fibers run in the cerebrospinal nerves. Some of the parts of the body with visceral afferent fibers are the face, scalp, nose, mouth, descending colon, lungs, abdomen, and rectum.

visceral pain, pain that results from the activation of nociceptors of the thoracic, pelvic, or abdominal viscera. It is felt as a poorly localized aching or cramping sensation and is often referred to cutaneous sites.

W

waking imagined analgesia (WIA), [AS, *wacian,* to awaken; L, *imaginari,* to picture oneself; Gk, *a* + *algos,* without pain], the pain relief experienced by a patient who uses the psychological technique of concentrating on previous pleasant personal experiences that produced tranquility, such as lying on a summer beach beside cooling ocean water or drifting down a quiet river in a canoe. The patient using the WIA technique is encouraged to verbalize such experiences, thereby reinforcing recollection with attendant soothing biological responses. This technique is often effective in reducing mild to moderate pain, especially when used with a mild nonopioid analgesic and the compassionate interaction of an attending health care professional. *See also* pain assessment, pain intervention.

wean, [AS, *wenian,* to accustom], 1. To induce a child to give up breastfeeding and accept other food in place of breast milk. Many children are ready for weaning during the second half of the first year; some wean themselves. 2. To withdraw a person from something on which he or she is dependent. 3. To remove a patient gradually from dependency on mechanical ventilation.

wear-and-tear theory, /wer/, one theory of biological aging in which structural and functional changes occur during the aging process (e.g., osteoarthritis). Damage accumulates when the body fails to repair itself.

weight loss, a reduction in body weight. The loss may be the result of a change in diet or lifestyle or a febrile disease. To lose 1 lb a week a person must consume 500 fewer calories daily and/or expend 500 more calories daily through physical activity.

weight-reduction diet, a diet used to decrease body weight. It must supply fewer calories than the individual expends each day while supplying all the essential nutrients for maintaining health.

wet tap, accidental puncture of the dura mater during injection of epidural anesthesia, so-called from the leakage of cerebrospinal fluid from the needle hub.

whiplash injury, [ME, *whippen* + *lasshe* + L, *ijuria*], (informal) an injury to the cervical vertebrae or their supporting ligaments and muscles marked by pain and stiffness. It usually results from sudden acceleration or deceleration, such as in a rear-end car collision that causes violent back-and-forth movement of the head and neck.

white noise, a sound in which the intensity is the same at all frequencies within a designated band.

withdrawal symptoms, the unpleasant, sometimes life-threatening physiologic changes that occur when some drugs are withdrawn after prolonged, regular use. The effects may occur after use of an opioid, antipsychotic, stimulant, sedative-hypnotic, alcohol, corticosteroid, or other substance to which the person has become physiologically or psychologically dependent or addicted. Other drug therapy may be used to relieve symptoms of withdrawal, such as methadone, used for heroin withdrawal, or chlordiazePOXIDE, used for alcohol withdrawal. Withdrawal symptoms also can be managed by gradually reducing the drug dose over time, as with the tapering of corticosteroids.

withdrawn behavior, a condition in which there is a blunting of the emotions and a lack of social responsiveness.

work tolerance, the kind and amount of work that a physically or mentally ill person can or should perform.

X

xeno-, /zē′ne-, zen′ō-/, combining form meaning "strange or pertaining to foreign matter": xenodiagnosis, xenogenous, xenology.

Y

yin/yang, a Chinese philosophy that each entity is one, but contains two equal and opposite forces. The forces of yang include maleness, the sun, and heat. The forces of yin include femaleness, darkness, and cold. Macrobiotic diets are based on the division of food into yin and yang properties. Many holistic care practices are rooted in the belief that there must be a balance between yin and yang forces for health and that illness is the result of imbalance. *See also* ch'i, yin/yang principle.

yin/yang principle, in Chinese philosophy, the concept of polar complements existing in dynamic equilibrium and always present simultaneously. In traditional Chinese medicine, a disturbance of the proper balance of yin and yang causes disease, and the goal is to maintain or to restore this balance.

yoga, a discipline that focuses on the body's musculature, posture, breathing mechanisms, and consciousness. The goal of yoga is attainment of physical and mental well-being through mastery of the body, achieved through exercise, holding of postures, proper breathing, and meditation.

Z

zone therapy, a complementary therapy in which there is treatment of a disorder by mechanical stimulation and counterirritation of a body area in the same longitudinal zone as the affected organ or region.

Zung Self-Rating Depression Scale, a "self-report test" of 20 descriptors of depression on which clients rate themselves on a 4-point scale ranging from "a little of the time" to "most of the time." The scale is useful in determining the depth or intensity of a client's depression.

Definitions for this appendix have been selected from Mosby. (2020). *Mosby's dictionary of medicine, nursing, and health professions* (10th ed.). St. Louis, MO: Elsevier.

Index

Note: Page numbers followed by *f* indicate figures, *t* indicate tables, and *b* indicate boxes.

A

Abdominal breathing, 592
Abnormal processing
    central mechanisms, 42–43
    peripheral mechanisms, 41–42, 42*t*
Acceptance and commitment therapy (ACT), 625–626
Accurate pain assessment, 73
Acetaminophen
    adverse effects, 212–213
    dosing, 212
    FDA warnings, 213–214
    formulations, 212, 212*t*
    hepatotoxicity, 213
    history, 210
    indications for use, 211–212
    monitoring of patients, 214
    pharmacologic effects, 210–211
    routes, 212
    use in special populations, 214
        impaired renal function, 214
        liver disease patients, 214
        older adults, 214
Acetyl-l-carnitine, 707–708
Acoustic comfort, 748
ACT-UP, psychosocial assessment, 80*b*
Acupressure, 647
Acupuncture, 642–644
Acute pain
    assessment, conducting, 84–85, 87–88*t*
    classifications of, 31
    symptoms, 19
Adult nonverbal pain score (NVPS) tool, 124
Affordable Care Act (ACA), 770
Agitation, unrelieved pain, 21
Alberta Breakthrough Pain Assessment Tool
        for Cancer Patients (ABPAT), 103–104,
        103*f*
Alfentanil, 259
Alpha₂-adrenergic agonists, 494–495
Alpha-adrenergic receptor agonists,
        398–401
Alternate nostril breathing, 592
Alternating/contrasting temperature therapy,
        759–760
American Medical Association (AMA), 1
American Music Therapy Association (AMTA),
        597
American Pain Society (APS), 384
American Society for Anesthesiology, 22
American Society for Pain Management Nursing
        (ASPMN), 22
American Society of Anesthesiologists (ASA),
        384–385
American Society of Regional Anesthesia and
        Pain Medicine (ASRA), 384–385

A3 methodology
    clinical application, 785*b*
    pitfalls, 783–786
    quality improvement, 783–786, 788–789*t*
    template, 783
    using plan-do-study-act (PDSA) cycles, 784*t*
Amitriptyline, 442
Analgesia
    Beer's criteria, medications in, 165–166*t*
    definition, 8
    dosing considerations
        around-the-clock dosing, 182–184
        awakening patients, 184
        comorbidities, 181
        dosing to pain intensity using numbers,
                184–187
        equianalgesic dosing, 181–182
        individualized dose selection, 188*f*
        opioid dose requirement, 186*t*
        pain intensity, 187*t*
        prescription and implementation, 189*b*
        range order, 187–190
        therapeutic duplication, 190
    route selection, medications, 168–170*t* (*see
            also* Medication administration)
        gastrointestinal stomal route, 172
        intramuscular route, 178
        intravenous route, 173–174
        medications administered by, 173*t*
        neuraxial and peripheral nerve routes, 181
        oral, 167–171
        rectal route, 172
        subcutaneous route, 175–178, 175*f*, 176*b*
        sublingual, buccal, and intranasal, 171–172
        topical, 178–179
        transdermal, 179–181
        transmucosal route, 171–173
        vaginal route, 173
Animal-assisted activity (AAA), 600
Animal-assisted therapy
    cautions, 603
    definitions, 600
    indications for, 600–601
    pain management, 601–603
    relaxation response, 602*t*
    research, 602–603
Antidepressants, tricyclic, 394–396, 394*t*
Antiinflammatory diet
    cautions, 747
    pain management, 745–747
    patient handout, 746*f*
Anxiety
    assessment of, 147–149
    catastrophizing, 147
    definition, 146
    discomfort intolerance, 146
    generalized anxiety disorder (GAD-7), 156*f*
    hospital anxiety and depression scale (HADS),
            148, 148*f*
    pain, 146–147

Anxiety (*Continued*)
    pain catastrophizing scale, 148–149
    patient health questionnaire-4 (PHQ-4),
            147–148, 147*f*
    sensitivity, 146
    unrelieved pain, 20–21
Aquatic exercise, 568–569, 569*b*
Aromatherapy
    cautions, 740–741
    lavender, 739
    massage, 739–740
    pain management evidence, 739–740
    sweet orange, 739
Around-the-clock dosing, 182–184
Art, 588–589
Aspirin, 198
    indications for use, 197*b*, 199–200
    pharmacologic effects, 197–199
Assessment of pain
    acute *vs.* chronic pain, 63
    aims of, 62*b*
    behavioral indicators, 69*b*
    breakthrough pain assessment
        Alberta Breakthrough Pain Assessment Tool
                for Cancer Patients (ABPAT), 103–104,
                103*f*
        breakthrough pain assessment tool (BAT),
                107, 107*f*
        Italian Questionnaire for Breakthrough
                Pain (IQ-BTP), 108
        screening tool, 102*f*
    classification of, 62–64
    components of comprehensive, 76–84
    conducting
        acute pain assessment, 84–85, 87–88*t*
        chronic pain assessment, 85, 88–89*t*
    context of care, 82
    in culturally diverse patient populations, 66*b*
    discrepancies in, 65–67
    environmental factors, 81
    hierarchy of, 67–70, 68*b*
    importance of, 61–62
    initial pain assessment tool, 75*f*
    mechanisms, 63–64
    mnemonics for use in, 76
    mnemonic tools, comprehensive pain
            assessment, 76*t*
    multidimensional pain assessment tools
        brief pain inventory (BPI), 95, 96*f*
        chronic pain grade scale (CPGS), 98
        clinically aligned pain assessment tool, 94,
                94*f*
        defense and veterans pain rating scale 2.0
                (DVPRS), 94, 95*f*
        functional pain scale (FPS), 95–97, 97*f*
        McGill Pain Questionnaire (MPQ), 94–95
        PEG scale tool, 95, 97*f*
        short form 36 bodily pain score (SF-36 BPS)
                tool, 98
    neuropathic pain assessment, 98*t*

Assessment of pain *(Continued)*
　Leeds assessment of neuropathic symptoms and signs (LANSS) tool, 99–100, 99*f*
　neuropathic pain questionnaire (NPQ), 101–102, 101*f*
　pain rating scale, 86*b*
　pertinent history
　　clinical opiate withdrawal scale, 83*f*
　　medical history, 82
　　mental health history, 82
　　patient goal, 84
　　substance use disorder risk and history, 82–84
　physiologic and sensory aspects
　　aggravating and alleviating factors, 77
　　cognition, 80–81
　　effects of pain, 77–80
　　intensity, 76–77
　　location, 76
　　mental status, 81
　　onset and duration (temporal aspects), 77
　　pain affect, 80
　　pain control diary, 78–79*f*
　　psychosocial, 80
　　quality, 77
　roles of health team, 64
　routine nursing admission assessment questions, 74*t*
　sociocultural factors, 81
　sources of inaccurate, 66*b*
　stoicism, 67
　timing
　　and extent, 73–76
　　and frequency, 64–70
　tools for
　　clinically important changes, 90–91
　　daily clinical practice, 90*b*
　　effective pain scales, 85
　　use with older adults, 89*t*
　unidimensional pain assessment tools
　　colored analogue scale (CAS), 93–94
　　FACES Pain Scale (Revised) (FPS-R) tool, 92–93
　　Iowa pain thermometer (IPT) tool, 93
　　numeric rating scale, 91
　　verbal descriptor scale, 92
　　vertical version, 91*f*
　　visual analogue scale, 91–92
　　Wong-Baker FACES pain rating scale, 92, 93*f*
Auricular acupuncture (AA), 644–647, 645–646*f*
Autogenic training (AT), 604–605, 605*b*
Autonomy, 23
Avocado and soybean unsaponifiables (*Persea gratissma* and *Glycine max*) (Piascledine), 702–704
Awakening patients, 184
Awareness through movement (ATM), 565

B
Baclofen, 412–415, 443
Barriers, effective pain management
　access issues
　　finances, 54
　　residential area, 54–55
　　transportation, 54
　clinical application, 52
　family, 53–54
　fear, 52
　　of side effects, 52–53
　　of substance abuse or misuse, 53
　health care literacy, 53
　opportunities, 57
　past experiences with pain, 52
　patient expectations of pain and pain control, 52
　provider barriers

Barriers, effective pain management *(Continued)*
　clinician experience, 56
　culture, 55
　education, 55–56
　golden rule *vs.* platinum rule, 56
　perception, 55
　system barriers
　　continuing education of clinicians, 56–57
　　culture of organization, 56
　　insurance coverage, 57
　　time, 57
Beck depression inventory (BDI), 151
Behavioral activation (BA), 621. *See also* Cognitive-behavioral therapy
Behavioral pain scale (BPS), 124–125
Beneficence, 23
Benzomorphans, 235
Biodanza, 566
Biofeedback (Applied Psychophysiology), 626–627, 626*t*
Biopsychosocial factors, 614*t*
Biopsychosocial model, 30, 30*f*
Bispectral (BIS) index, 131
Botanicals and herbs
　avocado and soybean unsaponifiables (*Persea gratissma* and *Glycine max*) (Piascledine), 702–704
　Brazilian arnica (*Solidago chilensis*), 701
　bromelain (*Ananas comosus*) (pineapple plant), 704–705
　butterbur (*Petasites hybridus*), 701
　cannabis (*Cannabis sativa, Cannabis indica,* and *Cannabis indica*), 688–692
　cat's claw (*Uncaria tomentosa*), 692–693
　cayenne (*Capsicum frutescens*), 693
　comfrey (*Symphytum officinale L.*), 701
　devil's claw (*Harpagophytum procumbens, Harpagophytum zoyhori*), 693
　feverfew (*Tanacetum parthenium L.*), 694
　flavocoxid (limbrel), 705
　frankincense/olibanum (*Boswellia serrata*), 694–696
　ginger (*Zingiber officinale Roscoe*), 696–698, 696*f*
　ginseng (*Panax ginseng*), 701–702
　green tea (*Camellia sinensis*), 705–706
　honey, 706–707
　myrrh (*Commiphora molmol*), 702
　nutritional modulators of pain, 703*t*
　pharmaconutrients, 702–707
　St. John's Wort (*Hypericum perforatum*), 702
　supplements
　　acetyl-l-carnitine, 707–708
　　coenzyme Q$_{10}$ (ubiquinone-10), 708–709
　　glucosamine hydrochloride/sulfate and chondroitin sulfate, 709–710
　　hyaluronic acid (HA), 710–711
　　lactic acid-producing bacteria, 711–712
　　magnesium, 712–713, 712*b*
　　methylsulfonylmethane (MSM), 713–714
　　omega-3 polyunsaturated fatty acids, 714–716, 715*t*
　turmeric (*Curcuma longa/Curcuma domestica*), 698–700
　vitamins
　　vitamin B, 716–719
　　vitamin D, 719–721, 719–720*f*
　　vitamin E, 721–722
　white willow bark (*Salix alba*), 700–701
　willow bark (*Salicis cortex*), 700–701
Brazilian arnica (*Solidago chilensis*), 701
Breakthrough pain (BTP), 31
　assessment
　　Alberta Breakthrough Pain Assessment Tool for Cancer Patients (ABPAT), 103–104, 103*f*

Breakthrough pain (BTP) *(Continued)*
　　breakthrough pain assessment tool (BAT), 107, 107*f*
　　Italian Questionnaire for Breakthrough Pain (IQ-BTP), 108
　　screening tool, 102*f*
Breakthrough pain assessment tool (BAT), 107, 107*f*
Breathing technique
　abdominal breathing, 592
　alternate nostril breathing, 592
　diaphragmatic breathing, 592
　Lamaze breathing, 593
　square breathing, 592–593, 593*f*
　yogic breathing/pranayama, 592
Brief pain inventory (BPI), 95, 96*f*
Bromelain (*Ananas comosus*) (pineapple plant), 704–705
Buprenorphine, 264–266, 286–287, 367–368
　acute pain management, 372*t*
　chronic pain management, 375
Butterbur (*Petasites hybridus*), 701

C
Cannabidiol, 416–418
Cannabis (*Cannabis sativa, Cannabis indica,* and *Cannabis indica*), 688–692
　cautions, 692
　contraindications, 692
　pain management, 690–691
　potential interactions with medications, 692
Capnography, 352, 463–464
Capsaicin, 431–436
Caring by caregivers, 742–743
　cautions, 743
　clinician-patient communication, 743*b*
　pain management evidence, 743
Catabolic metabolic activity, 19
Cat's claw (*Uncaria tomentosa*), 692–693
Cayenne (*Capsicum frutescens*), 693
Center for epidemiologic studies depression scale (CES-D), 151, 152*f*
Centering prayer (spiritual meditation), 678–679
Centers for disease control and prevention guidelines, 9
Centers for Medicare and Medicaid Services (CMS), 770–771
Central pain, multimodal approaches, 45
Checklist of nonverbal pain indicators (CNPI), 129, 130*f*
Chiropractic practice
　active release techniques (ARTs), 664
　cautions, 665–666
　contraindications, 665*f*
　pain management, 664–665
　research, 665
　subgroups, 664*b*
Chronic neuropathic pain, guideline for treatment, 388*t*
Chronic pain
　assessment, conducting, 85, 88–89*t*
　movement with, 565
Chronic pain grade scale (CPGS), 98
Chronic postsurgical pain (CPSP), 31
Chronic regional pain syndrome (CRPS), 45–46, 45*t*
　Budapest clinical diagnostic criteria, 45*t*
　management, 46
　pathophysiology, 45–46
　type I, 45
　type II, 45
Classification of pain
　abnormal processing
　　central mechanisms, 42–43
　　peripheral mechanisms, 41–42, 42*t*
　acute pain, 31

Classification of pain *(Continued)*
  assessment of, 62–64
  based on duration, 31
  based on mechanism, 31–35
  breakthrough pain, 31
  chemicals involved in transmission, 40*f*
  chronic/persistent pain, 31
  chronic postsurgical pain (CPSP), 31
  dorsal horn and rexed laminae, 40*f*
  inflammatory mediators, 38*t*
  mixed pain states, 35
  modulation, 41
  neuroinflammation and immune system, 43–45
  neuropathic pain, 34–35
  nociceptive pain, 32–34, 32–33*t*, 34*b*, 36*f*,
    36–37*t*
  perception, 39–41
  physical and psychological symptoms, 32*t*
  physiologic processing of pain
    spinal and supraspinal pain pathways, 35*f*
    transduction, 35–37
  and prevalence, 33*t*
  primary afferent nerve fibers, 37*t*
  transmission, 37–39
Clinical care, 772
Clinically aligned pain assessment tool, 94, 94*f*
Clinical nursing efforts, organizational initiatives
    support
  A3 process using plan-do-study-act (PDSA)
    cycles, 784*t*
  nursing shared governance, 787–788
  pain resource nurse program, 788–789
  staged competencies, effective nursing practice
    councils, 787*f*
CloNIDine, 398–400, 400*t*, 442
  adverse effects, 400–401
Coanalgesic medications
  chronic neuropathic pain, 388*t*
  clinical benefits, 387*t*
  misconceptions about, 385–386*t*
  role of, 385*b*
  selection of, 386–388
Codeine
  adverse effects, 242–243
  indications and uses, 242
  pharmacologic considerations, 242
  routes and formulations, 242
Coenzyme Q$_{10}$ (ubiquinone-10), 708–709
Cognitive-behavioral therapy, 617–622
  activating event belief consequence model,
    624–625
  barriers, 623*t*
  behavioral activation (BA), 621
  cautions and contraindications, 624
  cognitive restructuring, 620
  components, 619*b*
  coping skill development, 621–622
  coping with trigger factors, 622
  exposure therapy (graded exposure therapy),
    621
  for insomnia (CBT-I), 144
  negative pattern, 620*b*
  for pain management, 622–624
  problem solving, 620–621
  relapse prevention and maintenance of skills,
    622
  research, 624
Cold therapy, 759
Colored analogue scale (CAS), 93–94
Coloring, 588–589
Columbia Suicide Severity Rating Scale
    (C-SSRS), 152–155
Comfrey (*Symphytum officinale L.*), 701
Compassion by caregivers, 742–743
  attention, 744
  behavior, 744

Compassion by caregivers *(Continued)*
  cautions, 745
  feeling, 744
  imagery, 744
  mind training, 744
  pain management evidence, 744–745
  reasoning, 744
  second psychology of, 744
  sensory, 744
Compound analgesics, 441–443
  amitriptyline, 442
  baclofen, 443
  CloNIDine, 442
  diclofenac, 439–440*b*
  gabapentin, 442
  ketamine, 441–442
  ketamine and amitriptyline combination,
    442
  opioids, 443
Connection dance, 566
Constipation, 306–311, 307*b*, 308*f*, 309*t*, 310*f*
Continuous quality improvement (CQI), 771
Corticosteroids, 401–403, 402*t*
Counter-irritants, topical analgesics
  capsaicin, 431–436
  menthol, 436
  salicylates, 436
Craniosacral therapy
  cautions, 655
  clinical application, 655*b*
  pain management, 654–655, 654*f*
  research, 655
Creatinine values and clearance calculations,
    230*b*
Critical care in pain observation tool (CPOT),
    125
Critically ill adults, pain assessment, 124–125
Crossing hands and/or arms over the midline
  care for well-being, 744
  distress tolerance, 744
  empathy, 744
  nonjudgement, 744
  sensitivity to distress, 744
  sympathy, 744
Cryoablation, 759
Current good manufacturing practice (CGMPs),
    688
Customer satisfaction, 771
Cyanocobalamin/cobalamin, 718
Cyclooxygenase 1 (COX-1) and COX-2 enzyme
    pathway, 199*f*
Cytochrome P450, 228
  enzymes CYP3A4 and CYP2D6 interactions,
    231*t*
  induction, 229*b*
  inhibition, 229*b*

D

Dance movement therapy (DMT), 565–566
Defense and veterans pain rating scale 2.0
    (DVPRS), 94, 95*f*
Delirium, patients with, 125
Dementia
  assessment tools of patients with, 122–123*t*
  pain assessment, self-report pain, 126
  patients with, 125–126
Depression
  assessment of, 149–151
  beck depression inventory (BDI), 151
  center for epidemiologic studies depression
    scale (CES-D), 151
  geriatric depression scale (GDS), 151
  prevalence, 149
  suicide ideation, 152–155
  unrelieved pain, 21
  vulnerability and resilience factors, 149*t*

Devil's claw (*Harpagophytum procumbens,
    Harpagophytum zeyheri*), 693
Dexmedetomidine, 399–400, 400*t*
  adverse effects, 401
Dextromethorphan, 403–404
Diaphragmatic breathing, 592
Diclofenac, 208*t*, 439–441, 439–440*b*
Dietary choices, antiinflammatory diet, 745–747
Dietary supplements, 688
  evidence-based resources, 691*t*
  and herbal products, 690*t*
Diphenylheptane, 234
Distraction
  art, 588–589
  coloring, 588–589
  doodling, 588–589
  drawing, 588–589
  electronic games, 589
  humor, 587–588
  types of, 587
Docosahexaenoic acid, 714–716
Doctrine of double effect, 24
Doodling, 588–589
Drawing, 588–589
Dronabinol, 416–418
Dry mouth. *See* Xerostomia

E

Education of clinicians, 789–790
  opportunities, 790*b*
  proactive education, 789
  reactive education, 789
Effective pain management barriers
  access issues
    finances, 54
    residential area, 54–55
    transportation, 54
  clinical application, 52
  family, 53–54
  fear, 52
    of side effects, 52–53
    of substance abuse or misuse, 53
  health care literacy, 53
  opportunities, 57
  past experiences with pain, 52
  patient expectations of pain and pain control,
    52
  provider barriers
    clinician experience, 56
    culture, 55
    education, 55–56
    golden rule *vs.* platinum rule, 56
    perception, 55
  system barriers
    continuing education of clinicians, 56–57
    culture of organization, 56
    insurance coverage, 57
    time, 57
Eicosapentaenoic acid, 714–716
Electronic games, 589
Electronic monitoring devices, 348
Empathy by caregivers, 742–743
Endorphins, 739
Enhanced Recovery After Surgery (ERAS)
    Society 2012, 22
Environmental modifications
  caution, 749
  hospital setting, 747–749
  lighting, 748
  pain management, 749
  positions, 749
  sound, 748
  temperature, 748–749
Epidural analgesia
  catheter insertion level recommendations, 483*t*
  caudal anesthesia, 485

Epidural analgesia *(Continued)*
combined, 485
combined spinal-epidural technique, 485*b*
lumbar, 485
misconceptions, 480–481*t*
patient-controlled, 495
technique for administration, 483*b*
thoracic, 484–485
verification, 484*b*
Epidural corticosteroid injections, 538–539
Epidural route, patient-controlled analgesia, 459
Epinephrine, neuraxial analgesia, 494
Epworth sleepiness scale, 143*f*
Equianalgesic dosing, 181–182, 486–487
Essential oil, 739. *See also* Aromatherapy
characteristics, 740*b*
overdose with, 741–742*t*
storing and controlling quality, 740*b*
Ethical considerations, multimodal analgesia
autonomy, 23
beneficence, 23
doctrine of double effect, 24
fidelity, 24
justice, 24
nonmaleficence, 23–24
principles, 23
veracity, 24
Exercise
aquatic, 568–569, 569*b*
goldfish, 569
isometric, 566–567
land aerobic, 568
patient education, 576, 577*t*
Pilates, 567–568, 567*t*
strengthening, 569
therapeutic, 572–573, 572–573*b*
biophysical agents used in, 575*t*
electrotherapeutic modalities, 574–576
mechanical modalities, 573
passive therapies, 573–574
Exercise-induced hypoalgesia (EIH), 564
Exposure therapy (graded exposure therapy),
621
Extended-release epidural morphine (EREM),
489, 489*b*

F
FACES Pain Scale (Revised) (FPS-R) tool, 92–93
Facet injections, interventional pain
management, 539–541, 539*b*
Family assessment, 158
Family-controlled/caregiver-controlled analgesia,
465–466
Fascial distortion model (FDM), 667–668
Fear avoidance model, 31
Fear of pain with movement. *See also* Exercise
assessment of, 562–563, 563*f*
fear-avoidance model, 561–562, 562*f*
treatment of, 563–564
Feldenkrais method (FM), 565
FentaNYL, 490
parenteral
indications and uses, 243
pharmacologic considerations, 243–244
transdermal, 245–247, 278–279*b*
transmucosal, 244–245
Feverfew (*Tanacetum parthenium* L.), 694
FICA tool, 675*f*
Fidelity, 24
Financial assessment, 158
Flavocoxid (limbrel), 705
Folate/folic acid, 718
Frankincense/olibanum (*Boswellia serrata*),
694–696
Functional Occupational Restoration Treatment
(FORT) program, 615–616

Functional pain scale (FPS), 95–97, 97*f*
Functional restoration programs (FRPs), 615
clinical application, 616*b*
components, 616*b*, 618*t*

G
Gabapentin, 442
Gabapentinoids, 389–394, 389–390*t*
adverse effects, 393
chronic postsurgical neuropathic pain, 392
dosing and routes, 393
monitoring of patients, 394
and neuropathic pain, 391
and perioperative pain, 391–392
pharmacokinetics, 392–393
Gastrointestinal stomal route, medication
administration, 172
Gate control theory of pain, 28–29, 29*f*
Generalized anxiety disorder (GAD-7), 156*f*
Geriatric depression scale (GDS), 151, 153–154*f*
Ginger (*Zingiber officinale* Roscoe), 696–698,
696*f*
Ginseng (*Panax ginseng*), 701–702
Global sleep assessment questionnaire (GSAQ),
142–143*f*
Glucosamine hydrochloride/sulfate and
chondroitin sulfate, 709–710
Glutamate, 39
Goldfish exercise, 569
Good manufacturing practice (GMP) code, 688
Granulocyte-colony stimulating factor (G-CSF),
418
Green tea (*Camellia sinensis*), 705–706
Guided imagery, 603–604
cautions and contraindications, 604
pain management, 603–604
research, 604

H
Healing touch (HT), 642
Health care quality, IOM definition, 771
Herbal medicine (HM), 689*t*. *See also* Botanicals
and herbs
Honey, 706–707
Hospital and Health system Association of
Pennsylvania-Hospital Improvement
Innovation Network (HAP HIIN), 779
Hospital anxiety and depression scale (HADS),
148, 148*f*
Humor, 587–588
Hyaluronic acid (HA), 710–711
HYDROcodone
benzhydrocodone, 248
indications and uses, 247
pharmacologic considerations, 247–248
routes and formulations, 247
HYDROmorphone, 490
indications and uses, 248
pharmacologic considerations, 249
routes and formulations, 248–249
Hyperalgesia, 326–327
Hypnosis
analgesia, 750
benefits, 751*b*
caution, 751
in clinical settings, 750
components, 749
in emergency department, 751*b*
pain management, 750–751
variables influencing quality, 750*b*
Hypogonadism, 321–323, 323*b*

I
Illuminance, 748
Immersive virtual reality (IVR), 589–590, 590*f*
Immune suppressing effect, 328–329

Incidence, 2
Index of Professional Nursing Governance
(IPNG) tool, 788
Individualized numeric rating scale (INRS), 130
Infusion tubing, 464
Insomnia disorder, 137. *See also* Sleep
Institute of Medicine (IOM), 10, 771
Intellectual disabilities (IDs), 127*f*, 129–131
Interdisciplinary pain oversight committee,
772–778
Interdisciplinary pain rehabilitation programs
(IPRPs), 615
Intermittent nursing assessment, opioids
capnography, 352
continuous electronic monitoring, 352
interventions after assessment, 353
level of sedation, 348–351
minute ventilation, 352–353
pulse oximetry, 352
respiratory rate, 351–353
International Association for the Study of Pain
(IASP), 1, 28
Interventional pain management
central nervous system anatomy, 533
cervical facet referral patterns, 536*f*
diagnostic imaging, 537–538
epidural corticosteroid injections, 538–539
facet injections, 539–541, 539*b*
intrathecal drug delivery system, 549–554,
550*b*, 552*b*
lumbar facet referral patterns, 536*f*
spinal cord stimulators, implantable therapies,
543–549, 543–545*b*, 544*f*, 548–549*b*
spinal injections, 538–543
spinal pain, 533–537
anatomy, 534*b*
cord and spinal nerves, 535*f*
facet joint arthropathy, 534–536
radicular pain, 534
vertebral body augmentation (VBA), 541–543,
541*f*
Intramuscular route, medication administration,
178
Intranasal route, patient-controlled analgesia,
461
Intravenous route, 173–174
patient-controlled analgesia, 459
Iowa pain thermometer (IPT) tool, 93
Isometric exercise, 566–567
Italian Questionnaire for Breakthrough Pain
(IQ-BTP), 108

J
Joint commission, 9
Justice, 24

K
Kabat-Zinn attitudes and behaviors, 627*t*
Kabbalah (qabalah) meditation, 679
Ketamine, 404–408, 441–442
acute pain, 405
administration protocols, 406*t*
and amitriptyline combination, 442
chronic pain, 405
patient monitoring parameter, 408*t*
Ketogenic diet, 747
Ketorolac, 206

L
Labyrinth walking meditation, 680
Lactic acid-producing bacteria, 711–712
Lamaze breathing, 593
Land aerobic exercise, 568
Lean methodology, 782–783
Leeds assessment of neuropathic symptoms and
signs (LANSS) tool, 99–100, 99*f*

Levorphanol
   indications and uses, 255–256
   pharmacologic considerations, 256
   routes and formulations, 256
Lidocaine, 409–411, 411t, 437, 438b
Local anesthetics, 491–493
   absorption, 492–493
   chemical structure, 491–492
   choices, 493
   classifications, 492t
   distribution, 492–493
   effects, 491
   for epidural analgesia, 493t
   excretion, 493
   lidocaine, 437
   mechanism of action, 491
   metabolism, 493
   physiologic and chemical activity, 492
   vasodilatation, 491
Loving kindness meditation (LKM), 679–680
Low-threshold neurons, 39

M
Magnesium, 408–409, 712–713, 712b
Maladaptive thinking, 619–620
Manual therapy, 652
Massage therapy
   cautions, 658
   pain management, 656–658
   premassage and postmassage plus topical
      analgesia session measures, 658t
   research, 658
   types of, 655–656, 656–657t
   Wilai massage stick, 658f
McGill Pain Questionnaire (MPQ), 94–95
Medication administration
   analgesic dosing considerations
      around-the-clock dosing, 182–184
      awakening patients, 184
      comorbidities, 181
      dosing to pain intensity using numbers,
         184–187
      equianalgesic dosing, 181–182
      individualized dose selection, 188f
      opioid dose requirement, 186t
      pain intensity, 187t
      prescription and implementation, 189b
      range order, 187–190
      therapeutic duplication, 190
   patient considerations
      age, 163–166, 164t
      genetics, 166–167
   route selection, 168–170t
      gastrointestinal stomal route, 172
      intramuscular route, 178
      intravenous route, 173–174
      medications administered by, 173t
      neuraxial and peripheral nerve routes, 181
      oral, 167–171
      rectal route, 172
      subcutaneous route, 175–178, 175f, 176b
      sublingual, buccal, and intranasal, 171–172
      topical, 178–179
      transdermal, 179–181
      transmucosal route, 171–173
      vaginal route, 173
Medication safety committee, 778
Meditation
   cautions and precautions, 682–683
   centering prayer (spiritual meditation),
      678–679
   definition, 675–678
   kabbalah (qabalah), 679
   labyrinth walking, 680
   loving kindness, 679–680
   mindfulness, 680

Meditation (Continued)
   movement, 680
   reflective walking, 680
   Ridhwan School Diamond Approach,
      680–681
   self-realization fellowship (SRF), 681
   systems of, 676–677t
   Tibetan Buddhist meditation, 681
   transcendental, 681
   Zen Buddhism/Ch'an, 682
Menthol, 436
Meperidine, 249
Methadone, 234, 283b, 286b, 365–367, 375
   advantages and disadvantages, 250–251t
   characteristics, 253b
   dosing, 280b
   drug-drug interactions, 254–255
   indications and uses, 249–251
   morphine to, 281–282t
   outpatient initiation, 253b
   pharmacokinetics, 252b
   pharmacologic considerations, 251–252
   recommendations, 254b
   rotation to, 285b, 285t
   routes and formulations, 251
   safety guidelines, 252
N-Methyl-d-aspartate receptor antagonists,
   403–409
Methylsulfonylmethane (MSM), 713–714
Mexiletine, 411–412
Michigan Opioid Safety Score (MOSS), 349,
   350f
Mindfulness-based stress management, 627–630,
   627t, 629–630f
Mindfulness meditation, 680
Mirror visual feedback therapy (MVFT)/mirror
   therapy, 752f
   cautions for, 754
   with chronic pain conditions, 753
   in home settings, 753
   painful/paralyzed limb, 751–752
   painful/phantom limb, 752
   pain management, 752
   personal computer-based desktop, 753f
   and referred sensation, 753–754
   virtual reality, 753
Mixed alpha antagonist opioids, 266
Mixed pain states, 35
Morphine
   indications and uses, 238–241
   pharmacologic considerations, 242
   routes and formulations, 241–242
Movement, 680. See also Exercise
   paleo, 565
   recovering with acute pain, 565
   symptoms, 564
Multidimensional objective pain assessment tool
   (MOPAT), 131
Multidimensional pain assessment tools
   brief pain inventory (BPI), 95, 96f
   chronic pain grade scale (CPGS), 98
   clinically aligned pain assessment tool, 94, 94f
   defense and veterans pain rating scale 2.0
      (DVPRS), 94, 95f
   functional pain scale (FPS), 95–97, 97f
   McGill Pain Questionnaire (MPQ), 94–95
   PEG scale tool, 95, 97f
   short form 36 bodily pain score (SF-36 BPS)
      tool, 98
Multimodal analgesia (MMA)
   acute perioperative setting, 19
   chronic pain management, 22
   clinical application, 24–25
   ethical considerations
      autonomy, 23
      beneficence, 23

Multimodal analgesia (MMA) (Continued)
   doctrine of double effect, 24
   fidelity, 24
   justice, 24
   nonmaleficence, 23–24
   principles, 23
   veracity, 24
   perioperative setting, 22
   plan
      acetaminophen, 166
      analgesic administration, 164–166
Multimodal pain management
   components, 11–12t
   evolution
      action of broad-analgesics, 6f
      early support, 5
      opioid prescribing, 5–7
      opioid-related complications, 7
      resurgence of support, 7
   historical perspective of, 2–4
      early national efforts to address pain, 3–4
      growth in pain research, 3
   institutional assessment checklist, 774f
   integrative health care themes, 8t
   interdisciplinary pain oversight committee,
      772–778
   medication safety committee, 778
   naloxone availability, 779–781
   opioid risk initiatives and safety interventions,
      778–781
   opioid-sparing approaches
      centers for disease control and prevention
         guidelines, 9
      challenges and opportunities, 10
      enhanced recovery after surgery society
         guidelines, 9
      institute of medicine report, 10
      joint commission, 9
      national pain strategy, 10
      professional organizations, 8–9
   organizational strategies recommendations,
      773b
   pain assessment as foundation, 4–5
   postoperative pain interventions, 12–14t
   quality improvement, 772
Mu opioid agonist medications, 239–240t
Muscle energy technique (MET), 667
Muscle relaxants, 412–416, 413–414t
Music therapy, 598f
   cautions, 600
   concerns, 600
   contraindications, 600
   indications, 598–599
   and multimodal pain management, 598
   vs. music interventions, 597b
   pain management, 599
   as profession, 597
Myoclonus, 325–326
Myofascial trigger points (MTrPs), 666–667
Myrrh (Commiphora molmol), 702

N
Nabilone, 416–418
Naloxone, 267–269, 268b
   availability, 779–781
Naltrexone, 368–369
   acute pain management for patients on, 373
   chronic pain management for patients on, 375
National Institutes of Health (NIH) report, 2
National pain strategy, 10
Nausea and vomiting, opioid-induced, 312–314
Neuraxial analgesia
   administration, 495–496
   alpha$_2$-adrenergic agonists, 494–495
   anatomy, 475–477
   beneficial effects of, 478–482

Neuraxial analgesia *(Continued)*
bioavailability, 486
catheter placement
epidural needle and, 478f
patient position, 478f
spinal (subarachnoid/intrathecal) needle
and catheter, 479f
clinician-administered intermittent bolus, 495,
496b
coanalgesic medications used in, 494–495
continuous infusion, 495
contraindications to, 482
dermatomes, 477f
distribution, 487
epidural analgesia
catheter insertion level recommendations,
483t
caudal anesthesia, 485
combined, 485
combined spinal-epidural technique, 485b
lumbar, 485
misconceptions, 480–481t
opioid regimens, 488t
technique for administration, 483b
thoracic, 484–485
verification, 484b
epinephrine, 494
equianalgesic dose conversions, 486–487
extended-release epidural morphine (EREM),
489, 489b
FentaNYL, 490
HYDROmorphone, 490
interventions, 477–478
intrathecal opioid analgesic regimens, 489t
local anesthetics, 491–493
absorption, 492–493
chemical structure, 491–492
choices, 493
classifications, 492t
distribution, 492–493
effects, 491
for epidural analgesia, 493t
excretion, 493
mechanism of action, 491
metabolism, 493
physiologic and chemical activity, 492
vasodilatation, 491
medications used in, 486–493
misconceptions, 480–481t
multimodal analgesia, neuraxial opioids and
local anesthetics, 493–494
opioid adverse effects, 497
patient-controlled, 494t
patient-controlled epidural analgesia, 495
patient selection, 479b
principles of, 475
programmed intermittent epidural bolus,
495–496
properties, 488t
recommended minimum monitoring, 498t
selected opioid analgesics, 487–491
solubility, 486
spinal anatomy, 476f
spinal nerves, 476–477
SUFentanil, 491
techniques
for administration of spinal anesthesia,
482b
preparation and education, 481b
spinal (subarachnoid/intrathecal) analgesia,
482
unintended effects, 496–497
unintended effects, neuraxial local anesthetics
allergic reaction, 498
American Society of Anesthesiologists
recommendations, 506b

Neuraxial analgesia *(Continued)*
assessment, 499t
bradycardia, 501
cardiovascular unintended effects, 500–502
direct needle trauma, 503
dural puncture, 502–503
epidural catheter migration, 503, 504b
epidural hematoma, 508–509, 509b
hypotension, 500–501
local anesthetic neurotoxicity, 498–500
local anesthetic systemic toxicity, 500, 501b
modified Bromage scale, 502b
motor block, 501–502
neurologic complications, 504–509
postdural puncture headache, 502–503,
502b
prevention of neurotoxicity, 505b
procedure-related complications, 502–503
signs and symptoms, 507b
urinary retention, 501
vertebral column, 475–476, 476f
Neuraxial and peripheral nerve routes,
medication administration, 181
Neuraxial local anesthetics, unintended effects
allergic reaction, 498
American Society of Anesthesiologists
recommendations, 506b
assessment, 499t
bradycardia, 501
cardiovascular unintended effects, 500–502
direct needle trauma, 503
dural puncture, 502–503
epidural catheter migration, 503, 504b
epidural hematoma, 508–509, 509b
hypotension, 500–501
local anesthetic neurotoxicity, 498–500
local anesthetic systemic toxicity, 500, 501b
modified Bromage scale, 502b
motor block, 501–502
neurologic complications, 504–509
postdural puncture headache, 502–503, 502b
prevention of neurotoxicity, 505b
procedure-related complications, 502–503
signs and symptoms, 507b
urinary retention, 501
Neuraxial opioids and local anesthetics, 493–494
Neuroinflammation and immune system, 43–45
Neuromatrix, theories of pain, 29
Neuropathic pain, 34–35, 98t
Leeds assessment of neuropathic symptoms
and signs (LANSS) tool, 99–100, 99f
neuropathic pain questionnaire (NPQ),
101–102, 101f
Nociception level index, 132
Nociceptive pain, 32–34, 32–33t, 34b, 36f,
36–37t
Nociceptive-specific neurons, 39
Non-communicating adult pain checklist
(NCAPC), 130–131
Nonmaleficence, 23–24
Nonopioid analgesic medications
acetaminophen
adverse effects, 212–213
dosing, 212
FDA warnings, 213–214
formulations, 212, 212t
hepatotoxicity, 213
history, 210
indications for use, 211–212
monitoring of patients, 214
pharmacologic effects, 210–211
routes, 212
use in special populations, 214
aspirin, 198
indications for use, 197b, 199–200
pharmacologic effects, 197–199

Nonopioid analgesic medications *(Continued)*
cyclooxygenase 1 (COX-1) and COX-2
enzyme pathway, 199f
history, 195–197
multimodal use, 214–215
NSAIDs *see also* Nonsteroidal
antiinflammatory drugs (NSAIDs)
adverse effects, 200–205
indications for use, 197b, 199–200
misconceptions about, 196t
pharmacologic effects, 197–199, 198f
Nonsteroidal antiinflammatory drugs (NSAIDs),
438–441
adverse effects, 200–205
bleeding and gastrointestinal, 200–202
blood pressure, 205
cardiovascular homeostasis, 202–204
cognitive, 205
FDA warnings, 205
hepatic, 205
renal, 204–205
safety summary, 205
treatment and prevention, 201b
diclofenac product descriptions, 208t
dosing and formulations, 206t
oral, 206
parenteral, 206
indications for use, 197b, 199–200
intranasal (IN) route, 207–208
misconceptions about, 196t
monitoring patients receiving therapy, 208–209
nanopharmacology, 205–206
ophthalmic route, 207
parenteral, 207t
protective strategies, 204t
risk factors, 203t
topical analgesics types, 438–441
topical salicylates and, 207
use in special populations
bariatric surgery patients, 209–210
older adults, 209
orthopedic patients, 210
patients with end-stage renal disease
(ESRD), 209
surgical patients, 209
Nonverbal pain assessment tool (NPAT), 124
Numeric rating scale, 91
Nurse-controlled analgesia, 466
Nursing shared governance, 787–788

O

Obesity and weight management
BMI recommendations, 754–755
caloric intake, 754
cautions, 756
clinical application, 755b
pain management, 755
Objective assessment of risk, 348
Obstructive sleep apnea, 144–146
assessment of, 144–146
risk reduction precautions, 145b
Omega-3 polyunsaturated fatty acids, 714–716,
715t
Opioids
advancing sedation and, 338–339
adverse effects, 238, 304–306t
antagonists, 267
assessment and monitoring of patients, 238
associated pharmacologic factors
combining classes of medications, 346–347
formulations, 342–345
mechanisms of delivery, 345–346
postanesthesia care unit, 343b
classes
benzomorphans, 235
diphenylheptane, 234

Opioids (Continued)
methadone, 234
phenanthrenes, 232–233, 233t
phenylpiperadines, 233–234
phenylpropylamines, 235
tapentadol, 235
TraMADol, 235
clinical application, 351b
compound analgesics, 443
detection using electronic monitoring devices, 348
dose requirement, 186t
dosing practices
continuous intravenous infusions, 273
equianalgesic dose chart, 274–275t
modified-release, 272
otation/switch, 273–280
therapy initiation, 270
titration of short-acting, 270–272
driving, 290b
factors affecting drug response
pharmacodynamics, 226–227
formulations, 238
identification of risk factors
health care team and institutional policies and procedures, 342
modifiable risk factors, 341–342
naloxone administration, 340–341
nonmodifiable risk factors, 340
indications, 236–238
intermittent nursing assessment
capnography, 352
continuous electronic monitoring, 352
interventions after assessment, 353
level of sedation, 348–351
minute ventilation, 352–353
pulse oximetry, 352
respiratory rate, 351–353
Michigan Opioid Safety Score (MOSS), 349, 350f
Mu opioid agonist medications, 239–240t
objective assessment of risk, 348
OxyCODONE to morphine conversion, 278b
Pasero opioid-induced sedation scale (POSS), 349, 349b
patient assessment for risk, 347–348
patient monitoring, 348
pharmacogenomics, 230–232
pharmacokinetics
absorption, 227–228
clearance, 229–230
distribution, 228
drug-drug interactions, 228–229
metabolism, 228–230
renal excretion, 230
pharmacology, chemical classes, 223, 223–224t
receptors
activation, 225–226f
agonists/antagonists, 227t
clinical effects, 224–225t
discovery, 225
nomenclature, 226
signaling, 226
during renal failure and dialysis, 240–241t
respiratory depression, 338
incidence, 338
nonmodifiable risk factors, 339b
recommendations, 339
and respiratory function, 338
Richmond sedation scale (RASS), 350–351
risk initiatives and safety interventions, 778–781
safety for patients at risk, 347
safety in community, 288–289
selection, 235

Opioids (Continued)
subjective assessment of risk, 347–348
tapering and discontinuing, 287–289
unintended effects of
constipation, 306–311, 307b, 308f, 309t, 310f
hyperalgesia, 326–327
hypogonadism, 321–323, 323b
immune suppressing effect, 328–329
myoclonus, 325–326
opioid-induced nausea and vomiting, 312–314
physical dependence on, 327–328
pruritus, 314–319, 317–318t
sedation, 323–325, 325t
tolerance, 328
urinary retention, 319–321, 319b, 320f
xerostomia (dry mouth), 311
use of, 236–238, 237b
Opioid-sparing approaches
centers for disease control and prevention guidelines, 9
challenges and opportunities, 10
enhanced recovery after surgery society guidelines, 9
institute of medicine report, 10
joint commission, 9
national pain strategy, 10
professional organizations, 8–9
Opioid use disorder
acute care setting, 369–376
acute pain management, 371–374
caring for patients with pain and, 363–365
chronic pain management in patients with, 374
clinical challenge, 378b
clinical challenges of treating pain with, 363–364
discharge planning for patients with, 374
ethical principles and application, 364t
medication-assisted treatments, 367t
methadone maintenance therapy, 370–371
opioid-induced hyperalgesia, 363
overdose prevention, 377
physical dependence, 362
pseudoaddiction, 363
risk factors, 364–365, 365t
safe treatment plan designing, 376–377
selection of, 376
substance use disorder and
pathophysiology of, 361
terminology related to, 361–363, 362b
tolerance, 362
tools, 366t
treatment, 365–369
universal precautions approach, 376
withdrawal, 363
Oral/enteral route, patient-controlled analgesia, 460–461
Oral medication administration, 167–171
Osteopathic manipulative therapy, 653–654
Osteopathy, 653–654
manual medicine, 653–654
Overdose education and naloxone (OEN) rescue kits, 780
OxyCODONE
clinical trials, 258
indications and use, 256
pharmacologic considerations, 257
routes and formulations, 257
OxyMORphone, 258–259

P
PAINAD tool, 128f
Pain assessment and intervention notation (PAIN), 124
Pain assessment checklist for seniors with limited ability to communicate (PACSLAC) tool, 126

Pain assessment in advanced dementia tool (PAINAD), 131
Pain resource nurse (PRN) program, 782, 788–789
Paleo movement, 565
Partial Mu agonist, 264–266
Pasero opioid-induced sedation scale (POSS), 349, 349b
Pasero opioid sedation scale (POSS), 463b, 779–780
Patient barriers
culture and beliefs, 51–52
meaning of pain, 50–51
misconceptions, 50, 51t
Patient considerations, medication administration
age, 163–166, 164t
genetics, 166–167
Patient-controlled analgesia (PCA)
advantages of use, 448
appropriate prescription, 451
authorized agent-controlled analgesia, 465–466, 466t, 467b
education points, 450b
equipment evaluation, 464
indications for use, 448–449
intravenous, 452b
opioid naïve, 454b
opioid tolerant, 454b
optimize safety within, 449–455
overview, 453f
patient and family education, 450–451
patient assessment and monitoring, 458–461
prescription components, 455–458, 455t, 457t
routes of administration, 458–461
sources of, 449b
Patient health questionnaire-9 (PHQ-9), 150f
Patient safety, 772
PEG scale tool, 95, 97f
Perception, 39–41
Persistent postsurgical pain (PPSP), 31
Pharmacogenetics, 167
Pharmacogenomics, 167, 230–232
Pharmacokinetics
absorption, 227–228
clearance, 229–230
distribution, 228
drug-drug interactions, 228–229
metabolism, 228–230
renal excretion, 230
Pharmacologic factors, opioids associated
combining classes of medications, 346–347
formulations, 342–345
mechanisms of delivery, 345–346
postanesthesia care unit, 343b
Phenanthrenes, 232–233, 233t
Phenylpiperadines, 233–234
Phenylpropylamines, 235
adult dosing of, 235t
Physical dependence, opioids, 327–328
Physical therapy, 571–576
Physiologic and sensory aspects
aggravating and alleviating factors, 77
cognition, 80–81
effects of pain, 77–80
intensity, 76–77
location, 76
mental status, 81
onset and duration (temporal aspects), 77
pain affect, 80
pain control diary, 78–79f
psychosocial, 80
quality, 77
Physiologic processing of pain
spinal and supraspinal pain pathways, 35f
transduction, 35–37
Pilates exercise, 567–568, 567t

Pioid-related complications, 7
Pittsburgh sleep quality index (PSQI), 138f
Plan-do-study-act (PDSA) cycles
　A3 methodology, 784t
　change in system, 782f
　quality improvement, 781–782
Polymorphisms, 231
Prayer
　cautions, 674–675
　pain management, 674
Pregabalin, 389t
President's Commission on Combating Drug
　　Addiction and the Opioid Crisis
　　(PCCDOC), 779
Prevalence, 2
Primary afferent nerve fibers, 37t
Proactive education, 789
Programmed intermittent epidural bolus,
　495–496
Progressive muscle relaxation (PMR)
　cautions, 596
　pain management, 595–596
　procedures, 594b
　research, 596
　sample script, 595b
　technique, 594–595
Provider barriers
　clinician experience, 56
　culture, 55
　education, 55–56
　golden rule vs. platinum rule, 56
　perception, 55
Pruritus, 314–319, 317–318t
Psychoeducation, 630–631
Pulse oximetry, 352, 463
Pupillary reflex as physiologic measure, 132
Pyridoxine, 717–718

Q
Quality
　definition, 771
　domains of, 771f
Quality improvement (QI), 770
　A3 methodology, 783–786, 788–789t
　clinical research programs, 786–787
　continuous, 771
　improvement opportunities, 790
　innovation, 790
　lean methodology, 782–783
　multimodal pain management, 772
　plan-do-study-act, 781–782
　safe and effective pain management, 790

R
Range order, 187–190
Rapid Induction Analgesia (RIA) technique, 751
Reactive education, 789
Rectal route, medication administration, 172
Referred sensation, 753–754
Reflective walking, 680
Reflexology
　cautions, 663–664
　effectiveness, 662
　homuncular map, 659
　left foot, 661f
　left hand, 659f
　left palm, 660f
　left sole, 662f
　pain management, 660–663
　protocol, 663f
　research, 663
　right foot, 661f
　right hand, 659f
　right palm, 660f
　right sole, 661f
　thumb walking, 659–660

Regional analgesia
　dosing regimens, 510t
　epidural safety, 522b
　infusion systems, 518–520, 519b, 522–523t
　local infiltration analgesia, 520–524, 521t
　peripheral nerve blocks
　　adductor canal, 517–518
　　administration, 513
　　beneficial effects, 511
　　contraindications and risks associated with,
　　　511–512
　　interventions, 510–511
　　management, 513
　　medications for, 512–513
　　truncal approaches, 513–515
　　truncal and peripheral regional analgesia, 510
Regional anesthesia approaches, 475
Regional route, patient-controlled analgesia,
　459
Reiki, 637–638
Relaxation
　breathing activities, 592
　cautions, 593–594
　pain management, 593
　response, animal-assisted therapy, 602t
　techniques, 591
　types of, 592–593
　　abdominal breathing, 592
　　alternate nostril breathing, 592
　　diaphragmatic breathing, 592
　　Lamaze breathing, 593
　　square breathing, 592–593, 593f
　　yogic breathing/pranayama, 592
Remifentanil, 259–260
Respiratory assessment, 462, 462t
Respiratory depression, opioid- induced, 338
　incidence, 338
　nonmodifiable risk factors, 339b
　recommendations, 339
Respiratory function and opioids, 338
Restorative sleep, 136–146
Revised Faces, Legs, Activity, Cries,
　　Consolability Scale (r-FLACC) scale, 130
Riboflavin, 716–717
Richmond sedation scale (RASS), 350–351
Ridhwan School Diamond Approach, 680–681
Risk factors identification, opioids
　health care team and institutional policies and
　　procedures, 342
　modifiable risk factors, 341–342
　naloxone administration, 340–341
　nonmodifiable risk factors, 340
Routes of administration
　patient-controlled analgesia
　　epidural route, 459
　　intranasal route, 461
　　intravenous route, 459
　　oral/enteral route, 460–461
　　regional route, 459
　　subcutaneous route, 459–460
　　sublingual route, 461
　　transdermal route, 460
　selection, 168–170t
　　gastrointestinal stomal route, 172
　　intramuscular route, 178
　　intravenous route, 173–174
　　medications administered by, 173t
　　neuraxial and peripheral nerve routes, 181
　　oral, 167–171
　　rectal route, 172
　　subcutaneous route, 175–178, 175f, 176b
　　sublingual, buccal, and intranasal, 171–172
　　topical, 178–179
　　transdermal, 179–181
　　transmucosal route, 171–173
　　vaginal route, 173

S
Salicylates, 436
Sedation, 323–325, 325t
　assessment, 462
　and opioids, 338–339
Self-realization fellowship (SRF), 681
Self-report pain
　adult nonverbal pain score (NVPS) tool, 124
　assessment tools of patients with dementia,
　　122–123t
　behavioral pain scale (BPS), 124–125
　cautions, 132
　checklist of nonverbal pain indicators (CNPI),
　　129, 130f
　common behavioral tools, 121–122t
　critical care in pain observation tool (CPOT),
　　125
　individualized numeric rating scale (INRS),
　　130
　multidimensional objective pain assessment
　　tool (MOPAT), 131
　newer trends in pain assessment for patients
　　who cannot
　　bispectral (BIS) index, 131
　　nociception level index, 132
　　pupillary reflex as physiologic measure, 132
　non-communicating adult pain checklist
　　(NCAPC), 130–131
　nonverbal pain assessment tool (NPAT), 124
　PAINAD tool, 128f
　pain assessment
　　in advanced dementia, 126
　　in critically ill adults who cannot, 124–125
　　of patients who cannot, 120–124
　pain assessment and intervention notation
　　(PAIN), 124
　pain assessment checklist for seniors
　　with limited ability to communicate
　　(PACSLAC) tool, 126
　pain assessment in advanced dementia tool
　　(PAINAD), 131
　patients at the end of life who cannot, 131
　patients with delirium who cannot, 125
　patients with dementia who cannot,
　　125–126
　for patients with particular characteristics,
　　128–129t
　people with intellectual disabilities (IDs),
　　127f, 129–131
　Revised Faces, Legs, Activity, Cries,
　　Consolability Scale (r-FLACC) scale, 130
Serotonin, 739
Serotonin norepinephrine reuptake inhibitors
　(SNRIs), 396–398, 397t
Short form 36 bodily pain score (SF-36 BPS)
　tool, 98
Skin anatomy and physiology, 430f
Sleep
　assessment of sleep quality, 137
　cognitive-behavioral therapy for insomnia
　　(CBT-I), 144
　Epworth sleepiness scale, 143f
　global sleep assessment questionnaire (GSAQ),
　　142–143t
　hygiene, 144b
　insomnia disorder, 137
　obstructive sleep apnea, 144–146
　　assessment of, 144–146
　　risk reduction precautions, 145b
　Pittsburgh sleep quality index (PSQI), 138f
　restorative, 136–146
　stop bang, 145t
　treatment of disorders, 137–144
SMART goal setting, 617–619, 619b
Sodium channel blockers, 409–412
SOLAR/SOL acronym, 628b

Spinal pain, 533–537
  anatomy, 534b
  cord and spinal nerves, 535f
  facet joint arthropathy, 534–536
  radicular pain, 534
Spirituality definition, 673
Square breathing, 592–593, 593f
Static magnet therapy
  cautions, 756
  pain management, 756
St. John's Wort (*Hypericum perforatum*), 702
Stratification Tool for Opioid Risk Mitigation
    (STORM), 779
Subcutaneous route
  medication administration, 175–178, 175f,
    176b
  patient-controlled analgesia, 459–460
Subjective assessment of risk, 347–348
Sublingual, buccal, and intranasal medication
    administration, 171–172
Sublingual route, patient-controlled analgesia,
    461
Substance P, 39
Substance use disorder and opioid use disorder
  pathophysiology of, 361
  terminology related to, 361–363, 362b
SUFentanil, 260–261, 491
Suicide ideation, 152–155
System barriers
  continuing education of clinicians, 56–57
  culture of organization, 56
  insurance coverage, 57
  time, 57

T
Tai chi, 569–570
Tampa Scale for Kinesiophobia (TSK), 562–563
Tapentadol, 235, 263–264
Temperature modalities, 756–759
The Dietary Supplement Health and Education
    Act of 1994 (DSHEA), 688
Theories of pain
  biopsychosocial model, 30, 30f
  fear avoidance model, 31
  gate control theory of pain, 28–29, 29f
  neuromatrix, 29
Therapeutic cold, ice, cryotherapy, 758
Therapeutic duplication, 190
Therapeutic exercises, 572–573, 572–573b. *See
    also* Exercise
  biophysical agents used in, 575t
  electrotherapeutic modalities, 574–576
  mechanical modalities, 573
  passive therapies, 573–574
Therapeutics Goods Act of 1989, 688
Therapeutic superficial heat
  cautions, 757–759
  contraindications, 758–759, 758–759b
  pain management, 757–759
Therapeutic touch (TT), 638–642, 642b, 643t
The Joint Commission (TJC), 770–771
Thiamine, 716
Tibetan Buddhist meditation, 681
TiZANidine, 399–400
  adverse effects, 401

Topical analgesics
  benefits of, 429–431
  compound analgesics, 441–443
    amitriptyline, 442
    baclofen, 443
    CloNIDine, 442
    diclofenac, 439–440b
    gabapentin, 442
    ketamine, 441–442
    ketamine and amitriptyline combination, 442
    opioids, 443
  intraarticular and periarticular injections, 179
  for locally acting drugs, 430f
  opioids, 179
  pharmacokinetic properties, 431t
  types of, 432–433t
    counter-irritants, 431–436
    local anesthetics, 436–437
    nonsteroidal antiinflammatory drugs,
      438–441
TraMADol, 235, 261–263
Transcendental meditation (TM), 681
Transdermal (TD) drug delivery systems,
    179–181, 180f
Transdermal route
  formulation for systemically acting drugs,
    431f
  patient-controlled analgesia, 460
Transmission, 37–39
Transmucosal route, medication administration,
    171–173
Tricyclic antidepressants, 394–396, 394t
Turmeric (*Curcuma longa/Curcuma domestica*),
    698–700

U
Unidimensional pain assessment tools
  colored analogue scale (CAS), 93–94
  FACES Pain Scale (Revised) (FPS-R) tool,
    92–93
  Iowa pain thermometer (IPT) tool, 93
  numeric rating scale, 91
  verbal descriptor scale, 92
  vertical version, 91f
  visual analogue scale, 91–92
  Wong-Baker FACES pain rating scale, 92, 93f
Unintended effects, neuraxial local anesthetics
  allergic reaction, 498
  American Society of Anesthesiologists
    recommendations, 506b
  assessment, 499t
  bradycardia, 501
  cardiovascular unintended effects, 500–502
  direct needle trauma, 503
  dural puncture, 502–503
  epidural catheter migration, 503, 504b
  epidural hematoma, 508–509, 509b
  hypotension, 500–501
  local anesthetic neurotoxicity, 498–500
  local anesthetic systemic toxicity, 500, 501b
  modified Bromage scale, 502b
  motor block, 501–502
  neurologic complications, 504–509
  postdural puncture headache, 502–503, 502b
  prevention of neurotoxicity, 505b

Unintended effects, neuraxial local anesthetics
    (*Continued*)
  procedure-related complications, 502–503
  signs and symptoms, 507b
  urinary retention, 501
Unit-based practice committees (UBPCs), 787
Unrelieved pain
  harmful effects of, 20t
  physiologic complications, 19–20
  psychosocial implications
    agitation, 21
    anxiety, 20–21
    depression, 21
    reciprocal effect, 21f
Urinary retention, 319–321, 319b, 320f

V
Vaginal route, medication administration, 173
Valsalva maneuver, 760–761
Veracity, 24
Verbal descriptor scale, 92
Vertebral body augmentation (VBA), 541–543,
    541f
U.S. Veterans Health Administration (VHA), 779
Virtual reality (VR), 589–590
Virtual reality mirror visual feedback therapy
    (VRMVFT), 753
Visual analogue scale, 91–92
Vitamin B, 716–719
  complex and combinations, 718–719
  vitamin B$_1$ (thiamine), 716
  vitamin B$_2$ (riboflavin), 716–717
  vitamin B$_6$ (pyridoxine), 717–718
  vitamin B$_9$ (folate/folic acid), 718
  vitamin B$_{12}$ (cyanocobalamin/cobalamin), 718
Vitamin D
  cautions, 721
  contraindications, 721
  deficiency, 720f
  metabolic pathway, 719f
  pain management, 720–721
  role of, 720
Vitamin E
  cautions, 722
  contraindications, 722
  gamma-tocotrienol, 722
  interactions with medications, 722
  pain management, 721–722

W
White willow bark (*Salix alba*), 700–701
Wide dynamic range (WDR) neurons, 39
Willow bark (*Salicis cortex*), 700–701
Wong-Baker FACES pain rating scale, 92, 93f

X
Xerostomia (dry mouth), 311

Y
Yoga, 570–571
Yogic breathing/pranayama, 592

Z
Zen meditation, 682
Ziconotide overdose, 552b